TARGETED TREATMENT of the
RHEUMATIC DISEASES

TARGETED TREATMENT of the
RHEUMATIC DISEASES

Michael H. Weisman, MD
Director, Division of Rheumatology
Cedars-Sinai Medical Center
Professor of Medicine
David Geffen School of Medicine at UCLA
Los Angeles, California

Michael E. Weinblatt, MD
John R. and Eileen K. Riedman Professor of Medicine
Harvard Medical School
Division of Rheumatology, Immunology, and Allergy
Brigham and Women's Hospital
Boston, Massachusetts

James S. Louie, MD
Professor Emeritus of Medicine
Division of Rheumatology at CHS
David Geffen School of Medicine at UCLA
Los Angeles, California

Ronald F. van Vollenhoven, MD, PhD
Senior Rheumatologist
Karolinska University Hospital
Associate Professor of Rheumatology
The Karolinska Institute
Stockholm, Sweden

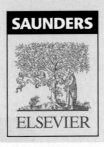

SAUNDERS

ELSEVIER

SAUNDERS
ELSEVIER

1600 John F. Kennedy Blvd.
Ste 1800
Philadelphia, PA 19103-2899

TARGETED TREATMENT OF THE RHEUMATIC DISEASES ISBN: 978-1-4160-9993-2
Copyright © 2010 by Saunders, an imprint of Elsevier Inc.

Cover photos:
Panel 2
The top figure shows TNF in its active trimer form with the monomers colored individually. Receptor binding occurs along the three monomer interfaces. The left figure models the TNF soluble receptor fusion protein comprised of two TNF receptor arms with their TNF binding sites (bright blue) attached to an Fc of IgG1 (cyan). The right figure models the TNF monoclonal antibodies with a complete IgG1 structure including the Fc (cyan) and its complementarity-determining regions which bind TNF (CDRs in bright blue).
Courtesy of the Journal of Investigative Dermatology Symposium Proceedings, volume 12, number 1, May 2007.

Library of Congress Cataloging-in-Publication Data

Targeted treatment of the rheumatic diseases / [edited by]
Michael H. Weisman ... [et al.]. -- 1st ed.
    p. ; cm.
   Includes bibliographical references and index.
   ISBN 978-1-4160-9993-2 (alk. paper)
1. Rheumatism--Treatment. 2. Arthritis--Treatment.
I. Weisman, Michael H.
   [DNLM: 1. Rheumatic Diseases--drug therapy.
2. Arthritis, Rheumatoid--drug therapy. WE 544 T1852 2009]
   RC927.T37 2009
   616.7'23--dc22   2009007823

Acquisitions Editor: Pamela Hetherington
Design Direction: Steven Stave
Marketing Manager: Courtney Ingram

Printed in China

Last digit is the print number: 9 8 7 6 5 4 3 2 1

This book is dedicated to our wonderful patients whose determination sustains us, and to our rheumatology colleagues whose devotion to the field energizes us.

As the understanding of pathogenic molecules and pathways, new genetics, and environmental triggers unfolds, our hope is that the use of targeted therapies for specific sub-populations of patients will bring us closer to the goal of optimal care for each and all.

We salute the engaged and knowledgeable clinician who will apply the subtleties of effective and prudent targeted therapies to the daily practice of rheumatology, hoping that this volume may help in that momentous task.

Contributors

Helene Alexanderson, PhD, RPT
Rheumatology Unit, Department of Medicine, The Karolinska Institute; Orthopedic/Rheumatology Unit, Department of Physical Therapy, Karolinska University Hospital, Solna, Stockholm, Sweden
Targeted Treatment of the Idiopathic Inflammatory Myopathies

Ralf Baron, MD
Sektion für Neurologische Schmerzforschung und Therapie, Klinik für Neurologie, Christian-Albrechts-Universität zu Kiel, Kiel, Germany
Mechanisms and Treatment Strategy of Complex Regional Pain Syndromes

Francis Berenbaum, MD, PhD
Professor, University Pierre and Marie Curie; Head, Department of Rheumatology, Assistance Publique Hôpitaux de Paris, Hôpital Saint-Antoine, Paris, France
Management of Osteoarthritis: Pharmacotherapy

Joel A. Block, MD
The Willard L. Wood, MD Professor, and Director, Section of Rheumatology, Rush Medical College, and Rush University Medical Center, Chicago, Illinois
Regional Disorders of the Neck, Shoulder, Arm, and Hand

Hendrika Bootsma, MD, PhD
Associate Professor of Rheumatology, Department of Rheumatology and Clinical Immunology, University Medical Center Groningen, Groningen, The Netherlands
Management of Sjögren's Syndrome

David G. Borenstein, MD
Clinical Professor of Medicine, The George Washington University Medical Center, Washington, DC
Management of Mechanical Lumbar Spine Disease

Johan Bratt, MD, PhD
Associate Professor, and Head, Department of Rheumatology, Karolinska University Hospital, Stockholm, Sweden
Management of Medium and Small Vessel Vasculitis, Including the Antineutrophil Cytoplasmic Antibody–Associated Diseases

Vivian P. Bykerk, MD, FRCP(C)
Assistant Professor of Medicine, University of Toronto; Director, Early Arthritis Program, and Assistant Director, Division of Advanced Therapeutics, Rebecca MacDonald Center for Arthritis and Autoimmune Disease; Staff Rheumatologist, Mount Sinai Hospital, University Health Network; Staff, Multidisciplinary Osteoporosis Program, Women's College Hospital, Toronto, Ontario, Canada
Management of Rheumatoid Arthritis: The Newly Diagnosed Patient

Grant W. Cannon, MD
Professor of Medicine, Division of Rheumatology, Department of Internal Medicine, University of Utah School of Medicine; Associate Chief of Staff for Academic Affiliations, George E. Whalen Veterans Affairs Medical Center, Salt Lake City, Utah
Management of Sarcoidosis, Behçet's Disease, and Other Rare Rheumatic Diseases

Hiok Hee Chng, MBBS(Singapore), MMed(Internal Medicine), FRCP(Glasg)
Clinical Professor, Yong Loo Lin School of Medicine, National University Singapore; Senior Consultant, Department of Rheumatology, Allergy and Immunology, Tan Tock Seng Hospital, Singapore
Principles in Management of Systemic Lupus Erythematosus

Leslie J. Crofford, MD
Gloria W. Singletary Professor of Internal Medicine, and Chief, Division of Rheumatology and Women's Health, University of Kentucky, Lexington, Kentucky
Management of Fibromyalgia and Unexplained Generalized Pain Syndromes

Maryam Dastmalchi, MD, PhD
Senior Consultant, Rheumatology Unit, Department of Medicine, The Karolinska Institute; Rheumatology Unit, Karolinska University Hospital, Stockholm, Sweden
Targeted Treatment of the Idiopathic Inflammatory Myopathies

William P. Docken, MD
Assistant Professor of Medicine, Harvard Medical
    School; Associate Physician, Brigham and
    Women's Hospital, Boston, Massachusetts
Polymyalgia Rheumatica and Giant Cell Arteritis

Doruk Erkan, MD
Assistant Professor of Medicine, Weill Medical
    College of Cornell University; Associate
    Physician-Scientist, The Barbara Volcker Center
    for Women and Rheumatic Disease; Assistant
    Attending Physician, Division of Rheumatology,
    Hospital for Special Surgery, New York, New York
Management of the Antiphospholipid Syndrome

Michael G. Feely, MD
Rheumatology Fellow, Section of Rheumatology
    and Immunology, Department of Internal
    Medicine, University of Nebraska Medical Center,
    Omaha, Nebraska
Management of Established Rheumatoid Arthritis

Dafna D. Gladman, MD, FRCP(C)
Professor of Medicine, University of Toronto;
    Senior Scientist, Toronto Western Research
    Institute, and Director, Psoriatic Arthritis
    Program, University Health Network, Toronto
    Western Hospital, Toronto, Ontario, Canada
Management of Psoriatic Arthritis

Merete Lund Hetland, MD, PhD
Associate Research Professor, University of
    Copenhagen, Copenhagen; Consultant in
    Rheumatology, Department of Rheumatology,
    Copenhagen University Hospital at Hvidovre,
    Hvidovre, Denmark
*Management of Rheumatoid Arthritis: Principles and
Strategies for Antirheumatic Pharmacotherapy*

Marc C. Hochberg, MD, MPH
Professor of Medicine and Epidemiology and
    Preventive Medicine, and Head, Division of
    Rheumatology and Clinical Immunology,
    University of Maryland School of Medicine,
    Baltimore, Maryland
Osteoporosis

Norman T. Ilowite, MD
Professor of Pediatrics, Albert Einstein College
    of Medicine; Division Chief, Pediatric
    Rheumatology, Children's Hospital at
    Montefiore, Bronx, New York
*Management of the Connective Tissue Diseases of
Childhood*

Wilfrid Jänig, MD
Department of Physiology, Christian-Albrechts-
    Universität zu Kiel, Kiel, Germany
*Mechanisms and Treatment Strategy of Complex Regional
Pain Syndromes*

Richard Keating, MD
Professor of Medicine, Pritzker School of
    Medicine, The University of Chicago; Attending
    Rheumatologist, Section of Rheumatology,
    Department of Medicine, The University of
    Chicago Medical Center, Chicago, Illinois
Management of CNS Vasculitis and Takayasu's Arteritis

Sonali Khandelwal, MD
Instructor, Section of Rheumatology, Rush
    University Medical Center, Chicago, Illinois
Regional Disorders of the Neck, Shoulder, Arm, and Hand

Gisela Kobelt, MBA, PhD
Department of Orthopedics, University of Lund,
    European Health Economics, Spéracèdes, France
*Economic Considerations in the Treatment of Rheumatic
Diseases*

James S. Louie, MD
Professor Emeritus of Medicine, Division of
    Rheumatology at CHS, David Geffen School of
    Medicine at UCLA, Los Angeles, California
Septic Arthritis

**Walter P. Maksymowych, MB, ChB, FRCP(C),
FACP, FRCP(UK)**
Scientist, Alberta Heritage Foundation for Medical
    Research, Consultant Rheumatologist, and
    Professor of Medicine, University of Alberta,
    Edmonton, Alberta, Canada
*Management of Ankylosing Spondylitis and Other
Spondyloarthropathies*

Brian F. Mandell, MD, PhD, FACR
Professor and Vice Chairman of Medicine,
    Cleveland Clinic Foundation Lerner College of
    Medicine of Case Western Reserve University;
    Center for Vasculitis Care and Research, and
    Editor in Chief, Cleveland Clinic Journal of
    Medicine, The Cleveland Clinic, Cleveland, Ohio
Gout and Crystal Deposition Disease

Kaisa Mannerkorpi, MD
Associate Professor, Department of Clinical
    Neuroscience and Rehabilitation/Occupational
    Therapy and Physiotherapy, Institute of
    Neuroscience and Physiology, Sahlgrenska
    Academy, University of Gothenburg; Specialist
    Physical Therapist, Sahlgrenska University
    Hospital, Göteborg, Sweden
Physical Activity and Exercise in Rheumatic Disease

Jiska M. Meijer, DMD, MD
Resident in Oral and Maxillofacial Surgery,
    Department of Oral and Maxillofacial Surgery,
    University Medical Center Groningen,
    Groningen, The Netherlands
Management of Sjögren's Syndrome

Petra M. Meiners, MD
Research Fellow, Department of Oral and
Maxillofacial Surgery, University Medical Center
Groningen, Groningen, The Netherlands
Management of Sjögren's Syndrome

Mathilde Michon, MD
Assistant, University Pierre and Marie Curie, Paris,
France
Management of Osteoarthritis: Pharmacotherapy

Ted R. Mikuls, MD, MSHP
Associate Professor, Section of Rheumatology and
Immunology, Department of Internal Medicine,
University of Nebraska Medical Center, Omaha,
Nebraska
Management of Established Rheumatoid Arthritis

Karla L. Miller, MD
Clinical Instructor, Division of Rheumatology,
University of Utah School of Medicine, Salt Lake
City, Utah
*Management of Sarcoidosis, Behçet's Disease, and Other
Rare Rheumatic Diseases*

Oscar D. Naidas, MD
Associate Professor and Chairman, Department
of Medicine, St. Luke's College of Medicine,
Quezon City, and University of Santo Tomas
Faculty of Medicine and Surgery, Manila;
Active Consultant, Section of Nephrology, and
Chairman, Department of Medicine, St. Luke's
Medical Center, Quezon City, Philippines
*Management of Systemic Lupus Erythematosus Renal
Disease*

Sandra V. Navarra, MD
Professor, University of Santo Tomas Faculty
of Medicine and Surgery, Manila; Chief,
Rheumatology, Clinical Immunology and
Osteoporosis, University of Santo Tomas, Manila;
Active Consultant, Rheumatology, St. Luke's
Medical Center, Quezon City, Philippines
*Management of Systemic Lupus Erythematosus Renal
Disease*

Perry M. Nicassio, MA, PhD
Clinical Professor, Department of Psychiatry, David
Geffen School of Medicine at UCLA, Los Angeles,
California
The Significance of Behavioral Interventions for Arthritis

Christina H. Opava, MD, PhD
Professor, Division of Physiotherapy, Department
of Neurobiology, Care Sciences and Society,
Karolinska University Hospital, Stockholm,
Sweden
Physical Activity and Exercise in Rheumatic Disease

Sonja Praprotnik, MD, PhD
Assistant Professor, Faculty of Medicine, University
of Ljubljana; Department of Rheumatology,
University Medical Centre Ljubljana, Ljubljana,
Slovenia
Septic Arthritis

Robert A.S. Roubey, MD
Associate Professor of Medicine, Division of
Rheumatology, Allergy and Immunology,
Thurston Arthritis Research Center, University of
North Carolina School of Medicine, Chapel Hill,
North Carolina
Management of the Antiphospholipid Syndrome

Lisa R. Sammaritano, MD
Associate Professor of Clinical Medicine, Weill
Medical College of Cornell University; Assistant
Attending Physician, Hospital for Special Surgery,
and New York Presbyterian Hospital, New York,
New York
*Management of the Patient with Rheumatic Disease During
and After Pregnancy*

Robert T. Schoen, MD, MBA
Clinical Professor of Medicine, Yale University
School of Medicine; Attending Physician, Yale-
New Haven Hospital, New Haven, Connecticut
Management of Lyme Disease

Jérémie Sellam, MD, PhD
Assistant Professor, University Pierre and Marie
Curie, Paris, France
Management of Osteoarthritis: Pharmacotherapy

Jeff Smith, MD
Senior Director, Medical Research, Alder
Pharmaceuticals, Bothell, Washington
Introduction of a Biologic Agent into the Clinic

Mary Beth F. Son, MD
Instructor in Medicine, Harvard Medical School;
Attending in Rheumatology, Children's Hospital
Boston, Boston, Massachusetts
Juvenile Arthritis

Vibeke Strand, MD
Adjunct Clinical Professor, Division of
Immunology and Rheumatology, Stanford
University School of Medicine, Palo Alto,
California
Introduction of a Biologic Agent into the Clinic

Robert P. Sundel, MD
Associate Professor of Pediatrics, Harvard Medical
School; Director of Rheumatology, Children's
Hospital Boston, Boston, Massachusetts
Juvenile Arthritis

Matija Tomšič, MD, PhD
Associate Professor, Faculty of Medicine,
　University of Ljubljana; Head, Department
　of Rheumatology, University Medical Centre
　Ljubljana, Ljubljana, Slovenia
Septic Arthritis

John Townes, MD
Associate Professor of Medicine, Division of
　Infectious Diseases, Oregon Health and Science
　University, Portland, Oregon
Septic Arthritis

Carl Turesson, MD, PhD
Associate Professor, Lund University, Malmö,
　Sweden
*Management of Rheumatoid Arthritis: The Patient with
Extra-Articular Disease*

Arjan Vissink, DMD, MD, PhD
Professor of Oral and Maxillofacial Surgery,
　Department of Oral and Maxillofacial Surgery,
　University Medical Center Groningen,
　Groningen, The Netherlands
Management of Sjögren's Syndrome

Dawn M. Wahezi, MD
Fellow, Pediatric Rheumatology, Children's
　Hospital at Montefiore, Bronx, New York
*Management of the Connective Tissue Diseases of
Childhood*

Daniel J. Wallace, MD, FACP, FACR
Clinical Professor of Medicine, Division of
　Rheumatology, Cedars-Sinai Medical Center,
　David Geffen School of Medicine at UCLA, Los
　Angeles, California
Management of Nonrenal Systemic Lupus Erythematosus 2

Fredrick M. Wigley, MD
Professor of Medicine, Johns Hopkins University
　School of Medicine; Professor of Medicine,
　Johns Hopkins Scleroderma Center, Baltimore,
　Maryland
*Management of Systemic Sclerosis and Raynaud's
Phenomenon*

Peter K. Wung, MD, MHS
Instructor of Medicine, Johns Hopkins University
　School of Medicine; Instructor of Medicine,
　Johns Hopkins Scleroderma Center, Baltimore,
　Maryland
*Management of Systemic Sclerosis and Raynaud's
Phenomenon*

Foreword

Targeted Therapies is an appropriate title for this textbook on the management of rheumatic diseases and painful musculoskeletal syndromes. Therapeutic targeting may be done on several levels. On the molecular level, increasing knowledge about the components of inflammation and immunity, and the interactions of these components with each other, has encouraged the development of agents that target specific aspects of these processes. Older examples include the xanthine oxidase inhibitor allopurinol to treat hyperuricemia and gout, and specific cyclo-oxygenase-2 inhibitors to decrease pain and inflammation. The perfection of recombinant technology has made possible the production of therapeutic proteins that mimic natural inhibitors of inflammatory cytokines, e.g., etanercept (TNF alpha soluble receptor) anakinra (IL-1 receptor antagonist); inactivate cytokines by a monoclonal antibody (infliximab, adalimumab); impair cell to cell signaling, e.g., abatacept; or destroy specific immunoactive cells, e.g., rituximab (CD-20 B cells). Successful and unsuccessful clinical trials of these specifically targeted therapeutic proteins increase knowledge about how pathogenic mechanisms differ in various chronic inflammatory diseases. Such mechanism targeted therapies are likely to be less toxic than general anti-metabolites such as cyclophosphamide or prednisone.

The increasing availability of more effective, less toxic targeted agents has encouraged the clinical application of a second level of targeting: treatment to achieve a pre-defined disease state. This philosophy has been incorporated in guidance documents for rheumatoid arthritis that advise adjusting therapies every 3 months as needed to achieve and maintain DAS remission or low disease activity state. Similar clinical targets for treatment regimens for other rheumatologic diseases will become possible as more effective agents become available. These outcomes-targeted regimens help compensate for individual variability in responses to initial agents, and adjust for the frequent loss of benefit from initially successful treatments.

A third level of targeting applies to the nuances involved in the management of clinical situations that are uniquely associated with certain rheumatic diseases, but are often unanticipated or missed in routine medical practices. Experts with special interests and experience in such diseases are often able to anticipate and avoid or manage these problems, and thus improve the quality of life for their patients.

This book has assembled an impressive group of international experts who have studied specific aspects of certain rheumatic diseases and have extensive experience with the in-depth management of patients with these diseases. They communicate their knowledge and experience to the reader in chapters that are keyed to illustrative case reports. The current best practices are described and future developments are anticipated.

Targeted Therapies is a useful text for anyone who manages patients with rheumatic diseases. Its expert contributors provide state of the art insight into the management of specific rheumatic diseases and build a solid foundation for understanding the avalanche of new targeted therapies currently being developed, that will markedly improve the quality of life and prognosis of patients with these chronic illnesses.

Harold E. Paulus, MD
Professor Emeritus
Division of Rheumatology
UCLA David Geffen School of Medicine
Los Angeles, California

Contents

Section I Management of Inflammatory Arthritis

Chapter 1

Management of Rheumatoid Arthritis: Principles and Strategies for Antirheumatic Pharmacotherapy

Merete Lund Hetland

CASE STUDY

Laura came into my office as the last patient that day. She had got an acute appointment. A bright, young woman of 25 years of age, university student, the future at her feet. Until suddenly one morning, she could not get out of bed and was unable to dress because her fingers and wrists were swollen, tender, and stiff. She had spent some days in bed, then moved back to her parents because she was unable to manage on her own. When I first saw her, she had been ill for about a month, and was just getting worse and worse day-by-day. She had lost 3 kg of body weight and was pale, desperate, and tired.

She had rheumatoid arthritis (RA). Tender synovitis was present in several joints of the hands. She was rheumatoid factor positive, had elevated C-reactive protein and slight anemia. Erosions appeared on her radiographs. No one else in the family had the disease.

Without delay, she was included in our then ongoing study of early, disease-modifying antirheumatic drugs (DMARD)-naïve RA, the CIMESTRA study.[1] I injected the four most swollen and tender finger joints with glucocorticoids and started methotrexate (MTX) 7.5 mg per week. A fortnight later, when I saw her in the clinic, she was smiling. She was no longer staying in her parents' home and had returned to the university. She had, she said, still one swollen joint, which she would like me to inject, because the four that had been injected the previous time had gone into remission. She got the injection, and we increased the dosage of MTX. The following months, the specially

trained nurses and I saw Laura monthly in the clinic to ensure treatment compliance and complete disease suppression with no evidence of inflammation. She also knew that she could request an appointment within 2 days in case of any swollen joints.

Two years passed quickly. She was in remission. No disease activity apart from one swollen joint 6 months later, which was silenced with an intra-articular injection. MTX 20 mg weekly gave her some discomfort, so she was switched to subcutaneous administration, which she handled herself. No progression was shown on radiographs. She lived a normal life, resumed her fitness training and enjoyed her life as a student.

And then her condition became worse the fall she had graduated from university. She had morning stiffness, fatigue, and new swollen and tender joints at each visit. We added sulfasalazine (SSZ) and hydroxychlorochine, but they had no effect. She was facing sick leave in her new job. She was lucky; the tumor necrosis factor (TNF) inhibitors had been marketed by then, and she was started on etanercept (Enbrel) in combination with MTX. It worked. She went into remission again. The patient still needed a single joint injection once every 1 or 2 years. Apart from that, there were no symptoms and no progression of joint damage. Four years passed, and the disease flared again. Many joints were affected, and the patient had severe problems in her daily life. She was switched to infliximab (Remicade), which was efficacious for 18 months, and then the arthritis showed its ugly face again.

For many rheumatologists, this case is not atypical. RA is a challenge to treat because it lasts life-long, so although a treatment works at some time point, there is no guarantee that it will continue to do so.

The treatment strategy that is outlined in this case focuses on disease-modifying treatment right after diagnosis with MTX in monotherapy or in combination with other DMARDs, intensive care with frequent visits in the clinic, individualized treatment aiming at remission, biologic therapies

as second-line drugs, intra-articular glucocorticoids as bridging therapy, and parental MTX in patients with poor tolerance for oral treatment.

Among the factors that have the greatest impact on prognosis in RA, pharmacologic intervention is probably the most significant. Treatment strategies have changed dramatically during the past decades from a concept of symptom control (with the rheumatologist in a "reactive" position) to one of disease control, in which the rheumatologist is proactive and aims at bringing the patient into remission, that is without any sign of the disease being active. This shift is the result of several significant advances in the field. These include move away from toxic or nonefficaceous DMARDs to the use of MTX as the anchor drug in RA treatment, better designed and conducted randomized controlled trials (RCTs), and biologic drugs with high efficacy (but also a potential for severe side effects and a substantial burden on economic resources in health care systems around the world).

In this chapter, I review some of the evidence found in the literature for the treatment principles and strategy that was illustrated in the case. Such a review cannot be complete; rather, I have instead selected some studies to illustrate my points. My focus is on the prevention of structural joint damage and clinical treatment response in early RA. Other important aspects, such as the impact of treatment strategy on cardiovascular disease, early death, malignancies and osteoporosis, and treatment of established RA, are outside the scope of this chapter.

EARLY VERSUS DELAYED TREATMENT?

The principle of early treatment is based on the concept of a therapeutic window of opportunity early in the disease.[2] By acting in this window, it is assumed that one gets a short-term effect of better treatment response and a long-term effect altering the disease permanently to a milder course. Even a delay of 8 to 9 months in starting DMARD therapy has a significant impact on disease parameters years later.[2]

A recent meta-analysis addressed this issue.[3] A total of 12 studies met the inclusion criteria. The pooled estimate of effects from these studies demonstrated a significant reduction of radiographic progression in patients treated early (standardized mean difference) of −0.19 (Fig. 1-1), which corresponded to a 33% reduction in long-term progression rates compared with patients treated later. Patients with more aggressive disease seemed to benefit most from early DMARD initiation. It was concluded that the effect size from early DMARD initiation was almost half the effect size observed from MTX therapy, and that it was sustained for several years regardless of subsequent treatment. This is an impressive impact and strongly supports the importance of early intervention in newly diagnosed RA.

There is little or no controversy in the rheumatologic field regarding the importance of early intervention. However, the referral of patients to a rheumatologist is often delayed several months for several reasons (patient-related factors, general practitioner hesitation and waiting lists at the hospitals). Therefore, although the establishment of "early arthritis" clinics has been beneficial, it has proven difficult to implement this important aspect of treatment into common clinical practice.

MONO- OR COMBINATION TREATMENT WITH CONVENTIONAL DRUGS?

Some earlier trials of mono- versus combination therapy such as the COBRA[4] and the FinRACo[5] studies showed that SSZ as monotherapy was inferior to SSZ in combination with other conventional drugs (DMARDs). SSZ as monotherapy is now used less

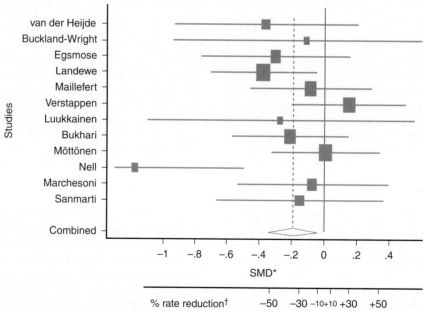

Figure 1-1. Meta-analysis of the evidence for a sustained effect of early treatment intervention on long-term joint damage. SMD, standardized mean difference. (Redrawn from Finckh A, Liang MH, van Herckenrode CM, de Pablo P. Long-term impact of early treatment on radiographic progression in rheumatoid arthritis: A meta-analysis. Arthritis Rheum 2006;55:864-72, Figure 3.)

frequently (but is still the first choice in women with a pregnancy wish), and MTX has become the first drug of choice in the treatment of RA. Therefore, a clinically more relevant question is whether MTX in combination with other conventional drugs is superior to MTX given alone as first-line therapy. The answer remains open, because studies that compare MTX as monotherapy to combinations of MTX with other conventional drugs (DMARDs) are scarce. Many of the studies do not reflect modern treatment strategy, either because the MTX dosage is too low (maximum dosages 5–10 mg per week)[6–10] or because they include obsolete drugs such as oral or parenteral gold.[11]

The CIMESTRA trial investigated the issue in a strategic study aimed at remission with intra-articular glucocorticoids, together with either MTX (up to 20 mg) alone or MTX combined with cyclosporine (2.5–4 mg/kg) (Fig. 1-2).[1,12] All patients were closely monitored (monthly visits with joint counts and adjustment of therapy in case of any swollen joints). The major finding was a very rapid and good clinical response in both groups, with 60% achieving 50% improvement or more (Fig. 1-3), and minimal radiographic progression (Fig. 1-4) with no progression after 2 years in two thirds of the patients (Table 1-1). The clinical response was higher in the combination therapy group, but there was no difference in radiographic progression between the two groups. All in all, the results are comparable to what is achieved with TNF inhibitors.

A major strength of the study was that the strategy with maximum inflammatory suppression was applied to both treatment arms. Thereby the isolated impact of combination treatment could be identified. This is in contrast to most other studies of combination therapy, in which the design is either open or the two treatment groups differ with respect to certain factors, such as visit frequency or use of concomitant prednisolone.[13–16] The weaknesses of the study included the use of cyclosporine, which is very limited in today's treatment palette due to a fear of toxicity, although the low-dose regimen was well tolerated (Table 1-2).

The MASCOT study reported that the combination of MTX and SSZ was more effective than the use of either drug alone in patients, who had a suboptimal response to SSZ (Table 1-3), but there was no difference in radiologic progression.[16] One study investigated patients with an inadequate response to MTX and found, not surprisingly, that combination with leflunomide[17] was more efficacious than continuing MTX alone.

If the clinician decides on combination therapy, one question that arises is whether to combine MTX with SSZ, hydroxychloroquine (HCQ), or both. A double-blinded, randomized study of DMARD-naïve patients addressed this question.[18] Triple therapy was demonstrated to be well tolerated and superior to the double combination of MTX and SSZ or MTX and HCQ with regard to clinical efficacy (ACR20 and ACR50, but not ACR70) (Fig. 1-5). Despite the fact that this well-performed study did not include radiology, it is often cited as an argument for triple therapy as first line therapy in early RA.

The BeSt study captured some of the central questions regarding treatment strategy in early RA. The study was Disease Activity Score (DAS) driven (i.e., treatment was intensified if a certain DAS goal was not achieved) and compared four different treatment strategies given head to head in an open-label, randomized design: (1) Sequential monotherapy with MTX (7.5–30 mg weekly); (2) step-up combination therapy (MTX initially, addition of SSZ 2 g/day and HCQ 200 mg/day); (3) initial combination therapy (MTX and SSZ) with prednisone (60–7.5 mg daily) and (4) initial combination therapy with MTX and infliximab (3 mg/kg). The treatments during the 4 years are shown in Figure 1-6. Initial combination therapies (3 and 4) seemed to provide earlier clinical improvement, but all treatment strategies eventually showed similar clinical improvements after 4 years. Progression of joint damage after 2 years (Fig. 1-7), and 4 years (Fig. 1-8) was significantly lower in the two initial combination therapy groups compared with initial monotherapy, although the differences were small. A major weakness of this study is the open design, which may have biased the clinical

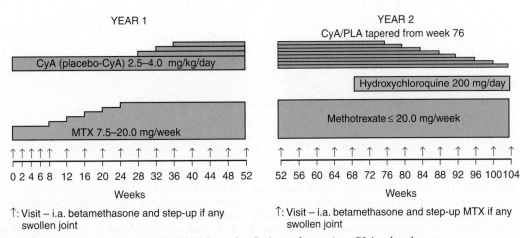

Figure 1-2. Treatment strategy in the CIMESTRA study. CyA, cyclosporine; PLA, placebo.

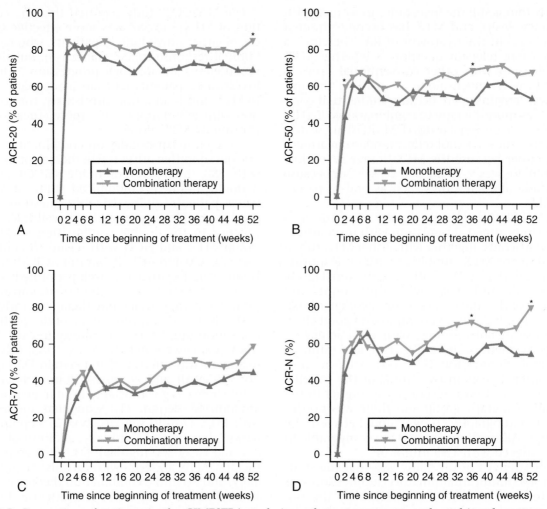

Figure 1-3. Proportion of patients in the CIMESTRA study in each treatment group who achieved responses at each study visit relative to baseline, according to the American College of Rheumatology (ACR) improvement criteria. **A,** ACR 20% response. **B,** ACR 50% reponse. **C,** ACR 70% response. **D,** Individual overall ACR response (ACR-N) at 52 weeks. * = $P < 0.05$ for difference between the two treatment groups. (Redrawn from Hetland ML, Stengaard-Pedersen K, Junker P, Lottenburger T, Ellingsen T, Andersen LS, et al; CIMESTRA Study Group. Combination treatment with methotrexate, cyclosporine, and intraarticular betamethasone compared with methotrexate and intraarticular betamethasone in early active rheumatoid arthritis: an investigator-initiated, multicenter, randomized, double-blind, parallel-group, placebo-controlled study. Arthritis Rheum 2006;54:1401-9, Figure 2.)

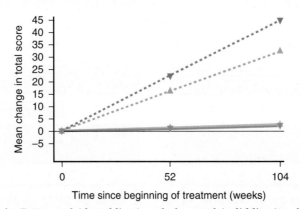

Figure 1-4. The CIMESTRA study. Estimated (*dotted lines*) and observed (*solid lines*) radiographic changes in the mono- (Δ) and the combination therapy (∇) groups during 2 years. (Redrawn from Hetland ML, Stengaard-Pedersen K, Junker P, Lottenburger T, Hansen I, Andersen LS, et al; CIMESTRA study group. Aggressive combination therapy with intra-articular glucocorticoid injections and conventional disease-modifying anti-rheumatic drugs in early rheumatoid arthritis: second-year clinical and radiographic results from the CIMESTRA study. Ann Rheum Dis 2008;67;815-22, Figure 3.)

Table 1-1. *Clinical Outcome Measures, Drug Doses and Disease Activity at Baseline, After 1 Year and After 2 Years in the CIMESTRA Study*

	Baseline (Week 0)			Year 1 (Week 52)			Year 2 (Week 104)		
	MTX + Cyclosporine	MTX + Placebo-Cyclosporine	p Value*	MTX + Cyclosporine	MTX + Placebo-Cyclosporine	p Value*	MTX + Cyclosporine	MTX + Placebo-Cyclosporine	p Value*
No. of tender joints, range 0–10	14 (1–20)	14 (8–20)	0.48	0 (0–1)	1 (0–5)	0.004	0 (0–2)	1 (0–4)	0.23
No. of swollen joints, range 0–40	12 (6–14)	11 (6–15)	0.47	0 (0–0)	0 (0–2)	0.11	0 (0–0)	0 (0–1)	0.61
Doctor's global assessment, 0–100 mm VAS	54 (37–65)	61 (39–71)	0.15	1 (0–7)	5 (0–18)	0.02	2 (0–6)	3 (0–11)	0.60
Patient's assessment of gain, 0–100 mm VAS	46 (28–70)	48 (29–63)	0.96	11 (2–23)	15 (5–35)	0.13	8 (3–23)	10 (1–29)	0.80
Patient's global assessment, 0–100 mm VAS	50 (28–70)	52 (32–73)	0.31	11 (2–27)	15 (4–43)	0.20	12 (2–25)	8 (1–34)	1.00
Serum CRP, mg/L	21 (10–42)	19 (8–46)	0.54	7 (3–10)	8 (4–13)	0.07	7 (3–13)	7 (4–13)	0.61
ESR, mm/h	28 (10–48)	27 (10–47)	0.67	13 (7–23)	10 (5–23)	0.42	10 (6–19)	10 (4–19)	0.26
DAS28 score, ESR based	5.4 (4.6–5.1)	5.7 (4.7–6.2)	0.35	2.1 (1.6–2.9)	2.4 (1.6–3.5)	0.33	2.0 (1.6–3.0)	2.2 (1.5–3.2)	0.92
HAQ score, range 0–3	1.0 (0.4–1.5)	0.9 (0.5–1.4)	0.51	0.1 (0–0.5)	0.4 (0–0.8)	0.18	0 (0–0.4)	0.1 (0–0.8)	0.17
ACR20, % of patients	–	–	–	85	68	0.02	88	73	0.04
ACR50, % of patients	–	–	–	58	53	0.08	79	62	0.03
ACR70, % of patients	–	–	–	59	44	0.08	59	54	0.6
EULAR remission, % of patients	0	0	–	43	34	0.33	51	50	1.00
ACR remission, % of patients	0	0	–	35	28	0.39	41	35	0.52
Max. MTX dose, mg/week	0	0	–	12.5 (10–17.5)	15 (12.5–20)	0.08	17.5 (12.5–20)	17.5 (12.5–20)	–
Max. cyclosporine/Placebo-cyclosporine dose, mg/kg	0	0	–	2.5 (2.5–2.5)	2.5 (2.5–2.5)	–	2.5 (2.5–2.5)	2.5 (2.5–3.0)	–
Cumulated dose of intra-articular betamethasone (ml)	0	0	–	9 (6–17)	12 (6–18)	0.09	1.5 (0–5.125)	2 (0–7.25)	0.18
Blood pressure, mmHg	130/50 (120–140/78–88)	130/50 (120–139/72–85)	0.14–0.35	135/82 (120–140/77–88)	127/81 (117–140/75–88)	0.10–0.63	130/81 (120–140/74–86)	131/80 (120–140/77–86)	0.68–0.71
Serum creatinine, µmol/L mean (SD)	75.4 (11.0)	75.3 (12.2)	0.90	81.5 (13.6)	78.0 (14.1)	0.008	81.0 (13.7)	76.5 (12.9)	0.09

Values are median (integrated range) unless otherwise stated.
*Mann Whitney U test for non-dichotomous variables, X³ test for dichotomous variables.
ACR, American College of Rheumatology; CRP, C-reactive protein; DAS28, Disease Activity Score in 28 points; ESR, erythrocyte sedimentation rate; EULAR, European League Against Rheumatism; HAQ, Health Assessment Questionnaire, MTX, methotrexate; VAS, visual analogus scale.
From Hetland ML, Stengaard-Pedersen K, Junker P, Lottenburger T, Hansen I, Andersen LS, et al; CIMESTRA study group. Aggressive combination therapy with intra-articular glucocorticoid injections and conventional disease-modifying anti-rheumatic drugs in early rheumatoid arthritis: second-year clinical and radiographic results from the CIMESTRA study. Ann Rheum Dis 2008;67;815-822, Table 1.

Table 1-2. Adverse Events in the CIMESTRA Study

Type of Adverse Event	Methotrexate Plus Cyclosporine (n = 80)	Methotrexate Plus Placebo-Cyclosporine (n = 80)	P
Dyspepsia	18 (23)	16 (20)	0.85
Hypertrichosis	26 (33)	6 (8)	<0.001
Constipation	3 (4)	9 (11)	0.13
Insomnia	4 (5)	9 (11)	0.25
Antihypertensive agent added due to hypertension (BP > 140/90 mm Hg)	17 (21)	9 (11)	0.13
> 10% decrease in serum albumin versus baseline	6 (8)	9 (11)	0.59
> 30% increase in serum creatinine versus baseline	15 (19)	5 (6)	0.03

Shown are the number (%) of adverse events that occurred in > 10% of patients in either treatment group. P values were determined by Fisher's exact test. BP, blood pressure.
From Hetland ML, Stengaard-Pedersen K, Junker P, Lottenburger T, Ellingsen T, Andersen LS, et al; CIMESTRA Study Group. Combination treatment with methotrexate, cyclosporine, and intraarticular betamethasone compared with methotrexate and intraarticular betamethasone in early active rheumatoid arthritis: an investigator-initiated, multicenter, randomized, double-blind, parallel-group, placebo-controlled study. Arthritis Rheum 2006;54:1401-9, Table 2.

response rates and the incentive in patient and physician to change treatment. Furthermore, the design does not allow us to identify whether the improved response in group 3 should be attributed to SSZ and HCQ or to high-dose prednisolone. Scatter plots of radiographic change after 2 years (Fig. 1-9) reveal that the poorer outcome in the monotherapy group was driven by a number of patients with high baseline

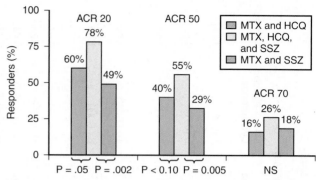

Figure 1-5. ACR20, 50 and 70 responses after 2 years in methotrexate combined with hydrochloroquine, sulfasalazine, or both. (Redrawn from O'Dell JR, Leff R, Paulsen G, Haire C, Mallek J, Eckhoff PJ, et al. Treatment of rheumatoid arthritis with methotrexate and hydroxychloroquine, methotrexate and sulfasalazine, or a combination of the three medications: results of a two-year, randomized, double-blind, placebo-controlled trial. Arthritis Rheum 2002;46:1164-70.)

joint damage. The combination groups had been assigned fewer patients with high baseline scores.

A meta-analysis of efficacy and toxicity of combining conventional drugs in RA concluded that overall combination therapy was more effective than monotherapy, although the risk of toxicity was also slightly higher.[19] Combinations of MTX with SSZ or antimalarials showed good efficacy/toxicity ratios. A severe drawback of this meta-analysis is that it included both obsolete drugs and biologics, and therefore does not adequately address the subject in question here.

In conclusion, the issue of initial combination therapy or not in early RA has not been settled. Combination

Table 1-3. The MASCOT Study: Change in Clinical Outcomes Since Baseline in Combination Therapy (MTX and SSZ) and SSZ and MTX Alone

Variable	Combination (n = 56)	SASP (n = 55)	MTX (n = 54)	Comb v SASP* p Value	Comb v MTX* p Value	SASP v MTX* p Value
DAS	−0.67 (−1.38 to −0.21)	−0.3 (−0.8 to 0)	−0.26 (−0.99 to 0)	0.039	0.023	0.29
HAQ	−0.5 (−10.25 to 0.06)	−0.25 (−9.13 to 0.13)	−0.19 (−10.25 to 0.13)	0.51	0.57	0.99
Ritchie articular index	−4 (−7.5 to −0.5)	−3 (−9 to 1)	0 (−6 to 3)	0.43	0.019	0.13
Swollen joint count	−3 (−4 to −0.5)	−3 (−6 to 0)	−2 (−6 to 0)	0.94	0.81	0.74
Pair score	−8 (−27.5 to 2)	0 (−13 to 7)	0 (−23 to 11)	0.071	0.25	0.58
Patient global	−11.5 (−27.5 to 0.5)	0 (−15 to 5)	−7 (−26 to 2)	0.06	0.72	0.14
Physician global	−12.5 (−25 to 0)	−4 (−15 to 5)	−5 (−22 to 0)	0.044	0.62	0.13
ESR	0 (−8.5 to 1)	0 (−4 to 9)	1 (−3 to 6)	0.087	0.033	0.86
CRP	0 (−5.5 to 1)	0 (−1 to 2)	0 (−3 to 2)	0.18	0.24	0.90

CRP, C-reactive protein; DAS, disease activity score; ESR, erythrocyte sedimetation rate; HAQ health assessment questionnaire; MTX, methotrexate; SASP, sulfasalazine.
A positive value indicates an increase in the variable over the final period. Data are median (IQR) increase in score. Changes are 18-month values minus 6-month values.
*Mann Whitney U test used.
From Capell HA, Madhok R, Porter DR, Munro RA, McInnes IB, Hunter JA, et al. Combination therapy with sulfasalazine and methotrexate is more effective than either drug alone in patients with rheumatoid arthritis with a suboptimal response to sulfasalazine: results from the double-blind placebo-controlled MASCOT study. Ann Rheum Dis 2007;66:235-41, Table 3.

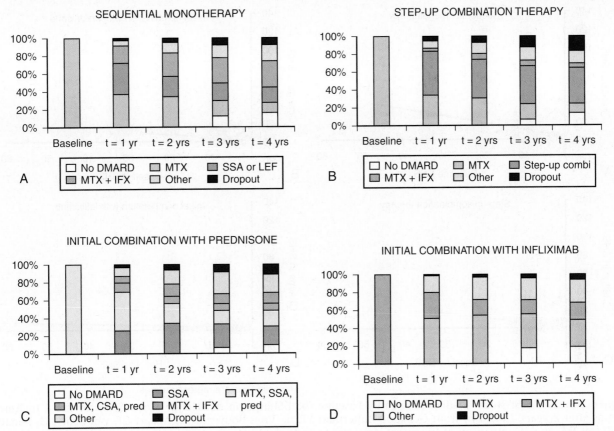

Figure 1-6. The BeSt study. Percentage of patients on different treatment steps during the 4-year study. (Redrawn from Van der Kooij SM, Goekoop-Ruiterman YP, de Vries-Bouwstra JK, Guler-Yuksel M, Zwinderman AH, Kerstens PJ, et al. Drug-free remission, functioning and radiographic damage after 4 years of response-driven treatment in patients with recent onset rheumatoid arthritis. Ann Rheum Dis 2009;68:914-21.)

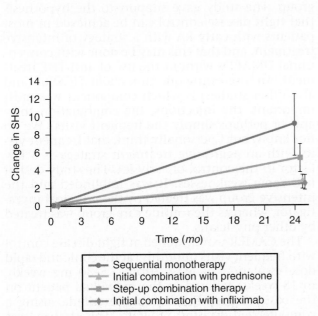

Figure 1-7. The BeSt study. Radiographic outcome after 2 years. (Redrawn from Goekoop-Ruiterman YP, de Vries-Bouwstra JK, Allaart CF, van Zeben D, Kerstens PJ, Hazes JM, et al. Comparison of treatment strategies in early rheumatoid arthritis: a randomized trial. Ann Int Med 2007;146:406-15.)

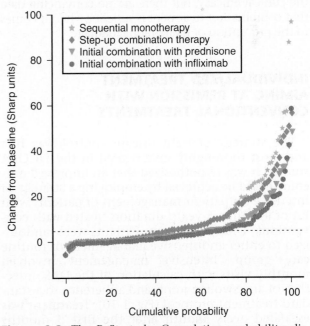

Figure 1-8. The BeSt study. Cumulative probability distribution of radiographic score over 4 years of treatment. (Redrawn from Van der Kooij SM, le Cessie S, Goekoop-Ruiterman YP, de Vries-Bouwstra JK, van Zeben D, Kerstens PJ, et al. Clinical and radiological efficacy of initial versus delayed treatment with infliximab plus methotrexate in patients with early rheumatoid arthritis. Ann Rheum Dis 2009;68:1153-8.)

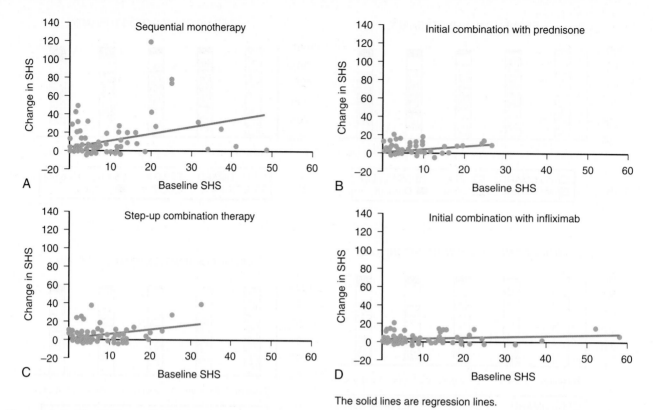

The solid lines are regression lines.

Figure 1-9. The BeSt study. Median change by baseline total Sharp-van der Heijde score (SHS) for the 4 treatment groups after 2 years. (Redrawn from Goekoop-Ruiterman YP, de Vries-Bouwstra JK, Allaart CF, van Zeben D, Kerstens PJ, Hazes JM, et al. Comparison of treatment strategies in early rheumatoid arthritis: a randomized trial. Ann Int Med 2007;146:406-15.)

of MTX with other conventional drugs may increase the clinical efficacy, but there are no convincing data that combination treatment is superior when it comes to the prevention of radiographic damage.

INDIVIDUALIZED TREATMENT AIMING AT REMISSION WITH CONVENTIONAL TREATMENTS

The strategy of tight disease control was first and most thoroughly investigated in the TICORA study.[13] It was hypothesized that an improved outcome could be achieved by employing a strategy of intensive outpatient management of patients with RA of less than 5 years' duration treated with conventional DMARD therapy. Patients were randomized to either an intensive management or routine care group. Intensive management involved monthly visits with calculation of the DAS, injection of any swollen joint, and adherence to a standard treatment protocol (Fig. 1-10). Treatment was escalated every month after the first 3 months if the DAS was higher than 2.4. The routine care group was seen in the clinic every 3 months, treated according to the physician's decision, and the DAS was not systematically assessed. The results were impressive (Tables 1-4 and 1-5). The odds for achieving a good response after 18 months were

5.8 in favor of the group who underwent intensive therapy, and radiographic progression was reduced by nearly 50%. Sixty-five percent were in remission, in contrast to 16% in the routine care group. The study gave support to the hypothesis that tight disease control can be achieved in most patients with early RA with a strategy of intensive treatment, and that this may be done with conventional DMARDs without the use of anti-TNF treatment. An interesting question about TICORA (and also other studies) is which component was most important: the injections, the combination therapy, or perhaps simply the frequent visits? We do not know, but I personally think that frequent visits with an aggressive treatment strategy is a key factor in the control of early RA. The study design had some weaknesses: It was unblinded and the intensive group was treated by the principal investigator, whereas the routine care group was treated by other physicians.

The CAMERA study aimed at tight disease control with frequent visits (monthly) at the clinic and rapid dose escalation of MTX (from 7.5–30 mg weekly in 18 weeks) tailored to the individual patient on the basis of predefined response criteria, using a computerized decision program. This strategy was compared with a group who received standard care (3 monthly visits) with MTX (from 7.5–30 mg in 52 weeks).[14] The protocol and response criteria are

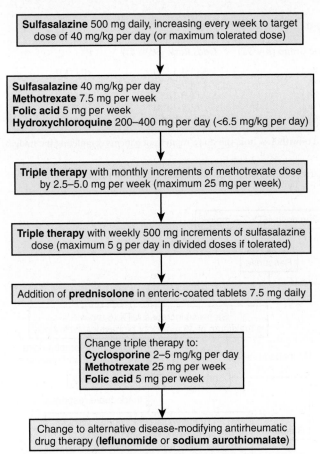

Sulfasalazine 500 mg daily, increasing every week to target dose of 40 mg/kg per day (or maximum tolerated dose)

Sulfasalazine 40 mg/kg per day
Methotrexate 7.5 mg per week
Folic acid 5 mg per week
Hydroxychloroquine 200–400 mg per day (<6.5 mg/kg per day)

Triple therapy with monthly increments of methotrexate dose by 2.5–5.0 mg per week (maximum 25 mg per week)

Triple therapy with weekly 500 mg increments of sulfasalazine dose (maximum 5 g per day in divided doses if tolerated)

Addition of prednisolone in enteric-coated tablets 7.5 mg daily

Change triple therapy to:
Cyclosporine 2–5 mg/kg per day
Methotrexate 25 mg per week
Folic acid 5 mg per week

Change to alternative disease-modifying antirheumatic drug therapy (leflunomide or sodium aurothiomalate)

Figure 1-10. The TICORA study. Protocol for escalation of disease-modifying antirheumatic therapy in patients with persisting disease activity. (Redrawn from Grigor C, Capell H, Stirling A, McMahon AD, Lock P, Vallance R, et al. Effect of a treatment strategy of tight control for rheumatoid arthritis [the TICORA study]: a single-blind randomised controlled trial. Lancet 2004;364: 263-9, Figure 1.)

shown in Figure 1-11. The main finding was that after 2 years, 50% of the intensive strategy group had been in remission for at least 3 months, in contrast to 37% in the conventionally treated group. However, it should be noted that the effect was most pronounced in the first months after inclusion (Fig. 1-12), and after 2 years, the clinical and functional changes from baseline were similar between the two groups. In both groups, approximately 50% did not progress radiographically. We do not know how much the use of a computerized decision algorithm contributed to the results, but it may be an interesting idea for future on-line registration of patients.

In the CIMESTRA study, treatment was individualized, aiming at tight inflammatory control.[20] After 2 years, 50% of the patients in each group were in remission, and two thirds had not progressed radiographically since baseline (see Table 1-1).

My interpretation of the studies is that the goal of disease control can be achieved with MTX as the anchor drug in a much larger proportion of patients than was previously thought. Frequent visits (monthly) allow frequent dose adjustments, and partial responders to MTX (who should be considered for other treatments) are identified earlier.

BIOLOGICS OR DISEASE-MODIFYING ANTIRHEUMATIC DRUGS AS FIRST-LINE THERAPY?

The effect of biologic therapies in both early and established RA has been documented in a number of well-performed RCTs. The TNF inhibitors, as well as other biologics, show best radiographic results when given in combination with MTX[21-23]

Table 1-4. *The TICORA Study. Change in Disease Activity, Radiographic Damage, Physical Function, and Quality of Life Between 0 And 18 Months*

	Intensive Group (n = 53)	Routine Group (n = 50)	Difference (95% CI)	P*
Disease activity score	–3.5 (1.1)	–1.9 (1.4)	1.6 (1.1 to 2.1)	<0.0001
Joint swelling count	–11 (5)	–8 (5)	3 (1 to 5)	0.0028
Joint tenderness count	–20 (9)	–12 (12)	8 (4 to 12)	0.0003
Patient global assessment	–51 (30)	–21 (34)	30 (17 to 42)	<0.0001
Assessor global assessment	–58 (22)	–34 (28)	24 (14 to 34)	<0.0001
Pain score	–45 (24)	–20 (31)	25 (14 to 36)	<0.0001
Erythrocyte sedimentation rate	–30 (28)	–12 (24)	18 (8 to 28)	0.0007
C-reactive protein	–30 (53)	–14 (40)	16 (–3 to 34)	0.09
Health assessment questionnaire	–0.97 (0.8)	–0.47 (0.9)	0.5 (0.2 to 0.8)	0.0025
Shortform-12 physical summary score	9.3 (12)	4.0 (11)	5.3 (0.8 to 9.8)	0.021
Short form-12 mental health summary score	10.9 (16)	6.0 (18)	5.0 (–1.6 to 11.6)	0.138
Erosion score†	0.5 (0–3.375)	3 (0.5–8.5)	n/a	0.002‡
Joint space narrowing†	3.25 (1.125–7.5)	4.5 (1.5–9)	n/a	0.331‡
Total Sharp score†	4.5 (1–9.875)	8.5 (2–15.5)	n/a	0.02‡

Data are mean (SD) unless otherwise indicated.
n/a, not applicable.
*Students test used.
†Median (IQR) increase in score.
‡Mann-Whitney U test used.
From Grigor C, Capell H, Stirling A, McMahon AD, Lock P, Vallance R, et al. Effect of a treatment strategy of tight control for rheumatoid arthritis [the TICORA study]: a single-blind randomised controlled trial. Lancet 2004;364:263-9, Table 3.

Table 1-5   *The TICORA Study (Number of patients responding at 18 month assessment)*

	Intensive Group (n = 55)	Routine Group (n = 55)	Odds Ratio (95% CI)	P*
EULAR good response	45 (82%)	24 (44%)	5.8 (2.4-13.9)*	<0.0001
EULAR remission	36 (65%)	9 (16%)	9.7 (3.9-23.9)*	<0.0001
ACR 20 response	50 (91%)	35 (64%)	5.7 (1.9-16.7)*	<0.0001
ACR 50 response	46 (84%)	22 (40%)	6.1 (2.5-14.9)*	<0.0001
ACR 70 response	39 (71%)	10 (18%)	11 (4.5-27)*	<0.0001

Intention-to-treat analysis of all patients randomized, including those who died or withdrew from the study. Analysis of patients completing the study is very similar (data not shown).
*Mantel-Haenszel procedure used.
From Grigor C, Capell H, Stirling A, McMahon AD, Lock P, Vallance R, et al. Effect of a treatment strategy of tight control for rheumatoid arthritis [the TICORA study]: a single-blind randomised controlled trial. Lancet 2004;364:263-9, Table 2.

Figure 1-11. The CAMERA study. Protocol and response criteria for the intensive and conventional strategy group are shown separately. The sustained response criteria had to be fulfilled for 6 months (three subsequent visits) in the conventional strategy group and for 12 weeks (four subsequent visits) in the intensive strategy group. (Redrawn from Verstappen SM, Jacobs JW, van der Veen MJ, Heurkens AH, Schenk Y, ter Borg EJ, et al; Utrecht Rheumatoid Arthritis Cohort study group. Intensive treatment with methotrexate in early rheumatoid arthritis: aiming for remission. Computer Assisted Management in Early Rheumatoid Arthritis [CAMERA, an open-label strategy trial]. Ann Rheum Dis 2007;66:1443-9, Figure 1.)

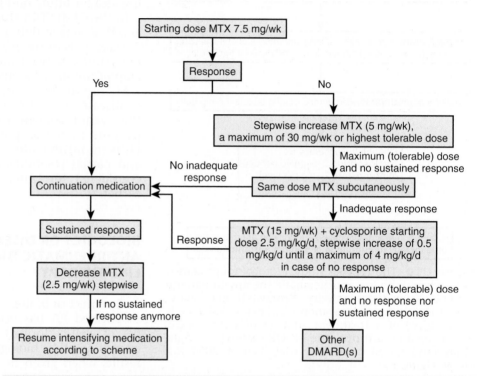

	Response compared to previous visit	Inadequate response	Sustained response
Intensive strategy group	>20% improvement of number of swollen joints and >20% improvement in 2 out of 3 criteria: ESR, number of tender joints, and VAS general well-being.	≤50% improvement from baseline for number of swollen joints and ≤50% improvement from baseline for 2 out of 3 variables: ESR, number of tender joints, and VAS general well-being.	No swollen joints and 2 out of 3 criteria: number of painful joints ≤3, ESR ≤20 mm/h1st, VAS general well-being ≤20 mm.
Conventional strategy group	• Decrease of number of swollen joints • If number of swollen joints unchanged, decision of response depended on assessors' judgment, looking at number of tender joints, ESR, and VAS general well-being.	Number of swollen joints ≥6, number of painful joints ≥3, ESR ≥28 mm/h1st, and morning stiffness ≥45 min.	

compared with biologics given as monotherapy. The drawback of the biologics is that they are very expensive and associated with an increased rate of serious infections.

In the BeSt study, at 4 years follow-up,[24] the group that received infliximab initially (in combination with high-dose MTX) did not perform better clinically or radiographically than the group that

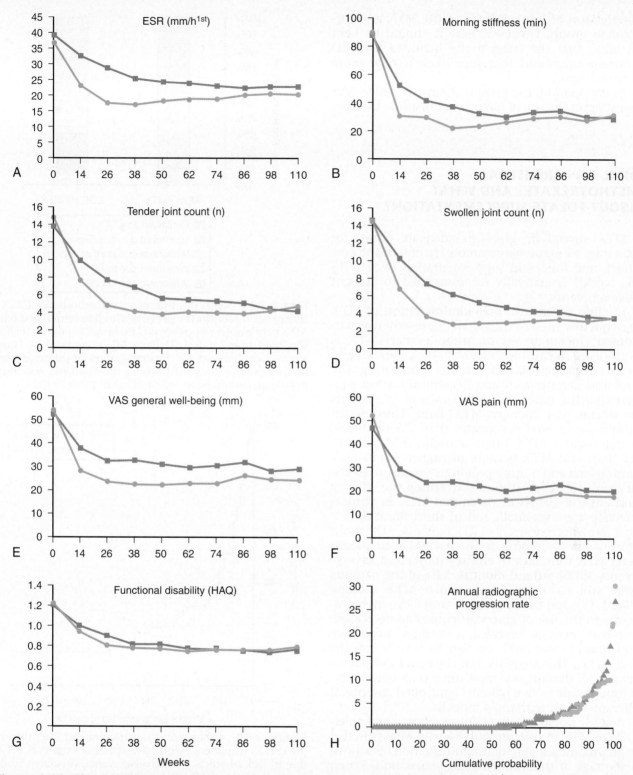

Figure 1-12. The CAMERA study. Mean scores over time for all clinical variables for the intensive strategy group (*red line*) and the conventional strategy group (*blue line*). (Redrawn from Verstappen SM, Jacobs JW, van der Veen MJ, Heurkens AH, Schenk Y, ter Borg EJ, et al; Utrecht Rheumatoid Arthritis Cohort study group. Intensive treatment with methotrexate in early rheumatoid arthritis: aiming for remission. Computer Assisted Management in Early Rheumatoid Arthritis [CAMERA, an open-label strategy trial]. Ann Rheum Dis 2007;66:1443-9, Figure 3.)

received initial combination therapy with MTX, SSZ, and prednisolone (see Fig. 1-7).

In a post-hoc analysis of the BeSt study, the authors compared the patients who received

MTX and infliximab for the initial treatment with those who started it after failing traditional DMARDs.[25] They found more Health Assessment Questionnaire (HAQ) improvement and less progression of joint damage in the MTX and infliximab group. However, here it should be kept in mind that the latter group included DMARD nonresponders and, therefore, likely to have more severe disease.

In my opinion, the present clinical evidence does not support the use of biologics as first-line therapy.

ORAL OR PARENTERAL METHOTREXATE? AND WHAT ABOUT FOLATE SUPPLEMENTATION?

MTX should be given in adequate doses, for example, 15 mg weekly or more, to obtain the best effect, and folic acid supplementation of 5 to 15 mg weekly is generally recommended to prevent adverse events.

In clinical practice, oral administration of MTX is frequently used in the initial phase, whereas parenteral (subcutaneous or intramuscular) MTX is considered in cases with lack of efficacy or adverse events. Pharmacokinetic studies comparing the oral and parenteral routes of administration suggest that the latter may be efficacious in patients in whom oral therapy MTX fails. Thus, when administered in doses greater than 7.5 mg/week, intramuscular MTX offers a higher bioavailability than oral MTX because of higher serum concentrations and a more prolonged exposure to the drug.[26,27] However, studies concerning the efficacy and adverse events of parenteral MTX in clinical practice are few, small, and of short duration.[28-32] In a retrospective study of 212 patients,[33] the main reasons for switching from oral MTX to parenteral MTX were lack of efficacy (66%) and adverse events (28%). After 6 months, 54% of the patients were still receiving intramuscular MTX therapy (Fig. 1-13), and their median serum C-reactive protein and the use of glucocorticoids had decreased. Survival analysis revealed a median adherence to intramuscular MTX therapy of 6 to 8 months (Fig. 1-14). This suggests that the benefit of parenteral MTX therapy was most often only temporary, although one in five patients continued parenteral therapy for more than 24 months.

A study compared the clinical efficacy and tolerance of MTX in patients with RA who were switched from intramuscular to oral administration because of a shortage of the intramuscular preparation. When MTX was first switched from intramuscular to oral administration, increased disease activity, exacerbation of morning pain and hand stiffness, duration of morning stiffness, increased joint pain, and increased joint swelling were observed (Table 1-6). There were more gastrointestinal symptoms, but no increase in liver abnormalities. When intramuscular MTX became available again, one third of the 143 patients were switched back with subsequent improved disease manifestations and reduced side effects.

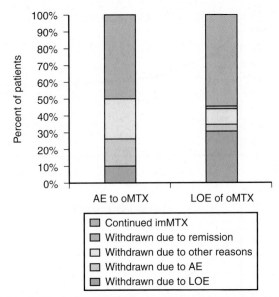

Figure 1-13. Status of intramuscular methotrexate (MTX) therapy at 6 months for patients who had terminated oral MTX because of adverse events (AEs) or lack of efficacy (LOE). (Redrawn from Linde L, Hetland ML, Ostergaard M. Drug survival and reasons for discontinuation of intramuscular methotrexate: a study of 212 consecutive patients switching from oral methotrexate. Scand J Rheum 2006;35:102-6.)

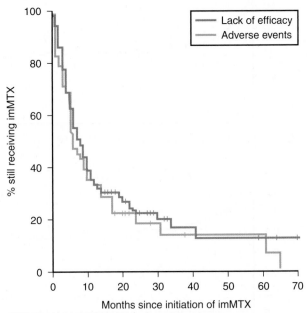

Figure 1-14. Adherence to intramuscular methotrexate (MTX) in patients who had switched from oral MTX due to lack of efficacy or adverse events. (Redrawn from Linde L, Hetland ML, Ostergaard M. Drug survival and reasons for discontinuation of intramuscular methotrexate: a study of 212 consecutive patients switching from oral methotrexate. Scand J Rheum 2006;35:102-6.)

Thus, MTX given parenterally had improved clinical efficacy with fewer side effects than given orally. Parenteral MTX administration should be considered when RA remains active in spite of high-dose oral MTX. To my knowledge, any parenteral

Table 1-6. *Effects of a Switch from Intramuscular to Oral Methotrexate in 143 Patients*

	Increase	No Change	Decrease	No Answered
Morning pain	70 (49)	59 (41)	0	14 (10)
Hand morning stiffness	92 (64)	49 (34)	0	2 (2)
Duration of morning joint stiffness	89 (63)	49 (34)	0	5 (3)
Joint pain	102 (71)	41 (29)	0	0
Joint swelling	85 (59)	49 (34)	0	9 (7)
Consumption of analgesics	94 (66)	45 (31)	0	4 (3)
Eye dryness	19 (14)	82 (57)	0	42 (29)
Mouth dryness	27 (19)	71 (50)	0	45 (31)
Nausea after taking methotrexate	69 (48)	32 (22)	0	42 (29)
Transaminase levels	23 (16)	89 (62)	1	30 (22)

Results are expressed as n (%).
From Wegrzyn J, Adeleine P, Miossec P. Better efficacy of methotrexate given by intramuscular injection than orally in patients with rheumatoid arthritis. Ann Rheum Dis 2004;63:1232-4.

route of administration (subcutaneous or intramuscular) offer similar benefits regarding both efficacy and toxicity.

Most rheumatologists acknowledge the use of supplemental folates, including folic and folinic acid, in RA patients treated with MTX, for example, 5 mg of oral folic acid given 1 to 3 days following the day of MTX administration. This is supported in a review that showed supplementation to improve continuation rates by reducing the incidence of liver function test abnormalities and gastrointestinal intolerance.[34] Folate supplements did not appear to significantly reduce the effectiveness of MTX. However, some clinicians believe that folinic acid (in contrast to folic acid) does decrease the efficacy of MTX.

GLUCOCORTICOIDS AS PART OF TREATMENT STRATEGIES IN RHEUMATOID ARTHRITIS

The euphoria that prednisolone first caused, when its dramatic effect on disease activity in RA patients was discovered, was followed by rational—and irrational—fears of side effects. During the last decade or so, low-dose glucocorticoids have regained some of their good reputation, both as bridging therapy initially in the disease course and as an important supplement in periods with disease exacerbation.[35] Glucocorticoids rapidly relieve signs and symptoms of RA, and they also reduce joint destruction.[35-37] Intra-articular administration, which ensures a high concentration of glucocorticoids at the site of inflammation and reduces synovitis more than MTX alone, has been used successfully in studies of early RA.[13,36,38] Despite this, many rheumatologists are reluctant to inject small joints. In the CIMESTRA study, intra-articular injections with betametasone had a rapid onset of anti-inflammatory action, the need for additional injections was low, and the cumulative dose was moderate.[1] During the 2-year study, 1579 joints were injected blindly, that is, without aid from ultrasonography. The effect lasted for 96 weeks (median time before relapse of synovitis) in proximal interphalangel (PIP) and metacarpophalangeal (MTP) joints. For other joint groups, the time before relapse of synovitis was as follows: shoulders, 88 weeks; knees, 68 weeks; elbows, wrists and ankles, 36 to 42 weeks. Seventy-five percent of the PIP joints and 64% of the MTP joints injected once, and 64% of MTP joints injected twice stayed in remission (Hørsley-Peterson K, under preparation). I hope this study will stimulate more rheumatologists to give intra-articular injections. Patients are reluctant the first time they get an injection, but later when they again experience a swollen joint, they will request an injection again.

IDENTIFYING PATIENTS AT RISK

Modern treatment strategies have raised concern that there is a risk of "overtreating" the patients who have a milder disease. Therefore, identification and development of biomarkers, genetic factors, algorithms, or imaging techniques that may assess us in identifying correctly the patients at risk for progressive disease may help the clinician to optimize treatment in the individual patient.

The past years have brought some promising news in the field. Antibodies against cyclic citrullinated peptide (anti-CCP) is a promising prognostic marker of erosive disease in RA. A recent meta-analysis concluded that anti-CCP–positive patients had a greater risk of radiographic progression than anti-CCP–negative patients.[39] In a study with 10 years' follow-up, anti-CCP, immunoglobulin M rheumatoid factor, erythrocyte sedimentation rate, and female gender were found to be independent predictors of radiographic progression and could be combined into an algorithm for better prediction (Fig. 1-15).[40]

Human leukocyte antigen (HLA)–DRB1 genotyping for shared epitope (HLA-SE) has been associated with the presence of anti-CCP antibodies in early RA, thus playing an indirect role as a risk factor for

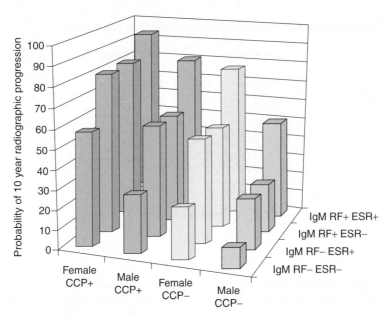

Figure 1-15. The probability of radiographic progression according to different combinations of the independent predictors. ESR, erythrocyte sedimentation rate; RF, rheumatoid factor; CCP, cyclic citrullinated peptide. (From Syversen SW, Gaarder PI, Goll GL, Ødegård S, Haavardsholm EA, Mowinckel P, et al. High anti-cyclic citrullinated peptide levels and an algorithm of four variables predict radiographic progression in patients with rheumatoid arthritis: results from a 10-year longitudinal study. Ann Rheum Dis 2008;67:212-7, Figure 2.)

erosive disease.[41] In a mortality study of 767 patients with early RA, those with DRB1*0101/0401 genotype were found to develop more radiographic damage by the second year compared with all patients with genotypes other than DRB1*0401/*0401.[42] In the future, we can expect identification of genetic markers that can predict treatment response in individual patients. This will open the door to truly personalized medicine in the treatment of RA.

A multicenter study of early RA patients treated in a randomized controlled trial with DMARDs and intra-articular glucocorticoids aiming at maximal inflammatory control showed that the baseline magnetic resonance imaging (MRI) bone edema score of MCP and wrist joints, as well as of wrist joints only, was a strong independent predictor of radiographic progression in hands, wrists, and forefeet during the subsequent 2 years. DAS (DAS28), anti-CCP, smoking, shared epitope, MRI synovitis score, MRI erosion score, and radiographic score at baseline were not independent risk factors.[43] There is growing evidence that bone marrow edema on MRI scan represents inflammatory infiltrates in the bone marrow in established RA.[44] In contrast to radiographic erosions, which reflect bone damage that has already occurred, bone marrow edema thus may represent an important part of the early immunopathologic development in RA.[44]

Smoking is a well-established risk factor for the development of anti-CCP–positive RA,[45] but its influence on RA disease progression is unclear. In 2000 RA patients with variable disease duration, radiographic joint damage progressed at an equivalent rate in smokers and nonsmokers,[46] and in

200 patients with early RA, smoking status did not influence radiographic progression after 2 years.[47]

In conclusion, several promising potential predictors of severe RA have been identified, and the development in this field may lead to improved treatment strategies in the future.

MONEY MATTERS

A cross-sectional study from the collaborative database QUEST-RA (Sokka T, under preparation), involving more than 6000 patients from 25 countries across the world, has found that the DAS (DAS28) ranged from 6.0 in countries with low gross domestic product (GDP) to 3.1 in countries with high GDP per capita. DAS was associated with GDP (r^2 = 72%) among 18 European countries. In univariate models, the use of medications explained 25%, GDP 61%, and psychosocial distress 75% of the variation of the DAS28 among the 25 countries. A multivariable model with all three variables explained 83% of DAS28. This suggests that the burden of RA is substantially greater in poor countries compared with rich countries.

SUMMARY

In this chapter, I have presented evidence that supports the emerging principles of RA treatment with aggressive use of DMARDs, combination therapies, frequent follow-up visits, intra-articular glucocorticoid injections, steadfastly pursuing low disease activity or remission with radiographic monitoring and consideration of biologics in patients with an inadequate treatment response.

References

1. Hetland ML, Stengaard-Pedersen K, Junker P, Lottenburger T, Ellingsen T, Andersen LS, et al. Combination treatment with methotrexate, cyclosporine, and intraarticular betamethasone compared with methotrexate and intraarticular betamethasone in early active rheumatoid arthritis: an investigator-initiated, multicenter, randomized, double-blind, parallel-group, placebo-controlled study. Arthritis Rheum 2006;54:1401-9.
2. O'Dell JR. Treating rheumatoid arthritis early: a window of opportunity? Arthritis Rheum 2002;46(2):283-5.
3. Finckh A, Liang MH, van Herckenrode CM, de Pablo P. Long-term impact of early treatment on radiographic progression in rheumatoid arthritis: a meta-analysis. Arthritis Rheum 2006;55:864-72.
4. Boers M, Verhoeven AC, Markusse HM, van de Laar MA, Westhovens R, van Denderen JC, et al. Randomised comparison of combined step-down prednisolone, methotrexate and sulphasalazine with sulphasalazine alone in early rheumatoid arthritis. Lancet 1997;350:309-18.
5. Mottonen T, Hannonen P, Leirisalo-Repo M, Nissila M, Kautiainen H, Korpela M, et al. Comparison of combination therapy with single-drug therapy in early rheumatoid arthritis: a randomised trial. FIN-RACo trial group. Lancet 1999;353:1568-73.
6. Haagsma CJ, van Riel PL, de Jong AJ, van de Putte LB. Combination of sulphasalazine and methotrexate versus the single components in early rheumatoid arthritis: a randomized, controlled, double-blind, 52 week clinical trial. Br J Rheumatol 1997;36:1082-8.
7. Dougados M, Combe B, Cantagrel A, Goupille P, Olive P, Schattenkirchner M, et al. Combination therapy in early rheumatoid arthritis: a randomised, controlled, double blind 52 week clinical trial of sulphasalazine and methotrexate compared with the single components. Ann Rheum Dis 1999;58:220-5.
8. Willkens RF, Urowitz MB, Stablein DM, McKendry Jr RJ, Berger RG, Box JH, et al. Comparison of azathioprine, methotrexate, and the combination of both in the treatment of rheumatoid arthritis. A controlled clinical trial. Arthritis Rheum 1992;35:849-56.
9. Willkens RF, Sharp JT, Stablein D, Marks C, Wortmann R. Comparison of azathioprine, methotrexate, and the combination of the two in the treatment of rheumatoid arthritis. A forty-eight-week controlled clinical trial with radiologic outcome assessment. Arthritis Rheum 1995;38:1799-806.
10. Ferraz MB, Pinheiro GR, Helfenstein M, Albuquerque E, Rezende C, Roimicher L, et al. Combination therapy with methotrexate and chloroquine in rheumatoid arthritis. A multicenter randomized placebo-controlled trial. Scand J Rheumatol 1994;23:231-6.
11. Lehman AJ, Esdaile JM, Klinkhoff AV, Grant E, Fitzgerald A, Canvin J. A 48-week, randomized, double-blind, double-observer, placebo-controlled multicenter trial of combination methotrexate and intramuscular gold therapy in rheumatoid arthritis: results of the METGO study. Arthritis Rheum 2005;52:1360-70.
12. Hetland ML, Stengaard-Pedersen K, Junker P, Lottenburger T, Hansen I, Andersen LS, et al. Aggressive combination therapy with intra-articular glucocorticoid injections and conventional disease-modifying anti-rheumatic drugs in early rheumatoid arthritis: second-year clinical and radiographic results from the CIMESTRA study. Ann Rheum Dis 2008;67:815-22.
13. Grigor C, Capell H, Stirling A, McMahon AD, Lock P, Vallance R, et al. Effect of a treatment strategy of tight control for rheumatoid arthritis (the TICORA study): a single-blind randomised controlled trial. Lancet 2004;364:263-9.
14. Verstappen SM, Jacobs JW, van der Veen MJ, Heurkens AH, Schenk Y, ter Borg EJ, et al. Intensive treatment with methotrexate in early rheumatoid arthritis: aiming for remission. Computer Assisted Management in Early Rheumatoid Arthritis (CAMERA, an open-label strategy trial). Ann Rheum Dis 2007;66:1443-9.
15. Goekoop-Ruiterman YP, de Vries-Bouwstra JK, Allaart CF, van Zeben D, Kerstens PJ, Hazes JM, et al. Clinical and radiographic outcomes of four different treatment strategies in patients with early rheumatoid arthritis (the best study): a randomized, controlled trial. Arthritis Rheum 2005;52:3381-90.
16. Capell HA, Madhok R, Porter DR, Munro RA, McInnes IB, Hunter JA, et al. Combination therapy with sulfasalazine and methotrexate is more effective than either drug alone in patients with rheumatoid arthritis with a suboptimal response to sulfasalazine: results from the double-blind placebo-controlled MASCOT study. Ann Rheum Dis 2007;66:235-41.
17. Kremer JM, Genovese MC, Cannon GW, Caldwell JR, Cush JJ, Furst DE, et al. Concomitant leflunomide therapy in patients with active rheumatoid arthritis despite stable doses of methotrexate. A randomized, double-blind, placebo-controlled trial. Ann Intern Med 2002;137:726-33.
18. O'Dell JR, Leff R, Paulsen G, Haire C, Mallek J, Eckhoff PJ, et al. Treatment of rheumatoid arthritis with methotrexate and hydroxychloroquine, methotrexate and sulfasalazine, or a combination of the three medications: results of a two-year, randomized, double-blind, placebo-controlled trial. Arthritis Rheum 2002;46:1164-70.
19. Choy EH, Smith C, Dore CJ, Scott DL. A meta-analysis of the efficacy and toxicity of combining disease-modifying anti-rheumatic drugs in rheumatoid arthritis based on patient withdrawal. Rheumatology (Oxford) 2005;44:1414-21.
20. Hetland ML, Stengaard-Pedersen K, Junker P, Lottenburger T, Hansen I, Andersen LS, et al. Aggressive combination therapy with intraarticular glucocorticoid injections and conventional dmards in early rheumatoid arthritis Two year clinical and radiographic results from the CIMESTRA Study. Ann Rheum Dis 2008;67:815-22.
21. St Clair EW, van der Heijde DM, Smolen JS, Maini RN, Bathon JM, Emery P, et al. Combination of infliximab and methotrexate therapy for early rheumatoid arthritis: a randomized, controlled trial. Arthritis Rheum 2004;50:3432-43.
22. Emery P, Breedveld FC, Hall S, Durez P, Chang DJ, Robertson D, et al. Comparison of methotrexate monotherapy with a combination of methotrexate and etanercept in active, early, moderate to severe rheumatoid arthritis (COMET): a randomised, double-blind, parallel treatment trial. Lancet 2008;372:375-82.
23. Breedveld FC, Weisman MH, Kavanaugh AF, Cohen SB, Pavelka K, van Vollenhoven R, et al. The PREMIER study: a multicenter, randomized, double-blind clinical trial of combination therapy with adalimumab plus methotrexate versus methotrexate alone or adalimumab alone in patients with early, aggressive rheumatoid arthritis who had not had previous methotrexate treatment. Arthritis Rheum 2006;54:26-37.
24. Van der Kooij SM, Goekoop-Ruiterman YP, de Vries-Bouwstra JK, Guler-Yuksel M, Zwinderman AH, Kerstens PJ, et al. Drug-free remission, functioning and radiographic damage after 4 years of response-driven treatment in patients with recent onset rheumatoid arthritis. Ann Rheum Dis 2009;68:914-21.
25. Van der Kooij SM, le Cessie S, Goekoop-Ruiterman YP, de Vries-Bouwstra JK, van Zeben D, Kerstens PJ, et al. Clinical and radiological efficacy of initial versus delayed treatment with infliximab plus methotrexate in patients with early rheumatoid arthritis. Ann Rheum Dis 2009;68:1153-8.
26. Freeman-Narrod M, Gerstley BJ, Engstrom PF, Bornstein RS. Comparison of serum concentrations of methotrexate after various routes of administration. Cancer 1975;36:1619-24.
27. Hamilton RA, Kremer JM. Why intramuscular methotrexate may be more efficacious than oral dosing in patients with rheumatoid arthritis. Br J Rheumatol 1997;36:86-90.
28. Wegrzyn J, Adeleine P, Miossec P. Better efficacy of methotrexate given by intramuscular injection than orally in patients with rheumatoid arthritis. Ann Rheum Dis 2004;63:1232-4.

29. Bingham SJ, Buch MH, Lindsay S, Pollard A, White J, Emery P. Parenteral methotrexate should be given before biological therapy. Rheumatology (Oxford) 2003;42:1009-10.

30. Osman A, Mulherin D. Is parenteral methotrexate worth trying? Ann Rheum Dis 2001;60:432.

31. Burbage G, Gupta R, Lim K. Intramuscular methotrexate in inflammatory rheumatic disease. Ann Rheum Dis 2001;60:1156.

32. Rozin A, Schapira D, Balbir-Gurman A, Braun-Moscovici Y, Markovits D, Militianu D, et al. Relapse of rheumatoid arthritis after substitution of oral for parenteral administration of methotrexate. Ann Rheum Dis 2002;61:756-7.

33. Linde L, Hetland ML, Ostergaard M. Drug survival and reasons for discontinuation of intramuscular methotrexate: a study of 212 consecutive patients switching from oral methotrexate. Scand J Rheumatol 2006;35:102-6.

34. Whittle SL, Hughes RA. Folate supplementation and methotrexate treatment in rheumatoid arthritis: a review. Rheumatology (Oxford) 2004;43:267-71.

35. Kirwan JR. The effect of glucocorticoids on joint destruction in rheumatoid arthritis. The Arthritis and Rheumatism Council Low-Dose Glucocorticoid Study Group. N Engl J Med 1995;333:142-6.

36. Conaghan PG, O'Connor P, McGonagle D, Astin P, Wakefield RJ, Gibbon WW, et al. Elucidation of the relationship between synovitis and bone damage: a randomized magnetic resonance imaging study of individual joints in patients with early rheumatoid arthritis. Arthritis Rheum 2003;48:64-71.

37. Svensson B, Boonen A, Albertsson K, van der Heijde D, Keller C, Hafstrom I. Low-dose prednisolone in addition to the initial disease-modifying antirheumatic drug in patients with early active rheumatoid arthritis reduces joint destruction and increases the remission rate: a two-year randomized trial. Arthritis Rheum 2005;52:3360-70.

38. Proudman SM, Conaghan PG, Richardson C, Griffiths B, Green MJ, McGonagle D, et al. Treatment of poor-prognosis early rheumatoid arthritis. A randomized study of treatment with methotrexate, cyclosporin A, and intraarticular corticosteroids compared with sulfasalazine alone. Arthritis Rheum 2000;43:1809-19.

39. Nishimura K, Sugiyama D, Kogata Y, Tsuji G, Nakazawa T, Kawano S, et al. Meta-analysis: diagnostic accuracy of anti-cyclic citrullinated peptide antibody and rheumatoid factor for rheumatoid arthritis. Ann Intern Med 2007;146: 797-808.

40. Syversen SW, Gaarder PI, Goll GL, Odegard S, Haavardsholm EA, Mowinckel P, et al. High anti-cyclic citrullinated peptide levels and an algorithm of four variables predict radiographic progression in patients with rheumatoid arthritis: results from a 10-year longitudinal study. Ann Rheum Dis 2008;67:212-7.

41. Berglin E, Johansson T, Sundin U, Jidell E, Wadell G, Hallmans G, et al. Radiological outcome in rheumatoid arthritis is predicted by presence of antibodies against cyclic citrullinated peptide before and at disease onset, and by IgA-RF at disease onset. Ann Rheum Dis 2006;65:453-8.

42. Mattey DL, Thomson W, Ollier WE, Batley M, Davies PG, Gough AK, et al. Association of DRB1 shared epitope genotypes with early mortality in rheumatoid arthritis: results of eighteen years of followup from the early rheumatoid arthritis study. Arthritis Rheum 2007;56:1408-16.

43. Hetland ML, Ejbjerg BJ, Horslev-Petersen K, Jacobsen S, Vestergaard A, Jurik AG, et al. MRI bone oedema is the strongest predictor of subsequent radiographic progression in early rheumatoid arthritis. Results from a 2 year randomized controlled trial (CIMESTRA). Ann Rheum Dis 2008;68:384-90.

44. McQueen FM, Ostendorf B. What is MRI bone oedema in rheumatoid arthritis and why does it matter? Arthritis Res Ther 2006;8:222.

45. Pedersen M, Jacobsen S, Garred P, Madsen HO, Klarlund M, Svejgaard A, et al. Strong combined gene-environment effects in anti-cyclic citrullinated peptide-positive rheumatoid arthritis: a nationwide case-control study in Denmark. Arthritis Rheum 2007;56:1446-53.

46. Finckh A, Dehler S, Costenbader KH, Gabay C. Cigarette smoking and radiographic progression in rheumatoid arthritis. Ann Rheum Dis 2007;66:1066-71.

47. Manfredsdottir VF, Vikingsdottir T, Jonsson T, Geirsson AJ, Kjartansson O, Heimisdottir M, et al. The effects of tobacco smoking and rheumatoid factor seropositivity on disease activity and joint damage in early rheumatoid arthritis. Rheumatology (Oxford) 2006;45:734-40.

Chapter 2

Management of Rheumatoid Arthritis: The Newly Diagnosed Patient

Vivian P. Bykerk

CASE STUDY   New-Onset Rheumatoid Arthritis

A 32-year-old woman presents with a 4-month duration of pain rated at 8 on a scale of 1 to 10 and swelling in her hands, wrists, left elbow, right knee, ankles, and forefeet. This started initially with 2 months of bilateral wrist and forefoot pain and progressed over time to involve more joints. She is currently 10 months postpartum, after having given birth to her third child. She has a history of 3 cesarian births and an appendectomy. She is an ex-smoker, having stopped 7 years ago, and uses no alcohol. She had no associated history of photosensitivity, alopecia, nasal mucosal ulcers, rashes, fevers or weight loss. She is experiencing many difficulties in performing homemaking tasks, particularly in lifting and bathing her young son. The general physical examination revealed no rashes, nodules, adenopathy, or other findings. The musculoskeletal exam revealed eight swollen and tender, and two tender-only joints out of 28, as revealed in Figure 2-1. Her metatarsal phalangeal joints were also noted to be very tender and swollen. She rated her disease activity as an 8 on a scale of 1 to 10. Initial investigations revealed that she had an antinuclear antibody test score (ANA) of 1:80, a positive rheumatoid factor (RF) of 53 IU, and a normal chest radiograph. The anti–cyclic citrillinated peptide (anti-CCP) test was 100 IU. Radiographs of the hands and feet showed soft tissue swelling at the proximal interphalangeal joint and wrist joints, and periarticular osteopenia of the hands. No erosions or joint space narrowing were noted. Her baseline liver function tests were normal; Hepatitis B and C status were negative. The C-reactive protein (CRP) was elevated at 23.5 mg/L. We rated her disease activity as a 7 on a scale of 1 to 10.

When a patient presents with new onset inflammatory polyarthritis consistent with rheumatoid arthritis (RA), initial principles of management are to (1) confirm a diagnosis, (2) provide the patient with an understanding of his or her disease process and potential prognosis, (3) provide opportunities for physical/occupational therapies and information about exercise. You also need to discuss factors that the patient may be able to control (e.g., dietary and lifestyle changes) and advise how to learn about self-management. These are important aspects of therapy, as is a complete investigation and initiation of pharmacotherapy.

INITIAL EVALUATION AND INVESTIGATION

Patients presenting with a history of at least 12 weeks of synovitis, fulfill the American College of Rheumatology (ACR) criteria for the classification of RA, and would be considered to have newly diagnosed or early RA. It is important to note that the ACR criteria are worthwhile for classification purposes but not for diagnostic purposes in clinical practice. If a patient is seen very early in the course of disease (within 12 weeks of onset of symptoms), disease-modifying antirheumatic drug (DMARD) therapy will be recommended once other causes of inflammatory arthritis are excluded. When faced with patients with early disease such as in our case, it is important to characterize the extent of disease severity and look at predictors of prognosis to determine if they are at risk for rapid radiographic deterioration. To this end, initial investigations to consider include radiographs of the hands and feet, as well as acute-phase reactants (erythrocyte sedimentation rate, CRP), a tender and swollen joint count, and a RF and anti-CCP antibody. In the future, there may also be a potential role of magnetic resonance imaging (MRI) or musculoskeletal ultrasound (US) with power Doppler (PD) studies to characterize the extent and severity of synovitis and identify early bony erosions unrecognized on baseline radiographs.

Recent guidelines from the ACR[1] and the European League Against Rheumatism (EULAR)[2] recommend the use of standardized composite outcome measures to aid in therapeutic decisions with regard to the treatment of RA. In the absence of having a full questionnaire completed inquiring more detailed information based on patient-reported outcomes, the simplest outcome measures include the Disease Activity Score 28 (DAS28) (erythrocyte sedimentation rate [ESR] or CRP)[3,4] the Simplified Disease Activity Index (SDAI) or the clinical disease

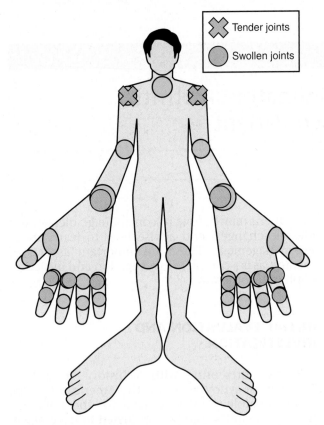

Tender joints

Swollen joints

Figure 2-1. A representation of the patient's swollen and tender joints as drawn on a homunculus.

Table 2-1. *Calculation of Clinical Outcome Measures*

	DAS 28	SDAI	CDAI
Swollen joint count	$0.28 \times \sqrt{(0-28)}$	0–28	0–28
Tender joint count	$0.56 \times \sqrt{(0-28)}$	0–28	0–28
Patient global score	$0.014 \times (0-100)$	0–10	0–10
Physician global score		0–10	0–10
ESR	$0.70 \times Ln(ESR)$		
CRP (mg/dL)		0.1–10	
Range of score values		0.1–86	0–76

DAS, Disease Activity Score; CDAI, Clinical Disease Activity Index; ESR, erythrocyte sedimentation rate; CRP, C-reactive protein; SDAI, Simplified Disease Activity Index.

activity index when a CRP level is not available.[5,6] The calculation of these and value ranges indicating remission, low, moderate, and high disease activity are shown in Tables 2-1 and 2-2.[3,7,8]

Based on these scoring instruments, our patient's pretreatment DAS28 was 5.8, her SDAI was 36, and her CDAI was 33, confirming that her disease activity was moderate to high after 4 months of symptoms of inflammatory arthritis consistent with RA.

DISCUSSION OF PROGNOSTIC FACTORS

Patients with new-onset RA can have a variable disease course. Anywhere from 10% to 30% of patients are at risk for developing rapid and potentially

Table 2-2. *Current and Proposed Definitions of Disease Activity*

Index	Disease Activity State	Original Definition	Newly Proposed Definition
SDAI	Remission	≤5	≤3.3
	Low disease activity	≤20	≤11
	Moderate disease activity	≤40	≤26
	High disease activity	>40	>26
CDAI	Remission		≤2.8
	Low disease activity		≤10
	Moderate disease activity		≤22
	High disease activity		>22
DAS28	Remission	≤2.6	≤2.4
	Low disease activity	≤3.2	≤3.6
	Moderate disease activity	≤5.1	≤5.5
	High disease activity	>5.1	>5.5

CDAI, Clinical Disease Activity Index; DAS, Disease Activity Score; SDAI, Simplified Disease Activity Index.
From Aletaha D, Smolen J. The Simplified Disease Activity Index (SDAI) and the Clinical Disease Activity Index (CDAI): a review of their usefulness and validity in rheumatoid arthritis. Clin Exp Rheumatol 2005;23(Suppl 39):S100-8.

Table 2-3. *Markers of Poor Prognosis in Patients Presenting with Early Rheumatoid Arthritis*

Young age
Female gender
High titers of rheumatoid factor (RF), and/or anticyclic citrullinated peptide antibodies (anti-CCP)
Evidence of early erosive disease
Elevated acute phase reactants: ESR or CRP
High disease activity measure by the DAS28, SDAI, or CDAI
Extra-articular disease (Sjögren's, pulmonary disease)

CDAI, Clinical Disease Activity Index; CRP, C-reactive protein; DAS, Disease Activity Score; ESR, erythrocyte sedimentation rate; SDAI, Simplified Disease Activity Index.

severe deterioration. Selected markers of poor prognosis have been identified (Table 2-3). When more than one of these poor prognostic factors is present, it is possible that even with effective nonbiologic DMARDs, patients will have suboptimal responses. Patients who do not reach a low disease activity state by month 4 will continue to have more radiographic damage. Thus, it is important to estimate the patient's prognosis based on available clinical tools to identify which patients merit close follow-up in the initial stages, to identify earlier than later those who may need an adjustment in their treatment paradigm.

An anti-CCP test was performed on this patient to provide more information on the prognosis of her inflammatory arthritis. Lee et al. summarized the emerging data that a positive anti-CCP can provide prognostic information on the severity of the disease, and the likelihood that the arthritis will rapidly worsen.[9] They note that in numerous studies, patients with anti-CCP antibodies have more radiographic damage and progression than those without anti-CCP. This patient had high titers of anti-CCP levels (100 IU), indicating that her disease may not respond well to initial treatment with DMARDs and that she merits a treatment approach that will rapidly result in full control of her synovitis so as to reduce the risk of rapid radiographic progression.

ROLE OF HIGH-SENSITIVITY IMAGING IN THE INITIAL EVALUATION OF PATIENTS WITH NEWLY DIAGNOSED RHEUMATOID ARTHRITIS

Despite the normal radiographic findings in our case, there may be a potential benefit to know if she has subclinical erosions. This would be of particular importance had there not been other features of poor prognosis such as a high CRP or positive anti-CCP antibodies. Researchers are now evaluating the role of high-sensitivity imaging including MRI or US with PD studies of the dominant wrist or metacarpophalangeal joints (MCPs) to provide more information as to the patient's risk of further disease progression based on presence or absence of early subclinical erosions.

To further investigate whether there is a rationale for MRI using either high-resolution MRI machines ($\geq$ 1.5 Tesla) with or without gadolinium or lower Tesla (0.2–1.0) office-based units on the dominant wrist or MCPs, a limited number of studies have been performed. To date, these studies have involved only small numbers of patients and have not yet fully evaluated the role of this technology in clinical practice. A recent review by the American College of Rheumatology Extremity Magnetic Resonance Imaging Task Force concluded that there is currently insufficient evidence for employing MRI in patients with early-stage inflammatory arthritis.[10] This was based on the paucity of longitudinal trials to show prognostic capabilities of this technique, poor positive and negative predictive capacity of this modality, and the lack of trials to show that information obtained with peripheral MRI may alter the clinical decision-making process or impact clinical outcomes. Nonetheless, as further studies are undertaken, this viewpoint may change.

GOALS OF THERAPY IN THE NEWLY TREATED PATIENT WITH RHEUMATOID ARTHRITIS

The goal of medical treatment in RA patients is to achieve a state of low disease activity and, if possible, a state of remission, in order to minimize structural damage and improve functional status.[11] Our patient has a number of clinical features to suggest that she could have a poor clinical outcome including young age, female gender, high disease activity as noted by a high number of tender and swollen joints, a high CRP, and a positive RF and anti-CCP antibody. A number of treatment strategies are discussed, including how they can be implemented to achieve this goal.

Joint damage can be viewed from two perspectives: (1) soft tissue damage seen as deformities that occur rapidly as a result of nature's forces acting on joints whose capsules have undergone prolonged distention causing ligamentous laxity, and (2) radiographic damage defined as joint space narrowing and marginal bony erosions. The latter is more easily measured, with validated scores measuring radiographic damage becoming a key outcome along with clinical and functional measures to evaluate the success of either DMARD or biologic therapy.[12] While progression of radiographic abnormalities has limited effects on function initially, over time, accumulation of destruction is associated with a decline of functional capacity and quality of life,[13,14] making the elimination of radiographic progression a key goal in therapy.

Debates remain as to whether the goal of reaching, at minimum, a state of low disease activity and, at best, a state of EULAR clinical remission is sufficient. Recent studies suggest that more stringent outcomes should be targeted in terms of goals of treatment, indicating that true remission will be achieved only when synovitis is fully eliminated and only then will radiographic progression be halted. In a recent study evaluating the frequency of inflamed joints in patients thought to be in clinical remission, 42 of 102 patients defined as being in sustained clinical remission using the DAS28 score of less than 2.6 followed for 1 year, 87% still had synovial hypertrophy and 56% had increased PD signals on musculoskeletal ultrasound.[15] Despite being in clinical remission, 19% of the patients displayed deterioration in joint damage using high sensitivity imaging instruments over the study period. Whether or not these high-sensitivity imaging techniques should be routinely incorporated into daily practice to determine whether achieving a state of true remission yields better functional outcomes remains to be proven. The current trend among rheumatologists is to use an optimal treatment strategy to eliminate synovitis. To that end, our patient was immediately started on methotrexate (MTX) therapy (by subcutaneous injections) at 15 mg weekly and increasing over 2 to 4 weeks to 25 mg subcutaneously, and her knee, elbow and wrists were injected with glucocorticoids. The rationale for this particular treatment regimen is explained in the next section.

INITIAL TREATMENT STRATEGY IN THE PATIENT WITH NEWLY DIAGNOSED RHEUMATOID ARTHRITIS

Treatment goals of RA have changed significantly over the past decade. Previously, a conservative strategy was used in which DMARDs were initiated only when the diagnosis was established and a trial of nonsteroidal anti-inflammatory drugs had failed. Now, a preventive strategy is used in which DMARDs are initiated from the first recognition of synovitis in conjunction with typical features of RA such that the current standard of care is to immediately initiate DMARD therapy in the newly diagnosed RA patient to ideally induce a remission and halt joint damage. It is still not known why some patients even with early institution of DMARD therapy continue to have active disease. Studies are in progress to determine if serum biomarkers, genetic profiling, and proteomic studies will help identify those patients who continue to experience progression of damage despite drug therapy. What also remains inconsistent among clinicians is determining what should be the ideal initial treatment approach. Recent treatment guidelines and recommendations are not consistent as to which DMARD should be the first chosen for patients such as ours.[1,2,16] Conventional nonbiologic DMARDs, meaning small molecules that reduce inflammation and have structure-modifying properties, are used as monotherapy or in combination during the long-term therapy of RA. The most frequently used DMARD is MTX, which is now considered the anchor drug of RA treatment.[2]

In light of the many published clinical trials studying recently diagnosed patients with RA, it has become clear that the most effective initial therapy is MTX. The ACR has recently published recommendations for the use of nonbiologic and biologic DMARDs.[1] Following a systematic review of the scientific evidence, a series of treatment algorithms were developed based on disease duration and features of poor prognosis, which were validated using a series of clinical scenarios (Fig. 2-2).

Although such recommendations are useful to help guide therapy, they require that each rheumatologist implement the use of a composite outcome instrument to determine the extent of disease activity and make treatment decisions accordingly. This will require a shift in practice patterns for those rheumatologists and arthritis practitioners who do not routinely perform joint counts in their practice.

Benefits of Earlier Disease-Modifying Antirheumatic Drug Intervention in the Patient with Newly Diagnosed Rheumatoid Arthritis

Mottonen et al.[17] studied the effect of delaying DMARD therapy in patients with early RA in the FIN-RACo (FINnish Rheumatoid Arthritis Combination therapy) trial. In this study, 195 patients with recent-onset RA (median duration 6 months) were randomly assigned to receive either combination DMARDs (sulfasalazine [SSZ], MTX, hydroxychloroquine [HDQ], and prednisolone) or a single DMARD with or without prednisolone. The authors noted that a delay in therapy of 4 months was a predictor for patients who would not reach a state of remission when treated with DMARD monotherapy. More patients in the combination-DMARD group after 2 years reached remission (42%) compared with patients on DMARD monotherapy; 35% of patients in the early group and only 11% of those with delayed treatment reached remission. Thus, when employing initial monotherapy, a delay in

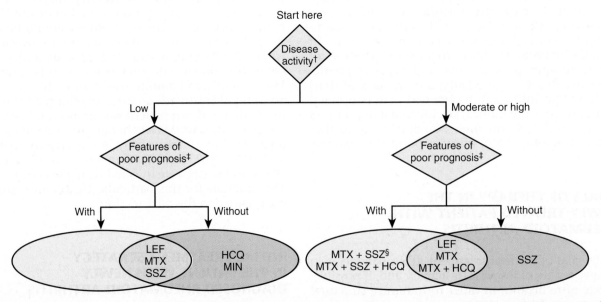

Figure 2-2. A treatment algorithm to facilitate the first choice of nonbiologic disease-modifying antirheumatic drug (DMARD) for the patient with new-onset rheumatoid arthritis. (From Saag KG, Teng GG, Patkar NM, Anuntiyo J, Finney C, Curtis JR, et al. American College of Rheumatology 2008 Recommendations for the use of nonbiologic and biologic disease-modifying antirheumatic drugs in rheumatoid arthritis. Arthritis Rheum 2008;59:762-84.)

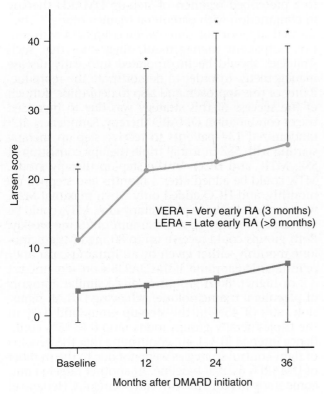

Figure 2-3. Radiographic benefit for patients when treated very early with disease-modifying antirheumatic drugs in patients with early rheumatoid arthritis. (Adapted with permission from Nell VPK, Machold KP, Eberl G, Stamm TA, Uffmann M, Smolen JS. Benefit of very early referral and very early therapy with disease-modifying anti-rheumatic drugs in patients with early rheumatoid arthritis. Rheumatology 2004;43:906-14.)

treatment can affect the ability to achieve remission in the long term. Others have shown that a delay in treatment will result in worse radiographic outcomes. The benefits of early DMARD intervention were demonstrated in a study by Nell et al. in which patients started very early (within 3 months) on DMARDs had less radiographic progression than in those whose DMARDs were started later (>9 months) (Fig. 2-3).[18]

Is There an Advantage to Using Initial Combination Disease-Modifying Antirheumatic Drug Therapy in the Patient with Newly Diagnosed Rheumatoid Arthritis?

The question of whether patients with new-onset RA should be treated initially with more than one DMARD is still controversial. Several recent studies do not support this approach, but in most of these studies, glucocorticoids were used frequently and may have confounded their ability to answer to this question. Dougados et al. performed a randomized

trial in 205 patients with ERA (fulfilling 1987 ACR criteria for the classification of RA) comparing initial SSZ and MTX monotherapies versus SSZ and MTX combination therapies.[19] Although there were no significant differences at 24 weeks among the groups, patients receiving the combination treatment showed a trend toward better improvements in their DAS score, but had greater numbers of adverse events. The real impetus behind the use of earlier combination DMARD therapy may be based on recommendations from practice guidelines. A recent systematic review of all guidelines on the use of Biologic Agents in Rheumatoid Arthritis reported that 8 out of 10 of the guidelines recommended that a patient have high disease activity and should have an inadequate response for at least 3 to 6 months of combination DMARD therapy before initiating biologic DMARDs.[16] Many of these recommendations are based on formulary and country-specific requirements and are not derived from evidence-based data. To satisfy many of the arbitrary formulary requirements, clinicians may start with combination DMARD therapy rather than monotherapy so that they can access biologic therapies sooner for their patients.

Is There an Optimal Use of Methotrexate in the Newly Diagnosed Rheumatoid Arthritis Patient?

MTX has become recognized as the most important drug for the treatment of RA.[20,21] In recent guidelines for the treatment of early RA, it has been recommended as the initial and mainstay of therapy.[2] Based on current understanding of the metabolism of MTX,[22] a recent meta-analysis of the use of MTX in RA,[23] and its performance in recent trials comparing it to biologic therapies in early RA,[24-26] new observations have provided insights on the optimal use of MTX. These insights include starting MTX at a higher initial dose of 10 to 15 mg weekly, more rapid dose escalation up to 25 mg weekly (if tolerated), and parenteral administration of higher dose MTX to ensure maximal bioavailability. Better outcomes may be reached when patients using higher weekly doses of MTX administer it subcutaneously.[27] This presumably is based on better absorption. Several recent studies have supported higher doses of MTX in patients with early arthritis. In randomized controlled trials comparing MTX monotherapy to MTX with biologic DMARDs, impressive improvements in swollen and tender joint counts, function, patient and physician global assessments, DAS28 responses, and improvement in radiographic progression were seen with MTX monotherapy.[24,25,28,29] Typically 15% to 20% of patients will achieve responses akin to remission when MTX alone is initiated. For example, in one study (COMET) comparing MTX monotherapy (rapid dose escalation to 20 mg/wk) as compared with etanercept plus MTX in early RA, the MTX monotherapy group achieved a DAS remission in 50% of patients, 80% of patients did not have radiographic progression, and 24% of patients on MTX monotherapy had stopped work at 52 weeks, but only 9% had done so in the combination group.[29] Moreover, other studies report higher rates of remission using MTX in combination with intra-articular or intramuscular corticosteroids (at the initial visits) to initiate a more rapid improvement, with remission rates higher than 50%.[30,31] At present, I start patients on MTX at a dose of 10 to 15 mg per week (except in older patients in whom I start MTX therapy at 7.5 to 10 mg per week). Within the next two to four weeks, the dose of MTX is increased to 20 mg per week (or to 15 mg in older patients and then to 20 mg weekly after another 4 weeks). The MTX dose may be increased to 25 mg per week administered subcutaneously if the patient's disease activity does not reach a low disease activity state after a total of 4 to 8 weeks of 20 mg of oral MTX. If the disease remains active despite this approach, I will consider adding either another DMARD or a biologic if there has been a suboptimal response to MTX. Using this rapid dose escalaton regimen we are making a decision about adding additional therapies to MTX after only 8 to 12 weeks of maximally escalated MTX monotherapy. About 40% of patients will do very well with only MTX monotherapy using this treatment approach and will not require biologics. Furthermore rapidly escalating the dose of MTX (ideally 20–25 mg per week if tolerated) reduces the risk of inadequate response to MTX monotherapy, thus lessening the risk of radiographic progression.

Thus, based on what is known about the optimal use of MTX and the benefits of adjunctive intra-articular glucocorticoids, we opted to choose this initial treatment algorithm for our patient. Based on studies evaluating frequent assessments and treating to an activity target, as explained in the next section, we also planned to see our patient every 3 months until she reaches a state of remission.

Treating to a Target: Should Patients with Early Rheumatoid Arthritis Undergo Frequent Assessments and Treatment Adjustments?

Several recent studies have provided evidence to support intensive care of patient with new-onset RA by frequently assessing patients every 1 to 3 months, and adjusting therapies such that the physician treats to a defined target. Such a target might be zero swollen joints or to a remission state based on a validated outcome measure. Two such studies have shown very positive outcomes using such a treatment strategy. Grigor et al. examined the effect of intensive management of early RA in the Tight Control of Rheumatoid Arthritis (TICORA) study by regularly assessing patients every 3 months, targeting persistent disease activity of a DAS

greater than 2.4 and intensifying therapy according to a prescribed regimen of step-up DMARD therapy in conjunction with parenteral triamcinolone.[31] They showed superior outcomes when compared with routine outpatient management, suggesting that such strategies should be incorporated into early disease management. In order to demonstrate the reproducibility of this approach and also to determine if much of the success of this strategy was due to increased use of combination DMARD therapy, Saunders et al.[32] randomized 134 patients to receive step-up therapy starting with SSZ or initial triple therapy consisting of SSZ, MTX, and HCQ. In the step-up therapy group, MTX could be added after 3 months and stepped up monthly, and HCQ added only when maximal MTX was reached. In the triple-therapy arm, MTX could be increased monthly to a maximum of 25 mg weekly. Both groups could receive up to 80 mg of triamcinolone monthly, either given by an intramuscular and/or intra-articular route, if the DAS28 score remained at 3.2 or higher. Both groups received similar amounts of parenteral triamcinolone, achieving EULAR remission rates of 45% in the step-up group and 33% in the triple-therapy groups (odds ratio 0.6; 95% confidence interval [0.3–1.4]), confirming that the benefits of tight-control strategies were not due to the number of DMARDs used at baseline. In another targeted outcome study in patients with early-onset RA, Hetland et al.[30] demonstrated high DAS remission rates of 51 and 50% in the CIMESTRA study. In the study, patients were assessed monthly and treated to a target of zero swollen joints whereby all swollen joints were injected with intra-articular betamethasone. Patients received either MTX plus cyclosporine or MTX monotherapy plus placebo. Addition of cyclosporine during the first year improved clinical outcomes after 2 years, but did not have any additional effect on the remission rate and radiographic outcome.

In the CAMERA study, clinical remission rates of 50% could be achieved using MTX alone initially with adjustment of doses and the addition if needed of cyclosporine A in patients who were assessed monthly as opposed to every 3 months.[33]

IS THERE A ROLE FOR INDUCTION REGIMENS IN THE TREATMENT OF THE NEWLY DIAGNOSED RHEUMATOID ARTHRITIS PATIENT?

Martin Du Pan et al.[34] reviewed six clinical trials comparing the combination of MTX-infliximab (IFX) and MTX-placebo in early RA. These studies examined the effects of upfront induction therapy using IFX for a fixed period of time at the outset on radiographic joint damage, composite disease activity measures, and functional disability scores when used in patients with early RA. The authors concluded that initial limited use of IFX was associated with an acceptable safety profile but noted that as yet there has been no study that demonstrated the cost-effectiveness of initial short-term IFX use in early RA. In the BeST study, the early use of an IFX-MTX combination was reported to be more effective in preventing radiographic damage and functional disability progression.[35] However, although they found superiority of this combination in improving disease activity compared with nonbiologic DMARDs alone, they did not find superiority of this combination as an initial induction therapy when it was compared with an initial course of high-dose steroids.

THE ROLE OF GLUCOCORTICOIDS IN THE NEWLY TREATED RHEUMATOID ARTHRITIS PATIENT

Glucocorticoids are not considered to be conventional DMARDs, but they are are widely used based on their effectiveness in controlling inflammation as well as their low cost.[36] There is also evidence for their effectiveness in reducing radiographic damage in some studies, and confirmed in a recent meta-analysis.[37,38] Even the use of initial parenteral steroids has been found to be effective, albeit moderately so, in halting radiographic progression in patients randomized to receive intramuscular glucocorticoids monthly in addition to the usual DMARDs as compared with placebo[39]; however, the radiographic benefits of initial steroids are less pronounced than those seen with tumor necrosis factor (TNF) inhibitors.[40] However, glucocorticoids have numerous adverse effects with long-term use, including negative effects on glucose and bone metabolism,[41] an increased risk of infection such as pneumonia,[42] being associated with an increased mortality rate.[43] They are not recommended for long-term use but rather for initial transient use (EULAR guidelines on use of glucocorticoids). Short-term use of moderate-to-high doses of glucocorticoids provide rapid initial control of active synovitis in early RA, helping to prevent further accumulation of structural damage, as demonstrated in the Combinatietherapie Bij Reumatoide Artritis (COBRA) study.[44] Based on data from studies showing improved outcomes with subcutaneous use of MTX when used at higher doses and when treatment is adjusted frequently according to a predetermined target,[27,30,31] we opted to implement a regimen of frequent assessment, intra-articular glucocorticoids, and maximal subcutaneous MTX treatment to a target of zero swollen joints. Despite our patient having presented with several poor prognostic indicators, she initially responded very well, and was in remission by 6 months and remained in sustained remission. At her 18-month follow-up examination, she presented with a flare of her disease after having opted to stop her MTX 3 months earlier. However 4 months of retreatment with MTX in combination with HCQ and intra-articular steroids failed to regain control of her disease. She was subsequently offered a TNF inhibitor to control her RA.

TREATMENT OF THE NEWLY DIAGNOSED PATIENT IF EARLY REMISSION NOT REACHED— INITIATING BIOLOGIC RESPONSE MODIFIERS (ALTERNATIVE TREATMENT OF THE DMARD NONRESPONDER)

When Should Biologic Therapies Be Initiated in the Patient with Newly Diagnosed Rheumatoid Arthritis?

As noted earlier, 10% to 30% of patients with new-onset RA will have an inadequate response to a combination of nonbiologics with or without some form of glucocortiocoid therapy. This raises the question as to when biologic DMARDs should be offered to patients with RA. Most rheumatologists recommend their use only after a trial of at least one or two synthetic DMARDs in patients who continue to have active synovitis. The most recent practice recommendation by Saag et al.[1] uses a decision algorithm for initiating biologic DMARDs, promoting the use of a biologic (TNF inhibitor or abatacept) in cases in which nonbiologic DMARDs have failed patients and the patients still have high disease activity and poor prognostic indicators.

No practice guideline or recommendation has recommended the initial use of a TNF inhibitor except in extenuating circumstances (e.g., pregnancy, hepatitis C infection). This is despite several randomized controlled studies (RCTs)[24-26] demonstrating superiority in group scores in clinical, radiographic outcomes, improved work productivity, and function when initiating therapy with a combination of MTX plus a TNF inhibitor as opposed to MTX monotherapy. There are a number of reasons for this. In a substantial number of patients in each of these studies, their RA improved substantially and radiographic progression was halted using MTX monotherapy, even in some patients with more severe disease characteristics, such as high CRP levels at baseline, high tender and swollen joint counts, presence of RF, or anti-CCP. To date, there is no way of predicting which patient will respond well to MTX monotherapy alone and which truly should have started with the combination therapy. The cost of therapy must be considered in the treatment decision process.

The current cost of biologics precludes in most patients initial institution of biologics, particularly if they need to be dosed chronically and not as induction therapy. Research is underway to determine which patients would benefit from initial biologic DMARDs, and it is hoped that as yet undiscovered soluble biomarkers will help to direct therapy in an optimal and cost-effective fashion.

Applying Safety Concerns of Treatment (Hepatic or Renal Disease, Diabetes, Osteoporosis, Latent Tuberculosis Infection, History of Malignancy, Congestive Heart Failure, Chronic Obstructive Pulmonary Disease, and History of Recurrent Infection)

Many patients we treat with new-onset RA will have other comorbidities. These will pose relative contraindications for the use of either nonbiologic DMARDs or biologic DMARDs. For example, TNF inhibitors should be avoided in patients with recurrent infections, congestive heart failure, untreated latent or active tuberculosis (TB) infection, or untreated hepatitis B infection. Full vaccinations should be up to date for any patient starting immunosuppressive therapy, and patients should be screened for latent TB before starting anti-TNF therapies. For example, MTX should also be avoided in patients with liver disease, hepatitis B or C infection or significant renal impairment, significant alcohol consumption, or untreated chronic infections. Recommendations for the safe implementation of nonbiologic and biologic DMARDs have been extensively reviewed by the ACR.[1] Physicians and other health care providers involved in the care of patients with RA are encouraged to review these recommendations in detail.

SUMMARY

In order to optimally treat patients with RA, it is important to implement early intervention with DMARDs. The initial DMARD chosen needs to be effective, and there is consensus based on the current literature that this agent should be MTX. This should be initiated at doses of 10 to 15 mg weekly and rapidly escalated as tolerated to 25 mg weekly (if tolerated), ideally given parenterally by subcutaneous self-injection if the higher dose of MTX is required.[45] Folic acid at a minimum dose of 1 mg per day and at least 5 mg weekly, or folinic acid given 8 to 24 hours after MTX at a dose of 5 mg weekly[46] should also be provided to reduce side effects of MTX. Additional use of corticosteroids or other DMARDs appears to yield better clinical and radiographic responses. Glucocorticoids have been shown to be effective in rapidly reducing disease activity in patients with early RA and should be considered either as temporary oral therapy or implemented by intermittent parenteral therapy as intramuscular or intra-articular injections, until nonbiologic and, if need be, biologic DMARDs have become fully effective.

Patients with multiple poor prognostic markers (including a high number of involved joints, high acute-phase response, high-titer RF and anti-CCP) starting with MTX have a much higher risk of rapid radiographic progression,[47] and warrant frequent assessments. If they are inadequate responders, by 3 to 4 months, they should be considered for initiation of early biologic therapy. There is no consensus yet as to which biologic should be chosen initially, because all currently approved TNF inhibitors have evidence of superior efficacy in patients with active early synovitis. During the first year (and if need be longer) of any therapeutic strategy for the newly diagnosed RA patient, frequent assessments (every 1–3 months) while treating patients to a predetermined target will optimize their clinical response. This may be as simple as treating by targeting to zero swollen joints, or targeting to a remission score using a composite measure of disease activity.

OUR CASE

In the case of our patient, her initial presentation of multiple swollen joints including large joints, presence of several poor prognostic or risk factors, we used an evidence-based approach consisting of initial DMARD, in this case MTX monotherapy, with parenteral glucocorticoids, subsequent combination DMARDs, and ultimately, a biologic DMARD. My own clinical experience has shown that this has been an effective approach for many newly diagnosed patients, because the adverse events are generally manageable and the therapeutic outcomes relatively predictable and positive. Careful monitoring of newly diagnosed patients is essential to success, including follow-up visits every 4 to 12 weeks for the first 3 to 12 months, and regular laboratory monitoring, not only for safety but including acute phase reactants for effectiveness, and radiographs initially every 12 months to verify the efficacy of the chosen treatment regimen.

References

1. Saag KG, Teng GG, Patkar NM, Anuntiyo J, Finney C, Curtis JR, et al. American College of Rheumatology 2008 Recommendations for the use of nonbiologic and biologic disease-modifying antirheumatic drugs in rheumatoid arthritis. Arthritis Rheum 2008;59:762-84.
2. Combe B, Landewe R, Lukas C, Bolosiu HD, Breedveld F, Dougados M, et al. EULAR recommendations for the management of early arthritis: report of a task force of the European Standing Committee for International Clinical Studies Including Therapeutics (ESCISIT). Ann Rheum Dis 2007;66:34-45.
3. Prevoo ML, van't Hof MA, Kuper HH, van Leeuwen MA, van de Putte LBA, van Riel PLCM. Modified disease activity scores that include twenty-eight-joint counts. Development and validation in a prospective longitudinal study of patients with rheumatoid arthritis. Arthritis Rheum 1995;38:44-8.
4. Fransen JWP, De Keijzer RMH, Van Riel PLCM. Disease activity scores using C reactive protein: CRP may replace ESR in the assessment of RA disease activity. Ann Rheum Dis 2003;62(Suppl. 1):151.
5. Smolen JS, Breedveld FC, Schiff MH, Kalden JR, Emery P, Eberl G, et al. A simplified disease activity index for rheumatoid arthritis for use in clinical practice. Rheumatology 2003;42:244-57.

6. Aletaha D, Ward MM, Machold KP, Nell VPK, Stamm T, Smolen JS. Remission and active disease in rheumatoid arthritis. Defining criteria for disease activity states. Arthritis Rheum 2005;52:2625-36.

7. Aletaha D, Smolen J. The Simplified Disease Activity Index (SDAI) and the Clinical Disease Activity Index (CDAI): a review of their usefulness and validity in rheumatoid arthritis. Clin Exp Rheumatol 2005;23(Suppl. 39):S100-8.

8. Fransen J, van Riel PL. The Disease Activity Score and the EULAR response criteria. Clin Exp Rheumatol 2005;23(Suppl. 39):S93-9.

9. Lee W, Weisman MH. The predictive power of anti-cyclic citrullinated peptide antibodies: window into understanding gene/environment/immunity interactions. J Rheumatol 2006;33:1216-8.

10. Anonymous. Report of the American College of Rheumatology Extremity Magnetic Resonance Imaging Task Force. Arthritis Rheum 2006;54:1034-47.

11. Breedveld FC, Kalden JR. Appropriate and effective management of rheumatoid arthritis. Ann Rheum Dis 2004;63:627-33.

12. van der Heijde D. Impact of imaging in established rheumatoid arthritis. Best Pract Res Clin Rheumatol 2003;17:783-90.

13. Drossaers-Bakker KW, de Buck M, van Zeben D, Zwinderman AH, Breedveld FC, Hazes JM. Long-term course and outcome of functional capacity in rheumatoid arthritis: the effect of disease activity and radiologic damage over time. Arthritis Rheum 1999;42:1854-60.

14. Scott DL, Symmons DP, Coulton BL, Popert AJ. Long-term outcome of treating rheumatoid arthritis: results after 20 years. Lancet 1987;1:1108-11.

15. Brown AK, Conaghan PG, Karim Z, Quinn MA, Ikeda K, Peterfy CG, et al. An explanation for the apparent dissociation between clinical remission and continued structural deterioration in rheumatoid arthritis. Arthritis Rheum 2008;58:2958-67.

16. Lopez-Olivo MA, Kallen MA, Ortiz Z, Skidmore B, Suarez-Almazor ME. Quality appraisal of clinical practice guidelines and consensus statements on the use of biologic agents in rheumatoid arthritis: a systematic review. Arthritis Rheum 2008;59:1625-38.

17. Mottonen T, Hannonen P, Korpela M, Nissilä M, Kautiainen H, Ilonen J, et al. Delay to institution of therapy and induction of remission using single-drug or combination-disease-modifying antirheumatic drug therapy in early rheumatoid arthritis. Arthritis Rheum 2002;46:894-8.

18. Nell VPK, Machold KP, Eberl G, Stamm TA, Uffmann M, Smolen JS. Benefit of very early referral and very early therapy with disease-modifying anti-rheumatic drugs in patients with early rheumatoid arthritis. Rheumatology 2004;43:906-14.

19. Dougados M, Combe B, Cantagrel A, Goupille P, Olive P, Schattenkirchner M, et al. Combination therapy in early rheumatoid arthritis: a randomised, controlled, double blind 52 week clinical trial of sulphasalazine and methotrexate compared with the single components. Ann Rheum Dis 1999;58:220-5.

20. Kremer JM. Methotrexate treatment of rheumatic diseases: can we do better? Arthritis Rheum 2008;58:3279-82.

21. Weinblatt ME, Kaplan H, Germain BF, Block S, Solomon SD, Merriman RC, et al. Methotrexate in rheumatoid arthritis. A five-year prospective multicenter study. Arthritis Rheum 1994;37:1492-8.

22. Dalrymple JM, Stamp LK, O'Donnell JL, Chapman PT, Zhang M, Barclay ML. Pharmacokinetics of oral methotrexate in patients with rheumatoid arthritis. Arthritis Rheum 2008;58:3299-308.

23. Visser K, van der Heijde D. Optimal dosage and route of administration of methotrexate in rheumatoid arthritis: a systematic review of the literature. Ann Rheum Dis 2009;68:1094-9.

24. St. Clair EW, van der Heijde DM, Smolen JS, Maini RN, Bathon JM, Emery P, et al. Combination of infliximab and methotrexate therapy for early rheumatoid arthritis. Arthritis Rheum 2004;50:3432-43.

25. Breedveld FC, Weisman MH, Kavanaugh AF, Cohen SB, Pavelka K, van Vollenhoven R, et al. The PREMIER study: a multicenter, randomized, double-blind clinical trial of combination therapy with adalimumab plus methotrexate versus methotrexate alone or adalimumab alone in patients with early, aggressive rheumatoid arthritis who had not had previous methotrexate treatment. Arthritis Rheum 2006;54:26-37.

26. Emery P, Breedveld FC, Hall S, Durez P, Chang DJ, Robertson D, et al. Comparison of methotrexate monotherapy with a combination of methotrexate and etanercept in active, early, moderate to severe rheumatoid arthritis (COMET): a randomised, double-blind, parallel treatment trial. Lancet 2008;372:375-8.

27. Braun J, Kästner P, Flaxenberg P, Wahrisch J, Hanke P, Demary W, et al. Comparison of the clinical efficacy and safety of subcutaneous versus oral administration of methotrexate in patients with active rheumatoid arthritis: results of a six-month, multicenter, randomized, double-blind, controlled, phase IV trial. Arthritis Rheum 2008;58:73-81.

28. Bathon JM, Martin RW, Fleischmann RM, Tesser JR, Schiff MH, Keystone EC, et al. A comparison of etanercept and methotrexate in patients with early rheumatoid arthritis.[see comment][erratum appears in N Engl J Med 2001 Jan 18;344(3):240]. N Engl J Med 2000;343:1586-93.

29. Emery P, McInnes IB, van Vollenhoven R, Kraan MC. Clinical identification and treatment of a rapidly progressing disease state in patients with rheumatoid arthritis. Rheumatology 2008;47:392-8.

30. Hetland ML, Stengaard-Pedersen K, Junker P, Lottenburger T, Hansen I, Andersen LS, et al. Aggressive combination therapy with intra-articular glucocorticoid injections and conventional disease modifying anti-rheumatic drugs in early rheumatoid arthritis: second-year clinical and radiographic results from the CIMESTRA study. Ann Rheum Dis 2008;67:815-22.

31. Grigor C, Capell H, Stirling A, McMahon AD, Lock P, Vallance R, et al. Effect of a treatment strategy of tight control for rheumatoid arthritis (the TICORA study): a single-blind randomised controlled trial. Lancet 2004;364:263-9.

32. Saunders SA, Capell HA, Stirling A, Vallance R, Kincaid W, McMahon AD, et al. Triple therapy in early active rheumatoid arthritis. Arthritis Rheum 2008;58:1310-7.

33. Verstappen SM, Jacobs JW, van der Veen MJ, Heurkens AHM, Schenk Y, ter Borg EJ, et al. Intensive treatment with methotrexate in early rheumatoid arthritis: aiming for remission. Computer Assisted Management in Early Rheumatoid Arthritis (CAMERA, an open-label strategy trial). Ann Rheum Dis 2007;66:1443-9.

34. Martin Du Pan S, Gabay C, Finckh A. A systematic review of infliximab in the treatment of early rheumatoid arthritis. Ther Clin Risk Manag 2007;3:905-11.

35. Goekoop-Ruiterman YP, de Vries-Bouwstra JK, Allaart CF, van Zeben D, Kerstens PJ, Hazes JM, et al. Clinical and radiographic outcomes of four different treatment strategies in patients with early rheumatoid arthritis (the best study): a randomized, controlled trial. Arthritis Rheum 2005;52:3381-90.

36. Carette S. All patients with rheumatoid arthritis should receive corticosteroids as part of their management (editorial). J Rheumatol 2007;34:656-60.

37. Boers M, Verhoeven AC, Markusse HM, van de Laar MA, Westhovens R, van Denderen JC, et al. Randomised comparison of combined step-down prednisolone, methotrexate and sulphasalazine with sulphasalazine alone in early rheumatoid arthritis. Lancet 1997;350:309-18.

38. Kirwan JR, Bijlsma JW, Boers M, Shea BJ. Effects of glucocorticoids on radiological progression in rheumatoid arthritis. Cochrane Database Syst Rev 2007;CD006356.

39. Choy EH, Smith CM, Farewell V, Walker D, Hassell A, Chau L, Scott DL; CARDERA (Combination Anti-Rheumatic Drugs in Early Rheumatoid Arthritis) Trial Group. Factorial randomised controlled trial of glucocorticoids and combination disease modifying drugs in early rheumatoid arthritis glucocorticoids and combination disease. Ann Rheum Dis 2007;67:656-63.

40. Durez P, Malghem J, Nzeusseu Toukap A, Depresseux G, Lauwerys BR, Westhovens R, et al. Treatment of early rheumatoid arthritis: a randomized magnetic resonance imaging

study comparing the effects of methotrexate alone, methotrexate in combination with infliximab, and methotrexate in combination with intravenous pulse methylprednisolone. Arthritis Rheum 2007;56:3919-27.

41. Van Staa TP. The pathogenesis, epidemiology and management of glucocorticoid-induced osteoporosis. Calc Tissue Int 2006;79:129-37.

42. Wolfe F, Caplan L, Michaud K. Treatment for rheumatoid arthritis and the risk of hospitalization for pneumonia associations with prednisone, disease-modifying antirheumatic drugs, and anti-tumor necrosis factor therapy. Arthritis Rheum 2006;54:628-34.

43. Wolfe F, Michaud K. The risk of myocardial infarction and pharmacologic and nonpharmacologic myocardial infarction predictors in rheumatoid arthritis. Arthritis Rheum 2008;58:2612-21.

44. van Tuyl LH, Lems WF, Voskuyl AE, Kerstens PJ, Garnero P, Dijkmans BA, et al. Tight control and intensified COBRA combination treatment in early rheumatoid arthritis: 90% remission in a pilot trial. Ann Rheum Dis 2008;67: 1574-7.

45. Katchamart W, Trudeau J, Phumethum V, Bombardier C. Efficacy and toxicity of methotrexate (MTX) monotherapy vs. MTX combination therapy with non-biologic disease-modifying anti-rheumatic drugs in rheumatoid arthritis: A systematic review and metaanalysis. Ann Rheum Dis 2009;68:1105-12.

46. Visser K, Katchamart W, Loza E, Martinez-Lopez JA, Salliot C, Trudeau J, et al. Multinational evidence-based recommendations for the use of methotrexate in rheumatic disorders with a focus on rheumatoid arthritis: integrating systematic literature research and expert opinion of a broad international panel of rheumatologists in the 3E Initiative. Ann Rheum Dis 2009;68:1086-93.

47. Smolen JS, Van Der Heijde DM, St. Clair EW, Emery P, Bathon JM, Keystone E, et al. Predictors of joint damage in patients with early rheumatoid arthritis treated with high-dose methotrexate with or without concomitant infliximab: results from the ASPIRE trial. Arthritis Rheum 2006;54:702-10.

Management of Established Rheumatoid Arthritis

Michael G. Feely and Ted R. Mikuls

A 27-year-old school teacher with a 6-year history of rheumatoid arthritis (RA) is seen for routine follow-up. She was recently married, and her disease had previously been well controlled with 20 mg of weekly oral methotrexate and folic acid 1 mg daily. She currently reports 90 minutes of morning stiffness that is new, and she is having difficulty writing on the chalkboard at school due to worsening pain and stiffness in her hands and wrists. On examination, she has marked synovitis involving the wrists and small joints in both hands.

CONSIDERATIONS WITH A SUBOPTIMAL RESPONSE TO METHOTREXATE

Methotrexate has revitalized the treatment of RA over the past 20 years, and is widely considered to be the cornerstone of active therapy for the disease. It is frequently the first disease-modifying antirheumatic drug (DMARD) prescribed following RA diagnosis. Although an effective treatment for many, a substantial number of patients (20%–53%)[1,2] do not adequately respond to methotrexate monotherapy. A number of factors may be implicated in the etiology of an incomplete methotrexate response, including poor gastrointestinal (GI) absorption and reduced bioavailability, possible antagonism by concomitantly administered folate or caffeine intake, and poor patient adherence.

Although a direct relationship exists between methotrexate dose and clinical response, the bioavailability of oral methotrexate has been thought to be a limiting factor in its efficacy. There is significant intra- and interpatient variability in the absorption of orally administered methotrexate.[3] Although much of the pharmacokinetic data specific to methotrexate relate to its use in the treatment of solid tumors, it has been suggested that at a dose of 20 to 25 mg per week or greater (typical dosing in RA) oral administration results in limited bioavailability. With higher doses of methotrexate, the intestinal folate transport system is saturated

and a parenteral route (typically subcutaneous) may be required to achieve higher circulating drug levels. The problem of decreased absorption with high-dose oral methotrexate can also potentially be overcome through the use of a split oral dose regimen (e.g., half of prescribed dose in morning and remaining half on evening of same day), a dosing strategy that has been demonstrated to be beneficial in the treatment of solid tumors.[4] Hoekstra et al.[5] demonstrated in 10 RA patients treated with high doses of oral methotrexate (median weekly dose of 30 mg) that improvements in bioavailability could be achieved with a split-dose regimen, recognizing that data supporting the clinical efficacy of this approach are limited.

Alternatively, increased bioavailability of methotrexate can be achieved by switching from an oral route to subcutaneous or intramuscular administration.[6] A small improvement in disease control was achieved by switching to intramuscular administration in patients with active disease despite 15 to 20 mg of oral weekly methotrexate.[7] Using parenteral methotrexate in patients with suboptimal response to maximum oral dosages, may obviate the need for biologics[8] or other forms of step-up therapy. In a retrospective study of 61 patients with juvenile inflammatory arthritis who failed oral methotrexate, a majority (76%) demonstrated significant clinical improvement after being switched to subcutaneous methotrexate.[9] In patients with a suboptimal response to weekly methotrexate at dosages of 20 mg or more, consideration should be given to switching to a split-dose regimen or switching to a parenteral route of administration.

Rheumatologists often prescribe folate supplementation concomitant with methotrexate therapy to minimize or prevent dose-related toxicity. Although the mechanism of action for methotrexate in RA is incompletely understood, some of its adverse effects (e.g., stomatitis, alopecia, and so on) are believed to be related to its effect on folate antagonism. Although folate administration has been associated with a lower incidence of methotrexate-related liver transaminase elevations, and GI and mucosal side effects, it is unknown whether folate supplementation reduces the effectiveness of methotrexate in the treatment of RA.[10,11] Folate supplementation (1 mg folic acid or 2.5 mg folinic acid) was not associated with significant differences in treatment response with weekly methotrexate in the trial by Van Ede and colleagues, but this study (with 434 patients divided among the three treatment arms) may have been underpowered to detect small, but potentially relevant differences in disease activity. In this study, the group treated with folate supplementation was characterized by a statistically significant higher dose of methotrexate achieved at the end of the study, suggesting that with folate supplementation, higher dosages of methotrexate may be required to achieve a clinical response similar to that without folate supplementation. A separate post hoc analysis of two randomized control trials demonstrated that 9% to 21% fewer patients receiving methotrexate in conjunction with folic acid, achieved an American College of Rheumatology -20, -50 or -70 response when compared with patients who did not receive folic acid.[12] This analysis was limited by the fact that neither of the two studies included in the analysis were performed with the primary goal of determining the effect of folic acid supplementation on disease activity. A randomized, double-blind, placebo-controlled study examining the effect of two different dosages of supplemental folic acid versus placebo on disease activity and toxicity found that the folic acid groups had similar response rates to those receiving placebo.[13] Although there is no consensus on the effect of folate supplementation on the efficacy of methotrexate, there is evidence that appropriate supplementation minimizes the risk of select toxicities. If there is a detrimental impact of folate on the efficacy of methotrexate in RA, it appears to be small and this risk is likely outweighed by the protection conferred against side effects.

Methylxanthines, such as caffeine, have been hypothesized to attenuate the anti-inflammatory effects of methotrexate due to their inhibitory effect on extracelluar adenosine. Although the mechanism of action of methotrexate is not completely understood, it is thought to work in part by increasing the extracellular expression of adenosine, which has potent anti-inflammatory effects.[14] Data on caffeine consumption in a series of 39 newly diagnosed RA patients receiving initial weekly methotrexate suggested that caffeine in excess of 180 mg/day (equivalent to approximately one to two cups of coffee or four servings of caffeinated soda) was associated with decreased response relative to methotrexate-treated patients with a daily caffeine intake of less than 120 mg.[15] In contrast, caffeine consumption in a larger cohort of 264 RA patients was not shown to impact methotrexate response, although there was a trend toward higher disease activity scores in the moderate and high caffeine consumption groups.[16] Although the evidence has not consistently demonstrated a relationship between caffeine consumption and the efficacy of methotrexate, it may be reasonable to counsel patients on the need for moderation in terms of caffeine intake (especially in those patients consuming in excess of 180 mg of caffeine per day).

With suboptimal response to methotrexate (and other DMARDs), issues of patient adherence must be taken into consideration. In a recent study of the Tennessee Medicaid database, Grijalva and colleagues[17] examined the long-term use of several DMARD/DMARD combinations in the treatment of RA, examining patient adherence using a medication possession ratio (MPR; total days supply of medication/total time of observation). Although adherence with methotrexate compared favorably with other DMARDs and DMARD combinations, approximately half of all patients treated with methotrexate monotherapy were nonadherent (corresponding to an MPR $\leq$ 0.8). These data underscore the importance of patient education and optimal patient-provider communication to successfully address and overcome the potential barriers of treatment adherence.

When faced with a patient with RA who has not achieved the desired clinical response to methotrexate monotherapy, it is important to take into consideration the aforementioned factors that might deleteriously affect the effectiveness of this treatment. Even after careful consideration of these factors, many patients will still not achieve an optimal treatment response to methotrexate and additional DMARD/DMARD combinations will be required to achieve improved disease control.

STRATEGIES FOR PHARMACOLOGIC MANAGEMENT OF PATIENTS WITH RHEUMATOID ARTHRITIS WITH A SUBOPTIMAL RESPONSE TO METHOTREXATE

Although the goal of treatment for patients with established RA was once merely improvement, treatment expectations have expanded with the availability of new and highly effective therapies. Increasingly, the treatment goal in established RA is best characterized by clinical remission.[18] Recognizing that a significant proportion of patients treated with initial DMARD monotherapy will not achieve remission, it is important that RA patients undergo frequent assessments of disease activity in order to best optimize treatment. Several therapeutic strategies, including escalation to triple therapy (methotrexate, sulfasalazine, and hydroxychloroquine) and the addition of biologic agents have been associated with improved clinical responses in patients with a suboptimal response to methotrexate (Fig. 3-1).[19] The availability of agents targeting tumor necrosis factor-α (TNF-α) (etanercept, infliximab, adalimumab) has revolutionized the treatment approach for such patients, because these agents appear to be particularly potent in protecting patients from radiographic disease progression and its associated disability.[20–22] The treatment armamentarium in established disease has expanded even further in recent years with the availability of agents targeting both B-cell (rituximab) and T-cell

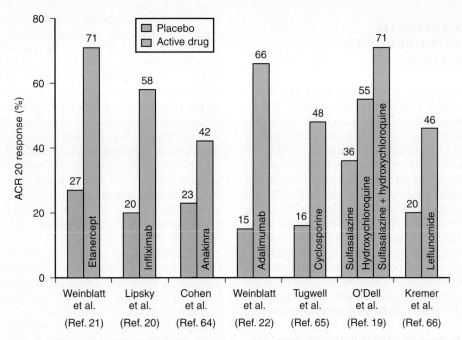

Figure 3-1. American College of Rheumatology -20 (corresponding to overall improvement of 20% or greater) response rates with various disease-modifying antirheumatic drug (DMARD) combinations in patients with a suboptimal response to methotrexate. Does not include all combinations studied to date. All patients were taking methotrexate in combination with above DMARD/DMARD combinations. (From O'Dell JR. Therapeutic strategies for rheumatoid arthritis. N Engl J Med 2004;350:2591-602).

costimulation (abatacept)—the first agents shown to be effective in anti-TNF failures.[23,24]

Although there are many effective treatment strategies from which to choose, recent studies have emphasized that the goal of therapy is as important or more important than the specific therapies used.[25] The goal of therapy should be remission—a disease state characterized by the elimination of joint pain and swelling, the maintenance of employability, a normalization of disability and mortality risk, and the slowing or even reversal of joint damage. The Tight Control in the Treatment of RA Study demonstrated that an intense management strategy with predefined goals and thresholds for escalation of therapy, resulted in substantial improvement in disease activity.[26] Patients exposed to this intensive regimen were approximately 10 times more likely (odds ratio = 9.7; 95% confidence interval [CI] 3.9 to 23.9) than RA patients randomized to routine care to achieve clinical remission. The BeSt (Dutch acronym for Behandel-Strategieen, "treatment strategies") study expanded on this approach, demonstrating that with implementation of an intensive strategy of monitoring disease activity and rapid escalation to combination DMARD/biologic therapies, 80% of patients achieved a target Disease Activity Score (DAS) of less than 2.4, and 42% achieved clinical remission (DAS < 1.6).[25] Once disease activity was controlled, most patients in this study were able to tolerate a de-escalation of therapy with either elimination of prednisolone or infliximab.

Despite the recent advances in the treatment of established RA, several questions remain. What

is the optimal initial strategy (e.g., triple therapy versus the addition of biologic versus other drugs) for patients with established RA and a suboptimal response to methotrexate or other DMARD monotherapy? What is the best strategy for patients with suboptimal treatment responses to second-line agents and various DMARD/biologic combinations? What is the role for newly available and evolving therapies in RA for patients with established disease? Is there an accurate and reproducible way to tailor therapy for individual patients? Can we predict efficacy and toxicity of available treatments? The answers to these and other questions are urgently needed, underscoring the need for additional investigations in this patient population.

CASE 2: Addressing Comorbid Illness

A 61-year-old man with long-standing seropositive RA is seen for follow-up examination. He is on subcutaneous weekly methotrexate (25 mg) in addition to daily sulfasalazine and hydroxychloroquine. He was recently hospitalized with newly diagnosed congestive heart failure (CHF: New York Heart Association Class II) with impaired left ventricular function (ejection fraction of 35%). He was successfully treated for a nosocomial pneumonia during his hospitalization. His renal function has also declined (Cr. 1.8 mg/dL, estimated GFR 42 mL/min). His RA is active with six tender and four swollen joints, an elevated erythrocyte sedimentation rate (54 mm/h), and several hours of morning stiffness.

RHEUMATOID ARTHRITIS–ASSOCIATED COMORBIDITIES AND COMPLICATIONS

Several RA-associated comorbidities have been identified including cardiovascular disease (coronary artery disease and CHF), infection, osteoporosis leading to fracture, and lymphoproliferative malignancies. RA-related comorbidities and preventive strategies to address them are summarized in Table 3-1 (although not all will be directly discussed here). Management of RA patients is further complicated by treatment-related toxicities including glucocorticoid-induced hyperglycemia, peptic ulcer disease related to nonsteroidal anti-inflammatory agents (NSAIDs), infections related to immunosuppression, and glucocorticoid-induced osteoporosis (GIOP). Additionally, comorbid illnesses not directly related to RA, such as renal or hepatic dysfunction, can substantially affect the available therapeutic options.

Cardiovascular disease (CVD) is the leading contributor to excess mortality in RA, accounting for one third to one half of all RA-related deaths.[27,28] The risk for incident myocardial infarction and CHF are significantly increased in patients with RA (40%, 60% respectively).[29] The increased morbidity and mortality of CVD in the setting of RA cannot be accounted for by an increase in the prevalence of traditional cardiac risk factors including dyslipidemia, hypertension, diabetes mellitus, family history, and cigarette smoking. Atherosclerosis (and resulting CVD) has been shown to be an inflammatory disease, or at least to have a core inflammatory component in its complex pathogenesis. Proinflammatory cytokines, elevated serum levels of acute phase reactants, neoangiogenesis, T-cell activation, expression of leukocyte adhesion molecules and endothelin, and collagen degradation with localized metalloproteinase expression via activated monocytes are all common pathogenic features to both RA and atherosclerosis.[30-34] The clinical associations of these two diseases, coupled with their histopathologic similarities, have led some authors to suggest that CVD should be considered an extra-articular manifestation of RA.[35]

In addition to the increased CVD risk inherent to RA, treatments used in managing RA have also been speculated to play a role in the development of CVD. For instance, methotrexate use leads to increased levels of circulating homocysteine, an independent risk factor for accelerated atherosclerosis and thrombotic events.[36,37] Both NSAID and glucocorticoid use may result in hypertension or worsen pre-existing hypertension, the former being associated with the risk of incident thromboembolic event and heart failure. TNF inhibitors have been associated with increased rates of mortality and need for hospitalization when given to patients with moderate to severe heart failure.[38] In addition to the effects on blood pressure, glucocorticoids

Table 3-1. *Rheumatoid Arthritis (RA)–Related Comorbidities and Preventive Strategies Used to Minimize Their Impact*

	RA Specific Factors	*Preventive Measures*
Cardiovascular disease	Severe disease with elevated inflammatory markers	Lifestyle modification (diet, exercise, smoking cessation) Prophylactic low-dose ASA Aggressive anti-inflammatory treatments Folate supplementation for methotrexate users Treatment of diabetes, dyslipidemia, hypertension Minimize glucocorticoid and NSAID use
Infection	Severe long-standing disease, immunosuppressive therapy	Minimize immunosuppressive exposure Routine influenza and pneumococcal vaccines TB screening before TNF inhibition Routine surveillance Patient education
Osteoporosis	Glucocorticoid use, severe disease, and immobility	Lifestyle modification (diet, exercise, smoking cessation) Minimize glucocorticoid exposure Calcium/Vitamin D supplementation BMD measurement Bisphosphonate and human recombinant parathyroid hormone (teriparatide) as appropriate
Peptic ulcer disease	NSAID use with or without glucocorticoid use	Minimize NSAID exposure Proton pump inhibitors High-dose H2 receptor antagonists Misoprostol COX-2 selective NSAIDs
Lymphoproliferative disease	Severe long-standing disease	Aggressive anti-inflammatory treatments, disease control (?)

ASA, aspirin; BMD, bone mineral density; COX, cyclooxygenase; H2, histamine type 2; NSAID, nonsteroidal anti-inflammatory drug; RA, rheumatoid arthritis; TB, tuberculosis; TNF, tumor necrosis factor.

may also promote hyperglycemia, increased adiposity, and hyperlipidemia-all independent risk factors for CVD. Recognizing the seminal role of inflammation in CVD, the benefit of select disease-modifying therapies may far outweigh any risk relevant to long-term cardiovascular outcomes. For instance, methotrexate use has been associated with a 70% reduction in cardiovascular mortality (HR = 0.3; 95% CI 0.2 to 0.7) after accounting for differences in RA disease severity, emphasizing the potential importance of disease control in RA patients as a means of reducing CVD burden.[39] Whether other DMARDs and biologic agents share the protective properties of methotrexate remains to be seen.

The increased risk for CVD in patients with RA should prompt aggressive primary and secondary preventive measures including smoking cessation, aggressive control of hyperlipidemia, the appropriate management of hypertension and co-morbid diabetes, and the routine use of prophylactic low-dose aspirin. There is evidence that 3-hydroxy-3-methylglutaryl coenzyme A reductase inhibitors (statins) have anti-inflammatory properties in addition to their lipid-lowering effect, underscoring that these treatments are important adjunctive therapies in RA.[40] Attempts should be made to achieve maximal control of the patient's RA, while minimizing the use of NSAIDs (particularly those that are highly selective inhibitors of cyclooxygenase-2) and glucocorticoids. Additionally, patients should be frequently screened for symptoms of CVD, helping to identify and intervene early in the course of this comorbid condition.

A significant increase in infection-related morbidity and mortality has been described in RA with an increased disease-related incidence in pulmonary infections, septic arthritis, cellulitis and soft tissue infections, osteomyelitis, and systemic sepsis.[28,41,42] The increased infection risk observed in established RA does not appear to be completely attributable to known risk factors including leukopenia, diabetes mellitus, smoking, lung disease, and glucocorticoid use. Alterations in cellular immunity, including decreased numbers of T-suppressor and natural killer cells, which may predispose to infection, are characteristic of RA. Infection risk in RA has been associated with increasing age, extra-articular disease, leukopenia, and select comorbidity (alcoholism, diabetes mellitus, organic brain disease, chronic lung disease).[43]

Similar to CVD, distinguishing between the effects of RA disease severity and its treatments in RA-related infection risk is difficult. Conflicting data have emerged regarding the increased risk of infection with TNF inhibition. A meta-analysis of randomized clinical trials demonstrated an increased risk for serious infections in RA patients treated with monoclonal anti-TNF antibodies, adalimumab or infliximab (relative risk [RR] 2.0; 1.3–3.1) versus placebo.[44] In contrast, large observational registries have not demonstrated an overall increased risk of serious infection related to TNF inhibition, although suggesting that there may be a period of heightened infection risk during the first three to six months of anti-TNF therapy (Fig. 3-2).[45] Although the effects of anti-TNF therapy on risk of infection are not currently fully understood, it is prudent to counsel patients on the risk of infection while receiving any immunomodulators. TNF-α plays a critical role in the development and maintenance of granulomas that are central in host defense against disseminated fungal and mycobacterial infections. All patients should be screened for latent tuberculosis prior to initiation of anti-TNF therapies, and appropriate surveillance should be undertaken during therapy. With first signs of infection, TNF inhibitors and other potent immunosuppressants should be discontinued until the infection has been satisfactorily treated.

In light of the increased infection risk associated with RA, preventive vaccinations represent an important preventive health care measure in this patient population (Table 3-2). Both the pneumococcal and influenza vaccines are indicated for patients on immunosuppressive medications, including the vast majority of patients with established RA.[46] Both vaccines (in their inactive form) have been shown to be safe and effective in RA, although antibody responses may be attenuated in the context of immunomodulating treatments. There are currently no data to suggest that the receipt of these vaccines results in increased disease activity in RA or any other connective tissue disease. The varicella zoster vaccine has recently been approved for patients at risk for herpes zoster infection. However, because the varicella zoster vaccine is a live attenuated vaccine and has not been approved for use in patients who are immunosuppressed, it should be used cautiously (as well as with other live vaccines) in RA until further data are available. It is recommended that all RA patients should be up to date on all indicated vaccinations before or at the time of initiating treatment with immunosuppressives.[46] With increasing immunosuppression, it is important to recognize that many vaccines including hepatitis B (given routinely to healthcare professionals and other at risk populations) may not induce immunity.

Osteoporosis is prevalent in RA, with up to one third of affected women experiencing a fracture within just 5 years of follow-up examination.[47] Factors implicated in the development of osteoporosis in RA include increased expression of proinflammatory cytokines mediating increased bone resorption, reductions in weight-bearing activity, and the deleterious effects on bone due to exogenous glucocorticoids. Bone mineral density (BMD), measured by dual-energy x-ray absorptiometry (DXA), remains one of the best clinical predictors of fracture risk. Patients with RA should undergo baseline DXA measurement, with measurements repeated serially (every 1 to 2 years) to monitor for progression and response to therapeutic interventions. Behavioral modifications should be encouraged for all patients, including smoking cessation,

CUMULATIVE INCIDENCE OF INFECTIONS, BY DRUG

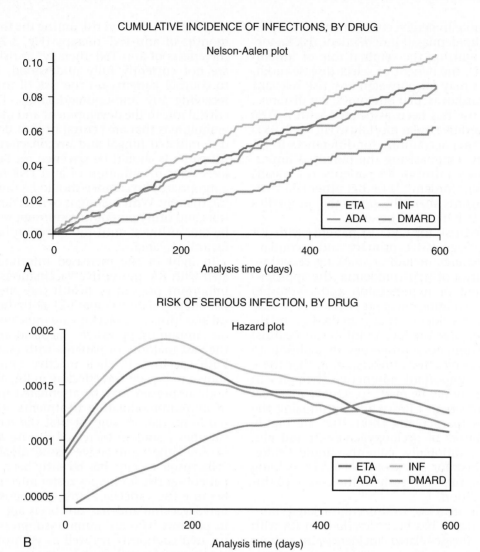

Figure 3-2. Cumulative incidence (**A**) of infection and hazard plot examining the risk of serious infection (**B**) over time among patients with rheumatoid arthritis (RA) receiving adalimumab, etanercept, infliximab, and conventional disease-modifying anti-rheumatic drug (DMARD). (From Dixon WG, Symmons DP, Lunt M, Watson KD, Hyrich KL; British Society for Rheumatology Biologics Register Control Centre Consortium, Silman AJ; British Society for Rheumatology Biologics Register. Serious infection following anti-tumor necrosis factor alpha therapy in patients with rheumatoid arthritis: lessons from interpreting data from observational studies. Arthritis Rheum 2007;56:2896-904.)

increased weight-bearing activity, and appropriate dietary changes. Attempts should be made to minimize glucocorticoid exposure, and supplementation with calcium (1500 mg/day) and vitamin D (800 IU/day) should be considered in all patients. Bisphosphonates are highly effective in preventing bone loss in the setting of glucocorticoid therapy, as well as in treating RA-associated osteoporosis.[48-50] Teriparatide has shown superior improvements in BMD relative to alendronate in patients with GIOP, suggesting that this agent may have an important role in RA.[51] Given the substantial morbidity and mortality associated with fracture, it is imperative that patients with established RA are screened for associated osteoporosis, and that preventive and therapeutic measures be employed early to help minimize the associated fracture risk.

In addition to associations with CVD, infection, and osteoporosis, RA is associated with an increase in the occurrence of lymphoproliferative malignancies, particularly Hodgkin's disease and aggressive forms of non-Hodgkins lymphoma. Observational studies have demonstrated approximately a two-fold increase of these malignancies in RA patients.[52] In a large Swedish population-based study, higher levels of RA disease activity, but not conventional DMARD therapy, were found to correlate with increased lymphoma risk.[53] These data suggest that any deleterious impact of DMARDs in terms of lymphoma risk may be offset by their anti-inflammatory properties and tight RA disease control may be important in lymphoma prevention.

As with other RA-related comorbidities, discriminating between the effect of unchecked disease activity and use of disease-modifying agents as

Table 3-2. *Recommendations for the Use of Routine Vaccinations in Patients with Rheumatoid Arthritis*

Vaccine	Recommendations
Influenza	Indicated for all patients with RA Only inactivated vaccine should be given Normal response to vaccine with methotrexate therapy (no need to hold before administration) Modest reduction in immunologic response with anti-TNF therapies and abatacept; marked reduction in immunologic response with rituximab (should be dosed before initiation of biologic therapy whenever possible)
Pneumococcal (23-valent)	Indicated for all patients with RA Modest reduction in immunologic response with methotrexate (should be given before initiation of methotrexate whenever possible) Modest reduction in immunologic response with anti-TNF therapies and abatacept, marked reduction in immunologic response with rituximab (should be dosed before initiation of biologic therapy whenever possible)
Hepatitis B	Should be given, based upon risk factors, prior to therapy with biologic agents
Herpes zoster/ other live vaccines	Live vaccines should be avoided in immunosuppressed patients

RA, rheumatoid arthritis; TNF, tumor necrosis factor.
From Saag KG, Teng GG, Patkar NM, Anuntiyo J, Finney C, Curtis JR, et al, American College of Rheumatology. American college of rheumatology 2008 recommendations for the use of nonbiologic and biologic disease-modifying antirheumatic drugs in rheumatoid arthritis. Arthritis Rheum 2008;59:762-84.

they pertain to lymphoma risk is difficult due to confounding by indication and channeling bias. Indeed, in a recent observational cohort study, glucocorticoid use was associated with a significantly decreased risk of lymphoma in RA.[53,54] There have been several case reports of Epstein-Barr virus–related lymphomas developing in RA patients receiving methotrexate, with some patients achieving spontaneous remission of the tumor simply with methotrexate withdrawal.[55,56] Despite these intriguing reports, large observational cohort studies have revealed no significant associations of methotrexate with increased lymphoma risk.[57]

Since an initial post-marketing report by the U.S. Food and Drug Administration,[58] there has been substantial speculation regarding the possible associations of anti-TNF therapies with lymphoma risk in RA. In a meta-analysis of randomized clinical trials studying monoclonal anti-TNF antibodies (adalimumab and infliximab), Bongartz and colleagues observed a more than three-fold increased risk of malignancy (RR = 3.3; 95% CI 1.2–9.1) among those receiving active drug versus placebo. Of the malignancies

observed in the nine trials included, there were nine lymphomas in patients receiving anti-TNF treatments versus zero in the placebo-treated patients.

In contrast, large, observational studies to date have failed to demonstrate a significant association between adalimumab, infliximab, and etanercept use (the latter not examined in the study of Bongartz et al) with lymphoma risk.[57,59,60] From the data available, it appears that lymphoma risk is predominantly associated with 'unchecked' disease activity in RA–an absolute risk that is low and that may be modified slightly by select antirheumatic treatments.

NONPHARMACOLOGIC MANAGEMENT STRATEGIES

In addition to pharmacologic treatment, nonpharmacologic modalities also play an important role in the treatment of established RA. Orthoses and splints are often used in RA patients to decrease pain, swelling, and deformity. Commonly prescribed orthoses include wrist supports, hand splints, molded insoles, and extra-depth shoes with metatarsal support. Despite frequent use, there are relatively few well-designed studies examining the efficacy of nonpharmacologic treatments in RA. A Cochrane review of 10 studies examining the efficacy and utility of orthoses and splints concluded that there was insufficient evidence to support the effectiveness of wrist splints in reducing either pain or disability associated with RA.[61] However, extra-depth shoes and molded insoles were associated with a reduction in pain during weight-bearing exercises. Although evidence is limited regarding the efficacy of orthotic devices and splints, they remain a safe and reasonable option for many patients because they may provide pain relief at a relatively low cost.

Referral to physical and occupational therapy may also be a beneficial component of the management strategy in established RA. Physical and occupational therapy can help to maintain and improve muscle strength, flexibility, and mobility. Patients can be educated on energy conservation, the appropriate use of assistive devices (canes, walkers), pacing of exercises, and techniques to protect the joints. Through a structured therapy program, physical and occupational therapists help empower patients in self-management of arthritis symptoms.

With the development of effective disease-modifying therapies and a more aggressive approach to the management of early RA, surgical modalities are less commonly indicated than in the past.[62] Commonly used surgical approaches in the treatment of RA are summarized in Figure 3-3. Disability in the advanced stages of RA frequently results from progressive joint destruction and resulting degenerative changes, which leads to reduced quality of life. Surgical interventions remain a viable option for many patients with RA symptoms that are refractory to available pharmacologic options.

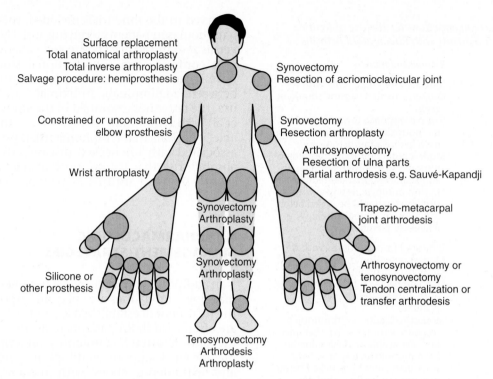

Surface replacement
Total anatomical arthroplasty
Total inverse arthroplasty
Salvage procedure: hemiprosthesis

Synovectomy
Resection of acriomioclavicular joint

Constrained or unconstrained
elbow prosthesis

Synovectomy
Resection arthroplasty

Arthrosynovectomy
Resection of ulna parts
Partial arthrodesis e.g. Sauvé-Kapandji

Wrist arthroplasty

Synovectomy
Arthroplasty

Trapezio-metacarpal
joint arthrodesis

Synovectomy
Arthroplasty

Silicone or
other prosthesis

Arthrosynovectomy or
tenosynovectomy
Tendon centralization or
transfer arthrodesis

Tenosynovectomy
Arthrodesis
Arthroplasty

Figure 3-3. Schematic demonstrating joint-specific surgical interventions used for the treatment of established rheumatoid arthritis (RA). Prosthetic replacement options shown on the left; soft tissue and corrective procedures shown on the right. (From Simmen BR, Bogoch ER, Goldhahn J. Surgery Insight: orthopedic treatment options in rheumatoid arthritis. Nat Clin Pract Rheumatol 2008;4:266-73).

Surgical intervention for RA seeks to achieve the following goals: (1) restore function; (2) relieve pain; (3) prevent further joint destruction; (4) correct deformity; and (5) improve appearance (generally limited to hands/feet).[62]

Synovectomy was previously a commonly used procedure to alleviate joint swelling and pain, and was associated with good outcomes at 2 to 5 years.[62] With effective DMARDs, synovectomy is currently indicated less frequently. However, persistent synovitis refractory to DMARDs without articular surface destruction remains an indication for synovectomy, with the goal of relieving pain and swelling while improving range of motion.

Arthroplasty (joint replacement) is currently the mainstay of surgical options for many patients whose RA has led to progressive joint destruction. Most commonly, the hips and knees are the joints that are replaced, although elbow, ankle, and shoulder arthroplasty are being performed with increasing frequency. Total joint arthroplasty has been associated with significant improvements, both in terms of pain and quality of life, for patients with established RA.[63] Arthrodesis is an option for joints in which the resulting limitation in range of motion can be compensated for by adjacent joints (most commonly performed in wrists, metacarpophalangeal joints, interphalangeal joints, ankles and feet). Arthrodesis does not limit progression of destruction of the articular surfaces but may increase stability and overall mobility.

CASE 1 REVISITED: A 27-YEAR-OLD FEMALE SCHOOL TEACHER WITH RHEUMATOID ARTHRITIS AND A SUBOPTIMAL RESPONSE TO WEEKLY METHOTREXATE

This patient has evidence of active disease despite oral methotrexate 20 mg per week. In light of her worsening disease activity, it would be important to review factors that could attenuate her treatment response, factors such as caffeine intake, medication adherence, and folate supplementation. In the absence of poor adherence, escalation of therapy would likely be indicated to achieve better disease control and help prevent the long-term sequelae of her RA. Reasonable approaches might include the addition of low-dose bridging glucocorticoids (generally ≤10 mg of prednisone daily) or changes in methotrexate administration that could include dose escalation to 25 mg weekly, the use of split-dose oral regimen, or advancing to parenteral administration. Alternatively, another approach might include the addition of hydroxychloroquine 200 mg twice daily and sulfasalazine, titrated up to 1 g twice daily (triple therapy). As shown in Figure 3-1, several other alternative approaches have been shown to be highly effective in this population including the addition of newer biologic therapies. Intra-articular corticosteroids may also be beneficial, particularly if the patient localizes her complaints to one or two joints. This is also an opportunity to review risk factors for osteoporosis, and establish a baseline BMD if not done previously (particularly in older patients or those taking chronic glucocorticoid therapy). Formal data are lacking, but most would advocate that this patient receive adequate supplementation with both calcium and vitamin D. The immunization history of this patient should be reviewed and any deficiencies be updated, including a seasonal influenza vaccine.

As is the case with this patient, it is important to recognize that RA frequently affects women of reproductive age. It is necessary to elicit patients' desires for pregnancy, and provide education on the importance of involving both a rheumatologist and obstetrician in their preparation for childbearing. DMARDs such as methotrexate, leflunomide, and several others, should not be used in pregnancy and should be discontinued well in advance of conception. Data on the safety of newer biologic therapies (along with many of the traditional non-biologic therapies) in pregnancy are incomplete. Pregnancy can (and should) be successful in RA, but it requires advanced planning to minimize or eliminate the use of agents that are associated with teratogenicity and adverse fetal outcome.

CASE 2 REVISITED: A 61-YEAR-OLD MAN WITH LONG-STANDING ACTIVE RHEUMATOID ARTHITIS (DESPITE TREATMENT WITH COMBINATION DMARDS) IN THE CONTEXT OF SIGNIFICANT COMORBID ILLNESS INCLUDING NEWLY DIAGNOSED CONGESTIVE HEART FAILURE, RENAL INSUFFICIENCY, AND A NOSOCOMIAL PNEUMONIA

This case demonstrates the complexity of treating active RA in the setting of multiple comorbidities. A predisposition to infection and CHF are common to RA. Although renal dysfunction is not inherent to RA itself, it can complicate the course of RA treatment and is a well-recognized adverse effect of select arthritis treatments (e.g., NSAIDs). Renal impairment leads to increased circulating levels of methotrexate, increasing the risk of dose-related toxicity. Thus, renal dosing of his methotrexate and close laboratory surveillance for toxicity are warranted. It is important to note that current surveillance guidelines do not account for combination therapy or patient comorbidity, both present in this patient.

This patient was hospitalized with incident CHF, described as New York Hospital Association (NYHA) class II. Given the increased incidence of coronary artery disease in RA, this may represent an ischemic cardiomyopathy, but the differential diagnosis also includes dilated cardiomyopathy, infiltrative diseases such as amyloidosis (particularly with longstanding, active RA), pericardial disease, or cardiomyopathy associated with hydroxychloroquine (rarely reported). A review of the patient's recent chest radiographs and laboratory data is also warranted to substantiate the diagnosis of bacterial pneumonia, and ensure that the pulmonary process was not secondary to methotrexate-induced lung injury.

This patient has active RA despite the administration of triple DMARD therapy. Although many would escalate to anti-TNF therapy patients failing a combination of non-biologic DMARDs, it is important to note that TNF-inhibition is contraindicated in NYHA Class III, and IV heart disease, and must be used with caution in all classes of heart failure. One possible approach for this patient is to replace methotrexate with leflunomide or azathioprine, recognizing that there are limited data for these treatments in this patient population. This patient may require bridging low-dose glucocorticoids to help temper active disease, although this would need to be done with caution given the possible fluid retention associated with corticosteroids. The addition of minocycline may improve control of RA, with a relatively favorable side effect profile, recognizing that minocycline has been shown to be most effective in patients with limited disease duration (< 1 to 2 years). New biologic modalities that do not inhibit TNF, including abatacept and rituximab, may also represent viable treatment options in this difficult-to-treat patient, again recognizing that data for these agents in the context of these comorbidities are limited.

SUMMARY

RA is a chronic systemic inflammatory illness with an unpredictable disease course. Given the systemic and complex nature of RA, it is critical that a comprehensive approach to disease management is adopted; one that incorporates structured goals for therapy and one that accounts for disease-related comorbidity. Adopting such an approach, disease activity should be frequently assessed and treatments modified with clinical remission as a goal. Significant advances in the treatment of RA have been made in the past 20 years, and recent evidence suggests that goal-oriented treatment approach leads to improved outcomes. In addition to the arthritic manifestations of RA, practitioners need to have a heightened awareness of comorbid illnesses such as infection, coronary vascular disease, osteoporosis, and lymphoproliferative malignancy.

References

1. Pincus T, Yazici Y, Sokka T, Aletaha D, Smolen JS. Methotrexate as the "anchor drug" for the treatment of early rheumatoid arthritis. Clin Exp Rheumatol 2003;21:S179-85.
2. Wessels JAM, van der Kooij SM, Sjoerd M, le Cessie S, Kievit W, Barerra P, et al. A clinical pharmacogenetic model to predict the efficacy of methotrexate monotherapy in recent-onset rheumatoid arthritis. Arthritis Rheum 2007;56:1765-75.

3. Hillson JL, Furst DE. Pharmacology and pharmacokinetics of methotrexate in rheumatic disease. Practical issues in treatment and design. Rheum Dis Clin North Am 1997;23:757-78.

4. Steele WH, Stuart JF, Lawrence JR, McNeill CA, Sneader WE, Whiting B, et al. Enhancement of methotrexate absorption by subdivision of dose. Cancer Chemother Pharmacol 1979;3:235-7.

5. Hoekstra M, Haagsma C, Neef C, Proost J, Knuif A, van de Laar M. Splitting high-dose oral methotrexate improves bioavailability: a pharmacokinetic study in patients with rheumatoid arthritis. J Rheumatol 2006;33:481-5.

6. Hoekstra M, Haagsma C, Neef C, Proost J, Knuif A, van de Laar M. Bioavailability of higher dose methotrexate comparing oral and subcutaneous administration in patients with rheumatoid arthritis. J Rheumatol 2004;31:645-8.

7. Lambert CM, Sandhu S, Lochhead A, Hurst NP, McRorie E, Dhillon V. Dose escalation of parenteral methotrexate in active rheumatoid arthritis that has been unresponsive to conventional doses of methotrexate: a randomized, controlled trial. Arthritis Rheum 2004;50:364-71.

8. Bharadwaj A, Agrawal S, Batley M, Hammond A. Use of parenteral methotrexate significantly reduces the need for biological therapy. Rheumatology (Oxford) 2008;47:222.

9. Alsufyani K, Ortiz-Alvarez O, Cabral DA, Tucker LB, Petty RE, Malleson PN. The role of subcutaneous administration of methotrexate in children with juvenile idiopathic arthritis who have failed oral methotrexate. J Rheumatol 2004;31:179-82.

10. Ortiz Z, Shea B, Suarez-Almazor ME, Moher D, Wells GA, Tugwell P. The efficacy of folic acid and folinic acid in reducing methotrexate gastrointestinal toxicity in rheumatoid arthritis. A metaanalysis of randomized controlled trials. J Rheumatol 1998;25:36-43.

11. van Ede AE, Laan RF, Rood MJ, Huizinga TW, van de Laar MA, van Denderen CJ, et al. Effect of folic or folinic acid supplementation on the toxicity and efficacy of methotrexate in rheumatoid arthritis: A forty-eight week, multicenter, randomized, double-blind, placebo-controlled study. Arthritis Rheum 2001;44:1515-24.

12. Khanna D, Park GS, Paulus HE, Simpson KM, Elashoff D, Cohen SB, et al. Reduction of the efficacy of methotrexate by the use of folic acid: Post hoc analysis from two randomized controlled studies. Arthritis Rheum 2005;52:3030-8.

13. Morgan SL, Baggott JE, Vaughn WH, Austin JS, Veitch TA, Lee JY, et al. Supplementation with folic acid during methotrexate therapy for rheumatoid arthritis. A double-blind, placebo-controlled trial. Ann Intern Med 1994;121:833-41.

14. Montesinos MC, Yap JS, Desai A, Posadas I, McCrary CT, Cronstein BN. Reversal of the antiinflammatory effects of methotrexate by the nonselective adenosine receptor antagonists theophylline and caffeine: Evidence that the antiinflammatory effects of methotrexate are mediated via multiple adenosine receptors in rat adjuvant arthritis. Arthritis Rheum 2000;43:656-63.

15. Nesher G, Mates M, Zevin S. Effect of caffeine consumption on efficacy of methotrexate in rheumatoid arthritis. Arthritis Rheum 2003;48:571-2.

16. Benito-Garcia E, Heller JE, Chibnik LB, Maher NE, Matthews HM, Bilics JA, et al. Dietary caffeine intake does not affect methotrexate efficacy in patients with rheumatoid arthritis. J Rheumatol 2006;33:1275-81.

17. Grijalva CG, Chung CP, Arbogast PG, Stein CM, Mitchel EF, Griffin MR. Assessment of adherence to and persistence on disease-modifying antirheumatic drugs (dmards) in patients with rheumatoid arthritis. Med Care 2007;45:S66-76.

18. Sokka T, Mäkinen H, Puolakka K, Möttönen T, Hannonen P. Remission as the treatment goal—the FIN-RACo trial. Clin Exp Rheumatol 2006;24:S74-6.

19. O'Dell JR, Leff R, Paulsen G, Haire C, Mallek J, Eckhoff PJ, et al. Treatment of rheumatoid arthritis with methotrexate and hydroxychloroquine, methotrexate and sulfasalazine, or a combination of the three medications: results of a two-year, randomized, double-blind, placebo-controlled trial. Arthritis Rheum 2002;46:1164-70.

20. Lipsky PE, van der Heijde DM, St. Clair EW, Furst DE, Breedveld FC, et al. Infliximab and methotrexate in the treatment of rheumatoid arthritis. Anti-tumor necrosis factor trial in rheumatoid arthritis with concomitant therapy study group. N Engl J Med 2000;343:1594-602.

21. Weinblatt ME, Kremer JM, Bankhurst AD, Bulpitt KJ, Fleischmann RM, Fox RI, et al. A trial of etanercept, a recombinant tumor necrosis factor receptor:Fc fusion protein, in patients with rheumatoid arthritis receiving methotrexate. N Engl J Med 1999;340:253-9.

22. Weinblatt ME, Keystone EC, Furst DE, Moreland LW, Weisman MH, Birbara CA, et al. Adalimumab, a fully human anti-tumor necrosis factor alpha monoclonal antibody, for the treatment of rheumatoid arthritis in patients taking concomitant methotrexate: The ARMADA trial. Arthritis Rheum 2003;48:35-45.

23. Emery P, Fleischmann R, Filipowicz-Sosnowska A, Schechtman J, Szczepanski L, Kavanaugh A, et al. The efficacy and safety of rituximab in patients with active rheumatoid arthritis despite methotrexate treatment: results of a phase IIB randomized, double-blind, placebo-controlled, dose-ranging trial. Arthritis Rheum 2006;54:1390-400.

24. Kremer JM, Dougados M, Emery P, Durez P, Sibilia J, Shergy W, et al. Treatment of rheumatoid arthritis with the selective costimulation modulator abatacept: Twelve-month results of a phase iib, double-blind, randomized, placebo-controlled trial. Arthritis Rheum 2005;52:2263-71.

25. Allaart CF, Goekoop-Ruiterman YPM, de Vries-Bouwstra JK, Breedveld FC, Dijkmans BAC. Aiming at low disease activity in rheumatoid arthritis with initial combination therapy or initial monotherapy strategies: the BeSt study. Clin Exp Rheumatol 2006;24:S77-82.

26. Grigor C, Capell H, Stirling A, McMahon AD, Lock P, Vallance R, et al. Effect of a treatment strategy of tight control for rheumatoid arthritis (the TICORA study): a single-blind randomised controlled trial. Lancet 2004;364:263-9.

27. Reilly PA, Cosh JA, Maddison PJ, Rasker JJ, Silman AJ. Mortality and survival in rheumatoid arthritis: a 25 year prospective study of 100 patients. Ann Rheum Dis 1990;49:363-9.

28. Wolfe F, Mitchell DM, Sibley JT, Fries JF, Bloch DA, Williams CA, et al. The mortality of rheumatoid arthritis. Arthritis Rheum 1994;37:481-94.

29. Gabriel SE, Crowson CS, O'Fallon WM. Comorbidity in arthritis. J Rheumatol 1999;26:2475-9.

30. Firestein GS. Starving the synovium: angiogenesis and inflammation in rheumatoid arthritis. J Clin Invest 1999;103:3-4.

31. Oppenheimer-Marks N, Lipsky PE. Adhesion molecules in rheumatoid arthritis. Springer Semin Immunopathol 1998;20:95-114.

32. Pasceri V, Yeh ET. A tale of two diseases: atherosclerosis and rheumatoid arthritis. Circulation 1999;100:2124-6.

33. Ross R. Atherosclerosis is an inflammatory disease. Am Heart J 1999;138:S419-20.

34. van der Wal AC, Becker AE, van der Loos CM, Das PK. Site of intimal rupture or erosion of thrombosed coronary atherosclerotic plaques is characterized by an inflammatory process irrespective of the dominant plaque morphology. Circulation 1994;89:36-44.

35. Van Doornum S, McColl G, Wicks IP. Accelerated atherosclerosis: an extraarticular feature of rheumatoid arthritis? Arthritis Rheum 2002;46:862-73.

36. Morgan SL, Baggott JE, Lee JY, Alarcón GS. Folic acid supplementation prevents deficient blood folate levels and hyperhomocysteinemia during longterm, low dose methotrexate therapy for rheumatoid arthritis: implications for cardiovascular disease prevention. J Rheumatol 1998;25:441-6.

37. Clarke R, Daly L, Robinson K, Naughten E, Cahalane S, Fowler B, et al. Hyperhomocysteinemia: an independent risk factor for vascular disease. N Engl J Med 1991;324:1149-55.

38. Chung ES, Packer M, Lo KH, Fasanmade AA, Willerson JT. Randomized, double-blind, placebo-controlled, pilot trial of infliximab, a chimeric monoclonal antibody to tumor necrosis factor-alpha, in patients with moderate-to-severe heart failure: results of the anti-TNF therapy against congestive heart failure (ATTACH) trial. Circulation 2003;107:3133-40.

39. Choi HK, Hernán MA, Seeger JD, Robins JM, Wolfe F. Methotrexate and mortality in patients with rheumatoid arthritis: a prospective study. Lancet 2002;359:1173-7.

40. Leung BP, Sattar N, Crilly A, Prach M, McCarey DW, Payne H, et al. A novel anti-inflammatory role for simvastatin in inflammatory arthritis. J Immunol 2003;170:1524-30.

41. Symmons DP, Jones MA, Scott DL, Prior P. Long-term mortality outcome in patients with rheumatoid arthritis: early presenters continue to do well. J Rheumatol 1998;25:1072-7.

42. Doran MF, Crowson CS, Pond GR, O'Fallon WM, Gabriel SE. Frequency of infection in patients with rheumatoid arthritis compared with controls: a population-based study. Arthritis Rheum 2002;46:2287-93.

43. Doran MF, Crowson CS, Pond GR, O'Fallon WM, Gabriel SE. Predictors of infection in rheumatoid arthritis. Arthritis Rheum 2002;46:2294-300.

44. Bongartz T, Sutton AJ, Sweeting MJ, Buchan I, Matteson EL, Montori V. Anti-TNF antibody therapy in rheumatoid arthritis and the risk of serious infections and malignancies: systematic review and meta-analysis of rare harmful effects in randomized controlled trials. JAMA 2006;295:2275-85.

45. Dixon WG, Symmons DPM, Lunt M, Watson KD, Hyrich KL, Silman AJ. Serious infection following anti-tumor necrosis factor alpha therapy in patients with rheumatoid arthritis: lessons from interpreting data from observational studies. Arthritis Rheum 2007;56:2896-904.

46. Saag KG, Teng GG, Patkar NM, Anuntiyo J, Finney C, Curtis JR, et al. American College of Rheumatology. American college of rheumatology 2008 recommendations for the use of nonbiologic and biologic disease-modifying antirheumatic drugs in rheumatoid arthritis. Arthritis Rheum 2008;59:762-84.

47. Michel BA, Bloch DA, Fries JF. Predictors of fractures in early rheumatoid arthritis. J Rheumatol 1991;18:804-8.

48. Reid DM, Hughes RA, Laan RF, Sacco-Gibson NA, Wenderoth DH, Adami S, et al. Efficacy and safety of daily risedronate in the treatment of corticosteroid-induced osteoporosis in men and women: a randomized trial. European corticosteroid-induced osteoporosis treatment study. J Bone Miner Res 2000;15:1006-13.

49. Saag KG, Emkey R, Schnitzer TJ, Brown JP, Hawkins F, Goemaere S, et al. Alendronate for the prevention and treatment of glucocorticoid-induced osteoporosis. Glucocorticoid-induced osteoporosis intervention study group. N Engl J Med 1998;339:292-9.

50. Solomon DH, Katz JN, Jacobs JP, La Tourette AM, Coblyn J. Management of glucocorticoid-induced osteoporosis in patients with rheumatoid arthritis: Rates and predictors of care in an academic rheumatology practice. Arthritis Rheum 2002;46:3136-42.

51. Saag KG, Shane E, Boonen S, Marín F, Donley DW, Taylor KA, et al. Teriparatide or alendronate in glucocorticoid-induced osteoporosis. N Engl J Med 2007;357:2028-39.

52. Gridley G, McLaughlin JK, Ekbom A, Klareskog L, Adami HO, Hacker DG, et al. Incidence of cancer among patients with rheumatoid arthritis. J Natl Cancer Inst 1993;85:307-11.

53. Baecklund E, Iliadou A, Askling J, Ekbom A, Backlin C, Granath F, et al. Association of chronic inflammation, not its treatment, with increased lymphoma risk in rheumatoid arthritis. Arthritis Rheum 2006;54:692-701.

54. Baecklund E, Iliadou A, Hellgren K, Ekbom A, Backlin C, Sundström C, et al. Long-term steroid treatment may decrease lymphoma risk in rheumatoid arthritis. Results from a Swedish case-control study of 400 RA-lymphomas. Ann Rheum Dis 2007;66(Suppl. II):65.

55. Bachman TR, Sawitzke AD, Perkins SL, Ward JH, Cannon GW. Methotrexate-associated lymphoma in patients with rheumatoid arthritis: report of two cases. Arthritis Rheum 1996;39:325-9.

56. Kingsmore SF, Hall BD, Allen NB, Rice JR, Caldwell DS. Association of methotrexate, rheumatoid arthritis and lymphoma: report of 2 cases and literature review. J Rheumatol 1992;19:1462-5.

57. Wolfe F, Michaud K. The effect of methotrexate and anti-tumor necrosis factor therapy on the risk of lymphoma in rheumatoid arthritis in 19,562 patients during 89,710 person-years of observation. Arthritis Rheum 2007;56:1433-9.

58. Brown SL, Greene MH, Gershon SK, Edwards ET, Braun MM. Tumor necrosis factor antagonist therapy and lymphoma development: twenty-six cases reported to the food and drug administration. Arthritis Rheum 2002;46:3151-8.

59. Askling J, Fored CM, Baecklund E, Brandt L, Backlin C, Ekbom A, et al. Haematopoietic malignancies in rheumatoid arthritis: lymphoma risk and characteristics after exposure to tumour necrosis factor antagonists. Ann Rheum Dis 2005;64:1414-20.

60. Setoguchi S, Solomon DH, Weinblatt ME, Katz JN, Avorn J, Glynn RJ, et al. Tumor necrosis factor alpha antagonist use and cancer in patients with rheumatoid arthritis. Arthritis Rheum 2006;54:2757-64.

61. Egan M, Brosseau L, Farmer M, Oiumet M, Rees S, Tugwell P, et al. Splints/orthoses in the treatment of rheumatoid arthritis. Cochrane Database Syst Rev (CDSR) 2001;CD004018.

62. Simmen BR, Bogoch ER, Goldhahn J. Surgery insight: orthopedic treatment options in rheumatoid arthritis. Nat Clin Pract Rheumatol 2008;4:266-73.

63. Michaud K, Mikuls TR, O'Dell JR, Garvin K, Fehringer E, Wolfe F. The impact of total knee replacement (TKR) on patient reported pain and health-related quality of life in subjects with rheumatoid arthritis (RA). Arthritis Rheum 2007;56(Suppl.):S407.

64. Cohen S, Hurd E, Cush J, Schiff M, Weinblatt ME, Moreland LW, et al. Treatment of rheumatoid arthritis with anakinra, a recombinant human interleukin-1 receptor antagonist, in combination with methotrexate: Results of a twenty-four-week, multicenter, randomized, double-blind, placebo-controlled trial. Arthritis Rheum 2002;46:614-24.

65. Tugwell P, Pincus T, Yocum D, Stein M, Gluck O, Kraag G, et al. Combination therapy with cyclosporine and methotrexate in severe rheumatoid arthritis. the methotrexate-cyclosporine combination study group. N Engl J Med 1995;333:137-41.

66. Kremer JM, Genovese MC, Cannon GW, Caldwell JR, Cush JJ, Furst DE, et al. Concomitant leflunomide therapy in patients with active rheumatoid arthritis despite stable doses of methotrexate. A randomized, double-blind, placebo-controlled trial. Ann Intern Med 2002;137:726-33.

Management of Rheumatoid Arthritis: The Patient with Extra-Articular Disease

Carl Turesson

CASE STUDY 1 Systemic Rheumatoid Vasculitis

The patient was a 62-year-old woman with long-standing rheumatoid arthritis (RA), who was admitted to a tertiary center because of increasing disability and fatigue. She had been diagnosed with RA 10 years ago. A rheumatoid factor (RF) test at diagnosis had been positive, but there was no information on anticitrullinated peptide antibodies (ACPA). Her family history was unremarkable, and she was previously healthy apart from her RA. Previous antirheumatic treatment included sulfasalazine, which had been stopped because of gastrointestinal side effects, and hydroxychloroquine, which had been stopped because of lack of efficacy. The patient had been reluctant to start methotrexate because of fear of side effects. She was on long-term treatment with low-dose glucocorticoids (prednisolone 5 mg daily). She had mild disability, with limited hand function, but was able to work part time as a seamstress.

During the last year, she had experienced increasing tingling and numbness in the hands and feet, followed by severe pain that was not relieved by rest. Increasing doses of analgesics had only a moderate effect on this. There were also recurrent ulcers on the lower legs and the feet, which occurred without major trauma. She reported gradual, unintentional weight loss over 1 year of approximately 20 kg (from 68 kg to 48 kg). Finally, she had developed trouble walking due to a foot drop on the left side.

On admission, the patient looked thin but was in no immediate distress. There was no peripheral lymphadenopathy. Examination of the heart, lungs and the abdomen were unremarkable. There was synovitis of several proximal interphalangeal and metacarpophalangeal joints of both hands, and moderate ulnar deviation of the fingers. There were several small, well-defined, ulcers in various stages of healing on the tibial aspect of both legs, as well as on the heels and on the toes of the left foot. Neurologic examination revealed decreased sensibility to touch and pain in both lower extremities, and a foot drop on the left side.

Routine laboratory tests revealed a mild normochromic anemia, thrombocytosis and a slightly elevated C-reactive protein level. Liver function tests and white blood cell counts were normal.

Differential Diagnosis

Patients with severe, long-standing RA have an increased risk of comorbidities. The differential diagnoses in a patient who develops constitutional symptoms, such as weight loss, should include malignancies and chronic infections. Patients with poorly controlled RA are at an increased risk of non-Hodgkin lymphoma[1] and severe infections.[2] Overall, such complications in patients with RA are more likely to be due to the burden of inflammation than to side effects of immunosuppressive drugs.[2,3] Early diagnosis, based on a careful evaluation of signs and symptoms, leading to appropriate treatment, is of major prognostic importance. In the present case, malignancy should be excluded, but the signs of neuropathy and the lower extremity ulcers are strongly suggestive of vasculitis. Lower leg ulcers in patients with RA may be associated with trivial trauma, and influenced by other factors including arterial insufficiency, repeated trauma, dependent edema, chronic glucocorticosteroid use, and smoking. Chronic or recurrent infection may also lead to impaired healing and should be excluded. In typical cases of systemic rheumatoid vasculitis, the ulcers are associated with an extensive rash and mononeuritis multiplex (Fig. 4-1). Mononeuritis usually involves the peroneal or radial nerves. Initially, the mononeuritis is asymmetric but may become symmetrical. However, most cases of peripheral neuropathy in patients with RA are not due to vasculitis but rather to conditions such as local nerve compression and diabetes.[4,5] Electroneurography should be performed, and a sural nerve biopsy may sometimes be helpful. Again, a pattern of nerve involvement with mononeuritis accompanied by polyneuropathy with neuropathic pain, additional extra-articular organ involvement, and signs of uncontrolled inflammation may all suggest vasculitis. A history of long-standing RA that was not aggressively treated with disease-modifying antirheumatic drugs (DMARDs) should also alert the physician to the possibility of extra-articular organ involvement. Low serum complement levels, indicating systemic complement consumption, is helpful in the diagnosis and indicates a poor prognosis in patients with systemic rheumatoid vasculitis.[6]

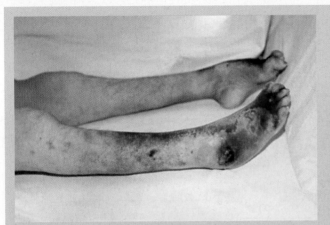

Figure 4-1. Systemic rheumatoid vasculitis. Bilateral foot drop due to mononeuritis multiplex and bilateral lower extremity vasculitis is seen.

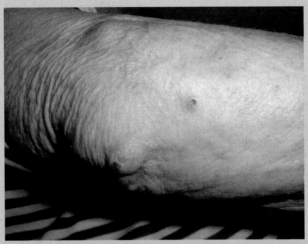

Figure 4-2. Subcutaneous rheumatoid nodule with microinfarcts in a patient with complicated extra-articular RA.

RA-associated vasculitis occurs more frequently among smokers[7] and among patients with rheumatoid nodules.[8] Sometimes, the development of small ulcerations overlying a rheumatoid nodule may herald the presentation of more extensive vasculitic lesions (Fig. 4-2).

Systemic rheumatoid vasculitis can affect other internal organs, although clinically evident vasculitic lesions in the coronary vessels or the central nervous system are rare. In the kidney, renal artery involvement, as occurs in polyarteritis nodosa with vasculitis, may cause renal failure, although the pathology is distinct from polyarteritis nodosa.[9,10] More frequently, a pauci-immune glomerulonephritis occurs in RA, usually of the mesangioproliferative type.[9] Furthermore, although systemic vasculitis associated with RA may affect the gastrointestinal tract,[11] it is not usually associated with the development of microaneurysms.[12]

Patients may be antinuclear antibody or perinuclear antineutrophilic cytoplasmic antibody (P-ANCA) positive in about one third of cases. A positive cytoplasmic antineutrophilic cytoplasmic antibody test (C-ANCA) is rarely seen, and especially if the ANCA is directed against proteinase-3 in a patient with RA, a second disease, such as primary systemic necrotizing vasculitis, should be suspected. However, the coexistence of RA and a primary systemic vasculitis in the same patient is rare.

CASE STUDY 2 Rheumatoid Arthritis Presenting with Rheumatoid Lung Disease

The patient was a previously healthy 57-year-old male warehouseman. He had been smoking at least 10 cigarettes per day since his late teens. His uncle had recently died from pulmonary carcinoma, but there was no history of lung disease among his first-degree relatives. The patient presented to a primary care physician with reports of increasing shortness of breath on moderate exertion and migratory joint pain. An initial physical examination was unremarkable, and a chest radiograph showed only suspected thickening of the right pleura and nonspecific interstitial abnormalities. The patient was referred to a pulmonary disease specialist. When evaluated, the patient reported rapid worsening with severe dyspnea, left-sided thoracic pain, and stiffness of the hands. A new chest radiograph revealed a pleural effusion and progression of basal reticular pulmonary changes. The erythrocyte sedimentation rate and the C-reactive protein were moderately elevated, but there was no increased white blood cell count. Analysis of pleural fluid from a diagnostic thoracocentesis indicated an exudate with a low glucose level and a mixed pattern of inflammatory cells. On physical examination performed by a rheumatologist, symmetric polyarthritis of the hands and feet was noted. Serum tests for RF and ACPA were both positive at high antibody concentrations.

Differential Diagnosis

RA associated lung involvement may precede the clinical onset of arthritis, or the presentation of manifestations such as pleuritis and interstitial pneumonitis may occur simultaneously with rapidly progressing joint symptoms. Differential diagnoses include pulmonary infections and malignancies. In the present case, with a long history of smoking, a pulmonary carcinoma must be excluded. In particular, pleural effusions that are asymptomatic and only noted on clinical examination or radiographs may be due to malignancy. Cytologic evaluation of aspirated pleural fluid is of major importance. The presence of multinucleated giant cells is highly specific for rheumatoid pleuritis, but such cells are seen in less than 50% of these cases.[13] A low glucose level[14] and a high level of the soluble form of the interleukin-2 receptor[15] in the pleural fluid compared with serum levels may also be helpful in distinguishing RA-associated pleuritis from other causes of chronic pleural exudates. In patients with lung manifestations due to RA and other connective diseases, an infectious origin is often initially suspected, but an atypical course with a poor response to antibiotics may suggest an underlying inflammatory disorder. High-resolution computed tomography and open lung biopsy are considered the gold standard for diagnosing interstitial lung disease. Histologic features from tissue obtained at lung biopsy include an inflammatory infiltrate with lymphocytes, plasma cells, and histiocytes with varying degrees of fibrosis, and may be classified as usual interstitial pneumonitis (IP) or nonspecific IP. Specific stainings have suggested a particular role for CD4+ T cells in patients with RA-associated IP, but not in patients with idiopathic IP (Figs. 4-3 and 4-4). RA-specific dysregulation of T cells may be important in the pathogenesis of rheumatoid lung disease, with potential implications for targeted therapies.[16] Furthermore, quantification of the CD20+ B-cell (Fig. 4-5) infiltrates reveals them to be significantly greater in patients with RA-associated IP compared with those with idiopathic IP.[17]

In patients with established RA treated with methotrexate, RA-associated IP must be distinguished from methotrexate-induced toxicity, which usually has a subacute onset with rapidly progressive respiratory symptoms, less radiographic evidence of fibrosis, and a histologic pattern dominated by eosinophilia and type II pneumocyte hyperplasia.[18] In practice, the distinction between rheumatoid lung disease and methotrexate-related toxic pneumonitis may be possible only after extensive follow-up investigations, and many cases of chronic RA

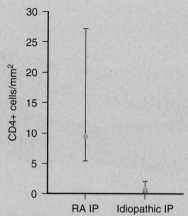

Figure 4-4. Higher number of CD4+ T cells in lung biopsy specimen from patients with rheumatoid arthritis–associated interstitial pneumonitis (RA IP) compared with idiopathic interstitial pneumonitis (idiopathic IP). Computer image analysis. Medians, interquartile ranges. (Data from Turesson C, Matteson EL, Vuk-Pavlovic Z, Colby TV, Vassallo R, Weyand CM, et al. Increased CD4+ T cell infiltrates in rheumatoid arthritis-associated interstitial pneumonitis compared with idiopathic interstitial pneumonitis. Arthritis Rheum 2005;52:73-9.)

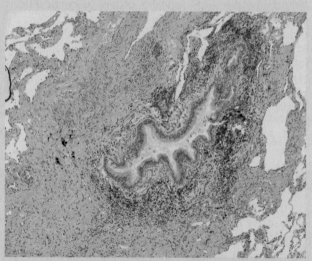

Figure 4-5. Peribronchial infiltrates with CD20+ cells (red stain) in a patient with RA associated non-specific interstitial pneumonitis. Immunohistochemistry. Magnification ×50. (From Turesson C, Matteson EL. Extra-articular manifestations in rheumatoid arthritis. Int J Adv Rheumatol 2007;5:72-7 with permission.)

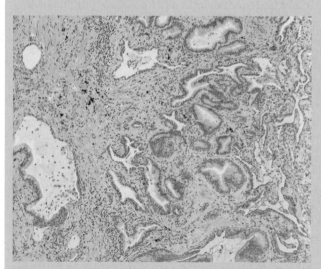

Figure 4-3. CD4+ cells (red stain) in a patient with rheumatoid arthritis–associated usual interstitial pneumonitis. Immunohistochemistry. Magnification ×100.

related IP are incorrectly suspected to be methotrexate induced at first presentation. Possible toxic drug reactions have also been reported in patients treated with leflunomide and tumor necrosis factor (TNF) inhibitors. The possibility of a superimposed respiratory tract infection must be considered in the setting of rapid progression of pulmonary symptoms in patients with suspected RA-associated or treatment related lung disease.

TREATMENT OF RHEUMATOID ARTHRITIS–ASSOCIATED VASCULITIS

Management of rheumatoid vasculitis remains largely empirical (Table 4-1). Two open-label studies,[19,20] as well as long-term clinical experience, favor the use of cyclophosphamide and high-dose glucocorticoids in patients with severe systemic rheumatoid vasculitis. Scott and Bacon[19] compared intermittent bolus intravenous cyclophosphamide plus methylprednisolone, followed by maintenance therapy with azathioprine or oral cyclophosphamide, with other treatments in a non-randomized, open trial of 45 patients. The control group received continuous treatment with other drugs, mainly azathioprine, continuous oral corticosteroids (20–60 mg/day), D-penicillamine or chlorambucil. The age and sex distributions were similar in the two treatment arms, but the patients treated with pulsed cyclophosphamide tended to have more extensive organ involvement. Response to treatment in the first four months was more frequent in the cyclophosphamide group (Fig. 4-6), which also had a lower rate of relapses over the following 4 years (24% versus 54%). Early improvements in the healing of leg ulcers as well as clinically significant improvements in sensory neuropathy occurred at higher rates in the cyclophosphamide group (see Fig. 4-5). Long-term clinical experience corroborates these findings. In particular, early and substantial reduction in neuropathic pain is often seen in RA patients, with vasculitis-related neuropathy treated with high doses of cyclophosphamide and methylprednisolone. In the study reported by Scott and Bacon, there was a striking improvement in mononeuritis, with complete resolution in all three patients treated with intravenous cyclophosphamide. However, in patients with long-standing motor deficits, only partial resolution may be possible due to irreversible neural damage. Serial measurements have indicated that clinical

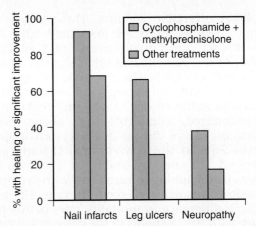

Figure 4-6. Response to treatment within 4 months after starting pulsed intravenous cyclophosphamide and methylprednisolone (MP) compared with other treatments. (Data from Scott DG, Bacon PA. Intravenous cyclophosphamide plus methylprednisolone in treatment of systemic rheumatoid vasculitis. Am J Med 1984;76:377-84.)

improvement following treatment with cytotoxic agents is associated with a decrease in immunoglobulin G RF levels and an increase in complement,[21] which confirms the importance of immune complexes in this subset.

The patient discussed in the case presentation was treated with intravenous cyclophosphamide (15 mg/kg) and methylprednisolone (500 mg) every 3 weeks. There was a rapid reduction of the painful neuropathic sensations in the hands and feet, and the patient was able to taper and stop all analgesics. After 10 infusions, there was complete healing of the lower extremity ulcers, but some numbness of the feet and a partial foot drop remained.

Foster and colleagues[20] compared cytotoxic treatment with conventional DMARD therapy in 34 patients with RA with necrotizing scleritis or

Table 4-1.   *Evidence-Based Therapies in Severe Extra-Articular Rheumatoid Arthritis*

Manifestation/Disease Subset	Treatment	Evidence Base	References
Systemic rheumatoid vasculitis	Cyclophosphamide (pulsed or oral) with high dose glucocorticosteroids	Nonrandomized, open label trials	(19,20)
Systemic rheumatoid vasculitis refractory to cyclophosphamide	TNF-inhibitors	Case series	(32,33)
Interstitial lung disease	Cyclosporin A	Case reports	(36–38)
Rapidly progressing interstitial lung disease	Cyclophosphamide (pulsed or oral) with high-dose glucocorticosteroids	Extrapolation from trials of patients with scleroderma associated alveolitis	(39)
Felty's syndrome	Methotrexate	Case reports	(53,54)
	Intramuscular gold		(52)
Systemic AA amyloidosis	Chlorambucil	Randomized controlled trial	(59)
Systemic AA amyloidosis	Cyclophosphamide	Retrospective cohort study	(60)

TNF, tumor necrosis factor.

peripheral ulcerative keratitis. These severe ophthalmic manifestations are associated with other extra-articular organ involvement, and a substantial number of the patients had other signs of systemic rheumatoid vasculitis. The cytotoxic therapy group was treated with oral cyclophosphamide (100–200 mg/day) or methotrexate (15–25 mg/week). In this nonrandomized, open-label trial, there was no progression of eye disease in the cytotoxic group, whereas 76% in the conventional therapy group progressed. The effect on healing of scleritis or keratitis was better among those treated with cyclophosphamide compared with methotrexate. There was a striking difference in mortality rates between the groups, with 9/17 patients in the conventional therapy group dying within 10 years (all from cardiovascular events), compared with 1/17 in the cytotoxic therapy group. Although these figures should be interpreted with caution due to the small number of patients and the lack of randomized controlled trials, the results are compatible with data from observational studies indicating a poor prognosis in patients with severe extra-articular RA,[22-24] and they favor aggressive therapy for such cases.

There have been no studies directly comparing daily oral continuous cyclophosphamide and pulsed cyclophosphamide in patients with rheumatoid vasculitis. Based on studies of patients with ANCA-associated vasculitis and clinical experience of patients with RA-associated vasculitis, pulsed intravenous cyclophosphamide may be less toxic than daily oral therapy,[25,26] although the risk of relapse in ANCA-associated vasculitis may be higher with pulsed therapy.[25] Based on current data and experience, a rational approach is to use intravenous cyclophosphamide as the treatment of choice in systemic rheumatoid vasculitis and to reserve oral continuous cyclophosphamide for nonresponders to this therapy. Chlorambucil may also be effective, but documentation of its use in rheumatoid vasculitis is scarce.

There is limited information on the efficacy of other immunosuppressive drugs in this setting. A small randomized controlled trial failed to demonstrate a benefit in patients with RA and vasculitic leg ulcers for azathioprine (2 mg/kg/day) and high-dose oral corticosteroids (60 mg/day) compared with conventional DMARD therapy (mainly D-penicillamine and gold).[27] Overall, azathioprine is usually insufficient as primary therapy in patients with severe vasculitis, and its use should be limited to patients with mild lesions and those who are intolerant to cytotoxic therapy. Based on the experience from treatment of patients with primary systemic vasculitides and the trial of rheumatoid vasculitis reported by Scott and Bacon,[19] azathioprine may be used as maintenance therapy. However, in patients with RA, methotrexate is probably a better option, because of its better long-term efficacy when used as therapy for RA in general.

Anti-TNF agents have been reported to be helpful in many cases of severe RA,[28] and TNF is thought to be an important cytokine in the pathogenesis of rheumatoid vasculitis.[29] Unfortunately, patients with severe extra-articular RA have been excluded from large controlled trials of TNF inhibitors. Because these agents have become available in clinical practice, many patients with treatment-resistant extra-articular RA or extra-articular manifestations and severe polyarthritis have received TNF-blocking therapy. There are more than 20 published cases of systemic rheumatoid vasculitis in which anti-TNF agents were found to be helpful.[30-32] The largest of these is a retrospective study from France on nine cases of patients with refractory rheumatoid vasculitis who had been treated with high-dose glucocorticosteroids and cyclophosphamide, with a mean cumulative dose of cyclophosphamide of 8.4 g and a mean prednisone dose of 29.6 mg/day before the use of anti-TNF agents.[33] The authors report that for 6 months, six patients were in remission (complete remission in five, partial in one), treatment failed in one patient, and two patients discontinued anti-TNF treatment because of side effects. The mean prednisone dose could be reduced to 11.2 mg/day. Relapse did occur in two patients, and in only one of these patients could remission be re-established by reintroduction of the anti-TNF agent. Serious infections occurred in three of the patients.[33] Taken together, the experience today suggests that although anti-TNF agents may be helpful in such patients, there is a substantial risk of disease progression and complications with any treatment of rheumatoid vasculitis.

TREATMENT OF RHEUMATOID ARTHRITIS–ASSOCIATED LUNG DISEASE

Whereas idiopathic pulmonary fibrosis responds poorly to immunosuppressive treatment,[34] the treatment outcomes and long-term prognosis in patients with interstitial lung disease in the context of RA and other collagen vascular diseases are better.[35] The treatment of RA-associated lung disease has traditionally focused on short-term high doses of glucocorticosteroids, although there are no controlled studies demonstrating the benefit of glucocorticoids or other antirheumatic drugs in rheumatoid lung disease. Case series have suggested a response to cyclosporin A in individual patients, compatible with a pathogenic role for T cells.[36-38] Based on experience from treatment of patients with severe interstitial lung disease in the setting of scleroderma,[39] there is a rationale for using cyclophosphamide in patients with RA and rapidly progressing interstitial lung disease, and some patients respond to this treatment, although documentation in the literature is limited. Clinical experience and case series[40] suggest that treatment with methotrexate is effective in some patients, although the risk of methotrexate-induced toxic pneumonitis is a concern, in particular among patients with severely impaired respiratory function. Again, the overall benefits of successful treatment with methotrexate in RA must be taken into account when making treatment decisions in individual patients with a complicated disease.

The patient with lung manifestations at RA onset discussed in the case presentation was treated with high-dose glucocorticosteroids and methotrexate, after a high-resolution computer tomography scan and an open lung biopsy confirmed the diagnosis of chronic interstitial pneumonitis. There was rapid improvement of both respiratory symptoms and arthritis, and pulmonary function tests remained stable during long term treatment with methotrexate.

Pleuritis in RA may occur in isolation or, as in this case, in association with interstitial lung disease. Large pleural effusions usually respond to high dose glucocorticosteroid treatment, but thoracocentesis or continuous suction drainage may sometimes be necessary. Patients with treatment-resistant pleural effusions may benefit from intralesional methylprednisolone after adequate drainage.[41]

There is no consensus on the role of TNF-inhibitors in the treatment of RA-associated lung disease. Although there have been reports on excellent responses in refractory patients,[42] worsening of interstitial lung disease after treatment with TNF inhibitors has also been reported,[43] and experimental models suggest that TNF may play a role in preventing pulmonary fibrosis.[44] Observational studies have yielded conflicting results. In a recent survey of a large US sample of patients with RA, there was no association between current treatment with TNF blockers and hospitalization for RA associated IP.[45] In a preliminary report from the British Society for Rheumatology database for biologic treatment of RA, physician-reported RA-associated lung disease was strongly associated with mortality both in patients treated with TNF blockers and traditional DMARDs, but there was a trend toward a worse survival rate in the anti-TNF treated subset.[46] There is a need for more data regarding the effects of TNF blockers on pulmonary disease.

TREATMENT OF OTHER EXTRA-ARTICULAR MANIFESTATIONS

Rheumatoid pericarditis may occasionally lead to life-threatening tamponade, which requires emergency pericardiocentesis.[47] Most patients with RA and clinically evident pericarditis may, however, be treated by the addition of a moderate dose (15–20 mg/day) of glucocorticosteroids to ongoing DMARD treatment. When pericardial effusions recur, more intensive immunosuppressive treatment with cyclophosphamide or other agents may be necessary. Chronic constrictive pericarditis may develop in this setting, leading to chronic heart failure without

major systolic dysfunction.[48,49] Pericardectomy is the treatment of choice for this condition, and the removal of the thickened pericardium should be as extensive as possible.[50]

Patients with Felty's syndrome often have other extra-articular organ manifestations, including vasculitis and sicca syndrome. Progression of joint damage has been demonstrated in neutropenic patients, in spite of the limited synovitis that is often associated with neutropenia.[51] Consequently, these patients should receive aggressive antirheumatic therapy. Clinical improvement and amelioration of neutropenia have been shown in patients treated with parenteral gold and methotrexate.[52-55] The idiosyncratic methotrexate-induced bone marrow failure seen in some patients is completely uncoupled from RA associated neutropenia, and most patients with Felty syndrome treated with methotrexate have stable or improved neutrophil levels (Fig. 4-7). Granulocyte-macrophage colony stimulating factor and granulocyte colony stimulating factor may also be of benefit,[56] although rapid normalization of neutrophils in the absence of adequate anti-rheumatic treatment may lead to flares of arthritis and vasculitis.[57] Hyperviscosity syndrome may occur in patients with Felty's syndrome or other patients with seropositive RA and elevated serum globulin levels. This has been successfully treated with a combination of plasmapheresis and cyclophosphamide.[58]

Systemic amyloidosis is a complication of long-standing, poorly controlled RA. In patients with clinical organ manifestations of amyloidosis, such as renal failure, cytotoxic therapy is warranted. A randomized controlled trial demonstrated that chlorambucil was efficient in inhibiting progression

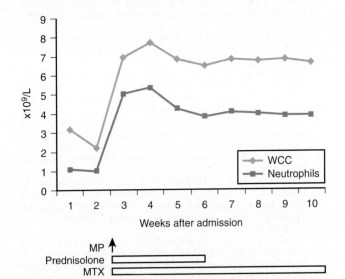

Figure 4-7. Response to treatment with pulsed intravenous methylprednisolone, oral prednisolone, and methotrexate in a patient with Felty's syndrome, with stabilization of the white cell count (WCC) and neutrophil count at normal levels during treatment with methotrexate. (From Turesson C. Arthritis with fever of unknown origin. Int J Adv Rheumatol 2006;4:72-5.)

of renal disease and mortality in patients with RA associated amyloidosis.[59] Case reports and a retrospective cohort study suggest that cyclophosphamide may be equally effective.[60]

TREATMENT OF EXTRA-ARTICULAR RHEUMATOID ARTHRITIS—EXPERIMENTAL APPROACHES

There are several published reports on cases of rheumatoid vasculitis responding to treatment with rituximab.[61,62] Given the role of high level RF:s, immune complexes, and ACPA in rheumatoid vasculitis, and the observed abnormalities in the T-cell repertoire, there is a rationale for treatment with agents directed against B cells or T cells. Rituximab may be an alternative in patients with severe rheumatoid vasculitis when cytotoxic agents and TNF inhibitors are unsuccessful or contraindicated. Because extensive infiltrates of B cells (see Fig. 4-5) and CD4+ T cells (see Figs. 4-3 and 4-4) distinguish RA-associated interstitial pneumonitis from idiopathic interstitial pneumonitis, agents such as rituximab and abatacept may be a more rational choice than TNF-inhibitors in patients with severe RA-associated lung disease. Future studies and increasing long-term clinical experience will help to define the role of rituximab, abatacept, and other new biologics in the treatment of severe extra-articular RA.

References

1. Baecklund E, Ekbom A, Sparén P, Feltelius N, Klareskog L. Disease activity and risk of lymphoma in patients with rheumatoid arthritis: nested case-control study. BMJ 1998;317:180-1.
2. Doran MF, Crowson CS, Pond GR, O'Fallon WM, Gabriel SE. Predictors of infection in rheumatoid arthritis. Arthritis Rheum 2002;46:2294-300.
3. Baecklund E, Iliadou A, Askling J, Ekbom A, Backlin C, Granath F, et al. Association of chronic inflammation, not its treatment, with increased lymphoma risk in rheumatoid arthritis. Arthritis Rheum 2006;54:692-701.
4. Agarwal V, Singh R, Wicla S, Tahlan A, Ahuja CK, et al. A clinical, electrophysiological, and pathological study of neuropathy in rheumatoid arthritis. Clin Rheumatol 2008;27:841-4.
5. Said G, Lacroix C. Primary and secondary vasculitis neuropathy. J Neurol 2005;252:633-41.
6. Puéchal X, Said G, Hilliquin P, Coste J, Job-Deslandre C, Lacroix C, et al. Peripheral neuropathy with necrotizing vasculitis in rheumatoid arthritis: A clinicopathologic and prognostic study of thirty-two patients. Arthritis Rheum 1995;38:1618-29.
7. Turesson C, Schaid DJ, Weyand CM, Jacobsson LT, Goronzy JJ, Petersson IF, et al. Association of smoking and HLA-C3 with vasculitis in patients with rheumatoid arthritis. Arthritis Rheum 2006;54:2276-83.
8. Turesson C, McClelland RL, Christianson T, Matteson E. Clustering of extraarticular manifestations in patients with rheumatoid arthritis. J Rheumatol 2008;35:179-80.
9. Boers M, Croonen AM, Dijkmans BAC, Breedveld FC, Eulderink F, Cats A, et al. Renal findings in rheumatoid arthritis: clinical aspects of 132 necropsies. Ann Rheum Dis 1987;46:658-63.
10. Ball J. Rheumatoid arthritis and polyarteritis nodosa. Ann Rheum Dis 1954;13:277-90.
11. Achkar A, Stanson AW, Johnson CM, Srivatsa SS, Dale LC, Weyand CM. Rheumatoid vasculitis manifesting as intra-abdominal hemorrhage. Mayo Clin Proc 1995;70:565-9.
12. Pagnoux C, Mahr A, Cohen P, Guillevin L. Presentation and outcome of gastrointestinal involvement in systemic necrotizing vasculitides: analysis of 62 patients with polyarteritis nodosa, microscopic polyangiitis, Wegener granulomatosis, Churg-Strauss syndrome, or rheumatoid arthritis-associated vasculitis. Medicine (Baltimore) 2005;84:115-28.
13. Boddington MM, Spriggs AI, Morton JA, Mowat AG. Cytodiagnosis of rheumatoid pleural effusions. J Clin Pathol 1971;24:95-106.
14. Walker WC, Wright V. Pulmonary lesions in rheumatoid arthritis. Medicine 1968;47:501-20.
15. Pettersson T, Söderblom T, Nyberg P, Rishu H, Linho L, Klockars M. Pleural fluid soluble interleukin-2 receptor in rheumatoid arthritis patients and systemic lupus erythematosus. J Rheumatol 1994;21:1820-4.
16. Turesson C, Matteson EL, Vuk-Pavlovic Z, Colby TV, Vassallo R, Weyand CM, et al. Increased CD4+ T cell infiltrates in rheumatoid arthritis-associated interstitial pneumonitis compared with idiopathic interstitial pneumonitis. Arthritis Rheum 2005;52:73-9.
17. Atkins SR, Turesson C, Myers JL, Tazelaar HD, Ryu JH, Matteson EL, et al. Morphological and quantitative assessment of CD20+ B-cell infiltrates in rheumatoid arthritis associated nonspecific interstitial pneumonia and usual interstitial pneumonia. Arthritis Rheum 2006;54:635-41.
18. Kremer JM, Alarcon GS, Weinblatt ME, Kaymakcian MV, Macaluso M, Cannon GW, et al. Clinical, laboratory, radiographic, and histopathologic features of methotrexate-associated lung injury in patients with rheumatoid arthritis: a multicenter study with literature review. Arthritis Rheum 1997;40:1829-37.
19. Scott DG, Bacon PA. Intravenous cyclophosphamide plus methylprednisolone in treatment of systemic rheumatoid vasculitis. Am J Med 1984;76:377-84.
20. Foster CS, Forstot SL, Wilson LA. Mortality rate in rheumatoid arthritis patients developing necrotizing scleritis or peripheral ulcerative keratitis. Effects of systemic immunosuppression. Ophthalmology 1984;91:1253-63.
21. Scott DG, Bacon PA, Allen C, Elson CJ, Wallington T. IgG rheumatoid factor, complement and immune complexes in rheumatoid synovitis and vasculitis: comparative and serial studies during cytotoxic therapy. Clin Exp Immunol 1981;43:54-63.
22. Erhardt CC, Mumford PA, Venables PJ, Maini RN. Factors predicting a poor life prognosis in rheumatoid arthritis: an eight year prospective study. Ann Rheum Dis 1989;48:7-13.
23. Turesson C, Jacobsson L, Bergström U. Extra-articular rheumatoid arthritis: prevalence and mortality. Rheumatology 1999;38:668-74.
24. Turesson C, O'Fallon WM, Crowson CS, Gabriel SE, Matteson EL. Occurrence of extra-articular disease manifestations is associated with excess mortality in a community based study of rheumatoid arthritis. J Rheumatol 2002;29:62-7.
25. de Groot K, Adu D, Savage CO. The value of pulse cyclophosphamide in ANCA-associated vasculitis: meta-analysis and critical review. Nephron Dial Transplant 2001;16:2018-27.
26. Guillevin L, Cohen P, Mahr A, Arène JP, Mouthon L, Puéchal X, et al. Treatment of polyarteritis nodosa and microscopic polyangiitis with poor prognostic factors: a prospective trial comparing glucocorticoids and six or twelve cyclophosphamide pulses in sixty-five patients. Arthritis Rheum 2003;49:93-100.
27. Heurkens AH, Westedt ML, Breedveld FC. Prednisone plus azathioprine treatment in patients with rheumatoid arthritis complicated by vasculitis. Arch Intern Med 1991;151:2249-54.
28. Lipsky PE, van der Heijde DM, St Clair EW, Furst DE, Breedveld FC, Kalden JR, et al. Infliximab and methotrexate in the treatment of rheumatoid arthritis. Anti-Tumor Necrosis Factor Trial in Rheumatoid Arthritis with Concomitant Therapy Study Group. N Engl J Med 2000;343:1594-602.

29. Turesson C, Englund P, Jacobsson L, Nennesmo I, Sturfelt G, Lundberg I. Increased endothelial expression of HLA-DQ and Interleukin-1-α in extra-articular rheumatoid arthritis—results from immunohistochemical studies of skeletal muscle. Rheumatology 2001;40:1346-54.

30. Den Broeder AA, van den Hoogen FH, van de Putte LB. Isolated digital vasculitis in a patient with rheumatoid arthritis: good response to tumour necrosis factor alpha blocking treatment. Ann Rheum Dis 2001;60:538-9.

31. Bartolucci P, Ramanoelina J, Cohen P, Mahr A, Godmer P, Le Hello C, et al. Efficacy of the anti-TNF-alpha antibody infliximab against refractory systemic vasculitides: an open pilot study on 10 patients. Rheumatology (Oxford) 2002;41:1126-32.

32. Unger L, Kayser M, Nussein HG. Successful treatment of severe rheumatoid vasculitis with infliximab. Ann Rheum Dis 2003;62:587-8.

33. Puéchal X, Miceli-Richard C, Mejjad O, Lafforgue P, Marcelli C, Solau-Gervais E, et al. Anti-tumour necrosis factor treatment in patients with refractory systemic vasculitis associated with rheumatoid arthritis. Ann Rheum Dis 2008;67:880-4.

34. Davies HR, Richeldi L, Walters EH. Immunomodulatory agents for idiopathic pulmonary fibrosis. Cochrane Database Syst Rev 2003;CD003134.

35. Agusti C, Xaubet A, Roca J, Agusti AG, Rodriguez-Roisin R. Interstitial pulmonary fibrosis with and without associated collagen vascular disease: results of a two year follow up. Thorax 1992;47:1035-40.

36. Puttick MP, Klinkhoff AV, Chalmers A, Ostrow DN. Treatment of progressive rheumatoid interstitial lung disease with cyclosporine. J Rheumatol 1995;22:2163-5.

37. Ogawa D, Hashimoto H, Wada J, Ueno A, Yamasaki Y, Yamamura M, et al. Successful use of cyclosporin A for the treatment of acute interstitial pneumonitis associated with rheumatoid arthritis. Rheumatology (Oxford) 2000;39:1422-4.

38. Chang HK, Park W, Ryu DS. Successful treatment of progressive rheumatoid interstitial lung disease with cyclosporine: a case report. J Korean Med Sci 2002;17:270-3.

39. Bérezné A, Valeyre D, Ranque B, Guillevin L, Mouthon L. Interstitial lung disease associated with systemic sclerosis: what is the evidence for efficacy of cyclophosphamide? Ann N Y Acad Sci 2007;1110:271-84.

40. Scott DG, Bacon PA. Response to methotrexate in fibrosing alveolitis associated with connective tissue disease. Thorax 1980;35:725-31.

41. Chapman PT, O'Donnell JL, Moller PW. Rheumatoid pleural effusion: response to intrapleural corticosteroid. J Rheumatol 1992;19:478-80.

42. Vassallo R, Matteson E, Thomas Jr CF. Clinical response of rheumatoid arthritis-associated pulmonary fibrosis to tumor necrosis factor-α inhibition. Chest 2002;122:1093-6.

43. Chatterjee S. Severe interstitial pneumonitis associated with infliximab therapy. Scand J Rheumatol 2004;33:276-7.

44. Kuroki M, Noguchi Y, Shimono M, Tomono K, Tashiro T, Obata Y, et al. Repression of bleomycin-induced pneumopathy by TNF. J Immunol 2003;170:567-74.

45. Wolfe F, Caplan L, Michaud K. Rheumatoid arthritis treatment and the risk of severe interstitial lung disease. Scand J Rheumatol 2007;36:172-78.

46. Dixon WD, Watson KD, Lunt M, Hyrich KL, Symmons DPM. Rheumatoid arthritis, interstitial lung disease, mortality and anti-TNF therapy: results from the BSR biologics register (BSBR). Ann Rheum Dis 2007;66(Suppl. II):55.

47. Escalante A, Kaufman RL, Quismoro Jr FP, Beardmore TD. Cardiac compression in rheumatoid pericarditis. Semin Arthritis Rheum 1990;20:148-63.

48. Thould AK. Constrictive pericarditis in rheumatoid arthritis. Ann Rheum Dis 1986;45:89-94.

49. Yurchak PM, Deshpande V. Case records of the Massachusetts General Hospital. Weekly clinicopathological exercises. Case 2-2003. A 60-year old man with mild congestive heart failure of uncertain cause. N Engl J Med 2003;348:243-9.

50. Blake S. The clinical diagnosis of constrictive pericarditis. Am Heart J 1983;106:432-3.

51. Campion G, Maddison PJ, Goulding N, James I, Ahern MJ, Watt I, et al. The Felty syndrome: a case-matched study of clinical manifestations and outcome, serologic features, and immunogenetic associations. Medicine (Baltimore) 1990;69:69-80.

52. Dillon AM, Luthra HS, Conn DL, Ferguson RH. Parenteral gold therapy in the Felty syndrome: experience with 20 patients. Medicine (Baltimore) 1986;65:107-12.

53. Fiechtner JJ, Miller RD, Starkebaum G. Reversal of neutropenia with methotrexate treatment in Felty's syndrome: correlation of response with neutrophil reactive IgG. Arthritis Rheum 1989;32:194-201.

54. Wassenberg S, Herborn G, Rau R. Methotrexate treatment in Felty's syndrome. Br J Rheumatol 1998;37:908-11.

55. Turesson C. Arthritis with fever of unknown origin. Int J Adv Rheumatol 2006;4:72-5.

56. Wagner DR, Combe C, Gresser U. GM-CSF and G-CSF in Felty's syndrome. Clin Invest 1993;71:168-71.

57. Hazenberg BP, van Leuwen MA, van Rijswijk MH, Stern AC, Vellenga E. Correction of granulocytopenia by granulocyte-macrophage colony-stimulating factor: simultaneous induction of interleukin-6 release and flare-up of the arthritis. Blood 1989;74:2769-70.

58. Zakzook SI, Yunus MB, Mulconrey DS. Hyperviscosity syndrome in rheumatoid arthritis with Felty's syndrome: case report and review of the literature. Clin Rheumatol 2002;21:82-5.

59. Ahlmen M, Ahlmen J, Svalander C, Bucht H. Cytotoxic drug treatment of reactive amyloidosis in rheumatoid arthritis with special reference to renal insufficiency. Clin Rheumatol 1987;6:27-38.

60. Chevrel G, Jenvrin C, McGregor B, Miossec P. Renal type AA amyloidosis associated with rheumatoid arthritis: a cohort study showing improved survival on treatment with pulse cyclophosphamide. Rheumatology (Oxford) 2001;40:821-5.

61. Maher LV, Wilson JG. Successful treatment of rheumatoid vasculitis-associated foot drop with rituximab. Rheumatology (Oxford) 2006;45:1450-1.

62. Hellmann M, Jung N, Owczarczyk K, Hallek M, Rubbert A. Successful treatment of rheumatoid vasculitis-associated cutaneous ulcers using rituximab in two patients with rheumatoid arthritis. Rheumatology (Oxford) 2008;47:929-30.

Chapter 5

Management of Ankylosing Spondylitis and Other Spondyloarthropathies

Walter P. Maksymowych

Ankylosing spondylitis (AS) is the most prototypic of a group of arthritides collectively known as spondyloarthritis (SpA) that are associated with the human leukocyte antigen B27 (HLA B27). The hallmarks of disease include sacroiliitis, spinal inflammatory lesions around intervertebral discs, costovertebral joints, facet joints and entheses, extraspinal inflammation in large joints as well as entheses, and extra articular manifestations such as psoriasis, inflammatory bowel disease (IBD) and acute anterior uveitis (AAU). A defining feature of disease is the development of ankylosis in the sacroiliac joints, across intervertebral discs, and in the facet joints. Disease onset is typically in the third and fourth decades of life, although it may present in children either with asymmetric involvement of large joints in the lower limbs or a syndrome of enthesopathy and involvement of the tarsal joints. Males are affected twice as frequently as females, and there is marked geographic diversity in prevalence and phenotypic manifestations. By far, the commonest presentation is lower back or buttock pain that may be difficult to distinguish from other causes of spinal pain, particularly in primary care practice. This may be the primary reason why diagnostic delay averages 8 to 9 years from onset of symptoms, even in countries with advanced health care systems. This chapter provides an integrated case-focused and evidence-based overview of the treatment of AS from its earliest manifestations to the most recalcitrant disease likely to be encountered in the clinic. A dominant theme, regardless of clinical presentation, is that this is a disease that requires decades of management for most patients and a comprehensive treatment plan that may include educational, physical, medical, and even surgical treatment modalities.

UNCOMPLICATED EARLY AKYLOSING SPONDYLITIS

CASE STUDY 1

A 25-year-old woman presents with a 2-year history of lower back and right buttock pain radiating into the posterior thigh associated with stiffness that is most prominent in the mornings, lasting 2 to 4 hours, and recurring after sitting for prolonged periods at her secretarial desk. Getting out of her chair and moving for 10 to 15 minutes alleviates her stiffness, as will exercise at her local gym. She is fatigued and often wakes up in the second half of the night with pain and stiffness alleviated by getting out of bed and walking around the house for 5 minutes. Her symptoms are interfering with her work. She is otherwise in good health. In the family history, she recalled that her grandmother had back trouble throughout her life. She has tried several over-the-counter analgesics and is now taking ibuprofen 200 mg 4 times a day on a regular basis for the past month. Physical examination shows no abnormalities. Laboratory analysis shows that she is HLA-B27 positive and her C-reactive protein (CRP) is slightly elevated at 12 mg/dL. Pelvic x-ray study indicates abnormal right sacroiliac joint with indistinct iliac subchondral bone and widening of the joint space in the lower one third of the joint.

This case highlights characteristic features of early disease, namely a typical history of inflammatory back pain, unremarkable physical examination, acute phase reactants that may be normal or only slightly elevated, positive screening test for HLA-B27, and minimal plain radiographic features so that more sensitive imaging modalities such as magnetic resonance imaging (MRI) may be warranted. Self-medication for spinal symptoms even before the primary care physician visit is typical, and patients often prefer analgesics with anti-inflammatory properties rather than acetaminophen alone. This patient continues to have significant symptoms of pain and stiffness despite having taken maximum recommended doses of ibuprofen for over-the-counter use and further therapy is warranted.

What are the key principles of management for patients with newly diagnosed AS?

At this stage of disease, the primary objectives are to reduce symptoms of pain, stiffness, and fatigue, and to maintain function and mobility, thereby preventing disability and improving work productivity and the quality of life. A comprehensive treatment plan for this patient should be recommended under the following headings.

Patient Education

Most patients are typically unaware of this disease and require counseling on several themes related to prognosis, impact on work and family life, an approach to regular exercise, and appropriate use of nonpharmacologic pain management techniques, relaxation, and cognitive distraction. Moreover, young patients are particularly distraught to learn that this is a genetic condition and often express anxieties regarding transmission of disease to offspring. In addition to the reassurance provided by the physician, patients should be encouraged to attend group educational programs where available specifically for patients with AS. These have been shown to improve depression, self-efficacy, psychological well-being, and self-efficacy for exercise.[1] There are limited data on the effectiveness of these programs. No comparisons between studies are possible owing to the heterogeneous nature of these programs. However, there appears to be general agreement that they promote coping with the emotional consequences of disease diagnosis and participating in decisions concerning treatment. Increasingly patients seek help through the electronic media and patient support groups such as The Spondylitis Association of America (www.spondylitis.org) provide extensive resources that help patients manage their disease.

Physical Modalities

Physiotherapy aimed at improving mobility of the spine and peripheral joints, and strengthening the axial and proximal musculature, and improvement in general fitness is an essential component of the management of all stages of disease. A vital role for the physiotherapist is also to promote an overall understanding of the necessity and appropriateness of regular exercise. Several exercise regimens have been described in the literature that include unsupervised individual exercise prescribed by a physiotherapist according to a predefined protocol of instruction, supervised individual exercises performed either at home or at a physiotherapy center, supervised group physical therapy, and in-patient physiotherapy typically consisting of a 2- to 4-week program of more intensive exercise aimed at correcting posture, improving flexibility, and motivating patients to pursue regular exercise when they leave the program.

It is difficult to recommend any particular approach due to their heterogeneous nature and their limited evaluation in controlled studies where interventions are poorly described. There is also a lack of consistency in outcomes assessed and use of independent blinded assessors. A Cochrane Review and a subsequent modification considered 43 studies of which only six trials met the criteria for inclusion in the review.[2] These included a total of 561 participants enrolled in two trials that compared individualized home exercise programs with no intervention, three trials that compared weekly supervised group physiotherapy with an individualized home exercise program, and a single spa therapy clinical trial that assessed a program of physical exercises, walking, postural correction, hydrotherapy, sports, bathing in thermal water or sauna received at a spa compared with a home-based program of weekly group therapy.[3] It was concluded that there was some benefit for group physiotherapy with small improvements in spinal mobility and patient global assessment, which could be due to mutual motivation and exchange of experience with similarly affected participants. Spa therapy was also beneficial for pain, although most studies were generally consistent in demonstrating that no approach is of benefit for treating symptoms, especially pain. Longitudinal study has shown that exercise intervention should be regularly reinforced and consistently applied by the patient to prevent functional disability and is most useful among those who have had AS for 15 years or less.[4]

Disease-Modifying Antirheumatic Drugs

These agents are primarily used to improve pain, stiffness, function, mobility, and overall patient well-being. Two categories of drugs are available; nonsteroidal anti-inflammatory drugs (NSAIDs) and adjuvant therapies such as analgesics and antidepressants.

NSAIDs have been the cornerstone of pharmacologic intervention for AS since their introduction in the 1950s. Their ability to suppress the production of proinflammatory prostaglandins through inhibition of cyclo-oxygenase is well known, although additional properties have been described, including suppression of neutrophil functions, which may lead to reduction of free oxygen radicals, reduced adhesion to endothelium, and decreased chemotaxis. These agents also inhibit both constitutively expressed cyclo-oxygenase-1 (COX-1), which is responsible for the physiologic production of cytoprotective prostaglandins in the gastric mucosa, as well as the highly regulated cyclo-oxygenase-2 (COX-2), which is increased in inflammatory tissues. Although these agents express varying degrees of inhibition of the cellular and enzymatic pathways leading to inflammation, this appears to have relatively little relevance with respect to their efficacy in AS. However, it is likely that the minimal efficacy of aspirin and salicylates for AS is due to their low potency in inhibiting COX-2. A total of six randomized placebo-controlled trials have shown that NSAIDs are effective for alleviating pain and stiffness and improving function and mobility.[5-10] These studies evaluated two agents that are not commonly used in clinical practice, namely piroxicam and ximoprofen, and were generally of only 2 to 6 weeks in duration. One study compared piroxicam with meloxicam over 52 weeks after a 6 week placebo-controlled phase. Two more recent studies examined COX-2–selective agents, celecoxib and etoricoxib, and suggested that these agents might be more effective than nonselective NSAIDs.[9,10] What all studies have shown is that maximal efficacy is attained by 2 weeks, which constitutes an appropriate trial of therapy. The clinical benefit of attempting second and third trials of treatment with alternative NSAIDs cannot be determined from the controlled studies performed to date which have typically enrolled patients experiencing a flare following withdrawal of NSAID and have therefore preselected for NSAID responsive patients. Nevertheless, several treatment recommendations support the use of at least two to three courses of different NSAIDs over 2 to 4 weeks before patients are considered NSAID refractory.[11,12]

Between 10% and 60% of patients receiving NSAIDs experience minor gastrointestinal symptoms such as nausea, dyspepsia, epigastric pain, and diarrhea, whereas more serious effects such as ulcers, upper gastrointestinal bleeding, and perforation occur in 2% to 4% of patients using NSAIDs for 12 months. Increasing age, use of NSAID combinations, and comorbidity increase the risk for such adverse events. Although COX-2–selective agents are associated with significantly decreased risk of major gastrointestinal side effects, the risk of less serious and more common gastrointestinal symptoms (dyspepsia, abdominal pain, nausea, flatulence, diarrhea) are not significantly reduced. An increased risk for significant cardiovascular events is now well established for COX-2–selective agents. One study of etorocoxib that recruited 387 patients who received treatment for up to a year recorded five serious cardiovascular thrombotic events in patients receiving this agent.[10] Additional concerns include hypertension, peripheral edema and congestive heart failure, and compromise of renal function in patients with pre-existing renal dysfunction.

Summary of Management Recommendations for Prototypic Case of Early Uncomplicated Ankylosing Spondylitis

This patient was reassured that satisfactory disease control could be achieved in up to two thirds of patients with a conservative regime of regular daily exercise aimed at maintaining spinal flexibility and core muscle strength, together with the use of NSAIDs such as naproxen taken in doses up to 500 mg twice daily as required for the relief of symptoms of pain and stiffness (Table 5-1). Review of the patient's background medical history verified no propensity to gastrointestinal side effects. The patient was referred to group physiotherapy and an educational program aimed at patients with AS and provided with the website address for The Spondylitis Association of America (www.spondylitis.org).

ESTABLISHED AS UNRESPONSIVE TO CONSERVATIVE THERAPIES

CASE STUDY 2

A 45-year-old man presents with a 16-year history of AS that has until the past 6 months been symptomatically well controlled with diclofenac 75 mg twice daily. He has morning stiffness of 2 hours' duration that is alleviated when he works as a construction laborer. He sleeps poorly due to frequent nocturnal awakening with pain and stiffness and is fatigued throughout the day. He is increasingly taking days off work due to sick leave. In his past medical history, he had a prolapsed lumbar disc associated with heavy lifting at work. Physical examination showed restricted lumbar flexion, with Schober's test being 2.5 cm, chest expansion being 3 cm, and cervical rotation measured with a goniometer being 50 degrees to left and right. Laboratory evaluation showed that he is HLA-B27 positive and has normal acute phase reactants but elevated serum metalloproteinase 3. Radiography showed sacroiliitis and several syndesmophytes in the thoracic and lumbar spine with fusion of several of the facet joints. The attending physician discontinued diclofenac and instituted naproxen 500 mg bd. One month later, the patient reported no significant benefit.

This patient has ongoing symptoms of pain and stiffness despite an adequate trial of 2 NSAIDs at maximum recommended dosage, has impaired spinal mobility, and x-rays indicate progression

Table 5-1. *Management of Uncomplicated Early Ankylosing Spondylitis*

Principal Clinical Features	Objectives of Treatment	Management Considerations	Key References

Spinal and buttock pain
Stiffness
Fatigue
Increased CRP
B27 positive
Sacroiliitis on plain
  x-ray study
	Reduce pain, stiffness, fatigue,
	  anxiety, depression
	Maintain function
	Prevent disability
	Improve self-efficacy, sleep,
	  work productivity, quality
	  of life
		Patient education
		Group physiotherapy
		NSAIDs
			Barlow and Barefoot. 1996 (1)
			www.spondylitis.org
			Dagfinrud et al. 2004 (2)
			Dougados et al. 2001 (9)
			Van der Heijde et al. 2005 (10)
			Braun et al. 2003 (11)
			Maksymowych et al. 2007 (12)

NSAIDs, nonsteroidal anti-inflammatory drugs; CRP, C-reactive protein.

of disease from the sacroiliac joints to the spine. It would be appropriate to monitor this patient's progress in a systematic manner using validated outcome instruments such as the Bath AS Disease Activity Index (BASDAI)[13] and the Bath AS Function Index (BASFI).[14] Both are self-reported questionnaires, the former having 6 items and the latter having 10 items. Each has a scoring range from 0 to 100, using a 0 to 100 Visual Analogue Scale for each item. Treatment recommendations call for the re-evaluation of treatment in AS patients who have active symptoms as recorded by a BASDAI score of at least 40 despite the use of at least 2 different NSAIDS.[11,12] Additional evidence of disease activity is desirable such as an elevated CRP, which may be normal in up to a half of all patients, or active inflammation on MRI of the spine and/or sacroiliac joints.

What should be the approach to the management of established AS when patients have active disease and are refractory to NSAIDs?

Only anti-tumor necrosis factor-α (anti-TNF-α)–directed therapies are of proven efficacy in this category of patient.

Anti-Tumor Necrosis Factor-α– Directed Therapies

The introduction of anti-TNF-α–directed therapies for the treatment of AS constitutes a significant advance in the treatment of this disease, particularly for patients who are refractory to NSAIDs. TNF-α is a pivotal cytokine associated with inflammation and has been demonstrated in mononuclear cells invading cartilage in both sacroiliac joints and entheses, whereas over-expression in mice is associated with the development of sacroiliitis. Inhibition of TNF-α has been achieved by the development of either monoclonal antibodies that bind both circulating and cell membrane bound forms of TNF-α or by soluble receptor proteins that primarily bind circulating TNF-α. Currently available monoclonal antibodies include infliximab, a chimeric monoclonal IgG1 that has a variable portion that is murine in origin while the remainder is of human origin, and adalimumab which is completely human in origin. Etanercept is a complex recombinant protein whereby two 75-kDa TNF receptor moieties are bound by an IgG1 Fc portion, which prolongs the half life of the receptor portion from a few minutes to about 16 hours. Infliximab is administered as an intravenous infusion over 2 hours at baseline, and 2 weeks, 6 weeks and every 6 to 8 weeks thereafter. Clinical trials primarily evaluated a dose of 5 mg/kg, although a lower dose of 3 mg/kg may also be effective and considered at the start of treatment with dose escalation for suboptimal responses. Etanercept is administered as a dose of 50 mg by once-weekly subcutaneous injection. Adalimumab is also given by subcutaneous injection at a dose of 40 mg on alternate weeks.

A total of nine randomized placebo-controlled trials have demonstrated substantial symptomatic benefit in NSAID refractory patients with reduction in pain, stiffness, function, and fatigue, which may be seen as soon as 2 weeks after the start of therapy while improvement in spinal mobility is also evident from 12 weeks onward.[15-23] Maximal benefit is seen by 12 weeks and is sustained over prolonged periods of several years. Other benefits include improved quality of life, reduced sick leave, improvement in work productivity, reduced acute phase reactants, improvement in synovial histopathology and reduction in MRI features of inflammation that are sustained over several years.[22,24-26] These agents appear to be of similar clinical efficacy for axial and peripheral joint inflammation with clinically evident responses being observed in about 60% of patients. All categories and subgroups of patients appear to respond, although younger patients with shorter disease duration, minimal impairment of function, elevated CRP, and MRI features of inflammation appear to respond best. However, even patients with complete spinal ankylosis report significant symptomatic improvement.

Despite the circumstantial data cited above suggesting that these agents might have a beneficial impact on the progression of radiographic changes, recent studies do not support such an effect in the spine. Radiographic change in the spine is measured using the modified Stoke AS Spinal Score (mSASSS), which records sclerosis, squaring, erosion, syndesmophytes, and ankylosis in the anterior vertebral corners of the cervical and lumbar spine. Changes in the thoracic spine are not recorded owing to lack of adequate visibility caused by overlapping soft tissues. The rate of progression in patients on standard therapy is slow and requires 2 years before change can be reliably detected, which is problematic for clinical trials where ethical considerations require that patients receiving only background NSAID treatment switch to open label anti-TNF therapy after 12 to 24 weeks. Consequently, patients in the long term open label extensions of placebo-controlled randomized trials of anti-TNF agents have been compared with a historical cohort of patients on standard therapy. No differences in rates of radiographic progression have been observed with any of the three available anti-TNF agents.[27-29] It should be noted that the same comparator cohort was evaluated in all three studies, and AS patients had long-established disease so that potential for reversibility may have been limited.

Potential adverse events of anti-TNF agents are similar to those that have been reported in patients with rheumatoid arthritis (RA). Tuberculosis and other forms of sepsis may be less common in AS patients in view of the younger demographic and lack of concomitant immunosuppressive therapy. There is little information on malignancies, and the reported higher frequency of lymphoma in RA patients receiving these therapies may not necessarily be observed in AS, which has not been associated with increased rates of lymphoma. Infusion reactions have been noted in patients with AS receiving infliximab, although less commonly than anticipated, considering the lack of use of concomitant methotrexate therapy. Nevertheless higher rates of infusion reactions and loss of efficacy are related to the development of antichimeric antibodies.[30]

Summary of Management Recommendations for Prototypic Case of Established Ankylosing Spondylitis Unresponsive to Conservative Therapies

In view of this patient's occupation and prior history of disc prolapse, an MRI was ordered and showed active inflammation in the spine and sacroiliac joints. A BASDAI was completed, and the patient scored 7.8, indicating highly symptomatic AS. The use of any one of the three available anti-TNF agents is appropriate, the choice of specific agent being dictated largely by patient preference with respect to mode of administration. The patient was sent for another course of group physiotherapy. NSAID therapy should be continued on a regular basis because one 2-year study has shown that continuous therapy was associated with less radiographic progression than on demand treatment.[31] This patient has already developed syndesmophytes on x-ray study, and this is a risk factor for further progression, together with elevated serum metalloproteinase-3.[32,33] This recommendation has to be weighed against individual patient risk for gastrointestinal and cardiovascular adverse events (Table 5-2).

ESTABLISHED AS COMPLICATED BY EXTRASPINAL MANIFESTATIONS

CASE STUDY 3

A 16-year-old boy presents with a 2-year history of Crohn's disease, which is currently inactive, and a 6-year history of AS that has been causing progressively more neck pain, stiffness, and limitation of motion. He also has painful knees and has had three episodes of acute anterior uveitis over the past 3 years. Current treatment includes celecoxib 100 mg twice daily, pentasa 250 mg daily and prednisone 7.5 mg daily. Physical examination shows active synovitis in both knees, Achilles' enthesitis and plantar fasciitis, restricted internal rotation of the hip, restricted spinal flexion, Schober's test being 2.5 cm, and rotation of the neck being 40 degrees bilaterally. Laboratory investigation indicates that he is HLA-B27 positive, has a CRP of 69 mg/dL, whereas x-ray studies show bilateral sacroiliitis, vertebral ankylosis in the cervical and lumbar spine, and concentric narrowing of the left hip joint.

NSAIDs have been associated with the onset or exacerbation of IBD which raises the question as to whether they should be used at all in these patients and whether COX-2–selective agents offer any advantages over nonselective agents.[34] Although there have been no controlled studies, a prospective open-label study of rofecoxib 12.5 mg/day in 45 patients with inactive IBD showed that relapse and drug withdrawal was more frequent in these patients than in a control group of 30 patients with dyspepsia.[35] Therefore, it is preferable to avoid NSAIDs in patients even with inactive disease.

In view of the presence of active peripheral synovitis, should second line therapies proven to be useful in RA such as salazopyrin (SSPN) and methotrexate be considered in the management of this patient?

Second-Line Therapies

In this category of therapies, the agent that has been studied most extensively in AS is salazopyrin, a therapeutic widely used for disease modification in RA. Its first reported use was in those AS patients who had concomitant peripheral arthritis. The rationale for this treatment is based on the well-documented association between AS and IBD, the demonstration of inflammatory lesions in the intestine of up to 60% of AS patients, the success of SSPN in the management of IBD, and its potential antimicrobial properties on intestinal bacteria thought to be involved in the pathogenesis of AS. A total of 10 double-blind, placebo controlled trials have been published, of which, two large multicenter studies

Table 5-2. *Management of Established Ankylosing Spondylitis Unresponsive to Conservative Therapies*

Principal Clinical Features	Objectives of Treatment	Management Considerations	Key References
Pain, stiffness, fatigue despite NSAID therapy	Reduce pain, stiffness, fatigue Improve sleep, quality of life	Reinstitute group physiotherapy	Van der Heijde et al. 2005 (17)
Poor sleep	Improve function and spinal mobility	Maintain NSAID therapy	Davis et al. 2003 (21)
Reduced spinal mobility	Increase work productivity and reduce sick leave	Anti-TNF therapy	Van der Heijde et al.
Reduced work productivity and increased sick leave	Prevent disease progression	Infliximab	2006 (23)
Spinal syndesmophytes and ankylosis on radiography		Etanercept Adalimumab	Wanders et al. 2005 (31)

NSAID, nonsteroidal anti-inflammatory drug; TNF, tumor necrosis factor.

have shown modest benefit for alleviating peripheral joint symptoms and synovitis but not the axial component of disease.[36,37] Most patients had longstanding disease, suggesting a lack of responsiveness. However, a recent study has shown a complete lack of benefit even in patients with very early disease.[38] Published treatment protocols recommend the use of this agent in doses of up to 3 g/day if tolerated over a period of 3 months in AS patients with concomitant peripheral synovitis.[11,12] A meta-analysis of salazopyrin in AS selected five trials and concluded that four clinical outcomes reached levels of statistical significance in the pooled analysis, with reductions in duration of morning stiffness (28.2%), severity of morning stiffness (30.6%), patient global (7.5%) and severity of pain (26.7%).[39] Adverse events consist mostly of diarrhea and upper abdominal pain, although the occasional development of anemia and neutropenia requires monthly complete blood count assessment.

Methotrexate has been widely used as a disease modifying agent in RA. Limited study suggests benefit in those AS patients with concomitant peripheral arthritis, although this has not been verified in controlled studies and none used more than 10 mg weekly. Canadian treatment recommendations indicate that it may be considered in patients with peripheral arthritis in doses of up to 25 mg weekly, if tolerated, over a period of at least 3 months, although this should be primarily aimed at centers where access to anti-TNF therapies is limited.[12]

Leflunomide is a disease-modifying agent used in RA that has also been studied in AS. One open-label study that was conducted over 24 weeks demonstrated improvement in patients with concomitant peripheral arthritis, although a small placebo-controlled study revealed no benefit. There are currently insufficient data to recommend its use in AS.

Unlike RA, there is minimal evidence that systemic steroids are useful for the treatment of AS. Studies have been confined to the examination of pulse intravenous steroids, which have generally been beneficial for symptom relief in open-label studies. There have been no controlled studies of oral steroid therapy, and this approach is not recommended for AS.

Intra-articular steroid injections may be beneficial for AS, particularly when administered using several imaging techniques into the sacroiliac joints. Fluoroscopically guided injections relieved pain in one placebo-controlled study and allowed a 50% reduction in the use of NSAIDs.[40] A significant drawback of fluoroscopy is its relatively low resolution and potential difficulty in accurate placement of the needle into the synovial portion of the joint. A second controlled study using fluoroscopy showed benefit even from periarticular injection, suggesting that intrasynovial injection may not be a prerequisite for a satisfactory therapeutic response.[41] Open-label studies have also described benefit following computed tomography (CT)–guided injection of the sacroiliac joints, although the relatively high exposure to ionizing radiation favors the use of fluoroscopy. Intra-articular injection into peripheral joints has a long established record of efficacy and safety for various forms of inflammatory arthritis.

Summary of Management Recommendations for Prototypic Case of Established Ankylosing Spondylitis Complicated by Extraspinal Manifestations

The patient's celecoxib was discontinued, and he was started on salazopyrin at a dose of 500 mg daily, escalated by 500 mg/week to 2 g/day. Group physiotherapy was reinstituted. He also received intra-articular injections of triamcinolone hexacetonide into both knees and a fluoroscopically guided injection of the same agent into the left hip. At 4 months, he had experienced only temporary relief from the steroid injections and continued to have significant back pain and stiffness. Salazopyrin was discontinued, and he was started on a monoclonal antibody anti-TNF-α agent. Etanercept has been shown to lack efficacy in Crohn's disease and does not appear to reduce flares of bowel disease in patients with AS. In contrast, both infliximab and adalimumab are beneficial for Crohn's and reduce flares of colitis in patients with AS.[42,43] Pooled analysis of anti-TNF controlled trials in AS and open-label data also support a beneficial effect of monoclonal antibodies to TNF in reducing flares of acute anterior uveitis in AS (Table 5-3).[44]

Table 5-3. *Management of Established Ankylosing Spondylitis Complicated by Extraspinal Manifestations*

Principal Clinical Features	Objectives of Treatment	Management Considerations	Key References
Pain, stiffness, fatigue despite NSAID therapy	Reduce pain, stiffness, fatigue	Reinstitute group physiotherapy	Hanauer and Sandborn. 2001 (34)
Reduced hip and spinal mobility	Reduce peripheral joint inflammation and enthesitis	Reduce NSAID therapy	Dougados et al. 1995 (36)
Peripheral synovitis	Improve quality of life	Intra-articular steroids	Clegg et al. 1996 (37)
Enthesitis	Improve function and spinal mobility	Salazopyrin	Braun et al. 2007 (42)
Crohn's disease		Anti-TNF therapy	Rudwaleit et al. 2008 (43)
Acute anterior uveitis	Prevent flares of Crohn's disease and anterior uveitis	Infliximab	Braun et al. 2005 (44)
Increased CRP		Adalimumab	
Spinal ankylosis and narrowing of hip joint on radiography	Prevent disease progression		

CRP, C-reactive protein; NSAID, nonsteroidal anti-inflammatory drug; TNF, tumor necrosis factor.

TREATMENT OF OTHER SPONDYLOARTHROPATHIES

CASE STUDY 4

A 28-year-old man presents with a 6-month history of right heel and left knee pain and swelling over 6 months that is unresponsive to NSAID therapy and orthotics. He has skin lesions of psoriasis over the elbows and knees, and in the past 3 months, he has developed right buttock pain with morning stiffness of 2 hours' duration and alleviation with activity. The family history is positive for AS in his mother. Physical examination shows tenderness at the insertion of the Achilles tendon into the calcaneum. Laboratory investigation shows that he is HLA-B27 positive. Pelvic x-ray study shows normal sacroiliac joints.

The diagnosis of AS very much rests on the finding of definite sacroiliitis on plain radiography. However, x-ray changes may not be apparent for many years in patients with inflammatory-type back pain and the term preradiographic SpA has been proposed. Very few studies have specifically examined therapeutic agents in this category of patient. A recent placebo-controlled trial showed that adalimumab was effective for the alleviation of pain and stiffness and improvement in function in these patients.[45] Approximately two thirds had MRI features of inflammation, which improved 12 weeks after treatment with adalimumab. Salazopyrin does not appear to be effective in this category of SpA,[38] although it does appear to be effective for psoriatic spondyloarthritis.[36] Although pivotal phase 3 trials of anti-TNF agents in AS have included about 10% of patients who had either psoriatic or enteropathic AS,[16] no studies have specifically examined these categories of SpA. Nevertheless all available anti-TNF agents appear to be equally beneficial in these patients for symptoms, function, and quality of life comparable to primary AS. A placebo-controlled study of infliximab in juvenile SpA similarly showed substantial benefit evident from 2 weeks onward.[46] Only case reports and small series describe benefits of anti-TNF therapy in patients with chronic reactive arthritis. There appears to be no evidence for benefit from second-line therapies such as salazopyrin.

Specific Management of Prototypic Case of Pre-radiographic Spondyloarthropathy

This patient was started on adalimumab, and NSAID therapy was continued.

REFRACTORY ANKYLOSING SPONDYLITIS

CASE STUDY 5

A 54-year-old man with a history of AS for 23 years was responding well to an anti-TNF agent until he developed congestive heart failure. He has morning stiffness of 2 hours' duration and scores 7.4 on the BASDAI and 6.5 on the BASFI. Physical examination shows restricted mobility in all segments of the spine and bilateral knee synovitis. His CRP is 65, and x-ray studies show several syndesmophytes with fusion of the sacroiliac joints. He has tried intra-articular steroid injections into the knees, but the benefit lasted only 3 weeks. His cardiologist has advised him not to take any NSAID or anti-TNF therapy.

Approximately 30% of AS patients either do not respond to anti-TNF therapy or develop side effects that preclude their use. Limited open-label data and one controlled study have shown that intravenously administered bisphosphonates, specifically pamidronate, given in a dose of 60 mg once monthly, may benefit patients with spinal pain and stiffness if given over a 6-month period but is not beneficial in the presence of peripheral synovitis.[47] Evidence from open-label studies would also support an empirical trial of either methotrexate or leflunomide therapy.

Several agents are under development targeting inflammatory cells and mediators thought to be important in patients with AS. These include B-cell–directed therapies such as rituximab, inhibitors of T-cell costimulation such as abatacept and interleukin-6 receptor–directed therapies. Recent work has identified a distinct group of T cells that produce the cytokine interleukin-17 as a defining phenotype. A major regulator of these T cells is interleukin-23, and early trials of antibodies directed toward the interleukin-23 receptor appear promising in patients with psoriasis and Crohn's disease, suggesting this is a promising target for further study in AS.

Management of Complications of Ankylosing Spondylitis

The commonest complication of AS is AAU occurring in up to 40% of patients with long-standing AS. Most attacks respond readily to steroids and mydriatic eye drops, but occasionally, systemic steroids are required for persistent inflammation. Attacks occur sporadically with intervening periods that may last several years, although occasionally, attacks occur much more frequently. Several therapeutic strategies may then be employed. NSAID therapy may diminish the severity and duration of an attack, and dosing may be increased at the immediate onset of an attack. Should this fail, prophylactic therapy may be necessary. Limited open-label data suggest that salazopyrin may be beneficial in reducing the frequency of attacks.[48] Pooled data from placebo-controlled trials and open-label studies indicate a reduced frequency of attacks in patients who receive anti-TNF therapy.[44] Open-label data support a preference for the use of infliximab and adalimumab over etanercept.[49]

The development of osteoporosis is under-recognized in AS and may lead to vertebral fracture. Vitamin D supplementation should be encouraged, as well as screening for low bone mineral density, particularly when disease has been active for many years requiring continuous NSAID therapy. Recommendations for treatment of osteoporosis complicating AS do not differ from those for primary osteoporosis, although there have been no controlled studies that have addressed the effects of oral bisphosphonates on the development of osteoporosis and fractures in patients with AS.

Rarer complications include cauda equina syndrome, pulmonary fibrosis, and amyloidosis. Cauda equina syndrome is characterized by a slow onset of neurologic deficits in the lower limbs, sphincter dysfunction, and the development of dural ectasia. A review of 86 patients concluded that surgical treatment of the dural ectasia, either by lumboperitoneal shunting or laminectomy, was the best treatment approach.[50] There is no effective therapy for pulmonary fibrosis. Case reports have described beneficial effects of anti-TNF therapy in patients with amyloidosis secondary to AS.

CONCLUDING COMMENTS

Significant strides have been made in the development of new therapeutic approaches for patients with AS and related spondyloarthropathies. Fewer than 10% of patients remain refractory to currently available therapies, although agents that alter the natural course of disease remain elusive. Moreover, there is little convincing evidence that any therapeutic approach, with the possible exception of NSAID therapy, can ameliorate the progression of structural changes on radiography. Nevertheless, accumulating genetic and pathophysiologic data offers optimism that even these challenges will soon be addressed.

References

1. Barlow JH, Barefoot J. Group education for people with arthritis. Patient Educ Couns 1996;27:257-67.
2. Dagfinrud H, Kvien TK, Hagen KB. Physiotherapy inventions for ankylosing spondylitis. Cochrane Dababase Syst Rev 2004;4:Cd002822.pub2.
3. Van Tubergen A, Landewe R, van der Heijde D, Hidding A, Wolter N, Asscher M, et al. Combined spa-exercise therapy is effective in patients with ankylosing spondylitis: a randomized controlled trial. Arthritis Rheum 2001;45:430-8.
4. Uhrin Z, Kuzis S, Ward MM. Exercise and changes in health status in patients with ankylosing spondylitis. Arch Intern Med 2000;160:2969-75.
5. Dougados M, Gueguen A, Nakache JP, Nguyen M, Mery C, Amor B. Evaluation of a functional index and an articular index in ankylosing spondylitis. J Rheumatol 1988;15:302-7.
6. Dougados M, Caporal R, Doury P, Thiesce A, Pattin S, Laffez B, et al. A double blind crossover placebo controlled trial of ximoprofen in AS. J Rheumatol 1989;16:1167-9.
7. Dougados M, Nguyen M, Caporal R, Legeais J, Bouxin-Sauzet A, Pellegri-Guegnault B, et al. Ximoprofen in ankylosing spondylitis. A double blind placebo controlled dose ranging study. Scand J Rheumatol 1994;23:243-8.
8. Dougados M, Gueguen A, Nakache JP, Velicitat P, Veys EM, Zeidler H, et al. Ankylosing spondylitis: What is the optimum duration of a clinical study? A one year versus 6 weeks non-steroidal anti-inflammatory drug trial. Rheumatology 1999;38:235-44.
9. Dougados M, Behier JM, Jolchine I, Calin A, van der Heijde D, Olivieri I, et al. Efficacy of celecoxib, a cyclo-oxygenase 2-specific inhibitor, in the treatment of ankylosing spondylitis: A six week controlled study with comparison against placebo and against a conventional nonsteroidal anti-inflammatory drug. Arthritis Rheum 2001;44:180-5.
10. Van der Heijde D, Baraf HSB, Ramos-Remus C, Calin A, Weaver AL, Schiff M, et al. Evaluation of the efficacy of etoricoxib in ankylosing spondylitis. Arthritis Rheum 2005;52:1205-15.
11. Braun J, Pham T, Sieper J, Davis J, van der Linden S, Dougados M, et al. On behalf of the ASAS Working Group. International ASAS consensus statement for the use of anti-tumour necrosis factor agents in patients with ankylosing spondylitis. Ann Rheum Dis 2003;62:817-24.
12. Maksymowych WP, Gladman D, Rahman P, Boonen A, Bykerk V, Choquette D, et al. The Canadian Rheumatology Association/Spondyloarthritis Research Consortium of Canada treatment recommendations for the management of spondyloarthritis: a national multidisciplinary stakeholder project. J Rheumatol 2007;34:2273-84.
13. Garrett S, Jenkinson T, Kennedy LG, Whitelock H, Gaisford P, Calin A. A new approach to defining disease status in ankylosing spondylitis: the Bath Ankylosing Spondylitis Disease Activity Index. J Rheumatol 1994;21:2286-91.
14. Calin A, Garrett S, Whitelock H, Kennedy LG, O'Hea J, Mallorie P, et al. A new approach to defining functional ability in ankylosing spondylitis: The development of the Bath Ankylosing Spondylitis Functional Index. J Rheumatol 1994;21:2281-5.
15. Braun J, Brandt J, Listing J, Zink A, Alten R, Golder W, et al. Treatment of active ankylosing spondylitis with infliximab: a randomized controlled multicentre trial. Lancet 2002;359:1187-93.
16. Van den Bosch F, Kruithof E, Baeten D, Herssens A, de Keyser F, Mielants H, et al. Randomised double-blind comparison of chimeric monoclonal antibody to tumor necrosis factor α (infliximab) versus placebo in active spondyloarthropathy. Arthritis Rheum 2002;46:755-65.
17. Van der Heijde D, Dijkmans B, Geusens P, Sieper J, DeWoody K, Williamson P, et al. Efficacy and safety of infliximab in patients with ankylosing spondylitis. Results of a randomized placebo-controlled trial (ASSERT). Arthritis Rheum 2005;52:582-91.
18. Gorman JD, Sack KE, Davis JC. Treatment of ankylosing spondylitis by inhibition of tumor necrosis factor a. N Engl J Med 2002;346:1349-56.
19. Brandt J, Khariouzov A, Listing J, Haibel H, Sörensen H, Grassnickel L, et al. Six-month results of a double-blind, placebo-controlled trial of etanercept treatment in patients with active ankylosing spondylitis. Arthritis Rheum 2003;48:1667-75.
20. Calin A, Dijkmans BA, Emery P, Hakala M, Kalden J, Leirisalo-Repo M, et al. Outcomes of a multicentre randomised clinical trial of etanercept to treat ankylosing spondylitis. Ann Rheum Dis 2004;63:1594-600.

21. Davis JC Jr, van der Heijde D, Braun J, Dougados M, Cush J, Clegg DO, et al. Recombinant human tumor necrosis factor receptor (Etanercept) for treating ankylosing spondylitis. Arthritis Rheum 2003;48:3230-6.

22. Lambert RGW, Salonen D, Rahman P, Inman RD, Wong RL, Einstein SG, et al. Adalimumab significantly reduces both spinal and sacroiliac joint inflammation in patients with ankylosing spondylitis. Arthritis Rheum 2007;56:4005-14.

23. van der Heijde D, Kivitz A, Schiff MH, Sieper J, Dijkmans BA, Braun J, et al. Efficacy and safety of adalimumab in patients with ankylosing spondylitis: results of a multicenter, randomized, double-blind, placebo-controlled trial. Arthritis Rheum 2006;54:2136-46.

24. Braun J, Baraliakos X, Golder W, Brandt J, Rudwaleit M, Listing J, et al. Magnetic resonance imaging examinations of the spine in patients with ankylosing spondylitis, before and after successful therapy with infliximab: evaluation of a new scoring system. Arthritis Rheum 2003;48:1126-36.

25. Braun J, Landewe R, Hermann K-GA, Han J, Yan S, Williamson P, et al.; ASSERT Study Group. Major reduction in spinal inflammation in patients with ankylosing spondylitis after treatment with infliximab. Arthritis Rheum 2006;54:1646-52.

26. Baraliakos X, Davis J, Tsuji W, Braun J. Magnetic resonance imaging examinations of the spine in patients with ankylosing spondylitis before and after therapy with the tumor necrosis factor alpha receptor fusion protein etanercept. Arthritis Rheum 2005;52:1216-23.

27. van der Heijde D, Landewé R, Einstein S, Ory P, Vosse D, Ni L, et al. Two-year etanercept therapy does not inhibit radiographic progression in patients with ankylosing spondylitis. Arthritis Rheum 2008;58:1324-31.

28. van der Heide D, Landewe R, Baraliakos X, Houben H, van Tubergen A, Williamson P, et al. Radiographic progression in patients with ankylosing spondylitis after 2 years of treatment not inhibited with infliximab. Arthritis Rheum 2008;58:3063-70.

29. van der Heijde DM, Landewe RDM, Maksymowych WP, Weissman B, Salonen D, Ballal S, et al. Adalimumab therapy for ankylosing spondylitis over 2 years does not demonstrate significant inhibition of radiographic progression compared with a historical control group. Arthritis Rheum 2008;57:670

30. de Vries MK, Wolbink GJ, Stapel SO, de Vrieze H, van Denderen JC, Dijkmans BA, et al. Decreased clinical response to infliximab in ankylosing spondylitis is correlated with anti-infliximab formation. Ann Rheum Dis 2007;66:1252-4.

31. Wanders A, Heijde D, Landewé R, Béhier JM, Calin A, Olivieri I, et al. Nonsteroidal anti-inflammatory drugs reduce radiographic progression in patients with ankylosing spondylitis: a randomized controlled trial. Arthritis Rheum 2005;52:1756-65.

32. van der Heijde DMFM, Wanders A, Mielants H, Dougados M, Landewe RB. Prediction of progression of radiographic damage over 4 years in patients with ankylosing spondylitis. Ann Rheum Dis 2004;63:132.

33. Maksymowych WP, Landewé R, Conner-Spady B, Dougados M, Mielants H, van der Tempel H, et al. Serum matrix metalloproteinase 3 is an independent predictor of structural damage progression in patients with ankylosing spondylitis. Arthritis Rheum 2007;56:1846-53.

34. Hanauer SB, Sandborn W. The Practice Parameters Committee of the American College of Gastroenterology. Am J Gastroenterol 2001;96:635-43.

35. Biancone L, Tosti C, Geremia A, Fina D, Petruzziello C, Emerenziani S, et al. Rofecoxib and early relapse of inflammatory bowel disease: An open-label trial. Aliment Pharmacol Ther 2004;19:755-64.

36. Dougados M, van der Linden S, Leirisalo-Repo M, Huitfeldt B, Juhlin R, Veys E, et al. Sulfasalazine in the treatment of spondyloarthropathy. Arthritis Rheum 1995;38:618-27.

37. Clegg DO, Reda DJ, Weisman MH, Blackburn WD, Cush JJ, Cannon GW, et al. Comparison of sulfasalazine and placebo in the treatment of ankylosing spondylitis. Arthritis Rheum 1996;39:2004-12.

38. Braun J, Zochling J, Baraliakos X, Alten R, Burmester G, Grasedyck K, et al. Efficacy of sulfasalazine in patients with inflammatory back pain due to undifferentiated spondyloarthritis and early ankylosing spondylitis: a multicentre randomized controlled trial. Ann Rheum Dis 2006;65:1147-53.

39. Ferraz MB, Tugwell P, Goldsmith CH, Atra E. Meta-analysis of sulfasalazine in ankylosing spondylitis. J Rheumatol 1990;17:1482-6.

40. Maugars Y, Mathis C, Berthelot JM, Charlier C, Prost A. Assessment of the efficacy of sacroiliac corticosteroid injections in spondyloarthropathies: a double-blind study. Br J Rheumatol 1996;35:767-70.

41. Luukkainen R, Nissilä M, Asikainen E, Sanila M, Lehtinen K, Alanaatu A, et al. Periarticular corticosteroid treatment of the sacroiliac joint in patients with seronegative spondylarthropathy. Clin Exp Rheumatol 1999;17:88-90.

42. Braun J, Baraliakos X, Listing J, Davis J, van der Heijde D, Haibel H, et al. Differences in the incidence of flares or new onset of inflammatory bowel diseases in patients with ankylosing spondylitis exposed to therapy with anti-tumor necrosis factor agents. Arthritis Rheum 2007;57:639-47.

43. Rudwaleit M, Claudpierre P, Loza E, Wordsworth P, Olivieri I, Wong R, et al. Adalimumab improves inflammatory bowel disease and psoriasis and prevents anterior uveitis flares in patients with ankylosing spondylitis. Arthritis Rheum 2008;57:675

44. Braun J, Baraliakos X, Listing J, Sieper J. Decreased incidence of anterior uveitis in patients with ankylosing spondylitis treated with the anti-tumor necrosis factor agents infliximab and etanercept. Arthritis Rheum 2005;52:2447-51.

45. Haibel H, Rudwaleit M, Listing J, Heldmann F, Wong RL, Kupper H, et al. Efficacy of adalimumab in the treatment of axial spondylarthritis without radiographically defined sacroiliitis. Arthritis Rheum 2008;58:1981-91.

46. Burgos-Vargas R, Casasola-Vargas J, Gutierrez-Suarez R, Vazquez-Mellado J. Efficacy, safety, and tolerability of infliximab in juvenile-onset spondyloarthropathies (JO-SpA): results of the three-month, randomized, double-blind, placebo-controlled trial phase. Arthritis Rheum 2007;56:749

47. Maksymowych WP, Jhangri GS, Fitzgerald AA, LeClercq S, Chiu P, Yan A, et al. A six-month randomized, controlled, double-blinded, dose response comparison of intravenous pamidronate (60 mg versus 10 mg) in the treatment of NSAID-refractory AS. Arthritis Rheum 2002;46:766-73.

48. Munoz-Fernandez S, Hidalgo V, Fernandez-Melon J, Schlincker A, Bonilla G, Ruiz-Sancho D, et al. Sulfasalazine reduces the number of flares of acute anterior uveitis over a one-year period. J Rheumatol 2003;30:1277-9.

49. Guignard S, Gossec L, Salliot C, Ruyssen-Witrand A, Luc M, Duclos M, et al. Efficacy of tumour necrosis factor blockers in reducing uveitis flares in patients with spondylarthropathy: A retrospective study. Ann Rheum Dis 2006;65:1631-4.

50. Ahn N, Ahn UM, Nallamshetty L, Springer BD, Buchowski JM, Funches L, et al. Cauda equina syndrome in ankylosing spondylitis (The CES-AS Syndrome): Meta-analysis of outcomes after medical and surgical treatments. J Spinal Dis 2001;14:427-33.

Management of Psoriatic Arthritis

Dafna D. Gladman

A 28-year-old man was referred to the psoriatic arthritis (PsA) clinic because of swollen toes. He developed a swollen left toe 6 to 7 years prior and was seen by a podiatrist who injected the toe with a corticosteroid with total resolution of the problem. However, there was a recurrence several months later. He was subsequently treated with orthotics with some improvement, but then noticed the right toe becoming swollen and painful. Nail changes were noticed in the left first toe which did not resolve with lemasil treatment. There were no other joint complaints and no family history of psoriasis, although the patient's father was diagnosed with spondylitis at age 60 years. His blood tests including serum uric acid were normal. He was given indomethacin 100 mg daily, with some improvement in pain, but the toes remained swollen. On examination at the clinic he had evidence of dactylitis—diffusely swollen and tender first toes bilaterally with evidence of inflammation in the metatarsophalangeal (MTP) joint, as well as in the interphalangeal joints of the toe bilaterally (Fig. 6-1). There was also swelling in the distal interphalangeal joint of the third right toe. He had active psoriasis with a psoriasis area severity index (PASI) score of 7.8. He also had nail pits and onycholysis. Laboratory tests were normal including negative rheumatoid factor and antinuclear factor. Radiographs revealed some periosteal reaction and a small erosion in the MTP joint. The chest x-ray study was normal.

Differential Diagnosis

The differential diagnosis of a swollen toe in a patient with psoriasis includes PsA, as well as gout and, less commonly, sarcoidosis. On occasion, a patient may present with a swollen toe secondary to trauma. Gout should be considered, but this patient did not have an elevated serum uric acid, and the pattern of the inflammation did not follow the usual course of gout. There was no evidence to support a diagnosis of sarcoidosis, and his chest radiograph was normal. There was no history of trauma, and none was detected on radiographs. A diagnosis of PsA was based on the presence of inflammatory arthritis, psoriasis, nail lesions and dactylitis. The patient was given a higher dose of indomethacin (150 mg/day) and was to be followed in a month's time.

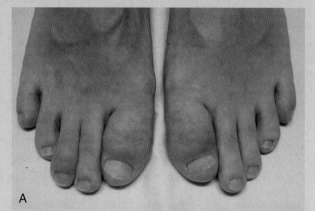

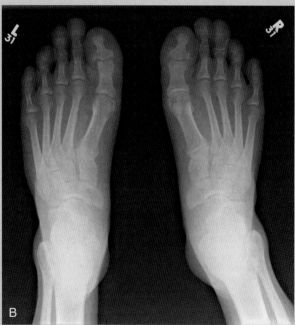

Figure 6-1. A, Case 1, both feet, clinical showing dactylitis of both big toes and swelling and redness over the third right toe distal interphalangeal joint. **B,** Case 1, both feet, radiographs demonstrating erosions and mild periosteal reaction.

CASE 2   Patient with Psoriasis and Joint Pain

A 32-year-old man presented with pain and occasional swelling in shoulders, wrists, hands, and right knee over the past 6 months. He had morning stiffness of over an hour. He complained of fatigue, and although he had managed most of his activities of daily living, it is with extreme discomfort. On functional enquiry, he related that he has had psoriasis for 13 years. He denied any other complaints. There was family history of psoriasis, arthritis, and Crohn's disease. The general physical examination was normal. Musculoskeletal examination revealed 20 tender and seven swollen joints. Schober's test was limited to 2.5 cm, cervical rotation to 55 degrees, and lateral spinal flexion was 10 cm. Skin examination revealed active psoriasis with a Psoriasis Area and Severity Index (PASI) score of 6.4, and there were nail pits. Laboratory investigations revealed an elevated erythrocyte sedimentation rate (ESR) at 25 mm/hour. Both rheumatoid factor and antinuclear factor tests were negative. Radiographs revealed bilateral sacroiliitis, grade 2 on the right, grade 3 on the left. There were syndesmophytes in the thoracic spine. There were entheseal spurs at the Achilles and plantar fascia insertions. An erosion was noted in the first metatasophalangeal joint.

Differential Diagnosis

This patient presents with an inflammatory arthritis associated with psoriasis. The most likely diagnosis is PsA. However, the differential diagnosis includes other forms of inflammatory arthritis, as well as seronegative rheumatoid arthritis (RA), reactive arthritis, and spondyloarthritis (SpA). The presence of SpA makes the diagnosis of RA unlikely (Table 6-1). There is no evidence in the history to support a diagnosis of reactive arthritis. A diagnosis of ankylosing spondylitis (AS) may be entertained on the basis of the presence of sacroiliitis and thoracic syndesmophytes, but he has not had significant inflammatory axial disease and the peripheral arthritis is more than one usually expects in AS (Table 6-2). Indeed, if radiographs were not taken, the limitation in his back movements might have been attributed to degenerative disease.

Table 6-1. *Differential Diagnosis of Psoriatic Arthritis: Comparison with Rheumatoid Arthritis, Gout, and Osteoarthritis*

Manifestation	Psoriatic Arthritis	Rheumatoid Arthritis	Gout	Osteoarthritis
Age at onset	36	40s	Any age	Older than 50 years of age
Male-to-female ratio	1.1:1	1:3	3:1	1:1
Joint affected	Proximal and distal, small and large	Proximal	Toes, knees, ankles	Weight bearing, distal hands
Symmetry	Usually asymmetric	Symmetric	Usually asymmetric	May be symmetric
Redness over joint	Yes	No	Yes	No
Spinal disease	Yes	No	No	Degenerative
Dactylitis	Yes	No	Podagra may look like dactylitis	No
Enthesitis	Yes	No	No	No
Nodules	No	Yes	Tophi	Heberden's and Bouchard's nodules
Psoriasis	100%	1%–3%	1%–3%	1%–3%
Nail lesions	87%	No	No	No

Table 6-2. *Differential Diagnosis of Psoriatic Arthritis (PsA): Comparison with Other Types of Spondyloarthritis*

Manifestation	PsA	AS	ReA	IBD Arthritis
Age	36	20	30	30
Male-to-female ratio	1.1:1	3:1	3:1	2:1
Peripheral joints	96%	30%	90%	30%
Axial joints	50%	100%	100%	30%
Dactylitis	Common	No	Uncommon	No
Enthesitis	Common	Common	Uncommon	Uncommon
Psoriasis	100%	10%	10%	10%
Nail lesions	87%	Uncommon	Uncommon	Uncommon
HLA-B*27	40-50%	90%	70%	30%

AS, ankylosing spondylitis; IBD, irritable bowel disease; REA, reactive arthritis.

CLASSIFICATION CRITERIA FOR PSORIATIC ARTHRITIS

The Classification of Psoriatic Arthritis (CASPAR) group studied 588 patients with PsA and 536 patients with other forms of inflammatory arthritis collected in 30 centers according to a set protocol that included clinical evaluation, radiographs, and laboratory tests.[1] Although the gold standard was the physician diagnosis, this was confirmed by an external team and a latent class analysis. The CASPAR criteria were derived from both logistic regression and classification and regression tree analyses, which yielded similar results. The resultant criteria can be applied to individuals with an inflammatory musculoskeletal disease including peripheral arthritis, spondylitis or enthesitis. To be classified as having PsA, a patient must score at least 3 points from the following criteria: Current psoriasis provides 2 points. If psoriasis is not present on the current assessment but the patient has a history of psoriasis, they score 1 point, or in the absence of personal psoriasis, if there is a family history of psoriasis, they may score 1 point. The following each provide 1 point: nail lesions; a negative rheumatoid factor; presence of dactylitis or history of dactylitis documented by a rheumatologist; presence of fluffy periostitis on hand or feet radiographs (excluding osteophytes) (Table 6-3). According to these criteria, a patient may be classified as PsA with 91.4% sensitivity and 98.8% specificity. Using these criteria, 99% of the patients in a large PsA clinic would be classified as PsA. Moreover, the criteria were 99% sensitive in an early PsA (less than 2 years of disease).[2] In addition, the criteria were very sensitive and specific in a family medicine clinic,[3] as well as in an early arthritis clinic.[4] Thus, these criteria may actually function well as diagnostic criteria.

In applying the CASPAR criteria to the patient in Case 1 who clearly had inflammatory arthritis, we can determine that the patient had dactylitis, nail lesions, a negative rheumatoid factor, psoriasis, and periosteal reaction, thus he scores 5 on the CASPAR criteria. The patient in Case 2 also clearly had an inflammatory musculoskeletal disease; he had current psoriasis, nail lesions, a negative rheumatoid factor, and dactylitis, thus scoring 5 on the CASPAR criteria.

SCREENING TOOLS FOR PSORIATIC ARTHRITIS

Because the CASPAR criteria require the recognition of inflammatory arthritis, which may not be apparent to a dermatologist or a general practitioner, a number of screening questionnaires have been developed to identify patients who might have PsA. The Psoriasis and Arthritis Questionnaire (PAQ) was developed by Peloso et al.[5] This 12-item questionnaire was administered to 108 psoriasis patients, of whom 70 patients (37 with low PAQ scores [3/12]

Table 6-3. *CASPAR Criteria*

Inflammatory musculoskeletal disease (joint, spine, or entheseal) with three or more of the following:

1. Evidence of psoriasis (one of a, b, c)
  a. Current psoriasis*
  b. Personal history of psoriasis
  c. Family history of psoriasis
	Psoriatic skin or scalp disease present today as judged by a dermatologist or rheumatologist
	A history of psoriasis that may be obtained from patient, family doctor, dermatologist or rheumatologist
	A history of psoriasis in a first or second degree relative according to patient report

2. Psoriatic nail dystrophy	Typical psoriatic nail dystrophy including onycholysis, pitting and hyperkeratosis observed on current physical examination
3. A negative test for rheumatoid factor	By any method except latex but preferably by ELISA or nephelometry, according to the local laboratory reference range

4. Dactylitis either a or b
  a. Current dactylitis
  b. History of dactylitis
	Swelling of an entire digit
	Recorded by a rheumatologist

5. Radiologic evidence of juxta-articular new bone formation	Ill-defined ossification near joint margins (but excluding osteophyte formation) on plain x-ray studies of hand or foot

CASPAR, Classification of Psoriatic Arthritis; ELISA, enzyme-linked immunosorbent assay.
*Current psoriasis scores 2, others 1.
Specificity 98.7%, sensitivity 91.4%.
Modified with permission from Taylor WJ, Gladman DD, Helliwell PS, Marchesoni A, Mease P, Mielants H. Classification criteria for psoriatic arthritis: development of new criteria from a large international study. Arthritis Rheum 2006;54:2665-73.

and 33 with high PAQ scores [>7/12]) were clinically evaluated by a rheumatologist. The PAQ score predicted PsA with a sensitivity of 0.85 and a specificity of 0.88 for a score of 7 or higher.

Alenius et al.[6] evaluated the PAQ in a study of prevalence of joint disease in 202 patients with psoriasis, all of whom underwent a clinical examination. The majority (82%) of the patients with joint or axial complaints also had radiographs, as did 20 individuals without musculoskeletal complaints. Although a large proportion of their patients (48%) turned out to have joint manifestations, they did not find the PAQ to be as sensitive in identifying patients with PsA as was detected in the first study. They identified a score of 4 as the best cutoff, providing a sensitivity of 0.60 and a specificity of 0.62. They then weighted the questions, and the weighted score did not provide better sensitivity, although the specificity increased to 0.73. They concluded that the use of that questionnaire was not helpful in identifying arthritis in their group of psoriatic patients.

The Psoriatic Arthritis Screening and Evaluation (PASE) questionnaire was recently published by Husni et al.[7] This questionnaire was developed primarily as a screening tool for dermatologists to identify patients with PsA because it was recognized that to have every patient with psoriasis evaluated by a rheumatologist would be impossible. PASE consists of two subscales, a symptom subscale and a function subscale. The instrument was tested in 69 patients, including 17 patients with PsA and 52 patients with psoriasis without arthritis. PsA was diagnosed by a rheumatologist on the basis of the Moll and Wright criteria. There were statistically significant differences in scores between patients with and without PsA, both in terms of symptoms and function components. Patients with PsA had higher scores than patients with psoriasis and osteoarthritis. Patients with more severe PsA had higher scores than those with milder disease. PASE scores ranged from 28 to 63. A cutoff of 47 proved to be optimal for differentiating patients with and without PsA. Using this cutoff, the sensitivity of PASE for PsA was 82% (95% confidence interval, 57–96) and the specificity was 73% (59–84).

The Toronto Psoriatic Arthritis Screening tool (ToPAS) was designed as a screening tool for PsA regardless of whether or not a patient was followed for psoriasis.[8] In that respect, it is different from the other screening tools. It was applied to patients in a PsA clinic, psoriasis clinic, general dermatology clinic, general rheumatology clinic and a family medicine clinic, and it was found to be highly sensitive and specific in all groups of patients in whom it was tested. ToPAS includes pictures of psoriasis and nail lesions. The latter were a major issue for the PAQ, because the agreement between physician and patient was very poor.[5] ToPAS addresses the issue of whether the patient has ever had joint symptoms or skin lesions. Although these screening questionnaires still require validation in other centers, they may be used to detect patients who should be seen by rheumatologists.

EPIDEMIOLOGY OF PSORIATIC ARTHRITIS

The exact prevalence and incidence of PsA are unknown. Estimates have varied from 0.04% to 0.37%. A recent systematic review of incidence and prevalence studies in PsA highlights the wide variation in estimates, as well as the importance of having widely accepted classification criteria.[9] Now that the CASPAR criteria are available, as well as the screening questionnaires, better epidemiologic studies can be carried out that provide more accurate estimates of the incidence and prevalence of PsA. PsA occurs in men and women almost equally. The average age at diagnosis in most series in the 4th decade, usually 7 to 10 years after the onset of psoriasis. Although in almost 85% of the patients the psoriasis either precedes or has a simultaneous onset with PsA, about 15% of the patients present with PsA before the onset of psoriasis. The clinical features outlined in the following sections help identify the correct diagnosis in these patients.

CLINICAL PICTURE OF PSORIATIC ARTHRITIS

Patients with PsA may present with peripheral arthritis, with or without dactylitis and enthesis, with or without spinal involvement.

Peripheral Arthritis

The arthritis of PsA is inflammatory in nature, presenting with pain, swelling, and stiffness in the affected joints. There is often a purplish discoloration of the affected joint.[10] About half of the patients have morning stiffness of more than 45 minutes' duration. The onset is often oligoarticular, but over time, many patients develop polyarticular disease.[11] Although initially the arthritis tends to be asymmetric, with the accrual of more joints, it may become more symmetric. As the number of affected joints increases, the arthritis is more likely to become symmetric.[12] A typical feature of PsA is the "ray distribution." This refers to the involvement of all three joints of a particular digit, as opposed to the same joints being involved in both sides (Figs. 6-2 through 6-6).

Any joint may be affected in PsA, including both small and large joints. Distal joint disease is common, occurring in more than 50% of the patients. The distal joints of the hands and feet may be affected. At the same time, knees, hips, shoulders, elbows, and ankles may be affected, with or without more distal joint disease (Table 6-4).

Dactylitis

Dactylitis, or sausage digit, reflects inflammation of the whole digit (Figs. 6-1 and 6-7). It likely results from inflammation in both tendons and the individual joints of the digit,[13] although magnetic

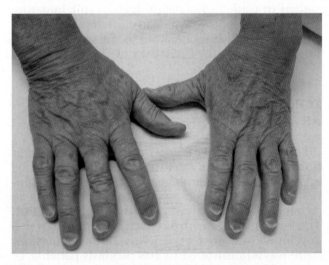

Figure 6-2. Psoriatic arthritis, distal involvement.

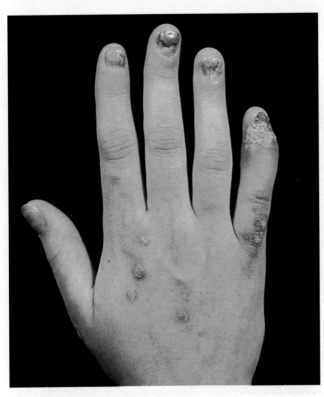

Figure 6-3. Psoriatic arthritis, oligoarthritis.

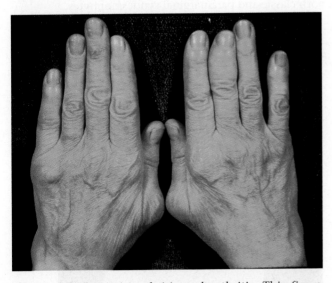

Figure 6-4. Psoriatic arthritis, polyarthritis. This figure demonstrates the shortened digit, which is typical for psoriatic arthritis, as well as the "ray" phenomenon.

resonance imaging studies suggested that the major component is tenosynovitis.[14,15] Dactylitis occurred at least once in 48% of the patients, whereas almost a third had dactylitis at presentation to clinic.[16,17] Digits with dactylitis had more radiographic progression than those without dactylitis.[16] Perhaps an extreme case of dactylitis may be the distal limb edema, which was identified in 21% of patients with PsA and only 4.9% of patients with other forms of arthritis.[18]

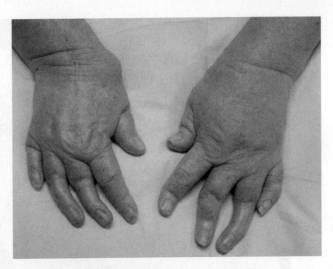

Figure 6-5. Psoriatic arthritis, arthritis mutilans, demonstrating severe deformities.

Enthesitis

Enthesitis is also a typical feature of PsA (Fig. 6-8). Fernández-Sueiro et al.[19] detected a higher prevalence of enthesitis in PsA than in AS (42.4% versus 12.1%, respectively, $P < 0.001$). Enthesitis was more common in patients with PsA who had axial disease, and the condition was associated with the activity of peripheral and axial disease. The Achilles and superior posterior iliac crest insertions are more common in PsA.

Spinal Disease

About 50% of patients with PsA have spinal involvement. The definition of axial disease in PsA has been controversial.[20] Depending on what definition was used, the prevalence of spinal disease has varied from 25% to 70% of PsA patients. It has been noted that patients with psoriatic spondylitis are not as tender as those with AS.[21] The majority of patients with psoriatic spondylitis are diagnosed by radiographs alone, have skip lesions in their spine, and often have asymmetric sacroiliitis.[22]

Skin Psoriasis

Psoriasis is a chronic inflammatory skin disease that may affect 1% to 3% of the population.[23] Several patterns have been recognized, but the one most commonly associated with PsA is psoriasis vulgaris, or plaque psoriasis, which presents with red scaly elevated lesions that occur primarily on the extensor surface of the arms and legs but may affect any part of the body.

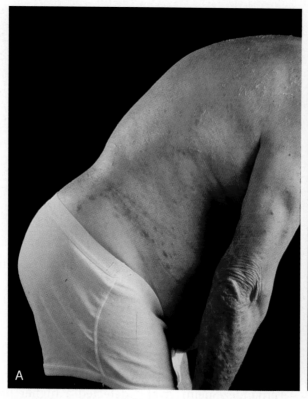

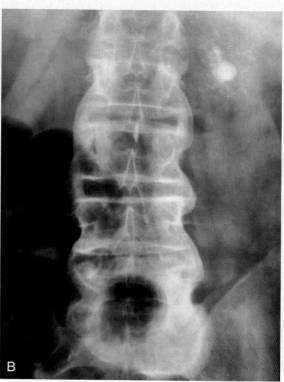

Figure 6-6. Psoriatic spondylitis. **A,** The figure demonstrates the inability of the patient to bend down. **B,** Radiographs demonstrate why the patient cannot bend, with evidence of both classic and paramarginal syndesmophytes.

Nail Lesions

Nail lesions are the only clinical feature that distinguished patients with PsA from those with psoriasis without arthritis.[24] The most common lesions include nail pits and onycholysis, but there are several other nail abnormalities detected in patients with psoriasis and PsA.

ASSESSMENT OF PATIENTS WITH PSORIATIC ARTHRITIS

In order to evaluate therapeutic intervention, proper assessment tools must be developed.[25] In PsA, the peripheral joints, dactylitis, enthesitis, spinal disease, as well as skin and nail assessments must be carried out to fully evaluate the patient. Joint

Table 6-4. *Joints Involved at Presentation to the Psoriatic Arthritis Clinic*

	Actively Inflamed Joints (%)	*Clinical Damage (%)*
Hands	71	10
Feet	64	8
Knees	33	1
Elbows/shoulders	32	1
Wrists	31	2
Ankles	17	0
Hips	9	1

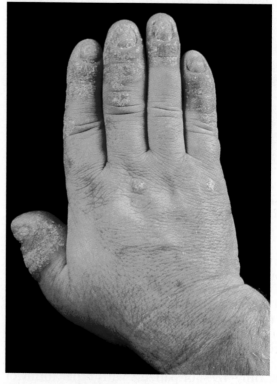

Figure 6-7. Dactylitis in a finger.

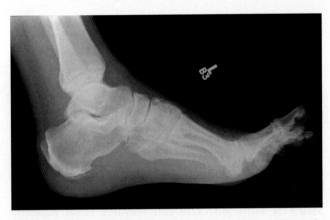

Figure 6-8. Enthesitis seen on radiographs with both Achilles and plantar fascia spurs.

inflammation is assessed by scoring 68 joints for tenderness, and 66 for swelling. These measures have been found to be sensitive to change in clinical trials. However, whereas the tender joint count is reliable, the swollen joint count is less reliable both among experts and physicians less experienced in joint assessment.[26,27] The assessment of dactylitis has been proven reliable by experts but not by non-experts,[21,22] whereas the assessment of enthesitis was found to be reliable among experts.[26] Spinal assessment tools used in AS have been found to be reliable in PsA.[28] Several tools have been developed for the assessment of skin and nail disease. The body surface area, physician global assessment of skin, and the PASI have been most commonly used in drug trials.[27,29] The nails can be evaluated using the Nail Psoriasis Severity Index (NAPSI) or the modified NAPSI.[30] Patient-reported outcomes are important in PsA becasue they provide additional information not included in the clinical assessment. These include the Medical Outcome Study Short Form 36 (SF-36); the Dermatology Life Quality Index, the Health Assessment Questionnaire (HAQ), which is a measure of function; the Fatigue Severity Scale, and the Functional Assessment of Chronic Illness Therapy-Fatigue (FACIT-F),[25] which measure fatigue. All of these instruments have proven reliable and sensitive to change in patients with PsA.

Response Criteria

Only the Psoriatic Arthritis Response Criteria (PsARC) were developed specifically for PsA.[25] These include tender and swollen joint scores, and a patient global and a physician global in a Likert scale.[31] In PsA, the joint score is usually equal to the joint count. Although this instrument did not function well in the study for which it was developed, it did function well in more recent studies in PsA. Most randomized controlled trials (RCTs) have used the American College of Rheumatology (ACR) response criteria originally developed for RA. A response is measured by a 20% improvement in tender and swollen joint counts and an additional 3 of: patient assessment of pain, patient global assessment of disease activity, physician global assessment of disease activity, the HAQ score, and an acute phase reactant. Additionally, a 50% and 70% improvement may be measured in the same manner. The Disease Activity Score (DAS), which was also developed for RA, assesses the state of the disease activity at any one point, and response is determined by the level of activity.[32] Although these measures have been found useful in PsA because they distinguish between drug-treated and placebo-treated patients, they do not include some of the other manifestations of the disease.[33] Skin disease is usually measured with a 75% improvement in the PASI score (PASI75 response). However, the physician global assessment of skin is an important outcome measure, as is the assessment of a target lesion, which is usually at least 2 cm in diameter, and is measured for changes in erythema, induration, and scale.

SHOULD PATIENTS WITH PSA BE TREATED AGGRESSIVELY?

PsA had been considered a mild form of arthritis. Wright's original description depicted a mild form of arthritis, with asymmetric oligoarticular pattern being most common.[11] However, over the past 2 decades, it has become clear that PsA is a more severe disease (than previously thought) and is at least as severe as RA.[34] Most recent studies indicate that PsA becomes polyarticular over time.[35-37] Indeed, in a study of early PsA, which included patients presenting to clinic within 5 months of onset of symptoms, 47% of the patients demonstrated at least one radiologic erosion by the 2-year follow-up.[38] Studies that included patients with more than 7 years of follow-up documented erosive disease in 67% of the patients at clinic entry.[15,34,36] Progression of clinical and radiologic damage has been demonstrated, and although polyarticular presentation is predictive for disease progression, the number of inflamed joints at any visit as well as current damage, predict progression of both clinical and radiologic damage at subsequent visits.[39,40] Patients with PsA are also at an increased mortality risk.[41] Although causes of death are similar to the general population, previously active and severe disease is associated with increased mortality risk.

In addition to the physical aspects of the disease, patients with PsA also suffer from reduced quality of life and function, which result from the inflammation and fatigue associated with PsA, as well as the discomfort associated with psoriasis.[42]

Thus, patients with PsA should be diagnosed and treated early in the course of their disease before there is any clinical or radiologic damage, to prevent progression of joint damage and reduce the mortality risk. Because the majority of patients with PsA have psoriasis, it is important for dermatologists and general physicians to recognize the symptoms and signs of arthritis and refer patients for rheumatologic consultation and management.

PATHOGENESIS OF PSORIATIC ARTHRITIS

The exact etiology of PsA is unknown. However, genetic, environmental and immunologic factors likely play a role. Understanding pathogenic mechanisms may help manage patients with this disease.

Genetic Factors

There is no doubt that genetic factors play a role in the susceptibility to PsA. Evidence comes from family studies showing a risk of 30 to 50 times for family members.[43,44] In addition, a number of genes have been identified as contributing to PsA susceptibility.[45] At present, recognizing these susceptibility genes does not help manage patients because we cannot alter the genes. However, genes may be identified that could either be modifiable or serve as targets for therapeutic intervention.

Environmental Factors

Prinz[46] highlighted the possibility that an infectious agent may have triggered the psoriatic process, and the immunological response seen in patients with both psoriasis and PsA may be the result of molecular mimicry between bacteria, antigens, and epidermal autoantigens. Viruses may also play a role,[47] supported by the observation that activating Killer Immunoglobulin-like Receptors (KIR) 2DS1 and 2DS2 in the absence of the appropriate human leukocyte antigen (HLA) ligand are associated with PsA.[48] Trauma may also trigger the disease.[49] It is proposed that the trauma-induced arthritis represents a deep Koebner phenomenon, therefore suggesting that trauma plays a role in the development of PsA. Substance P, a neuropeptide, and vasoactive intestinal peptide are overexpressed in psoriatic skin lesions and in psoriatic synovium, and may mediate the role of trauma in PsA.[50] However, both of these environmental factors are not amenable to a therapeutic intervention in PsA.

Immunologic Factors

The inflammatory nature of the joint lesions in PsA is demonstrated by synovial lining cell hyperplasia and mononuclear cell infiltration, resembling the histopathologic changes in RA.[51] However, the levels of Th1 cytokines (tumor necrosis factor-α [TNF-α], interleukin-1B [IL-1β] and IL-10) were higher in samples from PsA patients than RA patients suggesting that these two disorders may result from a different underlying mechanism.[52] Fibroblasts from the skin and synovia of patients with PsA have an increased proliferative activity and the capability to secrete increased amounts of IL-1, IL-6, and platelet-derived growth factors.[53,54] T lymphocytes, particularly CD8+ cells, are thought to play an important role in the pathogenesis of both the skin and joint manifestations of PsA.[55] These activated T cells likely contribute to the enhanced production of cytokines noted both in the synovial fluid and synovial cultures from patients with PsA.[56] These cytokines, including IL-1β, IL-2, IL-10, interferon-γ (IFN-γ) and TNF-α, induce proliferation and activation of synovial and epidermal fibroblasts, leading to the fibrosis reported in patients with long-standing PsA.[53,54] The proinflammatory cytokines IL-1 and TNF-α are regulators of not only the inflammatory response, but they also play an important role in bone metabolism; enhancing osteoclastogenesis via upregulation of osteoprotegerin ligand, a new member of the TNF receptor family of molecules, expressed by activated T cells.[57] Erosive disease in PsA is associated with increased osteoclast precursors in the peripheral circulation.[57] Recent observations indicate that IL-23 is overproduced in psoriatic plaques and is responsible for stimulating a newly recognized T cell—Th17, to release IL-17 as well as TNF, IL-21, and IL-22. These cytokines may also play a role in PsA.[58] Monocytes may also play an important role in the pathogenesis of PsA, likely through production of metalloproteinases (MMP).[59] MMP-2 and MMP-9 and their regulators MT-MMP and TIMP, as well as MMP-1 and MMP-3, were demonstrated in synovial tissue, and lesional and nonlesional skin from patients with PsA.[60,61] It is likely that many cell types interact to lead to the pathologic process in both the skin and the joints in PsA.[62]

Thus, it is likely that when an individual with the appropriate genetic background encounters an environmental factor, the resultant immunologic reaction leads to the development of psoriasis and PsA. Understanding these immune mechanisms may lead to therapeutic interventions.

MANAGEMENT OF PATIENTS WITH PSORIATIC ARTHRITIS

Patients should ideally be under the care of a multidisciplinary team composed of rheumatologists, dermatologists, physiotherapists and occupational therapists.

Symptom-Modifying Therapy

Nonsteroidal anti-inflammatory drugs (NSAIDs) are useful for symptomatic relief, but they do not prevent disease progression and may aggravate skin lesions.[63,64] NSAIDs should be used for mild non-erosive disease and for symptomatic management of pain, inflammatory swelling and morning stiffness. Both traditional NSAIDs and selective cyclooxygenase-2 (COX-2) inhibitors have been associated with an increased risk of cardiovascular events and should be used with caution.[65] If symptoms persist after adequate trial with two different NSAIDs, disease-modifying antirheumatic drug (DMARD) use should be considered. We often start a DMARD within 2 weeks of starting the NSAID. We wait a couple of weeks to make sure the NSAID is tolerated before adding another medication.

Intra-articular steroid injections (triamcinolone, methylprednisolone) are often used for rapid relief of symptoms in cases of mono- or oligoarthritis. A recent investigation has demonstrated that intra-articular injections lead to remission in 50% of the patients.[66] Systemic steroids are used occasionally for symptom relief when there is polyarthritis or when there is inadequate response to NSAIDs. However, it needs to be used with extreme caution with slow taper because psoriasis worsens in many instances and could occasionally evolve into pustular psoriasis.[67]

Traditional Disease-Modifying Antirheumatic Drugs

In patients with persistently active or erosive disease, traditional DMARDs are the first line of treatment and should be used early in the course of disease. Several drugs work for both the joints and skin. However, there have been few randomized control trials of DMARDs in PsA.[68]

Methotrexate

Although there are only a few studies on its efficacy, methotrexate (MTX) is the most widely used DMARD in PsA. It has a good risk-benefit ratio, based primarily on its use in RA, and has a relatively rapid onset of action. There are only two randomized controlled trials of its use in PsA.[69,70] The first study included 21 patients and used intravenous MtX (1–3 mg every 10 days). Although the drug reduced joint counts and the ESR compared with placebo, there were 3 deaths.[69] The other trial included 35 patients, used oral MTX (7.5–15 mg/week) for 12 weeks, and demonstrated improvement only in physician global assessment. The side effects were mild, and all patients completed the trial. However, the study was underpowered to demonstrate effect.[70] Thus, the evidence to support the use of MTX is not compelling; it has an effect size of 0.06 when the minimal therapeutic effect size is greater than 0.2.[71] Despite its widespread use, there is no evidence for any effect of MTX on radiographic progression. A case-control study demonstrated lack of effect,[72] although the number of patients in the study was small, the dose of MTX low (average 11 mg/week) and patients were treated at an average of 9 years of disease. A more recent study suggested that when patients are treated with higher doses and earlier in their course, the results may be better.[73] In the clinic, patients treated with MTX demonstrate clinical improvement, but there does not appear to be prevention of progression of damage.

Sulfasalazine

Unlike the case with MTX, there are several randomized controlled trials with sulfasalazine (SSZ).[71] Even the largest of the trials, including 221 patients, demonstrated only marginal response, with 55% of the drug-treated patients compared with 45% of placebo-treated patients considered responders.[31] The effect size for SSZ was 0.12, again much lower than the 0.2 required for effectiveness. Although there is level A evidence (because there are several RCTs) the evidence suggests that the drug does not work.

Cyclosporin A

Cyclosporin A (CsA) is effective in controlling psoriasis.[74] There are no RCTs comparing CsA with placebo in PsA, but there are trials comparing it with other DMARDs. An RCT comparing CsA 3 to 5 mg/kg/day added to standard therapy (NSAIDs and low-dose prednisone) with and without SSZ 2 g/day demonstrated improvement only in pain in CsA-treated patients.[75] Two studies compared CsA with MTX. In the first study, both arms showed improvement at 6 and 12 months, but more patients were withdrawn from CsA arm due to toxicity.[76] In the more recent RCT, CsA was compared with placebo as an add-on treatment in patients with PsA, demonstrating an incomplete response to MTX monotherapy. There was significant improvement at 12 months in the swollen joint count, C-reactive protein, PASI, and synovitis detected by high-resolution ultrasound. There was no improvement in the HAQ or pain scores.[77] Thus, CsA may have a role in patients with partial response to MTX. However, it is toxic and is not well tolerated. Moreover, its ability to prevent progression of damage is unknown.

Azathioprine

One RCT reported in an abstract form demonstrated improvement in patients treated with azathioprine (AZA) compared with patients on placebo.[78] A nested case-control study failed to show effectiveness or ability to prevent disease progression.[79] As demonstrated in that study, some patients do well on AZA both in terms of skin and joint disease.

Leflunomide

Leflunomide was shown to be an effective treatment of PsA in a multicenter double-blind controlled trial comparing it with placebo.[80] Leflunomide-treated patient had a better PsARC and ACR20 response, as well as improvement in PASI scores. The measures of quality of life also showed improvement in the leflunomide arm. It is an important addition to the therapeutic armamentarium that we have in treating psoriasis and PsA. Leflunomide works in only 40% of the patients, but when it works, it works well clinically. It is unknown whether it prevents progression of erosive disease.

Other Disease-Modifying Antirheumatic Drugs

Although not shown to protect from progression of joint damage, gold has been used, with intramuscular gold being more effective than oral gold.[81,82] Because of concern about toxicity, slow mode of action, problems with availability, and availability of more effective drugs, it is seldom used nowadays. Penicillamine use is limited due to its toxicity. There are some reports that mycophenolate mofetil may be efficacious.[83,84] Etretinate (a retinoic acid derivative) has been shown to be effective in an RCT.[85]

Biologic Agents

The majority of the traditional DMARDs used in PsA were "borrowed" from their use in RA. These have been used empirically, without particular relevance to the pathogenic mechanisms of the disease. Biologic agents, however, have been selected based on proposed mechanisms of disease, and include anti-cytokine agents and anti–T-cell agents (Table 6-5).

Anti–Tumor Necrosis Factor Agents

Etanercept

Etanercept is dimeric fusion protein consisting of the extracellular portion of the human p75 TNF receptor linked to the Fc portion of human immunoglobulin 1 (IgG1). It binds and inactivates TNF. It was initially administered as a subcutaneous injection of 25 mg twice weekly, although more recently doses of 50 mg once a week have been used. Results from the first phase 2 RCT in PsA showed that at 12 weeks, based on PsARC response 87% of etanercept-treated patients responded compared with 23% of placebo-treated patients.[86] ACR20 response was achieved by 73% of etanercept-treated patients compared to 13% of patients in the placebo arm. Only 26% of patients in the etanercept arm achieved a PASI75 response, compared with

none of those treated with placebo. The results were further confirmed in a phase 3 multicenter trial, which also demonstrated significant sustained improvement in quality of life, as well as a reduction in radiographic progression.[87] The only significant difference in the safety profile between etanercept and placebo was that there were a greater number of injection site reactions in the etanercept arm. Etanercept has been used successful to control both skin and joint manifestations in patients with PsA.

Infliximab

Infliximab is a chimeric monoclonal antibody that binds to human TNF. It is administered as an intravenous infusion at 0, 2 and 6 weeks, followed by once every 8 weeks. Results from the Infliximab Multinational PsA Controlled Trial (IMPACT) have shown that 65%, 46% and 29% of infliximab-treated patients achieved an ACR20, ACR50, and ACR70 response at week 16 compared to 10%, 0%, and 0% of placebo-treated patients, respectively.[88] Among patients who had PASI scores of 2.5 or higher at baseline, 68% of Infliximab-treated patients achieved PASI75 improvement by week 16 compared with none of the placebo-treated patients. Sustained improvement was seen through week 50. Dactylitis and enthesitis also improved. Adverse events were similar between the treatment groups. The larger IMPACT 2 trial showed similar results as the IMPACT trial, with significant improvement in active PsA, psoriasis, dactylitis and enthesitis.[89] Infliximab maintained the improvement through 1 and 2 years of therapy, was beneficial in terms of work and employment, and was also shown to retard radiographic progression.[90-95] Side effects included infusion reactions and development of human antimouse antibodies, which may lead to reduced efficacy.

Adalimumab

Adalimumab is a humanized anti-TNF-α antibody and is administered subcutaneously at biweekly

Table 6-5. Biologic Therapies in Psoriatic Arthritis—Effect on Joint Disease

Trial (ref)	No.	ACR 20%		ACR 50%		ACR 70%		PsARC %	
		Rx	P	Rx	P	Rx	P	Rx	P
Etanercept (86)[2]*	60	74	14	48	5	13	0	87	13
Infliximab (88)[2]+	100	69	8	49	9	28	0	76.5	18
Etanercept (87)[3]*	205	59	15	38	4	11	0	72	31
Etanercept (87)[3x]	205	50	13	37	4	9	1	70	24
Infliximab (89)[3]**	200	58	11	36	3	15	1	77	27
Infliximab (89)[3x]	200	54	16	41	4	27	2	60	32
Efalizumab (108)[2]+	107	28	19	NA	NA	NA	NA	NA	NA
Adalimumab (96)[2/3x]	315	58	14	36	4	20	1	62	26
Alefacept (106)[2x]	185	54	23	18	10	7	3	NA	NA
Golimumab (101)[3x]	405	52	8	32	3.5	18	0.9	NA	NA
Ustkinumab (105)[2]*	146	42	14	25	7	15	0	NA	NA

ACR, American College of Rheumatology; NA, not applicable; PsARC, Psoriatic Arthritis Response Criteria.
*12 weeks; **14 weeks + 16 weeks; [x]24 weeks.

intervals. A multicenter phase 3 placebo controlled double-blind study, which included 305 patients demonstrated efficacy.[96] ACR 20/50/70 responses were seen in 57%, 39%, and 23% of patients, respectively, in the adalimumab arm compared with placebo at week 24. In those with more than 3% of body surface area involvement with psoriasis, PASI 50/75/90 response was achieved in 75%, 59%, and 2% of patients, respectively. Adalimumab has also been reported to lead to clinically meaningful and statistically significant improvement in quality of life, and to inhibit radiographic disease progression over 1 year.[97,98] There was no difference in the adverse event profile between both treatment arms.

Golimumab

Golimumab is a human monoclonal anti-TNF antibody that may be administered either subcutaneously or intravenously. A large multicenter study of golimumab in PsA (in the GO-REVEAL study) demonstrated its efficacy for peripheral joint disease, dactylitis, enthesitis, skin and nail disease.[99,100] Doses of 50 and 100 mg once a month subcutaneously were proven effective, and the effect persisted through 1 year of treatment.[101] Quality of life and function also improved, and data on radiologic progression are currently being analyzed. There were no major safety concerns.[99]

Although during the trials these agents seemed safe, follow-up studies in patients with RA raise a number of safety issues, including infections and a possible increase in malignancies.[102] The latter concern comes primarily from studies in RA, in which an increased risk of malignancy exists, as opposed to PsA, in which there does not appear to be an increased malignancy risk.[103] A recent meta-analysis confirmed that all anti-TNF agents are effective for skin and joints manifestations of PsA.[104]

Ustekinumab

This is an anti–IL-23 human monoclonal antibody proven effective in psoriasis, which was recently tested in a phase 2 trial in PsA.[105] Although the ACR20 responses (42% in drug-treated patients compared with 14% in placebo) were not as impressive as the anti-TNF agents, it should be noted that the drug was given for 4 weeks whereas the response was measured at 12 weeks. Responses of more than 30% were maintained through week 36. The PASI75 response was 50%.

T-Cell–Directed Agents

Interactions such as those between lymphocyte function-associated antigen 1 (LFA-1) and its ligand intercellular adhesion molecule 1 (ICAM-1), and LFA-3 and CD2 are required for full T-cell activation. Molecules inhibiting these interactions have been developed recently, and clinical trials with these agents in the treatment of PsA have been performed, because T-cell activation is important in pathogenesis of PsA.

Alefacept

Alefacept is a fully human fusion protein comprising the first extracellular domain of LFA-3 fused to the hinge segment and constant regions of IgG1. It inhibits antigen driven activation of T cells and also causes selective apoptosis of memory T cells. Results from a double-blind, placebo-controlled RCT of alefacept in combination with MTX demonstrated efficacy.[106] Treatment with alefacept was provided for 12 weeks, and at 24 weeks, the ACR20 response was achieved in 54% of alefacept-treated patients compared with 23% of patients on placebo. In patients with psoriasis involving more than 3% body surface area, 53% of alefacept-treated patients achieved PASI50 compared with 17% of those receiving placebo. Adverse events were mild to moderate, and less than 2% of alefacept-treated patients discontinued treatment due to treatment-related adverse events.[106]

Efalizumab

Efalizumab is a humanized monoclonal IgG1 antibody against CD11a, one of the subunits of LFA-1. It is effective in the treatment of psoriasis.[107] Efalizumab was tested in a phase 2 randomized trial in 107 patients with PsA. After 12 weeks of treatment, 28% of the efalizumab treated patients achieved an ACR20 (primary endpoint) response compared with 19% of the placebo-treated patients.[108] The psoriasis response was similar to that previously reported and the medication was well tolerated. Although PsA was not worsened by the treatment during that study, there is concern that PsA may actually be precipitated by efalizumab in patients with psoriasis.[109] Efalizumab was recently taken off the market.

Treatment Guidelines

Guidelines for the treatment of psoriasis and PsA were recently published by the American Academy of Dermatology, and treatment recommendations were published by the Group for Research and Assessment of Psoriasis and Psoriatic Arthritis (GRAPPA).[110-112] Both recommend use of MTX before the use of biologics.

Generally both sets of recommendations are similar, suggesting use of topical psoriasis medications, psoralen and ultraviolet light A (PUVA), CsA, and MTX, as well as the use of biologic therapy for psoriasis. Generally the recommendations are to use biologic agents in patients with moderate to severe psoriasis. For PsA the recommendations are to treat the most severe manifestation according to a grid. For peripheral joints, there is some suggestion that DMARDs work at least clinically, but if there is severe disease with erosions and impaired function, biologics should be used. It should be noted that there is no evidence in the literature to support the use of DMARDs before biologics. However, there is a paucity of information on treatment of early PsA with DMARDs, and the trials performed in the past did not include the rigorous approach used for the recent biologic therapies. For spinal disease, dactylitis and enthesitis in which the only evidence for effect is from anti-TNF agents, those are recommended early. It should be noted, however, that none of the biologics work for more than 60% of the patients and new drugs are needed to better control the disease.

The University of Toronto Psoriatic Arthritis Clinic Approach

At the University of Toronto Psoriatic Arthritis Clinic, we work closely with our dermatology colleagues. If a patient is referred from a dermatologist, then the diagnosis of psoriasis is confirmed and we manage the patients together. When joint manifestations are the major issue, the dermatologist usually prefers that we take primary responsibility. However, when skin lesions become an issue, the dermatologist takes primary responsibility. There are several possible scenarios among patients with PsA. The first includes patients whose skin and joint disease are mild. Those would be treated with topical medications and NSAIDs. There are patients whose skin disease is mild, but the joint disease is persistently active. Those patients would be started on DMARDs, and may require biologic agents if their arthritis, spondylitis, enthesitis, or dactylitis is severe. Our first-line drug is MTX, which we usually start at a low dose of 7.5 to 10 mg per week and increase every week to 15 mg, following up the patient at 3 months. If there is no response, MTX is increased orally to 17.5 mg per week, and if a higher dose is required, we switch to subcutaneous administration. We quickly escalate to 25 mg per week. If there is no response, we generally add leflunomide 20 mg per day for 3 months. This approach is mainly based on the requirements for approval of a biologic through our government insurance plan. However, if we are not restricted by financial support, we proceed to an anti-TNF agent immediately after failure of MTX. Some of our patients, particularly those who could not take MTX, have responded to SSZ up to 4 g/day. We also have patients on AZA with good response. We still have a few patients on intramuscular gold who have done well.

There are patients who have severe skin and joint disease. Those patients require attention to both skin and joints and require systemic medications such as MTX or CsA, which work for both skin and joint manifestations, or biologic agents. For these patients anti-TNF agents would be most appropriate because they work for both skin and joints manifestations.

Finally there are patients whose joint disease is mild but the skin disease is severe. Those would also require systemic medications usually MTX, CsA, PUVA, or biologic agents. These patients may do well on anti–T-cell therapies, although anti-TNF agents would be considered more effective.

The evidence suggests that anti-TNF agents work much better than DMARDs for both signs and symptoms of the disease and to prevent progression of radiologic damage. Although these medications are expensive, there is now evidence to show that patients treated with anti-TNF agents are more likely to resume gainful employment, thus offsetting the expense to a certain degree. Economic evaluation studies have only just begun in patients with PsA, and it is hoped that they will demonstrate to insurers that it is an investment worth making patients better and to allow them to return to the workforce.

SUMMARY

PsA is a complex disease with skin and musculoskeletal manifestations. PsA may be severe, leading to significant functional limitation and impaired quality of life, and it is associated with an increased mortality risk. Therefore, patients with PsA should be diagnosed and treated early with the most appropriate medication to control inflammation and disease progression.

References

1. Taylor WJ, Gladman DD, Helliwell PS, Marchesoni A, Mease P, Mielants H. Classification criteria for psoriatic arthritis: development of new criteria from a large international study. Arthritis Rheum 2006;54:2665-73.
2. Chandran V, Schentag CT, Gladman DD. Sensitivity of the Classification of Psoriatic Arthritis (CASPAR) Criteria in early psoriatic arthritis. Arthritis Rheum 2007;57:1560-3.
3. Chandran V, Schentag CT, Gladman DD. Sensitivity and specificity of the CASPAR Criteria for Psoriatic Arthritis when applied to patients attending a Family Medicine Clinic. J Rheumatol 2008;35:2069-70.
4. D'Angelo S, Ferrante MC, Atteno M, Cauli A, Rotunno L, Vasile M, et al. The performance of CASPAR criteria in early psoriatic arthritis: preliminary results from an Italian prospective multicentre study. Ann Rheum Dis 2008;67(Suppl. 2):525.
5. Peloso PM, Behl M, Hull P, Reeder B. The Psoriasis & Arthritis Questionnaire (PAQ) in detection of arthritis among patients with psoriasis. Arthritis Rheum 1997;40(Suppl. 9):S64.
6. Alenius GM, Stenberg B, Stenlund H, Lundblad M, Dahlqvist Rantapää S. Inflammatory joint manifestations are prevalent in psoriasis: prevalence study of joint and axial involvement in psoriatic patients, and evaluation of psoriatic and arthritic questionnaire. J Rheumatol 2002;29:2577-82.
7. Husni ME, Meyer KH, Cohen DS, Mody E, Qureshi AA. The PASE questionnaire: pilot-testing a psoriatic arthritis screening and evaluation tool. J Am Acad Dermatol 2007;57:581-7.
8. Gladman DD, Schentag CT, Tom BD, Chandran V, Brockbank J, Rosen CF, et al. Development and initial validation of a screening questionnaire for psoriatic arthritis: the Toronto Psoriatic Arthritis Screen (ToPAS). Ann Rheum Dis 2009;68:497-501.
9. Alamanos Y, Voulgari PV, Drosos AA. Incidence and prevalence of psoriatic arthritis: a systematic review. J Rheumatol 2008;35:1354-8.
10. Jajic J. Blue-coloured skin over involved joints in psoriatic arthritis. Clin Rheumatol 2001;20:304-5.

11. Moll JM, Wright V. Psoriatic arthritis. Semin Arthritis Rheum 1973;3:55-78.

12. Helliwell PS, Hetthen J, Sokoll K, Green M, Marchesoni A, Lubrano E, et al. Joint symmetry in early and late rheumatoid and psoriatic arthritis: comparison with a mathematical model. Arthritis Rheum 2000;43:865-71.

13. Kane D, Greaney T, Bresnihan B, Gibney R, FitzGerald O. Ultrasonography in the diagnosis and management of psoriatic dactylitis. J Rheumatol 1999;26:1746-51.

14. Olivieri I, Barozzi I, Favaro L, Pierro A, de Matteis M, Borghi C, et al. Dactylitis in patients with seronegative spondyloarthropathy: assessment by ultrasonography and magnetic resonance imaging. Arthritis Rheum 1996;39:1524-8.

15. Olivieri I, Barozzi I, Pierro A, De Matteis M, Padula A, Pavlica P. Toe dactylitis in patients with spondyloarthropathy: assessment by magnetic resonance imaging. J Rheumatol 1997;24:926-30.

16. Brockbank J, Stein M, Schentag CT, Gladman DD. Characteristics of dactylitis in psoriatic arthritis (PsA). Ann Rheum Dis 2005;62:188-90.

17. Kane D, Stafford L, Bresniham B, Fitzgerald O. A prospective, clinical and radiological study of early psoriatic arthritis: an early synovitis clinic experience. Rheumatology 2003;42:1460-8.

18. Cantini F, Salvarani C, Olivieri I, Macchioni L, Niccoli L, Padula A, et al. Distal extremity swelling with pitting edema in psoriatic arthritis: a case-control study. Clin Exp Rheumatol 2001;19:291-6.

19. Fernández-Sueiro JL, Willisch A, Pinto J, Pertega S, Freire M, Aldo F, et al. Prevalence and location of enthesitis in ankylosing spondylitis and psoriatic arthritis. Ann Rheum Dis 2007;66(Suppl. 2):98.

20. Gladman DD. Axial disease in psoriatic arthritis. Current Rheumatology Report 2007;9:455-60.

21. Gladman DD, Brubacher B, Buskila D, Langevitz P, Farewell VT. Differences in the expression of spondyloarthropathy: a comparison between ankylosing spondylitis and psoriatic arthritis. Genetic and gender effects. Clin Invest Med 1993;16:1-7.

22. Helliwell PS, Hickling P, Wright V. Do the radiological changes of classic ankylosing spondylitis differ from the changes found in the spondylitis associated with inflammatory bowel disease, psoriasis, and reactive arthritis? Ann Rheum Dis 1998;57:135-40.

23. Griffiths CE, Barker JN. Pathogenesis and clinical features of psoriasis. Lancet 2007;370:263-71.

24. Gladman DD, Anhorn KB, Schachter RK, Mervart H. HLA antigens in psoriatic arthritis. J Rheumatol 1986;13:586-92.

25. Mease PJ. Assessment tools in psoriatic arthritis. J Rheumatol 2008;35:1426-30.

26. Gladman DD, Inman R, Cook R, Maksymowych WP, Braun J, Davis JC, et al. International spondyloarthritis interobserver reliability exercise—The Inspire Study: II. Assessment of peripheral joints, enthesitis and dactylitis. J Rheumatol 2007;34:1740-5.

27. Chandran V, Cook R, Helliwell P, Kavanaugh A, McHugh N, Mease P, et al. International Multi-centre Psoriasis and psoriatic Arthritis Reliability Trial (GRAPPA-IMPART): assessment of skin, joints, nails and dactylitis. Arthritis Rheum 2007;56(Suppl. 9):S798.

28. Gladman DD, Inman R, Cook R, van der Heijde D, Landewé RB, Braun J, et al. International spondyloarthritis interobserver reliability exercise—The Inspire Study: I. Assessment of spinal measures. J Rheumatol 2007;34:1733-9.

29. Menter A, Gottlieb A, Feldman SR, Van Voorhees AS, Leonardi CL, Gordon KB, et al. Guidelines of care for the management of psoriasis and psoriatic arthritis: Section 1. Overview of psoriasis and guidelines of care for the treatment of psoriasis with biologics. J Am Acad Dermatol 2008;58:826-50.

30. Cassell SE, Bieber JD, Rich P, Tutuncu ZN, Lee SJ, Kalunian KC, et al. The modified Nail Psoriasis Severity Index: validation of an instrument to assess psoriatic nail involvement in patients with psoriatic arthritis. J Rheumatol 2007;34:123-9.

31. Clegg DO, Reda DJ, Mejias E, Cannon GW, Weisman MH, Taylor T, et al. Comparison of sulfasalazine and placebo in the treatment of psoriatic arthritis. A Department of Veterans Affairs Cooperative Study. Arthritis Rheum 1996;39:2013-20.

32. Gladman DD, Helliwell P, Mease PJ, Nash P, Ritchlin C, Taylor W. Assessment of patients with psoriatic arthritis: a review of currently available measures. Arthritis Rheum 2004;50:24-35.

33. Fransen J, Antoni C, Mease PJ, Uter W, Kavanaugh A, Kalden JR, et al. Performance of response criteria for assessing peripheral arthritis in patients with psoriatic arthritis: analysis of data from randomised controlled trials of two tumour necrosis factor inhibitors. Ann Rheum Dis 2006;65:1373-8.

34. Gladman DD, Shuckett R, Russell ML, Thorne JC, Schachter RK. Psoriatic arthritis—clinical and laboratory analysis of 220 patients. Quart J Med 1987;62:127-41.

35. Gladman DD, Stafford-Brady F, Chang CH, Lewandowski K, Russell ML. Longitudinal study of clinical and radiological progression in psoriatic arthritis. J Rheumatol 1990;17:809-12.

36. McHugh NJ, Balachrishnan C, Jones SM. Progression of peripheral joint disease in psoriatic arthritis: a 5-yr prospective study. Rheumatology (Oxford) 2003;42:778-83.

37. Khan M, Schentag C, Gladman D. Clinical and radiological changes during psoriatic arthritis disease progression: working toward classification criteria. J Rheumatol 2003;30:1022-6.

38. Kane D, Stafford L, Bresniham B, Fitzgerald O. A prospective, clinical and radiological study of early psoriatic arthritis: an early synovitis clinic experience. Rheumatology 2003;42:1460-8.

39. Queiro-Silva R, Torre-Alonso JC, Tinture-Eguren T, Lopez-Lagunas I. A polyarticular onset predicts erosive and deforming disease in psoriatic arthritis. Ann Rheum Dis 2003;62:68-70.

40. Bond SJ, Farewell VT, Schentag CT, Gladman DD. Predictors for radiological damage in psoriatic arthritis. Results from a single centre. Ann Rheum Dis 2007;66:370-6.

41. Gladman DD. Mortality in psoriatic arthritis. Clin Exp Rheumatol 2008;26(Suppl. 51):S62-5.

42. Gladman DD. Disability and quality of life considerations. Psoriatic arthritis. In: Gordon GB, Ruderman E, editors. Psoriasis and psoriatic arthritis: an integrated approach. Heidelberg, Germany: Springer-Verlag; 2005. p. 118-23.

43. Moll JM, Wright V. Familial occurrence of PsA. Ann Rheum Dis 1973;32:181-201.

44. Chandran V, Schentag CT, Brockbank J, Pellett FJ, Shanmugrajah S, Toloza SMA, et al. Familial aggregation of psoriatic arthritis. Ann Rheum Dis 2009;68:664-7.

45. Callis Duffin K, Chandran V, Gladman DD, Krueger GG, Elder JT, Rahman P. Genetics of psoriasis and psoriatic arthritis: Update and Future Direction (GRAPPA 2007). J Rheumatol 2008;35:1449-53.

46. Prinz JC. Psoriasis vulgaris—a sterile antibacterial skin reaction mediated by cross-reactive T cells? An immunological view of the pathophysiology of psoriasis. Clin Exp Dermatol 2001;26:326-32.

47. Vasey FB, Seleznick MJ, Fenske NA, Espinoza LR. New signposts on the road to understanding psoriatic arthritis. J Rheumatol 1989;16:1405-7.

48. Martin MP, Nelson G, Lee J-H, Pellett F, Gao X, Wade J, et al. Susceptibility to psoriatic arthritis: influence of activating killer immunoglobulin-like receptor genes in the absence of their corresponding HLA ligands. J Immunol 2002;169:2818-22.

49. Olivieri I, Padula S, D'Angelo S, Scarpa R. Role of trauma in psoriatic arthritis. J Rheumatol 2008;35:2085-7.

50. Veale D, Barrell M, Fitzgerald O. Mechanisms of joint sparing in a patient with unilateral psoriatic arthritis and a long-standing hemiplegia. Br J Rheumatol 1993;32:413-6.

51. Veale D, Yanni G, Rogers S, Barnes L, Bresnihan B, Fitzgerald O. Reduced synovial membrane macrophage numbers, ELAM1 expression, and lining layer hyperplasia in psoriatic arthritis as compared with rheumatoid arthritis. Arthritis Rheum 1993;36:893-900.

52. Ritchlin C, Haas-Smith SA, Hicks D. Patterns of cytokine production in psoriatic synovium. J Rheumatol 1998;25:1544-52.
53. Espinoza LR, Aguilar JL, Espinoza CG, Cuéllar ML, Scopelitis E, Silveira LH. Fibroblast function in psoriatic arthritis. I: Alteration of cell kinetics and growth factor responses. J Rheumatol 1994;21:1502-6.
54. Espinoza LR, Aguilar JL, Espinoza CG, Scopelitis E, Silveira LH, Grotendorst GR. Fibroblast function in psoriatic arthritis. II: Increased expression of PDGF receptors and increased production of GF and cytokines. J Rheumatol 1994;21:1507-11.
55. Costello P, Bresnihan B, O'Farrell C, Fitzgerald O. Predominance of CD8+ T lymphocytes in psoriatic arthritis. J Rheumatol 1999;26:1117-24.
56. Anandarajah AP, Ritchlin CT. Pathogenesis of psoriatic arthritis. Curr Opin Rheumatol 2004;16:338-43.
57. Ritchlin CT, Haas-Smith SA, Li P, Hicks DG, Schwarz EM. Mechanisms of TNF-alpha- and RANKL-mediated osteoclastogenesis and bone resorption in psoriatic arthritis. J Clin Invest 2003;111:821-31.
58. Blauvelt A. T-helper 17 cells in psoriatic plaques and additional genetic links between IL-23 and psoriasis. J Invest Dermatol 2008;128:1064-7.
59. Neumüller J, Dunky A, Burtscher H, Jilch R, Menzel JE. Interaction of monocytes from patients with psoriatic arthritis with cultured microvascular endothelial cells. Clin Immunol 2001;98:143-52.
60. Fraser A, Fearon U, Reece R, Emery P, Veale DJ. Matrix metalloproteinase 9, apoptosis, and vascular morphology in early arthritis. Arthritis Rheum 2001;44:2024-8.
61. Hitchon CA, Danning CL, Illei GG, El Gabalawy HS, Boumpas DT. Gelatinase expression and activity in the synovium and skin of patients with erosive psoriatic arthritis. J Rheumatol 2002;29:107-17.
62. Hueber AJ, McInnes IB. Immune regulation in psoriasis and psoriatic arthritis—recent developments. Immunol Lett 2007;114:59-65.
63. Sarzi-Puttini P, Santandrea S, Boccassini L, Panni B, Caruso I. The role of NSAIDs in psoriatic arthritis: evidence from a controlled study with nimesulide. Clin Exp Rheumatol 2001;19:S17-S20.
64. Griffiths CE. Therapy for psoriatic arthritis: sometimes a conflict for psoriasis. Br J Rheumatol 1997;36:409-10.
65. Chan FK. The David Y. Graham lecture: use of nonsteroidal anti-inflammatory drugs in a COX-2 restricted environment. Am J Gastroenterol 2008;103:221-7.
66. Eder L, Chandran V, Ueng J, Bhella S, Schentag CT, Lee KA, et al. Predictors of response to intra-articular steroids in psoriatic arthritis. Arthritis Rheum 2008;58:3991.
67. Baker H, Ryan TJ. Generalized pustular psoriasis: a clinical and epidemiological study of 104 cases. Br J Dermatol 1968;80:771-93.
68. Nash P, Clegg DO. Psoriatic arthritis therapy: NSAIDs and traditional DMARDs. Ann Rheum Dis 2005;64(Suppl. 2):274-7.
69. Black RL, O'Brien WM, Vanscott EJ, Auerbach R, Eisen AJ, Bunim JJ. Methotrexate therapy in psoriatic arthritis; double-blind study on 21 patients. JAMA 1964;189:743-7.
70. Willkens RF, Williams HJ, Ward JR, Egger MJ, Reading JC, Clements PJ, et al. Randomized, double blind, placebo controlled trial of low-dose pulse methotrexate in psoriatic arthritis. Arthritis Rheum 1984;27:376-81.
71. Soriano ER, McHugh NJ. Therapies for peripheral joint disease in psoriatic arthritis. A systematic review. J Rheumatol 2006;33:1422-30.
72. Abu-Shakra M, Gladman DD, Thorne JC, Long J, Gough J, Farewell VT. Longterm methotrexate therapy in psoriatic arthritis: clinical and radiological outcome. J Rheumatol 1995;22:241-5.
73. Chandran V, Schentag CT, Gladman DD. Reappraisal of the effectiveness of methotrexate in psoriatic arthritis: results from a longitudinal observational cohort. J Rheumatol 2008;35:469-71.
74. Ellis CN, Fradin MS, Messana JM, Brown MD, Siegel MT, Hartley AH, et al. Cyclosporine for plaque-type psoriasis. Results of a multidose, double-blind trial. N Engl J Med 1991;324:277-84.
75. Salvarani C, Macchioni P, Olivieri I, Marchesoni A, Cutolo M, Ferraccioli G, et al. A comparison of cyclosporine, sulfasalazine, and symptomatic therapy in the treatment of psoriatic arthritis. J Rheumatol 2001;28:2274-82.
76. Spadaro A, Riccieri V, Sili-Scavalli A, Sensi F, Taccari E, Zoppini A. Comparison of cyclosporin A and methotrexate in the treatment of psoriatic arthritis: a one-year prospective study. Clin Exp Rheumatol 1995;13:589-93.
77. Fraser AD, van Kuijk AW, Westhovens R, Karim Z, Wakefield R, Gerards AH, et al. A randomised, double blind, placebo controlled, multicentre trial of combination therapy with methotrexate plus ciclosporin in patients with active psoriatic arthritis. Ann Rheum Dis 2005;64:859-64.
78. Levy JJ, Paulus HE, Barnett EV, et al. A double blind controlled evaluation of azathioprine treatment in rheumatoid arthritis and psoriatic arthritis. Arthritis Rheum 1972;15:116-7.
79. Lee JCT, Gladman DD, Schentag CT, Cook RJ. The long-term use of azathioprine in patients with psoriatic arthritis. J Clin Rheumatol 2001;7:160-5.
80. Kaltwasser JP, Nash P, Gladman D, Rosen CF, Behrens F, Jones P, et al. Efficacy and safety of leflunomide in the treatment of psoriatic arthritis and psoriasis: a multinational, double-blind, randomized, placebo-controlled clinical trial. Arthritis Rheum 2004;50:1939-50.
81. Carette S, Calin A, McCafferty JP, Wallin BA. A double-blind placebo-controlled study of auranofin in patients with psoriatic arthritis. Arthritis Rheum 1989;32:158-65.
82. Palit J, Hill J, Capell HA, Carey J, Daunt SO, Cawley MI, et al. A multicentre double-blind comparison of auranofin, intramuscular gold thiomalate and placebo in patients with psoriatic arthritis. Br J Rheumatol 1990;29:280-3.
83. Schrader P, Mooser G, Peter RU, Puhl W. [Preliminary results in the therapy of psoriatic arthritis with mycophenolate mofetil]. Z Rheumatol 2002;61:545-50.
84. Grundmann-Kollmann M, Mooser G, Schraeder P, Zollner T, Kaskel P, Ochsendorf F, et al. Treatment of chronic plaque-stage psoriasis and psoriatic arthritis with mycophenolate mofetil. J Am Acad Dermatol 2000;42:835-7.
85. Hopkins R, Bird HA, Jones H, Hill J, Surrall KE, Astbury C, et al. A double-blind controlled trial of etretinate (Tigason) and ibuprofen in psoriatic arthritis. Ann Rheum Dis 1985;44:189-93.
86. Mease PJ, Goffe BS, Metz J, VanderStoep A, Finck BK, Burge DJ. Etanercept in the treatment of psoriatic arthritis and psoriasis: a randomised trial. Lancet 2000;356:385-90.
87. Mease PJ, Kivitz AJ, Burch FX, Siegel EL, Cohen SB, Ory P, et al. Etanercept treatment of psoriatic arthritis: safety, efficacy, and effect on disease progression. Arthritis Rheum 2004;50:2264-72.
88. Antoni CE, Kavanaugh A, Kirkham B, Tutuncu Z, Burmester GR, Schneider U, et al. Sustained benefits of infliximab therapy for dermatologic and articular manifestations of psoriatic arthritis: results from the infliximab multinational psoriatic arthritis controlled trial (IMPACT). Arthritis Rheum 2005;52:1227-36.
89. Antoni C, Krueger GG, de Vlam K, Birbara C, Beutler A, Guzzo C, et al. Infliximab improves signs and symptoms of psoriatic arthritis: results of the IMPACT 2 trial. Ann Rheum Dis 2005;64:1150-7.
90. Kavanaugh A, Antoni C, Krueger GG, Yan S, Bala M, Dooley LT, et al. Infliximab improves health related quality of life and physical function in patients with psoriatic arthritis. Ann Rheum Dis 2006;65:471-7.
91. Kavanaugh A, Krueger GG, Beutler A, Guzzo C, Zhou B, Dooley LT, et al. Infliximab maintains a high degree of clinical response in patients with active psoriatic arthritis through 1 year of treatment: results from the IMPACT 2 trial. Ann Rheum Dis 2007;66:498-505.
92. Antoni CE, Kavanaugh A, van der Heijde D, Beutler A, Keenan G, Zhou B, et al. Two-year efficacy and safety of infliximab treatment in patients with active psoriatic arthritis: findings of the Infliximab Multinational Psoriatic Arthritis Controlled Trial (IMPACT). J Rheumatol 2008;35:869-76.
93. Kavanaugh A, Antoni C, Mease P, Gladman D, Yan S, Bala M, et al. Effect of infliximab therapy on employment, time

lost from work, and productivity in patients with psoriatic arthritis. J Rheumatol 2006;33:2254-9.

94. Kavanaugh A, Krueger GG, Beutler A, Guzzo C, Zhou B, Dooley LT, et al. Infliximab maintains a high degree of clinical response in patients with active psoriatic arthritis through one year of treatment: results from the IMPACT 2 trial. Ann Rheum Dis 2007;66:498-505.

95. van der Heijde D, Kavanaugh A, Gladman DD, Antoni C, Krueger CC, Guzzo C, et al. IMPACT 2 Study Group Infliximab inhibits progression of radiographic damage in patients with active psoriatic arthritis through one year of treatment: results from the induction and maintenance psoriatic arthritis clinical trial 2. Arthritis Rheum 2007;66:2698-707.

96. Mease PJ, Gladman DD, Ritchlin CT, Ruderman EM, Steinfeld SD, Choy EH, et al. Adalimumab in the treatment of patients with moderately to severely active psoriatic arthritis: results of The ADEPT Trial. Arthritis Rheum 2005;52:3279-89.

97. Gladman DD, Mease PJ, Cifaldi MA, Perdok RJ, Sasso E, Medich J. Adalimumab improves joint- and skin-related functional impairment in patients with psoriatic arthritis: functional outcomes of the Adalimumab Effectiveness in Psoriatic Arthritis Trial (ADEPT). Ann Rheum Dis 2007;66:166-8.

98. Gladman DD, Mease PJ, Ritchlin CT, Choy EHS, Sharp JT, Ory PA, et al. Adalimumab for long-term treatment of psoriatic arthritis: 48-week data and subanalysis from ADEPT. Arthritis Rheum 2007;56:476-88.

99. Kavanaugh A, McInnes I, Mease P, Krueger GG, Gladman D, Gomez-Reino J, et al. Golimumab, a new human TNF-alpha antibody, administered every 4 weeks as a subcutaneous injection in psoriatic arthritis: 24-week efficacy and safety results of the randomized, placebo-controlled GO-REVEAL study. Arthritis Rheum 2009;60:976-86.

100. Gladman D, Kavanaugh A, McInnes I, Mease P, Gomez-Reino JJ, Papp K, et al. Golimumab, a new human TNF-alpha antibody administered every 4 weeks as a subcutaneous injection in psoriatic arthritis: nail enthesitis, and dactylitis response in the randomized placebo-controlled Go-Reveal study. Ann Rheum Dis 2008;67(Suppl. 2):526.

101. Kavanaugh A, Mease P, Krueger GG, Gladman D, Gomez-Reino JJ, Papp K, et al. Golimumab, a new human TNG alpha antibody administered subcutaneously every 4 weeks in psoriatic arthritis patients: 52 week efficacy and safety

results of the randomized placebo-controlled Go-Reveal study. Ann Rheum Dis 2008;67(Suppl. 2):99.

102. Askling J, Bongartz T. Malignancy and biologic therapy in rheumatoid arthritis. Curr Opin Rheumatol 2008;20:334-9.

103. Rohekar S, Tom BD, Hassa A, Schentag C, Farewell VT, Gladman DD. Malignancy in psoriatic arthritis. Arthritis Rheum 2008;58:82-7.

104. Saad AA, Symmons DPM, Noyce PR, Ashcroft DM. Risk and benefits of tumour necrosis factor-α inhibitors in the management of psoriatic arthritis: systematic review and metaanalysis of randomized controlled trials. J Rheumatol 2008;35:883-90.

105. Gottlieb AB, Mendelsohn A, Shen YK, Menter A. Randomized, placebo-controlled phase 2 study of ustekinumab, a human IL-12/23 monoclonal antibody in psoriatic arthritis. Ann Rheum Dis 2008;67(Suppl. 2):99.

106. Mease PJ, Gladman DD, Keystone EC. Alefacept in combination with methotrexate for the treatment of psoriatic arthritis: results of a randomized, double-blind, placebo-controlled study. Arthritis Rheum 2006;54:1638-45.

107. Lebwohl M, Tyring SK, Hamilton TK, Toth D, Glazer S, Tawfik NH, et al. A novel targeted T-cell modulator, efalizumab, for plaque psoriasis. N Engl J Med 2003;349:2004-13.

108. Papp KA, Caro I, Leung HM, Garovoy M, Mease PJ. Efalizumab for the treatment of psoriatic arthritis. J Cutan Med Surg 2007;11:57-66.

109. Viguier M, Richette P, Aubin F, Beylot-Barry M, Lahfa M, Bedane C, et al. Onset of psoriatic arthritis in patients treated with efalizumab for moderate to severe psoriasis. Arthritis Rheum 2008;58:1796-802.

110. Menter A, Gottlieb A, Feldman SR, Van Voorhees AS, Leonardi CL, Gordon KB, et al. Guidelines of care for the management of psoriasis and psoriatic arthritis: Section 1. Overview of psoriasis and guidelines of care for the treatment of psoriasis with biologics. J Am Acad Dermatol 2008;58:826-50.

111. Gottlieb A, Korman NJ, Gordon KB, Feldman SR, Lebwohl M, Koo JY, et al. Guidelines of care for the management of psoriasis and psoriatic arthritis: Section 2. Psoriatic arthritis: overview and guidelines of care for treatment with an emphasis on the biologics. J Am Acad Dermatol 2008;58:851-64.

112. Ritchlin CT, Kavanaugh A, Gladman DD, Mease PJ, Boehncke WH, de Vlam K, et al. Treatment recommendations for psoriatic arthritis. Ann Rheum Dis epub ahead of print 24/10/08.

Chapter 7

Juvenile Arthritis

Mary Beth F. Son and Robert P. Sundel

Juvenile rheumatoid arthritis (JRA) is an umbrella term for a number of arthritides of unknown etiology that occur in children younger than 16 years of age.

It is the most common rheumatic disease of children in the developed world, occurs in all races and ethnic groups, and is an important cause of morbidity. Use of the term JRA implies that childhood arthritis has a uniform presentation, treatment, and prognosis. To the contrary, it is likely that the subtypes of juvenile arthritis are related but distinct disease processes with varying presentations that require different treatment approaches and have different prognoses.

The difficulty in accurately describing the subtypes of inflammatory arthritis of childhood has been reflected in the number of proposed nomenclature systems for the classification of JRA (Tables 7-1 through 7-3).[1,2] The most recent classification is the International League of Associations for Rheumatology criteria, which designates juvenile arthritis as juvenile idiopathic arthritis (JIA; Tables 7-4 and 7-5). Although widely used, this classification is relatively new and has yet to be validated. The earlier criteria published by the American College of Rheumatology (ACR) use the more familiar term JRA. Lastly, the European League Against Rheumatism has also published criteria for juvenile chronic arthritis (JCA). In addition to being a source of confusion for families and patients, the proliferation of classification schemes leads to great difficulty in comparing studies based on different systems. As with other clinically defined diseases, precise terminology will likely have to await a fuller genetic and pathogenic understanding of juvenile arthritis. For the purposes of this chapter, the general terms juvenile arthritis, oligoarthritis and polyarthritis will be used; in cases in which specific nomenclature is required, the ACR terms will be used because they are widely recognized by most practitioners.

DIFFERENTIAL DIAGNOSIS OF OLIGOARTHRITIS

The differential diagnosis of a child with oligoarthritis, defined as inflammation of fewer than five joints, includes infectious, traumatic, oncologic and

---

CASE 1

A 6-year-old previously healthy girl presents to her pediatrician with 3 months of left knee swelling. Her parents report that she limps when she gets out of bed, but her gait improves over the course of the day. Additionally, she has difficulty descending the steps from her bedroom in the morning, but does so easily at night. The family notes that the knee has appeared swollen but not warm or erythematous. The girl generally does not report knee pain, but she does not run as quickly in soccer practice as previously, volunteering that her knee hurts when she sprints. Her parents do not recall specific trauma or infections preceding the onset of symptoms. The child has been without fevers, rashes, weight loss, or visual changes. She has continued to go to school, and her energy level and appetite have remained normal. She sleeps through the night.

The child has had no joint complaints in the past, and in general has been healthy with normal growth and development. She has not had prior hospitalizations or surgeries and takes no long-term medications. Her family history is significant because a maternal aunt had hypothyroidism.

On examination, the patient is well appearing and afebrile. Her height is 50th percentile for age and her weight is 25th percentile. The only abnormal findings are limited to the musculoskeletal system: Her left knee is slightly warm and swollen with a ballotable effusion but no erythema. She has pain at the extremes of range of motion, and is unable to flex her knee beyond 75 degrees or extend it beyond 15 degrees. She has a leg length discrepancy of about 1 cm. Her other joints are normal, without evidence of inflammation or restricted motion. She does not have dactylitis or enthesitis.

Laboratory results include normal complete blood counts, an elevated erythrocyte sedimentation rate (ESR) of 23 mm/hour, and a positive antinuclear antibody (ANA) with a titer of 1:320. Rheumatoid factor (RF) and antibodies to cyclic citrullinated peptide are negative. Plain radiographs of the left knee reveal only an effusion.

Table 7-1. *Comparison of Classifications of Chronic Arthritis in Children*

Juvenile Rheumatoid Arthritis (ACR)	Juvenile Chronic Arthritis (EULAR)	Juvenile Idiopathic Arthritis (ILAR)
Systemic	Systemic	Systemic
Polyarticular	Polyarticular RF-negative	Polyarticular RF-negative
Pauciarticular	Juvenile rheumatoid arthritis RF-positive	Polyarticular RF-positive
	Pauciarticular	Oligoarticular Persistent Extended
	Juvenile psoriatic arthritis	Psoriatic arthritis
	Juvenile ankylosing spondylitis	Enthesitis-related arthritis Undifferentiated arthritis

RF, rheumatoid factor.
Adapted from Cassidy P, Petty R. Textbook of pediatric rheumatology. 5th ed. Philadelphia: Elsevier; 2005.

Table 7-2. *Characteristics of the ACR, EULAR, and ILAR Classifications of Chronic Arthritis in Children*

Characteristic	ACR	EULAR	ILAR
Onset types	3	6	6
Age at onset of arthritis	< 16 years	< 16 years	< 16 years
Duration of arthritis	≥ 6 weeks	≥ 3 months	≥ 6 weeks
Includes JAS	No	Yes	Yes
Includes JPsA	No	Yes	Yes
Includes inflammatory bowel disease	No	Yes	Yes
Other diseases excluded	Yes	Yes	Yes

ACR, American College of Rheumatology; EULAR, European League Against Rheumatism; ILAR, International League of Associations for Rheumatology; JAS, juvenile ankylosing spondylitis; JPsA, juvenile psoriatic arthritis.
Adapted from Cassidy P, Petty R. Textbook of pediatric rheumatology. 5th ed. Philadelphia: Elsevier; 2005.

Table 7-3. *Characteristics of Chronic Arthritis in Children by Type of Onset*

Characteristic	Polyarthritis	Oligoarthritis	Systemic Disease
Percent of cases	30	60	10
Number of joints involved	≥5	≤4	Variable
Age at onset	Bimodal peak: 2–5 years 10–14 years	Peak: 1–2 years	Throughout childhood
Male-to-female ratio	3:1	5:1	1:1
Systemic involvement	Occasional fevers, uveitis	Uveitis	Fevers and rash
Occurrence of chronic uveitis	5%	5–15%	Rare
Frequency of seropositivity:			
ANA	40–50%	75–85%	10%
RF	10%	Rare	Rare
Prognosis	Variable in severe joint disease; otherwise good.	Excellent unless vision loss	Moderate to poor

ANA, antinuclear antibody; RF, rheumatoid factor.
Adapted from Cassidy P, Petty R. Textbook of pediatric rheumatology. 5th ed. Philadelphia: Elsevier; 2005.

rheumatologic etiologies (Table 7-6). In general, infectious arthritis is less likely to cause a gelling phenomenon, in which the joints are stiff following a period of inactivity, and is more likely to present with pain. Furthermore, in a previously healthy child, the more joints involved, the less likely the process is to be infectious. Septic arthritis caused by virulent organisms such as *staphylococcus* or *streptococcus* presents acutely, with fever and a single red, warm, swollen, and painful joint. Septic monoarthritis is more common in children than septic polyarthritis.[3] Lyme arthritis typically has a less fulminant presentation, although at times, it may mimic a bacterial arthritis, including elevated markers of inflammation. A history of a preceding tick bite or rash may be elicited in fewer than 50% of children with Lyme arthritis. Indolent organisms such as kingella, on the other hand, may present with

a more gradual onset of discomfort and no joint erythema. Children with an immune deficiency, whether primary or acquired, can develop an oligoarthritis due to opportunistic organisms including mycobacteria, *Bartonella henselae* and ureaplasma. Lastly, patients with oligoarthritis may have a reactive arthritis secondary to arthritogenic bacteria such as *Salmonella, Shigella, Yersinia, Campylobacter,* and *Chlamydia.*

Cases of monoarthritis caused by trauma usually have a clear preceding history. Similarly, a traumatic hemarthropathy can occur in patients with known bleeding diatheses. Less commonly encountered diagnoses to consider include venous or arterial malformations.

Childhood malignancies can present as arthritis,[4-7] and consideration of cancer is important before initiating treatment, which may obscure the underlying condition. Leukemia is the most common cancer of childhood, and it presents with reports of musculoskeletal symptoms in up to 20% of cases. Primary malignant joint tumors are extremely rare, but pigmented villonodular synovitis, a benign but locally invasive tumor, should be considered when the child has an inflamed joint with significant pain or nighttime symptoms. Neuroblastoma metastasizes to periarticular areas of bone, but the child's reports of limp and pain may appear to originate in joints. In all such conditions, a history of weight loss and fatigue, or

Table 7-4. *Categories of Juvenile Idiopathic Arthritis (ILAR Classification)*

Systemic onset
    Arthritis in one or more joints
    2 weeks of fever with at least 3 days of a quotidian pattern
    Plus one or more of
        Evanescent erythematous rash
        Generalized lymphadenopathy
        Hepato and/or splenomegaly
    Exclusions 1 to 4 (See Table 7-5)
Oligoarthritis
    Persistent oligoarthritis
        Affecting four or fewer joints throughout the disease course
        Exclusions 1 to 5
    Extended oligoarthritis
        Affecting more than four joints after the first 6 months of disease
        Exclusions 1 to 5
Polyarthritis, rheumatoid factor negative
    Arthritis affecting five or more joints during the first 6 months of the disease
    Rheumatoid factor negative
    Exclusions 1 to 5
Polyarthritis, rheumatoid factor positive
    Arthritis affecting five or more joints during the first 6 months of the disease
    Rheumatoid factor positive two or more times, at least 3 months apart
    Exclusions 1,2,3,5
Psoriatic arthritis
    Arthritis and psoriasis or
    Arthritis and two of the following
        Dactylitis
        Nail pitting or onycholysis
        Psoriasis in a first-degree relative
Enthesitis-related arthritis
    Arthritis and enthesitis or
    Arthritis or enthesitis and two of the following
        SI joint tenderness and inflammatory lumbosacral pain
        HLA-B27 positive
        Arthritis in a boy older than 6 years of age
        Acute anterior uveitis
        History of ankylosing spondylitis, enthesitis-related arthritis, sacroiliitis with inflammatory bowel disease, Reiter's syndrome or acute anterior uveitis in a first-degree relative
    Exclusions 1,4,5
Undifferentiated arthritis
    Fulfills criteria in none of the above categories
    Fulfills criteria for more than one of the above-mentioned categories

HLA, human leukocyte antigen; ILAR, International League of Associations for Rheumatology.

Table 7-5. *Exclusion Criteria for Categories of Juvenile Idiopathic Arthritis*

Psoriasis or a history of psoriasis in a first-degree relative

Arthritis in an HLA-B27–positive boy beginning after his 6th birthday

History of ankylosing spondylitis, enthesitis-related arthritis, sacroiliitis with inflammatory bowel disease, Reiter's syndrome, or acute anterior uveitis in a first-degree relative

IgM rheumatoid factor on two or more occasions 3 months apart

Systemic Juvenile Idiopathic Arthritis in the patient

HLA, human leukocyte antigen; IgM, immunoglobulin M.

Table 7-6. *Differential Diagnosis of Monoarthritis in Children*

Infections
Septic arthritis (acute bacterial infection with agents such as *staphylococcus* or *streptococcus*)
Lyme arthritis
Tuberculosis arthritis
Viral associated arthritis (mumps, varicella, human immunodeficiency virus)
Reactive arthritis secondary to arthritogenic bacteria

Traumatic Arthritis
Hemarthropathy in hemophilia

Tumors
Malignant:
    Acute lymphoblastic leukemia
    Neuroblastoma
    Ewing's sarcoma
    Synovial sarcoma
Benign:
    Pigmented villonodular synovitis

Inflammatory Arthropathies
Oligoarthritis
Psoriatic arthritis
Sarcoidoisis

physical examination findings of an ill-appearing child, should suggest the possibility of a nonrheumatologic condition. Plain films may reveal metaphyseal rarefaction or "leukemia lines" in the case of a hematologic malignancy, or periosteal elevation or an abdominal mass in cases of neuroblastoma or bony tumors. Complete blood counts with cytopenias or even normal platelet counts in the face of systemic inflammation should also raise concern for a tumor.[8]

Rheumatologic diseases that can present with oligoarthritis include JRA, other forms of juvenile arthritis such as psoriatic arthritis, and sarcoidosis. Children with psoriatic arthritis often have a remarkably large, swollen knee with a massive effusion. Other characteristic findings that are distinct from those in JRA include asymmetric arthritis involving both large and small joints, dactylitis, and stigmata of psoriasis including nail pits or onycholysis. In the absence of a characteristic psoriasiform rash, a family history of a first-degree relative with psoriasis is necessary for a definitive diagnosis. Sarcoidosis in a child typically presents with the triad of arthritis, uveitis, and rash; pulmonary involvement is less common than in adults, so angiotensin converting enzyme (ACE) levels may be misleading. Joint involvement is characterized by thick, boggy synovitis and often tendinitis, and it typically begins in an oligoarticular pattern, later evolving to involve numerous joints. Drug-induced autoimmune disease as seen with minocycline does not generally cause an oligoarthritis.[9]

TREATMENT OF JUVENILE ARTHRITIS: OLIGOARTHRITIS

As with adult rheumatoid arthritis (RA), the medical management of JRA has changed dramatically during the past two decades. Although nonsteroidal anti-inflammatory drugs (NSAIDs) are helpful in treating the symptoms of arthritis, they no longer form the foundation of the therapeutic pyramid. Rather, early introduction of disease-modifying agents aimed at preventing joint damage has become the norm. Most recently, biologic response modifiers have been added to the armamentarium for treating recalcitrant disease. A particular patient's regimen is determined by risk-benefit calculations, with more intensive (and potentially more toxic) therapies reserved for children with the most aggressive forms of arthritis. For example, seropositive polyarticular JRA is similar to the adult form of RF-positive rheumatoid arthritis, with a tendency for early and diffuse erosions. Accordingly a more aggressive approach is indicated compared with those patients with pauciarthritis or reactive arthritis.

First-line treatment for patients with oligoarthritis includes NSAIDs (Tables 7-7 and 7-8) or intra-articular corticosteroid injections. Most practitioners choose naproxen as the initial NSAID, given its extensive experience in JRA and the convenience of twice-daily administration. Numerous other agents are also approved for the treatment of JRA, including most recently celecoxib.[10] Patients should be encouraged to take all NSAIDs with food,

and children should wear sunscreen while taking naproxen to avoid pseudoporphyria. With the exception of anti-cycloogenase-2–specific agents, all NSAIDs have similar adverse side effects, including gastritis, peptic ulcer disease, transaminitis, and dermatologic complications. Duffy and colleagues[11] studied central nervous system toxicity in children taking NSAIDs and found that up to 33% reported headache. There were rare reports of seizures in patients taking indomethacin in this case series. Finally, the impact of chronic NSAID use on a child's cardiovascular risk remains to be determined. However, NSAIDs are generally well tolerated by children, with the major limitation to their use being lack of efficacy.

Intra-articular steroid injections are an efficient and effective approach to treating pauciarthritis in children.[12,13] Response rates are up to 90%, benefits persist for more than 12 months in up to 80%, and onset of action is more rapid than with systemic agents. The risks of intra-articular steroids, including infection and subcutaneous atrophy at the site of the injection, are generally outweighed by the benefits. Most practitioners inject the same joint no more than twice in the same year to avoid possible adverse effects on cartilage and growth plates. Triamcinolone hexacetonide at a dose of approximately 1 mg/kg has the longest duration of action and is generally well tolerated, although some practitioners prefer methylprednisolone acetate or triamcinolone acetonide.

Treatment of arthritis in children is predicated on complete control of articular inflammation. Even low-grade ongoing synovitis may result in life-long consequences, including leg length discrepancies, valgus or varus deformities, and a learned preference to avoid physical activities. Further management of children with oligoarthritis who continue to have active arthritis after use of NSAIDs or intra-articular steroids depends upon a variety of diagnostic, prognostic, and therapeutic considerations. A percentage of such children go on to develop polyarticular disease, so-called extended pauciarthritis. They should be treated in the same way as children with polyarticular involvement from disease onset (see the section on Management of Polyarthritis). Risk factors for developing extended joint involvement include ankle and/or wrist arthritis, systemic inflammation on laboratory studies, and symmetric synovitis at disease onset.[14] Sedimentation rates that are significantly elevated at diagnosis should prompt evaluation for uveitis, inflammatory bowel disease, or concomitant infection, because most patients with isolated pauciarthritis generally do not have evidence of systemic inflammation, as illustrated in Case 1.

Once a patient has failed to respond completely to NSAIDs and intra-articular corticosteroid injections, consideration of a disease-modifying antirheumatic drug (DMARD) is warranted. Knees, hips, and wrists are particularly prone to debilitating complications with prolonged inflammation, so

Table 7-7. Selected NSAIDs used in the Treatment of Juvenile Rheumatoid Arthritis

Drug	Dose (mg/kg/day)	Doses per day	Maximum dose/day
Ibuprofen	30–40	3–4	2400
Naprosyn	10–20	2	1000
Meloxicam	0.25	1	15
Piroxicam	0.2–0.3	1	20
Indomethacin	1.5–3.0	3	200
Tolmetin	20–30	3–4	1800
Celecoxib	10–25 kg: 50 mg/dose	2	100
	> 25 kg: 100 mg/dose	2	200
	> 40 kg: 200 mg/dose	2	400

Table 7-8. Relative Toxicities of Nonsteroidal Anti-Inflammatory Drugs

Toxicity	Ibuprofen	Naprosyn	Indomethacin	Tolmetin
GI irritation	+	++	+++	++
Peptic ulcer	+	++	++	+
Hepatitis	+	+	+	?
Asthma	+	+	+	+
CNS	±	+	+++	+

+, rare; ++, occasional; +++, common; CNS, central nervous system; GI, gastrointestinal.
Adapted from Cassidy P, Petty R. Textbook of pediatric rheumatology. 5th ed. Philadelphia: Elsevier; 2005.

DMARDs should be started earlier in children with such involvement, even when they are asymptomatic. Involvement of ankles, on the other hand, may persist for months or years without leading to significant chronic changes. Thus, practitioners take into account a child's age, the severity of the inflammation, and the speed with which control must be achieved, when choosing among disease-modifying agents.

Sulfasalazine is most often used in children with inflammatory bowel disease or a spondyloarthropathy. It has been used to treat arthritis for more than 70 years, so unexpected side effects are rare. Nonetheless, sulfasalazine does not halt erosive disease, so it is most appropriately used in milder cases of JRA, particularly oligoarticular disease. Sulfasalazine is administered at a dose of 40 to 70 mg/kg/day divided bid or tid. Headache and gastrointestinal upset—especially with preparations that are not enteric coated—are the most common side effects. More severe toxicity is common to the family of sulfa drugs, including bone marrow suppression, agranulocytosis, photosensitive eruptions, and hypersensitivity reactions such as Stevens-Johnson syndrome. Sulfasalazine is contraindicated in children with known intolerance of sulfa drugs, as well as in children younger than 2 years of age, in whom neurotoxicity may occur. Finally, children with systemic onset JRA should not be treated with sulfasalazine, because use of this medication can precipitate macrophage activation syndrome and other severe complications.[15,16]

TREATMENT OF JUVENILE ARTHRITIS: UVEITIS

The risk of uveitis in children with JRA requires special emphasis. Ocular inflammation may occur independent of the activity of articular disease, and without appropriate monitoring and treatment, this condition can have devastating effects.[17,18] Therefore, regular ophthalmologic screening with slit lamp examinations and aggressive therapy of uveitis once it is detected are of utmost importance in the care of children with arthritis. This is particularly true in cases of ANA-positive pauciarticular JRA, in whom the lifetime risk of developing uveitis may approach 90%. The American Academy of Pediatrics has published guidelines on screening for uveitis in arthritis patients that takes into account the age of the child, the child's ANA status, and the subtype of JRA (Table 7-9).[19]

Although DMARDs and biologic response modifiers may decrease the likelihood of developing uveitis, failsafe prevention is not available. Consequently, current recommendations emphasize diagnosis and treatment of uveitis before the development of irreversible complications such as cataracts, synechiae, glaucoma, band keratopathy, macular edema, and visual loss. Of the approximately one quarter of

Table 7-9. Guidelines for Screening of Uveitis from the American Academy of Pediatrics

Age and Serology Status	Disease Duration	Eye Examination
Age at Onset < 6 years, +ANA	Duration of disease ≤ 4 years	Every 3 months
	Duration of disease > 4 years	Every 6 months
	Duration of disease >7 years	Every 12 months
Age at Onset > 6 years, +ANA	Duration of disease ≤ 4 years	Every 6 months
	Duration of disease > 4 years	Every 12 months
Age at Onset < 6 years, −ANA	Duration of disease ≤ 4 years	Every 6 months
	Duration of disease > 4 years	Every 12 months
Age at Onset > 6 years, −ANA		Every 12 months

ANA, antinuclear antibody.

patients with pauciarthritis who develop uveitis, up to 50% have complications.[20,21] Ophthalmologic treatment begins with topical steroids and mydriatics. Should inflammation in the eye persist, methotrexate should be added.[22,23] The poor outcome of children with persistent uveitis has led to trials of tumor necrosis factor inhibitors for treatment of refractory uveitis. Monoclonal antibodies against TNF (i.e., infliximab and adalimumab) are generally efficacious,[24-26] whereas the TNF receptor antagonist etanercept appears to be less effective.[27,28] When ocular inflammation persists despite use of these agents, recent case reports suggest that mycophenolate mofetil, rituximab and abatacept may be effective in at least some cases.[29-32] Regardless of the medications chosen, successful management of persistent uveitis relies on a close collaboration between rheumatologist and ophthalmologist.

CASE 2

A 12-year-old girl presents to the rheumatology clinic with 2 months of increasing joint pain and swelling. She began having difficulty writing and typing at the start of the school year and at about the same time noted the gradual development of stiffness and swelling in the small joints of her hands, then in her knees and ankles. Recently, she has been asking to skip her weekly dance class because the movements are painful. She takes ibuprofen intermittently, with some relief. She has not had fevers or rashes. Her bowel movements have been normal and without blood. She denies mouth sores, hair loss, Raynaud's phenomenon, photosensitivity, hematuria, and sicca symptoms. She has been feeling less energetic for the past several weeks, at times having to nap after getting home from school. Her appetite has decreased as well, and her jeans now fit more loosely. She has no other medical problems and takes no regular medications. Her family history is negative for autoimmune or rheumatologic diseases.

On examination, the young lady is thin and anxious appearing. Her weight is at the 10th percentile and her height is in the 25th percentile. She is afebrile. Pertinent negative findings include no rashes, normal nailbed capillaries, and a benign abdomen without tenderness, masses or hepatosplenomegaly. Her extremities are warm and well perfused. Musculoskeletal examination is notable for symmetric swelling and tenderness of the wrists, 2nd and 3rd metacarpophalangeal (MCP) joints, and 1st through 4th proximal interphalangeal (PIP) joints bilaterally. Range of motion is restricted by pain. Her elbows are tender and full and are held in 15 degrees of flexion with only 60 degrees of extension. Her shoulders move normally, although there is mild acromioclavicular tenderness. Her temporomandibular joints move well and her interincisor gap is 4.0 cm. Her neck rotates normally but has decreased extension and is tender posteriorly. On lower extremity examination, she has swelling and pain in her bilateral ankles and knees with decreased range of motion. MTP joints are slightly swollen and tender to palpation. She does not have enthesitis or dactylitis. Her hips have full painless range of motion. Examination of her spine is also unremarkable, including a normal modified Schober test.

Laboratory studies include normal white blood cell counts, a mild normocytic anemia with a hematocrit of 33%, and a minimal thrombocytosis (476×10^9/L). Her sedimentation rate is 52 mm/hour and C-reactive protein (CRP) is 4.3 mg/dL. ANA is negative; RF is positive at a titer of 21 IU/mL and antibodies to cyclic citrullinated peptide are positive.

DIFFERENTIAL DIAGNOSIS OF POLYARTHRITIS

The differential diagnosis of a child with polyarthritis, defined as inflammation of more than four joints, includes infectious and postinfectious entities as well as other rheumatologic conditions (Table 7-10). Septic arthritis in immunocompetent children very rarely involves multiple joints apart from rare infections with salmonella or *Neisseria gonorrhoeae*. In one of the largest series of septic arthritis in children, Fink and associates[3] reported that only one of

Table 7-10. *Differential Diagnosis of Polyarthritis in Children*

Infectious Arthritis
Bacteria
  Borrelia burgdorferi
  Tuberculosis (Poncet's disease)
  Neisseria gonorrhoeae
  Mycoplasma pneumoniae
  Bartonella henselae
Viruses
  Parvovirus
  Human immunodeficiency virus
  Rubella

Postinfectious Arthritis
  Acute rheumatic fever
  Campylobacter

Inflammatory Arthritis
Polyarthritis
  Rheumatoid factor positive
  Rheumatoid factor negative
Oligoarthritis, extended
Systemic lupus erythematosus
Systemic juvenile rheumatoid arthritis
Psoriatic arthritis
Minocycline-induced autoimmunity with polyarthritis
Inflammatory bowel disease–related arthritis
Celiac-related arthritis
Enthesitis-related arthritis

every 20 cases involved four joints compared with 93.4% having a single infected joint. Viral arthritis, on the other hand, is more similar to polyarticular JRA and commonly involves multiple joints including the small joints of the hands. In fact, up to 5% of cases of arthritis due to parvovirus or rubella go on to have a chronic arthropathy indistinguishable from rheumatoid arthritis. Some forms of reactive arthritis, specifically *Campylobacter*-related arthropathy, can involve multiple joints. Acute rheumatic fever is also characterized by polyarthritis, but joints typically become involved in an additive or migratory fashion and the inflamed joints are characteristically more painful than those of JRA.

Rheumatologic processes other than JRA tend to be distinguishable on the basis of associated systemic features. Children with systemic lupus erythematosus commonly present with rashes, nephritis, and cytopenias, and they often have abnormal nailbed capillaries on examination. The condition is common enough that testing for autoantibodies to nuclear antigens, double-stranded DNA, and extractable nuclear antigens should be considered in adolescents, particularly girls, presenting with polyarthritis. Systemic JRA can present in children of any age and the arthritis has a distribution similar to that of polyarticular JRA. However, by definition patients have associated systemic features including a salmon pink evanescent rash, double quotidian fevers, diffuse lymphadenopathy, hepatosplenomegaly, and pericarditis. Patients with psoriatic arthritis tend to have large and small joint involvement that is asymmetric as compared with the symmetry of polyarticular JRA. Less commonly, polyarteritis nodosa, dermatomyositis, and sarcoidosis may present as polyarthritis. Associated findings of abnormal pulses, a livedo reticularis rash, muscle weakness, or sicca symptoms should alert the clinician to consider these rarer entities.

Minocycline, most commonly prescribed to treat acne, may trigger autoimmune phenomena including arthritis, hepatitis and vasculitis. Although multiple joints may be involved, the degree of discomfort tends to be more marked than in JRA.[9] Patients with occult or confirmed inflammatory bowel disease can present with a polyarthritis that tends to reflect the activity of the gastrointestinal disease. Isolated or multiple joints may be involved in a symmetric or asymmetric pattern, so any child with arthritis and evidence of systemic inflammation or poor growth should be screened for inflammatory bowel disease. Enthesitis-related arthritis is also on the differential of patients with polyarthritis; as its name indicates, enthesitis in addition to arthritis is found on exam.

TREATMENT OF JUVENILE ARTHRITIS: POLYARTHRITIS

Treatment of patients with polyarticular disease, as well as severe cases of oligoarthritis, usually involves more potent anti-inflammatory agents. NSAIDs may be used for relief of stiffness and pain, but they are rarely, if ever, adequate for disease control and do not prevent joint damage. As in adult inflammatory arthritis, methotrexate is typically the first DMARD considered for treating severe or erosive arthritis in children. Its use has been evaluated in juvenile arthritis,[33] including both extended oligoarthritis[34] and polyarticular disease.[35-39] Dosing is usually 10 to 15 mg/m² body surface area per week (Table 7-11); higher doses have not been shown to be more effective.[37] The subcutaneous route is preferred for improved absorption as compared with oral administration, particularly at doses greater than 0.5 mg/kg). However, weekly injections can be problematic for young children. Use of numbing creams such as lidocaine/prilocaine preparations may provide some relief. Nonetheless, anticipatory anxiety can become a significant issue and may necessitate a change in the medication regimen. Nausea and abdominal pain are more pronounced side effects when methotrexate is taken orally. Increased dosing of folic acid or concurrent administration of a histamine type 2 blocker such as ranitidine may be helpful in alleviating these symptoms.

Laboratory studies to screen for hepatotoxicity and bone marrow suppression should be performed within the first month of therapy, then every 2 to 4 months once the child is receiving a stable dose. Adjustments in the dose are warranted if even minor hepatic abnormalities are detected. Conversely, studies of liver biopsies in children receiving up to 8 years of treatment with methotrexate suggest that as long as the aspartate aminotransferase (AST) and alanine aminotransferase (ALT) remain normal, occult hepatotoxicty does not appear to be a concern.[40-43] However, the number of patients enrolled in these studies was small and other reports have highlighted the presence of hepatic fibrosis in patients treated with methotrexate.[44] Overall, the risk of serious toxicity from methotrexate appears to be less in children than in adults, possibly because children are not exposed to other toxins such as alcohol or cigarettes. Thus, there is only a single case report of a pediatric patient with JRA who developed pneumonitis while being treated with methotrexate.[45] Nonetheless, adolescents taking methotrexate need to be apprised of the risks of life-threatening liver toxicity when combined with alcohol ingestion, as well as potential detrimental effects that methotrexate may have on a fetus.

Leflunomide, a pyrimidine synthesis inhibitor, appears to be similar to methotrexate in mechanism of action, but its administration as a daily oral tablet at a dose of 5 to 20 mg/day (see Table 7-11) may be preferable. The risk profile is also similar to methotrexate, and includes gastrointestinal upset, hepatotoxicity, hematologic toxicity, and teratogenicity. Studies of the use of leflunomide in patients with JRA by Silverman and coworkers[46] have generally been positive. An open-label trial revealed that the majority of patients who had failed or become intolerant of methotrexate achieved an ACR Pedi 30[47] (Table 7-12) when taking leflunomide. Leflunomide was then compared directly to methotrexate in a blinded, randomized controlled trial.[48] Both medications provided good disease control, because the majority of patients in both groups achieved an ACR Pedi 30 at 4 months. Methotrexate was more effective than leflunomide, although it was more frequently associated with elevations of transaminases. Both findings may be related to the fact that dosing of leflunomide in the study was proportionally lower than that of methotrexate. Another consideration in prescribing leflunomide is its persistence in the circulation and tissues, posing concerns of teratogenicity for months or years after the medication is stopped. Some clinicians require documentation of effective contraception before prescribing leflunomide to adolescent females. In cases in which pregnancy does occur, cholestyramine can be used for more rapid elimination of the drug but there are no data that this decreases fetal risk. Fortunately, despite these concerns, the number of documented cases of leflunomide fetopathy is small.

Other immunosuppressive agents, including azathioprine[49] and cyclosporine,[50] have been used for treating refractory childhood arthritis. For the most part, they no longer have a role unless biologic agents are contraindicated or unavailable. Azathioprine can be started at a dose of 1 mg/kg/day with slow escalation after 6 to 8 weeks in increments of 0.5 mg/kg/day to a maximum dose of 2.5 mg/kg/day (see Table 7-11). Patients taking azathioprine

Table 7-11. *Advanced Medications for the Treatment of Polyarthritis in Children*

	Mechanism of Action	Dose	Principal Toxicities	Monitor
DMARDs				
Methotrexate	Block folate metabolism and purine synthesis Increase adenosine levels (anti-inflammatory mediator)	25–30 mg/m² qwk PO/SQ/IV, escalate as tolerated	Hepatitis, nausea, oral ulcers, bone marrow suppression, pneumonitis (rare in children)	LFTs q2–4 mo, periodic CBCs; folate can limit GI and hematologic toxicity.
Hydroxy-chloroquine	? block lysosome antigen processing	<7.0 mg/kg/d PO, max 400 mg daily, divided qd-bid	Retinopathy, nausea, rash, agranulocytosis	Ophthalmology eval q6 mo, CBC, LFTs q3–6 mo
Sulfasalazine	? increase adenosine levels	Goal 40–70 mg/kg/d PO divided bid-tid, max 3 g daily, start slowly	Rash, nausea, leukopenia, hepatitis, headache/CNS, Stevens-Johnson syndrome	CBC + LFTs q month × 3–4 months, then periodically
Leflunomide	Block pyrimidine synthesis	< 20 kg: 5 mg qD; adult: 10–20 mg qD	Diarrhea, hepatitis, bone marrow suppression, alopecia/rash	LFTs q month until stable, then q2–3 mo
Biologic Response Modifiers				
Etanercept	TNF-α and lymphotoxin receptor antagonist	0.4 mg/kg SQ 2/wk, max 25 mg 2/wk	Injection site reactions, infections, cytopenias, CNS demyelination, ? malignancies	CBC, LFTs, document negative TB status before use
Infliximab	Chimeric anti-TNF monoclonal antibody	3–5 mg/kg IV q6–8 wk	Hypersensitivity, infections (esp. reactivation TB), hepatic necrosis, cytopenias, ? malignancies	CBC, LFTs, document negative TB status before use; use with low-dose MTX to inhibit antibodies against drug.
Adalimumab	Humanized anti-TNF monoclonal antibody	20 mg SQ q 2 wk (15–30 kg); 40 mg SQ q 2 wk (>30 kg)	Infections, injection site pain, cytopenias, ? malignancies	CBC, LFTs, document negative TB status before use
Abatacept	Anti-CTLA4 Ig (T-cell costimulatory inhibitor)	10 mg/kg IV q 4 wk to maximum of 750 mg	Hypersensitivity, infections, ? malignancies	Hepatitis panel, PPD at baseline
Immunosuppressive Agents				
Azathioprine	Active metabolite 6-MP blocks purine synthesis	1–2.5 mg/kg/d PO qD	Bone marrow suppression, infection (esp. zoster), nausea, hepatitis, rash	CBC, LFTs
Cyclosporine A	Block synthesis of IL-2 and other cytokines by inhibiting calcineurin	1–3 mg/kg/d PO divided bid	Hypertension, nephrotoxicity, hyperlipidemia, diabetes, tremor, seizures, gingival hyperplasia, hirsutism, skin cancer, lymphoma	Blood pressure, U/A, CBC, BUN/Cr, glucose, LFTs, K, Mg (not CsA levels) q2 wk × 3 mo then q2–3 mo; *multiple drug interactions*.

BUN, blood urea nitrogen; CBC, complete blood count; CNS, central nervous system; Cr, creatinine; CsA, cyclosporine A; CTLA, cytotoxic T lymphocyte antigen 4; DMARDs, disease-modifying antirheumatic drugs; GI, gastrointestinal; IL-2, interleukin-2; LFTs, liver function tests; MP, mercaptopurine; MTX, methotrexate; TB, tuberculosis; TNF, tumor necrosis factor.

Table 7-12. *Core Set Criteria for Improvement in Juvenile Idiopathic Arthritis*

Number of active joints
Number of joints with loss of motion
Physician's Global Assessment
Parent's Global Assessment
Childhood Health Assessment Questionnaire
Erythrocyte sedimentation rate

Patients must have at least a 30% improvement in 3/6 items and a worsening of 30% in no more than 1 item to achieve an ACR Pedi 30. ACR Pedi 50 and 70 require a 50% or 70% improvement in 3/6 items with worsening of 30% in no more than 1 item.

may experience gastrointestinal upset, hepatotoxicity or hematologic toxicity. Patients with decreased activity of thiopurine methyl transferase may develop severe marrow suppression while taking azathioprine; genetic testing for enzymatic activity can be performed before starting therapy. The dosing of cyclosporine is 1 to 3 mg/kg/day (see Table 7-11). Side effects include hirsutism and headaches. Additionally, monitoring for hepatotoxicity, nephrotoxicity, hematologic toxicity, and hypertension is an important part of ongoing care in patients who take cyclosporine.

Tumor necrosis factor-α (TNF-α) inhibitors are revolutionizing the care of adults with rheumatoid arthritis.[51] Effects on juvenile arthritis are similarly promising, although definitive pediatric trials have been slowed by concerns about use of parenteral placebos in children.

Etanercept was the first TNF inhibitor approved for clinical use, and it is the most thoroughly studied in children. Coincident with early trials in adults, the first study of etanercept in children illustrated both efficacy, with nearly 75% of patients achieving an ACR Pedi 30 after three months of treatment, and safety, because adverse events did not differ significantly between the treatment and placebo groups.[52] Follow-up studies showed that improvements were durable with etanercept, and patients taking prednisolone were able to taper their steroid dose. Serious bacterial infections were slightly increased, occurring at a rate of 0.04 per patient-year with a total etanercept exposure of 225 patient-years.[53,54] However, it is important to note that this cohort of patients has been followed for only 8 years, making estimates of long-term safety difficult. The dosing of etanercept is usually 0.4 mg/kg/dose given subcutaneously twice weekly. Some practitioners give a single weekly dose of 0.8 mg/kg/week, with a maximum dose of 50 mg/week. Etanercept is approved by the US Food and Drug Administration (FDA) for use in juvenile arthritis in children older than 2 years of age.

Adalimumab also has been approved by the FDA for use in children older than four years of age with moderately to severely active polyarticular juvenile arthritis. Adalimumab was evaluated in a large trial of 171 children with active polyarthritis; the population was stratified according to methotrexate use.[55] Following a 16-week open-label phase, patients receiving adalimumab were less likely to have a disease flare as compared with patients receiving placebo, regardless of methotrexate use. Dosing of adalimumab is based on weight: 20 mg subcutaneously every other week in children from 15 to 30 kg, and 40 mg subcutaneously every other week in children weighing more than 30 kg.

The other TNF inhibitor effective in adult rheumatoid arthritis, infliximab, is not approved for use in children. Ruperto and colleagues[56] studied infliximab in combination with methotrexate in a withdrawal trial in 122 children. The infliximab group did not achieve improved outcomes when compared with placebo, and the children receiving the TNF inhibitor had a higher rate of adverse events. Nonetheless, many smaller case series support the impression of most pediatric rheumatologists that infliximab is a useful tool in treating recalcitrant juvenile arthritis, particularly in conjunction with methotrexate. Dosing of infliximab is usually 3 to 5 mg/kg intravenously every 4 to 6 weeks following loading doses at 0, 2, and 6 weeks.

Just as lack of efficacy of one TNF-α inhibitor in treating adult RA does not preclude effectiveness of other members of this drug class, so, too, children might do better on one TNF inhibitor than another. Infliximab is associated with human anti-chimeric antibodies (HACAs) that can lead to anaphylactic reactions as well as decreased efficacy.[57] Patients who develop HACAs with infliximab may be treated with either adalimumab or etanercept, because both are fully humanized molecules. Similarly, a study by Radstake and associates[58] found that clinical responses to infliximab and adalimumab are related to both trough levels of the drugs as well as to the presence of antibodies to the medications. Thus, patients who fail one agent may respond well to a different member of the TNF-α inhibitor family.

The most significant risk common to all TNF inhibitors is an increased frequency and severity of infections, especially reactivation or dissemination of tuberculosis. This immunosuppressive effect is most commonly manifested by somewhat more persistent viral upper respiratory infections; however, occasional serious bacterial infections can occur. Children who take TNF inhibitors should be evaluated by a physician if they have a temperature greater than 101.5° F without a clear source. Lastly, the FDA has recently added a warning to all TNF inhibitors regarding the risk of unrecognized invasive fungal infections and the dangers of these infections if therapy with TNF antagonists is continued.

TNF inhibitors block a molecule important for immune surveillance, and concern about a possible increase in malignancies with use of these medications dates back to the earliest days of their development. This subject has been studied in adults,[59,60] but there are far fewer data for children. In 2005, the first case of hepatosplenic lymphoma in an adolescent patient treated with infliximab and 6-mercaptopurine was published.[61] Since then, postmarketing surveillance of infliximab has revealed other cases of hepatosplenic lymphoma, a rare but usually fatal form of non-Hodgkin's lymphoma.[62] In 2008, the FDA launched an Ongoing Safety Review to evaluate the use of TNF-α inhibitors in children following MedWatch reports of 30 cases of malignancies in children prescribed TNF-α inhibitors. These cases included children with a wide variety of conditions in addition to JRA, receiving a broad spectrum of concurrent medications, so no conclusions are possible. Nonetheless, caution is appropriate when prescribing TNF inhibitors to children. The potentially serious risks of such therapy should be extensively discussed with families and deemed to be warranted. Even as the Safety Review is ongoing, the FDA's statement acknowledges that: "At the current time, the FDA believes that the potential benefits of the use of TNF blockers outweigh the potential risks in certain children and young adults having one of the diseases for which the TNF blockers are approved to treat."[63]

The biologic agent most recently approved by the FDA for children aged 6 years and older with severe polyarthritis is abatacept, a CTLA-4 antagonist that interferes with costimulation of T lymphocytes. The pivotal pediatric study enrolled nearly 200 children with polyarthritis who had failed at least one DMARD.[64] After an open-label lead in of 4 months, patients were randomized to receive monthly infusions of active drug or placebo. Children who received abatacept at a dose of 10 mg/kg experienced fewer disease flares compared with those receiving placebo. Additionally, there was no significant difference in adverse events between the treatment and placebo groups. Use of this agent is limited to date, and longer term studies are needed to clarify its safety and efficacy in childhood arthritis.

Rituximab, an anti-CD20 agent that has been approved for use in adult rheumatoid arthritis, has been little studied in children. Personal communications among pediatric rheumatologists suggest a role for rituximab in treatment of seropositive polyarticular JRA. Similarly, there is anecdotal evidence that rituximab is effective in recalcitrant uveitis. For example, one single case report describes a 26-year-old woman with a history of juvenile arthritis resistant to multiple other therapies since 8 years of age. She had remittance of disease with B-cell depletion via rituximab.[65] Although this agent appears to have promise, more studies are needed before its potential role in childhood inflammatory diseases can be defined. Caution using rituximab off label is supported by recent reports of patients developing progressive multifocal leukoencephalopathy after receiving rituximab.

Corticosteroids have a long history in the treatment of juvenile arthritis. Use of intra-articular injections is discussed earlier. Patients with polyarthritis occasionally require systemic steroids to achieve rapid relief of disabling symptoms while waiting for longer acting agents, such as methotrexate, to take effect. Evidence in the adult population that early treatment of inflammatory arthritis with corticosteroids may lead to improved outcomes,[66,67] has led to an ongoing trial of early aggressive therapy, including corticosteroids, in children with polyarthritis. The deleterious effects of long-term exposure to corticosteroids in childhood are well documented and include growth retardation, hypertension, cataracts, and excessive weight gain with its concomitant morbidity. Thus, corticosteroids must be used judiciously; doses less than 0.20 mg/kg/day have fewer side effects and allow for at least some growth while providing potent anti-inflammatory activity.

CASE 3

A 16-month-old girl presents to her pediatrician's office with diffuse rash and fever. Her mother reports that the rash began on her trunk about a week ago, but appears on her arms, legs, trunk, and face intermittently over the course of the day. The rash is composed of large, red blotches. It does not appear to be pruritic or painful, and is more prominent when the girl has a fever. Her mother also has noted daily temperatures for the past 2 weeks that are typically in the 102° to 103° F range. The fevers tend to improve with ibuprofen, and between fevers she behaves almost normally. The child had one episode of nonbloody, nonbilious emesis, but has not had other localizing signs such as rhinorrhea, nasal congestion, or cough. Her mother notes that she has been quite irritable, and although she has been walking since the age of 13 months, she now often asks to be carried.

The patient was the product of a full-term gestation and uneventful delivery. Previously she has been well without medical problems. Her only medications include ibuprofen and acetaminophen on an as-needed basis for the fevers. She has received all of her immunizations to date. Her family history is negative for autoimmune or inflammatory disorders.

On examination, she is a fussy child. She has a temperature of 39.5° C and is mildly tachycardic, but the remainder of her vital signs are normal. Her weight is 9.8 kg (50th percentile for age) and her height is 77 cm (25th percentile for age). On skin examination, she has erythematous papules 1 to 4 cm in diameter on her trunk. Her heart examination is significant for tachycardia but no rub or gallop. A liver edge is palpable just beneath the costal margin. Splenomegaly is not detected. Musculoskeletal examination is remarkable for fullness and limited range of motion in her left wrist. Additionally, she has small effusions in her knees bilaterally. Her right ankle is significantly swollen, tender and has a limited range of motion. The remainder of her exam is normal.

Laboratory studies demonstrate leukocytosis with a white blood cell count of 19,000 cells/µL, anemia with hemoglobin of 7.8 g/dL, and thrombocytosis with platelets of 670×10^9/L. A sedimentation rate is 98 mm/hour. Her CRP is 4.5 mg/dL. Mild transaminitis is noted with an ALT of 45 units/L and an AST of 60 units/L. A ferritin is elevated at 4150 ng/mL. Her triglycerides and coagulation studies are normal.

TREATMENT OF JUVENILE ARTHRITIS: SYSTEMIC ONSET DISEASE

The polyarthritis associated with systemic onset JRA (SoJRA) may have a different pathogenesis than other forms of juvenile inflammatory arthritis[68] and may require a different therapeutic approach. SoJRA is more likely to be in the spectrum of autoinflammatory diseases, such as familial Mediterranean fever or other cryopyrin-associated periodic syndromes, a theory supported by the finding of an increased frequency of MEFV alleles in a small study of patients with SoJRA.[69] The spectrum of SoJRA can vary from mild disease that responds to NSAIDs to life-threatening illness with macrophage activation syndrome. Mortality among children with JRA is largely limited to this subtype, so patients with moderate to severe SoJRA should be referred to a pediatric rheumatologist with experience in managing these difficult patients.

SoJRA is defined as arthritis in children younger than 16 years of age accompanied by daily fevers of at least 2 weeks' duration and one or more of the following: evanescent erythematous rash, generalized lymphadenopathy, or hepatosplenomegaly. Commonly encountered laboratory findings include leukocytosis, anemia, and elevated inflammatory markers. SoJRA affects boys and girls equally and may have its onset in children of any age; overall, it accounts for no more than 10% of cases of JRA. Other more common entities such as infection or malignancy must be excluded before confirming the diagnosis and initiating therapy.

As with other forms of juvenile arthritis, NSAIDs are useful for relief of pain and stiffness in patients with SoJRA. In most cases of SoJRA, these are inadequate for regaining of normal functioning, and patients generally require relatively rapid escalation of therapy. Corticosteroids have been the mainstay of treatment, traditionally given both orally and as intravenous boluses of 30 mg/kg in patients who have severe systemic symptoms. Until recently, most children had to remain on high doses of steroids for long periods of time, with predictably poor outcomes. Prognosis has improved with the addition of agents such as methotrexate,[70] other DMARDs, and finally biologic response modifiers.

TNF-α inhibitors have been used in SoJRA, but they are inconsistently helpful in decreasing disease activity.[71,72] Thalidomide has also been used effectively in patients with SoJRA.[73] The most commonly reported side effect of thalidomide is somnolence, which is avoided by administration at bedtime. Additionally, thalidomide's antiangiogenesis effects on the vasa nervorum can lead to a permanent peripheral neuropathy. This adverse side effect typically occurs at daily doses higher than 3 mg/kg and cumulative doses greater than 20 g.[74,75] Some practitioners obtain regular screening electromyography and nerve conduction studies because nerve damage initially can be subclinical; others rely on patient reports of neurologic symptoms. Development of a neuropathy necessitates cessation of treatment with thalidomide. In addition, prescribing of thalidomide is tightly controlled to ensure that the severe limb defects associated with thalidomide use during pregnancy in the 1960s are not allowed to recur.

Anakinra, a recombinant interleukin-1 (IL-1) receptor antagonist, has been studied in juvenile polyarthritis, with favorable results in children with SoJRA.[76-78] Reiff and colleagues[77] reported that 11 of 15 SoJRA patients had significant improvement with anakinra. In a study by Pascual and coworkers, seven of nine patients with SoJRA had an excellent response to IL-1 inhibition. However, the feasibility of using anakinra is limited by the fact that it is currently available only as a daily subcutaneous injection that causes significant burning and pain. Tocilizumab, an anti-IL-6 receptor antibody, has also been found effective in patients with SoJRA.[79] However, the drug has been delayed in its approval by the FDA; the company has been asked to conduct an animal study examining effects of the molecule on reproductive issues.

Macrophage activation syndrome is a life-threatening complication that occurs in 5% to 8% of patients with SoJRA.[68] It is heralded by the presence of high fevers, hepatosplenomegaly, evidence of disseminated intravascular coagulation, and neurologic symptoms. Laboratory studies reveal pancytopenia, a precipitous fall in the sedimentation rate due to consumption of fibrinogen, coagulopathy, triglyceridemia, and massively elevated levels of ferritin. Bone marrow aspiration reveals hemophagocytosis. Treatment is with pulsed doses of methylprednisolone and fresh frozen plasma to correct the coagulopathy. Cyclosporine may be used in refractory cases.

JUVENILE ARTHRITIS: PROGNOSIS

Before the development and appropriate use of DMARDs, children with inflammatory arthritis suffered from long-term disability and pain. Children with seropositive polyarthritis and SoJRA in particular frequently became wheelchair bound. Prospects for productive employment, successful marriage, and normal life expectancy were guarded. Fortunately, the prognosis has changed significantly during the past 20 years, first as a result of the introduction of methotrexate, and more recently with the development of biologic therapies. Wallace and coworkers[80] studied the outcomes of children with arthritis before the advent of biologic agents. The prognosis depended on the subtype of arthritis; patients with extended oligoarthritis were most likely to have inactive disease during most of their disease course. Children with other forms of inflammatory arthritis, on the other hand, seldom experienced drug-free remissions. Nonetheless, nearly 90% of patients were able to achieve inactive disease while on medications. Thus, despite the dramatic advances since treatment was limited to prednisone, aspirin, and bed rest little more than a half century ago, currently available therapies are not curative. Caregivers can realistically expect to achieve full disease control in most cases of JRA, but it is a respite dependent on continued use of maintenance medications. Still, discussions with families of children with inflammatory arthritis should focus on the fact that medical management of JRA is generally successful. More than ever before, the vast majority of children with arthritis should anticipate full, productive lives.

REFERENCES

1. Cassidy JT. What's in a name? Nomenclature of juvenile arthritis. A North American view. J Rheumatol Suppl 1993;40:4-8.
2. Schneider R, Passo MH. Juvenile rheumatoid arthritis. Rheum Dis Clin North Am 2002;28:503-30.
3. Fink CW, Nelson JD. Septic arthritis and osteomyelitis in children. Clin Rheum Dis 1986;12:423-35.
4. Cabral DA, Tucker LB. Malignancies in children who initially present with rheumatic complaints. J Pediatr 1999;134:53-7.
5. Goncalves M, Terreri MT, Barbosa CM, Len CA, Lee L, Hilario MO. Diagnosis of malignancies in children with musculoskeletal complaints. Sao Paulo Med J 2005;123:21-3.
6. Listernick R. A 2-year-old boy with fever and a limp. Pediatr Ann 2003;32:11-4.
7. Thapa R, Mallick D, Mandal P, Ghosh A. Neuroblastoma masquerading as juvenile idiopathic arthritis. Indian J Pediatr 2007;74:421-2.
8. Jones OY, Spencer CH, Bowyer SL, Dent PB, Gottlieb BS, Rabinovich CE. A multicenter case-control study on predictive factors distinguishing childhood leukemia from juvenile rheumatoid arthritis. Pediatrics 2006;117:e840-4.
9. El-Hallak M, Giani T, Yeniay BS, Jacobs KE, Kim S, Sundel RP, et al. Chronic minocycline-induced autoimmunity in children. J Pediatr 2008;153:314-9.
10. Celebrex Approved to Treat Juvenile Rheumatoid Arthritis. http://www.fda.gov/bbs/topics/NEWS/2006/NEW01530.html
11. Duffy CM, Gibbon M, Yang H, et al. Non-steroidal anti-inflammatory drug-induced central nervous system toxicity in a practice-based cohort of children with juvenile arthritis. J Rheumatol 2000;27(Suppl 58):73.
12. Padeh S, Passwell JH. Intraarticular corticosteroid injection in the management of children with chronic arthritis. Arthritis Rheum 1998;41:1210-4.
13. Sherry DD, Stein LD, Reed AM, Schanberg LE, Kredich DW. Prevention of leg length discrepancy in young children with pauciarticular juvenile rheumatoid arthritis by treatment with intraarticular steroids. Arthritis Rheum 1999;42:2330-4.
14. Al-Matar MJ, Petty RE, Tucker LB, Malleson PN, Schroeder ML, Cabral DA. The early pattern of joint involvement predicts disease progression in children with oligoarticular (pauciarticular) juvenile rheumatoid arthritis. Arthritis Rheum 2002;46:2708-15.
15. Jung JH, Jun JB, Yoo DH, Kim TH, Jung SS, Lee IH, et al. High toxicity of sulfasalazine in adult-onset Still's disease. Clin Exp Rheumatol 2000;18:245-8.
16. Silva CA, Silva CH, Robazzi TC, Lotito AP, Mendroni Jr A, et al. [Macrophage activation syndrome associated with systemic juvenile idiopathic arthritis]. J Pediatr (Rio J) 2004;80:517-22.
17. Reiff A. Ocular complications of childhood rheumatic diseases: uveitis. Curr Rheumatol Rep 2006;8:459-68.
18. Petty RE, Smith JR, Rosenbaum JT. Arthritis and uveitis in children. A pediatric rheumatology perspective. Am J Ophthalmol 2003;135:879-84.
19. American Academy of Pediatrics Section on Rheumatology and Section on Ophthalmology. Guidelines for ophthalmologic examinations in children with juvenile rheumatoid arthritis. Pediatrics 1993;92:295-6.
20. Saurenmann RK, Levin AV, Feldman BM, Rose JB, Laxer RM, Schneider R, et al. Prevalence, risk factors, and outcome of uveitis in juvenile idiopathic arthritis: a long-term followup study. Arthritis Rheum 2007;56:647-57.
21. Heiligenhaus A, Niewerth M, Ganser G, Heinz C, Minden K. Prevalence and complications of uveitis in juvenile idiopathic arthritis in a population-based nation-wide study in Germany: suggested modification of the current screening guidelines. Rheumatology (Oxford) 2007;46:1015-9.
22. Heiligenhaus A, Mingels A, Heinz C, Ganser G. Methotrexate for uveitis associated with juvenile idiopathic arthritis: value and requirement for additional anti-inflammatory medication. Eur J Ophthalmol 2007;17:743-8.
23. Galor A, Jabs DA, Leder HA, Kedhar SR, Dunn JP, Peters 3rd GB, et al. Comparison of antimetabolite drugs as corticosteroid-sparing therapy for noninfectious ocular inflammation. Ophthalmology 2008;115:1826-32.
24. Richards JC, Tay-Kearney ML, Murray K, Manners P. Infliximab for juvenile idiopathic arthritis-associated uveitis. Clin Exp Ophthalmol 2005;33:461-8.
25. Tugal-Tutkun I, Mudun A, Urgancioglu M, Kamali S, Kasapoglu E, Inanc M, et al. Efficacy of infliximab in the treatment of uveitis that is resistant to treatment with the combination of azathioprine, cyclosporine, and corticosteroids in Behcet's disease: an open-label trial. Arthritis Rheum 2005;52:2478-84.
26. Vazquez-Cobian LB, Flynn T, Lehman TJ. Adalimumab therapy for childhood uveitis. J Pediatr 2006;149:572-5.
27. Saurenmann RK, Levin AV, Feldman BM, Laxer RM, Schneider R, Silverman ED. Risk of new-onset uveitis in patients with juvenile idiopathic arthritis treated with anti-TNFalpha agents. J Pediatr 2006;149:833-6.
28. Saurenmann RK, Levin AV, Rose JB, Parker S, Rabinovitch T, Tyrrell PN, et al. Tumour necrosis factor alpha inhibitors in the treatment of childhood uveitis. Rheumatology (Oxford) 2006;45:982-9.
29. Teoh SC, Hogan AC, Dick AD, Lee RW. Mycophenolate mofetil for the treatment of uveitis. Am J Ophthalmol 2008;146:752-60.
30. Thorne JE, Jabs DA, Qazi FA, Nguyen QD, Kempen JH, Dunn JP. Mycophenolate mofetil therapy for inflammatory eye disease. Ophthalmology 2005;112:1472-7.
31. Angeles-Han S, Flynn T, Lehman T. Abatacept for refractory juvenile idiopathic arthritis-associated uveitis—a case report. J Rheumatol 2008;35:1897-8.
32. Tappeiner C, Heinz C, Specker C, Heiligenhaus A. Rituximab as a treatment option for refractory endogenous anterior uveitis. Ophthalmic Res 2007;39:184-6.
33. Takken T, Van Der Net J, Helders PJ. Methotrexate for treating juvenile idiopathic arthritis. Cochrane Database Syst Rev 2001;(4):CD003129.
34. Woo P, Southwood TR, Prieur AM, Doré CJ, Grainger J, David J, et al. Randomized, placebo-controlled, crossover trial of low-dose oral methotrexate in children with extended oligoarticular or systemic arthritis. Arthritis Rheum 2000;43:1849-57.
35. Wallace CA, Bleyer WA, Sherry DD, Salmonson KL, Wedgwood RJ. Toxicity and serum levels of methotrexate in children with juvenile rheumatoid arthritis. Arthritis Rheum 1989;32:677-81.
36. Ravelli A, Martini A. Methotrexate in juvenile idiopathic arthritis: answers and questions. J Rheumatol 2000;27:1830-3.
37. Ruperto N, Murray KJ, Gerloni V, Wulffraat N, de Oliveira SK, Falcini F, et al. A randomized trial of parenteral methotrexate comparing an intermediate dose with a higher dose in children with juvenile idiopathic arthritis who failed to respond to standard doses of methotrexate. Arthritis Rheum 2004;50:2191-201.
38. Giannini EH, Brewer EJ, Kuzmina N, Shaikov A, Maximov A, Vorontsov I, et al. Methotrexate in resistant juvenile rheumatoid arthritis. Results of the U.S.A.-U.S.S.R. double-blind, placebo-controlled trial. The Pediatric Rheumatology Collaborative Study Group and The Cooperative Children's Study Group. N Engl J Med 1992;326:1043-9.
39. Giannini EH, Cassidy JT, Brewer EJ, Shaikov A, Maximov A, Kuzmina N. Comparative efficacy and safety of advanced drug therapy in children with juvenile rheumatoid arthritis. Semin Arthritis Rheum 1993;23:34-46.
40. Graham LD, Myones BL, Rivas-Chacon RF, Pachman LM. Morbidity associated with long-term methotrexate therapy in juvenile rheumatoid arthritis. J Pediatr 1992;120: 468-73.
41. Hashkes PJ, Balistreri WF, Bove KE, Ballard ET, Passo MH. The relationship of hepatotoxic risk factors and liver histology in methotrexate therapy for juvenile rheumatoid arthritis. J Pediatr 1999;134:47-52.
42. Hashkes PJ, Balistreri WF, Bove KE, Ballard ET, Passo MH. The long-term effect of methotrexate therapy on the liver in patients with juvenile rheumatoid arthritis. Arthritis Rheum 1997;40:2226-34.

43. Lahdenne P, Rapola J, Ylijoki H, Haapasaari J. Hepatotoxicity in patients with juvenile idiopathic arthritis receiving long-term methotrexate therapy. J Rheumatol 2002;29:2442-5.

44. Keim D, Ragsdale C, Heidelberger K, Sullivan D. Hepatic fibrosis with the use of methotrexate for juvenile rheumatoid arthritis. J Rheumatol 1990;17:846-8.

45. Cron RQ, Sherry DD, Wallace CA. Methotrexate-induced hypersensitivity pneumonitis in a child with juvenile rheumatoid arthritis. J Pediatr 1998;132:901-2.

46. Silverman E, Spiegel L, Hawkins D, Petty R, Goldsmith D, Schanberg L, et al. Long-term open-label preliminary study of the safety and efficacy of leflunomide in patients with polyarticular-course juvenile rheumatoid arthritis. Arthritis Rheum 2005;52:554-62.

47. Giannini EH, Ruperto N, Ravelli A, Lovell DJ, Felson DT, Martini A. Preliminary definition of improvement in juvenile arthritis. Arthritis Rheum 1997;40:1202-9.

48. Silverman E, Mouy R, Spiegel L, Jung LK, Saurenmann RK, Lahdenne P, et al. Leflunomide or methotrexate for juvenile rheumatoid arthritis. N Engl J Med 2005;352:1655-66.

49. Lin YT, Yang YH, Tsai MJ, Chiang BL. Long-term effects of azathioprine therapy for juvenile rheumatoid arthritis. J Formos Med Assoc 2000;99:330-5.

50. Ruperto N, Ravelli A, Castell E, Gerloni V, Haefner R, Malattia C, et al. Cyclosporine A in juvenile idiopathic arthritis. Results of the PRCSG/PRINTO phase IV post marketing surveillance study. Clin Exp Rheumatol 2006;24:599-605.

51. Valesini G, Iannuccelli C, Marocchi E, Pascoli L, Scalzi V, Di Franco M. Biological and clinical effects of anti-TNFalpha treatment. Autoimmun Rev 2007;7:35-41.

52. Lovell DJ, Giannini EH, Reiff A, Cawkwell GD, Silverman ED, Nocton JJ, et al. Etanercept in children with polyarticular juvenile rheumatoid arthritis. Pediatric Rheumatology Collaborative Study Group. N Engl J Med 2000;342:763-9.

53. Lovell DJ, Giannini EH, Reiff A, Jones OY, Schneider R, Olson JC, et al. Long-term efficacy and safety of etanercept in children with polyarticular-course juvenile rheumatoid arthritis: interim results from an ongoing multicenter, open-label, extended-treatment trial. Arthritis Rheum 2003;48:218-26.

54. Lovell DJ, Reiff A, Jones OY, Schneider R, Nocton J, Stein LD, et al. Long-term safety and efficacy of etanercept in children with polyarticular-course juvenile rheumatoid arthritis. Arthritis Rheum 2006;54:1987-94.

55. Lovell DJ, Ruperto N, Goodman S, Reiff A, Jung L, Jarosova K, et al. Adalimumab with or without methotrexate in juvenile rheumatoid arthritis. N Engl J Med 2008;359:810-20.

56. Ruperto N, Lovell DJ, Cuttica R, Wilkinson N, Woo P, Espada G, et al. A randomized, placebo-controlled trial of infliximab plus methotrexate for the treatment of polyarticular-course juvenile rheumatoid arthritis. Arthritis Rheum 2007;56:3096-106.

57. Miele E, Markowitz JE, Mamula P, Baldassano RN. Human antichimeric antibody in children and young adults with inflammatory bowel disease receiving infliximab. J Pediatr Gastroenterol Nutr 2004;38:502-8.

58. Radstake TR, Svenson M, Eijsbouts AM, van den Hoogen FH, Enevold C, van Riel PL, et al. Formation of antibodies against infliximab and adalimumab strongly correlates with functional drug levels and clinical responses in rheumatoid arthritis. Ann Rheum Dis Nov 19 2008 [epub ahead of print].

59. Askling J, Bongartz T. Malignancy and biologic therapy in rheumatoid arthritis. Curr Opin Rheumatol 2008;20:334-9.

60. Nasir A, Greenberg JD. TNF antagonist safety in rheumatoid arthritis: updated evidence from observational registries. Bull NYU Hosp Jt Dis 2007;65:178-81.

61. Thayu M, Markowitz JE, Mamula P, Russo PA, Muinos WI, Baldassano RN. Hepatosplenic T-cell lymphoma in an adolescent patient after immunomodulator and biologic therapy for Crohn disease. J Pediatr Gastroenterol Nutr 2005;40:220-2.

62. Rosh JR, Gross T, Mamula P, Griffiths A, Hyams J. Hepatosplenic T-cell lymphoma in adolescents and young adults with Crohn's disease: a cautionary tale? Inflamm Bowel Dis 2007;13:1024-30.

63. Early communication about an ongoing Safety Review of Tumor Necrosis Factor (TNF) blockers. http://www.fda.gov/cder/drug/early_comm/TNF_blockers.htm

64. Ruperto N, Lovell DJ, Quartier P, Paz E, Rubio-Pérez N, Silva CA, et al. Abatacept in children with juvenile idiopathic arthritis: a randomised, double-blind, placebo-controlled withdrawal trial. Lancet 2008;372:383-91.

65. Kuek A, Hazleman BL, Gaston JH, Ostor AJ. Successful treatment of refractory polyarticular juvenile idiopathic arthritis with rituximab. Rheumatology (Oxford) 2006;45:1448-9.

66. Boers M. Understanding the window of opportunity concept in early rheumatoid arthritis. Arthritis Rheum 2003;48:1771-4.

67. Svensson B, Boonen A, Albertsson K, van der Heijde D, Keller C, Hafstrom I. Low-dose prednisolone in addition to the initial disease-modifying antirheumatic drug in patients with early active rheumatoid arthritis reduces joint destruction and increases the remission rate: a two-year randomized trial. Arthritis Rheum 2005;52:3360-70.

68. Ravelli A, Martini A. Juvenile idiopathic arthritis. Lancet 2007;369:767-78.

69. Ayaz NA, Ozen S, Bilginer Y, Ergüven M, Takiran E, Yilmaz E, et al. MEFV mutations in systemic onset juvenile idiopathic arthritis. Rheumatology (Oxford) 2009;48:23-5.

70. Wallace CA. The use of methotrexate in childhood rheumatic diseases. Arthritis Rheum 1998;41:381-91.

71. Kietz DA, Pepmueller PH, Moore TL. Clinical response to etanercept in polyarticular course juvenile rheumatoid arthritis. J Rheumatol 2001;28:360-2.

72. Takei S, Groh D, Bernstein B, Shaham B, Gallagher K, Reiff A. Safety and efficacy of high dose etanercept in treatment of juvenile rheumatoid arthritis. J Rheumatol 2001;28:1677-80.

73. Lehman TJ, Schechter SJ, Sundel RP, Oliveira SK, Huttenlocher A, Onel KB. Thalidomide for severe systemic onset juvenile rheumatoid arthritis: A multicenter study. J Pediatr 2004;145:856-7.

74. Zara G, Ermani M, Rondinone R, Arienti S, Doria A. Thalidomide and sensory neurotoxicity: a neurophysiological study. J Neurol Neurosurg Psychiatry 2008;79:1258-61.

75. Priolo T, Lamba LD, Giribaldi G, De Negri E, Grosso P, De Grandis E, et al. Childhood thalidomide neuropathy: a clinical and neurophysiologic study. Pediatr Neurol 2008;38:196-9.

76. Ilowite N, Porras O, Reiff A, Rudge S, Punaro M, Martin A, et al. Anakinra in the treatment of polyarticular-course juvenile rheumatoid arthritis: safety and preliminary efficacy results of a randomized multicenter study. Clin Rheumatol 2009;28:129-37.

77. Reiff A. The use of anakinra in juvenile arthritis. Curr Rheumatol Rep 2005;7:434-40.

78. Pascual V, Allantaz F, Arce E, Punaro M, Banchereau J. Role of interleukin-1 (IL-1) in the pathogenesis of systemic onset juvenile idiopathic arthritis and clinical response to IL-1 blockade. J Exp Med 2005;201:1479-86.

79. Yokota S, Imagawa T, Mori M, Miyamae T, Aihara Y, Takei S, et al. Efficacy and safety of tocilizumab in patients with systemic-onset juvenile idiopathic arthritis: a randomised, double-blind, placebo-controlled, withdrawal phase III trial. Lancet 2008;371:998-1006.

80. Wallace CA, Huang B, Bandeira M, Ravelli A, Giannini EH. Patterns of clinical remission in select categories of juvenile idiopathic arthritis. Arthritis Rheum 2005;52:3554-62.

Chapter 8

Principles in Management of Systemic Lupus Erythematosus

Hiok Hee Chng

INTRODUCTION

Systemic lupus erythematosus (SLE) is an inflammatory systemic autoimmune disorder that has a very wide ranging spectrum of clinical manifestations as well as varied clinical course.[1,2] It is characterized by the presence of autoantibodies, in particular the antinuclear antibodies (ANA) and a relapsing and remitting course. SLE affects mainly women in their childbearing years, although men, the very young, and the elderly are not spared. The disease presents subtly in many patients such as with intermittent mild photosensitive facial rashes (Fig. 8-1), malaise, or incidental findings of mild thrombocytopenia, anemia or elevated erythrocyte sedimentation rate (ESR). On the other hand, the presentation can be very acute as in a medical emergency of sudden dyspnea with or without hemoptysis, a change in mental status or coma, or even an acute abdomen. The Lupus in Minorities: Nature vs. Nurture (LUMINA) cohort study, a longitudinal outcome study, reported that acute disease onset is associated with higher levels of overall disease activity.[3]

The rheumatologist's first task when consulted is to decide whether the patient indeed has SLE or a nonrheumatologic condition, or not uncommonly, even both disorders concurrently. The next step is the assessment of disease severity, extent of organ involvement and damage, and disease activity. Patients with SLE have a nearly fivefold increased risk of death compared with the general population.[4,5] Several observational cohorts and case-control studies have identified infections,[6,7] diabetes mellitus,[8] hypertension,[8] dyslipidemia,[8,9] atherosclerosis,[9,10] coronary heart disease,[9,11] osteoporosis,[12] avascular bone necrosis,[6,13] and certain types of cancer (non-Hodgkin's lymphoma, lung cancer, hepatobiliary cancer)[14] as common causes of morbidity and mortality in SLE patients. Attention must be directed toward the presence or absence of these comorbidities when planning the patient's medical care. Treatment plans should be discussed and formulated with the patient and, when appropriate, with the family. Medical cost is often a concern to the patient faced with a chronic, potentially disabling illness and should be taken into consideration when planning investigations and treatment to encourage patient compliance. Socioeconomic determinants are important in the ultimate outcome of SLE as noted by several investigators, and poverty, not ethnicity, is a predictor of diminished survival in patients with lupus from the LUMINA cohort.[15,16]

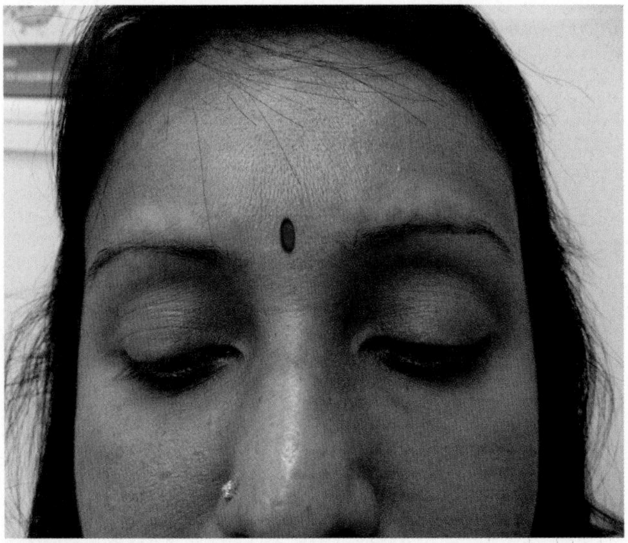

It is increasingly clear that successful management of a patient with lupus requires the rheumatologist to be well versed in internal medicine and practice a holistic approach, working closely with the family physician. Good outcome also often requires the participation of a team of other health care workers including the relevant specialists, nurse counselor, therapist, and social worker. Readers are to refer to the two chapters in this book for details on specific management of the different organ system manifestations. This chapter discusses the broad principles in the approach to the lupus patient and practical considerations in decisions on treatment, monitoring of the disease, and comorbidities.

INITIAL EVALUATION

Assessing patients with lupus requires attention to detail and becomes easier with experience. As in the evaluation of any other disease, the approach starts

Figure 8-1. Subtle acute lupus rashes on brows and nasal bridge.

with a good history and thorough physical examination, followed by well thought out investigations.

History and Physical Examination

It is essential to remember that the American College of Rheumatology (ACR) SLE classification[17] is not a set of diagnostic criteria. In addition, new clinical features and autoantibodies may develop in a patient over time.[18] In the case of a patient who has a prior diagnosis of SLE, it is advisable to go over the patient's history, investigations, and all available past medical records, to confirm that the diagnosis of SLE is appropriate. Cases of misdiagnosis of SLE based on a positive ANA or weak positive anti-dsDNA antibody (anti-dsDNA Ab) test carried out in a laboratory with less than satisfactory quality assurance occasionally happens. Primary Sjögren's syndrome may be mistaken for SLE when sicca symptoms are mild and overlooked.

History should include constitutional symptoms and inquiry into all organ systems. The patient is also asked about symptoms that suggest associated connective tissue diseases such as secondary Sjögren's syndrome and antiphospholipid syndrome (APS). Obtain details of other medical conditions in particular whether there is history of diabetes mellitus, hypertension, hyperlipidemia, cardiovascular and cerebrovascular events, and osteopenia/osteoporosis. In women, obtain menstrual and obstetric history, contraceptive practices and any pregnancy plan. Information on treatment received by the patient already known to have SLE is important and should include both conventional and alternative medications used as well as the disease response and any adverse drug reactions experienced.

In the physical examination, remember to examine the oral mucosa (oral ulcers are painless), feet and fingers for cutaneous vasculitis (Fig. 8-2), pinna for rashes (Fig. 8-3), and scalp for small areas of scarring alopecia that may not be reported by the patient. Fundi are examined for signs of retinal vasculitis. During the physical examination, take note of all organ involvement and any potentially irreversible damage such as scarring alopecia.

Investigations

Investigations can be grouped into those for diagnosis, monitoring disease activity, monitoring adverse effects of drug therapy; and monitoring comorbidity. Readers are to refer to the other chapters in this book on investigations of specific organ involvement.

There is no necessity to order a whole host of serologic tests for every patient. These tests are best ordered with a clinical question in mind and interpreted accordingly. The anti-dsDNA Ab test should not be used as a screening test for SLE because it is

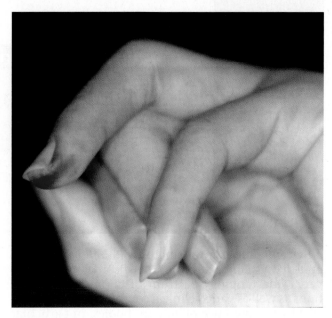

Figure 8-2. Nailfold and fingertip vasculitis.

present in only about 60% of patients with lupus even when repeated over time. Neither is its presence alone diagnostic of SLE. Besides reflecting active SLE, it is linked to renal involvement.[19-21] In clinical practice, the main value of the anti-dsDNA Ab is as an indicator of disease activity and in monitoring the patient's response to treatment especially in nephritis.[22,23] There are exceptions to this. Some patients have been reported to have high levels of this antibody without disease activity, and on the other hand, it may be negative during active disease, particularly when organs other than kidneys are affected. Prospective studies have also shown a rise in anti-dsDNA Ab levels well before a major SLE flare and a decrease at the time of or following a

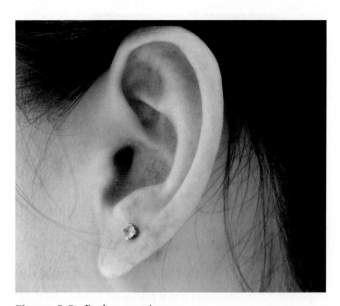

Figure 8-3. Rashes on pinna.

flare.[24] A patient with high anti-dsDNA Ab should be observed more closely. The trend of the anti-dsDNA Ab levels in a patient is more relevant in clinical practice than its absolute value.

The Anti-Ro/SSA Ab is ordered when suspecting the rare ANA-negative lupus or when secondary Sjögren's syndrome is considered. More commonly, it is ordered together with anti-La/SSB Ab and the antiphospholipid antibodies (aPLs) (immunoglobulin G [IgG] and immunoglobulin M [IgM] anticardiolipin antibodies [ACA], lupus anticoagulant [LA], anti-B2 glycoprotein I [anti-B2GP I]) when a patient plans to start a family.[25] Anti-Ro/SSA Ab and anti-La/SSB Ab are associated with neonatal lupus (NNL). The incidence of congenital heart block due to NNL in the offspring of a mother with anti-Ro Ab is about 2%, with a recurrence rate of 16% in subsequent pregnancies.[26] Antiphospholipid antibodies (aPLs) are ordered when secondary APS is suspected and before pregnancy to assess the risks in pregnancy to the fetus and mother and the need for closer monitoring and prophylactic treatment with aspirin.

Complete blood count and white blood cell differential are informative and inexpensive tests for assessing activity in clinical practice.[22] A normochromic and normocytic anemia is consistent with any chronic illness or an acute blood loss such as in pulmonary hemorrhage (note: hemoptysis may be clinically absent during pulmonary hemorrhage). A macrocytic anemia suggests hemolysis, and the reticulocyte count is high in this instance unless there is a vitamin B_{12} or folate deficiency. Data from the LUMINA study have shown that anemia/hematocrit is a predictor of not only disease activity but also damage accrual.[27] Leukopenia and lymphopenia indicate active SLE unless patient is already on immunosuppressive drugs such as cyclophosphamide when the possibility of adverse drug reactions has to be entertained.[28] Azathioprine often increases the mean corpuscular volume but rarely causes a pancytopenia. Thrombocytopenia indicates either active SLE or associated secondary APS (when platelets are often only slightly rather than markedly reduced). In a pregnant patient with lupus, thrombocytopenia may be due to active disease or a variety of other causes including secondary APS; pre-eclampsia; and hemolysis, elevated liver enzymes, and low platelet count (HELLP) syndrome associated with pregnancy; heparin therapy; and the gestational state itself.[29,30]

ESR and complements C3 and C4 are used in conjunction with anti-dsDNA Ab to assess disease activity. A high ESR indicates active disease,[31] although at times, it may remain persistently high without any evidence of lupus activity. In this instance, look for evidence of secondary Sjögren's syndrome, occult infection, or malignancy. In the presence of a high ESR, C-reactive protein (CRP) may help differentiate active SLE from infection when it is normal or slightly elevated. CRP is moderately raised in patients with SLE with manifestations of serositis and Jaccoud's arthropathy, and therefore, in

these instances, it is not useful in the exclusion of infection.[32-34]

Complements C3 and C4 are low in active lupus.[35,36] Rarely, patients may have persistent hypocomplementemia due to inherited complement deficiencies, such as the C4A/C4B null allele that is associated with lupus. During pregnancy, complements C3 and C4 may rise to supranormal levels, and a flare with complement activation may occur despite apparently normal levels of complements C3 and C4.[29,30] It is more helpful to follow the trend of the complement levels to predict disease flare in pregnancy.

Urine analysis for red and white blood cells, protein, and cellular casts are important tests of renal activity and may reveal clinically silent renal disease. During pregnancy, the patient with history of renal involvement may have a worsening of proteinuria due to physiologic response to pregnancy or pre-eclampsia and not necessarily a flare of lupus nephritis.[29,30] In this instance, there should not be any feature of active urinary sediments. Blood urea, electrolyte, and serum creatinine should be ordered at baseline. A high creatinine with active urinary sediments indicates active lupus nephritis and warrants prompt initiation of treatment and further investigations such as renal ultrasound and biopsy to avoid delay in instituting appropriate immunosuppressants.

A chest x-ray study is routinely ordered before starting corticosteroids or immunosuppressants. In countries in which the infection is endemic and when individuals are at high risk for hepatitis B, screening for this infection should be ordered because fulminant hepatitis may occur when high-dose corticosteroids or immunosuppressive drugs are used.[37] All patients should have a baseline assessment of fasting lipids and glucose, calcium, phosphate, and bone mineral densitometry (when indicated). When appropriate, electrocardiograms, stress echocardiography, or other cardiac screening measures and duplex scanning of the carotids may be ordered.

FORMULATING TREATMENT PLANS

Based on current knowledge and information, the aims in treatment of SLE should be early control of disease activity, prevention of disease relapse and good control of comorbidities (Table 8-1). The principles in management of SLE are outlined in Table 8-2, and keys to successful management are provided in Table 8-3.

In planning treatment, the doctor should take into consideration several issues including comorbidities and concurrent medications, patient's work and other daily activities, and whether the patient is planning or plans to have a child in the near future. There should be an assessment of the extent of disease damage. Both the doctor and the patient must be realistic in what can be achieved. It is also good to

Table 8-1. *Aims of Treatment of Systemic Lupus Erythematosus*

Control of disease activity—'induction therapy'—aim for remission as soon as possible.
Prevention of disease flare—'maintenance' therapy with minimum effective medication.
Prevention and management of morbidity from the chronic illness and from medications.

Table 8-2. *Principles in Management of Active Systemic Lupus Erythematosus*

Detailed assessment of patient and exclusion of disorders that could mimic active lupus
Therapy directed at specific disease manifestations that are active rather than irreversible damage
Severity of disease manifestation determines the intensity of management
Treatment for the shortest time and at lowest dose possible to avoid toxicity

Table 8-3. *Keys to Successful Management of Systemic Lupus Erythematosus*

Early recognition of disease
Timely and appropriate therapy
Good control of comorbidities
Prevention of complications
Counseling and education of patients and their caregivers/ family to ensure treatment compliance

Table 8-4. *Pregnancy in Systemic Lupus Erythematosus*

Patients with lupus can have successful pregnancies and healthy children
Pregnancy in lupus should be considered high risk
Plan before conception
Conceive when lupus is in remission
During pregnancy, close monitoring of maternal and fetal health is essential
Postpartum period is just as important

anticipate difficulties that may be encountered such as patient noncompliance with medication, use of alternative therapies, and the frequent defaulters.

Control of diabetes mellitus, hypertension, and hyperlipidemia must be optimized to reduce risk of atherosclerosis and its complications. If patients are taking drugs that predispose them to osteoporosis, bone mineralization should be regularly monitored and appropriate prophylaxis with calcium, vita-min D, bisphosphonate, or hormone replacement therapy (HRT) prescribed.[38-42] Patients with chronic hepatitis B should be comanaged with a hepatologist because special care is required to avoid fulminant hepatic failure in a patient on corticosteroid or immunosuppressants.[37] Although there are no randomized controlled trials (RCTs) to evaluate the effectiveness of lifestyle modifications, general health advice on adequate rest to relieve fatigue of active disease, exercise, weight reduction, and a healthy diet should be provided. Advise patients on avoidance of known trigger factors. Sun avoidance is encouraged, especially during midday, and sunscreens are recommended. Smoking must be stopped because not only does it worsen Raynaud's phenomenon but it also interferes with the efficacy of antimalarials and raises pulmonary pressures. Freemer and associates[43] demonstrated that cigarette smoke is an important risk factor for the occurrence of anti-dsDNA Abs in patients affected with SLE.

With regards to oral contraceptives, two RCTs have concluded that oral estrogen contraceptives do not increase the risk for flare in stable disease[44,45] although estrogen use has been associated with increased risk for developing SLE.[46] HRT results in significantly better change in bone mass density compared with placebo or calcitriol, without increasing the risk for flares.[41,42] HRT is contraindicated in patients with aPLs or thrombophilia, and the general guidelines for HRT should be taken into account, including the exclusion of hypertension, high cholesterol, obesity and smoking.

SLE is not in itself a contraindication to pregnancy, except when there is severe organ system complications such as pulmonary hypertension or renal failure, when it may be best avoided.[47-49] Pregnancy loss in patients with SLE is decreased if the patient has been in remission for 6 to 12 months before conception. Thus, pregnancy in SLE should be planned. A management strategy is decided with the patient, before conception (Table 8-4). Preconception counseling includes discussions on medication, a review of obstetric history, and history of hypertension. Drugs that are teratogenic and should be stopped at least 3 months before conception include methotrexate, mycophenolate mofetil, and cyclophosphamide. These drugs should be replaced with an alternative such as azathioprine, because withdrawal may cause a flare during pregnancy. Pregnancy should be postponed for 6 months after withdrawal of bisphosphonates.[50] Patients are also advised about possible exacerbations of SLE in the postpartum period.

EDUCATION AND COUNSELING

Treatment adherence is crucial to the successful management of patients with chronic diseases, and lack of adherence is directly associated with poor treatment outcomes. Table 8-5 lists four major barriers to treatment adherence. All new lupus patients should be provided with information on the disease to remove fear, encourage acceptance of illness, and

Table 8-5. *Barriers to Treatment Adherence*

Fear of medication side effects
Perceived lack of efficacy of therapy
Financial cost of drug therapy
Problems with the health system environment and logistics

improve compliance. This counseling session may be carried out by the doctor or a trained nurse. Provide patients with reading materials, and for those who are Internet savvy, a list of reliable websites they could visit for more information.

By recognizing the patient's experience of the illness and efforts at coping with the emotions related to the illness, a rapport can be established, which goes a long way to enhancing patient compliance. The rheumatologist should be aware of the discrepant appreciation of disease activity by himself or herself as the physician (scoring on physical and laboratory abnormalities) and the patient (subjective scoring of disease activity based on how he or she feels).[51] Efforts could be directed at enhancing coping skills, independence, and better self-management.

FOLLOW-UP CLINIC VISITS

The frequency of follow-up reviews depends on the disease activity and severity, and may vary from as short as one review every two weeks to a review every three months. At the earliest sign of disease relapse, the review interval should be shortened. This includes when there is appearance of laboratory evidence of disease relapsing before clinical symptoms appear, such as a trend of rising anti-dsDNA Ab levels or ESR, falling complement C3 or C4 values, a hemoglobin level that is drifting downward without any obvious reasons, or appearance of urinary sediments or protein in urine. It is much easier to control SLE early in the disease flare. Early and prompt treatment also reduces the morbidity that accompanies not only severe disease but also immunosuppressive drugs such as cyclophosphamide that have to be started as a result of progression of severity. Patients are also reviewed earlier when new therapies are instituted, and during pregnancy and puerperium. It is advisable to review pregnant patients every 4 weeks until 28 weeks, and then every 2 weeks till 36 weeks; thereafter weekly until delivery.

A thorough history including a review of medications and physical examination is undertaken at each clinic visit. Any new symptoms, signs, or changes since the patient's previous visit require further evaluation. It is important to ascertain that a clinical feature being recorded is actually due to lupus and not to a concomitant condition. If symptoms suggest a disease relapse, explore reasons such as medication noncompliance or precipitating factors such as sun exposure. The patient's blood pressure must be recorded each visit.

It is recommended that the following be checked at each visit: complete blood count and platelet count, urine analysis for cells, casts and protein, ESR, complement C3, and anti-dsDNA Ab. Because cost is often a concern, it is possible to decide for each individual patient which of the 3 (ESR, complement C3, anti-dsDNA Ab) are better markers of activity and to order one or more of them routinely. However when a disease relapse is suspected, then it is preferable all three tests are ordered. The argument for doing anti-dsDNA Ab test every visit is that studies indicate that increases in anti-dsDNA Abs can be used to initiate pre-emptive treatment to reduce disease flares and may be a more sensitive measure than complement 3 or 4 levels for predicting exacerbations.[52,53]

If urine analyses are abnormal and especially if serial tests are increasingly abnormal, further investigations including a 24-hour urinary protein estimation or the often preferred protein/creatinine ratio estimation and creatinine clearance test, should be ordered. Renal ultrasound looking for renal size, structural abnormalities, and renal vein thrombosis, and renal biopsy may be considered.

Regular screening of fasting glucose and lipids, serum calcium, and phosphate, as well as bone mineral density follows standard recommended guidelines.

DISEASE ACTIVITY INDICES

Many indices have been developed to objectively measure lupus disease activity, and several have been validated. Of these, four disease activity indices are more widely used and are used in RCTs: British Isles Lupus Assessment Group Index (BILAG), Systemic Lupus Erythematosus Disease Activity Index (SLEDAI), European Consensus Lupus Activity Measurement Index (ECLAM) and Systemic Lupus Activity Measure (SLAM).[54-57] These indices have good reliability, validity and responsiveness to change.

The SLEDAI, SLAM, and ECLAM are global indices. In global scoring indices, a clinical feature gets points if it is present and no points if it is absent. However, clinical features may get somewhat better or somewhat worse, and partial improvement or deterioration cannot be captured easily in a global scoring index. The BILAG, established on the principle of the physician's intention to treat, provides an overview of activity in eight organs or systems. The BILAG identifies "A" or major and "B" or moderate disease flares and identifies improvement. In the BILAG, the recorded clinical data are entered only if the physician is certain that the feature is due to SLE. The British Isles Lupus Assessment Group 2004 (BILAG-2004) index is a revision of the classic BILAG index.[58,59] The main difference between the two indices is the addition of ophthalmic and gastrointestinal manifestations in the BILAG-2004 index. Like the classic BILAG index, it is a transitional index that is able to capture changing severity of clinical manifestations and produces an overview of disease activity across nine body systems.

In the recently published EULAR recommendations for the management of SLE,[60] the committee suggested that at least one of these indices should be used in monitoring disease activity—BILAG, ECLAM, SLEDAI. To ensure optimal performance of any of the indices, a well-defined glossary must be followed and training of raters is essential. It takes between 10 to 15 minutes to complete a set of forms. In clinical practice, the rheumatologist has to decide on the feasibility of using one of these activity indices, weighing the advantage of an additional tool for patient care versus added costs in terms of time and for some indices, and the need to order specific investigations at every assessment.

ASSESSING EXTENT OF ORGAN SYSTEMS INVOLVEMENT AND DAMAGE

It has been shown by several groups that early acquisition of damage is a sign of a poor prognosis in SLE. Once damage occurs, it continues to accrue.[61] Permanent organ damage in SLE may be due to the disease itself, treatment of disease, or unrelated factors. All patients should be assessed for evidence of organ damage at presentation and ideally once yearly. It may be possible to prevent lupus damage by using hydroxychloroquine, particularly if used before damage starts.[62]

The Systemic Lupus International Cooperating Clinics/American College of Rheumatology (SLICC/ACR) Damage Index measures irreversible organ system damage that has been present for at least 6 months, due to either the disease or its treatment.[63] It assesses the cumulative effect of the disease since onset. The index records damage in 12 organs or systems and is ascertained clinically or by simple investigations. An assessment of damage using this instrument could be considered at baseline and yearly for the patient.

SUMMARY

Table 8-6 summarizes the key issues to be considered in the management of a patient with SLE. Delay in diagnosis, poor treatment compliance, persistent overall disease activity, and major organ involvement are by far the most important predictors of a poor outcome for patients with SLE. By paying careful attention and addressing these issues with a team comprising of other physicians and health care professionals, a good outcome is possible for all patients with lupus.

References

1. Boumpas DT, Austin 3rd HA, Fessler BJ, Balow JE, Klippel JH, Lockshin MD. Systemic lupus erythematosus: emerging concepts. Part 1: Renal, neuropsychiatric, cardiovascular, pulmonary, and hematologic disease. Ann Intern Med 1995;122:940-50.
2. Boumpas DT, Fessler BJ, Austin 3rd HA, Balow JE, Klippel JH, Lockshin MD. Systemic lupus erythematosus: emerging concepts. Part 2: Dermatologic and joint disease, the antiphospholipid antibody syndrome, pregnancy and hormonal therapy, morbidity and mortality, and pathogenesis. Ann Intern Med 1995;123:42-53.
3. Bertoli AM, Vila LM, Reveille JD, Alarcón GS. Systemic lupus erythaematosus in a multiethnic US cohort (LUMINA) LIII: disease expression and outcome in acute onset lupus. Ann Rheum Dis 2008;67:500-4.
4. Abu-Shakra M, Urowitz MB, Gladman DD, Gough J. Mortality studies in systemic lupus erythematosus. Results from a single center. II. Predictor variables for mortality. J Rheumatol 1995;22:1265-70.
5. Jacobsen S, Petersen J, Ullman S, Junker P, Voss A, Rasmussen JM, et al. Mortality and causes of death of 513 Danish patients with systemic lupus erythematosus. Scand J Rheumatol 1999;28:75-80.
6. Cervera R, Khamashta MA, Font J, Sebastiani GD, Gil A, Lavilla P, et al. Morbidity and mortality in systemic lupus erythematosus during a 10-year period: a comparison of early and late manifestations in a cohort of 1,000 patients. Medicine (Baltimore) 2003;82:299-308.
7. Mok CC, Mak A, Chu WP, To CH, Wong SN. Long-term survival of southern Chinese patients with systemic lupus erythematosus: a prospective study of all age-groups. Medicine (Baltimore) 2005;84:218-24.
8. Bruce IN, Urowitz MB, Gladman DD, Ibanez D, Steiner G. Risk factors for coronary heart disease in women with systemic lupus erythematosus: the Toronto Risk Factor Study. Arthritis Rheum 2003;48:3159-67.
9. Asanuma Y, Oeser A, Shintani AK, Turner E, Olsen N, Fazio S, et al. Premature coronary artery atherosclerosis in systemic lupus erythematosus. N Engl J Med 2003;349:2407-15.
10. Jimenez S, Garcia-Criado MA, Tassies D, Reverter JC, Cervera R, Gilabert MR, et al. Preclinical vascular disease in systemic lupus erythematosus and primary antiphospholipid syndrome. Rheumatology (Oxford) 2005;44:756-61.
11. Bjornadal L, Yin L, Granath F, Klareskog L, Ekbom A. Cardiovascular disease a hazard despite improved prognosis in patients with systemic lupus erythematosus: results from a Swedish population based study 1964-95. J Rheumatol 2004;31:713-9.
12. Gilboe IM, Kvien TK, Haugeberg G, Husby G. Bone mineral density in systemic lupus erythematosus: comparison with rheumatoid arthritis and healthy controls. Ann Rheum Dis 2000;59:110-15.
13. Gladman DD, Urowitz MB, Chaudhry-Ahluwalia V, Hallet DC, Cook RJ. Predictive factors for symptomatic osteonecrosis in patients with systemic lupus erythematosus. J Rheumatol 2001;28:761-5.
14. Bernatsky S, Boivin JF, Joseph L, Rajan R, Zoma A, Manzi S, et al. An international cohort study of cancer in systemic lupus erythematosus. Arthritis Rheum 2005;52:1481-90.
15. Duran S, Apte M, Alarcón GS. Poverty, not ethnicity, accounts for the differential mortality rates among lupus patients of various ethnic groups. J Natl Med Assoc 2007;99:1196-8.

Table 8-6. *Summary of Key Points in Management*

Patients with lupus should be diagnosed early
Early damage is an independent predictor of mortality
Lupus activity should be brought under control as early as possible
The management of systemic lupus erythematosus should aim at the prevention of major organ involvement
Avoid complications of therapy including infections by judicious use of medications
Manage comorbidities including risks for atherosclerosis and osteoporosis well and, if necessary, by coordinating care with the primary care physician
Patients who do not understand their illness or for various reasons are noncompliant do badly and need help early

16. Kasitanon N, Magder LS, Petri M. Predictors of survival in systemic lupus erythematosus. Medicine (Baltimore) 2006;85:147-56.

17. Hochberg MC. Updating the American College of Rheumatology revised criteria for the classification of systemic lupus erythematosus. Arthritis Rheum 1997;40:1725.

18. Alarcón GS, McGwin Jr G, Roseman JM, Uribe A, Fessler BJ, Bastian HM, et al. Systemic lupus erythematosus in three ethnic groups. XIX: Natural history of the accrual of the American College of Rheumatology criteria prior to the occurrence of criteria diagnosis. Arthritis Rheum 2004;51:609-15.

19. Kavanaugh AF, Solomon DH and the American College of Rheumatology Adhoc Committee on immunologic testing guidelines. Guidelines for immunologic laboratory testing in the rheumatic diseases: Anti-DNA antibody test. Arthritis Rheum 2002;47:546-55.

20. Illei GG, Tackey E, Lapreva L, Lipsky PE. Biomarkers in systemic lupus erythematosus. II. Markers of disease activity. Arthritis Rheum 2004;50:2048-65.

21. Linnik MD, Hu JZ, Heilbrunn KR, et al. Relationship between anti-double-stranded DNA antibodies and exacerbation of renal disease in patients with systemic lupus erythematosus. Arthritis Rheum 2005;52:1129-37.

22. Mirzayan MJ, Schmidt RE, Witte T. Prognostic parameters for flare in systemic lupus erythematosus. Rheumatology (Oxford) 2000;39:1316-9.

23. Swaak AJ, Groenwold J, Bronsveld W. Predictive value of complement profiles and antidsDNA in systemic lupus erythematosus. Ann Rheum Dis 1986;45:359-66.

24. Ho A, Magder LS, Barr SG, Petri M. Decreases in anti-double stranded DNA levels are associated with concurrent flares in patients with systemic lupus erythematosus. Arthritis Rheum 2001;44:2342-9.

25. Lockwood CJ, Romero R, Feinberg RF, Clyne LP, Coster B, Hobbins JC. The prevalence and biologic significance of lupus anticoagulant and anticardiolipin antibodies in a general obstetric population. Am J Obstet Gynecol 1989;161:369-73.

26. Buyon JP, Hiebert R, Copel J, et al. Autoimmune-associated congenital heart block: demographics, mortality, morbidity and recurrence rates obtained from a national neonatal lupus registry. J Am College Cardiol 1998;31:1658-66.

27. Bertoli AM, Vila LM, Apte M, et al. Systemic lupus erythematosus in a multiethnic US cohort LUMINA LI: anaemia as a predictor of disease activity and damage accrual. Rheumatology (Oxford) 2007;46:1471-6.

28. Vila LM, Alarcón GS, McGwin Jr G, Bastian HM, Fessler BJ, Reveille JD. Systemic lupus erythematosus in a multiethnic US cohort, XXXVII: association of lymphopenia with clinical manifestations, serologic abnormalities, disease activity, and damage accrual. Arthritis Rheum 2006;55:799-806.

29. Buyon JP, Kalunian KC, Ramsey-Goldman R, et al. Assessing disease activity in SLE patients during pregnancy. Lupus 1999;8:677-84.

30. Petri M. The Hopkins Lupus Pregnancy Center: ten key issues in management. Rheum Dis Clin N Am 2007;33:27-35.

31. Vila LM, Alarcon GS, McGwin Jr G, Bastian HM, Fessler BJ, Reveille JD. Systemic lupus erythematosus in a multiethnic cohort (LUMINA): XXIX. Elevation of erythrocyte sedimentation rate is associated with disease activity and damage accrual. J Rheumatol 2005;32:2150-5.

32. Zein N, Ganuza C, Kushner I. Significance of serum C-reactive protein elevation in patients with systemic lupus erythematosus. Arthritis Rheum 1979;22:7-12.

33. Ter Borg EJ, Horst G, Limburg PC, van Rijswijk MH, Kallenberg CG. C-reactive protein levels during disease exacerbations and infections in systemic lupus erythematosus: a prospective longitudinal study. J Rheumatol 1990;17:1642-8.

34. Spronk PE, ter Borg EJ, Kallenberg CG. Patients with systemic lupus erythematosus and Jaccoud's arthropathy: a clinical subset with an increased C reactive protein response? Ann Rheum Dis 1992;51:358-61.

35. Ho A, Barr SG, Magder LS, Petri M. A decrease in complement is associated with increased renal and hematologic activity in patients with systemic lupus erythematosus. Arthritis Rheum 2001;44:2350-7.

36. Illei GG, Takada K, Parkin D, Austin HA, Crane M, Yarboro CH, et al. Renal flares are common in patients with severe proliferative lupus nephritis treated with pulse immunosuppressive therapy: long-term follow-up of a cohort of 145 patients participating in randomized controlled studies. Arthritis Rheum 2002;46:995-1002.

37. Calabrese LH, Zein NN, Vassilopoulous D. Hepatitis B virus (HBV) reactivation with immunosuppressive therapy in rheumatic diseases: assessment and preventive strategies. Ann Rheum Dis 2006;65:983-9.

38. Sambrook P, Birmingham J, Kelly P, Kempler S, Nguyen T, Pocock N, et al. Prevention of corticosteroid osteoporosis. A comparison of calcium, calcitriol, and calcitonin. N Engl J Med 1993;328:1747-52.

39. Adachi JD, Bensen WG, Bianchi F, Cividino A, Pillersdorf S, Sebaldt RJ, et al. Vitamin D and calcium in the prevention of corticosteroid induced osteoporosis: a 3 year follow up. J Rheumatol 1996;23:995-1000.

40. Nzeusseu Toukap A, Depresseux G, Devogelaer JP, Houssiau FA. Oral pamidronate prevents high-dose glucocorticoid-induced lumbar spine bone loss in premenopausal connective tissue disease (mainly lupus) patients. Lupus 2005;14:517-20.

41. Bhattoa HP, Bettembuk P, Balogh A, Szegedi G, Kiss E. The effect of 1-year transdermal estrogen replacement therapy on bone mineral density and biochemical markers of bone turnover in osteopenic postmenopausal systemic lupus erythematosus patients: a randomized, double-blind, placebo-controlled trial. Osteoporos Int 2004;15:396-404.

42. Buyon JP, Petri MA, Kim MY, Kalunian KC, Grossman J, Hahn BH, et al. The effect of combined estrogen and progesterone hormone replacement therapy on disease activity in systemic lupus erythematosus: a randomized trial. Ann Intern Med 2005;142:953-62.

43. Freemer MM, King Jr TE, Criswell LA. Association of smoking with dsDNA autoantibody production in systemic lupus erythematosus. Ann Rheum Dis 2006;65:581-4.

44. Petri M, Kim MY, Kalunian KC, Grossman J, Hahn BH, Sammaritano LR, et al. Combined oral contraceptives in women with systemic lupus erythematosus. N Engl J Med 2005;353:2550-8.

45. Sanchez-Guerrero J, Uribe AG, Jimenez-Santana L, Mestanza-Peralta M, Lara-Reyes P, Seuc AH, et al. A trial of contraceptive methods in women with systemic lupus erythematosus. N Engl J Med 2005;353:2539-49.

46. Sanchez-Guerrero J, Karlson EW, Liang MH, Hunter DJ, Speizer FE, Colditz GA. Past use of oral contraceptives and the risk of developing systemic lupus erythematosus. Arthritis Rheum 1997;40:804-8.

47. Ruiz-Irastorza G, Khamashta MA, Hughes GRV. Heart disease, pregnancy and systemic autoimmune diseases. In: Oakley C, Warnes CA, editors. Heart disease in pregnancy. 2nd ed. Oxford, UK: Blackwell Publishing; 2007. p. 136-50.

48. Bonnin M, Mercier FJ, Sitbon O, Roger-Christoph S, Jaïs X, Humbert M, et al. Severe pulmonary hypertension during pregnancy. Mode of delivery and anesthetic management of 15 consecutive cases. Anesthesiology 2005;102:1133-7.

49. McMillan E, Martin WL, Waugh J, Rushton I, Lewis M, Clutton-Brock T, et al. Management of pregnancy in women with pulmonary hypertension secondary to SLE and antiphospholipid syndrome. Lupus 2002;11:392-8.

50. Oestensen M, Khamashta M, Lockshin M, Parke A, Brucato A, Carp H, et al. Antiinflammatory and immunosuppressive drugs and reproduction. Arthritis Res Ther 2006;8:209-28.

51. Alarcón GS, McGwin Jr G, Brooks K, Roseman JM, Fessler BJ, Sanchez ML, et al. Systemic lupus erythematosus in three ethnic groups: XI. Sources of discrepancy in perception of disease activity: a comparison of physician and patient visual analog scale scores. Arthritis Rheum 2002;47:408-13.

52. Walz LeBlank BAE, Gladman DD, Urowitz MB. Serologically active clinically quiescent systemic lupus erythematosus—predictors of clinical flares. J Rheumatol 1994;21:2239-41.

53. Bootsma H, Spronk P, Derksen R, et al. Prevention of relapses in systemic lupus erythematosus. Lancet 1995;345:1595-9.

54. Hay EM, Bacon PA, Gordon C, Isenberg DA, Maddison P, Snaith ML, et al. The BILAG index: a reliable and valid

instrument of measuring clinical disease activity in systemic lupus erythematosus. Q J Med 1993;86:447-58.

55. Bombardier C, Gladman DD, Urowitz MB, Caron D, Chang CH. Derivation of the SLEDAI A disease activity index for lupus patients. The Committee on Prognosis Studies in SLE. Arthritis Rheum 1992;35:630-40.

56. Vitali C, Bencivelli W, Isenberg DA, Smolen JS, Snaith ML, Sciuto M, et al. Disease activity in systemic lupus erythematosus: report of the Consensus Study Group of the European Workshop for Rheumatology Research. Clin Exp Rheumatol 1992;10:541-7.

57. Liang MH, Socher SA, Larson MG, Schor P. Reliability and validity of six systems for the clinical assessment of disease activity in SLE. Arthritis Rheum 1989;32:1107-18.

58. Isenberg DA, Rahman A, Allen E, Farewell V, Akil M, Bruce IN, et al. BILAG 2004. Development and initial validation of an updated version of the British Isles Lupus Assessment Group's disease activity index for patients with systemic lupus erythematosus. Rheumatology (Oxford) 2005;44:902-6.

59. Yee CS, Farewell V, Isenberg DA, Prabu A, Sokoll K, Teh LS, et al. Revised British Isles Lupus Assessment Group 2004 index: a reliable tool for assessment of systemic lupus erythematosus activity. Arthritis Rheum 2006;54:3300-5.

60. Bertsias GK, Ioannidis JP, Boletis J, Bombardieri S, Cervera R, Dostal C, et al. EULAR recommendations for the management of Systemic Lupus Erytematosus (SLE). Report of a Task Force of the European Standing Committee for International Clinical Studies Including Therapeutics (ESCISIT)*. Ann Rheum Dis 2008;67:195-205.

61. Alarcón GS, Roseman JM, McGwin Jr G, Uribe A, Bastian HM, Fessler BJ, et al. Systemic lupus erythematosus in three ethnic groups: XX. Damage as predictor of further damage. Rheumatology (Oxford) 2004;43:202-5.

62. Fessler BJ, Alarcón GS, McGwin Jr G, Roseman J, Bastian HM, Friedman AW, et al. Systemic lupus erythematosus in three ethnic groups: XVI. Association of hydroxychloroquine use with reduced risk of damage accrual. Arthritis Rheum 2005;52:1473-80.

63. Gladman DD, Urowitz MB, Goldsmith C, Fortin P, Ginzler E, Gordon C, et al. Assessment of the reliability of the Systemic Lupus Collaborating Clinics/American College of Rheumatology damage index in patients with systemic lupus erythematosus. Arthritis Rheum 1997;40:809-13.

Management of Nonrenal Systemic Lupus Erythematosus 2

Daniel J. Wallace

INTRODUCTION

Systemic lupus erythematosus (SLE) is a multi-system, inflammatory disorder. Its treatment warrants general anti-inflammatory measures as well as organ-specific, preventive, or focused measures concentrating on sets of commonalities. The author has chosen to use the eight organ/systemic components validated for use in clinical trials based on the BILAG. Otherwise known as the British Isles Lupus Assessment Group index, the third version of the BILAG compiled nearly 100 symptoms, signs, and imaging and laboratory findings and divided them into eight categories (Table 9-1).[1] The management of renal manifestations of SLE was covered in the previous chapter. This section provides an overview of a clinical approach toward managing the remaining seven systems using case presentations and discussion, differential diagnoses, and treatment overview. *The reader should be cautioned that other than for the kidney, there is no established, evidence-based treatment for any of the manifestations of the seven systems reviewed in this chapter.* Thus, this chapter constitutes a compilation of consensus-derived, eminence-based recommendations.

THE "GENERAL," OR CONSTITUTIONAL SYSTEM

CASE STUDY 1

Patricia is a 36-year-old black woman with an established diagnosis of SLE of 5 years' duration. The disease has been manifested by inflammatory arthritis, mild proteinuria, anemia, pleuritic pain, and rashes. Her current treatment includes hydroxychloroquine, methotrexate 15 mg weekly, 5 mg of prednisone daily, topical corticosteroids, and ibuprofen. At this visit, she relates having gone to the beach a few days before and relates that she is tired, achy, has lost her appetite, She appears toxic but denies any infection. Patricia's temperature is 100.6° F, cervical adenopathy is present, and a moderate amount of synovitis is evident in the wrists, hands, ankles, and feet. An acute cutaneous lupus rash is present on her cheeks, the "V" area of the chest, and forearms. Laboratory work includes sedimentation rate 85 (nL < 20), hemoglobin 9 mg/dL (nL > 12.0), C3 complement 39 mg/dL (nL 80–120), anti DNA (Farr) 300 (normal < 5). You conclude that the patient is experiencing a generalized flare. What is the best approach for managing this problem?

Symptoms and Signs: Fatigue, Fever, Adenopathy, Weight Loss

It is common for patients with lupus to feel "unwell." Generalized complaints of being tired and achy are present in the majority of patients who relate decreased stamina or endurance, malaise, a flu-like sensation, or "having the blahs."[2] The first matter a clinician needs to address is to ensure that these symptoms are not due to infection or a comorbidity. In other words, does the patient have cancer, hypothyroidism (up to 20% with SLE have thyroid antibodies), an opportunistic process, or severe anemia (e.g., heavy periods in a young woman with inflammatory activity suppressing the bone marrow)? Fatigue is highly subjective and can result from psychosocial stressors, malnutrition, substance abuse, or even an early pregnancy. Up to 30% of patients with SLE have concurrent fibromyalgia, and this syndrome can mimic lupus flares. In Patricia's case, the aggravation of rashes by exposure to the sun, elevation of acute phase reactants, and findings of adenopathy tend to rule out these considerations, but the situation is not always clear. If fatigue and aching due to inflammation are not addressed, systemic manifestations such as rashes, fevers, or swollen glands will follow shortly. Usually, generalized nonspecific lupus activity promptly responds to anti-inflammatory regimens such as moderate doses (0.5 mg/kg/day) of prednisone for several weeks, although milder flares may respond to nonsteroidal anti-inflammatory therapy.

The presence of temperatures above 99.6° F is by definition a fever. Active lupus is frequently associated with fevers and tachycardia.[3] Infection and drug-induced fevers need to be ruled out; most lupus-induced temperature elevations are nonfocal. Any persistent temperature

Table 9-1. *Characteristics of Lupus that Merit Mention in the BILAG*

General: pyrexia, weight loss, adenopathy, splenomegaly, fatigue, malaise, lethargy, anorexia

Mucocutaneous: Maculopapular rash, generalized or localized discoid lesions, alopecia, severe panniculitis, angioedema, mucosal ulceration, malar erythema, subcutaneous nodules, lupus pernio, periungual erythema, swollen fingers, sclerodactyly, calcinosis, telangiectasia

Neurologic: Deteriorating level of consciousness, acute psychosis, delerium, confusional state, seizures, stroke or stroke syndrome, aseptic meningitis, mononeuritis multiplex, ascending or transverse myelitis, peripheral or cranial neuropathy, chorea, disc swelling/cytoid bodies, cerebellar ataxia, severe unremitting or episodic migraine headache, organic brain syndrome or depression, pseudotumor cerebri

Musculoskeletal: arthralgia or arthritis, myalgia or myositis, tendonitis, aseptic necrosis

Cardiovascular and respiratory: pleuropericardial pain or effusion, dyspnea, cardiac failure, friction rub, electocardiographic or chest x-ray changes suggestive of SLE, abnormal pulmonary function, cytohistopathological evidence for inflammatory lung disease, cardiac arrhythmias including tachycardia without fever

Vasculitis: cutaneous (can include ulceration, purpura), abdominal, recurrent thromboemboli, Raynaud's livedo reticularis, superficial phlebitis

Renal: hypertension, proteinuria, decreased creatinine clearance, nephrosis, active urinary sediment, histologic evidence for nephritis

Hematology: anemia, leukopenia, lymphopenia, thrombocytopenia, hemolysis, Coombs' positivity, circulating anticoagulant.

SLE, systemic lupus erythematosus.

Table 9-2. *Constitutional Findings in SLE*

Finding	Comment/Management
Fever	Presents early or with flares Infection should be ruled out especially if on steroids/immune suppressive Responds to nonsteroidals, corticosteroids
Fatigue	Malaise present in most lupus patients Coexisting conditions should be ruled out: fibromyalgia, drug-related, metabolic Antimalarials/steroids help fatigue related to inflammation Ameliorated by good sleep hygiene, pacing, stress reduction
Adenopathy	Seen in 15% with SLE and associated with inflammation Generalized, nodes are movable and rubbery Responds to NSAIDs, antimalarials, steroids, immune suppressives
Weight loss	Often an initial presentation; responds to anti-inflammatory regimens Need to rule out steroid withdrawal, resolving nephrosis

NSAIDs, nonsteroidal anti-inflammory drugs; SLE, systemic lupus erythematosus.

higher than 100° F in a lupus patient who is on corticosteroids, salicylates, acetaminophen, or nonsteroidals should be taken seriously and may be a reason to admit the patient to the hospital.

Generalized adenopathy is present in 15% of patients with SLE during the course of disease.[4] The lymph nodes are rubbery and movable as opposed to malignancies in which they are matted and firm. Swollen glands usually quickly disappear with anti-inflammatory regimens, such as prednisone 0.25 mg/kg daily for several weeks.

Patients with lupus may initially present with weight loss in increments of up to 10% of their body weight. Involuntary weight loss from SLE is due to inflammation, resolving nephrotic syndrome, or steroid tapering. Underlying systemic processes such as a malignancy, malnutrition or a psychiatric disorder should be ruled out (Table 9-2).

MUCOCUTANEOUS LUPUS

Mr. Jenkins is a 50-year-old white man who has a long-standing history of chronic cutaneous lupus erythematosus (CCLE) with mild systemic complaints and leukopenia. He smokes two packs of cigarettes a day, and is employed in the moving and storage business. He took hydroxychloroquine for 10 years but has not been compliant with it recently. Mild flares have been treated with topical over-the-counter hydrocortisone creams. As a diabetic, he has been cautioned against using systemic steroids. Over the past 3 months, the patient reports that his skin has become gradually worse. You note that 80% of his body is covered with rash, which is more severe in sun-exposed regions. There are regions of chronic scarring, along with alopecia and acute cutaneous lesions. What therapeutic approaches would be optimal in this circumstance?

Seventy percent of patients with SLE have skin involvement, and individuals who do not fulfill criteria for systemic lupus but have pathologic evidence on skin biopsy for lupus have cutaneous lupus. Eighty percent of the latter group is termed chronic cutaneous (discoid) lupus (Fig. 9-1). (The remaining 20% of patients have urticarial lupus, bullous lupus, tumid, hypertrophic, lupus pernio, subacute cutaneous lupus erythematosus, lupus pemphigoid, or lupus panniculitis. These lesions can overlap with discoid lupus [Table 9-3].)[5] CCLE is histologically characterized by hyperkeratosis, follicular plugging, and dermal atrophy. Ultraviolet light exposure, sun-sensitizing medications, and tobacco abuse are the principal aggravating factors for chronic cutaneous lupus lesions (Table 9-4).[6] New rashes associated with systemic flares are termed "acute cutaneous lupus erythematosus."

Cutaneous lupus can coexist and be difficult to differentiate from other lesions. For example, malar rashes are prominent features of rosacea and polymorphous light eruption, but lupus uniquely

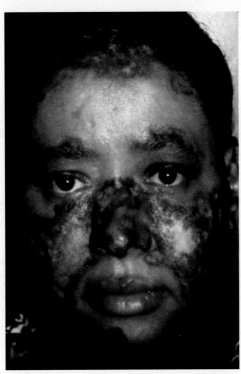

Figure 9-1. Chronic cutaneous lupus with discoid lesions, malar erythema and scarring alopecia. (Courtesy of the American College of Rheumatology Slide Collection.)

Table 9-3. *The Gilliam Classification of Lupus Erythematosus–Associated Skin Lesions*

I. Histopathologically specific (LE-specific)
  A. Acute cutaneous LE
    1) Localized
    2) Generalized
  B. Subacute cutaneous LE
    1) Annular
    2) Papulosquamous
  C. Chronic cutaneous LE
    1) "Classic" DLE
      a) Localized
      b) Generalized
    2) Hypertrophic (verrucous) DLE
    3) Lupus profundus (LE panniculitis)
    4) Mucosal LE
    5) LE tumidus
    6) Chilblains LE (perniotic LE)

DLE, discoid lupus erythematosus; LE, lupus erythematosus.

Table 9-4. *Examples of Drugs that May Precipitate or Exacerbate Lupus Erythematosus–Specific Skin Disease*

Subacute cutaneous lupus erythematosus: calcium channel blockers, thiazide diuretics, terbinafine

Chronic cutaneous lupus erythematosus: anti-tumor necrosis factor therapies

Tumid lupus: angiotensin converting enzyme inhibitors

Exacerbation of pre-existing lupus: sulfa (especially nonarylamine)-based agents, piroxicam, oral contraceptives, nonsteroidal anti-inflammatory agents

---

tends to spare the nasolabial folds.[7] Psoriasis and eczema can be mistaken for cutaneous lupus, and occasionally, a skin biopsy is performed. With the exception of urticarial lupus, the lesions tend not to itch.

Management of Acute Cutaneous Lupus Erythematosus

Mr. Jenkins has a mixed picture of both acute cutaneous lupus erythematosus (ACLE) and CCLE. Treating acute cutaneous lupus flares involves staging the degree of activity of systemic disease. This non-scarring rash usually responds quickly to moderate to high doses of corticosteroids (0.5 to 1 mg/kg/day of prednisone equivalent).[8] The range of involvement of ACLE varies from a transient flare secondary to imprudent sun exposure to the onset of new, serious organ-threatening disease. A complete blood chemistry panel, complete blood count, acute phase reactants, complement levels, anti-DNA should be obtained, along with a screen for specific organ involvement. This can include a chest x-ray study, electrocardiogram, two-dimensional echocardiogram, urinalysis, or viewing a peripheral blood smear, depending on the patient's symptoms or signs. Infections can also produce concomitant systemic flares. Steroid-sparing agents such as immune suppressants may be indicated.

Management of Chronic Cutaneous Lupus Erythematosus

As in the case of Mr. Jenkins, lifestyle can play an important role in following the activity of CCLE. His job involves some outdoor responsibilities, and ultraviolet light exposure can aggravate rashes. Two thirds of patients with SLE self-report sun sensitivity, of whom half have a "wheal and flare" reaction to the administration of ultraviolet light. Some patients observe aggravation of fatigue, fevers, or aching with ultraviolet light exposure. Sun avoidance is a key intervention for CCLE patients. They should minimize midday sun exposure and be careful at higher altitudes, where ultraviolet radiation is greater.[9] Sunscreens consist of agents that block ultraviolet A and B light and are shown in Table 9-5. Topical corticosteroids are best absorbed as ointments and vary widely according to potency (Table 9-6). Fluorinated steroids are available by prescription only, whereas hydrocortisone preparations are sold over the counter. The former should never be used on the face for more than 2 weeks, because they can produce cutaneous atrophy and accentuate telangiectasias. Occasionally, occlusive dressings or intralesional injections may be indicated. Tacrolimus or pinecrolimus represent alternative topical interventions to corticosteroids but are not as effective.[10]

Table 9-5. *General Photoprotective Treatment Approach to Subacute and Chronic Cutaneous Lupus Erythematosus*

Physical Protection

Schedule discretionary outdoor activities before 10 am and after 4 pm even on cloudy days because as much as 80% of ultraviolet (UV) rays penetrate the cloud cover. Limit exposure to reflected UV rays from surfaces such as water, concrete, sand, snow, tile, and reflective window glass in buildings. The window glass in homes blocks some UV rays, especially the sunburning UV rays (UVB). However, considerable amounts of long wavelength UV rays (UVA) may still pass through such glass. Plastic adherent films that can easily be applied to home window glass are available that block all UVB and UVA rays. Clothing can be an excellent form of sun protection. Cover up with loose-fitting and lightweight clothing (long pants and long sleeved shirt, when possible), sunglasses and 4-inch wide brimmed hats. Tightly woven fabric blocks UV rays best. UV protection drops significantly when the fabric becomes wet. Dark colors protect better than light colors. The average white t-shirt provides a sun protective factor (SPF) of only 6 to 8. Sun-protective clothing lines with a rating of SPF 30 or greater are available.

Sunscreens

Sunscreen products (sunblocks) should be applied 15–30 minutes before sun exposure to be most protective. Sunscreen should be reapplied after prolonged swimming or vigorous activity. *Water-resistant* sunscreens protect skin for 40 minutes of water exposure, and *waterproof* sunscreens protect for 80 minutes. Sunscreen needs to be applied liberally. As much as 1 oz may be needed to cover the entire body. Particular attention needs to be paid to the back of the neck, the ears, and the areas of the scalp with thin hair. Use sunscreens with at least a 30 SPF. Select a broad-spectrum sunscreen that contains ingredients that effectively block both UVB and UVA rays. Such ingredients include avobenzone (Parsol 1789), titanium dioxide, and zinc oxide. Mexoryl-containing sunscreens, not yet available in the United States but approved for use in Canada and Europe, may have some advantages over avobenzone (Parsol 1789)-containing sunscreens. Sunscreen gels work well on oily skin or when sweating. Sunscreen lotions help dry skin, and sunscreen sprays work best on the body. Stick type sunscreens can be used on the lips or around the eyes to avoid eye irritation or for maximal protection of the ears. UV light from sunlight exposure causes the skin to produce an important precursor of vitamin D. Adults who use sunscreens daily should consider taking a daily oral supplement of 400-800 units of vitamin D. Sunscreen should not be applied to broken skin or rash (allergies to sunscreen ingredients can develop in some people). Keep in mind that sunscreens are not meant to allow individuals to spend more time in the sun than they would otherwise. They are meant to protect the skin while you *must* be in the sun.

Table 9-6. *Examples of Topical Steroids Used to Manage Cutaneous Lupus*

Level of Potency	Generic and Trade Drug Names
High potency	Clobetasol, betamethasone, diflorasone, halobetasol, amcinonide (e.g., Temovate, Diprolene, Psorcon, Ultravate, Elcon)
Midpotent	Triamcinolone, fluocinonide, fluticasone, mometasone (e.g., Diprosone, Valisone, Kenalog, Lidex, Cyclocort)
Mild	Hydrocortisone, dexamethasone, prednisolone, methylprednisolone (e.g., Synalar, Westcort, Locorten, Aristocort, DesOwen)

Rules

Rule #1: Never use fluorinated steroids on the face for more than 2 weeks, or they can lead to accelerated cutaneous atrophy.

Rule #2: Ointments are 80% absorbed, lotions/gels 50%, and creams 20%, but the latter is the most comfortable vehicle. Occlusive dressings, sprays, or intralesional injections may be indicated in specialized circumstances.

Rule #3: Apply high-potency steroids for more active or inflamed lesions, and lower potency for maintenance or mild lesions.

Antimalarial remedies, especially hydroxychloroquine (HCQ; Plaquenil), are the cornerstone of managing CCLE. Doses of 5 mg/kg/day will heal 80% of lesions over a 3-month period. HCQ works by blocking TLR 7 and 9 (toll receptors) and raises intracellular pH, which interferes with cell signaling and decreases the area of surface receptor interactions with cytokines by invaginating them into the lysosome.[11,12] Tobacco smoke also diminishes the effectiveness of antimalarial therapies and is associated with more lupus activity in general.[13] Approximately 10% of patients cannot tolerate HCQ owing to cutaneous, musculoskeletal, or gastrointestinal reactions. Over a 10-year period, 3% of patients given HCQ develop macular changes, which is almost always reversible with the drugs discontinuation. Individuals unable to tolerate HCQ may respond to quinacrine (50–100 mg daily), an antimalarial that does not affect the eyes, or dapsone, retinoids, or thalidomide.[14,15] Chloroquine is much more toxic to the retina than HCQ but may be safely used for 1 to 3 months for severe, refractory CCLE lesions. All patients with CCLE lesions should be screened for systemic activity, and because CCLE also responds to methotrexate or azathioprine, these agents may be appropriate interventions in selected circumstances (Table 9-7).

Management of Other Forms of Cutaneous Lupus

Mucosal ulcerations are found in 20% of patients with SLE. They usually appear on the soft or hard palate, nasal mucosa, or vaginal wall.[16] These lesions respond to dental gels impregnated with steroids or lidocaine, buttermilk, or peroxide gargles. *Subacute cutaneous lupus erythematosus* is found in 10% of patients with SLE at any given time and may coexist with CCLE. This nonscarring papulosquamous lesion can appear in an annular or polycyclic form, especially in individuals who are anti SSA (Ro) positive

Table 9-7. *Medication Management of Cutaneous Lupus*

Sun protective measures (see Table 9-5)

Topical steroids: Nonfluorinated steroids on face, fluorinated steroids elsewhere (see Table 9-6)

Antimalarials: First choice—hydroxychloroquine 5 mg/kg/day for at least 6 months.

Alternatives: Chloroquine for marked activity. Start at 500 mg daily for 30 days and taper to 250 mg a day. Can transition to hydroxychloroquine after 2–3 months once there is a response. Compounded quinacrine 50–100 mg daily is synergistic with chloroquines and works in 30 days. Can be used as monotherapy if there is a contraindication or side effect from chloroquines.

Retinoids—useful for subacute cutaneous lupus for patients who are antimalarial resistant or intolerant. Options include isotretinoin (Accutane) or acitretin (Soriatene). These agents are sun sensitizing and teratogenic. Usually only needed for short term use.

Dapsone—ameliorative as a second-line agent for chronic cutaneous lupus erythematosus. Has been used as a first-line agent for bullous lupus, lupus panniculitis (profundus), and lupus pemphigoid. Doses range from 50–200 mg daily. G6PD screening advised.

Thalidomide—very effective for cutaneous lesions. Teratogenic and can lead to chronic neuropathies. Patients should use this drug short term (50–200 mg daily) and be transitioned to antimalarials.

Calcineurin inhibitors: Cyclosporine, tacrolimus (Protopic), pinecrolimus (Elidel)—systemic cyclosporine helps urticaria, and psoriasiform and eczematous lesions in doses of 100 mg bid; topical tarcolimus and pinecrolimus modestly effective for chronic cutaneous lupus that can be used on the face and with topical steroids.

Immune suppressive therapies: Methotrexate, azathioprine, cyclophosphamide and mycophenolate mofetil (for pemphigoid) show efficacy in case series.

and is hence observed in patients with Sjögren's syndrome. More resistant to antimalarials than CCLE, subacute cutaneous lupus rashes can also be induced by numerous prescription drugs and are ameliorated by retinoid derivatives.[17] *Lupus pemphigoid* responds to mycophenolate mofetil, *bullous lupus* to dapsone, *lupus profundus (panniculitis)* is a dermal lesion that can be ameliorated with dapsone and surprisingly nonsteroidal anti-inflammatory agents.[18]

Cutaneovascular Manifestations: Raynaud's Phenomenon, Livedo Reticularis, and Vasculitis

Raynaud's phenomenon is a feature noted in up to 25% of lupus patients. Usually independent of inflammatory activity, Raynaud's phenomenon represents vasomotor instability as a manifestation of dysautonomia. Patients with Raynaud's phenomenon respond to cold preventive measures (e.g., mittens, cold avoidance, hand warmers, not using beta blockers) and vasodilators. The latter include

nitrates, calcium channel blockers, alpha-adrenergic blockade, and 5-phosphodiesterase inhibitors.[19,20] Livedo reticularis is a common feature of SLE that does not warrant treatment but is associated with dysautonomia and the presence of antiphospholipid antibodies. Other uncommon cutaneovascular manifestations of SLE include erythromelalgia, leukocytoclastic vasculitis, cyroglobulinemic vasculitis, digital or peripheral vasculitis, cutaneous necrosis, vasculitis, or gangrene. They are associated with inflammation, and they can represent serious disease activity that warrants corticosteroid and immune suppressive interventions (discussed further in the vasculitis section).

CASE STUDY 2

You are called by the local emergency room regarding Mrs. Jones. She was diagnosed with SLE 15 years ago on the basis of acute central nervous system (CNS) disease manifested by seizures, psychosis, fever, and headache. After 2 weeks in the hospital where her disease was managed with high-dose corticosteroids and she was given the first of six monthly doses of intravenous cyclophosphamide, the disease went into remission for many years. Three weeks before admission, Mrs. Jones began complaining of numbness, burning, and tingling in her legs. Earlier tonight, she attended a concert. When the strobe lights went on, she had a grand mal seizure and paramedics transported her to your hospital. By the time you arrive, she is no longer postictal and feels well. You are asked by the hospital staff if she has had a recurrence of CNS SLE. How should her complaints be best evaluated?

NERVOUS SYSTEM MANIFESTATIONS

The American College of Rheumatology has delineated 19 specific presentations of SLE affecting the nervous system, which are listed in Table 9-8.[21] Twelve involve the CNS, of which five are behavioral (acute confusional state, mood disorder, anxiety disorder, psychosis, cognitive dysfunction). Just about any part of the brain can be affected by any of the lupus syndromes listed in the next section such as myelopathy, movement disorders, seizures, meningitis, and demyelination. Seven affect the peripheral nervous system (Table 9-9).

Central Nervous System Vasculitis and Organic Brain Syndrome

The differential diagnosis of nervous system manifestations of SLE is among the most problematic in the disease. CNS vasculitis is one of the most difficult to evaluate and manage. It can often be the initial presentation of lupus, and most patients with CNS

Table 9-8. *Neuropsychiatric Lupus Syndromes: American College of Rheumatology Classification*

Central
Behavioral: psychosis, mood disorder, cognitive dysfunction, anxiety disorder, acute confusional state
Function related: movement disorder, myelopathy, demyelinating state
Other: aseptic meningitis, cardiovascular state, headache, seizure disorders

Peripheral
Nerve related: mononeuropathy, cranial neuropathy, polyneuropathy, autonomic neuropathy
Other: Guillain-Barre syndrome, myasthenia gravis, plexopathy

Table 9-9. *Prinicipal Central Nervous System Syndromes in Patients with Systemic Lupus Erythematosus: Differential Diagnosis*

Due to SLE
   Cerebral vasculitis: seen in 10%, diagnosed by lumbar puncture (pleocytosis, elevated protein, oligoclonal bands, high IgG synthesis rate, neuronal antibodies)

   Stroke/TIA from antiphospholipid antibodies: diagnosed by prolonged PTT, lupus anticoagulant, antiphospholipid antibodies, seen in10%

   Vasomotor instability: dysautonomia producing lupus headache, cognitive dysfunction. SPECT, PET, or fMR imaging suggestive. Seen in most with SLE.

   Non-antiphospholipid related coagulopathies: TTP, thrombocytopenias producing bleeds, cryoglobulinemia, hyperviscosity syndrome, marked hypergammaglobulinemic states, found in 5%, can produce bleeding, clots, or symptoms from sludging

Statistically associated with lupus but not part of the disease process
   CNS infection: diagnosed by abscess on imaging or at lumbar puncture. Suspect in immunosuppressed patients

   Fibromyalgia: nervous system related complaints with normal blood, spinal fluid and unimpressive imaging studies.

   Medication related symptoms due to agents which can alter cognitive function, induce headache, influence mood, appearance or behavior (e.g., steroids, NSAIDs, methotrexate, antimalarials, antidepressants, antihypertensives)

CNS, central nervous system; fMR, functional magnetic resonance; IgG, immunoglobulin G; PET, positron emission tomography; PTT, partial thromboplastin time; SLE, systemic lupus erythematosus; SPECT, single photon emission computed tomography; TIA, transient ischemic attack; TTP, thrombotic thrombocytopenic purpura.

SLE have had the disease for less than 5 years.[22–24] The typical presentation is that of low-grade fevers, cognitive dysfunction, headache, malaise, and stiff neck that progresses to seizures, stupor, and coma. Patients are often initially diagnosed as having a flu-like illness. Fortunately, prompt performance of a lumbar puncture with findings of pleocytosis, elevated spinal fluid protein, increased IgG synthesis rate, oligoclonal bands, or the presence of antineuronal antibodies can accelerate confirming the diagnosis if cultures are negative.[25] Magnetic resonance imaging (MRI) can be normal or demonstrates diffuse, generalized changes.[26] In the case of Mrs. Jones, the emergency room physicians suspected CNS vasculitis and administered high doses of corticosteroids for what turned out to be an organic brain syndrome. Her lupus was long standing and under good control, and the seizure represented light-induced activation of a scar focus.

Organic brain syndrome is best managed with steroid avoidance, emotional support, and cognitive behavioral therapy. CNS vasculitis responds to pulse doses of steroids, cyclophosphamide, rituximab, or in serious cases, apheresis, but there is no established evidence based management strategies.[27-29] The most frequently used protocol is 1 g of methylprednisolone daily for several days followed by 1 mg/kg/day of prednisone equivalent for several weeks, followed by a slow tapering. Cyclophosphamide is usually given in doses of 750mg/m^2 monthly for 6 months and then discontinued. A 40 to 60 mL/kg plasma exchange can be added for the first few weeks every other day if there is no initial response. Recent reports suggest that rituximab or intrathecal methotrexate can be administered in lieu of cyclophosphamide.

Vasomotor Central Nervous System Lupus: Lupus Headache and Cognitive Dysfunction

Ten percent of the United States population suffers from migraine headaches; this prevalence is doubled in SLE. Single photon emission computed tomography (SPECT), positron emission tomography (PET), and functional MRI has documented the association of this phenomena with increased cerebral blood flow. Conversely, cognitive dysfunction in SLE correlates with intermittent diminished flow and Raynaud's phenomenon (Fig. 9-2).[30,31] This phenomon represents the dysautonomic aspects of SLE, which implicates sympathetic mediated vasomotor instability as the principal inciting factor of these symptoms. Headache and cognitive impairment are intermittent which distinguishes them from a brain tumor or dementia. They are worsened by anxiety and stress. High doses of corticosteroids are unnecessary but, unfortunately, temporarily often subjectively beneficial, which misleads clinicians. Neither vasodilator nor vasoconstrictive therapies are effective over the long run. Anxiolytics, psychotropic agents, antimalarials, antidepressants, cognitive behavioral therapy, and biofeedback represent the treatments of choice.[32,33]

PERIPHERAL NEUROPATHIES

Inflammation of cranial nerves or other peripheral neuritides respond quickly to moderate-dose corticosteroid therapy for several weeks.[22-24] Involvement of several single nerves (mononeuritis

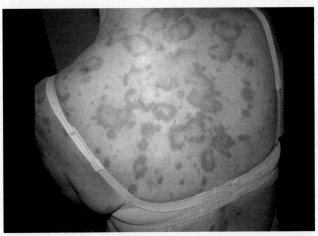

Figure 9-2. Subacute cutaneous lupus with epidermal and dermal, nonscarring lesions. Nervous system lupus.

multiplex) can be confirmed by electrical studies or nerve biopsy and requires high-dose corticosteroids for several months and intravenous immune globulin. Acute neuropathies, such as Guillain-Barré syndrome may benefit from apheresis or intravenous immune globulin.

RHEOLOGIC ABNORMALITIES: ANTIPHOSPHOLIPID SYNDROME, STROKE, CRYOGLOBULINEMIA, THROMBOTIC THROMBOCYTOPENIC PURPURA, HYPERVISCOSITY SYNDROME

Focal neurologic findings result from vascular events. Patients with SLE have an increased prevalence of stroke due to the presence of antiphospholipid antibodies (see Chapter xx) in addition to the risk factors for a cerebral event associated with migraine and accelerated atherogenesis.[34,35] These events occur suddenly and do not necessarily correlate with disease activity. Individuals with nonantiphospholipid coagulopathies (e.g., thrombocytopenic [TTP], immune thrombocytopenic purpura [ITP]) can also sustain strokes or cerebral bleeds. Antiplatelet regimens or anticoagulation may be indicated. High levels of circulating immune complexes and immunoglobulin are found in lupus patients with concurrent Sjögren's syndrome, some of whom complain of mental clouding due to sludging related to cryoglobulinemia or hyperviscosity.[36,37] This problem responds to apheresis, steroids, and immune suppressive therapies.

Differential Diagnosis

Up to 30% of patients with SLE have fibromyalgia, which produces symptoms and mimics CNS lupus

manifestations such as cognitive dysfunction, headache, fatigue, numbness, burning, and tingling.[38] CNS infections should be ruled out before prescribing anti-inflammatory therapies with immune suppressive, especially if fevers are present.[39] Medications used to manage SLE or aspects of the disease can cause CNS symptoms,[40] either through a drug reaction or producing pathologic changes (e.g., posterior reversible encephalopathic syndrome [PRES] in hypertensive hospitalized patients treated with immune suppressives). For example, corticosteroids can induce psychosis and other mental status changes, aseptic meningitis may result from ibuprofen, and headaches from indomethacin.

THE CARDIOPULMONARY SYSTEM

CASE STUDY 3

A young woman with recently diagnosed SLE presents to you as the covering rheumatologist in the Emergency Room. Her history is notable for sun-sensitive rashes, Raynaud's phenomenon, arthralgias, fatigue and pain on taking a deep breath with intermittent chest pains. Over the past week, she has developed a minimally productive cough, shortness of breath, and fevers. Her primary care physician prescribed erythromycin over the telephone 3 days earlier without benefit. A chest x-ray study reveals an interstitial infiltrate and a right-sided pleural effusion. An electrocardiogram demonstrated decreased voltage and nonreciprocal ST elevations. After deciding to admit her, what is the differential diagnosis and what interventions should be considered?

Low-grade fevers with pulmonary complaints are common occurrences in SLE. Making a correct, prompt diagnosis warrants a critical decision-making process (Table 9-10). First of all, our patient displayed a combination of fever with shortness of breath or pain on taking a deep breath. Cardiopulmonary manifestations of SLE are diverse, and their presentation can be challenging. One of the most common mistakes in managing this presentation is treating a presumptive infection when in fact it represents a lupus flare. As with our patient, all too often a prominent bronchial infection is managed over the telephone with antibiotics. Acute lupus pneumonitis should always be considered in the differential diagnosis of any patient with SLE who seems to have a fever, cough, and shortness of breath. This neutrophilic infiltrate loaded with immune complexes is present in 1% to 9% of patients with SLE and is best diagnosed at bronchoscopy.[41] Characterized by a rapid, downhill course, acute lupus pneumonitis has a 50% mortality rate if not treated with high-dose corticosteroids in the first 2 weeks.[42] It should always

Table 9-10. *Cardiopulmonary Manifestations of Systemic Lupus Erythematosus*

Manifestation	Prevalence	Comment and Management
Pleuritis	60%	Rarely serious, responds to NSAIDs, antimalarials, low dose steroids
Myocardial dysfunction	40%	Asymptomatic in most, frank myocarditis in 5-10% in disease course warrants moderate dose steroids
Hypertension	25%	Associated with renal disease, accelerated atherogenesis, ACE and ARB inhibitors drug of choice, calcium channel blocker also help Raynaud's while beta blockers worsen it
Effusions	25%	Pleural or pericardial: exudates respond to moderate dose steroids, drainage of diagnostic value, transudates respond to treating underlying cause
Interstitial lung	10%	Associated with Sjogren's and overlap syndromes, lymphocytic infiltrate. Treat if reversible with moderate dose steroids, immune suppressants
Pulmonary embolus	9%	Standard but long term treatment warranted Work up for coexisting antiphospholipid syndrome
Acute pneumonitis	5%	Serious, with 80% mortality without treatment in 2 weeks Aggressive work up to rule out infection Responds to high dose steroids
Pulmonary hypertension	5%	Associated with MCTD, overlap syndromes. Rule out pulmonary vasculitis and antiphospholipid syndrome. Managed with calcium channel blockers, 5 PDE antagonists, prostaglandins and endothelin blockade
Endocarditis	3%	Use preventive measures (platelet antagonists, anticoagulants) and antibiotic prophylaxis to prevent stroke, infection Valve replacement ultimately needed in 30%
Pulmonary hemorrhage	1%	Rare but causes up to 10% of deaths in lupus; alveolar infiltrates Treated aggressively with steroids, immune suppressants, apheresis

ACE, angiotensin-converting enzyme; ARB, angiotensin II receptor blockers; MCTD, mixed connective tissue disease; NSAIDs, nonsteroidal anti-inflammatory drugs; PDE, phosphodiesterase.

be considered in any lupus patient with chest-related symptoms and fevers, and can be readily identified with a screening chest x-ray study. Our patient's circumstance could also represent an infection, particularly an opportunistic one as well as being a lupus flare aggravated by a community-acquired infection. Patients with pulmonary infiltrates benefit from hospitalization, where due diligence can be undertaken to rule out infection versus a disease flare or a combination of the two.

MANAGING OTHER PRESENTATIONS OF PULMONARY LUPUS: PLEURISY, INTERSTITIAL LUNG DISEASE, PULMONARY EMBOLUS, PULMONARY HYPERTENSION, PULMONARY HEMORRHAGE

Pain on taking a deep breath is observed in 60% of patients and a frank effusion in 25% of patients with SLE during the course of their disease.[43-45] Inflammation of the pleura is not considered an organ-threatening manifestation of the disease. Pleuritic discomfort can also be a presentation of infections, allergy, occupational exposures, or scar-ring from previously active lupus. Pleural effusions may be exudates, which usually represent active disease, whereas transudates are associated with nephrosis, ascites, and concurrent pericardial effusions. Draining the effusion, under ultrasonic guidance if necessary, usually clarifies the cause of chest pains. Pleuritic pain without an effusion usually responds to nonsteroidal anti-inflammatory regimens, such as up to 1.5 g of naproxen daily. More intense discomfort is responsive to 20 to 40 mg of prednisone daily or the equivalent for 10 to 14 days, followed by tapering. Chronic pleuritis can be ameliorated with antimalarial therapies or immune suppressive regimens.

Interstitial lung infiltrates evolve slowly over several years and are more common in lupus patients with concurrent Sjögren's and overlap syndromes.[46,47] Interstitial lung disease is identified by a ground-glass appearance on a high-resolution computed tomography CT scan with a diminished diffusing capacity on pulmonary function testing, and affected patients have a mild cough with shortness of breath. Most do not have fevers, although concurrent infections are more common and always should be considered in the differential diagnosis. This manifestation responds to moderate-dose corticosteroids with immune suppressive (e.g., azathioprine, cyclophosphamide, mycophenolate mofetil) regimens. Untreated interstitial lung disease ultimately leads to irreversible pulmonary fibrosis and occasionally pulmonary hypertension.

One third of patients with SLE have antiphospholipid antibodies, and one third of these patients sustain a thromboembolic event as a consequence of this. This in part explains the 8% to 11% prevalence of pulmonary embolus in the disease.[48] All at-risk patients should be screened for thromboembolic factors such as anticardiolipin antibody, circulating lupus anticoagulant, and prolonged partial thromboplastin times. The management of pulmonary embolus is the same as with any non-lupus patient: heparin followed by warfarin. The only difference is that treatment with warfarin is usually not discontinued.

Elevated pulmonary pressures are prominent with those with mixed connective tissue disease (especially with high titer anti-ribonucleo protein [RNP]) and overlap syndromes as well as individuals with recurrent pulmonary emboli.[49,50] Rarely, pulmonary hypertension can be a consequence of pulmonary vasculitis. Diagnostic screening begins with a two-dimensional echocardiogram, followed by direct pressure measurements, if indicated. Endothelial cell hyperplasia–mediated pulmonary hypertension represents the overwhelming majority of cases in the 5% of patients with SLE who develop this complication. It is treated with prostaglandins, 5-phosphodiesterase blockers, endothelin receptor antagonists, and calcium channel blockers.[51,52]

Pulmonary hemorrhage is a catastrophic event seen in 1% of patients but causes up to 10% of lupus deaths owing to its delayed diagnosis.[53] It presents with hemoptysis, and imaging studies reveal alveolar infiltrates. Prompt treatment with apheresis, pulse doses of steroids, and cyclophosphamide can be life saving.

Chest Pain

Chest discomfort in SLE is widespread, problematic, frequently misdiagnosed, and inappropriately treated. The etiologies are diverse and include noncardiac causes (e.g., costochondritis, esophageal, anxiety), angina, pericarditis, dysautonomias (e.g., mitral valve prolapse in a patient who drinks a lot of caffeine), and myocarditis (Table 9-11).[54] An electrocardiogram, echocardiogram, blood testing with acute phase reactants, and a careful physical examination and history can usually clarify the issue.

Accelerated Atherogenesis and Hypertension

Premature atherosclerotic heart disease is the most common source of morbidity and mortality in patients with lupus who survive 20 years (Fig. 9-3).[55] Originally ascribed to corticosteroid therapy, this has been reported in patients who were not treated with

Table 9-11. *Conditions to Rule Out in Patients with Possible Cardiopulmonary Manifestations of Systemic Lupus Erythematosus*

Infection
Costochondritis
Fibromyalgia
Noncardiac chest pain (GERD, esophageal spasm, peptic ulcer disease)
Environmental
Allergies
Asthma
Chronic scarring from prior inflammation
Chronic obstructive pulmonary disease
Atherosclerotic heart disease
Non-lupus vasculitis (e.g., Churg-Strauss disease, Wegener's syndrome)
Eosinophilic lung syndromes
Lymphoma or carcinoma

GERD, gastrointestinal reflux disease.

prednisone. Patients with lupus are more likely to be hypertensive (25%, especially if renal involvement is present), hyperlipidemic, and have insulin resistance, metabolic syndrome, and hyperhomocystinemia. Approximately half with SLE have proinflammatory high-density lipoproteins (HDLs), or good cholesterol, which can be associated with oxidative stress, endothelial apoptosis, proinflammatory cytokines, elevated leptin levels, and dyslipidemias.[56]

The optimal management involves cardioprotective measures (Table 9-12).[57] This involves proactive screening for traditional risk factors such as blood pressure and blood sugar monitoring, lifestyle interventions (including diet, exercise, smoking cessation), and carotid duplex ultrasound, two-dimensional echocardiography, and stress testing, or 64-slice CT coronary artery imaging, when appropriate. Medication interventions include low-dose aspirin, statins, angiotensin-converting enzyme inhibitors, and antimalarials (which have antiplatelet activity and lower lipid levels).

Pericardial, Myocardial and Endocardial Involvement

At autopsy, 60% of patients with SLE have pericardial involvement, which is present incidentally and asymptomatically in 25% on two-dimensional echocardiography. Seen in 5% of lupus patients at any given time, pericardial effusions are associated with chest discomfort, which are alleviated by leaning forward and diagnosed by echocardiography or electrocardiographic changes.[58] Pericardial and pleural involvement often occur together. If other etiologies (e.g., pure cardiac, infectious) are ruled out and high-dose nonsteroidal anti-inflammatory therapies are not helpful, moderate-dose corticosteroid therapy for several weeks is ameliorative. Pericardial scarring may produce chest pain but is not responsive to anti-inflammatory regimens and

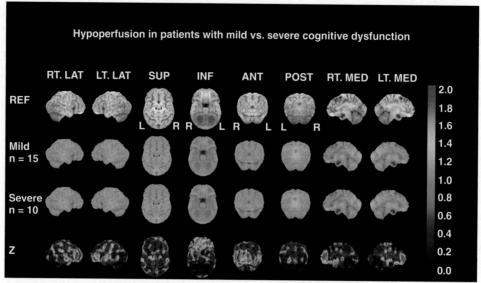

Figure 9-3. SPECT imaging in patients with SLE and cognitive impairment but without vasculitis. (From Driver CB, Wallace DJ, Lee JC, Forbess CJ, Pourrabbani S, Minoshima S, et al. Clinical validation of the watershed sign as a marker for neuropsychiatric systemic lupus erythematosus. Arthritis Rheum 2008;59:332-7.)

Table 9-12. *Cardioprotective Screening Measures that Can Decrease Morbidity and Mortality in Patients with Systemic Lupus Erythematosus*

Smoking cessation
Aggressive management of blood pressure
Weight reduction
Minimize use of corticosteroids
Screening for and proactive management of dyslipidemias
CT angiography/two-dimensional echo/carotid duplex
  scanning when indicated
Screen for and manage insulin resistance/metabolic
  syndrome, especially if on steroids
Anti-inflammatory regimens
Minimize use of nonsteroidal anti-inflammatory agents
Annual electrocardiogram
Promote adherence to medication
Engage in stress minimizing lifestyles

CT, computed tomography.

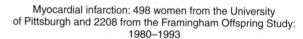

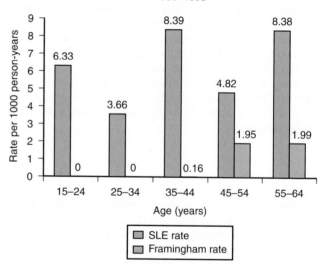

Figure 9-4. Incidence of myocardial infarction in women with SLE. (Adapted from Manzi S, Meilahn EN, Rairie JE, Conte CG, Medsger TA Jr, Jansen-McWilliams L, et al. Age-specific incidence rates of myocardial infarction and angina in women with systemic lupus erythematosus: comparison with the Framingham study. Am J Epidemiol 1997;145:408-15.)

necessitates stripping or pericardiectomy to prevent or manage constrictive pericarditis.

Although myocardial dysfunction is found in 40% of patients with lupus on stress echocardiography, frank noninfectious myocarditis is noted in less than 5% during the course of their disease (Fig. 9-4).[59] Coronary arteritis is an equally rare but serious complication of SLE. Suggested by elevation of acute phase reactants (e.g., sedimentation rate, C-reactive protein), muscle enzymes (e.g., creatine phosphokinase [CPK], troponin), and injury patterns on electrocardiography, more sophisticated interventional studies (e.g., myocardial biopsy) may be necessary to confirm the diagnosis of myocarditis. Most patients respond quickly to high-dose corticosteroids, but failure to completely resolve within a few weeks is an indication to implement immune suppressive therapies.

One to 5% of patients with SLE develop cellular debris, proliferative cells, or immune complexes on their heart valves. Historically known as "Libman Sacks endocarditis," these vegetations are associated with the presence of antiphospholipid antibodies or the lupus circulating anticoagulant.[60] Frequently a source of stroke or infectious endocarditis, patients with vegetations should be on thromboprophylactic measures ranging from antimicrobial dental prophylaxis to aspirin to clopidogrel or warfarin. Although only 30% of vegetations are seen on a routine two-dimensional echo, they are visible in 70% of patients using a transesophageal approach.

THE MUSCULOSKELETAL SYSTEM

CASE STUDY 4

Ms. Smith is a 24-year-old woman who presents with arthralgias, mostly in her hands and feet of 1 year duration. The discomfort is worse in the morning and is associated with stiffness. She initially consulted with her primary care physician, who noted a normal examination, sedimentation rate, CRP, rheumatoid factor, and ASO titer 6 months ago. The patient was told it could be postviral, and naproxen was prescribed. On examination, she shows definite but mild synovitis at the second and third metacarpophalangeal joints (MCPs) and metatarsophalangeal joints (MTPs) bilaterally. More recently, Mrs. Smith experienced fatigue and temperatures up to 100° F. A repeat rheumatoid factor and anti-cyclic citrullinated peptide (CCP) were negative, but the sedimentation rate is now 28 and an antinuclear antibody (ANA) is 1:160 speckled. The physical examination is otherwise normal. What is the diagnosis and how should it be treated?

INFLAMMATORY ARTHRITIS

Non–organ-threatening lupus arthritis can often be diagnosed when individuals who are too young to develop osteoarthritis report bilateral, symmetric pain in their hands and feet. Further inquiry reveals evidence for morning stiffness, involvement of the MCPs and MTPs (which are not seen with osteoarthritis), and response to nonsteroidal anti-inflammatory arthritis. Although 80% of patients with SLE have arthralgias, only half of these patients demonstrate an inflammatory arthritis.[61] In other words, the symptoms can be more profound than physical findings. The inflammatory process of lupus arthritis is similar histopathologically to that of rheumatoid arthritis (RA) but tends to be blander. Only 5% of patients ever develop erosions.[62] One characteristic feature is the presence of what is termed a Jaccoud's arthropathy. Long-standing inflammation of the MCPs leads to ulnar deviation. In RA, this process frequently produces a permanent deformity. However, in SLE, the Jaccoud's arthropathy refers to a reversible subluxation, which can be normalized with manipulation.[63] The differential diagnosis of Ms. Smith's presentation includes undifferentiated connective tissue disease (UCTD). There are probably

Table 9-13. *Classification of Undifferentiated Connective Tissue Disease*

Mandatory: inflammatory arthritis in more than one joint or Raynaud's phenomenon or keratoconjunctivitis sicca
Mandatory: positive antinuclear antibody, rheumatoid factor or anti-CCP
Need 3 of the following: myalgias, autoimmune rash, serositis, persistent fever without infection, adenopathy, elevated sedimentation rate or CRP, antiphospholipid antibody. Must not fulfill ACR definitions or criteria for any other rheumatic process

ACR, American College of Rheumatology; CCP, cyclic citrullinated peptide; CRP, C-reactive protein.

4-5 cases of UCTD for every one with RA and up to 10 for each case of SLE. Patients with UCTD can have a positive serology (ANA, rheumatoid factor, or anti-CCP) or Raynaud's phenomenon with inflammatory arthritis but do not fulfill the American College of Rheumatology criteria for any other rheumatic disorder (Table 9-13).[64] Other considerations could include primary Sjögren's or polymyalgia rheumatica (in an older patient), inflammatory osteoarthritis, or hemachromatosis.

The management of lupus arthritis involves staging the disease for extra-articular manifestations and simultaneously treating them (Table 9-14). If synovitis is the major focus of a patient's symptoms, then starting out with a nonsteroidal anti-inflammatory agent such as naproxen is recommended. Hydroxychloroquine is approved by the US Food and Drug Adminstration (FDA) for RA has had established disease-modifying potential. Lupus patients tend not to do well with sulfasalazine, gold salts, or d-penicillamine. Other agents approved for RA such as methotrexate, leflunomide and azathioprine are clearly beneficial in SLE as well (Table 9-15). Low doses of prednisone (less than 10 mg daily) are uniformly efficacious but should be used cautiously and for the shortest possible period of time. The role for anti-tumor necrosis factor (TNF) agents in lupus is controversial. Although they improve synovitis, these medications can raise anti-ds DNA and anti-cardiolipin levels, as well as aggravate certain manifestations of the disease. This writer uses anti-TNFs in lupus patients with synovitis who lack anti-ds DNA and anticardiolipin, and have minimal extra-articular activity.

Myalgias and Myositis

Whereas arthralgias and inflammatory arthritis are the most common musculoskeletal manifestations of SLE, muscles can be involved as well.[65,66] Seventy percent of patients report myalgias but myositis (defined as a CK greater than 500 IU) in the absence of other etiologies (e.g., hypothyroidism, statin therapy) has been reported in 5% to 10% of patients during the course of their disease. Proximal

Table 9-14. *Differential Diagnosis of Inflammatory Arthritis in Patients Suspected of Having Systemic Lupus Erythematosus*

Disease or Syndrome	Symptoms and Signs
Sjögren's syndrome	Older patients, anti SSA (Ro) positive, sicca symptoms
Polymyalgia rheumatica	Older patients, high sedimentation rate, affects proximal shoulder and hip girdle areas
Rheumatoid arthritis	Presence of anti CCP, RF, erosions, deformities, nodules, smoking history
Inflammatory osteoarthritis	Low-grade or local inflammation, involves PIPs, DIPs, IPs but not MCPs
Scleroderma	Early disease-hands are puffy, Raynaud's phenomenon, glossy appearance, positive anti Scl-70, anticentromere antibody
Inflammatory myositis	Elevated CKs, heliotrope rash, Gottron's papules, anti Jo or PM-1, proximal muscle weakness
Hepatitis C	Lifestyle risk factors, abnormal liver enzymes, hepatitis serologies positive along with evidence for viral load
Parvovirus	Positive serologies, sudden onset of polyarthritis with flu-like presentation with rash

CCP, cyclic citrullinated peptide; CKs, creatine phosphokinase; DIPs, distal interphalangeal joints; IPs, interphalangeal joints; MCPs, metacarpophalangeal joints; PIPs, peripheral interphalangeal joints; PM-1, polymyositis-1; RF, rheumatoid factor; SSA, Sjögren's syndrome A.

Table 9-15. *Management of Inflammatory Arthritis in Systemic Lupus Erythematosus*

Medication	Features
Topical NSAIDs	Diclofenac gels and patches are available, not tested in SLE but useful for mild, focal inflammation, little GI toxicity
Nonsteroidals	Naproxen and celecoxib studied and efficacious, gastroprotective measures may be indicated along with monitoring for hematologic, liver or renal effects
Hydroxychloroquine	FDA approved for SLE, effective after 3 months in most, ocular monitoring annually recommended
Methotrexate	RA doses used except with renal involvement, numerous studies document efficacy, liver and hematologic monitoring required
Leflunomide	RA doses used, controlled studies document efficacy in most
Prednisone	FDA approved for SLE, effective in doses of 5–10 mg daily, chronic daily requirement warrants evaluation for steroid-sparing alternatives if only used for arthritis
Azathioprine	FDA approved for RA, numerous studies document effectiveness in SLE, hematologic and hepatic monitoring every 2–3 months recommended, long term use associated with lymphoma risk
TNF blockade	Approved for RA, less effective in SLE but helpful in RA overlaps, use judiciously if anti-DNA present
Mycophenolate mofetil	RA studies showed no efficacy, no evidence it helps lupus arthritis

FDA, US Food and Drug Administration; GI, gastrointestinal; RA, rheumatoid arthritis; SLE, systemic lupus erythematosus; TNF, tumor necrosis factor.

upper and lower extremities tend to be targeted. Unlike polymyositis, the process usually responds to a few weeks of 20 mg of prednisone equivalent a day. An electromyogram can usually easily confirm the presence of myositis.

Associated Conditions: Fibromyalgia, Osteopenia, Osteoporosis, and Avascular Necrosis

A variety of other musculoskeletal disorders are commonly seen in patients with SLE but are not considered to be part of the inflammatory process. These include fibromyalgia, osteopenia and osteoporosis, and avascular necrosis. Fibromyalgia has been reported in 10% to 30% of patients with SLE.[67] Fibromyalgia is considered to be a syndrome and not a disease, and it is a disorder in which defects in sensory afferent processing lead to pain amplification. Muscle spasm and joint aches can be mistaken for inflammatory processes. Lupus activity may be clinically difficult to differentiate from fibromyalgia-related symptoms, but the latter complaints never elevate acute phase reactants (e.g., sedimentation rate, C-reactive protein), lower complement or white blood counts, or raise anti-ds DNA. Patients tapering steroids or who have significant psychosocial stressors are more susceptible to experiencing non-inflammatory myofascial discomfort.

Fibromyalgia is worsened by corticosteroids and does not respond to anti-inflammatory regimens. Inflammation by itself demineralizes bone, as do corticosteroids, methotrexate, and anticoagulants. As a consequence, up to 20% of patients with SLE at any given time have osteopenia or osteoporosis.[68] The American College of Rheumatology has recommended that any individual taking 5 mg of prednisone or greater for more than 1 month should be on antiresorptive therapy such as a bisphosphonate.[69] Finally, fat emboli from corticosteroid use increase the risk of lupus patients developing avascular necrosis, especially in the hip joint. Although a small number of patients with SLE can develop avascular necrosis from vasculitis, nearly all of the 8% with the disease who have this complication associate it with medication.[70,71] Medical treatment consists of bisphosphonates, calcium channel blockers, and analgesics. Most patients ultimately benefit from surgical approaches, which include revascularization in early stages and joint replacement.

VASCULITIS

CASE STUDY 5

Mrs. Walsh is a 34-year-old woman who was diagnosed with mild SLE 2 years before seeing you. Although she took hydroxychloroquine for a year, her family and acupuncturist convinced her that Eastern herbs and supplements could control her disease, and she went off all medication. One year later, she was referred to your office with a week of bloody diarrhea and fever. Your abdominal examination revealed generalized tenderness and guarding, diminished bowel sounds, and distention. It was decided that she should be admitted to the hospital. How should her abdominal pain be approached?

As in Mrs. Walsh's case, systemic vasculitis is one of the most feared manifestations of SLE. Although all caliber vessels can be affected, lupus vasculitis usually affects the small and medium-sized blood vessels.[72] Pathologically characterized by intimal proliferation, medial necrosis, and adventitial necrosis, patients with vasculitis are ill and often toxic appearing.[73,74] They tend to have multisystem activity, abnormal serologies such as low C3 complements, and high double-stranded anti-DNA, as well as elevated acute phase reactants.[75] A listing of the vasculidites seen with SLE are listed in Table 9-16, and its histopathology is shown in Figure 9-5.[76-78] Mesenteric vasculitis occurs in only 1% of patients with SLE, but it has at least a 50% mortality rate.[79] This is due to its often delayed recognition and the poor prognosis of infracted bowel. Our patient can be diagnosed with MRI or traditional angiography, "thumbprinting" on a gastrograffin enema, or biopsy.[80] Mesenteric thrombosis in patients with antiphospholipid antibodies can be concurrent or misdiagnosed as infarction, perforation, or infection.

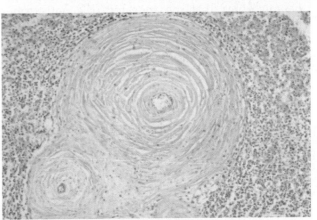

Figure 9-5. Vasculitis of a splenic arteriole in a lupus patient demonstrating intimal thickening, medial necrosis, and adventitial fibrosis.

Table 9-16. *Forms of Vasculitis Seen in Systemic Lupus Erythematosus*

Type of Vasculitis	Features
Retinal vasculitis	Occurs in 3-5% with SLE, presents with visual changes
Autoimmune vestibulitis	One case in 500; presents with hearing loss
Pulmonary vasculitis	Seen with alveolar hemorrhage, interstitial lung disease, can raise pulmonary pressures
Myocarditis	Occurs in 3–5%, includes coronary arteritis, presents with chest pain
Mesenteric vasculitis	Occurs in 1–3%, presents with bloody diarrhea and abdominal pain, has highest mortality rate of systemic vasculidites, variants include pancreatic vasculitis, hepatic vasculitis, renal arteritis
Cutaneous vasculitis	Only form in which small vessel arteritis and capillaritis predominate, is very responsive to steroids and has the best prognosis
CNS vasculitis	Occurs in up to 10%, best diagnosed at lumbar puncture, associated with seizures, psychosis, meningoencephalitis, prompt early treatment carries best prognosis

CNS, central nervous system; SLE, systemic lupus erythematosus.

Alternatively, many non–lupus-related causes of abdominal pain such as diverticulitis, cholecystitis, or pancreatitis need to be ruled out. Although pancreatitis can be caused by steroids, the principal treatment for pancreatic vasculitis is corticosteroids. Administering them for a few days in an uncertain clinical presentation outweighs potential risks. Surgical interventions for vasculitis (especially with mesenteric vasculitis or digital gangrene) may be needed to complement pulse dose steroids, followed by high-dose steroids for several weeks, along with the institution of an immune suppressive regimen and limb or organ salvage measures, if necessary.[81,82]

HEMATOLOGIC ABNORMALITIES

CASE STUDY 6

A 15-year-old high school sophomore reported that she was too tired to do her homework. Her parents noted that she appeared pale but attributed her appearance to recent heavy periods and gave her iron pills. Over the last week, she developed nosebleeds, bumps on her legs, and oozing from her gums. Testing revealed a platelet count of 10,000/mm³ and her hemoglobin was 8.0 g/dL. A diagnosis of Evan's syndrome was made, but when her ANA test returned with a value of 1:2560 homogenous, she was referred to you for definitive diagnoses and treatment. How should she be evaluated and managed?

Anemias are seen in 80% of patients with SLE. The most common causes include an anemia of chronic disease aggravated by factors associated with menstruating women such as heavy periods or iron deficiency (Table 9-17).[83,84] Other comorbidities such as vitamin B_{12} deficiency (seen in other autoimmune syndromes such as atrophic gastritis with antibodies to intrinsic factor), sickle cell anemia (since one in 250 black women have lupus), or thalassemia, or circulating factors inhibiting erythropoiesis should be considered as well. Ten percent of patients with lupus evolve end-stage renal disease, which is also associated with anemia. Nevertheless, consideration of a hemolytic anemia, as in the case of our patient, should always be contemplated as a cause of marked anemia, especially in young women, including children and adolescents.[85,86] Patients with autoimmune hemolytic anemia (AIHA) can be readily identified because they have most of the following: an elevated serum lactate dehydrogenase (LDH), reticulocyte count, low haptoglobin, and positive direct Coombs' test. Patients appear pale and tired. AIHA can be the presenting symptom of lupus. Attention is next focused on the platelet count. AIHA with autoimmune thrombocytopenia, or Evan's syndrome, is found in a significant minority of this group. Combinations of anemia and thrombocytopenia should warrant consideration of microangiopathic hemolytic anemia as part of thrombotic thrombocytopenic purpura (TTP).[87] This life-threatening combination consists of the pentad of hemolytic anemia, thrombocytopenia, renal impairment, CNS changes, and fever, and is often brought on by infection. Viewing a peripheral smear or bone marrow examination frequently helps make a definitive diagnosis, as well as obtaining ADAMTS13 levels (a von Willebrand factor protease). Also, approximately 15% of patients with lupus run low platelet counts as a manifestation of generalized inflammation. A subgroup of young women with SLE present with isolated idiopathic thrombocytopenic purpura (ITP) months to years before lupus develops.[88]

Leukopenia in SLE is almost always due to lymphopenia and results from antilymphocyte antibodies, medications such as corticosteroids (lymphocytosis with lymphopenia), or infection. It is rarely of clinical significance and only roughly correlates with inflammatory activity.[89]

Managing the cytopenias of SLE depends on the underlying cause. Repletion of vitamin B_{12}, iron, hormonal interventions, and dietary supplementation may be helpful. Hemolytic anemias mandate high-dose corticosteroids (1 mg/kg/day) for 4 to 12 weeks,

---

Table 9-17. *Differential Diagnosis of Cytopenias Associated with Systemic Lupus Erythematosus*

Anemias
Due to SLE: autoimmune hemolytic anemia, microangiopathic hemolytic anemia (seen with TTP), circulating inhibitory factors of erythropoiesis, bone marrow hypoplasia
Associated with lupus patients: iron deficiency (young women with concurrent heavy menses), vitamin B_{12} deficiency (with atrophic autoimmune gastritis), folic acid deficiency (with methotrexate), peptic ulcer disease (with NSAID therapy), sickle cell anemia (in African Americans), end-stage renal disease (lack of erythropoietin)

Leukopenias
Due to SLE: lymphopenia related to antilymphocyte antibodies and inflammation
Associated with lupus patients: immune suppressive medications, lymphopenia in patients taking corticosteroids

Thrombocytopenias
Due to SLE: ITP, TTP, active inflammation associated thrombocytopenias, marrow hypoplasia, qualitative platelet defects (rare), Evan's syndrome, antiphospholipid syndrome
Associated with lupus patients: immune suppressive medications

ITP, idiopathic thrombocytopenic purpura; NSAID, nonsteroidal anti-inflammatory drug; SLE, systemic lupus erythematosus; TTP, thrombotic thrombocytopenic purpura.

along with the institution of an immunosuppressive agent. Case reports and case series have suggested that mycophenolate mofetil, cyclophosphamide, azathioprine, and rituximab are efficacious.[90] The agent of choice should depend on whether or not other manifestations (e.g., liver, renal, pulmonary) of SLE are present.

Thrombocytopenias are rarely treated unless platelet counts drop below 60,000/mm³. As with anemias, the management of thrombocytopenias depends in part on the presence of extrahematologic disease. ITP quickly responds to moderate-dose corticosteroids, but refractory cases may benefit from the addition of azathioprine, cyclophosphamide, or rituximab.[91] Life-threatening ITP with platelet counts below 10,000/mm³ are usually managed with intravenous immune globulin. About 70% of refractory cases respond to splenectomy.[92]

References

1. Gordon C, Sutcliffe N, Skan J, Stoll T, Isenberg DA. Definition and treatment of lupus flares measured by the BILAG index. Rheumatology (Oxford) 2003;42:1372-9.
2. Bruce IN, Mak VC, Hallett DC, Gladman DD, Urowitz MB. Factors associated with fatigue in patients with systemic lupus erythematosus. Ann Rheum Dis 1999;58:379-81.
3. Stahl NI, Klippel JH, Decker JL. Fever in systemic lupus erythematosus. Am J Med 1979;67:935-40.
4. Shapira Y, Weinberger A, Wysenbeek AJ. Lymphadenopathy in systemic lupus erythematosus. Prevalence and relation to disease manifestations. Clin Rheumatol 1996;15:335-8.
5. Gilliam JN, Sontheimer RD. Distinctive cutaneous subsets in the spectrum of lupus erythematosus. J Am Acad Dermatol 1981;4:471–5.
6. Norris DA. Pathomechanisms of photosensitive lupus erythematosus. J Invest Dermatol 1993;100:58S-68S.
7. Wallace DJ, Pistiner M, Nessim S, Metzger AL, Klinenberg JR. Cutaneous lupus erythematosus without systemic lupus erythematosus. Clinical and laboratory features. Semin Arthritis Rheum 1992;21:221-6.
8. Sontheimer RD, Mc Cauliffe DP. Lupus specific skin disease (cutaneous LE). In: Wallace DJ, Hahn BH, editors. Dubois' lupus erythematosus. 7th ed. Philadelphia: Lippincott Williams & Wilkins; 2007. p. 576-620.
9. Lowe NJ. Photoprotection. Semin Dermatol 1990;9:78–83.
10. Kanekura T, Yoshi N, Terasaki K, Miyoshi H, Kanzaki T. Efficacy of topical tacrolimus for treating the malar rash of systemic lupus erythematosus. Br J Dermatol 2003;148:353-6.
11. Wallace DJ. Antimalarial therapies. In: Wallace DJ, Hahn BH, editors. Dubois' lupus erythematosus. 7th ed. Philadelphia: Lippincott Williams & Wilkins; 2007. p. 1152-74.
12. Esdaile J for the Canadian Cooperative Clinics. A randomized study of the effect of withdrawing hydroxychloroquine sulfate in systemic lupus erythematosus. Canadian Hydroxychloroquine Study Group. N Engl J Med 1991;324:150-4.
13. Rahman P, Gladman DD, Urowitz MB. Smoking interferes with efficacy of antimalarial therapy in cutaneous lupus. J Rheumatol 1998;25:1716-9.
14. Wallace DJ. The use of quinacrine (Atabrine). In rheumatic diseases: a re-examination. Semin Arthritis Rheum 1989;18:282-97.
15. Duong DJ, Spigel GT, Moxley RT, Gaspari AA. American experience with low-dose thalidomide therapy for severe cutaneous lupus erythematosus. Arch Dermatol 1999;135:1079-87.
16. Yell JA, Mbuagbaw J, Burge SM. Mucosal involvement in systemic and chronic cutaneous lupus erythematosus. Br J Dermatol 1989;121:727-41.
17. Sontheimer RD, Maddison PJ, Reichlin M, Jordon RE, Stastny P, Gilliam JN. Serologic and HLA associations in subacute cutaneous lupus erythematosus, a clinical subset of lupus erythematosus. Ann Intern Med 1982;97:664-71.
18. Lindskov R, Reymann F. Dapsone in the treatment of cutaneous lupus. Dermatologica 1986;172:214-7.
19. Wigley F. Raynaud's phenomenon. N Engl J Med 2002;347:1001-8.
20. Herrick AL. Treatment of Raynaud's phenomenon: new insights and developments. Curr Rheum Rep 2003;5:168-74.
21. ACR Ad Hoc Committee on Neuropsychiatric Lupus Nomenclature. The American College of Rheumatology nomenclature and case definitions for neuropsychiatric syndromes. Arthritis Rheum 1999;42:599-608.
22. Feinglass EJ, Arnett FC, Dorsch CA, Zizic TM, Stevens MB. Neuropsychiatric manifestations of systemic lupus erythematosus: diagnosis, clinical spectrum and relationship to other features of the disease. Medicine 1976;55:3230-9.
23. West SG, Emlen W, Wener MH, Kotzin BL. Neuropsychiatric lupus erythematosus: a 10-year prospective study on the value of diagnostic tests. Am J Med 1995;99:153-63.
24. Hanly JG, Mc Curdy G, Fougere L, Douglas JA, Thompson K. Neuropsychiatric events in systemic lupus erythematosus: attribution and clinical significance. J Rheumatol 2004;31:2156-62.
25. Hirohata S, Hirose S, Miyamoto T. Cerebrospinal fluid IgM, IgA, and IgG indexes in systemic lupus erythematosus. Their use as estimates of central nervous systemc disease activity. Arch Intern Med 1985;145:1843-6.
26. Hanly JG, Kuznetsova A, Fisk JD. Psychopathology of lupus and neuroimaging. In: Wallace DJ, Hahn BH, editors. Dubois' lupus erythematosus. 7th ed. Philadelphia: Lippincott Williams & Wilkins; 2007. p. 747-74.
27. Sanna G, Bertolaccini ML, Mathieu A. Central nervous system lupus: a clinical approach to therapy. Lupus 2003;12:935-42.
28. Boumpas DT, Yamada H, Patronas NJ, Scott D, Klippell JH, Bralow JE, et al. Pulse cyclophosphamide in severe neuropsychiatric lupus. Q J Med 1991;296:975-84.
29. Saito K, Nawata K, Nakayamada S, Tokunaga M, Tsukada J, Tanaka Y. Successful treatment of anti-CD20 monoclonal antibody (rituximab) of life-threatening refractory systemic lupus erythematosus with renal and central nervous system involvement. Lupus 2003;12:798-800.
30. Huang WS, Chiu PY, Tsai CH, Kao A, Lee CC. Objective evidence of abnormal cerebral blood flow in patients with systemic lupus erythematosus on Tc-99, ECD SPECT. Rheumatol Int 2002;22:178-81.
31. Driver CB, Wallace DJ, Lee JC, Forbess CJ, Pourrabbani S, Minoshima S, et al. Clinical validation of the watershed sign as a marker for neuropsychiatric systemic lupus erythematosus. Arthritis Rheum 2008;59:332-7.
32. Omdal R, Jorde R, Mellgren SL, Husby G. Autonomic function in systemic lupus erythematosus. Lupus 1994;3:413-7.
33. Gomex-Nava JL, Gonzalez-Lopez L, Ramos-Remus C, Fonseca-Gomez MM, Cardona-Muñoz EG, Suarez-Almazor ME. Autonomic dysfunction in patients with systemic lupus erythematosus. J Rheumatol 1998;25:1092-6.
34. Katav A, Chapman J, Shoenfeld Y. CNS dysfunction in the antiphospholipid antibody syndrome. Lupus 2003;12:903-7.
35. Toubi E, Khamashta MA, Panarra A, Hughes GR. Association of antiphospholipid antibodies with central nervous system disease in systemic lupus erythematosus. Am J Med 1995;99:397-401.
36. Jara LJ, Capin NR, Lavalle C. Hyperviscosity syndrome as the initial manifestation of systemic lupus erythematous. Am J Med 1989;16:225-30.
37. Ionnidis JP, Moutsopoulos HM. Sjogren's syndrome: too many associations, too little evidence. The enigma of central nervous system involvement. Semin Arthitis Rheum 1999;29:1-3.
38. Buskila D, Press J, Abu-Shakra M. Fibromyalgia in systemic lupus erythematosus. Clin Rev Allergy Immunol 2003;25:25-8.

39. Illopoulos AG, Tsokos GC. Immunopathogenesis and spectrum of infections in systemic lupus erythematosus. Semin Arthritis Rheum 1996;25:318-36.

40. Hoppman RA, Peden JG, Ober SK. Central nervous system side effects of nonsteroidal anti-inflammatory drugs. Arch Intern Med 1991;151:1309-13.

41. Elser AR, Shanies HM. Treatment of lupus interstitial lung disease with intravenous cyclophosphamide. Arthritis Rheum 1994;37:428-31.

42. Matthay RA, Schwartz MI, Petty TL, Stanford RE, Gupta RC, Sahn SA, et al. Pulmonary manifestations of systemic lupus erythematosus: review of twelve cases of acute lupus pneumonitis. Medicine 1975;54:397-409.

43. Good JT, King TE, Antony VD, Sahn SA. Lupus pleuritis: clinical features and pleural fluid characteristics with special reference to pleural fluid antinuclear antibodies. Chest 1983;84:714-8.

44. Murin S, Wiedmann HP, Matthay PA. Pulmonary manifestations of systemic lupus erythematosus. Clin Chest Med 1998;19:641-65.

45. Sant SM, Doran M, Fenlon HM, et al. Pleuropulmonary abnormalities in patients with systemic lupus erythematosus: assessment with high resolution computed tomography, chest radiography, and pulmonary function tests. Clin Exp Rheumatolol 1997;15:507-13.

46. Weinrib L, Sharma OP, Quirmorio FP. A long term study of interstitial lung disease in systemic lupus erythematosus. Semin Arthritis Rheum 1990;16:479-91.

47. Eichaker PQ, Pinsker K, Epstein A, Schiffenbauer J, Grayzel A. Serial pulmonary function testing in patients with systemic lupus erythematosus. Chest 1988;94:129-32.

48. Gladman DD, Urowitz MB. Venous syndromes and pulmonary embolism in systemic lupus erythematosus. Ann Rheum Dis 1980;39:340-3.

49. Asherson RA, Higgenbottom TW, Dihn Xuan AT, Khamashta MA, Hughes GR. Pulmonary hypertension in a lupus clinic: experience with 24 patients. J Rheumatol 1990;17:1291–8.

50. Pope J. An update in pulmonary hypertension in systemic lupus erythematosus—do we need to know about it? Lupus 2008;17:274-7.

51. Yoshio T, Masuyama J, Sumiya M, Minota S, Kano S. Antiendothelial cell antibodies and their relation to pulmonary hypertension in systemic lupus erythematosus. J Rheumatol 1994;21:2058-63.

52. Rubin LJ, Badesch DB, Barst JR, Galie N, Black CM, Keogh A, et al. Bosentan therapy for pulmonary arterial hypertension. N Engl J Med 2002;346:896-903.

53. Zamora MR, Warner ML, Tuder R, et al. Diffuse alveolar hemorrhage and systemic lupus erythematosus. Clinical presentation, histology, survival and outcome. Medicine 1997;76:192-202.

54. Wallace DJ. Pants and pulses: The lungs and heart. The lupus book. 3rd ed. New York: Oxford University Press; 2005. p. 85-103.

55. Manzi S, Meilahn EN, Rairie JE, Conte CG, Medsger TA, Jansen-McWilliams L, et al. Age-specific incidence rates of myocardial infarction and angina in women with systemic lupus erythematosus: comparison with the Framingham study. Am J Epidemiol 1997;145:408-15.

56. McMahon M, Grossman J, FitzGerald J, Dahlin-Lee E, Wallace DJ, Thong BY, et al. Proinflammatory high-density lipoprotein as a biomarker for atherosclerosis in patients with systemic lupus erythematosus and rheumatoid arthritis. Arthritis Rheum 2006;54:2541-49.

57. Wallace DJ. Are there models for predicting accelerated atherogenesis in systemic lupus erythematosus? Nature Clin Pract Rheumatol 2008;4:450-1.

58. Sturfelt G, Eskilsson F, Nived O, Truedsson L, Valind S. Cardiovascular disease in systemic lupus erythematosus. A study of 75 patients from a defined population. Medicine 1992;71:216-23.

59. Wijetunga M, Rockson S. Myocarditis in systemic lupus erythematosus. Am J Med 2002;113:419-23.

60. Bulkley BH, Roberts WC. The heart in systemic lupus erythematosus and the changes induced by it in corticoster-oid therapy. A study of 36 necropsy patients. Am J Med 1975;38:243-64.

61. Petri M. Musculoskeletal complications of systemic lupus erythematosus in the Hopkins Lupus Cohort: an update. Arthritis Care Res 1995;8:137-45.

62. Richter Cohen M, Steiner G, Smolen JS, Isenberg DA. Erosive arthritis in systemic lupus erythematosus: analysis of a distinct clinical and serological subset. Br J Rheumatol 1998;37:421-4.

63. Szczepanski L, Targonska B, Piotrowski M. Deforming arthropathy and Jaccoud's syndrome in patients with systemic lupus erythematosus. Scand J Rheumatol 1992;21:308-9.

64. Williams HJ, Alarcon GS, Joks R, Steen VD, Bulpitt K, Clegg DO, et al. Early undifferentiated connective tissue disease (CTD): VI. An inception cohort after 10 years: disease remissions and changes in diagnoses in well established and undifferentiated CTD. J Rheumatol 1999;26:816-25.

65. Isenberg DA, Snaith ML. Muscle disease in systemic lupus erythematosus: a study of its nature, frequency and cause. J Rheumatol 1981;8:917-24.

66. Dayal NA, Isenberg DA. SLE/myositis overlap: are the manifestations of SLE different in overlap disease? Lupus 2002;11:293-8.

67. Staud R. Are patients with systemic lupus erythematosus at increased risk for fibromyalgia? Curr Rheumatol Rep 2006;8:430-5.

68. Almehed K, Forsblad d'Elia H, Kvist G, Ohlsson C, Carlsten H. Prevalence and risk factors of osteoporosis in female SLE patients-extended report. Rheumatology (Oxford) 2007;46:1185-90.

69. American College of Rheumatology Ad Hoc Committee on Glucocorticoid-Induced Osteoporosis. Recommendations for the prevention and treatment of glucocorticoid-induced osteoporosis. Arthritis Rheum 2001;44:1496-503.

70. Gladman DD, Urowitz MB, Chaudhry-Ahluwalia V. Predictive factors for symptomatic osteonecrosis in patients with systemic lupus erythematosus. J Rheumatol 2001;28:761-5.

71. Cozen L, Wallace DJ. Avascular necrosis in systemic lupus erythematosus: clinical associations and a 47-year perspective. Am J Orthop 1998;27:352-4.

72. Takeuchi T. Systemic lupus erythematosus and vasculitis. In: Tsokos GC, Gordon C, Smolen JS, editors. Systemic lupus erythematosus, a companion to rheumatology. Philadelphia: Elsevier; 2007. p. 310-6.

73. Drenkard C, Villa AR, Reyes E, Abello M, Alarcon-Segovia D. Vasculitis in systemic lupus erythematosus. Lupus 1997;6:236-42.

74. Fauci AS, Haynes BF, Katz P. The spectrum of vasculitis. Clinical, pathological, immunologic and therapeutic considerations. Ann Intern Med 1978;89:660-76.

75. Calmia KT, Balbanova M. Vasculitis in systemic lupus erythematosus. Clin Dermatol 2004;22:148-56.

76. Howare TW, Iannini MJ, Burge JJ, Davis 4th JS. Rheumatoid factor, cryoglobulinemia, anti DNA and renal disease in patients with systemic lupus erythematosus. J Rheumatol 1991;18:826-30.

77. Read RW, Chong LP, Rao NA. Occlusive retinal vasculitis associated with systemic lupus erythematosus. Ann Ophthalmol 2000;118:588-9.

78. Andonopoulos AP, Naxakis S, Gumas P, Lygatsikas C. Sensorineural hearing disorders in systemic lupus erythematosus. A controlled study. Clin Exp Rheumatol 1995;13:137-41.

79. Mc Collum CN, Sloan ME, Davidson AM, Giles GR. Ruptured hepatic aneurysm in systemic lupus erythematosus. Ann Rheum Dis 1979;38:396-8.

80. Zizic TM, Classen JN, Stevens MB. Acute abdominal complications of systemic lupus erythematosus and polyarteritis nodosa. Am J Med 1982;73:525-31.

81. Ko SF, Lee TY, Cheng TT, Ng SH, Lai HM, Cheng YF, et al. CT findings at lupus mesenteric vasculitis. Acta Radiol 1997;38:115-20.

82. Ho MS, The LB, Goh HS. Ischemic colitis in systemic lupus erythematosus of case and review of the literature. Ann Acad Med Singapore 1987;16:501-3.

83. Lian TY, Edwards CJ, Chan SP, Chng HH. Reversible acute gastrointestinal syndrome associated with active systemic lupus erythematosus in patients admitted to the hospital. Lupus 2003;12:612-6.

83. Voulgarelis M, Kokori S, Ioannidis JPA, Tzioufas AG, Kyriaki D, Moutsopoulos HM. Anaemia in systemic lupus erythematosus aetiological profile and role of erythropoietin. Ann Rheum Dis 2000;59:217-22.

84. Richert-Boe KE. Hematologic complications of rheumatic disease. Hematol Oncol Clin North Am 1987;1:301-19.

85. Sultan SM, Begum S, Isenberg DA. Prevalence, patterns of disease and outcome in patients with systemic lupus erythematosus who develop hematologic problems. Rheumatology (Oxford) 2003;42:230-4.

86. Nossent JC, Weaak AJG. Prevalence and significance of haematological abnormalities in patients with systemic lupus erythematosus. Q J Med 1991;80:605-12.

87. Fox DA, Faix JD, Coblyn J, Fraser P, Smith B, Weinblatt ME. Thrombotic thrombocytopenic purpura and systemic lupus erythematosus. Ann Rheum Dis 1986;45:319-22.

88. Rivero SJ, Diaz-Jouanen E, Alarcon-Segovia D. Lymphopenia in systemic lupus erythematous. Arthritis Rheum 1978;21: 295-305.

89. Mestanza-Peralta M, Ariza-Ariza R, Cardiel MH, Alcocer-Varela J. Thrombocytopenic purpura as intitial manifestation of systemic lupus erythematosus. J Rheumatol 1997;24:867-70.

90. King KE, Ness PM. Treatment of autoimmune hemolytic anemia. Semin Hematol 2005;42:131-6.

91. Arnal C, Piette JC, Léone J, Taillan B, Hachulla E, Roudot-Thoraval F, et al. Treatment of severe immune thrombocytopenia associated with systemic lupus erythematosus: 59 cases. J Rheumatol 2002;29:75-83.

92. Hakim AJ, Machin SJ, Isenberg DA. Autoimmune thrombocytopenia in primary antiphospholipid syndrome and systemic lupus erythematosus: the response to splenectomy. Semin Arthritis Rheum 1998;28:20-5.

Management of Systemic Lupus Erythematosus Renal Disease

Sandra V. Navarra and Oscar D. Naidas

INTRODUCTION

Renal involvement is one of the most serious clinical manifestations of systemic lupus erythematosus (SLE), contributing significantly to overall morbidity and mortality. Its prevalence in lupus varies from 31% to 75%, typically presenting within the first year of SLE diagnosis.[1-5] If present at SLE diagnosis, it is also a major predictor for future disease exacerbations.[6] It has direct and indirect socioeconomic effects, as well as a significant impact on quality-of-life measures,[7] due to both the disease itself and the side effects of therapies. It is important to recognize that lupus kidney disease has an extremely broad spectrum of clinical manifestations, and there is no single standard of care appropriate for all patients with lupus nephritis. Although more recent attempts at clarification of the various histologic patterns and clinical correlations provide useful guidelines in clinical decision-making, such characteristics can vary over time, requiring careful monitoring for progression, response to treatment, as well as complications of therapy.

CASE STUDY 1

A 26-year-old female executive presents with a faint malar rash, alopecia, arthralgias, and fevers of 2 months' duration. Laboratory tests show mild anemia, leukopenia, 2+ proteinuria (1.2 g/day) with granular casts and dysmorphic erythrocytes, hypocomplementemia, high titers anti-nuclear antibody (ANA) and moderate titer anti-dsDNA. The 24-hour creatinine clearance and serial blood pressure determinations are normal.

CLINICAL PRESENTATION AND DIAGNOSIS

Renal involvement in lupus is highly variable and may occur as any or a combination of the following: occult or "silent," active nephritis, nephrotic syndrome, rapidly progressive nephritis, and chronic kidney disease. This may follow a protracted course with periods of remissions and exacerbations, and tendency for worse prognosis in certain racial groups.[6,8]

Because renal involvement in lupus is largely asymptomatic, it is important to specifically elicit symptoms such as foamy urine (proteinuria) and edema, and monitor closely for new-onset or worsening hypertension.

Laboratory Tests

Laboratory tests are used to assess the degree of glomerular inflammation and renal function. The urinalysis is the most important and cost-effective method to detect and monitor lupus nephritis. For accurate results, a fresh midstream clean-catch urine specimen, preferably the first morning urine sample, must be expeditiously processed and examined at the clinic or laboratory particularly for dipstick protein and sediments. Hematuria with dysmorphic erythrocytes (Fig. 10-1) indicates inflammatory glomerular or tubulointerstitial disease, granular casts reflect proteinuria, cellular (red blood cell, white blood cell, mixed cellular) casts (Fig. 10-2) reflect nephritic states, and broad and waxy casts reflect chronic renal damage. Serum creatinine alone crudely reflects renal function, and more precise evaluation should include estimation of glomerular filtration rate (GFR) by 24-hour creatinine clearance measurement, or calculating from formulas such as the traditional Cockroft-Gault,[9] or the Modification of Diet in Renal Disease study formula, the latter being less precise but more closely approximating GFR changes in older subjects.[10] Several clinical laboratories now routinely incorporate formula-based GFR estimates with serum creatinine values. Once a patient demonstrates significant proteinuria (>300–500 mg/day) or has a urinary dipstick proteinuria (+1 or greater), the measurement of the protein to creatinine (P/C) ratio should be performed on a random urine sample. Random urine P/C ratio is highly sensitive (92%–97%) and specific (87%–94%), and correlates well with 24-hour urinary protein.[11,12] Because of diurnal variations, urinary P/C ratios obtained at certain timed collections (3–6 PM and 6 AM–6 PM)

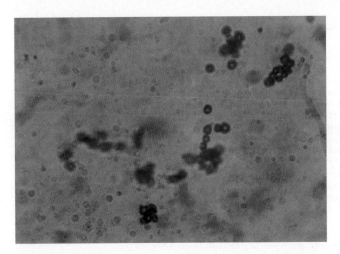

Figure 10-1. Dysmorphic red blood cells on urinalysis. (With permission from Daysog AO, Moral GA, Marcial MR. Daysog's Atlas of Urinary Sediments. Manila, Philippines: Anvil Publishing, Inc.; 2001.)

were shown to be more reliable than spot urine samples, and may be more convenient for the patient than a 24-hour collection.[13]

Measurements of complement components are useful in evaluating the extent of glomerular inflammation. SLE patients with renal involvement were more frequently found to have markedly reduced serum levels of C3 and C4 than patients with extrarenal involvement only. Moreover, low C3 levels were predictive of persistently active glomerular disease and associated with progression to end-stage renal disease (ESRD). Detection of high titers antidsDNA is useful not only in the diagnosis of SLE, but also suggests high risk for renal disease flares, especially when associated with low levels of serum complement.[14]

Levels of plasma and urinary cytokines or chemokines such as monocyte chemoattractant protein-1, soluble vascular cell adhesion molecule-1, soluble tumor necrosis factor receptor-1 (sTNFR-1), osteoprotegerin, and neutrophil gelatinase-B–associated lipocalin (lipocalin-2)[15-18] have been shown to correlate with renal disease activity and predict renal flares. Because they are noninvasive and relatively sensitive, these biomarkers provide an attractive tool for monitoring therapeutic response and are being explored for potential use in clinical practice.

Renal Biopsy

Renal biopsies rarely help in the diagnosis of lupus but are useful in determining the treatment choice and prognosis, especially when weighing the benefits versus risks of vigorous immunosuppressive therapy. The morphologic classification of SLE nephritis has evolved over the past 4 decades as more lesions were identified and defined, with the increasing challenge to make each classification and index relevant to clinical practice. The original 1974 World Health Organization (WHO) classification of lupus nephritis (Table 10-1) has been modified and further supplemented by the development of activity and chronicity indices (Table 10-2) of the National Institutes of Health.[19] High activity scores are often reversible with aggressive treatment, whereas high chronicity scores reflect irreversible changes that lack response to immunosuppression. The most current International Society of Nephrology/Renal Pathology Society (ISN/RPS) 2003 classification (Table 10-3) incorporates and combines the basic elements of the

Table 10-1. *Original World Health Organization (WHO) Classification of Lupus Nephritis (1974)*

Class	Description
Class I	Normal glomeruli (by light microscopy, immunofluorescence and electron microscopy)
Class II	Purely mesangial disease Normocellular mesangium by light microscopy but mesangial deposits by immunofluorescence or electron microscopy Mesangial hypercellularity with mesangial deposits by immunofluorescence or electron microscopy
Class III	Focal proliferative glomerulonephritis (< 50%)
Class IV	Diffuse proliferative glomerulonephritis (≥ 50%)
Class V	Membranous glomerulonephritis

Modified from Appel GB, Silva FG, Pirani CL. Renal involvement in systemic lupus erythematosus (SLE): A study of 56 patients emphasizing histologic classification. Medicine 1978;75:371-410; and Weening JJ, D'Agati VD, Schwartz MM, Seshan SV, Alpers CE, Appel GB, et al. The classification of glomerulonephritis in systemic lupus erythematosus revisited. J Am Soc Nephrol 2004;15:241-50.

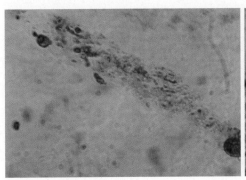 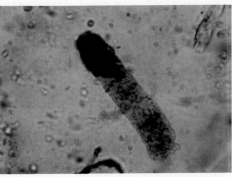

Figure 10-2. Coarse granular casts on urinalysis. (With permission from Daysog AO, Moral GA, Marcial MR. Daysog's Atlas of Urinary Sediments. Manila, Philippines: Anvil Publishing, Inc.; 2001.)

Table 10-2. *Activity and Chronicity Scoring Indices in Lupus Nephritis*

ACTIVITY INDEX (maximum score 24 points)

Hypercellularity: endocapillary proliferation compromising glomerular capillary circulation*
Leukocyte exudation: polymorphonuclear leukocytes in glomeruli*
Karyorrhexis/fibrinoid necrosis (weighted ×2): necrotizing changes in glomeruli†
Cellular crescents (weighted ×2): layers of proliferating epithelial cells and monocytes lining Bowman's capsule†
Hyaline deposits: eosinophilic materials lining (wire loops) or PAS-positive filling (hyaline thrombi) in capillary loops*
Interstitial inflammation: infiltration of leukocytes (predominantly mononuclear cells) among tubules*

CHRONICITY INDEX (maximum score 12 points)

Glomerular sclerosis: collapse and fibrosis of capillary tufts†
Fibrous crescents: layers of fibrous tissue lining Bowman's capsule†
Tubular atrophy: thickening of tubular basement membranes, tubular epithelial degeneration, with separation of residual tubules*
Interstitial fibrosis: deposition of collagenous connective tissue among tubules*

PAS, periodic acid-Sciff stain.
*Scored on a scale of 0 to 3 representing either absent, mild, moderate and severe lesions, respectively.
†Scored on a scale of 0 to 3 according to presence of lesions in none, <25%, 25-50%, and >50% of glomeruli, respectively.
Modified from Balow JE, Boumpas DT, Austin HA. Systemic lupus erythematosus and the kidney. In: Lahita RG, editor. Systemic lupus erythematosus. San Diego: Academic Press; 1999. p. 657-85.

Table 10-3. *International Society of Nephrology/Renal Pathology Society (ISN/RPS) 2003 Classification of Lupus Nephritis*

Class I	**Minimal mesangial lupus nephritis** Normal glomeruli by light microscopy, with mesangial immune deposits by immunofluorescence
Class II	**Mesangial proliferative lupus nephritis** Purely mesangial hypercellularity of any degree or mesangial matrix expansion by light microscopy, with mesangial immune deposits. A few isolated subepithelial or subendothelial deposits visible by immunofluorescence or electron microscopy, but not by light microscopy
Class III	**Focal lupus nephritis*** Active or inactive focal, segmental or global endo- or extracapillary glomerulonephritis involving <50% of all glomeruli, typically with focal subendothelial immune deposits, with or without mesangial alterations
Class III(A)	Active lesions: focal proliferative LN
Class III(A/C)	Active and chronic lesions: focal proliferative and sclerosing LN
Class III(C)	Chronic inactive lesions with glomerular scars: focal sclerosing LN
Class IV	**Diffuse lupus nephritis†** Active or inactive diffuse, segmental or global endo- or extracapillary glomerulonephritis involving ≥50% of all glomeruli, typically with diffuse subendothelial immune deposits, with or without mesangial alterations. This class is divided into diffuse segmental (IV-S) LN when ≥50% of involved glomeruli have segmental lesions, and diffuse global (IV-G) LN when ≥50% of involved glomeruli have global lesions. Segmental is defined as a glomerular lesion that involves less than half of the glomerular tuft, and includes cases with diffuse wire loop deposits but with little or no glomerular proliferation
Class IV-S(A)	Active lesions: diffuse segmental proliferative LN
Class IV-G(A)	Active lesions: diffuse global proliferative LN
Class IV-S(A/C)	Active and chronic lesions: diffuse segmental proliferative and sclerosing LN
Class IV-G(A/C)	Active and chronic lesions: diffuse global proliferative and sclerosing LN
Class IV-S(C)	Chronic inactive lesions with scars: diffuse segmental sclerosing LN
Class IV-G(C)	Chronic inactive lesions with scars: diffuse global sclerosing LN
Class V	**Membranous lupus nephritis** Global or segmental subepithelial immune deposits or their morphologic sequelae by light microscopy and by immunofluorescence or electron microscopy, with or without mesangial alterations Class V LN may occur in combination with class III or IV in which case both will be diagnosed Class V LN show advanced sclerosis
Class VI	**Advanced sclerosis lupus nephritis** ≥ 90% of glomeruli globally sclerosed without residual activity

LN, lupus nephritis.
*Indicate the proportion of glomeruli with active and with sclerotic lesions.
†Indicate the proportion of glomeruli with fibrinoid necrosis and/or cellular crescents.
From Weening JJ, D'Agati VD, Schwartz MM, Seshan SV, Alpers CE, Appel GB, et al. The classification of glomerulonephritis in systemic lupus erythematosus revisited. J Am Soc Nephrol 2004;15:241-50.

WHO classification with the activity and chronicity indices and aims to standardize definitions, emphasize clinically relevant lesions, and encourage uniform and reproducible reporting among centers.[20]

The usual indications for renal biopsy in lupus nephritis include unexplained hematuria, cellular casts or proteinuria (>0.5 to 1 g/day), or unexplained worsening of renal function. Renal biopsy is also indicated to establish the specific class and severity of lesions, which correlate to some degree with clinical findings and require different approaches to therapy.[21] Patients with established clinical and laboratory evidence of lupus nephritis or nephrotic syndrome may not require a renal biopsy before treatment with cytotoxic drugs. On the other hand, patients with persistent clinically active disease despite previous immunosuppressive treatment may be candidates for renal biopsy.[22]

The pathologist must provide an accurate and detailed description of all the biopsy findings by light microscopy, immunofluorescence and electron microscopy (Fig. 10-3A to D), with a summary diagnosis that includes the class (or classes) of lupus nephritis, and percentage of glomeruli with active and chronic lesions. The extent, severity and type of tubulointerstitial and vascular involvement should also be documented and graded.[20] The renal biopsy findings must be interpreted by the clinician in the context of the patient's clinical presentation, serologic findings and clinical course.

TREATMENT

General Approach

Current strategies for management of lupus nephritis include an induction phase intended to aggressively suppress glomerular inflammation and

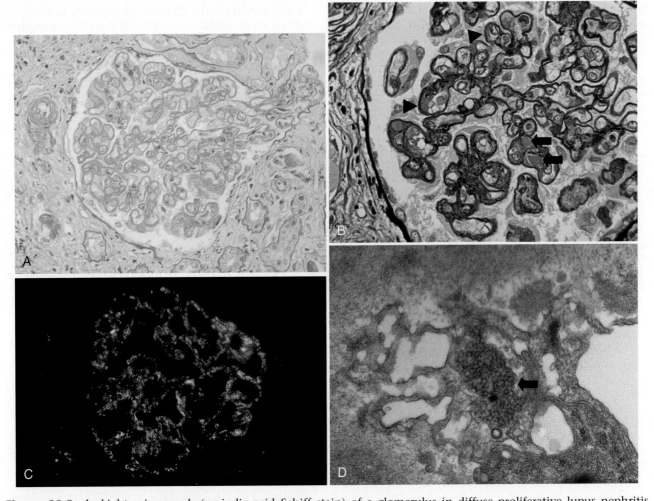

Figure 10-3. A, Light micrograph (periodic acid–Schiff stain) of a glomerulus in diffuse proliferative lupus nephritis showing endocapillary proliferation with infiltrating leukocytes. **B,** Light micrograph (with silver staining) of a glomerulus in diffuse proliferative lupus nephritis ISN/RPS Class IV Global-Active, showing wire loops produced by subendothelial deposits (*arrowheads*) and hyaline thrombi (*arrow*). **C,** Immunofluorescence photomicrograph of diffuse proliferative lupus nephritis ISN/RPS Class IV Global-Active, showing "full house" immunofluorescence with mesangial and glomerular basement membrane staining for immunoglobulin G (IgG), immunoglobulin A (IgA), immunoglobulin M (IgM), C3, and C1q. **D,** Electron microscopic finding in lupus nephritis ISN/RPS Class IV Global-Active, showing tubuloreticular inclusion (*arrow*) in the endothelium highly suggestive of lupus nephritis. (Photomicrographs courtesy of Dr. Sonia Chicano.)

achieve disease remission, and a maintenance phase, which aims to consolidate and sustain the therapeutic effect. The main issue with the induction phase is the achievement of an effective therapeutic response, whereas the maintenance phase aims toward an acceptable balance between sustaining the therapeutic response and minimizing adverse effects of medications.

Corticosteroids

Corticosteroids, particularly in high doses, have remained the mainstay of therapy for active lupus nephritis. Although there have been no controlled clinical trials proving the benefit of corticosteroids over supportive therapy alone, widespread clinical experience has established its value, especially for active renal disease. For induction therapy or renal flares, it is used at a high daily dose, for example, prednisone 0.5 to 1.0 mg/kg/day, or as pulse intravenous therapy, for example, methylprednisolone 0.5 to 1.0 g/day for 1 to 3 days. The main limitation of corticosteroids consists of a waning of effectiveness over time, with side effects eventually outweighing benefits. Thus, it is common practice to combine corticosteroids with other "steroid-sparing" immunosuppressive regimens during the induction phase, especially for proliferative lupus nephritis. It is also important to prevent or minimize steroid side effects, which further contribute to morbidity, for example, calcium 1.2 g/day plus vitamin D

800 IU/d, bisphosphonates and teriparatide to prevent or treat glucocorticoid-induced osteoporosis (see Chapter 24).

Immunosuppressive Regimens

A meta-analysis of early trials showed that the addition of immunosuppressive drugs like cyclophosphamide (CY) or azathioprine (AZA) to corticosteroids lowered the risk of renal insufficiency and dialysis.[23] Since then, effective immunosuppressive therapy has been established in several controlled clinical trials for lupus nephritis. Although most trials have been limited by diverse study variables such as small populations, racial mixtures, and short follow-up, these studies have provided the templates by which physicians make clinical decisions. It is not unusual practice to shift or combine the various regimens, because each management program has to be tailored for the individual patient.

Cyclophosphamide

Early studies have shown the superior efficacy of oral CY over corticosteroids alone in lupus nephritis.[23-25] However, the higher risks of toxicity like hemorrhagic cystitis and bladder cancer has strongly favored the use of intravenous (IV) CY pulse over oral therapy.

The National Institutes of Health pulse CY regimen (Table 10-4), established in a series of controlled trials over several decades,[26-28] has provided

Table 10-4. *The National Institutes of Health (NIH) Pulse Cyclophosphamide Regimen for Lupus Nephritis*

Initial dose of cyclophosphamide (CY)	Administer 0.75 g/m² of body surface area (BSA) if glomerular filtration rate (GFR) is greater than one third of normal value, or 0.5 g/m² of BSA if GFR is less than one-third of normal value.
Administration of CY	Use 500 ml of 5% dextrose in 0.3% to 0.9% saline, and infuse 250 ml over 1 to 2 hours. To remaining 250 ml, incorporate CY and infuse over 1 to 2 hours.
Diuresis	Administer 500 ml of 5% dextrose in 0.3% to 0.9% saline and infuse for ≥ 3 hours (± 250 mL/h). Increase oral fluid intake to 2 liters in 24 hours. Use diuretics, e.g., furosemide for edema, fluid retention, hypertension or signs and symptoms of impending pulmonary congestion
2-Mercaptoethane sulfonate sodium (Mesna) [optional]	To minimize the risk of hemorrhagic cystitis, Mesna® orally (with fruit juice) or IV (with infusions), each Mesna dose being 20% of the CY dose
Antiemetic therapy	Single dose of dexamethasone (5 to 10 mg) orally or IV, followed by any of the following over the next 1 to 2 days: (a) 5HT3 antagonists, e.g., ondansetron, tropisetron, or granisetron, orally or IV, or (b) oral metoclopramide (watch for extrapyramidal side effects). Antihistamine and benzodiazepine can be used as alternatives
White blood cell (WBC) count monitoring	Measure WBC counts between day 10 and 14 after CY pulse
Subsequent CY doses	If nadir WBCs > 4000/µL, increase subsequent dose to a maximum of 1.0 g/m² of BSA. If nadir WBCs < 1500/µL, reduce subsequent dose of CY by 0.25 g/m² of BSA
Pulse timing	Administer CY pulses monthly for six months for induction; may extend to seven months for very active disease. Then administer CY pulses quarterly for maintenance for at least 1 year beyond remission, defined by: inactive urinalysis, reduction of proteinuria to less than nephrotic range (ideally <1 g/day), normalization of serum complement titers (and ideally anti-dsDNA antibodies), and minimal extrarenal lupus activity)

Modified from Balow JE, Boumpas DT, Austin HA. Systemic lupus erythematosus and the kidney. In: Lahita RG, editor. Systemic lupus erythematosus. San Diego: Academic Press; 1999. p. 657-68.

the standard against which other regimens have been compared. In this regimen, IV-CY pulses are given monthly for 6 months, with the starting dose (0.75–1 g/m^2) increased to achieve a white blood cell count nadir between 1500/μL and 4000/μL on day 14. Hydration with forceful diuresis is required, and antiemetics are coadministered. Dexamethasone (oral or IV) or pulse IV methylprednisolone administered immediately before CY also has antiemetic effects. Mesna (20% of total CY dose) may be used to avoid bladder toxicity, especially in patients who cannot tolerate hyperhydration, and leuprolide acetate (3.75 mg subcutaneously 2 weeks before each CY dose) can be used to prevent ovarian failure (special precautions in patients with thrombotic diathesis), or testosterone (100 mg intramuscularly every 2 weeks) to prevent male infertility.[28]

Extended follow-up of patients who received both methylprednisolone and CY pulses demonstrated greater efficacy of the combination therapy compared with CY alone, without significant risk of toxicity.[29]

The Euro-Lupus nephritis trial (ELNT) compared the high-dose IV-CY regimen (six monthly pulses and two quarterly pulses with doses increased according to the white blood cell count nadir), to a low-dose IV-CY regimen (six fortnightly pulses at a fixed dose of 500 mg), each regimen followed by AZA, in 90 European SLE patients with proliferative glomerulonephritis (Table 10-5). The data showed comparable number of patients who achieved renal remission (54% to 71%) in both regimens, with a trend (but not statistically different) toward more infections in the high-dose group.[30]

The overall data support the use of high dose steroids, for example, pulse IV methylprednisolone plus CY. The subtle differences in the efficacy, safety, and long-term outcomes of the various CY regimens including the high rate of renal relapse despite intensive therapy,[31] reiterates the need to individualize therapy, closely monitor the patient's response and treatment side effects, and consider alternative therapies in the patient with severe, aggressive disease.

Alternatives to Pulse Induction Therapy

AZA, a cytotoxic drug mainly used for steroid-sparing and maintenance therapy, has been proposed as an alternative to CY for the induction phase. However, the Dutch Lupus Nephritis study comparing a standard NIH IV-CY regimen (CY arm) with combined AZA (2 mg/kg/day) plus pulse IV methylprednisolone (AZA/MP arm) showed more relapses and doubling of creatinine (albeit unsustained) in the AZA/MP arm at median 5.7 years follow-up.[32] We recommend induction with AZA only in patients with mild disease or those who refuse to risk the side effects of more proven effective agents like CY.

Mycophenolate mofetil (MMF) has recently become an important alternative drug for induction therapy in lupus nephritis.[33,34] The initial study conducted among Chinese patients with class IV nephritis compared MMF 2 g/day for 6 months decreased to 1 g/day for the next 6 months, with oral CY 2.5 mg/kg/day for 6 months followed by AZA 1.5 mg/kg/day in the next 6 months. At 1 year, MMF was found comparable to CY for inducing remission. However, with longer

Table 10-5. *The Euro-Lupus Nephritis Trial (ELNT) Low-Dose Intravenous Cyclophosphamide Regimen*

Dose of cyclophosphamide (CY)	500 mg (fixed dose)
Administration of CY	Use 500 mL 5% dextrose in 0.3% to 0.9% saline, infuse 250 ml over 1 to 2 hours. To remaining 250 mL, incorporate 500 mg CY and infuse 1 to 2 hours.
Diuresis	Infuse 100 to 500 mL of 5% dextrose in 0.3% to 0.9% saline over 1 to 3 hours. Increase oral fluid intake to 2 liters in 24 hours. Use diuretics, for example, furosemide for edema, fluid retention, hypertension or signs and symptoms of impending pulmonary congestion
2-Mercaptoethane sulfonate sodium (Mesna) [optional]	To minimize the risk of hemorrhagic cystitis, give Mesna orally (with fruit juice) or IV (with infusions), each Mesna dose being 20% of the CY dose
Antiemetic therapy	Single dose of dexamethasone 5 to 10 mg orally or intravenously, followed by: metoclopramide (10–20 mg orally or IV), or alizapride (50–100 mg orally or IV) If needed, prescribe 5HT3 antagonists such as ondansetron, tropisetron or granisetron over the next 1–2 days
White blood cell (WBC) count monitoring	No need to monitor WBC count
Subsequent CY doses	Always 500 mg
Timing	Administer CY pulses every 2 weeks for six times (six doses of 500 mg)

Modified from Houssiau FA, Vasconcelos C, D'Cruz D, Sebastiani GD, Garrido EE, Danieli MG, et al. Immunosuppressive therapy in lupus nephritis: the Euro-Lupus Nephritis Trial, a randomized trial of low-dose versus high-dose intravenous cyclophosphamide. Arthritis Rheum 2002;46:2121-31.

follow-up, patients treated with MMF relapsed more often than the CY/AZA group (46% versus 17%, respectively). These observations led to a modified protocol using MMF given initially at 2 g/day for 6 months, then 1.5 g/day for 6 months and finally 1 g/day for at least a year before further tapering; CY/AZA was administered as in the first study. Using this modified protocol also in Chinese patients with a median follow-up of 63 months, the complete and partial remission rates were comparable at greater than 90% for both groups. Side effects such as amenorrhea and infections were more common in the CY group.[34]

A multicenter study[35] among 140 SLE patients (56% blacks) with class III to V nephritis compared MMF at initial dose 1 to 3 g/day with the NIH IV CY pulse regimen (IV-CY). At 24 weeks, more patients in the MMF compared with the IV-CY group achieved complete (16% versus 4%) or partial (21% versus 17%) remission. The more recent Aspreva Lupus Management Study (ALMS) trial randomized 370 patients to either MMF (<3 g/day) or IV-CY (0.5–1.0 g/m[2]/month), in combination with prednisone for 24 weeks. Although this trial did not meet its primary endpoint to demonstrate superiority of MMF over IV-CY, MMF appeared more consistently effective across racial/ethnic and geographic groups than IV-CY.[36] It is also important to note that the therapeutic response depended on the dose of MMF, and only about 40% of patients had improvement of proteinuria with MMF doses below 1 g/day.[35] Moreover, MMF was withdrawn from some patients because of adverse side effects, particularly diarrhea and abdominal discomfort.[37] For patients unable to tolerate the recommended doses of MMF, enteric-coated mycophenolate sodium has recently been shown to be a useful alternative.[38] Despite the limited number of patients and short follow-up time, these results support the use of MMF as an alternative for induction therapy in lupus nephritis.

A recent observational study compared leflunomide given at a loading dose of 1 mg/kg/day for 3 days, followed by 30 mg/day in combination with prednisone, to IV-CY at a dose of 0.5 g/m[2] body surface area administered monthly for 6 months as induction therapy in 110 Chinese patients with proliferative lupus nephritis. After 6 months, the total response rate was 73% for both treatment groups, with similar rates of adverse events.[39]

Although IV immunoglobulin (IVIg) therapies have been used successfully with dramatic response in treating clinical manifestations of SLE like refractory thrombocytopenia, the beneficial effects are often of limited duration. Moreover, nephrotoxicity is a potentially serious complication of IVIg therapy, and patients with lupus nephritis who receive IVIg should be adequately hydrated and closely monitored.[40] High-dose immunoablative chemotherapy (HDIC) with autologous hematopoietic stem cell transplantation (HSCT) has been used to treat patients with severe disease refractory to standard immunosuppressive treatment[41] with vari-

able results. A recent trial compared HDIC therapy (200 mg/kg CY administered over 4 days with or without HSCT) with the standard NIH monthly CY pulse therapy, followed by quarterly maintenance dosing over 2 years. Interestingly, the results still showed superior efficacy of the traditional CY regimen over HDIC.[42] A few trials evaluating the role of plasmapheresis in lupus nephritis have shown variable results. Overall, the most impressive results were reported in patients with active disease and minimal scarring, and when combined with high-dose immunosuppressive therapy. At this time, plasmapheresis can be recommended only for patients with renal disease who are resistant to corticosteroid and cytotoxic drug therapy.[43,44]

The increasing use of biologic agents such as rituximab in clinical practice has fueled the conduct of randomized clinical trials of these agents in lupus nephritis. These are more extensively discussed toward the end of this chapter.

Maintenance Therapy

A sequential study[45] compared IV-CY, AZA, and MMF as maintenance therapy after inducing remission with pulse IV-CY (seven pulses) in 59 patients with lupus nephritis (95% Hispanic or blacks). Response to pulse IV-CY induction occurred in 83%. During maintenance therapy, although there were no significant differences in actuarial renal survival, the 72-month event-free survival (based on a composite endpoint of death and renal failure) was significantly better in both the AZA and the MMF groups than in the IV-CY group, although the small sample size, suboptimal IV-CY doses, and high doses of concomitant corticosteroids may have biased the results in favor of AZA and MMF. Analysis of pooled data on 445 patients in eight controlled trials showed that MMF conferred a significant survival benefit with the ability to induce renal remissions and prevent ESRD comparable to CY, and with a more favorable safety profile.[46] These studies demonstrate that AZA and MMF provide good alternative options for maintenance therapy.

Cyclosporine A (CsA), a calcineurin inhibitor, has been used in lupus nephritis, particularly in those refractory to cytotoxic therapy.[40,47] In a randomized controlled trial, CsA (2.5 to 4 mg/kg/day) was comparable to AZA (1.5 to 2 mg/kg/day) as induction and maintenance therapy in proliferative lupus nephritis for up to 4 years.[48] Another controlled study of CsA and oral CY in nephritic children with proliferative lupus nephritis and nephrotic syndrome demonstrated a corticosteroid-sparing effect of CsA.[49] Although there is no permanent nephrotoxicity in patients treated with low dose (<5 mg/kg/day) CsA, serum creatinine should be checked at baseline and every 2 to 4 weeks on treatment.[50] For patients who fail to respond to these regimens, other less extensively studied drugs like tacrolimus (FK506) at 0.06 to 0.1 mg/kg/day[51] may be tried, with strict monitoring for adverse effects.

These multiple studies across various centers and different racial groups offer and compare various regimens currently used in lupus nephritis. Obviously, there is no single regimen suitable for all patients. While maintaining some degree of flexibility in the management of individual patients, there is general consensus advocating early aggressive therapy during the "window of opportunity" (induction phase), including liberal use of moderate- to high-dose corticosteroids. During the maintenance phase, the predominant factors likely to affect clinical decisions include patient preference, long-term side effects such as fertility issues, and overall cost-benefit ratio. Patient choices are particularly important, with studies demonstrating an unwillingness of patients to opt for the best therapy (a regimen containing cytotoxic agents) when confronted with the potential side effects.[52] Patients at high risk for ESRD should be counseled not to compromise future health by rejecting timely effective therapy for lupus nephritis. Close monitoring and strict patient adherence are crucial to achieving renal remission and preventing recurrences.

Adjunct Therapies

Patients with lupus nephritis are at heightened risk for accelerated atherosclerosis and cardiovascular events, and it is essential to aggressively control contributory factors such as hypertension and dyslipidemia by both pharmacologic and nonpharmacologic measures such as diet and exercise.[53-55]

Hypertension, particularly a mean diastolic blood pressure exceeding more than 85 mm Hg, is a strong independent factor for occurrence of arterial thrombosis. Moreover, lupus nephritis patients who achieve optimum blood pressure control have a greater decline in proteinuria. Among the antihypertensive agents, angiotensin-converting enzyme (ACE) inhibitors, angiotensin-receptor blockers (ARBs), either singly or combined, have the additional benefit of reducing proteinuria and slowing the progression of renal disease.[22,54,55] Although serum creatinine may increase with these drugs, a mild increase may reflect a reduction in glomerular capillary pressure associated with extended preservation of renal function. The risk of hyperkalemia may be reduced by a loop diuretic and avoidance of potassium-rich foods. Combination antihypertensive regimens are frequently necessary in patients with chronic renal insufficiency, and the ACE inhibitors or ARBs can be effectively combined with other anti-hypertensives including diuretics, calcium channel antagonists, and beta blockers.[21]

Patients with lupus are prone to urinary tract infections (UTI), usually caused by *Escherichia coli*. Some other associated risk factors include elderly age, previous UTI, thrombocytopenia, leukopenia, and methotrexate treatment.[56] It is also important to distinguish UTI, which predominantly presents as isolated pyuria, from active nephritis which presents with pyuria accompanied by proteinuria and other urine sediments. Lupus nephritis frequently coexists and exacerbates with any infection including UTI.

Dietary protein restriction (0.3 to 0.6 g/kg/day) delays the progression of chronic kidney disease in nondiabetics, including those with lupus nephritis, and decreases the risk of need for dialysis, kidney transplantation, or death.[57] However, a low-protein diet is usually not palatable, making it difficult for most patients to adhere to this dietary prescription. The benefits of a low-protein diet among chronic kidney disease patients (creatinine clearance <60 ml/min) should be weighed against the risk of protein-calorie malnutrition, and these patients should be closely monitored to assess compliance, nutritional status, and progression of kidney disease. On the other hand, the overall benefit and safety of dietary protein restriction or supplementation among patients with nephrotic syndrome (proteinuria >3.5 g/day and hypoalbuminemia) remains uncertain.

Membranous Nephropathy

Membranous lupus nephritis (MLN) represents about 20% of clinically significant renal involvement in lupus. The course and prognosis of MLN is variable, but the coexistence of proliferative changes generally confers a worse prognosis compared with pure membranous lupus nephritis. The effects of adding alternate-month pulse CY (<1 g/m²/infusion) or low-dose CsA (<5 mg/kg/day) to alternate-day prednisone in 42 patients with MLN were evaluated in a prospective randomized controlled trial, the results of which support the use of combination prednisone with either pulse CY or CsA over prednisone alone.[58] For patients who cannot receive or tolerate CY, CsA may be an alternative, although extended follow-up has shown remissions to be more enduring with CY than with CsA. A recent open-label study showed tacrolimus at 0.1 to 0.2 mg/kg/day to be effective and safe in the treatment of MLN, with faster resolution of proteinuria and lower risk of lupus flare within 1 year, compared with conventional cytotoxic therapy.[59]

Monitoring Disease Activity

The term "remission" has been used for inactive extrarenal disease, absence of urine sediments even with small amounts of proteinuria (<1g/d), normal serum complement, and low steroid dose requirement (<10 mg/day).[22,54] Complete renal remission is defined by the Lupus Nephritis Collaborative Group as serum creatinine less than 1.4 mg/dL, inactive urine sediment, and protein excretion less than 330 mg/day. On the other hand, partial remission is defined as a 50% reduction in proteinuria (<1.5 g/ day) and stable renal function.[60] Although partial remission in lupus nephritis was associated with a significantly better patient and renal survival compared with no remission,[61] the high rate of relapse with early discontinuation of cytotoxic drug therapy supports the continuation of maintenance treatment for several months beyond remission. Long-term follow-up of patients in the ELNT demonstrated that early response to immunosuppressive therapy predicted good renal outcome in lupus nephritis, enabling early identification of responders versus non-responders to cytotoxic drug therapy.[62]

Nephritic flares with active urine sediment and increasing serum creatinine portend a poor renal prognosis, and must be approached using any of the induction regimens discussed earlier. Milder nephritic flares may be treated less aggressively, but close monitoring is essential with intensification of therapy if patients do not respond promptly. It is also important to identify and control precipitating and exacerbating factors such as infection, dehydration, uncontrolled hypertension, and drugs.

CASE STUDY 2

A 33-year-old housewife developed active nephritis 2 years after the diagnosis of SLE. Renal histology disclosed ISN/RPS Class IV-G (A) with activity index 10 and chronicity 3. She achieved partial remission after 6 monthly pulses of CY, and was maintained on azathioprine 100 mg/day. Eighteen months later, she had rapidly progressive glomerulonephritis manifesting as hypertension, proteinuria, oliguria, and azotemia, requiring maintenance hemodialysis. A second biopsy showed ISN/RPS Class VI with activity index 3 and chronicity 10. Two years later, with clinically quiescent disease, she underwent allograft kidney transplantation.

Dialysis and Kidney Transplantation

Even with aggressive immunosuppressive treatment, lupus nephritis still leads to renal failure in at least 10% of patients. ESRD is also associated with a decrease in the extrarenal manifestations of SLE in most patients. Although there are guidelines in the choice of dialysis, hemodialysis is theoretically more effective than peritoneal dialysis in reducing circulating immune complexes and ameliorating disease activity. Lupus nephritis patients on peritoneal dialysis also tend to have higher SLEDAI scores, primarily due to higher levels of anti-dsDNA and lower C3 and C4 levels compared with those on hemodialysis.[44,63]

Newer studies suggest that patients with SLE are suitable candidates for kidney transplantation, and that the overall graft survival in patients with lupus nephritis is similar to those in patients with other causes of chronic kidney disease. Review of data has also demonstrated superiority of kidney transplantation over dialysis in terms of long-term patient survival.[53] A recent study has demonstrated recurrent lupus nephritis in 20 (11%) of 177 patients during a mean follow-up of 6 years, with the majority of the transplanted kidneys showing mesangial glomerulonephritis (WHO II), and only four of 20 patients developing extrarenal manifestations of lupus activity.[64]

Transplantation is most successful if the lupus activity is quiescent, with a low risk for graft failure and disease recurrence. Risk factors for native kidney disease recurrence include black race, antiphospholipid antibodies, prior peritoneal dialysis, comorbidities at the time of transplantation, and poor compliance to immunosuppressive drugs. Furthermore, the combined presence of hypocomplementemia and proteinuria may indicate disease recurrence and adversely affect graft survival.[65] In a retrospective study of the United States Renal Disease System from 1995 to 2003, other factors affecting graft failure in patients with lupus nephritis include multiple pregnancies, multiple blood transfusions, greater comorbidity index, higher body weight, advanced age and black race of the donor or recipient, prior transplantation, higher levels of panel reactive antibodies, lower human leukocyte antigen compatibility, and deceased donors.[66]

The definitive diagnosis of recurrent lupus nephritis post-transplantation requires a renal biopsy with light microscopy, immunofluorescence, and electron microscopy studies, particularly to rule out graft rejection. The most commonly observed lesions in recurrent post-transplant lupus nephritis were mesangial lupus nephritis, focal proliferative glomerulonephritis and membranous glomerulonephritis. Fortunately, lesions that portend a graver prognosis were rare and consistent with the low occurrence (5%) of ESRD in this subpopulation.[67]

CASE STUDY 3

A 25-year-old nulligravid female with lupus nephritis went into partial remission following 6 monthly pulses of CY. She was stable on maintenance prednisone 10 mg/day and AZA 100 mg/day over the next year, until she returned to the clinic with edema and new-onset hypertension (160/90) complicating the first trimester of an unplanned pregnancy.

SPECIAL SITUATIONS

Lupus Nephritis and Pregnancy

In addition to antiphospholipid antibodies, lupus nephritis is a risk factor for adverse pregnancy outcomes, including hypertensive complications, miscarriages, stillbirth, and premature delivery

Table 10-6. *Factors that Distinguish Between Pre-eclampsia and Systemic Lupus Erythematosus (SLE) Activity*

	Pre-eclampsia	SLE Activity
Risk Factors		
First pregnancy	Increases risk	No impact
Pre-eclampsia in prior pregnancy	Increases risk	No impact
Multifetal gestation	Increases risk	Unknown impact
History of lupus nephritis	Increases risk	Increases risk
Timing in pregnancy	Always after 20 weeks, usually after 30 weeks' gestation	Any time in pregnancy
Laboratory Findings		
Active urine sediment (white blood cells, red blood cells, casts)	Usually negative	Positive
Coombs test	Usually negative	May be positive
Antiplatelet antibody	Usually negative	May be positive
Complement (C3 and C4)	Usually normal or high	May be low
Anti-dsDNA antibody	Usually negative	May be positive
Serum uric acid	>5.5 mg/dL	No change
Urine calcium	Low	Normal
sFlt-1 (soluble FMS-like tyrosine kinase 1)	High	Unknown
Placental growth factor (PlGF)	Low	Unknown
Physical Findings: Signs and Symptoms of Active SLE		
Mucocutaneous, for example, vasculitic, discoid or subacute cutaneous rash, mouth ulcers, alopecia	Not present	Present
Arthritis	Not present	Present
Serositis	Not present	Present

Adapted from Clowse MEB. Lupus activity in pregnancy. Rheum Dis Clin N Am 2007;33:237-52.

(relative risks ranging from 2.2 to 5.8), and is associated with low birth weight and intrauterine growth restriction.[68-70] Moreover, lupus nephritis and pre-eclampsia can coexist, making it difficult to distinguish between both conditions. In addition to the presence of extrarenal manifestations of an SLE flare, active urine sediments like red blood cells and casts are more consistent with lupus nephritis. Low levels of complement C3 and C4 also suggest lupus nephritis rather than pre-eclampsia because complement levels are expected to increase during normal pregnancy and pre-eclampsia (Table 10-6).[71] Every patient must be counseled that SLE (renal and extrarenal) disease activity be quiescent and stable for at least 6 months before pregnancy. Pregnancy, particularly in uncontrolled lupus nephritis, is a high-risk situation requiring vigilant monitoring by an experienced team consisting of the obstetrician, perinatologist, rheumatologist, and nephrologist.

Antiphospholipid Syndrome and Renovascular Complications

The renal manifestations of antiphospholipid syndrome include cortical ischemia and infarction, thrombotic microangiopathy, and renal artery or vein thrombosis.[72] Renal vein thrombosis classically presents as flank pain, hematuria, a sudden increase in proteinuria, and rapid worsening of renal function. It also seems more common in nephrotic syndrome, which in itself is a hypercoagulable state.

Antiphospholipid antibodies are additional risk factors for graft loss in patients undergoing kidney transplantation. Prompt recognition and control of these microangiopathic abnormalities, as well as aggressive control of hypertension, are essential in the preservation of renal function. Antiphospholipid syndrome is more thoroughly discussed in Chapter 11.

NOVEL THERAPIES

Biologic Therapies

The successful experience with autoimmune diseases like rheumatoid arthritis and a better understanding of the molecular pathogenesis of lupus has led to the clinical use and development of trials for the more targeted and potentially safer biologic therapies (Table 10-7).

Cytokines, like tumor necrosis factor (TNF), are known to play a role in the pathogenesis of lupus nephritis, and some anticytokine therapies have been tried in small trials or case series of SLE patients. Infliximab, a chimeric anti-TNF monoclonal antibody, decreased proteinuria by more than 80% in six SLE patients in a small open-label study.[73] Follow-up data on the clinical course of these patients suggested long-term efficacy for lupus nephritis and acceptable safety for those treated with short-term (four infusions) infliximab, but increased complications with additional infliximab infusions.[74]

Table 10-7. *Some Biologic Agents* for Systemic Lupus Erythematosus*

Biologic Agent	Mechanism of Action
Rituximab (Rituxan, Mabthera)	Anti-CD20 chimeric monoclonal antibody
Ocrelizumab	Anti-CD20 humanized monoclonal antibody
Belimumab (Benlysta)	Anti-BLyS fully human monoclonal antibody
LJP394 or Abetimus sodium (Riquent)	B cell toleragen, blocks anti-dsDNA production
CTLA4-Ig or Abatacept (Orencia)	Recombinant fusion protein of modulating molecule CTLA-4
TACI-Ig or Atacicept	Recombinant fusion protein of inhibitory B-cell receptor TACI
Tocilizumab (Actemra)	Anti-Interleukin-6 (IL-6) receptor monoclonal antibody

BLyS, B-lymphocyte stimulator; CTLA-4, cytotoxic T-lymphocyte antigen 4; TACI, transmembrane activator and calcium modulator and cyclophilin ligand interactor.
*Ongoing or in development for clinical trials in systemic lupus erythematosus.

The experience with anakinra, a recombinant interleukin-1 (IL-1) receptor antagonist, is limited to a small case series,[75] with more notable efficacy for the arthritis involvement. Interleukin-6 (IL-6) levels are elevated in both human and murine lupus, and blocking IL-6 or its receptor had a beneficial effect in all murine models of lupus tested to date. A phase I clinical study using an anti-IL6 receptor monoclonal antibody (tocilizumab) is underway to address some of these questions.[76] Evidence from mice and humans demonstrate a higher expression of several interferon (IFN)–inducible genes and proteins such as chemokines, which correlate with disease activity, and a high IFN-γ–producing phenotype has been associated with diffuse proliferative nephritis.[77-79] IFN-β, which downregulates IFN-γ and modulates numerous other cytokine pathways, was highly effective in prolonging survival and ameliorating the clinical, serologic, and histologic parameters of lupus-like disease including nephritis in mice.[80] These beneficial effects of IFN-β may be due to the prevention of renal leukocytic infiltration, reduction of immunoglobulin deposition, and decrease in proteinuria via IL-10 release, reduced Th1 lymphocyte responses and promotion of regulatory T-cell functions. These imply that IFN-β therapy may find a place in treating patients with life-threatening forms of glomerulonephritis such as Goodpasture's syndrome or severe lupus nephritis.[80] Early phase trials evaluating anti-IFN-α in SLE are ongoing.

Rituximab, a chimeric monoclonal antibody directed against the B-cell–specific antigen CD20, has shown encouraging results in patients with SLE.[81-83] There is further evidence that rituximab treatment of patients with SLE has immunologic effects beyond autoantibody reduction, including increased apoptosis and deactivation of T cells and down-regulation of costimulatory molecule expression.[84,85] To date, experience with rituximab in SLE comes from uncontrolled trials and case series involving patients with various disease manifestations (renal, central nervous system [CNS], cytopenias) refractory to conventional immunosuppressive treatments.[81-87] Different protocols were used, ranging from the usual full-dose regimen (375 mg/m^2 rituximab weekly for 4 weeks) to various shorter and lower dosing schemes (two doses of 500 to 1000 mg rituximab given 2 weeks apart). Most, but not all, patients received simultaneous immunosuppressive therapy with CY or MMF and corticosteroids. In a review on the published experience with rituximab in SLE,[88] 33 out of 45 patients with lupus nephritis responded to rituximab, based on a variety of lupus activity indices. When the response was assessed by serum creatinine and proteinuria, out of 20 patients, six entered complete remission, eight had partial remission, and six failed to respond. For reasons that are still inadequately understood, response to treatment did not correlate consistently with the degree of B-cell depletion, although greater absolute numbers of CD19+ cells at baseline predicted a less impressive clinical and serologic response.[89] In most studies, rituximab was a useful alternative in refractory SLE, except in patients with rapidly progressive nephritis or renal impairment, likely because these latter patients were being treated too late in the course of their disease.[90,91] The Lupus Nephritis Assessment with Rituximab (LUNAR) trial evaluated the additive benefit of rituximab to MMF for induction therapy and maintenance in 144 patients with proliferative lupus nephritis. However, this study did not meet its primary endpoint of achieving a renal response (defined as improvement in renal function, urinary sediment and proteinuria) at 52 weeks. One concern is the development of human antichimeric antibodies in approximately 26% to 30% of lupus patients receiving rituximab,[81,92] which can potentially interfere with B-cell depletion and adversely affect clinical response. Ocrelizumab, a fully humanized monoclonal antibody also directed against the CD20 antigen, may address this latter issue,[93] and phase III trials are now ongoing for active lupus nephritis.

In murine models of SLE, serum levels of B-lymphocyte stimulator (BLyS), also known as BAFF, are increased, and treatment with soluble BLyS receptors significantly decreased proteinuria and increased survival of these mice.[94] Belimumab is a fully human anti-BLyS monoclonal antibody. A phase II study showed sustained improvement in disease activity across multiple clinical measures, decreased frequency of disease flares, and favorable safety profile over 4 years of belimumab in patients with active SLE (excluding active CNS or renal SLE).[95] Recently, results of the first of two global phase III trials in serologically active SLE (BLISS-52) showed that belimumab plus standard of care achieved a clinically and statistically significant improvement in patient response rate at week 52, compared with standard of care alone. BLyS also binds to the B-cell inhibitory receptor TACI, and treatment with the soluble construct TACI-Ig delayed disease progression and improved survival in experimental mouse models.[96] Atacicept (or TACI-Ig), a recombinant fusion protein of TACI, decreased B-lymphocyte and immunoglobulin levels in a phase I SLE trial.[97] However, a phase II/III clinical trial on atacicept in lupus nephritis (but not in other forms of lupus) was recently discontinued owing to an increased risk of severe infections when the drug was administered with immunosuppressives.

Anti-dsDNA have been implicated in the underlying pathogenesis of SLE renal disease, and changes in anti-dsDNA antibody levels were found to directly correlate with the risk of renal flare.[98] LJP394 (abetimus sodium) is a complex of four oligonucleotides with strong avidity to anti-dsDNA antibodies. In a double-blind, placebo-controlled study, 230 patients with SLE were randomized to receive 16 weekly doses of 100 mg of LJP394 or placebo, followed by alternating-week drug withdrawal and 12 weekly doses of 50 mg of LJP394 or placebo. In the intent-to-treat population, the time to renal flare was not significantly different between treatment groups. However, in patients with high-affinity antibodies to its DNA epitope, LJP394 prolonged the time to renal flare, decreased the number of renal flares, and required fewer high-dose corticosteroid or CY treatments compared with placebo.[99] An interim analysis of the ongoing phase III Abetimus Sodium in Patients with a History of Lupus Nephritis (ASPEN) study indicates that 300 mg and 900 mg doses of abetimus provided significant and sustained reductions in anti-dsDNA levels in patients with lupus nephritis.[100] Unfortunately, this trial has been terminated following an interim efficacy analysis which indicated it futile to continue the study.

A promising therapeutic strategy for the treatment of lupus nephritis is blockade of the interactions between B and T cells, based on the observation that T-cell activation requires a second signal other than the initial presentation of antigen in the context of major histocompatibility complex molecules. This second signal is provided by the interaction of the CD40:CD40L and CD28:B7 family

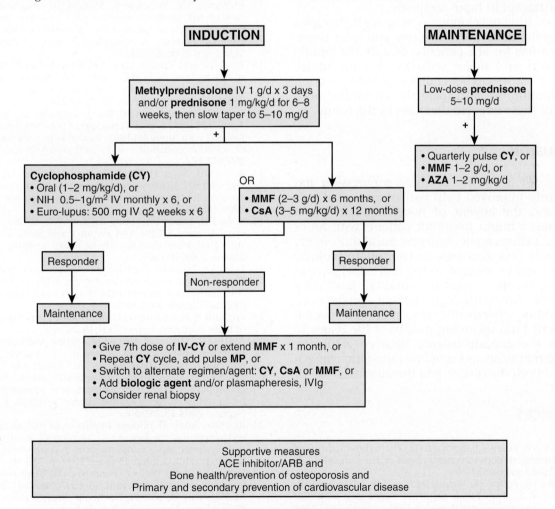

NIH-National Institutes of Health; CY-cyclophosphamide; MMF-mycophenolate mofetil; AZA-azathioprine; CsA-cyclosporine; MP-methylprednisolone; IVIg-IV immunoglobulin; ACE inhibitor-angiotensin converting enzyme inhibitor; ARB-angiotensin receptor blocker

Figure 10-4. Management algorithm for active (Class III or IV) lupus nephritis.

of costimulatory molecules on T-lymphocytes and antigen-presenting cells, and dysregulation of these interactions can contribute to loss of self-tolerance and development of SLE.[101] An open-label trial of a humanized anti-CD40L monoclonal antibody (riplizumab) did show reduction of serologic lupus activity and improvement in renal function; however, the high prevalence of life-threatening thromboembolic events led to the premature termination of trials with this agent.[102] The other well-characterized T-cell costimulatory signal is mediated through the CD28:B7 pathway. Cytotoxic T-lymphocyte antigen 4 (CTLA-4), a structural homolog of CD28, plays a crucial modulating role in T-cell response by competing with CD28 for the same B7 ligands and antagonizing CD28-dependent costimulation.[103] In humans, two preparations of the recombinant fusion protein molecule CTLA4-Ig—belatacept and abatacept—have found clinical use in transplantation and autoimmune diseases like rheumatoid arthritis.[104,105] Data from animal studies support the efficacy of CTLA4-Ig in lupus nephritis,[106] and clinical trials are underway to assess the role of abatacept in lupus nephritis.

These exciting developments in biologic therapies provide potentially more effective and safer therapeutic options for SLE patients. Despite the ambivalent results and major setbacks in some trials[92] spurring initiatives to better define patient selection and endpoints, we anticipate the increasing need and use of these targeted therapies in the future.[93]

CONCLUSION

The use of aggressive immune suppression has significantly improved both patient and renal outcomes, and the advent of novel biologic therapies heralds a bright future for patients with lupus nephritis. Management strategies must thoroughly include both pharmacologic and nonpharmacologic measures, and be tailored to the individual patient depending on the clinical presentation, laboratory parameters, histopathology, patient preferences, comorbidities, therapeutic response, and overall cost-benefit ratio including quality of life issues to maintain the delicate balance between achieving sustained remission and avoiding long-term complications of both the disease and therapies (Fig. 10-4).

REFERENCES

1. Pollack VE, Pirani CL, Schwatz FD. The natural history of renal manifestations of systemic lupus erythematosus. J Lab Clin Med 1964;63:537-50.
2. Wallace DJ, Podell TE, Weiner JM, Cox MB, Klinenberg JR, Forouzesh S, et al. Lupus nephritis. Experience with 230 patients in a private practice from 1950 to 1980. Am J Med 1982;72:209-20.
3. Pistiner M, Wallace DJ, Nessim S, Metzger AL, Klinenberg JR. Lupus erythematosus in the 1980s: a survey of 570 patients. Semin Arthritis Rheum 1991;21:55-64.
4. Navarra SV, King JO. Overview of clinical manifestations and survival of systemic lupus erythematosus patients in Asia. APLAR J Rheumatol 2006;9:336-41.
5. Dooley MA. Clinical and laboratory features of lupus nephritis. In: Wallace DJ, Hahn B, editors. Dubois' lupus Erythematosus. 7th ed. Philadelphia: Lippincott Williams & Wilkins; 2007. p. 1112-24.
6. Tomioka R, Tani K, Sato K, Suzuka C, Toyoda Y, Kishi J, et al. Observations on the occurrence of exacerbations in clinical course of systemic lupus erythematosus. J Med Invest 2008;55:112-9.
7. Appenzeller S, Clarke AE, Panopalis P, Joseph L, St. Pierre Y, Li T. The relationship between renal activity and quality of life in systemic lupus erythematosus. J Rheumatol 2009;36:947-52.
8. Appel GB, Radhakrishnan J, D'Agati VD. Secondary glomerular disease. In: Brenner B, editor. Brenner and Rector's The Kidney. 8th ed. Philadelphia: Elsevier; 2008. p. 1072-3.
9. Cockcroft DW, Gault MH. Prediction of creatinine clearance from serum creatinine. Nephron 1976;16:31-41.
10. Levey AS, Bosch JP, Lewis JB, Greene T, Rogers N, Roth D. A more accurate method to estimate glomerular filtration rate from serum creatinine: a new prediction equation. Ann Intern Med 1999;130:461-70.
11. Leung YY, Szeto CC, Tam LS. Urine protein-to-creatinine ratio in an untimed urine collection is a reliable measure of proteinuria in lupus nephritis. Rheumatology 2007;46:649-52.
12. Anutunes VV, Verunese F, Morales JV. Diagnostic accuracy of the protein/creatinine ratio in urine samples to estimate 24 hour proteinuria in patients with primary glomerulopathies: A longitudinal study. Nephrol Dial Transplant 2008;23:2242-6.
13. Ziegenbein M, Petri M, Carson K, Rovin B, Fine D. Reliability of shorter than 24-hr timed urine collections in estimating 24-hr total urine protein excretion in patients with lupus nephritis. Arthritis Rheum 2007;56:S214.
14. Cortés-Hernández J, Ordi-Ros J, Labrador M, Segarra A, Tovar JL, Balada E, et al. Predictors of poor renal outcome in patients with lupus nephritis treated with combined pulses of cyclophosphamide and methylprednisolone. Lupus 2003;12:287.
15. Rovin BH, Song H, Birmingham DJ, Hebert LA, Yu CY, Nagaraja HN. Urinary chemokines as biomarkers of human systemic lupus erythematosus activity. J Am Soc Nephrol 2005;16:467-73.
16. Kong KO, Leung BP, Thong BY, Law WG, Chia F, Lian TY, et al. Urinary MCP-1 and svcam-1 and urine and serum stnfr-1 correlate with activity of lupus nephritis. Arthritis Rheum 2008;58:S565.
17. Kiani AN, Diehl EE, Huaizhong H, Vasudevan G, Johnson K, Chen CJ, et al. Urine osteoprotegerin (OPG) and monocyte chemoattractant protein-1 (MCP-1) in lupus nephritis (LN). Arthritis Rheum 2008;58:S558-9.
18. Enghard P, Riemekasten G. Immunology and the diagnosis of lupus nephritis. Lupus 2009;18:287-90.
19. Austin HA, Muenz IR, Joyce KM. Diffuse proliferative lupus nephritis: identification of specific pathologic features affecting renal outcome. Kidney Int 1984;25:689-95.
20. Weening JJ, D'Agati VD, Schwartz MM, Seshan SV, Alpers CE, Appel GB, et al. The classification of glomerulonephritis in systemic lupus erythematosus revisited. J Am Soc Nephrol 2004;15:241-50.
21. Illei GG, Balow JE. Kidney involvement in systemic lupus erythematosus. In: Tsokos GC, Gordon C, Smolen JS, editors. Systemic lupus erythematosus. A companion to rheumatology. Philadelphia: Elsevier; 2007. p. 336-50.
22. Sidiropoulos PI, Illei G, Boumpas DT. Treatment—renal involvement. In: Hochberg M, Silman A, Smolen J, Weinblatt M, Weisman M, editors. Hochberg Rheumatology. 4th ed. Philadelphia: Elsevier; 2008. p. 1320-1.
23. Felson DT, Anderson J. Evidence for the superiority of immunosuppressive drugs and prednisone over prednisone alone in lupus nephritis. Results of pooled analysis. N Engl J Med 1984;311:1528-33.

24. Donadio JV Jr, Holley KE, Ferguson RH, Ilstrup DM. Treatment of diffuse proliferative lupus nephritis with prednisone and combined prednisone and cyclophosphamide. N Engl J Med 1978;299:1151-5.

25. Austin HA, Klippel JH, Balow JE, LeRiche NG, Steinberg AD, Plotz PH, et al. Therapy of lupus nephritis. Controlled trial of prednisone and cytotoxic drugs. N Engl J Med 1986;314:614-9.

26. Boumpas DT, Austin HA, Vaughn EM, Klippel JH, Steinberg AD, Yarboro CH, et al. Controlled trial of pulse methylprednisolone versus two regimens of pulse cyclophosphamide in severe lupus nephritis. Lancet 1992;340:741-5.

27. Gourley MF, Austin HA, Scott D, Yarboro CH, Vaughan EM, Muir J, et al. Methylprednisolone and cyclophosphamide, alone or in combination, in patients with lupus nephritis. A randomized controlled trial. Ann Intern Med 1996;125:549-57.

28. Balow JE, Boumpas DT, Austin HA. Systemic lupus erythematosus and the kidney. In: Lahita RG, editor. Systemic lupus erythematosus. San Diego: Academic Press; 1999. p. 657-85.

29. Illei GG, Austin HA, Crane M, Collins L, Gourley MF, Yarboro CH, et al. Combination therapy with pulse cyclophosphamide plus pulse methylprednisolone improves long-term renal outcome without adding toxicity in patients with lupus nephritis. A randomized controlled trial. Ann Intern Med 2001;135:248-57.

30. Houssiau FA, Vasconcelos C, D'Cruz D, Sebastiani GD, Garrido EE, Danieli MG, et al. Immunosuppressive therapy in lupus nephritis: The Euro-Lupus Nephritis Trial, a randomized trial of low-dose versus high-dose intravenous cyclophosphamide. Arthritis Rheum 2002;46:2121-31.

31. Illei GG, Takada K, Parkin D, Austin HA, Crane M, Yarboro CH, et al. Renal flares are common in patients with severe proliferative lupus nephritis treated with pulse immunosuppressive therapy: Long term follow-up of cohort of 145 patients participating in randomized controlled studies. Arthritis Rheum 2002;46:995-1002.

32. Grootscholten C, Ligtenberg G, Hagen EC, van den Wall B, de Glas-Vos JW, Bijl M, et al. Dutch Working Party on Systemic Lupus Erythematosus. Azathioprine/methylprednisolone versus cyclophosphamide in proliferative lupus nephritis: A randomized controlled trial. Kidney Int 2006;70:616-8.

33. Chan TM, Li FK, Tang CS, Wong RW, Fang GX, Ji YL, et al. Efficacy of mycophenolate mofetil in patients with diffuse proliferative lupus nephritis. Hongkong-Guangzhou Nephrology Study Group. N Engl J Med 2000;343:1156-62.

34. Chan TM, Tse KC, Tang CS, Mok MY, Li FK, for the Hong Kong Nephrology Study Group. Long-term study of mycophenolate mofetil as continuous induction and maintenance treatment for diffuse proliferative lupus nephritis. J Am Soc Nephrol 2005;16:1076-84.

35. Ginzler EM, Dooley MA, Aranow C, Kim MY, Buyon J, Merrill JT, et al. Mycophenolate mofetil or intravenous cyclophosphamide for lupus nephritis. N Engl J Med 2005;353:2219-28.

36. Dooley MA, Appel GB, Ginzler EM, Isenberg D, Jayne E, Solomons N, et al. Effects of race/ethnicity on response to mycophenolate mofetil (MMF) and intravenous cyclophosphamide (IVC) for lupus nephritis in the Aspreva Lupus Management Study (ALMS). Lupus 2008;17:455.

37. Karim MY, Alba P, Cuadrado MJ, Abbs IC, D'Cruz DP, Khamashta MA, et al. Mycophenolate mofetil for systemic lupus erythematosus refractory to other immunosuppressive agents. Rheumatology 2002;42:876-82.

38. Traitanon O, Avihingsanon Y, Kittikovit V, Townamchai N, Kanjanabuch T, Praditpornsilpa K, et al. Efficacy of enteric-coated mycophenolate sodium in patients with resistant-type lupus nephritis: A prospective study. Lupus 2008;17:744-51.

39. Wang HY, Cui TG, Hou FF, Ni ZH, Chen XM, Lu FM, et al. Induction treatment of proliferative lupus nephritis with leflunomide combined with prednisone: a prospective multi-centre observational study. Lupus 2008;17:638-44.

40. Ponticelli C. New therapies for lupus nephritis. Clin J Am Soc Nephrol 2006;1:863-8.

41. Jayne D, Passweg J, Marmont A, Farge D, Zhao X, Arnold R, et al. Autologous stem cell transplantation for severe and refractory lupus erythematosus. Lupus 2004;13:168-76.

42. Abou-Khamis T, Magder L, Jones R, Brodsky R, Petri M. High dose cyclophosphamide versus traditional regimen in lupus nephritis (LN). Arthritis Rheum 2007;56:S215.

43. Lewis EJ, Hunsicker LG, Lan SP, Rohde RD, Lachin JM. A controlled trial of plasmapheresis therapy in severe lupus nephritis. The Lupus Nephritis Collaborative Study Group. N Engl J Med 1996;326:1373-9.

44. Wallace DJ. Nonpharmacologic and complementary therapeutic modalities. In: Wallace DJ, Hahn B, editors. Dubois' lupus erythematosus. 7th ed. Philadelphia: Lippincott Williams & Wilkins; 2007. p. 1228-30.

45. Contreras G, Pardo V, Leclercq B, Lenz O, Tozman E, O'Nan P, et al. Sequential therapies for proliferative lupus nephritis. N Engl J Med 2004;350:971-80.

46. Mak A, Tan J, Su H, Ho R. Mycophenolate mofetil confers survival benefit and is safer than cyclophosphamide in the treatment of proliferative lupus nephritis: A comprehensive meta-analysis of 445 patients in 8 controlled trials. Arthritis Rheum 2008;58:S563.

47. Ferrario L, Bellone M, Bozzolo E, Baldissera E, Sabbadini MG. Remission from lupus nephritis resistant to cyclophosphamide after additional treatment with cyclosporin A. Rheumatology 2000;39:218-20.

48. Moroni G, Doria A, Mosca M, Della Casa Alberighi O, Ferraccioli G, et al. A randomized pilot trial comparing cyclosporine versus azathioprine for maintenance therapy in diffuse lupus nephritis. Clin J Am Soc Nephrol 2006;1:925-32.

49. Fu LW, Yang LY, Chen WP, Lin CY. Clinical efficacy of cyclosporine and neoral in the treatment of paediatric lupus nephritis with heavy proteinuria. Br J Rheumatol 1998;37:217-21.

50. Feutren G, Mihatsch MJ. Risk factors for cyclosporine-induced nephropathy in patients with autoimmune diseases. International Kidney Biopsy Registry of Cyclosporine in Autoimmune Diseases. N Engl J Med 1992;326:1654-60.

51. Mok CC, Tong KH, To CH, Siu YP, Au TC. Tacrolimus for induction therapy of diffuse proliferative lupus nephritis: an open-labeled pilot study. Kidney Int 2005;68:813-7.

52. Fraenkel L, Bogardus S, Concato J. Patient preferences for treatment of lupus nephritis. Arthritis Rheum 2002;47:421-8.

53. Bertsias G, Ioannidis J, Boletis J, Bombardieri S, Cervera R, Dostal C, et al. EULAR recommendations for the management of systemic lupus erythematosus. Report of a Task Force of the EULAR Standing Committee for International Clinical Studies Including Therapeutics. Ann Rheum Dis 2008;67:195-205.

54. Gordon C, Jayne D, Pusey C, Adu D, Amoura Z, Aringer M, et al. European consensus statement on the terminology used in the management of lupus glomerulonephritis. Lupus 2009;18:257-63.

55. Masood S, Jayne D, Karim Y. Beyond immunosuppression–challenges in the clinical management of lupus nephritis. Lupus 2009;18:106-15.

56. Hidalgo-Tenorio C, Jimenez-Alonzo J, de Dios Luna J, Tallada M, Martinez-Brocal A, Sabio JM. Urinary tract infection and systemic lupus erythematosus. Ann Rheum Dis 2004;63:431-7.

57. Fouque D, Laville M, Boissel JP. Low protein diets for chronic kidney disease in non-diabetic adults. Cochrane Database Syst Rev 2006;(2):CD001892.

58. Austin HA, Illei GG, Braun MJ, Balow JE. Randomized, controlled trial of prednisone, cyclophosphamide, and cyclosporine in lupus membranous nephropathy. J Am Soc Nephrol 2009;20:901-11.

59. Szeto CC, Kwan CH, Lai MM, Tam LS, Li KM, Chow KM, et al. Tacrolimus for the treatment of systemic lupus erythematosus with pure class V nephritis. Rheumatology 2008;47:1678-81.

60. Korbet SM, Louise EJ, Schwartz MM, Reichlin M, Evans J, Rohde RD, et al. Factors predictive of outcome in severe lupus nephritis. Lupus Nephritis Collaborative Study Group. Am J Kidney Dis 2000;35:904-14.

61. Chen YE, Korbet SM, Katz RS, Schwartz MM, Lewis EJ, for the Collaborative Study Group. Value of a complete or partial remission in severe lupus nephritis. Clin J Am Soc Nephro 2008;3:46-53.

62. Houssiau FA, Vasconcelos C, D'Cruz DP, Sebastiani GD, de Ramon Garrido E, Danieli MG, et al. Early response to immunosuppressive therapy predicts good renal outcome in lupus nephritis. Arthritis Rheum 2004;50:3934-40.

63. Dhillon M, Madger L, Petri M. Systemic lupus erythematosus disease activity: Effect of peritoneal dialysis vs hemodialysis. Arthritis Rheum 2008;58:S559.

64. Perkins EL, Burgos P, Liu J, Kendrick SA, Kendrick WA, Pons Estel GJ, et al. Recurrent lupus nephritis is infrequent and benign in renal transplant patients with SLE. ACR/ARHP 2008 Program Book Supplement: Abst F26(480):15.

65. Baracat ALS, Ribeiro-Alves MAV, Alves-Filho G, Mazzali M. Systemic lupus erythematosus after renal transplantation: Is complement a good marker for graft survival? Transplant Proc 2008;40:746-8.

66. Tang H, Chelamcharla M, Baird BC, Shihab FS, Koford JK, Goldfarb-Rumyantzev AS. Factors affecting kidney-transplant outcome in recipients with lupus nephritis. Clin Transplant 2008;22:263-72.

67. Ponticelli C, Moroni G. Renal transplantation in lupus nephritis. Lupus 2005;14:95-8.

68. Cortes-Hernandez J, Ordi-Ros J, Paredes F, Casellas M, Castillo F, Vilardell-Tarres M. Clinical predictors of fetal and maternal outcome in systemic lupus erythematosus: a prospective study of 103 pregnancies. Rheumatology (Oxford) 2002;41:643-50.

69. Moroni G, Ponticelli C. The risk of pregnancy in patients with lupus nephritis. J Nephrol 2003;16:161-7.

70. Wagner SJ, Craici I, Reed D, Norby S, Bailey K, Wiste HJ, et al. Maternal and foetal outcomes in pregnant patients with active lupus nephritis. Lupus 2009;18:342-7.

71. Clowse M. Lupus activity in pregnancy. Rheum Dis Clin N Am 2007;33:237-52.

72. D'Cruz DP. Renal manifestations of the antiphospholipid syndrome. Lupus 2005;14:45-8.

73. Aringer M, Smolen JS. Tumour necrosis factor and other proinflammatory cytokines in systemic lupus erythematosus: a rationale for therapeutic intervention. Lupus 2004;13:344-7.

74. Aringer M, Houssiau F, Graninger WB, et al. Severe adverse events under prolonged TNF blockade in SLE, but favourable efficacy and safety data of short-term infliximab therapy for lupus nephritis. Lupus 2008;17:463.

75. Moosig F, Zeuner R, Renck C, Schoder JO. Interleukin-1 receptor antagonist in refractory systemic lupus erythematosus. Lupus 2004;13:605-6.

76. Tackey E, Lipsky PE, Illei GG. Rationale for interleukin-6 blockade in systemic lupus erythematosus. Lupus 2004; 13:339-43.

77. Baechler EC, Gregersen PK, Behrens TW. The emerging role of interferon in human systemic lupus erythematosus. Curr Opinion Immunol 2004;16:801-7.

78. Wing-Yan Chan R, Mac-Moune Lai F, Kwok-Ming Li E, Tam LS, Chow KM, Lai KB, et al. Intra-renal cytokine gene expression in lupus nephritis. Ann Rheum Dis 2007;66: 886-92.

79. Fu Q, Chen X, Cui H, Guo Y, Chen J, Shen N, et al. Association of elevated transcript levels of interferon-inducible chemokines with disease activity and organ damage in systemic lupus erythematosus patients. Arthritis Res Ther 2008;10:R112.

80. Schwarting A, Paul K, Tschirner S, Menke J, Hansen T, Brenner W, et al. Interferon beta: a therapeutic for autoimmune lupus in MRL-Faslpr mice. J Am Soc Nephrol 2005;16: 3264-72.

81. Leandro MJ, Edwards JC, Cambridge G, Ehrenstein MR, Isenberg DA. An open study of B lymphocyte depletion in systemic lupus erythematosus. Arthritis Rheum 2002;46:2673-7.

82. Looney RJ, Anolik JH, Campbell D, Felgar RE, Young F, Arend LJ, et al. B cell depletion as a novel treatment for systemic lupus erythematosus: a phase I/II dose-escalation trial of rituximab. Arthritis Rheum 2004;50:2580-9.

83. Anolik JH, Barnard J, Cappione A, Pugh-Bernard AE, Felgar RE, Looney RJ, et al. Rituximab improves peripheral B cell abnormalities in human systemic lupus erythematosus. Arthritis Rheum 2004;50:3580-90.

84. Sfikakis PP, Boletis JN, Leonaki S, Vigklis V, Fragiadaki KG, Iniotaki A, et al. Remission of proliferative lupus nephritis following B cell depletion therapy is preceded by down-regulation of T-cell co-stimulatory molecule CD40 ligand: an open-label trial. Arthritis Rheum 2005;52:501-13.

85. Vigna-Perez AU, Hernandez-Castro B, Paredes-Saharopulos O, Portales-Perez D, Baranda L, Abud-Mendoza C, et al. Clinical and immunological effects of rituximab in patients with lupus nephritis refractory to conventional therapy: a pilot study. Arthritis Res Ther 2006;8:R83.

86. Leandro MJ, Cambridge G, Edwards JC, Ehrenstein MR, Isenberg DA. B-cell depletion in the treatment of patients with systemic lupus erythematosus: a longitudinal analysis of 24 patients. Rheumatology (Oxford) 2005;44:1542-5.

87. Gunnarsson I, Jonsdottir J, Sundelin B, Jacobson S, Henriksson E, van Vollenhoven R, et al. Histopathological and clinical outcome of rituximab treatment in patients with cyclophosphamide-resistant proliferative lupus nephritis. Arthritis Rheum 2007;56:1263-72.

88. Thatayatikom A, White AJ. Rituximab: A promising therapy in systemic lupus erythematosus. Autoimmunity Rev 2006;5:18-24.

89. Jónsdóttir T, Gunnarsson I, Risselada A, Henriksson EW, Klareskog L, van Vollenhoven R. Treatment of refractory SLE with rituximab plus cyclophosphamide: clinical effects, serological changes and predictors of response. Ann Rheum Dis 2008;67:330-4.

90. Sangle SR, Davies RJ, Aslam L, Lewis MJ, Wedgwood R, Hughes GR, et al. Rituximab in the treatment of resistant systemic lupus erythematosus: Failure of therapy in rapidly progressive crescentic lupus nephritis. Arthritis Rheum 2007;56:S215.

91. Navarra SV, Gerona JG, Vargas PJ, Torralba KD. Indications and responses to rituximab in Filipino patients with refractory systemic lupus erythematosus. Int J Rheumatic Dis 2008;11:A504.

92. Merrill JT, Neuwelt CM, Wallace DJ, Shanahan JC, Latinis KM, Oates JC, et al. Efficacy and safety of rituximab in patients with moderately to severely active systemic lupus erythematosus (SLE): Results from the randomized double-blind Phase II/III Study EXPLORER. ACR/ARHP 2008 Program Book Supplement: Abst L12: 57.

93. Isenberg D, Gordon C, Merrill J, Urowitz M. New therapies in systemic lupus erythematosus—trials, troubles and tribulations....working towards a solution. Lupus 2008;17: 967-70.

94. Zhang J, Roschke V, Baker KP, Wang Z, Alarcon GS, Fessler BJ, et al. Cutting edge: a role for B lymphocyte stimulator in systemic lupus erythematosus. J Immunol 2001;166:6-10.

95. Merrill JT, Furie R, Wallace DJ, McKay J, Ginzler EM, Wellborne F, et al. Four year experience of belimumab, a fully human monoclonal antibody, in the treatment of systemic lupus erythematosus (SLE). Ann Rheum Dis 2009;68:S254.

96. Liou W, Szalai A, Zhao L, Liu D, Martin F, Kimberly RP, et al. Control of spontaneous B lymphocyte autoimmunity with adenovirus-encoded soluble TACI. Arthritis Rheum 2004;50:1884-96.

97. Dall'Era M, Chakravarty E, Wallace D, Genovese M, Weisman M, Kavanaugh A, et al. Reduced B lymphocyte and immunoglobulin levels after atacicept treatment in patients with systemic lupus erythematosus. Arthritis Rheum 2007;56:4142-50.

98. Linnik MD, Hu JZ, Heilbrunn KR, Strand V, Hurley FL, Joh T, et al. and the LJP 394 Investigator Consortium. Relationship between anti-double-stranded DNA antibodies and exacerbation of renal disease in patients with systemic lupus erythematosus. Arthritis Rheum 2005;52:1129-37.

99. Alarcon-Segovia D, Tumlin JA, Furie RA, McKay JD, Cardiel MH, Strand V, et al. LJP 394 for the prevention of renal flare in patients with SLE: Results from a randomized double blind placebo-controlled study. Arthritis Rheum 2003;48:442-54.

100. Linnik MD, Tansey MJ, Joh T. Dose dependent reduction in anti-DNA antibody correlates with Abetimus sodium through 52 weeks in the phase 3 ASPEN Study (Abetimus sodium in patients with a history of lupus nephritis). Arthritis Rheum 2008;58:S567.

101. Wong CK, Lit LC, Tam LS, Li EK, Lam CW. Aberrant production of soluble co-stimulatory molecules CTLA-4, CD28, CD80 and CD86 in patients with systemic lupus erthematosus. Rheumatology 2005;44:989-94.

102. Boumpas DT, Furie R, Manzi S, Illei GG, Wallace DJ, Balow JE, et al., on behalf of the BG9588 Lupus Nephritis Trial Group. A short course of BG9588 (anti-CD40 ligand antibody) improves serologic activity and decreases hematuria in patients with proliferative lupus glomerulonephritis. Arthritis Rheum 2003;48:719-27.

103. Collins AV, Brodie DW, Gilbert RJ, Iaboni A, Manso-Sancho R, Walse B, et al. The interaction properties of costimulatory molecules revisited. Immunity 2002;17:201-10.

104. Vincenti F, Larsen C, Durrbach A, Wekerle T, Nashan B, Blancho G, et al. Costimulation blockade with belatacept in renal transplantation. N Engl J Med 2005;353:770-81.

105. Genovese MC, Becker JC, Schiff M, Luggen M, Sherrer Y, Kremer J, et al. Abatacept for rheumatoid arthritis refractory to tumor necrosis factor alpha inhibition. N Engl J Med 2005;353:1114-23.

106. Daikh DI, Wofsy D. Cutting edge: reversal of murine lupus nephritis with CTLA4Ig and cyclophosphamide. J Immunol 2001;166:2913-6.

INTRODUCTION

The antiphospholipid syndrome (APS) is the association of thrombosis, pregnancy loss, and morbidity, and certain other clinical manifestations with antiphospholipid antibodies (aPLs) (lupus anticoagulant [LA], anticardiolipin antibodies [aCL], and/or anti–β_2-glycoprotein I antibodies [aβ_2GPI]).[1] International consensus classification criteria for definite APS (Table 11-1) have been developed to facilitate research in the field. Although they were not designed for clinical use, these criteria highlight the need for appropriate documentation of clinical events and the importance of antibody titer and persistence. It should be kept in mind that certain clinical manifestations associated with aPL, for example, valvular heart disease (Libman-Sacks endocarditis), livedo reticularis, and thrombocytopenia, were not included in the classification criteria (Table 11-2). These manifestations can occur in patients with or without a history of thrombosis or pregnancy loss.

Using a case-based approach, this chapter reviews current recommendations for the treatment of APS. Management of APS is often challenging. Although there is general consensus on approaches to treatment, the application of these principles in clinical practice is often difficult. In other words, "the devil is in the details." In the initial evaluation of patients, the relative contribution of aPL to clinical events may not be clear. Positivity of aPL tests and antibody titers may vary over time. Also, patients with aPL may have other inherited and acquired risk factors for thrombosis and/or pregnancy loss. For patients in whom aPLs are clinically relevant, there are relatively few prospective clinical trials to provide therapeutic guidance and a number of important variables have not been studied.

MANAGEMENT OF ACUTE THROMBOSIS AND SECONDARY THROMBOSIS PREVENTION

Diagnostic Considerations

The differential diagnosis of acute peripheral arterial thrombosis in a young woman includes trauma, an embolic event, and a hypercoagulable state. A list

CASE STUDY 1

A 25-year-old white woman presents with a 2-day history of a blue, painful right index finger. Her past medical history is notable for two pregnancies, both of which were fetal deaths (at 15 and 17 weeks' gestation, 2 years and 6 months prior, respectively) and frequent headaches. She does not smoke cigarettes, has no prior history of blood clots, and is taking no medications. Physical examination is normal except for diffuse livedo reticularis (Fig. 11-1) of the upper and lower extremities, a decreased right radial artery pulse, and cyanosis of the right index finger distal to the distal interphalangeal joint. An arteriogram shows complete occlusion of the right radial artery at the navicular level. Significant laboratory tests include a positive antinuclear antibody (ANA), 1:160 in a nucleolar pattern, immunoglobulin G (IgG) aCL and aβ_2GPI greater than 80 units (high positive), negative immunoglobulin M (IgM) and immunoglobulin A (IgA) aCL and aβ_2GPI, negative LA test, normal complement levels, and a normal platelet count. A thorough evaluation for other hypercoagulable conditions is negative. Echocardiography is normal. Treatment with intravenous heparin followed by warfarin at a target international normalized ratio (INR) of 3.0 results in gradual improvement of her finger.

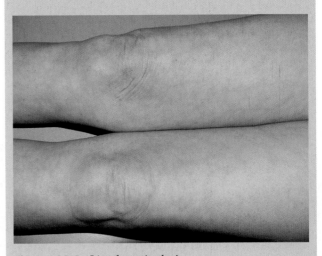

Figure 11-1. Livedo reticularis.

Table 11-1. *Revised Sapporo Classification Criteria for the Antiphospholipid Syndrome*

Clinical Criteria
1. Vascular thrombosis:
   One or more clinical episodes of arterial, venous, or small vessel thrombosis, in any tissue or organ.
2. Pregnancy morbidity:
   One or more unexplained deaths of a morphologically normal fetus at or beyond the 10th week of gestation, *or*

   One or more premature births of a morphologically normal neonate before the 34th week of gestation because of eclampsia, severe pre-eclampsia, or recognized features of placental insufficiency, *or*

   Three or more unexplained consecutive spontaneous abortions before the 10th week of gestation, with maternal anatomic or hormonal abnormalities and paternal and maternal chromosomal causes excluded.

Laboratory Criteria
1. Lupus anticoagulant present in plasma, on two or more occasions at least 12 weeks apart, detected according to the guidelines of the International Society on Thrombosis and Hemostasis or
2. Anticardiolipin antibody of IgG or IgM isotype in serum or plasma, present in medium or high titer (i.e., >40 GPL or MPL, or >the 99th percentile), on two or more occasions, at least 12 weeks apart, measured by a standardized enzyme-linked immunosorbent assay (ELISA) or
3. Anti-β_2 glycoprotein-I antibody of IgG or IgM isotype in serum or plasma (in titer higher than the 99th percentile), present on two or more occasions, at least 12 weeks apart, measured by a standardized ELISA.

   Definite APS is present if at least one of the clinical criteria and one of the laboratory criteria are met. Classification of APS should be avoided if less than 12 weeks or more than 5 years separate the positive aPL test and the clinical manifestation. In studies of populations of patients who have more than one type of pregnancy morbidity, investigators are strongly encouraged to stratify groups of subjects according to a, b, or c above.

Adapted from Miyakis S, Lockshin MD, Atsumi T, Branch DW, Brey RL, Cervera R, et al. International consensus statement on an update of the classification criteria for definite antiphospholipid syndrome. J Thromb Haemost 2006;4:295-306.

Table 11-2. *Major Noncriteria Features of Antiphospholipid Antibodies*

Cutaneous Manifestations
  Livedo reticularis
  Cutaneous ulcers
Hematologic Manifestations
  Thrombocytopenia
  Hemolytic anemia
Cardiac Manifestations
  Valve vegetation/thickening
Renal Manifestations
  Antiphospholipid antibody associated nephropathy
Nonstroke Neurological Manifestations (controversial)
  Chorea
  Cognitive dysfunction
  Headache
  Multiple sclerosis–like syndromes

Table 11-3. *Thrombosis Risk Factors Other than Antiphospholipid Antibodies*

Demographic characteristics
  Older age
Traditional cardiovascular risk factors
  Hypertension, diabetes mellitus, proatherogenic lipid profile, elevated homocysteine levels, obesity, sedentary lifestyle, early menopause, family history of early premature cardiovascular disease
Acquired thrombosis triggers
  Smoking, oral contraceptives, hormone replacement therapy, pregnancy, prolonged hospitalization, immobilization, surgical procedures, malignancy, nephrotic syndrome
Genetic hypercoagulable states
  Protein C deficiency, protein S deficiency, antithrombin deficiency, factor V Leiden mutation, prothrombin 20210 gene mutation, dysfibrinogenemia, methylenetetrahydrofolate reductase (*MTHFR*) gene mutation
Acquired lupus-related risk factors
  Chronic inflammation, renal disease, corticosteroid use (controversial), vasculitis

of thrombophilic conditions is shown in Table 11-3. This patient's history of pregnancy losses and the physical finding of livedo reticularis suggest the possibility of APS. It should be noted that other thrombophilic conditions, for example, factor V Leiden and inherited deficiencies of protein C and protein S, may also be associated with pregnancy loss. In the past, the association of livedo reticularis with arterial thrombosis (typically stroke) in young women has been termed Sneddon's syndrome. Studies indicate that many patients with Sneddon's syndrome have aPLs.

The location of this patient's thrombosis, a small peripheral artery, is somewhat uncommon in APS. Although thrombosis in almost every location in the vasculature has been reported in association

with aPL, stroke and transient ischemic attack (TIA) are the most common types of arterial thrombosis. Lower extremity deep vein thrombosis (DVT), with or without associated pulmonary embolism, is the most common type of venous events. In patients with APS, recurrent thrombotic events tend to be of the same type, that is, patients with an initial arterial event tend to have subsequent arterial events and patients with venous events tend to have subsequent venous events. That said, some patients with APS have both arterial and venous thromboses.

The characterization of this patient as having APS should be considered tentative at this stage in the clinical evaluation. The strongest association of aPLs with thrombosis is for a persistently positive LA or persistently positive IgG or IgM aCL/aβ$_2$PI at medium to high titer. Transient or low-titer aPLs may occur in apparently healthy individuals and in association with certain infections. In this patient, aPL positivity has been documented on only one occasion. The high titer and isotype of the antibody (in this case, IgG aCL and aβ$_2$GPI), suggests that this is a clinically significant finding; however, aPL testing should be repeated. The optimal time interval for repeat testing is not known. Current classification criteria require that positive tests be demonstrated at least 12 weeks apart,[1] whereas the original iteration of these criteria required a minimum interval of only 6 weeks.[2] Twelve weeks is reasonable due, in large part, to the fact that critical treatment decisions affected by repeat testing (e.g., how long to continue full anticoagulation after the acute thrombotic event) do not usually need to be made before 12 weeks.

Identification of persistent moderate- to high-titer aPLs in a patient with thrombosis does not obviate the need to evaluate the patient for additional causes of thrombophilia (inherited and acquired) and, importantly, to identify any reversible thrombotic risk factors (see Table 11-3). Approximately 50% of patients with APS with thrombotic events have one or more reversible or modifiable risk factors for thrombosis at the time of their acute events.[3,4]

Two other aspects of this patient's case are worth mentioning, that is, the positive ANA and the history of severe headache. A positive ANA, and occasionally more specific autoantibodies associated with systemic lupus erythematosus (SLE), may be present in patients with APS. APS may occur in association with SLE or other autoimmune diseases, or in the absence of these conditions (primary APS). Approximately a third of SLE patients have aPLs, and about a third of these (approximately 10%–15% of SLE patients) have clinical manifestations of APS. Primary APS and APS associated with SLE probably represent two extremes of a spectrum. It is not unusual for patients with primary APS to have some serologic features of SLE. Because of the association of APS with SLE, patients with APS should have a thorough history and physical examination to evaluate for SLE and other systemic autoimmune diseases. Secondly, an association between migraine headache and aPL has been reported but is controversial owing to the relatively high prevalence of headaches in the general population.

Therapy

There are no APS-specific recommendations for the management of acute thrombosis. Anticoagulation with intravenous unfractionated heparin or subcutaneous low-molecular-weight heparin, followed by warfarin, is the initial treatment strategy for both aPL-positive and aPL-negative patients with acute thrombosis.

An important issue in the long-term management of APS (prevention of recurrent thrombosis, that is, secondary thrombosis prevention), is the optimal intensity of anticoagulation with warfarin. Previous retrospective studies indicated that high-intensity treatment (INR = 3.0) warfarin was more effective than moderate-intensity warfarin or low-dose aspirin for the prevention of recurrent thrombosis in aPL-positive patients. More recently, two randomized controlled trials demonstrated that high-intensity anticoagulation (INR 3.1–4.0) was no better that moderate intensity (INR 2.0–3.0).[5,6] Based on these studies, moderate-intensity anticoagulation is the current standard of care. Several caveats to this recommendation should be considered. These studies did not separate patients with arterial and venous thrombosis. It is possible that larger studies of these patient subsets would yield different recommendations. Some clinicians assume that prevention of arterial thrombosis requires more intensive therapy, perhaps due to the clinical impact of arterial thrombi, for example, stroke or loss of a limb. This may or may not be the case, however. The Antiphospholipid Antibodies and Stroke Study found no difference between warfarin (INR 1.4–2.8) and aspirin (325 mg/day) for prevention of recurrent stroke or death in patients following an initial stroke.[7] Drawbacks to this study are that patients were tested only once for aPL and that most aPL were low-titer aCL. The use of newer antiplatelet agents, such as clopidogrel, to prevent recurrent arterial thrombosis associated with aPL is potentially interesting but has not been studied.

Duration of anticoagulation is another difficult issue. Although the optimal duration of therapy is not known, it is recommended that warfarin be continued indefinitely. Schulman and colleagues[8] found an increased incidence of recurrent venous thrombosis following a 6-month course of anticoagulation in patients with aCL as compared with those without aCL (29% versus 14%, risk ratio 2.1, 95% confidence interval [CI] 1.3–3.3, $P < 0.01$). It is not known whether it might be safe to discontinue or reduce the intensity of anticoagulation for patients whose aPL tests become persistently negative months or years after their last thrombotic event. In evaluating such a patient, it is important to consider whether there were reversible non-aPL thrombosis risk factors, for example, an estrogen oral contraceptive, at the time of the thrombotic event.

There may be difficulties in monitoring warfarin therapy in patients with aPLs. Antiphospholipid antibodies may interfere with the prothrombin time assay, causing an unreliable INR. This occurs in 6.5% to 10% of patients with positive LA tests.[9-11] Another, more general concern with using the INR to guide warfarin therapy is that not all vitamin K proteins affect the INR equally. The INR is affected by levels of factor II (prothrombin), factor VII, and factor X, with factor VII having the greatest impact.[12] In contrast, the prothrombin level is thought to be the most important determinant of the therapeutic effect of warfarin.[13,14] For these reasons, Kasthuri and Roubey have suggested the following approach.[15] Once a patient with APS has been started on warfarin and the INR is in the 2.0 to 3.0 range, a factor II activity assay should be checked simultaneously with an INR. If the INR is in the target range and the factor II level is therapeutic (15%–25%), the patient is adequately anticoagulated and the INR is a reliable indicator. In contrast, if the INR is in range but the factor II level is greater than 30%, the patient is not adequately anticoagulated. For subsequent monitoring, an INR range corresponding to a therapeutic factor II level should be established, or the factor II level could be followed in lieu of the INR. A chromogenic factor X level can also be used in a similar fashion. It should be noted that this approach, although rational, has not been studied in clinical trials.

Corticosteroids and other immunosuppressive agents are not effective and not recommended for prevention of recurrent thrombosis in APS.

MANAGEMENT OF PREGNANCY MORBIDITIES

Diagnostic Considerations

In general, pregnancy losses are classified into four main groups: *preembryonic loss* (conception through the 4th week of gestation); *embryonic loss* (5th through 9th weeks of gestation); *fetal loss* (10th week of gestation until delivery); and *neonatal loss*. Early pregnancy losses (less than 10 weeks) are common in the general population, and aPL testing should be interpreted cautiously in women with early losses. In the current classification criteria, embryonic deaths are considered as clinical evidence for definite APS only if there are three or more consecutive unexplained early losses.[1]

APS is most strongly associated with fetal losses, as in Case 2. Other pregnancy morbidity that can occur in aPL-positive patients includes premature birth, pre-eclampsia, eclampsia, and intrauterine growth restriction. *H*emolysis, *E*levated *L*iver Enzymes, *L*ow *P*latelet (HELLP) syndrome may also be associated with aPLs. HELLP syndrome in aPL-positive patients,

---

CASE STUDY 2

A 27-year-old white woman with past medical history of single fetal loss (28 weeks' gestation) 6 months prior (gravida: 1, para: 0) seeks advice regarding her future pregnancy options. She was asymptomatic during the pregnancy, and fetal death was detected on a routine sonogram. She is currently asymptomatic and denies any history of thrombosis. The workup within the last 6 months showed a positive LA (tested twice 3 months apart), negative aCL (IgG, IgM, and IgA), negative aβ$_2$GPI (IgG and IgM), normal uterine, karyotypic, and hormonal assessments, and no genetic hypercoagulable conditions (see Table 11-3). Histologic evaluation of the placenta demonstrated ischemic-hypoxic changes, extensive maternal floor infarction due to uteroplacental/spiral artery thrombosis, and decidual vasculopathy (Fig. 11-2B).

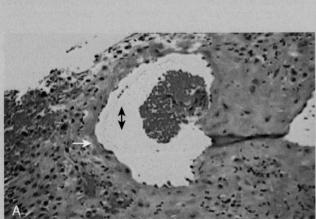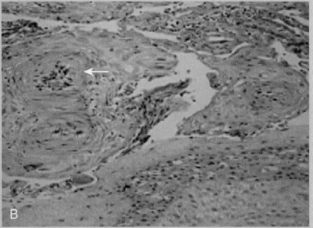

Figure 11-2. A, Placental biopsy specimen demonstrating the normal physiologic conversion of a decidual vessel. Note that the vessel has a large lumen (*double-headed arrow*) and that the vessel wall is composed of an endothelial layer but lacks a smooth muscle layer (*single-headed arrow*). **B,** Placental biopsy specimen demonstrating lack of physiologic conversion resulting in decidual vasculopathy. Arrow indicates spiral arterioles with smooth muscular walls and small lumen. (Reprinted from George D, Vasanth L, Erkan D, Bass A, Salmon J, Lockshin MD. Primary antiphospholipid syndrome presenting as HELLP syndrome. HSS J 2007;3:216-21.)

as compared with the aPL-negative population, occurs earlier in the second trimester of pregnancy, is more commonly associated with hepatic infarcts, and requires aggressive treatment, because the majority of patients develop severe thrombotic complications.[16]

Other factors that can predispose women to poor pregnancy outcome should be thoroughly investigated patients with a history of recurrent pregnancy loss, whether or not they have aPLs. These include uterine abnormalities (congenital, synechiae, fibroids, or cervical incompetence), chronic infections, systemic diseases (thyroid disorders, diabetes mellitus, or hypertension), hormonal imbalance (luteal phase defect or hypersecretion of luteinizing hormone), maternal and paternal karyotype abnormalities, fetal genetic abnormalities, and substance abuse.

This patient's placenta had extensive changes of malperfusion, hypoxia, and ischemia with lack of physiologic conversion of the decidua to uteroplacental tissue (decidual vasculopathy). Although these changes can also occur in pregnancy-induced hypertension, pre-eclampsia, HELLP syndrome, and APS, in the presence of persistent aPL and in the absence of other clinical findings (e.g., hypertension), aPL is the most likely cause of the fetal death. Of note, the conditions listed earlier may represent a continuum of similar processes and determining a clear cause of pregnancy loss can be a diagnostic challenge both clinically and pathologically.

Therapy

There are several key points in the management of pregnant aPL-positive patients. First, APS patients with history of vascular events require secondary thrombosis prophylaxis during pregnancy. The general recommendation is therapeutic dose low-molecular-weight heparin (LMWH) (e.g., enoxaparin 1 mg/kg twice a day or 1.5 mg/kg once a day) and low-dose (81 mg) aspirin during pregnancy; however, it is unknown if aspirin significantly affects outcome. Second, patients with APS with history of only pregnancy morbidities require prophylactic dose LMWH (e.g., enoxaparin 0.5 mg/kg once a day) and low-dose aspirin to decrease the risk of a recurrent pregnancy event. Based on controlled studies, the combination of heparin and aspirin is more effective than aspirin alone, and prophylactic dose heparin is equally as effective as therapeutic dose heparin. Third, there are no evidence-based data supporting the effectiveness or necessity of any medication in asymptomatic (no history of thrombosis or pregnancy morbidity) persistently aPL-positive pregnant women. These patients are usually treated with low-dose aspirin given the potential benefits and low risk of side effects.[17]

Keeping the above-mentioned key points in mind, this patient should be treated with prophylactic-dose heparin and low-dose aspirin during the next pregnancy. Aspirin is generally started before the pregnancy, and heparin is started when the pregnancy is confirmed. The heparin requirement may increase during pregnancy due to increased levels of heparin-binding proteins, increased heparin clearance, and larger volume of heparin distribution. Thus, especially in high-risk patients, factor Xa level monitoring during pregnancy may be helpful. It is also important that these patients should be followed by obstetricians who specialize in high-risk pregnancy with regular fetal ultrasound, echocardiography, and surveillance tests such as umbilical artery Doppler sonogram.

Finally, postpartum thrombosis prophylaxis is crucial in all persistently aPL-positive patients with or without history of thrombosis. The risk of thrombosis during the postpartum period is higher than the risk during pregnancy; LMWH should be continued for 8 to 12 weeks in persistently aPL-positive patients if they are not on life-long warfarin. Patients who were on warfarin before pregnancy can be switched back to warfarin after delivery. Warfarin is safe during breast-feeding.

CATASTROPHIC ANTIPHOSPHOLIPID SYNDROME

CASE STUDY 3

A 55-year-old man with active Crohn's disease and a history of APS (right lower extremity DVT one year ago and persistently positive LA and high-titer IgG aCL) presented with recurrent right lower extremity DVT. The DVT occurred while warfarin was being held before surgery for Crohn's disease. His admission platelet count was 124×10^9/L. He was started on heparin, which was stopped the next day due to thrombocytopenia of 47×10^9/L (there was no history of heparin-induced thrombocytopenia) and new-onset diffuse bilateral pulmonary infiltrates on chest x-ray study. Hemoglobin was 8.2 mg/dL, and schistocytes were present on the peripheral blood smear. Platelet serotonin release assay and anti–heparin-platelet factor 4 antibodies (anti-HPF4) were negative. Bronchoscopy with bronchoalveolar lavage showed bloody lavage fluid and hemosiderin-laden macrophages. The patient received daily intravenous pulse corticosteroids (1000 mg methylprednisolone) and plasma exchange for 3 days with stabilization of platelet counts and pulmonary hemorrhage. On the third day of the admission, he was started on heparin, and subsequently converted to warfarin.

Diagnostic Considerations

Catastrophic antiphospholipid syndromre (CAPS) is the most severe form of APS. It is characterized by the acute onset of multiple organ thromboses

(Table 11-4), commonly occurring with thrombotic microangiopathy, thrombocytopenia, and microangiopathic hemolytic anemia.[18] CAPS is fatal in approximately 50% of reported cases. Sepsis, disseminated intravascular coagulation, heparin-induced thrombocytopenia, or other thrombotic microangiopathies (such as thrombotic thrombocytopenic purpura or hemolytic uremic syndrome) should be included in the differential diagnosis of CAPS. There may be considerable overlap among these conditions, and in many cases, a definitive diagnosis may be difficult. Regardless, in a patient with history of APS, the new onset of multiple organ thromboses and characteristic hematologic manifestations should raise the possibility of CAPS and treatment should be started without any delay.

Based on an international consensus statement on the classification of CAPS, *Definite CAPS* is defined as the presence of all four criteria in Table 11-4 and *Probable CAPS* is defined as the presence of three of the four criteria.[19] The purpose of the "Probable CAPS" classification category is to facilitate early suspicion, diagnosis, and treatment, which significantly improve patient survival. It should be noted that aPL-positive patients may present with a "CAPS-like" picture without fulfilling the *Definite or Probable CAPS* criteria. These patients may progress to *Definite or Probable CAPS* over time. Owing to the high mortality rate associated with CAPS, aggressive treatment should not be delayed if the condition is suspected, whether or not criteria are met. Given that this patient had persistent aPL, one large and one small vessel thrombosis simultaneously (although there was no biopsy confirmation of the presumed microthrombosis of the lungs), thrombocytopenia, and microangiopathic hemolytic anemia, he should be managed as having CAPS.

Other diagnostic points that merit special attention in this case are as follows: (1) withdrawal of anticoagulation can trigger large vessel thrombosis or CAPS in persistently aPL-positive patients; (2) diffuse alveolar hemorrhage is relatively common in CAPS patients; (3) thrombocytopenia can occur in up to 60% of patients with CAPS[20]; (4) heparin-induced thrombocytopenia can present a diagnostic challenge in patients with APS; and (5) a subset of patients with CAPS present with thrombotic microangiopathic hemolytic anemia.[21]

Withdrawal of anticoagulation during a perioperative period is a well-known trigger of recurrent thrombosis (and rarely CAPS) in persistently aPL-positive patients. Bridging anticoagulation with heparin should be instituted between the withdrawal of warfarin and surgery. Usually, LMWH is stopped 12 hours before the surgery; however, low-dose aspirin can be continued in high-risk patients. Moreover, patients should be started on anticoagulation as soon as the postsurgical bleeding risk decreases to acceptable levels. Postoperatively, mechanical DVT prevention strategies should be instituted vigorously.

Diffuse alveolar hemorrhage due to microthrombosis and/or pulmonary capillaritis should be strongly considered in patients with APS with hemoptysis or acute pulmonary infiltrates.[22] In patients with APS, thrombocytopenia, overanticoagulation, and heparin-induced thrombocytopenia can also contribute to the risk of the bleeding. A lung biopsy may not be always feasible in patients with CAPS due to concurrent thrombocytopenia. As noted earlier, treatment may need to be instituted without a pathologic diagnosis.

Thrombocytopenia occurs in 20% of APS and 60% of CAPS patients. The differential diagnosis includes immune-mediated thrombocytopenia due to antibodies against glycoprotein IIb/IIIa complex[23] and thrombosis-induced platelet consumption. Severe thrombocytopenia compounding bleeding or

---

Table 11-4. *International Classification Criteria for Catastrophic Antiphospholipid Syndrome (CAPS)*

1. Evidence of involvement of three or more organs, systems, or tissues*
2. Development of manifestations simultaneously or in less than 1 week
3. Confirmation by histopathology of small vessel occlusion in at least one organ or tissue[†]
4. Laboratory confirmation of the presence of aPL[‡]

Definite CAPS
→ All 4 criteria

Probable CAPS
→ All 4 criteria, except for involvement of only two organs, systems, or tissues
→ All 4 criteria, except for the absence of laboratory confirmation at least 6 wk apart attributable to the early death of a patient never tested for aPL before CAPS
→ 1, 2, and 4
→ 1, 3, and 4 and the development of a third event in more than 1 week but less than 1 month, despite anticoagulation treatment

aPLs, antiphospholipid antibodies; APS, antiphospholipid syndrome.
*Usually, clinical evidence of vessel occlusions, confirmed by imaging techniques. Renal involvement is defined by 50% increase in serum creatinine, severe systemic hypertension (>180/100 mm Hg), and/or proteinuria (>500 mg/24 h).
[†]For histopathologic confirmation, significant evidence of thrombosis must be present, although vasculitis may coexist occasionally.
[‡]If the patient had not been previously diagnosed as having APS, the laboratory confirmation requires that presence of aPLs must be detected on 2 or more occasions at least 6 weeks apart (not necessarily at the time of the event).
Adapted from Asherson RA, Cervera R, de Groot PG, Erkan D, Boffa MC, Piette JC, Khamashta MA, Shoenfeld Y. Catastrophic antiphospholipid syndrome: International consensus statement on classification criteria and treatment guidelines. Lupus 2003;12:530-4.

thrombosis, as in this patient, brings multiple challenges to the management of CAPS, such as the need to stop anticoagulation despite ongoing thrombosis.

Heparin-induced thrombocytopenia (HIT) due to anti-HPF4 may represent an additional prothrombotic risk factor and diagnostic challenge in aPL-positive patients treated with heparin. Although HIT occurs within 4 to 10 days of heparin exposure in heparin-naïve patients, it can develop within hours in those with a history of heparin exposure (especially within the prior 3–4 months). Patients with a significant drop in their platelet counts are usually switched to a direct thrombin inhibitor while the results of HIT laboratory tests are pending. Given that heparin was used almost a year ago in this case and that confirmatory HIT laboratory tests were negative, thrombocytopenia in this patient was most likely related to aPL. He was restarted on heparin without any complications after the bleeding was controlled. Of note, Alpert and associates[24] demonstrated an association between anti-HPF4, aPLs, and APS (particularly arterial thrombosis), in heparin-naïve SLE patients.

Thrombotic microangiopathic hemolytic anemia is relatively common in CAPS. Patients with CAPS with thrombocytopenia, compared with those without thrombocytopenia, have a higher incidence of concomitant hematologic manifestations (hemolysis, schistocytes, disseminated intravascular coagulation and elevated fibrin degradation products).[21] Overlap between CAPS and other microangiopathic conditions such as thrombocytopenic purpura may exist. Thus, the term "microangiopathic aPL-associated APS" has been suggested for this group of patients.[25]

Therapy

Based on analysis of the international web-based CAPS registry, the best clinical outcomes are achieved when CAPS patients are treated with the combination of anticoagulation, corticosteroids, and plasma exchange or intravenous immunoglobulin. Cyclophosphamide can improve the survival in CAPS patients with lupus but not in those with primary CAPS.[26] Despite the limitations of the CAPS registry (e.g., retrospective data collection, ascertainment bias), it is an important source for systematic analysis of a relatively uncommon disease. Based on limited number of case reports, rituximab can be effective against thrombocytopenia and hemolytic anemia.[27] There are no data regarding the effects of rituximab on thrombosis. The choice or timing of medications used to treat CAPS varies among patients and depends on the severity of the presentation, thrombocytopenia, bleeding, and concomitant infections.

Diffuse alveolar hemorrhage in CAPS patients usually responds to corticosteroids; however, the recurrence risk is higher without immunosuppressive treatment.[22] Thus, intravenous pulse corticosteroids with plasma exchange or intravenous immunoglobulin is the most commonly used initial approach in aPL-positive patients presenting with diffuse alveolar hemorrhage. These patients should be started on anticoagulation as soon as bleeding is controlled because bleeding in aPL-positive patients does not protect against thrombosis. There are no evidence-based recommendations for the management of bleeding in APS patients. When bleeding occurs, the timing of anticoagulation is a difficult decision. In general, anticoagulation should be started as soon as bleeding is controlled, with the understanding that the risk of further bleeding remains high.[28]

Severe thrombocytopenia usually responds to corticosteroids. This patient was initially managed by corticosteroids and plasma exchange followed by anticoagulation. Based on anecdotal experience, both intravenous immunoglobulin and rituximab would be a reasonable next step if his thrombocytopenia had not improved even though there are no systematic data in the management of CAPS patients.

OTHER NONCRITERIA MANIFESTATIONS ASSOCIATED WITH ANTIPHOSPHOLIPID ANTIBODIES

CASE STUDY 4

A 21-year-old black woman is seen in consultation for management of Raynaud's phenomenon. She is usually asymptomatic in the summer but has experienced brief episodes of classic Raynaud's syndrome on cold exposure during the winter for several years. Her physical examination is normal except for diffuse livedo reticularis of the upper and lower extremities. Laboratory studies show a platelet count of 120×10^9/L, ANA positive at 1:320, antibodies to double-stranded DNA negative, LA test positive, and IgG aCL of 78 U (high positive). Repeat studies done 3 months later again show mild thrombocytopenia and confirm a positive LA test and high-positive IgG aCL.

Diagnostic Considerations

As listed in Table 11-3, a number of clinical manifestations other than thrombosis and pregnancy mortality and morbidity have been associated with aPLs. Although the authors of the most recent consensus classification criteria for definite APS recognized these associations, they elected not to include these clinical features in the criteria due to concerns about specificity.[1] These clinical manifestations may occur in association with aPLs in the patients with or without a history of thrombosis or pregnancy loss. The presence of one or more of these manifestations, in this case livedo reticularis and thrombocytopenia, should prompt testing for aPLs, particularly when no other etiology is evident. Similarly, in patients with established APS, these manifestations should be considered in the appropriate setting. For example, a heart murmur or cardiac symptoms should prompt evaluation for valvular disease.

Livedo reticularis is the most common skin condition associated with aPL (see Fig. 11-1) and has been defined as "the persistent, not reversible with rewarming, violaceous, red or blue, reticular or mottled, pattern of the skin of trunk, arms or legs."[1] Although the dermatologic literature varies on nomenclature, at least two patterns of livedo have been described.[29] One pattern (regular livedo reticularis) is characterized by unbroken circles or polygons. The other (livedo racemosa) is characterized by a more open pattern of irregular branching lines or "broken" shapes. Livedo racemosa may be associated with a greater risk of thrombosis than regular livedo reticularis.[30] Thrombocytopenia associated with aPLs is usually mild, as in the case presented earlier.

This case again highlights the close association between SLE and APS, as was discussed in the earlier section on thrombosis. SLE is obviously a diagnostic consideration in a patient with Raynaud's phenomenon, a positive ANA, and mild thrombocytopenia.

Therapy

In general, these nonthrombotic and non–pregnancy-related clinical manifestations do not require aPL-specific therapy. Thrombocytopenia, if it becomes severe enough to require treatment, usually responds to moderate doses of corticosteroids. As noted earlier, mild aPL-associated thrombocytopenia does not protect patients from the risk of thrombosis. Livedo reticularis does not generally cause pain or discomfort and there is no specific therapy for it. Valvular heart disease associated with aPL is usually asymptomatic but may occasionally require valve replacement. Anticoagulation or antiplatelet agents may be necessary if the involved valve is a source of emboli.

In certain instances, anticoagulation may be considered for some aPL-associated manifestations in the absence of overt or obvious thrombosis. For example, anecdotal reports suggest that anticoagulation may be helpful in treating refractory cutaneous ulcers associated with aPL.[31] However, anticoagulation is not always effective based on our experience and immunosuppressive treatment may be required. Antiphospholipid antibody-associated nephropathy is a form of small vessel vasculopathy, which may include intrarenal thrombi and microthrombi. In this condition, there is a good rationale for considering anticoagulation; however, it appears that nephropathy may slowly progress despite such treatment. It is tempting to consider anticoagulation for certain nonstroke neurologic manifestations, due to the absence of effective treatment for these conditions. There are, however, no convincing data to support the use of anticoagulants in this setting and there is a risk of bleeding. Anecdotal reports and noncontrolled trials may be misleading. For example, a small, noncontrolled case series suggested that heparin was effective in treating chronic severe headache in patients with aPLs.[32] In contrast, a subsequent randomized, placebo-controlled trial conducted by the same group of investigators showed no effect.[33]

A retrospective study of five patients provides evidence that B-cell depletion with rituximab is well tolerated and effective for refractory thrombocytopenia and skin ulcers in aPL-positive patients.[34] Based on this experience and in vitro evidence that B cells are involved in aPL-related clinical events,[35] an open-label phase IIa descriptive pilot study of rituximab for anticoagulation-resistant manifestations of aPL is in progress. Inclusion criteria for this study (in addition to the persistent aPL-positivity) are persistent thrombocytopenia, persistent autoimmune hemolytic anemia, cardiac valve disease, chronic skin ulcers, renal thrombotic microangiopathy, or cognitive dysfunction (with/without white matter changes). This trial will provide systematic data on the effects of rituximab on clinical, laboratory (including thrombocytopenia), and serologic parameters of aPL-positive patients (Clinical Trials. gov Identifier: NCT00537290).

Finally, primary thrombosis prevention strategies (discussed later) are also important in the management of patients with non-criteria aPL features.

PRIMARY THROMBOSIS PROPHYLAXIS IN ASYMPTOMATIC PERSISTENTLY ANTIPHOSPHOLIPID ANTIBODY–POSITIVE INDIVIDUALS

CASE STUDY 5

A 28-year-old white man was found to have an elevated activated partial thromboplastin time (aPTT) during a routine preoperative screening for knee arthroscopy. Further testing confirmed the presence of a LA, which has been persistently positive for the last year (IgG, IgM, and IgA aCL and aβ₂GPI are negative). He denies any history of thrombosis, other significant medical history, and cigarette smoking. Review of systems is negative. Physical examination is normal and basic laboratory studies (including platelet count) are within normal limits.

Diagnostic Considerations

Based on cross-sectional studies, up to 10% of the general healthy population can be positive for aPLs, which is usually low-titer transient aCL.[36] Isolated persistent LA positivity is relatively rare. These asymptomatic aPL-positive patients merit a careful history and physical examination to rule out systemic autoimmune diseases, especially lupus or lupus-like disease, in which the prevalence of aPLs is 30% to 40%. aPLs can also be associated with various malignancies.[37]

Prevention

At least 50% of patients with APS with thrombotic events possess one or more non-aPL reversible risk factors at time of thrombosis.[4] Therefore, identification and elimination of these risk factors, as well as aggressive prophylaxis during high-risk periods (such as surgical procedures), are crucial for the primary thrombosis prevention.

The effectiveness of aspirin in persistently aPL-positive patients without vascular events is not supported by a recent prospective controlled study. In this randomized, double-blind, placebo-controlled trial, low-dose aspirin appeared to be no better than placebo in preventing first thrombotic episodes in asymptomatic persistently aPL-positive patients.[38] The overall incidence rate of thrombosis in this study was relatively low. In addition, the majority of the patients who developed thrombosis had concomitant non-aPL thrombosis risk factors. Thus, the ideal primary thrombosis prevention strategy in asymptomatic persistently aPL-positive individuals should be risk stratified and determined based on age, traditional cardiovascular risk factors, other comorbidities, systemic autoimmune diseases, and the aPL profile. We suggest that cardiovascular disease prevention guidelines for the general population, such as those formulated based on the Framingham Heart Study,[39] should play a role in the decision whether or not to recommend low-dose aspirin therapy in asymptomatic persistently aPL-positive individuals. Hormone replacement therapy and estrogen-containing oral contraceptives should not be given to aPL-positive patients.

Perioperative thrombosis may occur despite prophylaxis in aPL-positive patients. Thus, pharmacologic and physical antithrombosis interventions should be vigorously employed and periods without anticoagulation should be kept to an absolute minimum. Importantly, intravascular manipulation for access and monitoring should be minimized. Any deviation from a normal course should be considered a potential aPL-related event until proven otherwise.[40]

Independently of aPL and traditional cardiovascular disease risk factors, patients with SLE (and most likely also those with other systemic autoimmune disease) are at significantly increased risk for premature atherosclerosis and thrombosis.[41] Thus, physicians should always keep in mind that thrombosis is a multifactorial process that requires a risk-stratified and patient-tailored prevention strategy.

Finally, hydroxychloroquine, based on experimental data and positive clinical experience in lupus patients, and the enzyme 3-hydroxy-3-methylglutaryl coenzyme (HMG-CoA) reductase inhibitors (statins), based on experimental data and positive clinical experience in aPL-negative general population[42] will potentially be part of APS management in the near future. However, in the absence of randomized controlled trials in aPL-positive patients, we do not currently recommend these agents for primary thrombosis prevention unless they are indicated for concomitant conditions.

References

1. Miyakis S, Lockshin MD, Atsumi T, Branch DW, Brey RL, Cervera R, et al. International consensus statement on an update of the classification criteria for definite antiphospholipid syndrome. J Thromb Haemost 2006;4:295-306.
2. Wilson WA, Gharavi AE, Koike T, Lockshin MD, Branch DW, Piette JC, et al. International consensus statement on preliminary classification criteria for definite antiphospholipid syndrome: Report of an international workshop. Arthritis Rheum 1999;42:1309-11.
3. Erkan D, Yazici Y, Peterson MG, Sammaritano L, Lockshin D. A cross-sectional study of clinical thrombotic risk factors and preventive treatments in antiphospholipid syndrome. Rheumatology 2002;41:924-9.
4. Kaul M, Erkan D, Sammaritano L, Lockshin MD. Assessment of the 2006 revised antiphospholipid syndrome classification criteria. Ann Rheum Dis 2007;66:927-30.
5. Crowther MA, Ginsberg JS, Julian J, Denburg J, Hirsh J, Douketis J, et al. A comparison of two intensities of warfarin for the prevention of recurrent thrombosis in patients with the antiphospholipid antibody syndrome. N Engl J Med 2003;349:1133-8.
6. Finazzi G, Marchioli R, Brancaccio V, Schinco P, Wisloff J, Musial J, et al. A randomized clinical trial of high-intensity warfarin vs. conventional antithrombotic therapy for the prevention of recurrent thrombosis in patients with the antiphospholipid syndrome. J Thromb Haemost 2005;3:848-53.
7. Levine SR, Brey RL, Tilley BC, Thompson JL, Sacco RL, Sciacca RR, et al. Antiphospholipid antibodies and subsequent thrombo-occlusive events in patients with ischemic stroke. JAMA 2004;291:576-84.
8. Schulman S, Svenungsson E, Granqvist S. Anticardiolipin antibodies predict early recurrence of thromboembolism and death among patients with venous thromboembolism following anticoagulant therapy. Duration of Anticoagulation Study Group. Am J Med 1998;104:332-8.
9. Moll S, Ortel TL. Monitoring warfarin therapy in patients with lupus anticoagulants. Ann Intern Med 1997;127:177-85.
10. Sanfelippo MJ, Sennet J, McMahon EJ. Falsely elevated inrs in warfarin-treated patients with the lupus anticoagulant. WMJ 2000;99:62-64, 43.
11. Rosborough TK, Shepherd MF. Unreliability of international normalized ratio for monitoring warfarin therapy in patients with lupus anticoagulant. Pharmacotherapy 2004;24:838-42.
12. Lind SE, Callas PW, Golden EA, Joyner Jr KA, Ortel TL. Plasma levels of factors II, VII and X and their relationship to the international normalized ratio during chronic warfarin therapy. Blood Coagul Fibrinolysis 1997;8:48-53.
13. Sise HS, Lavelle SM, Adamis D, Becker R. Relation of hemorrhage and thrombosis to prothrombin during treatment with coumarin-type anticoagulants. N Engl J Med 1958;259:266-71.
14. Zivelin A, Rao LV, Rapaport SI. Mechanism of the anticoagulant effect of warfarin as evaluated in rabbits by selective depression of individual procoagulant vitamin K-dependent clotting factors. J Clin Invest 1993;92:2131-40.

15. Kasthuri RS, Roubey RA. Warfarin and the antiphospholipid syndrome: does one size fit all? Arthritis Rheum 2007;57:1346-7.

16. George D, Vasanth L, Erkan D, Bass A, Salmon J, Lockshin MD. Primary antiphospholipid syndrome presenting as HELLP syndrome. HSS J 2007;3:216-21.

17. Derksen RH, Khamashta MA, Branch DW. Management of the obstetric antiphospholipid syndrome. Arthritis Rheum 2004;50:1028-39.

18. Vero S, Asherson RA, Erkan D. Critical care review: catastrophic antiphospholipid syndrome. J Intensive Care Med 2006;21:144-59.

19. Asherson RA, Cervera R, de Groot PG, Erkan D, Boffa MC, Piette JC, et al. Catastrophic antiphospholipid syndrome: International consensus statement on classification criteria and treatment guidelines. Lupus 2003;12:530-4.

20. Espinosa G, Bucciarelli S, Asherson RA, Cervera R. Morbidity and mortality in the catastrophic antiphospholipid syndrome: pathophysiology, causes of death, and prognostic factors. Semin Thromb Hemost 2008;34:290-4.

21. Bayraktar UD, Erkan D, Bucciarelli S, Espinosa G, Cervera R, Asherson R. Catastrophic antiphospholipid syndrome: comparison between CAPS patients with and without thrombocytopenia [abstract]. Clin Exp Rheumatol 2007;25:14.

22. Deane K, West SG. Antiphospholipid antibodies as a cause of pulmonary capillaritis and diffuse alveolar hemorrhage: a case series and literature review. Semin Arthritis Rheum 2005;35:154-65.

23. Galli M, Finazzi G, Barbui T. Thrombocytopenia in the antiphospholipid syndrome. Br J Haematol 1996;93:1-5.

24. Alpert D, Mandl LA, Erkan D, Yin W, Peerschke EI, Salmon JE. Anti-heparin platelet factor 4 antibodies in systemic lupus erythaematosus are associated with IgM antiphospholipid antibodies and the antiphospholipid syndrome. Ann Rheum Dis 2008;67:395-401.

25. Asherson RA, Cervera R. Microvascular and microangiopathic antiphospholipid-associated syndromes ("MAPS"): semantic or antisemantic? Autoimmun Rev 2008;7:164-7.

26. Bayraktar UD, Erkan D, Bucciarelli S, Espinosa G, Asherson R, Catastrophic Antiphospholipid Syndrome Project Group. The clinical spectrum of catastrophic antiphospholipid syndrome in the absence and presence of lupus. J Rheumatol 2007;34:346-52.

27. Erre GL, Pardini S, Faedda R, Passiu G. Effect of rituximab on clinical and laboratory features of antiphospholipid syndrome: a case report and a review of literature. Lupus 2008;17:50-5.

28. Silverberg M, Erkan D, Lockshin MD. Hemorrhage in the antiphospholipid syndrome: The challenge of anticoagulation abstract. Arthritis Rheum 2003;46:S52.

29. Uthman IW, Khamashta MA. Livedo racemosa: a striking dermatological sign for the antiphospholipid syndrome. J Rheumatol 2006;33:2379-82.

30. Frances C, Niang S, Laffitte E, Pelletier F, Costedoat N, Piette JC. Dermatologic manifestations of the antiphospholipid syndrome: two hundred consecutive cases. Arthritis Rheum 2005;52:1785-93.

31. Aguirre MA, Jurado A, Mujic F, Cuadrado MJ. Oral anticoagulation therapy of chronic skin ulcers in a patient with primary antiphospholipid syndrome. Clin Exp Rheumatol 1998;16:628-9.

32. Hughes GR, Cuadrado MJ, Khamashta MA, Sanna G. Headache and memory loss: rapid response to heparin in the antiphospholipid syndrome. Lupus 2001;10:778.

33. Cuadrado MJ, Sanna G, Sharief M, Khamashta MA, Hughes GRV. Double blind, crossover, randomized trial comparing low molecular weight heparin versus placebo in the treatment of chronic headache in patients with antiphospholipid antibodies [abstract]. Arthritis Rheum 2003;48:S364.

34. Tenedios F, Erkan D, Lockshin MD. Rituximab in the primary antiphospholipid syndrome [abstract]. Arthritis Rheum 2005;52:4078.

35. Youinou P, Renaudineau Y. The antiphospholipid syndrome as a model for B cell-induced autoimmune diseases. Thromb Res 2004;114:363-9.

36. Vila P, Hernández MC, López-Fernández MF, Batlle J. Prevalence, follow-up and clinical significance of the anticardiolipin antibodies in normal subjects. Thromb Haemost 1994;72:209-13.

37. Schved JF, Dupuy-Fons C, Biron C, Quéré I, Janbon C. A prospective epidemiological study on the occurrence of antiphospholipid antibody: the Montpelier Antiphospholipid (MAP) Study. Haemostasis 1994;24:175-82.

38. Erkan D, Harrison MJ, Levy R, Peterson M, Petri M, Sammaritano L, et al. Aspirin for primary thrombosis prevention in the antiphospholipid syndrome: A randomized, double-blind, placebo-controlled trial in asymptomatic antiphospholipid antibody-positive individuals. Arthritis Rheum 2007;56:2382-91.

39. Goldstein LB, Adams R, Alberts MJ, Appel LB, Brass LM, Bushnell CD, et al. Primary prevention of ischemic stroke: a guideline from the American Heart Association/American Stroke Association Stroke Council. Circulation 2006;113:e873-923.

40. Erkan D, Leibowitz E, Berman J, Lockshin MD. Perioperative medical management of antiphospholipid syndrome: hospital for special surgery experience, review of literature, and recommendations. J Rheumatol 2002;29:843-9.

41. Erkan D. Lupus and thrombosis. J Rheumatol 2006;33:1715-7.

42. Pierangeli SS, Vega-Ostertag ME, Gonzalez EB. New targeted therapies for treatment of thrombosis in antiphospholipid syndrome. Expert Rev Mol Med 2007;9:1-15.

Management of Sjögren's Syndrome

Petra M. Meiners, Jiska M. Meijer, Arjan Vissink, and
Hendrika Bootsma

INTRODUCTION

Sjögren's syndrome (SS) is an autoimmune inflammatory disorder of exocrine glands. It particularly affects the lacrimal and salivary glands. Dry mouth and dry eyes are frequently the presenting symptoms. Extraglandular manifestations, for example, arthritis and polyneuropathy can also be present (Table 12-1). In addition, many SS patients report functionally limiting chronic fatigue.

SS can be a primary idiopathic condition of unknown etiology (primary Sjögren's syndrome, pSS). SS may also occur in the presence of another autoimmune disorder such as rheumatoid arthritis (RA), systemic lupus erythematosus (SLE), scleroderma, or mixed connective tissue disease. In these cases, the condition is designated as secondary Sjögren's syndrome (sSS). The estimated prevalence of SS in the general population is between 0.5% and 1%, which makes SS, after RA, the most common systemic autoimmune disease. In RA, the prevalence of SS is around 30%, and 20% of patients with SLE fulfill the criteria for sSS. SS is more frequent in women (female-to-male ratio, 9:1). Furthermore, SS is associated with organ-specific autoimmune diseases such as autoimmune thyroid disease, primary biliary cirrhosis, and autoimmune gastritis. This underscores the autoimmune nature of the disease.[1,2] Like other rheumatologic conditions, SS exerts a major impact on patients' quality of life. Apart from the symptoms mentioned earlier, patients may be restricted in their activities and their participation in society, resulting in reduced health-related quality of life and impaired socioeconomic status.[3]

Because patients have concomitant oral, ocular, and systemic medical problems, the management of the patient with SS should ideally involve a multidisciplinary team of health care practitioners with good lines of communication between them. In a multidisciplinary team with a specialized rheumatologist, oral and maxillofacial surgeon, ophthalmologist, pathologist, hematologist, dentist and oral hygienist, SS patients can get the care they need. It is important that one physician, usually the rheumatologist, has overall responsibility for the care of the patient. The strategy followed at the University

Medical Center Groningen, The Netherlands is given in Figure 12-1.

Although there is as yet no curative or causal treatment for SS, various supportive and palliative treatment options are available, and targeted approaches (biologics) are in development or currently being tested in phase I or phase II trials. This chapter presents and discusses the management of both glandular and extraglandular manifestations of SS (including mucosa-associated lymphoid tissue [MALT] lymphoma), and discusses prospects focusing on better understanding of the progression and more effective treatment of SS.

Table 12-1. *Extraglandular Manifestations in Primary Sjögren's Syndrome*[3,14,94]

Anatomic System	Findings	Percentage*
Constitutional symptoms	Fatigue	80%
	Fever	5%
	Lymphadenopathy	15%
Joints/muscles	Articular involvement	50%
	Tendomyalgia	40%
	Myositis	2%
Skin	Raynaud's phenomenon	40%
	Cutaneous vasculitis	15%
	Skin involvement other than cutaneous vasculitis	5%
Endocrine	Autoimmune thyroiditis	10%
Respiratory tract	Pulmonary involvement	25%
	Serositis	2%
Gastrointestinal tract	Esophageal involvement	5%
	Autoimmune hepatitis	10%
	Acute pancreatitis	1%
Nervous system	Peripheral neuropathy	10%
	CNS involvement	2%
Urogenital tract	Renal involvement	10%
	Bladder involvement	15%
Hematology	Thrombocytopenia	2%
	Lymphoproliferative disease	5%

CNS, central nervous system.
*Percentages differ greatly between studies.

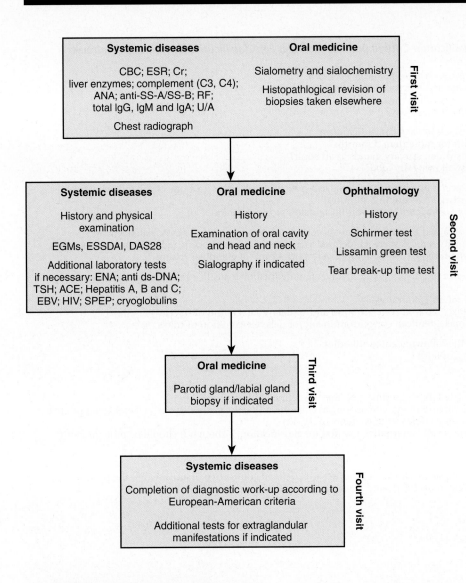

Figure 12-1. Diagnostic work-up strategy for patients referred under clinical suspicion of SS to the University Medical Center Groningen, The Netherlands. The referral may come from dentists, general practitioners, or other specialists. Before the first visit patients receive written information about the diagnostic procedure followed at our institution. ACE, angiotensin-converting enzyme; ANA, antinuclear antibody; CBC, complete blood cell count; Cr, creatinine; ds-DNA, double-stranded DNA; DAS28, disease activity score 28; EBV, Epstein-Barr virus; EGMs, extraglandular manifestations; ENA, extractable nuclear antigens; ESR, erythrocyte sedimentation rate; ESSDAI, Eular Sjögren's syndrome disease activity index; HIV, human immunodeficiency virus; RF, rheumatoid factor; SPEP, serum protein electrophoresis; TSH, thyroid stimulating hormone; U/A, urinalysis.

CLASSIFICATION AND DIAGNOSIS OF SJÖGREN'S SYNDROME

Many classification criteria for SS have been suggested. Presently, the revised American-European classification criteria for SS, which were proposed in 2002, are the most widely accepted and validated criteria (Table 12-2). These criteria combine subjective symptoms of dry eyes and dry mouth with objective signs of keratoconjunctivitis sicca and xerostomia.[4]

The subjective ocular and oral symptoms are obtained by history taking. Two tests are used to objectify reduced tear production. In the Schirmer's test a piece of filter paper is placed laterally on the lower eyelid, which results in wetting due to tear production. If less than 5 mm of paper is wetted after 5 minutes, the test result is positive (Fig. 12-2). In the Rose Bengal test, dye stains devitalized areas of the cornea and conjunctiva which can be scored using a slit lamp. A Rose Bengal score ≥4 according to the Van Bijsterveld scoring system is considered abnormal. Instead of Rose Bengal stain, lissamin green can be used, which shows comparable results but is less painful.

An additional test that is not accepted as a diagnostic technique for SS but provides a global assessment of the function of the tear film is the tear break-up time test. This test is performed by measuring break-up time and tear osmolarity after instillation of fluorescein. An interval of less than 10 seconds is considered abnormal.

To confirm the diagnosis of SS histopathologically, usually a biopsy from a labial salivary gland is taken. This should show focal lymphocytic sialoadenitis with a focus score of ≥ 1 (a focus is defined as an accumulation of 50 or more lymphocytes per 4 mm^2).[5] Recently it has been shown that parotid biopsy might serve as a proper alternative for labial biopsy in the diagnosis of SS (Fig. 12-3). Its morbidity is less than that of labial salivary gland biopsy. In addition, MALT/non-Hodgkin's lymphoma (NHL) pathology is easier to detect, because the labial glands are less commonly affected by MALT/NHL than the parotid glands.[6] Moreover, in contrast to a labial biopsy, parotid biopsies can be used to monitor various treatment methodologies since the same gland can be biopsied more than once.

Table 12-2. *Revised International Classification Criteria and Revised Rules For Classification of Sjögren's Syndrome*[4]

Ocular symptoms: a positive response to at least one of the following questions:
Have you had daily, persistent, troublesome dry eyes for more than 3 months?
Do you have a recurrent sensation of sand or gravel in the eyes?
Do you use tear substitutes more than three times a day?

Oral symptoms: a positive response to at least one of the following questions:
Have you had a daily feeling of dry mouth for more than 3 months?
Have you had recurrently or persistently swollen salivary glands as an adult?
Do you frequently drink liquids to aid in swallowing dry food?

Ocular signs–that is, objective evidence of ocular involvement defined as a positive result for at least one of the following two tests:
Schirmer's I test, performed without anesthesia (≤5 mm in 5 minutes)
Rose Bengal score or other ocular dye score (≥4 according to Van Bijsterveld's scoring system)

Histopathology: in minor salivary glands (obtained through normal-appearing mucosa) focal lymphocytic sialoadenitis,
   evaluated by an expert histopathologist, with a focus score ≥1, defined as a number of lymphocytic foci (which are adjacent to
   normal-appearing mucous acini and contain more than 50 lymphocytes) per 4 mm² of glandular tissue

Salivary gland involvement: objective evidence of salivary gland involvement defined by a positive result for at least one of the
   following diagnostic tests:
Unstimulated whole salivary flow (≤ 1.5 mL in 15 minutes)
Parotid sialography showing delayed uptake, reduced concentration and/or delayed excretion of tracer
Salivary scintigraphy showing delayed uptake, reduced concentration and/or delayed excretion of tracer

Autoantibodies: presence in the serum of the following autoantibodies:
Antibodies to Ro(SSA) or La(SSB) antigens, or both
Revised rules for classification

For Primary SS
In patients without any potentially associated disease, primary SS may be defined as follows:
The presence of any 4 of the 6 items is indicative of primary SS, as long as either item IV (Histopathology) or VI (Serology) is positive
The presence of any 3 of the 4 objective criteria items (that is, items III, IV, VI)
The classification tree procedure represents a valid alternative method for classification, although it should be more properly
   used in clinical-epidemiological survey

For Secondary SS
In patients with a potentially associated disease (for instance, another well defined connective tissue disease), the presence
   of item I or item II plus any 2 from among items III, IV, and V may be considered as indicative of secondary SS

Exclusion criteria:
Past head and neck radiation treatment
Hepatitis C infection
Acquired immunodeficienty disease (AIDS)
Pre-existing lymphoma
Sarcoidosis
Graft versus host disease
Use of anticholinergic drugs (since a time shorter than the 4-fold half life of the drug)

Currently, three diagnostic tests can be used to objectify salivary gland involvement, other than histopathology. The most commonly applied objective salivary gland diagnostic test is measuring the flow rate of unstimulated, whole saliva. Unstimulated whole saliva is a very useful indicator of salivary function and oral wetness. The patient is asked to expectorate once, then to collect all saliva into a graduated container. After 15 minutes, the volume of saliva is measured. These sialometric tests should be routinely performed regardless of whether the patient does or does not complain of oral disease, allowing later comparisons if the patient develops subjective oral dryness or presents with other symptoms or clinical signs of salivary dysfunction.[7] For research purposes, or if more specific functional information is required for a particular gland, individual gland collection techniques can be used. Collection of glandular saliva is not difficult but requires specialized equipment (e.g., a Lashley cup) and takes more time to perform. Other tests to evaluate salivary gland involvement are sialography and salivary gland scintigraphy. Sialography is the radiographic imaging of the salivary duct system through retrograde infusion of an oil- or water-based contrast fluid (Fig. 12-4).[8] Sialography has a low morbidity and is well accepted by patients.[9] The main sialographic characteristic of SS is a diffuse collection of contrast fluid at the terminal acini of the ductal tree, termed sialectasia.[10,11] Sialography has a high diagnostic accuracy. Finally, patients with SS demonstrate decreased uptake and release of technetium Tc 99m pertechnetate on scintigraphy.[12] At present, efforts are made to improve the diagnostic accuracy of scintigraphy.[13]

Approximately 80% of patients with SS display antinuclear antibodies (ANAs); about 40% to 60% of them have antibodies against anti-SS-A/Ro. This autoantibody is considered to be the most specific serologic marker for SS, even though it is also found in 25% to 35% of patients with SLE or other autoimmune connective tissue disorders, and in about 5%

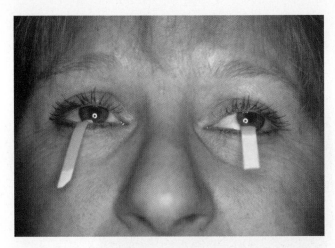

Figure 12-2. The Schirmer test can be used to assess lacrimal function in patients suspected of having SS. In SS the tear secretion of both eyes is reduced (< 5 mm/5 min). The case presented shows reduced tear secretion in the left eye and a normal function in the right eye (patients with SS usually show similar changes in both eyes).

of healthy subjects. Besides the presence of antibodies to Ro/SSA or La/SSB other laboratory blood studies are helpful in patients suspected of SS. The presence of nonspecific markers of autoimmunity, such as ANAs, rheumatoid factors, elevated immunoglobulins (particularly immunoglobulin G [IgG]), and elevated erythrocyte sedimentation rate are important contributors to the definitive diagnosis of SS.[14]

Diagnostic Work-Up

There is a large diversity in the initial clinical manifestation in patients with SS, and these manifestations are not always present at the same time. Therefore, physicians and dentists sometimes treat each symptom individually, unaware of an underlying systemic disease. In addition, patients with SS were frequently misdiagnosed in the past because their symptoms were considered minor or vague or mimicked those of other diseases. Consequently, delayed diagnosis in SS patients is frequent.

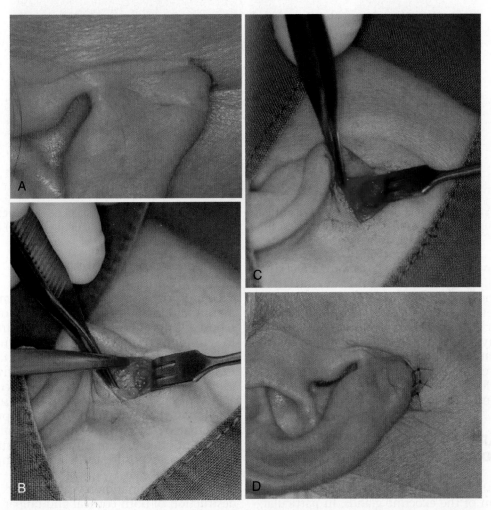

Figure 12-3. A parotid gland biopsy is performed under local anesthesia, according to the technique described by Kraaijenhagen (1975). **A,** The area to be incised is marked. **B,** The fibrous capsule surrounding the parotid gland is visualized. **C,** The capsule is opened. **D,** The skin is closed.

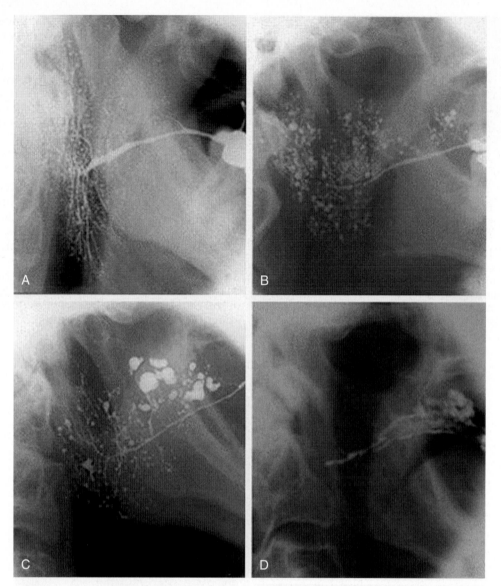

Figure 12-4. Sialography showing dilated and distorted ducts (sialectasis). Staging of sialectasia: punctate (< 1 mm) (**A**), globular (uniform, 1–2 mm) (**B**), cavitary (coalescent, > 2 mm) (**C**), destructive (no structure visible) (**D**).

An extensive delay in diagnosis can affect the patient's well-being if for no other reason than because of the anxiety that accompanies an undiagnosed illness. Early, accurate diagnosis of SS (see Fig. 12-1) can help prevent or ensure adequate treatment of many of the complications associated with the disease, and may contribute to prompt recognition and treatment of serious systemic complications of SS.[15] Management strategies are provided in Tables 12-3 and 12-4.

GLANDULAR MANIFESTATIONS: EXOCRINE DYSFUNCTION

Patients with SS have symptoms related to a diminished function of the exocrine glands, in particular, the lacrimal and salivary glands, although SS may also affect the glands in the upper respiratory tract, skin, and vagina.

Ocular Manifestations

Dryness of the eyes is the most prominent ocular manifestation of SS, and one fourth of SS patients report eye dryness as the first complaint.[16] It results in sensations of itching, burning, dryness, soreness and grittiness. Other ocular symptoms that may arise from ocular dryness are photosensitivity or photophobia, erythema, eye fatigue, decreased visual acuity, discharge in the eyes, and the sensation of a film across the visual field. These symptoms may be exacerbated by low humidity environments, such as air-conditioned or centrally heated buildings or dry climates, or exposure to irritants such as dust and cigarette smoke.

Physical examination reveals chronic irritation and destruction of both corneal and bulbar conjunctival epithelium (keratoconjunctivitis sicca) due to insufficient tear secretion. Accumulation of thick rope-like secretions along the inner canthus may be the result

Table 12-3. *Management Strategies for Ocular Manifestations of Sjögren's Syndrome*

Strategy	Approach	Description
Preventive measures	Avoidance of exacerbating factors	Avoiding low humidity atmospheres such as air-conditioned stores, centrally heated houses, airplanes, windy locations Avoiding irritants such as dust and cigarette smoke Avoiding activities that provoke tear film instability (e.g., prolonged reading or computer use)
	Avoidance of drugs that may worsen sicca symptoms	Caution when using antidepressants, antihistamines, anticholinergics, antihypertensives, neuroleptics
	Treatment of other medical conditions that result in dry eyes	Eyelid abnormalites (e.g., ectropion), meibomean gland disease
Symptomatic treatment	Tear substitution therapy	Low viscous eye drops (Schirmer ≤ 5 mm/5min) and high mucus secretions in the cul du sac High viscous eye drops (Schirmer >5 mm/5 min) and low mucus secretions in the cul du sac Opthalmic gels and ointments (at night)
	Blepharitis	Daily eyelid rubs with warm water and diluted baby shampoo Topical antibiotics if indicated
	Add mucolytic agents for mucus secretions/sticky eyes/mucus filaments in eye examination	N-acetylcysteine 5% eye drops (2-3 times daily)
	Tear retention measures	Use of air moisturizers Moisture glasses Lacrimal punctum occlusion (moderate to severe dry eyes)
	Topical immunomodulatory agents	Topical non-preserved corticosteroids (e.g., dexamethason 0.1% eyedrops 2 times daily; taper dose or discontinue drops based on clinical findings and eye pressure)
Tear stimulation	Systemic parasympathomimetic secretogogues	Pilocarpine (5–7.5 mg, 3–4 times/day) Cevimeline (30 mg, three times/day)
Treating underlying disorder	Systemic anti-inflammatory or immune-modulating therapies to treat the autoimmune exocrinopathy of Sjögren's syndrome	Anti-CD20 (rituximab)

Table 12-4. *Management Strategies for Oral Manifestations of Sjögren's Syndrome*

Strategy	Approach	Description
Preventive measures	Regular dental visits and radiographs	Usually every 3–4 months Intraoral photographs every 6–18 months in dentate subjects who frequently develop new and recurrent caries lesions
	Optimal oral hygiene	Guidance of team of oral health professionals (clinical instructions, written instructions)
	Topical fluorides and remineralizing solutions	Fluoride mouth rinse (0.1%, weekly) Neutral sodium fluoride gel (depending on the level of oral hygiene and residual level of salivary flow: from once a week to every second day; the gel is preferably applied with a custom made tray)
	Diet modifications	Noncardiogenic diet Minimize chronic use of alcohol and caffeine Use of nonfermentable dietary sweeters (xylitol, sorbitol, aspartame or saccharine), whenever possible
	Avoidance of drugs that may worsen sicca symptoms	Caution when using antidepressants, antihistamines, anticholinergics, antihypertensives, neuroleptics
	Treatment of other medical conditions that result in xerostomia	For example, endocrine disorders, metabolic diseases, viral infections
	Avoidance of exacerbating factors	Low humidity atmospheres such as air-conditioned stores, centrally heated houses, airplanes, windy locations Avoiding irritants such as dust and cigarette smoke
Local salivary stimulation	Masticatory stimulatory techniques	Sugar-free gums and mints
	Combined gustatory and masticatory stimulatory	Lozenges, mints, candies Water, with or without a slice of lemon

Table 12-4. *Management Strategies for Oral Manifestations of Sjögren's Syndrome—Cont'd*

Strategy	Approach	Description
Systemic salivary stimulation	Parasympathomimetic secretogogues	Pilocarpine (5-7.5 mg, three to four times/day)
		Cevimeline (30 mg, three times/day)
Symptomatic treatment	Relief of oral dryness (nonresponders on systemic salivary stimulation)	Use of air moisturizers
		Frequent sips of water
		Use of oral rinses, gels, and mouthwashes
		Use of saliva substitutes
		Increased humidification
	Oral candidiasis	Topical antifungal drugs:
		Nystatin oral suspension (100,000 U/mL: 400,000-600,000 units four to five times/day)
		Clotrimazole cream (1%, two times/day)
		Ketoconazole cream (2%, one to two times/day)
		Amphotericin B lozenge (10 mg, 4 times/day)
		Systemic antifungal drugs:
		Fluconazole tablets (200 mg on day 1, then 100 mg/day for 7–14 days)
		Itraconazole tablets (200 mg/day for 1–2 weeks)
		Ketoconazole (200–400 mg/day for 7–14 days)
		Dentures should be soaked in chlorhexine (2%) at night
	Angular cheilitis	Nystatin cream or ointment (100,000 U/g, four to five times/day)
		Clotrimazole cream (1%, two times/day)
		Miconazole cream (2%, one to two times/day)
Treating underlying disorder	Systemic anti-inflammatory or immune modulating therapies to treat the autoimmune exocrinopathy of Sjögren's syndrome	Anti-CD20 (rituximab)

of decreased tear film and an abnormal mucus component. At times, desiccation causes small superficial erosions of the corneal epithelium; in severe cases, slitlamp examination reveals filamentary keratitis, marked by mucus filaments that adhere to damaged areas of the corneal surface. Progressive keratitis can result in loss of vision. Blepharitis, which is the inflammation and infection of the meibomian glands of the eyelid, is a common problem in patients with dry eye, and conjunctivitis as a result of secondary infection with *Staphylococcus aureus* may also occur. Enlargement of the lacrimal glands is rare and should prompt a work-up for MALT. Ocular complications that may arise from SS include corneal ulceration, vascularization, opacification, and rarely perforation.[15]

Oral Manifestations

Autoimmune destruction of the salivary glands results in oral symptoms that accrue primarily as a result of salivary gland hypofunction and are due to the long-term effects of a decrease in oral fluids on mucosal hydration and oral function.

Loss of salivary gland function is already prominent in early onset SS. The submandibular and sublingual salivary glands, which are the most active glands under resting condition, are among the first glands to be involved in SS, whereas the parotid gland, the most active gland when stimulated, appears to be the last salivary gland to be affected. Patients with SS with long disease duration are characterized by severely reduced secretions of the parotid, submandibular, and sublingual glands. This results in a typical symptom pattern: in early SS, the sensation of dry mouth (xerostomia) is often present predominantly at rest and during the night. Over time, as the disease develops, the dryness is also present during the day and finally it gives rise to difficulties in chewing and swallowing food.[7]

Reduction in saliva production (Fig. 12-5) may also lead to difficulties in speaking and be related to burning sensations in the mouth. A diminished ability to taste foods and having problems with smell or a mucosa that is sensitive to spicy or coarse foods, are frequently mentioned symptoms. This limits the patient's enjoyment of meals and may compromise his or her nutrition.[17,18] Most patients carry bottles of water or other fluids with them at all times to aid speaking and swallowing and for their overall oral comfort, and many patients report about the decrease in their quality of life since the advent of oral dryness.

Patients with advanced salivary gland hypofunction as a result of SS have obvious signs of mucosal dryness (Fig. 12-6).[19,20] The lips often appear cracked, peeling and atrophic. They may even appear furrowed or pebbled, like dry soil in an arid climate. The buccal mucosa may be pale and corrugated in appearance, and the tongue may be smooth and reddened, with loss of some of the dorsal papillae or may have a fissured appearance. There is often a marked increase in erosion and dental caries. The decay may be progressive, even in the presence of vigilant oral

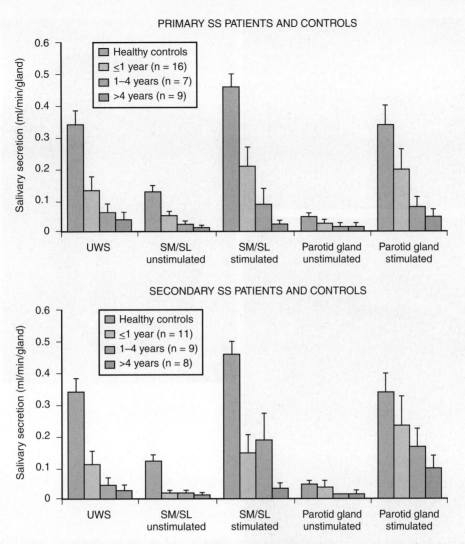

PRIMARY SS PATIENTS AND CONTROLS

SECONDARY SS PATIENTS AND CONTROLS

Figure 12-5. Relationship between disease duration, that is, the time from first complaints related to oral dryness until referral, and mean salivary flow rates (mean ± SEM). UWS, unstimulated whole saliva; SM/SL, submandibular/sublingual saliva. (From Pijpe J, Kalk WW, Bootsma H, Spijkervet FK, Kallenberg CG, Vissink A. Progression of salivary gland dysfunction in patients with Sjogren's syndrome. Ann Rheum Dis 2007;66:107-12.)

hygiene. With diminished salivary output, there is a tendency for greater accumulations of food debris at the so-called smooth surfaces and cervical regions, especially where recession has occurred (Fig. 12-7). Patients with a dry mouth as a result of SS also experience an increase in oral infections, particularly mucosal candidiasis (Fig. 12-8).[19,21] The patient may present with red, erythematous patches on the oral mucosa, for example, beneath dentures, or it may appear as white, curd-like mucocutaneous lesions on any surface (thrush), or the patient may complain of a burning sensation of the tongue or other intraoral soft tissues. Fungal lesions of the corners of the mouth (angular cheilitis) may also occur more frequently in patients with SS (see Fig. 12-6C).

Enlargement of the Salivary Glands

Enlargement of the salivary glands is seen frequently, in particular of the parotid and subman-

dibular glands. Enlargement is generally due to the presence of an autoimmune inflammatory process in these glands. In the parotid glands this inflammation process can be seen unilaterally but is most often present on both sides. Furthermore, salivary gland enlargement can be chronic or episodic. Stasis of saliva, which may occur due to distortion and narrowing of ducts, can result in secondary infection in cystic areas, leading to further swelling of the glands. Thirdly, glandular enlargement may be due to lymphoma development within, in most cases, the parotid gland. Most often these are MALT lymphomas but other NHLs may also develop.

Normally, palpation of the salivary glands is painless. Saliva can be "milked" from each major gland by compressing the glands, with bimanual palpation, and by pushing the fluid contained within them to the gland orifices. The expressed saliva should be clear, watery, and copious.

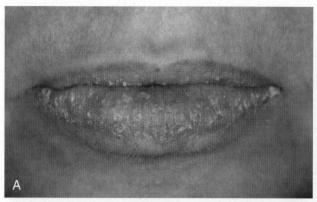

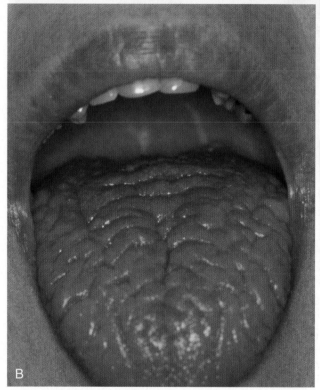

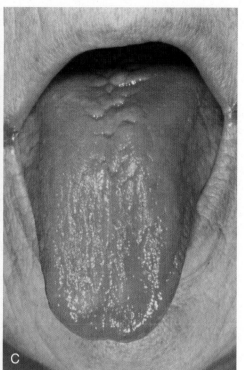

Figure 12-6. Some mucosal signs of oral dryness. **A,** Cracked, peeling and atrophic appearance of the lips. **B,** Dry and fissured tongue. **C,** Dry and smooth tongue. Note the signs of angular cheilitis, a common occurrence in dry mouth patients. (**A,** Courtesy Leo Sreebny.)

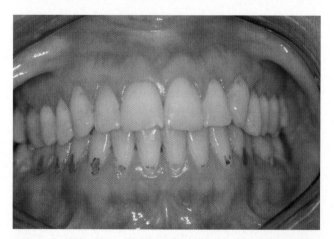

Figure 12-7. Hyposalivation-related dental caries. Note the cervical lesions. These lesions occur in an area that in healthy subjects is cleansed by the continuous flow of saliva, whereas accumulation of dental plaque and food debris occurs in patients with reduced salivary flow.

Diffuse swollen glands that are painful on palpation are indicative of infection or acute inflammation. Viscous saliva or scant secretions suggest chronically reduced function. A cloudy exudate may be a sign of bacterial infection. In these cases, there may be mucoid accretions and clumped epithelial cells, which account for the cloudy appearance of saliva. The exudate should be cultured if it does not appear clear, particularly in the case of an enlarged gland. Occasionally, a purulent secretion is observed, which makes the diagnosis of bacterial sialadenitis obvious.

Because the incidence of NHL lymphomas, including MALT lymphomas of the salivary glands, is about 40 times increased in SS patients, physicians should be alert for painless nodular masses, in particular in the parotid gland. Especially SS patients with risk factors for progression to lymphoma, namely those with persistent salivary gland enlargement, low levels of C4, and monoclonal cryoglobulinemia, should be monitored closely.[22,23]

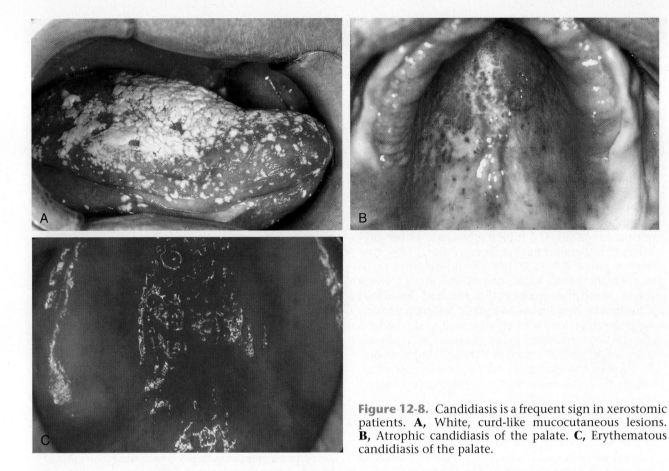

Figure 12-8. Candidiasis is a frequent sign in xerostomic patients. **A,** White, curd-like mucocutaneous lesions. **B,** Atrophic candidiasis of the palate. **C,** Erythematous candidiasis of the palate.

Additional Dry Surfaces

Dryness is not restricted to the eyes and mouth but also occurs at mucosal surfaces in the upper and lower airways, frequently leading to dryness of the nose, throat, and trachea resulting in persistent hoarseness and a chronic, nonproductive cough. Patients may also experience dermal dryness, and in female SS patients, desiccation of the vagina and vulva may result in dyspareunia and pruritus.[15]

MANAGEMENT OF GLANDULAR MANIFESTATIONS

In general, adequate explanation of the condition, including use of patient information brochures, will help in empowering patients to participate in their own care. Furthermore, various preventive measures and symptomatic treatments can be given in SS. It is possible that a single treatment modality may help; it is also possible that a combination of them may be necessary.

Management of Ocular Manifestations

Dry eye disease might be a sight threatening problem in SS patients, and many patients suffer from eye complaints all day. Treatment of ocu-

lar manifestations in these patients is difficult and often does not lead to satisfactory results.

The most widely used therapy for dry eye disease is tear substitution by topical artificial tears, to increase humidity at the ocular surface and to improve lubrication. However, the use of artificial tears has obvious limitations. Natural tears have a complex composition of water, salts, hydrocarbons, proteins, and lipids, which artificial tears cannot completely substitute. In addition, the integrity of the three-layered lipid, aqueous, and mucin structure, which is vital to the effective functioning of the tear film, cannot be reproduced by these artificial components. The majority of tear substitutions is not preservative free. Because many preservatives contain chemical substances that may damage the tear film stability and the corneal epithelium, use of preservative-free artificial tears is strongly recommended. Patients are advised not to use these tear substitutes as frequently as they want, because the substitutes dilute the small amount of natural tears that are still present, and because of the potential harmful effects of preservatives as mentioned earlier (see Table 12-3).

Preventive Measures

First of all, factors that can cause exacerbation of ocular symptoms should be avoided whenever possible. This includes windy or low-humidity environments and exposure to irritants such as dust and cigarette smoke. Patients can be instructed how to

This case describes a 35-year-old female with a 3-year history of pSS. The diagnosis had initially been confirmed by the absence of saliva secretion (unstimulated and stimulated), an abnormal sialography result, low Schirmer test values, an abnormal lissamin green test, anti-SS-A and anti-SS-B antibodies, and a positive labial biopsy. During follow-up she developed progressive, bilateral swelling of the parotid glands (Fig. 12-9) and the submandibular lymph nodes. Other signs were buccal petechiae and bilateral lower limb purpura. Laboratory examination revealed low complement C4 levels (0.05 g/L, normal range 0.1–0.4 g/L), a worsening of her pre-existent hypergammaglobulinemia (IgG 19.6 g/L, normal range 7.0–16.0 g/L) and an elevated rheumatoid factor (153 KIU/L, normal <11 KIU/L). These results raised the suspicion that she had developed a malignant lymphoma. Magnetic resonance imaging showed pronounced enlargement of the parotid glands with multiple cystic lesions. In addition, there were several enlarged cervical lymph nodes. To confirm the diagnosis, an excision biopsy of an enlarged lymph node and a parotid gland biopsy were performed.

Histopathologic and immunohistochemical examination of both biopsies showed an NHL lymphoma of the MALT. The B cells were monoclonal. Further staging investigations were not performed because the patient was pregnant at the time. During her pregnancy the patient was treated with 15 mg of prednisone once a day. After delivery, she was treated with anti-CD20 monoclonal antibodies (rituximab) because of increasing swelling of the parotids, a larger number of vasculitic lesions and progression

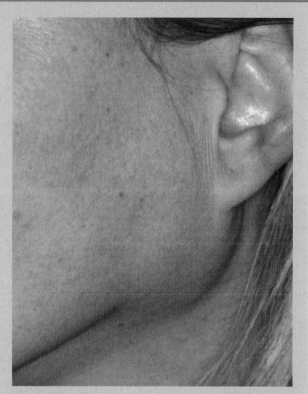

Figure 12-9. Patient with Sjögren's syndrome who has developed a mucosa-associated lymphoid tissue (MALT) lymphoma in the left parotid gland.

of the MALT-lymphoma. Treatment led to a reduction in size of the parotid glands and lymph nodes, improvement of the vasculitic lesions, and increasing complement C4 levels.

increase humidity in their own surroundings by installing room humidifiers. Activities that provoke tear film instability, such as prolonged reading or computer use should also be avoided or modified (e.g., taking regular breaks from reading or computer use, and lowering the computer monitor in a way that the gaze is directed downward).[24]

Several medical conditions and medications can result in keratoconjunctivitis sicca. Dry eyes can be caused by amyloidosis, inflammation (chronic blepharitis or conjunctivitis, pemphigoid, or Stevens-Johnson syndrome), neurologic conditions that impair eyelid or lacrimal gland function, sarcoidosis, toxicity (burns or drugs), and a variety of other conditions (corneal anesthesia, blink abnormality, hypovitaminosis A, eyelid scarring, or trauma). Antidepressants, antihistamines, anticholinergics, antihypertensives (diuretics, beta blockers) and neuroleptics may cause dry eyes as well.[15] The pathologic conditions should be ruled out or otherwise be promptly treated, and the use of drugs that may worsen sicca symptoms should be avoided.

Symptomatic Treatment

Substitution therapy is the main treatment modality. Patients with a Schirmer test of 5 mm/5 min or less and high mucus secretions in the cul du sac are treated with low-viscosity eye drops. In patients with a Schirmer test of more than 5 mm/5 min, with no or little mucus in the cul du sac, high-viscosity eye drops are prescribed. Patients are advised to use the drops three times a day, with a maximum of six times a day. Patients can test several different drops to determine which one is most suitable for their own individual needs. Ophthalmic gels and ointments may be used at night. Highly viscous drops, ophthalmic gels, and ointments last longer, but they may cause visual blurring. Blepharitis may worsen by the use of artificial tears, especially those with high viscosity or those containing preservatives. Treatment of blepharitis consists of cleansing of the eyelids (using warm water and diluted baby shampoo), and topical antibiotics, if needed.

If the patient reports mucus secretions in the eyes or of sticky eyes, a mucolytic agent, such as acetylcysteine 5% eye drops can be added to the medication, used two to three times a day. When successful, taper the dose; when no effect is seen, application of these drops should be discontinued. Mucolytic eye drops can also be prescribed when mucus filaments are found on eye examination.

Topical nonpreserved corticosteroids (e.g., dexamethason drops) can be used to suppress the associated inflammatory process. Their use should be restricted, because of their severe side effects, such as glaucoma, cataract and increased risk of secondary infections and epithelial defects.[24] Therefore their use should be either discontinued or the dose tapered as soon as possible, based on clinical findings and eye pressure.

To prevent drying out of the eyes, occluding glasses or moisture glasses can be tried. Tear preservation can also be achieved by closing of the orifice of the lacrimal duct, lacrimal punctum occlusion, a relatively common nonpharmacologic treatment for dry eye disease. Punctum occlusion can be achieved by temporary plugs, or by a permanent surgical procedure. This treatment can improve the quality and the quantity of the aqueous component of the tear film, relieving symptoms and signs of dry eye, making patients more comfortable and reducing the need for frequent administration of artificial tears. Nevertheless, these claims are controversial. Some authors have reported disadvantages to this technique including extrusion or loss of the plug, pruritis, discomfort, abrasion of the conjunctiva and cornea, tear overflow (epiphora), inflammation of the lacrimal duct (canaliculitis) and pyogenic granuloma. Furthermore, punctal occlusion may result in decreased tear production and clearance, and diminished ocular surface sensation. Therefore, most authors reserve this method for moderate to severe dry eyes and only in those patients in whom frequent use of unpreserved artificial tears and lubricants remains insufficient.[25]

Systemic Tear Stimulation

Two secretagogues, pilocarpine[26,27] and cevimeline[28,29] have been approved by the United States Food and Drug Administration for the treatment of dry mouth, and these drugs are also found to be effective for dry eye disease. Both drugs induce a transient increase in lacrimal and salivary output, and decrease their feeling of ocular and oral dryness in patients who have residual functional lacrimal and salivary gland tissue. These drugs are discussed in more detail in the management of oral manifestations section.

Systemic Anti-inflammatory or Immune-Modulating Therapies

In general, immune-modulating or immunosuppressive treatment has been disappointing for the glandular manifestations of SS. However, promising results have recently been reported with biologics. Relief of ocular and oral symptoms, fatigue, and other extraglandular manifestations was seen after treatment with anti-CD20 (rituximab), assessed with both subjective as well as objective measures.[30-35] These medications are discussed in the section on biologic agents.

Management of Oral Manifestations

Preventive and General Measures for Oral Complications

Because individuals with SS are at risk for a variety of oral complications, preventive measures are of great importance, in which the dentist plays a leading role.

SS patients require more frequent dental visits (usually every 3–4 months) and must work closely with their dentist and dental hygienist to maintain optimal dental health. Visits might be scheduled in alternating order: dentist–dental hygienist–dentist–dental hygienist. Prosthesis-wearing patients should have their prosthesis-bearing mucosal regions evaluated frequently (every 3–4 months) to help identify the early onset of oral mucosal lesions and infections. In dentate SS patients, periodic radiographs should be taken more frequently than in healthy individuals, to follow up on previous carious lesions and to trace new ones.

It is essential that SS patients maintain meticulous oral hygiene. Proper oral hygiene includes tooth brushing, flossing, the use of interproximal plaque-removing agents, and the use of mouth rinses. Interdental brushes and mechanical toothbrushes are helpful for those with oral-motor or behavioral complications. Regular brushing of the tongue with a toothbrush or a tongue scraper is also recommended. The team of oral-health professionals must play an important role in providing guidance (clinical instructions, written instructions) to the SS patient so that he or she is given every opportunity to prevent the onset of the common side effects of salivary hypofunction.

Furthermore, the use of topical fluorides in a patient with salivary gland hypofunction is absolutely critical to control dental caries.[36] There are many different fluoride therapies available, from low-concentration, over-the-counter fluoride rinses, to more potent highly concentrated prescription fluorides (e.g., 1.0% sodium fluoride). These are applied by brush or in a custom carrier. Oral health care practitioners may also use fluoride varnishes. The dosage chosen and the frequency of application (from daily to once a week) should be based on the severity of the salivary hypofunction and the rate of caries development.[37–39] A 5000-PPM fluoridated toothpaste, used twice daily, has been recommended for high-caries-risk patients with salivary dysfunction.[36]

When salivary function is compromised, the normal process of tooth remineralization is interrupted. This enhances demineralization and the consequent loss of tooth structure. Remineralizing solutions and fluorides (toothpaste, mouth rinse, neutral fluoride gel) should be used to alleviate some of these changes.[40]

Patients should be counseled to follow a diet that avoids cariogenic foods (especially fermentable carbohydrates) and beverages. The implementation of meticulous oral hygiene procedures after each meal is critical to help reduce the risk of developing new and recurrent carious lesions. Chronic use of alcohol and caffeine can increase oral dryness and should be minimized. Nonfermentable dietary sweeteners, such as xylitol, sorbitol, aspartame, or saccharine are recommended, whenever possible.[41] Polyols, such as xylitol, are considered to be anticariogenic because they decrease acid fermentation by *Streptococcus mutans*.[42]

Low-humidity atmospheres and irritants should be avoided whenever possible.

Local Salivary Stimulation

Dry mucosal surfaces, difficulty wearing dentures, accumulation of plaque and debris on surfaces normally cleansed by the mechanical washing action of saliva, difficulty speaking, tasting, and swallowing may all benefit from several techniques available to stimulate salivary secretions. These techniques work only if there are remaining viable salivary gland cells that are amenable to stimulation. In patients with long-term SS, the acinar fluid-producing cells may have already undergone atrophy. The atrophic tissue is generally replaced by non–fluid-producing connective tissue cells, which, clearly, do not respond to stimulation techniques.

Masticatory stimulatory techniques are the easiest to implement and have few side effects. The combination of chewing and taste, as provided by sugar-free gums or mints, can be very effective in relieving symptoms for patients who have remaining salivary function. Special gum bases have been developed for patients with dry mouth because regular chewing gums are often too sticky to handle by dry mouth patients.

Combined gustatory and masticatory stimulatory techniques, such as those that employ lozenges, mints, and candies, are easy to implement, generally harmless (assuming that they are sugar free), and easy to use by most patients. If an acid is added, malic acid is preferred because this has a less harmful effect on tooth substance and oral mucosa. Frequent sips of water during the day can be the easiest and most efficacious technique to improve symptoms of dry mouth in some patients. Many patients like such an approach, even though water is a bad moistener of the oral mucosa: it wets the mucosa when exposed, but the mucosa quickly gets dry again as water does not 'stick' to the mucosa.

Systemic Salivary Stimulation

The secretagogues pilocarpine and cevimeline are both muscarinic agonists that, in patients who have residual functional salivary gland tissue, induce a transient increase in salivary output and decrease the feeling of oral dryness.[26–29] Pilocarpine is a nonselective muscarinic agonist, whereas cevimeline reportedly has a higher affinity for M1 and M3 muscarinic receptor subtypes. Because M2 and M4 receptors are located on cardiac and lung tissues, cevimeline's M1 and M3 specificity suggests there will be fewer cardiac and/or pulmonary side effects.[43]

Common side effects of both medications include sweating, flushing, urinary urgency, and gastrointestinal discomfort. These side effects are frequent, but are rarely severe or serious. Parasympathomimetics are contraindicated in patients with uncontrolled asthma, narrow-angle glaucoma, or acute iritis and should be used with caution in patients with significant cardiovascular disease, Parkinson's disease, asthma, or chronic obstructive pulmonary disease. The best-tolerated doses for pilocarpine are 5 to 7.5 mg, given three or four times daily.[26,27] The duration of action is approximately 2 to 3 hours. Cevimeline is currently recommended at a dosage of 30 mg three times daily[20,28]; the duration of secretagogue activity is longer than pilocarpine (3 to 4 hours), whereas the onset is somewhat slower. In contrast to the United States, Canada, and Japan, cevimeline is not yet licensed in Europe.

Interferon-α has been tried via the oromucosal route. Initial studies looked promising, but later studies were less convincing. Furthermore, flu-like side effects and high costs make this way of treatment less attractive.[44]

Symptomatic Treatment

In patients who do not respond to the various stimulation techniques cited earlier, several symptomatic treatments are available. Water, although less effective then the patients' natural saliva, is by far the most important fluid supplement for individuals wth dry mouth. Patients should be encouraged to sip water and swish it around their mouth throughout the day. This will help to moisten the oral cavity, hydrate the mucosa, and clear debris from the mouth. Careful water drinking *with meals* is very important, because it will enhance taste perception, ease the formation of a bolus, and improve mastication and swallowing (particularly for hard and fibrous foods). It will also help prevent choking and possible pulmonary aspiration. Patients should be counseled, however, that aqueous solutions do not produce long-lasting relief from oral dryness. Water wets the mucosa, but its moisture is not retained, because the mucous membranes of xerostomic patients are inadequately coated by a protective glycoprotein layer.[45]

There are numerous oral rinses, mouthwashes and gels available for patients with dry mouth.[40,46-49] Patients should be cautioned to avoid products containing alcohol, sugar, or strong flavorings that may irritate the sensitive, dry oral mucosa. Saliva replacements (saliva substitutes or artificial salivas) are not well accepted over the long term by many patients, particularly when not instructed properly.[46] As a guide to choosing the best substitute for a patient, the following recommendations for the treatment of hyposalivation can be used[47]:

- *Slight hyposalivation:* Gustatory or pharmacologic stimulation of the residual secretion is the treatment of choice. Little amelioration is to be expected from the use of saliva substitutes.
- *Moderate hyposalivation:* If gustatory or pharmacologic stimulation of the residual salivary secretion does not ameliorate the dry mouth feeling, saliva substitutes with a rather low viscoelasticity, such as substitutes that have carboxymethylcellulose, hydroxypropylmethylcellulose, mucin (porcine gastric mucin), or low concentrations of xanthan gum as a base are indicated. During the night or other periods of severe oral dryness, the application of a gel is helpful.
- *Severe hyposalivation:* A saliva substitute with gel-like properties should be used during the night and when daily activities are at a low level. During the day, a saliva substitute with properties resembling the viscoelasticity of natural saliva, such as substitutes that have xanthan gum and mucin (particularly bovine submandibular mucin) as a base, should be applied.[48,49]

Saliva is critical for the retention and comfort in wearing removable prostheses.[19] Lack of saliva at the denture-mucosal interface can produce denture sores due to a lack of lubrication and prosthesis retention. Hyposalivation is also associated with a decrease in the concentration of immune factors conferred on the oral mucosa by the salivary film that usually coats its surface. Insufficient denture stability and retention can cause social embarrassment, because prostheses dislodge during ordinary usage and can impair a person's ability or willingness to speak or eat, particularly in public.[50] Patients with inadequate saliva should moisten their dentures before they place them in their mouths.[51] Salivary substitutes, artificial saliva, salivary stimulants, and water can be used. All of these agents help with the adhesion, cohesion, and retention of the denture. Patients can be advised to spray their prosthesis with artificial saliva before insertion of their dentures and before meals.

Prevention and Treatment of Oral Candidiasis

Secondary infection of the mucosa with *Candida albicans* is not uncommon in patients with SS. Therefore, a high index of suspicion for fungal disease should be maintained, and appropriate antifungal therapies should be instituted as necessary (see Table 12-4). Patients with salivary gland dysfunction may require prolonged treatment to eradicate oral fungal infections.[52]

To prevent candidiasis, patients should not wear dentures over night, and the dentures should be soaked in an aqueous solution of 0.2% chlorhexine to prevent reinfections of the oral cavity by Candida species living in the denture material. Nystatin or clotrimazole cream can be used to treat angular cheilitis.

Systemic Treatment for Glandular Manifestations

As mentioned for the treatment of ocular manifestations of SS, promising results have been reported with biologics. Relief of ocular and oral symptoms, fatigue, and other extraglandular manifestations was seen after treatment with anti-CD20 (rituximab), assessed with both subjective as well as objective measures.[30-35] These medications are discussed more extensively in the biologics section.

Management of Dry Surfaces Other than Mouth and Eyes

Sicca symptoms elsewhere are treated symptomatically. Dry lips can be treated with lip salves or petroleum jelly, whereas dryness of the skin may require the use of moisturizing lotions and bath additives. Vaginal dryness can be relieved with lubricant jellies.

The use of humidifiers may also be helpful for nasal and pharyngeal dryness. Saline nasal sprays are available to resolve blocked nasal passages, which may occur as a result of nasal dryness. These sprays should be used frequently, because nasal blockage increases mouth breathing and exacerbate oral dryness. Additional causes of nasal blockage, such as nasal polyps and sinus infection, should be excluded and treated appropriately.

MANAGEMENT OF EXTRAGLANDULAR DISEASE

Most of the traditional antirheumatic drugs used in RA and SLE have been tried in pSS with limited results, especially for the glandular manifestations. These drugs, however, may be of benefit in the management of extraglandular manifestations. Biologics such as tumor necrosis factor (TNF) inhibitors, interferon α, and B-cell depletion therapy have been tried in pSS with varying results, and research of their use is ongoing. The current treatment options available for extraglandular manifestations are summarized in Table 12-5.

Anti-inflammatory and Disease-Modifying Drugs

Fatigue, arthralgia, myalgia and low-grade fever are common nonexocrine manifestations of pSS.

Nonsteroidal anti-inflammatory drugs (NSAIDs) are the first-line therapy of the musculoskeletal and constitutional symptoms in pSS. However, pSS patients may have low tolerance of NSAIDs, resulting from dysphagia secondary to decreased salivary flow and esophageal dysmotility.

Table 12-5. *Management Strategies for Extraglandular Manifestations of Sjögren's Syndrome*

Symptom		Treatment
Severe fatigue		NSAIDs Hydroxychloroquine (400 mg/day) Prednisone (7.5–10 mg/day; max 15 mg)
Anorexia		Hydroxychloroquine (400 mg/day) Prednisone (7.5–10 mg/day; max 15 mg)
Arthralgia		NSAIDs
Myalgia		NSAIDs
Arthritis		NSAIDs Hydroxychloroquine (400 mg/day) Methotrextate (15 mg/week; max 25 mg) Prednisone (7.5–10 mg/day; max 15 mg)
Skin involvement	Mild vasculitis	Hydroxychloroquine (400 mg/day) and/or prednisone (7.5–10 mg/day; max 15 mg)
	Polymorphic erythema	Hydroxychloroquine (400/day; max 800 mg) and/or prednisone (7.5–10 mg/day; max 15 mg)
	Raynaud	Calcium channel blocker
Severe vasculitis		Prednisone (60 mg/day) with or without cyclophosphamide IV (750 mg/m²/monthly; 6–12 times)
Pulmonary involvement	Pleuritis / serositis	NSAIDs Prednisone (15–20 mg/day; max 30 mg)
	Interstitial pneumonitis	Prednisone (60 mg/day) with or without cyclophosphamide IV (750 mg/m²/monthly; 6–12 times)
Esophageal dysfunction		Omeprazol (20–40 mg/day)
Neurologic involvement	Severe PNS	Prednisone (60 mg/day) with or without cyclophosphamide IV (750 mg/m²/monthly; 6–12 times)
	CNS	Prednisone (60 mg/day) with or without cyclophosphamide IV (750 mg/m²/monthly; 6–12 times)
Interstitial cystitis		Pilocarpine (5–7.5 mg, three times/day) and/or prednisone (15 mg/day)
Renal involvement	Interstitial nephritis	Bicarbonate (individual dose) and/or potassium completion (individual dose) Prednisone (15–60 mg/day, depending on severity of proteinuria or renal impairment)
	Glomerulonephritis	Prednisone (60 mg/day) with or without cyclophosphamide IV (750 mg/m²/monthly; 6–12 times)
MALT lymphoma	With no active SS	Careful watching
	With symptomatic enlarged parotid gland(s), no active SS	Radiotherapy (2 × 2 Gy)
	With active SS	Rituximab IV (375 mg/m²; weekly; four times), cyclophosphamide IV (750 mg/m²; 3 weekly; 8 times), and prednisone (100 mg during 5 following days after cyclophosphamide infusions; eight times)

CNS, central nervous system; IV, intravenous; NSAIDs, nonsteroidal anti-inflammatory drugs; PNS, peripheral nervous system; SS, Sjögren's syndrome.

Corticosteroids are used in the treatment of arthritis, cutaneous symptoms, and severe constitutional manifestations of pSS. Low-dose prednisone up to 10 mg/day may relieve joint symptoms, pruritus, and mild leukocytoclastic vasculitis. A moderate dose of oral steroids up to 30 mg/day can be used in more severe cases of necrotic or ulcerating vasculitis. High-dose corticosteroids (1 mg/kg/day) are used mainly in combination with immunosuppressants (mostly cyclophosphamide) to treat severe manifestations of SS, for example, in case of central nervous system or kidney involvement. In a controlled trial, corticosteroids had no significant effect on salivary and lacrimal function.[53] Whether pSS patients should be treated over a long period with corticosteroids is debatable, because pSS patients are more prone to acceleration of parodontitis and development of candidiasis (oral, vaginal) besides the other well-known side effects of corticosteroids use.

Hydroxychloroquine (200–400 mg daily) has been reported to improve features of immunologic hyperreactivity in patients with SS; however, a demonstrated clinical benefit is lacking. Hydroxychloroquine is mostly used for the treatment of cutaneous, musculoskeletal, and constitutional symptoms. In some cases, it can be of benefit for lupus-like skin manifestations in pSS.[54] In all conducted clinical trials, a decrease of serologic parameters (IgG, erythrocyte sedimentation rate [ESR], ANA, rheumatoid factor [RF] and interleukin-6 [IL-6]) was seen. The long-term effect of this drug needs to be assessed further.[55]

Methotrexate is used for polyarticular inflammatory arthritis in pSS, even though data on efficacy regarding arthritis in association with pSS are lacking. Benefit on sicca symptoms but no improvement on objective parameters was reported in a small study. Furthermore, no effect on serologic parameters was found. A persistent elevation of hepatic transaminases was found more often in pSS compared with patients with RA and Wegener's granulomatosis.[56]

Azathioprine showed no effect on symptoms, signs, serology, histology, or disease activity in a controlled study. Even in low doses, a high frequency of adverse effects was seen. Azathioprine seems to have no place in the treatment of pSS.[57]

Sulfalazine has also failed to be effective in patients with pSS. It can result in various severe side effects such as meningitis and hepatitis, and it may also induce ulcerative colitis, systemic lupus erythematosus in pSS patients.[58]

Leflunomide was recently studied in a small open-label study. A modest but not significant improvement of salivary and lacrimal gland function was seen. The drug showed an acceptable safety profile in most patients; however, in several cases, an exacerbation of leukocytoclastic vasculitis was seen. A controlled study is needed to decide the place of this drug.[59]

Mycophenolate mofetil (MMF) has not yet been tested in pSS patients.

Other Systemic Drugs

Dehydroepiandrosterone (DHEA) was tried in women with pSS because of the female predominance in pSS, the demonstration of decreased serum levels of conjugated dihydrotestosterone in female pSS patients, and the finding that quality of life in pSS correlates with circulating levels of DHEA-sulfate. However, in a controlled trial, no evidence for efficacy of DHEA was found, except for subjective improvement of dry mouth.[60]

Biologic Agents

At present, biologic agents have been introduced in the treatment of various systemic autoimmune diseases, for example, RA and SLE. The biologic agents most frequently used in the treatment of autoimmune diseases are monoclonal antibodies, soluble receptors, and molecular imitators.[61] These biologic agents enhance or replace conventional immunosuppressive therapy. In contrast to RA and SLE, no biologic agent has yet been approved for the treatment of SS, but several phase II and III studies have been conducted or are currently being conducted. The biologic agents used in SS trials are interferon-α (IFN-α) and agents targeting TNF and B cells (anti-CD20, anti-CD22). Although no trials have yet been performed with B-cell activating factor (BAFF) antagonists, these antagonists are thought to be a promising therapy[62] and are also discussed in this chapter.

Interferon-α

IFNs are proteins with antiviral activity and potent immunomodulating properties. SS patients have an activated type I IFN system.[63] In a phase II study, treatment of pSS patients with IFN-α administered via the oromucosal route (by dissolving lozenges) demonstrated some efficacy and appeared safe.[64] Based on these promising results, a randomized, parallel group, double-blinded, placebo-controlled clinical trial (497 pSS patients) was designed. Patients were randomized into two groups and received 24 weeks of daily treatment with either 450 IU IFN-α (150 IU three times per day) or a placebo lozenge in a ratio 3:2, administered by the oromucosal route. This randomized controlled clinical trial failed to demonstrate a significant effect on the primary endpoints (Visual Analogue Scale [VAS] score for oral dryness and stimulated whole salivary flow) in the IFN-α group relative to the placebo group. However, there was a significant increase in unstimulated whole saliva in the patients treated with IFN-α, which correlated positively and significantly with improvement in seven of eight symptoms associated with oral and ocular dryness. No adverse events were observed.[44]

In conclusion, no clinical evidence for the efficacy of IFN-α treatment in pSS patients has been shown, although an increase in the secretion of unstimulated whole saliva was observed. Further research is needed to clarify the effects of IFN-α on salivary gland tissue.

Anti–Tumor Necrosis Factor Biologics

There are currently three biologic agents targeting TNF: the chimeric monoclonal antibody infliximab, the receptor fusion protein etanercept, and the fully human monoclonal antibody adalimumab.

In an open-label study, treatment with infliximab was reported to be effective in active pSS over a 3-month period.[65] In a follow-up study, retreatment of the patients induced an improvement of SS-related signs that was comparable with the effects from the first three infusions.[66] To confirm these promising results from an uncontrolled study, the Trial of Remicade In Primary Sjögren's Syndrome (TRIPPS) study was designed. In this double-blinded, placebo-controlled randomized clinical trial, 103 patients with active pSS were included and treated with infliximab (5 mg/kg) or placebo infusions at weeks 0, 2, and 6. The follow-up time was 22 weeks, and the primary endpoint was an improvement by greater than 30% in two of three VAS scores (joint pain, fatigue, and dry eyes). In contrast to the previously mentioned uncontrolled studies, no evidence for the efficacy of infliximab treatment on clinical or functional parameters could be demonstrated in this trial.[67] These disappointing results also underscore the difficulty of interpreting uncontrolled data in chronic autoimmune diseases.

In a pilot trial of etanercept, 25 mg subcutaneously twice a week for 12 weeks in 15 pSS patients (mean disease duration 3.6 years), no reduction of sicca symptoms or signs were seen, nor did continued treatment for up to 26 weeks show beneficial effects in the total group of patients.[68] Another trial evaluating etanercept versus placebo for 12 weeks in 28 patients also failed to show clinical efficacy.[69] No trials of adalimumab treatment in pSS have been reported in the literature.

In conclusion, TNF-targeting treatment could not be proven to be of benefit in reducing the signs and symptoms of pSS.

Anti-CD20 Monoclonal Antibodies

Anti-CD20 (rituximab) is a chimeric monoclonal antibody specific for the B-cell surface molecule CD20. CD20 is expressed on the surface of normal and malignant pre-B and mature B lymphocytes. Rituximab has been demonstrated to induce lysis of B cells by complement-dependent and antibody-dependent cytotoxicity mechanisms, as well as by direct induction of apoptosis.[70]

Rituximab is currently used for the treatment of low-grade B-cell lymphomas.[71] In controlled studies, it was shown to be safe and effective in the treatment of RA.[72-74] Moreover, some promising open label studies in SLE patients have been published.[75]

Two studies retrospectively evaluated the effect of rituximab (four infusions of 375 mg/m²) in 18 pSS patients (mean disease duration 10 years) with systemic features. Self-reported dryness improved in six patients (VAS scores not known for three patients,

no improvement in the other nine patients). Both studies reported good efficacy of the treatment on systemic features.[30,32]

In an open-label phase II study, 15 patients with pSS were treated with four infusions of rituximab (375 mg/m² once weekly) and followed for a 3-month period. Eight of the 15 patients were early pSS patients (mean disease duration 28 months, all had residual salivary gland function at baseline) and seven patients had a concomitant MALT lymphoma (mean disease duration 79 months). In the early pSS patients, rituximab treatment resulted in significant improvement of subjective symptoms and an increase in salivary gland function. All patients showed a rapid depletion of peripheral B cells within a few weeks, accompanied by a decrease in IgM-RF levels.[31] Repeated parotid gland biopsies in five of the early patients after treatment, showed redifferentiation of the lymphoepithelial duct lesions into normal striated ducts, possibly indicating regeneration of salivary gland tissue (Fig. 12-10).[76]

Five of the eight pSS patients without a MALT-lymphoma received a second course of rituximab (after 9–11 months) due to recurrence of symptoms. Retreatment resulted in the same significant improvement of the salivary flow rate and subjective symptoms compared with the results of the first treatment, together with a decrease in B cells and IgM-RF levels (Fig. 12-11).[77]

Six of the seven MALT/pSS patients were initially effectively treated with rituximab. The remaining MALT/pSS patient had progressive MALT disease and severe extraglandular SS disease within 3 months after the start of rituximab treatment. Cyclophosphamide was added, which led to stable disease of both MALT and SS. One of the six patients initially responding had a recurrence of

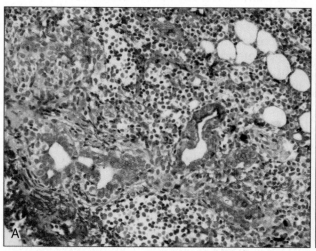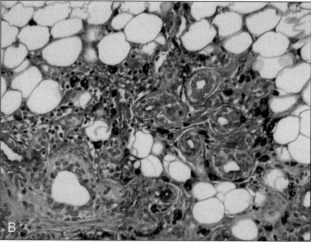

Figure 12-10. Biopsy from the parotid gland taken before starting rituximab and 12 weeks after rituximab treatment. Staining for immunoglobulin A (IgA). Before treatment a dense infiltrate and disordered ductal structures with a paucity of IgA plasma cells is present (**A**). After rituximab treatment, the infiltrate has almost disappeared with a more regular structure of ducts and a predominance of IgA plasma cells (**B**).

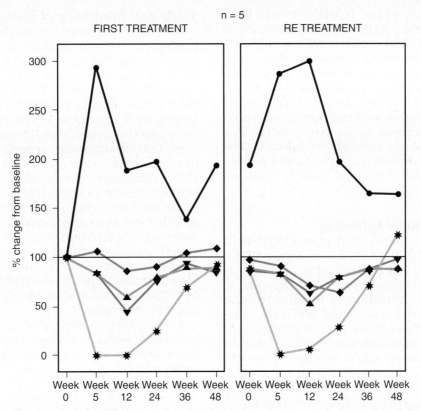

Figure 12-11. Increase and decrease (mean values of 5 pSS patients) in stimulated submandibular/sublingual flow rate, IgM-RF, B cells, VAS score for dry mouth during the night and MFI score for fatigue following rituximab (re)treatment (baseline is 100%). Baseline values (week 0 first treatment) were stimulated submandibular/sublingual flow rate 0.09 ± 0.07 mL/min, IgM-RF 339 ± 329 klU/l, B cells 0.19 ± 0.09 10^9/L, VAS score for dry mouth during the night 85 ± 12, MFI score for fatigue 16 ± 3. (From Meijer JM, Pijpe J, Vissink A, Kallenberg CG, Bootsma H. Treatment of primary Sjogren syndrome with rituximab: extended follow-up, safety and efficacy of retreatment. Ann Rheum Dis 2009;68:284-5.)
• Stimulated submandibular/sublingual salivary flow rate.
♦ IgM rheumatoid factor (IgM-RF).
* B cells.
▲ VAS score for dry mouth during the night.
▼ Multidimensional fatigue inventory (MFI) score for fatigue.

MALT lymphoma after 9 months and was successfully retreated with rituximab. The other patients are still in remission (unpublished data).

In another open-label study, 16 pSS patients received only 2 weekly rituximab infusions (375 mg/m²), with a follow-up of 36 weeks. Again, treatment resulted in rapid complete depletion of peripheral B cells. At week 12, a significant improvement of VAS scores for fatigue and dryness was recorded, and at week 36, a significant improvement in VAS scores for global disease, fatigue, dry mouth, dry eyes, and dry vagina, and also in the number of tender joint and tender points was reported.[33] Both in the study by Pijpe and associates[31] and the study by Devauchelle-Pensec and coworkers,[33] patients with a short disease duration showed more improvement than patients with longer disease duration.

Two double-blind randomized placebo-controlled trials have been performed. One trial focused on fatigue as the primary outcome parameter. In this trial with a total of 17 patients with pSS and a follow-up of 6 months, a significant improvement was seen from baseline on fatigue by VAS in the rituximab group in contrast to the placebo group. In addition, social functioning assessed with the short form 36 (SF-36) was also significantly different between the groups at 6 months.[34] The other trial focused on salivary gland function as the primary endpoint. In this trial with 30 patients and a follow-up of 12 months, salivary secretion improved in the rituximab group and decreased in the placebo group. The VAS score for oral dryness improved in the rituximab group and slightly deteriorated in the placebo group. The Multidimensional Fatigue Index (MFI) score for general fatigue improved in both groups; the largest improvement was observed in the rituximab-treated patients, with disease duration less than 4 years. The number of extraglandular manifestations decreased in the rituximab group, whereas the number of extraglandular manifestations increased in the placebo group. B cells were completely depleted in all patients treated with rituximab after the first infusion. IgM-RF (U/L) decreased in the rituximab group and slightly increased in the placebo group.[35]

In conclusion, in phase II trials, it has been shown that rituximab seems to be effective for at least 6 to 9 months in patients with active pSS, improving both subjective symptoms and objective signs of the disease. Retreatment with rituximab resulted in a similar good clinical response. In pSS patients with longer disease duration and lacking residual salivary gland function, rituximab treatment seemed to be effective for systemic features, but no recovery of salivary flow was observed. To confirm these promising results, randomized placebo-controlled clinical trials are needed.

Anti-CD22 Monoclonal Antibodies

Epratuzumab is a humanized monoclonal antibody specific for the B-cell surface molecule CD22, which is expressed on the surface of normal mature and malignant B lymphocytes. CD22 appears to be involved in the regulation of B cell activation through B-cell receptor signaling and cell adhesion.[78] In an open-label phase I and II study, safety and efficacy of epratuzumab was investigated in 16 pSS patients. Follow-up was 6 months. These pSS patients received four doses of 360 mg/m^2 epratuzumab intravenously. In contrast to rituximab, no complete depletion of peripheral B cells was induced, but a median decrease of 54% and 39% at 6 and 18 weeks, respectively. Improvements occurred in the Schirmer test, the level of unstimulated whole salivary flow, and the VAS score for fatigue. Remarkably, the number of responders was higher at 6 months after the treatment administration than at earlier time points. Epratuzumab seems to be a promising treatment, and randomized, placebo-controlled clinical trials are needed.[79]

Anti-BAFF

BAFF is a B-cell activating factor that acts as a positive regulator of B-cell function and expansion. BAFF levels were found to be elevated in serum and saliva in SS patients, but no correlation was observed between serum and saliva levels.[80] However, circulating levels of BAFF in pSS patients were shown to be a marker for disease activity.[81]

At present, two human BAFF antagonists have been developed: belimumab, a human antibody (anti-BLyS) that binds to soluble BAFF; and atacicept, a fusion protein of one of the BAFF receptors.[82,83] Especially SS patients with elevated BAFF levels, hypergammaglobulinemia, elevated levels of autoantibodies, and associated B cell lymphoma might be candidates for anti-BAFF treatment.[84] Levels of BAFF increase after B-cell depletion therapy, which could favor the re-emergence of autoreactive B cells. Therefore, BAFF antagonist treatment in combination with rituximab could be considered to prolong the period of remission after rituximab infusion.[85] Until now, no trials with anti-BAFF treatment in SS have been published.

Safety and Tolerability of Biologic Agents

The most important immediate side effects of treatment with infused biologic agents are infusion reactions. Most of these side effects are mild, but in SS, a more serious serum sickness–like disease has occurred with rituximab. This adverse effect of treatment occurred in 16% (eight of 49) of the patients treated with rituximab in the open-label study by Pijpe and colleagues,[31] and it may be related to the formation of antibodies against the biologic agent (human antichimeric antibodies [HACAs]), because HACA formation was indeed observed in these patients. Serum sickness–like disease occurred only in patients receiving low-dose corticosteroids and no other immunosuppressive drugs, whereas higher doses of corticosteroids during treatment might prevent the occurrence of this complication. Indeed, in the randomized placebo-controlled clinical trial by Meijer and associates,[35] which included higher doses of corticosteroids, the incidence of serum sickness was strongly reduced.

Some patients developed infections following treatment with a biologic agent, but some of these patients also used other immunosuppressive therapies.

Treatment Strategies in Severe Extraglandular Manifestations

The extraglandular manifestations of SS can be divided in two different categories; the peri-epithelial and the extraepithelial involvement, having different prognostic significance. Patients with periepithelial lesions, such as liver and lung involvement, interstitial cystitis, or interstitial nephritis (renal tubular acidosis), usually have more stable disease. If needed, these manifestations can be treated with a low or intermediate dose of prednisone. Patients suffering predominantly of extraepithelial manifestations of the disease have a higher morbidity and mortality. Examples of these manifestations are glomerulonephritis (mesangial or membranoproliferative), polyneuropathy, purpura (Fig. 12-12), and vasculitis. The more severe manifestations are associated with the following serologic parameters: lymphopenia, cryoglobulinemia, and low complement levels (C4).[86] These extraglandular manifestations, in combination with the serologic parameters and persistently swollen parotid glands, are predictors of MALT lymphoma. Close monitoring and sometimes aggressive treatment are needed in these patients. Treatment consists mostly of a combination of high-dose corticosteroids with cyclophosphamide, with or without B-cell depletion therapy.

Nephritis

Two types of kidney involvement are seen in pSS, namely interstitial nephritis and glomerulonephritis. Interstitial nephritis is seen in 30% of patients and leads to clinical symptoms in 5% to 10% of

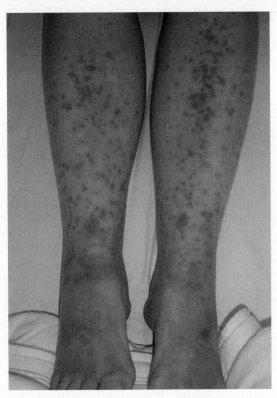

Figure 12-12. Purpura as an extraglandular manifestation.

patients. A distal or proximal renal tubular acidosis (RTA I or II) can result in clinical symptoms such as compromised renal function, proteinuria, nephrocalcinosis, kidney stones, hypokalemia, hypophosphatemia, polyuria, and nephrogenic diabetes insipidus. In mild cases, only supplementation with bicarbonate and potassium is recommended. In more severe cases, intermediate or high doses of prednisone are added. In 5% to 10% of the patients, an immune complex–mediated mesangial or membranoproliferative nephritis is seen, leading to clinical findings such as hypertension, proteinuria (mild to nephritic syndrome) and to an active urinary sediment with erythrocytes and casts. These patients are treated with a combination of high-dose prednisone (1 mg/kg/day) and cyclophosphamide (750/m²/month; 6–12 times). In cases of glomerulonephritis in combination with a MALT lymphoma, adding rituximab (375 mg/m²/week; four times), is recommended.

Neurologic Manifestations

Central nervous manifestations associated with pSS are either focal or diffuse. They are treated with high doses of corticosteroids. In case of diffuse symptoms based on vasculitis, pulse cyclophosphamide is added to the high doses of prednisone. In an acute setting or when symptoms are worsening, treatment with plasmapheresis or intravenous immunoglobulins (IVIG) may be considered.[87]

Involvement of the peripheral nervous system affects about 10% to 20% of the patients with pSS, mainly in the form of sensorimotor and sensory polyneuropathies and cranial neuropathies. These manifestations respond poorly to corticosteroids, but stabilization or spontaneous improvements were seen. Axonal neuropathy also responds badly to corticosteroids. Successful treatment with plasmapheresis and/or IVIG was described in anecdotal reports. On the contrary, in mononeuritis multiplex with nerve biopsies revealing vasculitis treatment with high doses of corticosteroids and pulse cyclophosphamide was found to be useful.

For neurologic manifestations, no studies of early treatment are available. The role of rituximab for the treatment of neurologic manifestations should be explored further.[88]

Vasculitis

Skin lesions based on vasculitis are seen in 10% of pSS patients. Most common are purpura, polymorphic erythema, urticarial lesions, and ulcers based on a leukocytoclastic vasculitis. Systemic vasculitis can lead to neuropathic, renal, pulmonary, and gastrointestinal symptoms. These manifestations are associated with cryoglobulinemia and low complement levels. Corticosteroids are the first step in treatment. In more severe cases, a combination of corticosteroids and intravenous cyclophosphamide is given. In life-threatening situations, treatment is started with plasmapheresis or IVIG, followed by intravenous corticosteroids and cyclophosphamide. Rituximab, especially in patients with cryoglobulinemia, may be successful; however, this has yet to be proved in controlled trials.[89]

Hematologic Complications

Most hematologic complications are asymptomatic and include mild autoimmune cytopenias and hyperglobulinemia. No specific therapy is necessary, but these patients need careful follow-up. For more severe cytopenias, aggressive treatment is indicated. Autoimmune hemolytic anemia, thrombocytopenia, and agranulocytosis are treated with corticosteroids. If the response is not sufficient, cyclophosphamide is added. Treatment with azathioprine is not recommended because it may facilitate the development of lymphoproliferative disorders in pSS patients who already are at increased risk for development of B-cell lymphomas. Plasmapheresis, IVIG, and rituximab are second- or third-line options in severe hemolytic anemia and thrombocytopenic purpura.

Mucosa-Associated Lymphoid Tissue Lymphoma

The therapeutic approach to SS patients with MALT lymphoma is still a matter of debate. Based on our experience[31] and that of others[90] the following approach seems justified. In patients with asymptomatic MALT lymphoma restricted to the salivary glands, a "wait-and-see" policy can be chosen. These localized MALT lymphomas, which are frequently diagnosed coincidentally by pathologists when evaluating parotid gland biopsies, show a benign course with a good prognosis. For a symptomatic localized MALT lymphoma, local radiotherapy, or eight cycles of R-CP (intermittent courses of IV rituximab, 375 mg/m²; IV cyclophosphamide, 750 mg/m²; and oral prednisone, 60 mg/m², for 5 days) are indicated. Disseminated MALT lymphoma should be treated with eight cycles of R-CP. In case of high-grade lymphoma, which is seen far less frequently than MALT lymphoma, cyclophosphamide/doxorubicin/vincristine/prednisone in combination with rituximab (CHOP-R) is the therapy of choice.

FUTURE PERSPECTIVES

Because many SS patients suffer from reduced health-related quality of life (HR-QOL) and are restricted in social and work related activities, there is a great need for development of adequate treatment modalities to reduce SS-related complaints and to intervene in the progression of SS.

Biologic agents are promising therapies for SS, but not all biologics studied were found to be effective. Thus, on the one hand randomized studies failed to show a clinical effect of anti-TNF and IFN-α in the treatment of SS, whereas B-cell depletion (both with rituximab and epratuzumab) seems promising. Other potential targets for biologic therapy include cytokines such as IL-6 and BlyS (BAFF), adhesion molecules, and chemokines. In patients with active autoimmune disease monoclonal antibodies may be more immunogenic, because HACAs have occurred at a higher rate, and serum sickness–like disease was observed in pSS patients with pSS but not in patients with pSS and MALT. Additional use of immunosuppressive therapy in SS patients with high disease activity might be mandatory to prevent serious side effects. These unwanted side effects might also be prevented by the use of fully humanized antibodies. The currently available humanized antibodies are promising but need further study.

Besides the availability of an effective treatment, there is still a need for improved assessment parameters to monitor treatment effects, both subjectively and objectively. For studies on intervention of SS, evaluation of the parotid gland might be of use because function, composition of saliva (repeated collections), and histology (repeated biopsies) can be evaluated on the same parotid gland at different time points. In addition, activity scores are currently being developed.[91-93] The development and widespread use of disease activity and disease damage indices may facilitate the evaluation of new treatment options in SS.

ACKNOWLEDGMENT

We would like to thank Cees G.M. Kallenberg, Nicole Kamminga, and Khaled Mansour for their contributions to this chapter.

References

1. Fox RI. Sjogren's syndrome. Lancet 2005;366:321-31.
2. Hansen A, Lipsky PE, Dorner T. Immunopathogenesis of primary Sjogren's syndrome: implications for disease management and therapy. Curr Opin Rheumatol 2005;17:558-65.
3. Meijer JM, Meiners PM, Huddleston-Slater JJR, Spijkervet FK, Kallenberg CG, Vissink A, et al. Health related quality of life, employment and disability in patients with Sjögren's syndrome. Rheumatology 2009 (in press).
4. Vitali C, Bombardieri S, Jonsson R, Moutsopoulos HM, Alexander EL, Carsons SE, et al. Classification criteria for Sjogren's syndrome: a revised version of the European criteria proposed by the American-European Consensus Group. Ann Rheum Dis 2002;61:554-8.
5. Daniels TE. Labial salivary gland biopsy in Sjogren's syndrome. Assessment as a diagnostic criterion in 362 suspected cases. Arthritis Rheum 1984;27:147-56.
6. Pijpe J, Kalk WW, van der Wal JE, Vissink A, Kluin PM, Roodenburg JL, et al. Parotid gland biopsy compared with labial biopsy in the diagnosis of patients with primary Sjogren's syndrome. Rheumatology (Oxford) 2007;46:335-41.
7. Pijpe J, Kalk WW, Bootsma H, Spijkervet FK, Kallenberg CG, Vissink A. Progression of salivary gland dysfunction in patients with Sjogren's syndrome. Ann Rheum Dis 2007;66:107-12.
8. Suzuki S, Kawashima K. Sialographic study of diseases of the major salivary glands. Acta Radiol Diagn (Stockh) 1969;8:465–78.
9. Kalk WW, Vissink A, Spijkervet FK, Moller JM, Roodenburg JL. Morbidity from parotid sialography. Oral Surg Oral Med Oral Pathol Oral Radiol Endod 2001;92:572-5.
10. Blatt IM, French AJ, Holt JF, Maxwell JH, Rubin P. Secretory sialography in diseases of the major salivary glands. Ann Otol Rhinol Laryngol 1956;65:295-317.
11. Blatt IM. On sialectasis and benign lymphosialdenopathy (the pyogenic parotitis, Gougerot-Sjoegren's Syndrome, Mikulicz's disease complex). A ten-year study. Laryngoscope 1964;74:1684-746.
12. Hermann GA, Vivino FB, Goin JE. Scintigraphic features of chronic sialadenitis and Sjogren's syndrome: a comparison. Nucl Med Commun 1999;20:1123-32.
13. Roescher N, Illei GG. Can quantified salivary gland scintigraphy results aid diagnosis of patients with sicca symptoms? Nat Clin Pract Rheumatol 2008;4:178-9.
14. Tzioufas AG, Mitsias DI, Moutsopoulos HM. Sjogren syndrome. In: Hochberg MC, Silman AJ, et al, editors. Rheumatology. Philadelphia: Elsevier; 2008. p. 1348-9.
15. Kassan SS, Moutsopoulos HM. Clinical manifestations and early diagnosis of Sjogren syndrome. Arch Intern Med 2004;164:1275-84.
16. Vissink A, Kalk WW, Mansour K, Spijkervet FK, Bootsma H, Roodenburg JL, et al. Comparison of lacrimal and salivary gland involvement in Sjogren's syndrome. Arch Otolaryngol Head Neck Surg 2003;129:966-71.
17. Dormenval V, Budtz-Jorgensen E, Mojon P, Bruyere A, Rapin CH. Associations between malnutrition, poor general health and oral dryness in hospitalized elderly patients. Age Ageing 1998;27:123-8.
18. Walls AW, Steele JG. The relationship between oral health and nutrition in older people. Mech Ageing Dev 2004;125:853-7.
19. Guggenheimer J, Moore PA. Xerostomia: etiology, recognition and treatment. J Am Dent Assoc 2003;134:61-9.

20. Fox PC, van der Ven PF, Sonies BC, Weiffenbach JM, Baum BJ. Xerostomia. Evaluation of a symptom with increasing significance. J Am Dent Assoc 1985;110:519-25.

21. Tanida T, Okamoto T, Okamoto A, Wang H, Hamada T, Ueta E, et al. Decreased excretion of antimicrobial proteins and peptides in saliva of patients with oral candidiasis. J Oral Pathol Med 2003;32:586-94.

22. Skopouli FN, Dafni U, Ioannidis JP, Moutsopoulos HM. Clinical evolution, and morbidity and mortality of primary Sjogren's syndrome. Semin Arthritis Rheum 2000;29:296-304.

23. Tzioufas AG, Boumba DS, Skopouli FN, Moutsopoulos HM. Mixed monoclonal cryoglobulinemia and monoclonal rheumatoid factor cross-reactive idiotypes as predictive factors for the development of lymphoma in primary Sjogren's syndrome. Arthritis Rheum 1996;39:767-72.

24. Lemp MA. Management of dry eye disease. Am J Manag Care 2008;14(Suppl.):S88-101.

25. Mansour K, Leonhardt CJ, Kalk WW, Bootsma H, Bruin KJ, Blanksma LJ. Lacrimal punctum occlusion in the treatment of severe keratoconjunctivitis Sicca caused by Sjogren syndrome: a uniocular evaluation. Cornea 2007;26:147-50.

26. Vivino FB, Al Hashimi I, Khan Z, LeVeque FG, Salisbury III PL, Tran-Johnson TK, et al. Pilocarpine tablets for the treatment of dry mouth and dry eye symptoms in patients with Sjogren syndrome: a randomized, placebo-controlled, fixed-dose, multicenter trial. P92-01 Study Group. Arch Intern Med 1999;159:174-81.

27. Papas AS, Sherrer YS, Charney M, Golden HE, Medsger Jr TA, Walsh BT, et al. Successful treatment of dry mouth and dry eye symptoms in Sjogren's syndrome patients with oral pilocarpine: a randomized, placebo-controlled, dose-adjustment study. J Clin Rheumatol 2004;10:169-77.

28. Petrone D, Condemi JJ, Fife R, Gluck O, Cohen S, Dalgin P. A double-blind, randomized, placebo-controlled study of cevimeline in Sjogren's syndrome patients with xerostomia and keratoconjunctivitis sicca. Arthritis Rheum 2002;46:748-54.

29. Fife RS, Chase WF, Dore RK, Wiesenhutter CW, Lockhart PB, Tindall E, et al. Cevimeline for the treatment of xerostomia in patients with Sjogren syndrome: a randomized trial. Arch Intern Med 2002;162:1293-300.

30. Seror R, Sordet C, Guillevin L, Hachulla E, Masson C, Ittah M, et al. Tolerance and efficacy of rituximab and changes in serum B cell biomarkers in patients with systemic complications of primary Sjogren's syndrome. Ann Rheum Dis 2007;66:351-7.

31. Pijpe J, van Imhoff GW, Spijkervet FK, Roodenburg JL, Wolbink GJ, Mansour K, et al. Rituximab treatment in patients with primary Sjogren's syndrome: an open-label phase II study. Arthritis Rheum 2005;52:2740-50.

32. Gottenberg JE, Guillevin L, Lambotte O, Combe B, Allanore Y, Cantagrel A, et al. Tolerance and short term efficacy of rituximab in 43 patients with systemic autoimmune diseases. Ann Rheum Dis 2005;64:913-20.

33. Devauchelle-Pensec V, Pennec Y, Morvan J, Pers JO, Daridon C, Jousse-Joulin S, et al. Improvement of Sjogren's syndrome after two infusions of rituximab (anti-CD20). Arthritis Rheum 2007;57:310-7.

34. Dass S, Bowman SJ, Vital EM, Ikeda K, Pease CT, Hamburger J, et al. Reduction of fatigue in Sjogren's syndrome with rituximab: results of a randomised, double-blind, placebo controlled pilot study. Ann Rheum Dis 2008;67:1541-4.

35. Meijer JM, Meiners PM, Vissink A, Spijkervet FK, Abdulahad W, Kamminga N, et al. Effective rituximab treatment in primary Sjögren's syndrome: a double-blind placebo controlled trial. submitted.

36. Chalmers JM. Minimal intervention dentistry: part 1. Strategies for addressing the new caries challenge in older patients. J Can Dent Assoc 2006;72:427-33.

37. Jansma J, Vissink A, Gravenmade EJ, Visch LL, Fidler V, Retief DH. In vivo study on the prevention of postradiation caries. Caries Res 1989;23:172-8.

38. Anusavice KJ. Dental caries: risk assessment and treatment solutions for an elderly population. Compend Contin Educ Dent 2002;23(10 Suppl.):12-20.

39. Kielbassa AM, Hinkelbein W, Hellwig E, Meyer-Luckel H. Radiation-related damage to dentition. Lancet Oncol 2006;7:326-35.

40. Zero DT. Dentifrices, mouthwashes, and remineralization/caries arrestment strategies. BMC Oral Health 2006;6(Suppl. 1):S9.

41. Walsh L. Lifestyle impacts on oral health. In: Mount G, Hume W, editors. Preservation and restoration of tooth structure. Middlesbrough, UK: Knowledgebooks and Software Ltd.; 2008. p. 83-110.

42. Van Loveren C. Sugar alcohols: what is the evidence for caries-preventive and caries-therapeutic effects? Caries Res 2004;38:286-93.

43. Chambers MS, Jones CU, Biel MA, Weber RS, Hodge KM, Chen Y, et al. Open-label, long-term safety study of cevimeline in the treatment of postirradiation xerostomia. Int J Radiat Oncol Biol Phys 2007;69:1369-76.

44. Cummins MJ, Papas A, Kammer GM, Fox PC. Treatment of primary Sjogren's syndrome with low-dose human interferon alfa administered by the oromucosal route: combined phase III results. Arthritis Rheum 2003;49:585-93.

45. Vissink A, De Jong HP, Busscher HJ, Arends J, Gravenmade EJ. Wetting properties of human saliva and saliva substitutes. J Dent Res 1986;65:1121-4.

46. Fox PC, Brennan M, Pillemer S, Radfar L, Yamano S, Baum BJ. Sjogren's syndrome: a model for dental care in the 21st century. J Am Dent Assoc 1998;129:719-28.

47. Regelink G, Vissink A, Reintsema H, Nauta JM. Efficacy of a synthetic polymer saliva substitute in reducing oral complaints of patients suffering from irradiation-induced xerostomia. Quintessence Int 1998;29:383-8.

48. Epstein JB, Emerton S, Le ND, Stevenson-Moore P. A double-blind crossover trial of Oral Balance gel and Biotene toothpaste versus placebo in patients with xerostomia following radiation therapy. Oral Oncol 1999;35:132-7.

49. Ship JA, McCutcheon JA, Spivakovsky S, Kerr AR. Safety and effectiveness of topical dry mouth products containing olive oil, betaine, and xylitol in reducing xerostomia for polypharmacy-induced dry mouth. J Oral Rehabil 2007;34:724-32.

50. Turner M, Jahangiri L, Ship JA. Hyposalivation, xerostomia and the complete denture: a systematic review. J Am Dent Assoc 2008;139:146-50.

51. Zarb G, Bolender C, Eckers S. Prosthodontic treatment for edentulous patients. 12th ed. St. Louis: Mosby; 2008.

52. Daniels TE, Fox PC. Salivary and oral components of Sjogren's syndrome. Rheum Dis Clin North Am 1992;18:571-89.

53. Fox PC, Datiles M, Atkinson JC, Macynski AA, Scott J, Fletcher D, et al. Prednisone and piroxicam for treatment of primary Sjogren's syndrome. Clin Exp Rheumatol 1993;11:149-56.

54. Dawson LJ, Caulfield VL, Stanbury JB, Field AE, Christmas SE, Smith PM. Hydroxychloroquine therapy in patients with primary Sjogren's syndrome may improve salivary gland hypofunction by inhibition of glandular cholinesterase. Rheumatology (Oxford) 2005;44:449-55.

55. Kruize AA, Hene RJ, Kallenberg CG, van Bijsterveld OP, van der Heide A, Kater L, et al. Hydroxychloroquine treatment for primary Sjogren's syndrome: a two year double blind crossover trial. Ann Rheum Dis 1993;52:360-4.

56. Skopouli FN, Jagiello P, Tsifetaki N, Moutsopoulos HM. Methotrexate in primary Sjogren's syndrome. Clin Exp Rheumatol 1996;14:555-8.

57. Price EJ, Rigby SP, Clancy U, Venables PJ. A double blind placebo controlled trial of azathioprine in the treatment of primary Sjogren's syndrome. J Rheumatol 1998;25:896-9.

58. Thanou-Stavraki A, James JA. Primary Sjogren's syndrome: current and prospective therapies. Semin Arthritis Rheum 2008;37:273-92.

59. van Woerkom JM, Kruize AA, Geenen R, van Roon EN, Goldschmeding R, Verstappen SM, et al. Safety and efficacy of leflunomide in primary Sjogren's syndrome: a phase II pilot study. Ann Rheum Dis 2007;66:1026-32.

60. Hartkamp A, Geenen R, Godaert GL, Bootsma H, Kruize AA, Bijlsma JW, et al. Effect of dehydroepiandrosterone administration on fatigue, well-being, and functioning in women with primary Sjogren syndrome: a randomised controlled trial. Ann Rheum Dis 2008;67:91-7.

61. Kourbeti IS, Boumpas DT. Biological therapies of autoimmune diseases. Curr Drug Targets Inflamm Allergy 2005;4:41-6.

62. d'Arbonneau F, Pers JO, Devauchelle V, Pennec Y, Saraux A, Youinou P. BAFF-induced changes in B cell antigen receptor-

containing lipid rafts in Sjogren's syndrome. Arthritis Rheum 2006;54:115-26.

63. Bave U, Nordmark G, Lovgren T, Ronnelid J, Cajander S, Eloranta ML, et al. Activation of the type I interferon system in primary Sjogren's syndrome: a possible etiopathogenic mechanism. Arthritis Rheum 2005;52:1185-95.

64. Ship JA, Fox PC, Michalek JE, Cummins MJ, Richards AB. Treatment of primary Sjogren's syndrome with low-dose natural human interferon-alpha administered by the oral mucosal route: a phase II clinical trial. IFN Protocol Study Group. J Interferon Cytokine Res 1999;19:943-51.

65. Steinfeld SD, Demols P, Salmon I, Kiss R, Appelboom T. Infliximab in patients with primary Sjogren's syndrome: a pilot study. Arthritis Rheum 2001;44:2371-5.

66. Steinfeld SD, Demols P, Appelboom T. Infliximab in primary Sjogren's syndrome: one-year followup. Arthritis Rheum 2002;46:3301-3.

67. Mariette X, Ravaud P, Steinfeld S, Baron G, Goetz J, Hachulla E, et al. Inefficacy of infliximab in primary Sjogren's syndrome: results of the randomized, controlled Trial of Remicade in Primary Sjogren's Syndrome (TRIPSS). Arthritis Rheum 2004;50:1270-6.

68. Zandbelt MM, de Wilde P, van Damme P, Hoyng CB, van de Putte L, van den Hoogen F. Etanercept in the treatment of patients with primary Sjogren's syndrome: a pilot study. J Rheumatol 2004;31:96-101.

69. Sankar V, Brennan MT, Kok MR, Leakan RA, Smith JA, Manny J, et al. Etanercept in Sjogren's syndrome: a twelve-week randomized, double-blind, placebo-controlled pilot clinical trial. Arthritis Rheum 2004;50:2240-5.

70. Salama AD, Pusey CD. Drug insight: rituximab in renal disease and transplantation. Nat Clin Pract Nephrol 2006;2:221-30.

71. McLaughlin P, Grillo-Lopez AJ, Link BK, Levy R, Czuczman MS, Williams ME, et al. Rituximab chimeric anti-CD20 monoclonal antibody therapy for relapsed indolent lymphoma: half of patients respond to a four-dose treatment program. J Clin Oncol 1998;16:2825-33.

72. Edwards JC, Szczepanski L, Szechinski J, Filipowicz-Sosnowska A, Emery P, Close DR, et al. Efficacy of B-cell-targeted therapy with rituximab in patients with rheumatoid arthritis. N Engl J Med 2004;350:2572-81.

73. Edwards JC, Cambridge G. B-cell targeting in rheumatoid arthritis and other autoimmune diseases. Nat Rev Immunol 2006;6:394-403.

74. Emery P, Fleischmann R, Filipowicz-Sosnowska A, Schechtman J, Szczepanski L, Kavanaugh A, et al. The efficacy and safety of rituximab in patients with active rheumatoid arthritis despite methotrexate treatment: results of a phase IIB randomized, double-blind, placebo-controlled, dose-ranging trial. Arthritis Rheum 2006;54:1390-400.

75. Looney RJ, Anolik JH, Campbell D, Felgar RE, Young F, Arend LJ, et al. B cell depletion as a novel treatment for systemic lupus erythematosus: a phase I/II dose-escalation trial of rituximab. Arthritis Rheum 2004;50:2580-9.

76. Pijpe J, Meijer JM, Bootsma H, van der Wal JE, Spijkervet FK, Kallenberg CG, et al. Clinical and histological evidence of salivary gland restoration supports the efficacy of rituximab treatment in Sjogren's syndrome. Arthritis Rheum 2009 (in press).

77. Meijer JM, Pijpe J, Vissink A, Kallenberg CG, Bootsma H. Treatment of primary Sjogren syndrome with rituximab: extended follow-up, safety and efficacy of retreatment. Ann Rheum Dis 2009;68:284-5.

78. Carnahan J, Wang P, Kendall R, Chen C, Hu S, Boone T, et al. Epratuzumab, a humanized monoclonal antibody targeting CD22: characterization of in vitro properties. Clin Cancer Res 2003;9(10 Pt 2):3982S-90S.

79. Steinfeld SD, Tant L, Burmester GR, Teoh NK, Wegener WA, Goldenberg DM, et al. Epratuzumab (humanised anti-CD22 antibody) in primary Sjogren's syndrome: an open-label phase I/II study. Arthritis Res Ther 2006;8:R129.

80. Pers JO, d'Arbonneau F, Devauchelle-Pensec V, Saraux A, Pennec YL, Youinou P. Is periodontal disease mediated by salivary BAFF in Sjogren's syndrome? Arthritis Rheum 2005;52:2411-4.

81. Szodoray P, Jellestad S, Alex P, Zhou T, Wilson PC, Centola M, et al. Programmed cell death of peripheral blood B cells determined by laser scanning cytometry in Sjogren's syndrome with a special emphasis on BAFF. J Clin Immunol 2004;24:600-1.

82. Ramanujam M, Davidson A. The current status of targeting BAFF/blys for autoimmune diseases. Arthritis Res Ther 2004;6:197-202.

83. Baker KP, Edwards BM, Main SH, Choi GH, Wager RE, Halpern WG, et al. Generation and characterization of lymphostat-B, a human monoclonal antibody that antagonizes the bioactivities of B lymphocyte stimulator. Arthritis Rheum 2003;48:3253-65.

84. Szodoray P, Jonsson R. The BAFF/APRIL system in systemic autoimmune diseases with a special emphasis on Sjogren's syndrome. Scand J Immunol 2005;62:421-8.

85. Lavie F, Miceli-Richard C, Ittah M, Sellam J, Gottenberg JE, Mariette X. Increase of B cell-activating factor of the TNF family (BAFF) after rituximab treatment: insights into a new regulating system of BAFF production. Ann Rheum Dis 2007;66:700-3.

86. Ramos-Casals M, Brito-Zeron P, Yague J, Akasbi M, Bautista R, Ruano M, et al. Hypocomplementaemia as an immunological marker of morbidity and mortality in patients with primary Sjogren's syndrome. Rheumatology (Oxford) 2005;44:89-94.

87. Wolfe GI, Nations SP, Burns DK, Herbelin LL, Barohn RJ. Benefit of ivig for long-standing ataxic sensory neuronopathy with Sjogren's syndrome. Neurology 2003;61:873.

88. Gorson KC, Natarajan N, Ropper AH, Weinstein R. Rituximab treatment in patients with ivig-dependent immune polyneuropathy: a prospective pilot trial. Muscle Nerve 2007;35:66-9.

89. Ferri C, Mascia MT. Cryoglobulinemic vasculitis. Curr Opin Rheumatol 2006;18:54-63.

90. Voulgarelis M, Dafni UG, Isenberg DA, Moutsopoulos HM. Malignant lymphoma in primary Sjogren's syndrome: a multicenter, retrospective, clinical study by the European Concerted Action on Sjogren's Syndrome. Arthritis Rheum 1999;42:1765-72.

91. Bowman SJ, Booth DA, Platts RG. Measurement of fatigue and discomfort in primary Sjogren's syndrome using a new questionnaire tool. Rheumatology (Oxford) 2004;43:758-64.

92. Oxholm P. Primary Sjogren's syndrome—clinical and laboratory markers of disease activity. Semin Arthritis Rheum 1992;22:114-26.

93. Seror R, Rauvaud P, Bowman SJ, Baron G, Gottenberg JE, Tzioufas AG, et al., for the EULAR Sjogren's Task Force. Elaboration of the EULAR Sjogren's Syndrome Disease Activity Index (ESSDAI). submitted.

94. Garcia-Carrasco M, Ramos-Casals M, Rosas J, Pallares L, Calvo-Alen J, Cervera R, et al. Primary Sjogren syndrome: clinical and immunologic disease patterns in a cohort of 400 patients. Medicine (Baltimore) 2002;81:270-80.

Chapter 13

Management of Systemic Sclerosis and Raynaud's Phenomenon

Peter K. Wung and Fredrick M. Wigley

Systemic sclerosis or scleroderma (SSc) is a rare and complicated autoimmune disease that presents with many challenging therapeutic quandaries. In this chapter, we will discuss and examine these frequently encountered treatment dilemmas through three illustrative cases. In general, we recommend adhering to five general principles in the everyday care of a patient with SSc.

PRINCIPLES OF MANAGING SCLERODERMA

- Define clinical phenotype: The disease expression is very heterogeneous.
- Evaluate for specific organ involvement: The disease is deeper than the skin.
- Define the clinical stage of the disease: The biology of the disease is dynamic and uniquely complex.
- Customize and redesign therapy: Specific focused therapy can make an impact.
- Complex patients with undefined therapies should be referred to specialty centers for novel therapeutic approaches.

CASE 1   Raynaud's Phenomenon

A 31-year-old chef with no significant past medical history was in good state of health until 4 months ago when she began to notice a cold, numb, and tingling sensation in her fingers after going into the freezer or working with frozen food. Her fingers would turn pale and occasionally blue upon exposure to cold temperatures. However, minutes after rewarming them under hot water, her fingers would return to their baseline color and temperature. Several months later, she developed severe pain in the right index finger and called urgently because of a persistently pale fingertip and local skin breakdown. Examination did not reveal evidence of sclerodactyly or fibrotic skin, but nailfold microscopy showed several capillary dilatations and telangietasias were noted on her fingertips, palms, and lips. All the fingers were cold to the touch, and the index finger was mottled with cyanosis surrounded by erythema. Pulses were strong but an Allen's test demonstrated compromised ulnar artery flow.

Differential Diagnosis

Raynaud's phenomenon (RP) is a vasospastic disorder that can be characterized clinically into primary and secondary forms (Table 13-1). Primary RP is suggested by the presence of a symmetric presentation, lack of tissue necrosis or gangrene, normal nailfold capillary examination, and a negative serologic status.[1] Our patient clearly presents with secondary RP with features of limited SSc and now severe critical digital ischemia requiring immediate attention. Patients with limited SSc, positive anti-centromere antibody, and evidence of microvascular disease on examination are more likely to have associated macrovascular disease resulting in digital ulcers or amputation.[2]

CASE 2   Cutaneous Manifestation

A 57-year-old woman with a 1-year history of RP treated with nifedipine and no other significant past medical history presents with a recent history of swollen hands and forearms. The skin is red, edematous, and pruritic and is rapidly progressing proximally over the past 2 months. On examination, she has sclerodactyly and erythematous swelling of her skin extending from her wrists to her elbows. Nailfold microscopy revealed several capillary dilatations and dropouts. Her antinuclear antibody status was positive with a titer of 1:320 in a nucleolar pattern.

Differential Diagnosis

Scleroderma can present in limited or diffuse form. The limited form involves area of the skin distal to the elbows or knees (with or without facial involvement), whereas the diffuse form presents with skin involvement extending above the knees or elbows or onto the trunk. Scleroderma must be differentiated from a wide range of rheumatologic and non-rheumatologic diseases that can mimic it[3] because the therapeutic strategy is vastly different in each case. The diseases that can be encountered in a patient initially thought to have SSc include scleredema adultorum, scleromyxedema, morphea, nephrogenic fibrosing dermopathy, eosinophilic fasciitis, myxedema

Table 13-1. *Diseases Associated with Secondary Raynaud's Phenomenon*

Systems	Association
Rheumatologic	Scleroderma, systemic lupus erythematosus, vasculitis, myositis, Sjögren's syndrome, undifferentiated connective tissue disease
Hematologic/oncologic	Paraneoplastic phenomenon, cryoglobulinemia, cryofibrinogenemia, paraproteinemia, cold agglutinin syndrome
Endocrine	Thyroid disorders
Vascular	Thoracic outlet syndrome
Neurologic	Carpal tunnel syndrome, migraine headache syndrome
Environmental	Vibration injury, frostbite, emotional stress
Drugs/Toxins	Sympathomimetic drugs, chemotherapeutic drugs, interferon, nicotine, cocaine, ergotamines, caffeine, polyvinyl chloride

secondary to hypothyroidism, systemic amyloidosis, graft-versus-host disease, and postradiation fibrosis. Careful history taking and physical examination alone often yield the correct diagnosis, whereas occasionally a skin or tissue biopsy and appropriate laboratory testing aid in confirming the diagnosis.

CASE 3   Pulmonary Manifestation

Seven years after our 31-year-old chef presented with limited SSc and RP (Case 1), she developed the insidious onset of shortness of breath. In the past 12 months, she experienced a significant decline in exercise tolerance and increasing fatigue. At present, she is dyspneic with moderate activity (e.g., climbing stairs). She denies having orthopnea, paroxysmal nocturnal dyspnea, cough, fever, chills, or weight loss. Six weeks ago, she noticed new-onset edema in her lower extremities.

Differential Diagnosis

The differential diagnosis for dyspnea in SSc is relatively broad, but the primary attention should be placed on the cardiac and pulmonary systems. Many cardiac complications are reported in SSc, including systolic and nonsystolic heart failure, conduction abnormalities, pericardial disease, myocardial inflammation, fibrosis, and coronary artery disease. The pulmonary complications are more commonly recognized in SSc, and they include pulmonary malignancy, bronchiectasis, pleura-based disease, drug-induced pneumonitis, pulmonary infections, pulmonary arterial hypertension (PAH), and interstitial lung disease (ILD). In the following discussion, we focus our attention on PAH and ILD because they are the most frequent pulmonary complications of SSc.

RAYNAUD'S PHENOMENON

Pathogenesis

There are three major biologic processes that occur in cases of SSc and digital ischemia. First, vasospasm occurs due to dysfunction in the thermoregulatory vessels of the skin and perturbation of small to medium arteries and arterioles of the peripheral circulation. This process presents clinically as RP (Fig. 13-1). Next, there is a nonvasculitic vasculopathy that is associated with endothelial dysfunction and a fibrotic thickening of the intimal layer of small arteries, which ultimately leads to narrowing of the vessel's lumen. Finally, there is occlusion of the involved vessels (arteries, arterioles, and capillaries) either secondary to advancing vasculopathy or thrombosis. These three processes result in critical ischemia, loss of digital tissue, and fibrosis. Management of critical ischemia attempts to address these underlying mechanisms.

Therapy

The primary goal in the management of RP is the prevention of digital ischemia (Fig. 13-2) through the use of nonpharmacologic and pharmacologic measures. In the setting of acute digital ischemia, as in our case, rapid intervention using both treatment modalities is required. Please refer to Table 13-2 for a summary of therapeutic options for RP.

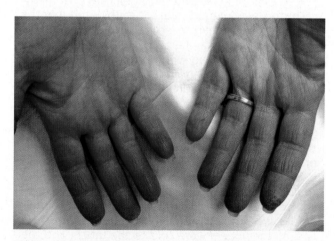

Figure 13-1. Raynaud's phenomenon induced by a change in ambient temperature. The fingers are acrocyanotic and cold to the touch. On rewarming, the fingers would return to their baseline color and temperature.

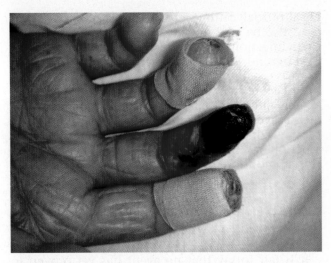

Figure13-2. Digital ischemia of the 3rd digit as a result of poor digital perfusion and lack of vasodilator therapy. The 2nd and 4th digits have skin breakdown, a finding associated with poor digital circulation.

Table 13-2. *Therapeutic Options for Raynaud's Phenomenon*

Class	Intervention
Nonpharmacologic	Avoidance of cold temperature
	Reduction of stress
	Behavioral therapies
	Biofeedback
	Autogenic training
	Classical conditioning
	Eliminating vasoconstrictive agents
	Tobacco
	Sympathomimetic drugs
Pharmacologic	Dihydropyridine calcium channel blockers
	Nifedipine (10–30 mg 3 times daily)
	Nifedipine XL (30–90 mg daily)
	Amplodipine (5–20 mg daily)
	Nisoldipine (17–34 mg daily)
	Isradipine (2.5–5 mg twice daily)
	Felodipine (2.5–5 mg twice daily)
	Non-dihydropyridine calcium channel blockers
	Diltiazem (30–120 mg 3 times daily)
	Prostaglandin
	Intravenous iloprost (0.5–2 ng/kg/min, 6–24 h for 2–5 days)
	Phosphodiesterase inhibitor
	Sidenafil (20 mg 3 times daily)
	Angiotensin receptor blocker
	Losartan (25–100 mg daily)
	Serotonin receptor uptake inhibitors
	Fluoxetine (20–40 mg daily)
	Vasodilator
	Topical nitroglycerin 2% (apply to affected digits)
	Sympatholytic agents
	Prazosin (2–5 mg 3 times daily)
	Antiplatelet agents
	Aspirin (81–325 mg daily)
	Cilostazol (100 mg twice daily)
Surgical	Sympathectomy
	Botulinum toxin injection

Nonpharmacologic Therapies

The primary and most important nonpharmacologic therapy for prevention is the avoidance of cold ambient temperatures, particularly transitioning from a warm or hot environment to a cold one. Additionally, strategies to keep the body and extremities warm (e.g., dressing warmly or wearing insulating gloves) should be employed. Patients who have an acute ischemic event are best treated by having them rest in a warm environment (home or hospital) while insulating them with additional warm blankets. Other potential therapies include minimizing emotional distress (reducing sympathetic tone) and eliminating any vasoconstricting agents (e.g., use of tobacco or sympathomimetic drugs). Although behavioral therapies (e.g., biofeedback, autogenic training, and classic conditioning) are reported to be helpful, their benefit is controversial and they play no role in the management of acute ischemia related to SSc. As for our patient (Case 1), she was admitted to a local hospital to rest, to keep her extremities warm, and to start pharmacologic therapy.

Pharmacologic Therapies

Calcium channel blockers are considered the first-line agents in the treatment of RP. This class of medication works by inducing arterial vasodilatation through stimulation of the smooth muscle cells, but they also reduce oxidative stress[4] and inhibit platelet activation.[5] Most published studies evaluating the efficacy of calcium channel blockers in RP have employed dihydropyridines including nifedipine, amlodipine, nisoldipine, isradipine, and felodipine. Both short- and long-acting formulations of calcium channel blockers decrease the intensity and frequency of ischemic attacks.[6] The current recommendation is to use an extended-release formulation of nifedipine (30–90 mg/day) or amlodipine (5–20 mg/day) for treatment of nonurgent RP. For urgent cases of RP, a short-acting formulation of the medication is preferred but the titration must be done in a carefully monitored setting in order to prevent worsening of digital ischemia due to "stealing" blood flow away from a structurally compromised digital vessel or an undue decrease in systemic blood pressure. In reference to our patient (Case 1), given the lack of vasodilator therapy, she was initiated on nifedipine 30 mg three times per day with dose titration.

Other Vasodilators

Sildenafil, a phosphodiesterase-5 inhibitor that has been well studied in the treatment of PAH, is thought to be effective in the prevention of RP attacks.[7-9] A recent 2007 study of quinapril suggests that angiotensin-converting enzyme inhibitors are not effective in treating SSc-related RP.[10] However, one study found that the angiotensin receptor blocker losartan (50 mg daily) was comparable to nifedipine (40 mg daily), showing a similar reduction in the severity and frequency of RP attacks.[11] Other agents that may be helpful include serotonin receptor uptake inhibitors,[12] topical nitrate,[13] other phosphodiesterase inhibitors (pentoxifylline,[14] cilostazol[15]), intermittent intravenous prostaglandins (iloprost), and sympatholytic agents (prazosin, an α1-adrenergic receptor blocker).[16,17]

Treating the Vasculopathy

The mechanism of SSc vascular disease is not completely understood, and therefore, intervention to prevent or reverse the vascular disease is not yet defined. Recent data suggest that the use of statins may be helpful by increasing the number of endothelial progenitor cells or by direct effects on vascular remodeling.[18,19] The vasoactive drugs (angiotensin receptor inhibitors, prostaglandins, calcium channel blockers, phosphodiesterase inhibitors, nitrates) are thought to aid in vascular remodeling as well. A controlled study reports that bosentan (62.5 mg twice daily), an endothelin-1 receptor inhibitor, can be effective in preventing new digital ulcers and improve hand function.[20] Antiplatelet agents (aspirin) may reduce thrombosis and further vascular injury. Chronic anticoagulation is not recommended unless there is a concomitant hypercoagulable disorder.

Surgical Interventions

Sympathectomy is a viable option for patients with RP who are unresponsive to medical therapy and should be used if a critical ischemic event is not quickly responding. Localized digital sympathectomy with lysis of fibrosis around the vessel is effective for acute ischemia[21-23] and has mostly replaced central sympathectomy. Improvement of RP after digital sympathectomy can be transient or prolonged. Last, careful assessment for reversible macrovascular disease should be conducted in the setting of RP with the aid of Doppler imaging if clinically warranted. If macrovascular disease is present, patient should be referred to vascular surgery to discuss potential procedures that may help to alleviate the occlusive process.

Treatment of Critical Digital Ischemia

Our patient (Case 1) has signs and symptoms of critical digital ischemia and immediate attention with medical intervention is most important to prevent ulceration or digital loss. In addition to initiating nonpharmacologic therapies, starting or maximizing a vasodilator such as a rapid-acting calcium channel blocker is strongly recommended. Antiplatelet therapy (daily aspirin) and unfractionated or low-molecular-weight heparin (1 mg/kg subcutaneously twice daily) should be initiated for 1 to 3 days if signs of larger vessel occlusion are present. Chemical sympathectomy performed by injection of lidocaine or bupivacaine locally at the base of a digit rapidly reduces pain and reverses vasospasm.

Local nitroglycerin gel applied to the affected areas may also be of some benefit. Although botulinum toxin injections are reported to improve digital ulcer healing and RP,[24,25] the experience with this treatment is too limited and thus not recommended during an acute crisis. A prostaglandin or prostaglandin analog can be initiated[26,27] if the above-mentioned measures are not helpful. Epoprostenol, iloprost, or prostacyclin analogs can be administered through a peripheral line continuously for 3 to 5 days in a closely monitored setting.[26-29]

Cutaneous Manifestation in Scleroderma

It is fair to say that no agent has yet proven to be effective in controlling SSc. There are two major treatment strategies for cutaneous manifestation of SSc. The first strategy is to employ immunosuppressive therapy during the initial phase of active cutaneous inflammation (Fig. 13-3) with tissue repair and before irreversible fibrosis occurs. The goal is to suppress the inflammatory cells that secrete proinflammatory cyokines (e.g., transforming growth factor-β) that activate and propagate the fibrotic pathway in skin and tissue. The second strategy is to employ an antifibrotic agent for the treatment of fibrotic skin (Fig. 13-4); however the efficacy of these agents is questionable. Examples of such antifibrotic agents that have yielded disappointing results in clinical trials include D-pencillamine, interferons, and relaxin. New agents that are promising include anticytokines (e.g., anti–transforming growth factor-β1; anti-interleukin 13) and tyrosine kinase inhibitors (e.g., imitanib, dasatanib).[30] So far, these agents are not yet fully studied, and thus, we will focus our discussion on the available immunosuppressive therapies used during the active inflammatory phase of the skin disease.

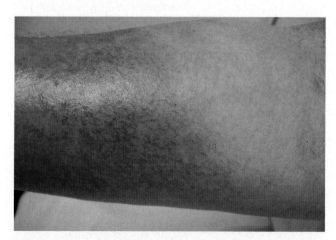

Figure 13-3. The forearm reveals both early active skin inflammation (*left*) and normal noninflamed skin (*right*) with a line of demarcation in the middle. The inflamed skin is warm, edematous and pruritic.

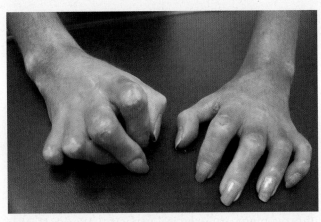

Figure 13-4. These hands reveal fibrotic skin changes seen in advanced scleroderma. As a result of the fibrosis in the skin and deeper tissue, contractures at the proximal interphalangeal joints are present.

Corticosteroids

There are uncontrolled reports of the benefits of corticosteroids for controlling the inflammatory phase of SSc, and many will use them alone or in conjunction with other immunosuppressive agents.[31] However, steroid use is known to increase the risk of SSc renal crisis, a problem that affects patients with early diffuse skin disease.[32,33] Corticosteroids help associated joint disease and myositis, but they do not appear to have an impact on advancing skin disease.

Methotrexate

Two randomized controlled studies have examined the effect of methotrexate on skin disease in early active diffuse SSc.[34,35] The 1996 and 2001 studies employed a subcutaneous (15–25 mg/week) and oral formulation (10–17.5 mg/week) of methotrexate, respectively. Both studies showed a small benefit associated with the use of methotrexate but concluded that methotrexate did not produce a clinically significant improvement.

Mycophenolate Mofetil

Mycophenolate mofetil (MMF) is a potent inhibitor of inosine-5 monophosphate dehydrogenase, which subsequently suppresses T- and B-lymphocyte proliferation. The effect of this agent on cutaneous disease was investigated in an open-label study that involved patients with early diffuse SSc.[36] These patients were first treated with antithymocyte globulin as an induction agent and were later maintained on MMF for at least 12 months. The patients showed statistically significant improvement in modified Rodnan skin score (MRSS) at 12 months. In a retrospective analysis of 172 SSc patients, of whom 109 were treated with MMF and the rest with other immunosuppressive agents, the MRSS improved similarly for both groups.[37] Our uncontrolled experience is that patients with early active skin disease who begin to improve on MMF usually do so in 6 to 12 weeks of therapy. If there is no improvement within this time frame then MMF is less likely to be helpful and a change in therapy should be considered.

Cyclophosphamide

Very little formal evidence is available to assess the safety and efficacy of cyclophosphamide in the treatment of active skin disease. It was investigated indirectly as a secondary analysis in the Scleroderma Lung Study,[38] which was a randomized placebo-controlled trial investigating its role in the treatment of SSc lung disease. Cyclophosphamide was given orally at a dose of 2 mg/kg. At 12 months, the change in MRSS from baseline between the two treatment groups was statistically significant; however, the effect was not observed at 18 or 24 months. Another study investigating the effect of monthly intravenous cyclophosphamide on skin disease found an improved skin score at study completion.[39] Immunoablation therapy with high-dose cyclophosphamide with or without autologous stem cell transplantation controls aggressive life-threatening disease with rapid skin progression.[40,41] This approach is still considered experimental and untested, and should be reserved only for those with severe life-threatening disease. Two prospective multicenter randomized trials[42] are underway to examine the effectiveness of this novel therapeutic approach. It is recommended that patients with early active and severe diffuse skin disease associated with evidence of internal organ involvement (e.g., low forced vital capacity [FVC] secondary to ILD) be considered for immunoablation therapy with or without stem cell rescue. If this course of therapy is elected, then the patient should either enter into a research protocol or be treated at a specialty center as the mortality using this aggressive approach can be high.

Intravenous Immunoglobulin

Several open-label studies demonstrate significant improvement in MRSS in patients with SSc treated with intravenous immunoglobulin (IVIG).[43,44] In these studies, patients with both limited and diffuse SSc in various stages of cutaneous disease were given 2 g/kg of IVIG divided over 4 to 5 days monthly for 6 months. Although it clearly benefits patients with scleromyxedema,[45] the use of IVIG in SSc is still being defined. At our center, we employ a 4- to 6-month trial to determine treatment efficacy. Patients with immunoglobulin A (IgA) deficiency may develop anaphylactic reactions toward IVIG, and thus, the IgA level should be checked before initial administration.

Other Therapies

Rapamycin, cyclosporin, antithymocyte globulin, oral type I collagen, anti–tumor necrosis factor, rituximab, and extracorporeal photopheresis have been studied in the treatment of SSc skin disease, but either the data is too sparse, the agent has not been effective, or significant side effects limit our ability to recommend their use. Emerging biologic therapies with tyrosine kinase inhibitors (e.g., imatinib, dasatinib)[46-48] are currently being studied, and the authors do not recommend their use in general settings; any off-label use should be considered only at specialty centers.

In reference to our patient (Case 2) with early active skin disease, she was initiated on MMF at 2 g/day with escalation to 3 g/day by 3 months. Her response at 3 months was excellent because she had no further progression of skin involvement.

PULMONARY MANIFESTATION IN SCLERODERMA

General Screening Guidelines

Pulmonary complications of SSc have become the leading causes of mortality in this patient population. As a result, careful and routine screening for such complications is now standard of care for these patients. All patients with SSc should obtain baseline and 6-month follow-up pulmonary function tests (PFTs) and a 12-month follow-up echocardiogram. If stable, both screening tests should be performed yearly. Scleroderma patients with new-onset dyspnea should obtain a high-resolution chest computed tomography (HRCT), PFT, echocardiogram, and electrocardiogram. In those asymptomatic patients with an abnormal baseline FVC or diffusion capacity for carbon monoxide (DLCO) (< 80%) or a significant change in FVC or DLCO compared with previous PFT, a HRCT should be performed. Last, right-sided heart catheterization is recommended for those patients with right-sided heart failure symptoms or an elevated estimated right ventricular systolic pressure (eRVSP) of greater than 40 to 45 mmHg. Recent unpublished data suggest that exercise echocardiogram may be able to detect nonsystolic heart failure in SSc patients.

Pulmonary Arterial Hypertension

Pulmonary arterial hypertension results from an increased resistance in the pulmonary vasculature. Although all patients are susceptible, isolated severe PAH is more common in patients with a limited form of SSc and those with a late age of disease onset; furthermore, it tends to occur late in the disease course. Early PAH may be asymptomatic and should be suspected if the patient has a decline in the DLCO on PFT. Early detection of PAH begins with a resting echocardiogram with particular attention on the eRVSP. Pulmonary arterial hypertension is suspected if the eRVSP is greater than 40 mm Hg with normal ejection fraction. This indirect method both underestimate and overestimate the true pulmonary pressure.[49] For lower eRVSP thresholds (> 25 mm Hg), the sensitivity for detecting PAH is

poor (58%).[50] Thus, the diagnosis of PAH can be made only with a confirmatory right-sided heart catheterization that directly measures right-sided heart and pulmonary arterial pressures.

Phosphodiesterase-5 Inhibitor

Sildenafil is an oral phosphodiesterase-5 antagonist that, in turn, relaxes and inhibits the growth of vascular smooth muscle cells. The effect of this drug was studied in a randomized double-blind, placebo-controlled trial involving 278 patients with symptomatic pulmonary hypertension, with nearly a third of the patients having connective tissue disease, including SSc.[51] The study showed significant improvement in exercise capacity, World Health Organization (WHO) functional class, and hemodynamics in patients with symptomatic PAH treated with varying doses of the study medication.

Endothelin-1 Inhibitors

Bosentan is a nonselective oral endothelin-1 receptor inhibitor. Its efficacy in the treatment of PAH was demonstrated in the large randomized placebo-controlled BREATHE-1 trial involving symptomatic patients, 30% of whom had concomitant diagnosis of SSc or systemic lupus erythematosus.[52] The patients were given one of two doses of bosentan (125 mg or 250 mg twice per day) or placebo for 16 weeks. During open-label extension study[53] of the previous trial, bosentan (either alone or with additional agents) was associated with improved survival rates compared with previous historical cases treated traditionally.[54] Bosentan also improved the exercise capacity of those patients with WHO class II symptoms as demonstrated in the EARLY study.[55] The selective (type A) endothelin-1 receptor antagonists ambrisentan[56] and sitaxsentan[57] also show good efficacy in the treatment of PAH.

Prostacyclins

Prostacyclin is a potent vasodilator by inducing cyclic adenosine monophosphate and inhibition of smooth muscle cells proliferation. Several prostacyclins in various formulations are available for the treatment of PAH. Epoprostenol is a intravenous prostacyclin that improves exercise capacity, symptoms, and cardiopulmonary hemodynamics in a randomized trial involving 111 patients with SSc.[58] The epoprostenol group had an associated 10% decrease in pulmonary artery pressure and decreased pulmonary vascular resistance. The common drawback of this medication is that it requires a continuous intravenous infusion and close monitoring during its administration.

Iloprost, a potent prostacyclin, is available in both the inhaled and intravenous formulation. Most current studies focus on inhaled iloprost because of the easier route of administration and its direct effect on the pulmonary vasculature. In a 2002 study, more than 200 patients with severe PAH were randomized to receive inhaled iloprost (median dose ~30 μg daily) or placebo. Seventeen percent of the treatment arm versus 4% of the placebo arm ($P = 0.007$) reached a primary endpoint that consisted of 10% improvement in 6-minute walk distance, improvement in New York Heart Association functional class, no deterioration, and no mortality.[59]

Treprostinil, a prostacyclin analog, is available in inhaled, subcutaneous, and intravenous formulations, but only the subcutaneous and intravenous administrations are approved for the treatment of PAH. In a large multicenter trial involving 470 patients with severe PAH, the efficacy of subcutaneous infusion of treprostinil (1.25–22.5 ng/kg/min) was comparable to placebo. The treatment arm led to clinically and statistically significant improvement in the 6-minute walk distance, dyspnea, cardiopulmonary hemodynamics, and quality of life at 12 weeks.[60] In a recent open-label study evaluating the efficacy of intravenous treprostinil, there was a substantial improvement in the 6-minute walk distance and pulmonary dynamics associated with the treatment arm.[61]

Our recommendation is start patients with proven PAH by right-sided heart catheterization with WHO class I, II, or III symptoms with sildenafil at 20 mg orally three times per day, in addition to diuretics to reduce preload. Alternatively, an oral endothelin-1 inhibitor (bosentan or ambrisentan) can be initially used as monotherapy. If the patient worsens or does not improve, then a second agent is added to the initial drug (e.g., sildenafil plus ambrisentan). For cases with progressive disease or WHO class IV symptoms the addition of either inhaled or IV prostaglandin is started alone or in addition to sildenafil or an endothelin-1 inhibitor. Despite ideal current therapy, patients with SSc still have a shortened life expectancy, and lung transplantation may be the only option. As for our patient (Case 3), she was diagnosed with PAH by right-sided heart catheterization and had WHO class II symptoms. She was started on sildenafil, and at 3-month follow-up, she demonstrated an improved 6-minute walk distance.

Interstitial Lung Disease

ILD is a broad term that encompasses a spectrum of pulmonary disorders that are associated with SSc, including pulmonary fibrosis, alveolitis, and interstitial pneumonitis. It carries a poor prognosis,[62,63] occurs in patients with early phase of the disease, and is more frequently seen in patients with diffuse skin disease, in nonwhites, and in those with antitopoisomerase antibodies. Although ILD is common and not always severe, it can progress to the severe form in approximately 20% of patients with diffuse SSc.[64] Suspicion of ILD occurs when there is a decline in lung volumes or DLCO on serial screening PFT. An HRCT can aid in the diagnosis by assessing for features of ground-glass opacification (Fig. 13-5), suggestive of interstitial and alveolar inflammation or reticular opacities and honeycombing patterns,

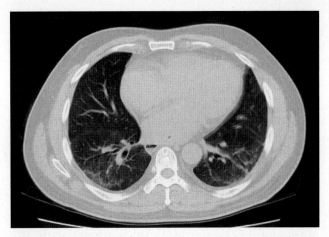

Figure 13-5. This high-resolution chest computed tomography reveals ground-glass opacities in the posterior portion of both lungs consistent with active interstitial lung disease.

suggestive of interstitial fibrosis. Evidence suggests that diagnostic testing with bronchoalveolar lavage (BAL) can define active alveolitis (neutrophilia of $\geq$ 3%, eosinophilia of $\geq$ 2%, or both in BAL).[64] However, recent studies have found that the BAL does not predict response to therapy or progression of disease.[65]

Cyclophosphamide

In the Scleroderma Lung Study, patients with SSc with active ILD defined by BAL and radiographic features were randomized to receive either oral cyclophosphamide ($\leq$ 2 mg/kg) or placebo for 1 year. The treatment arm was associated with a modest beneficial effect on lung function (FVC and total lung capacity) and severity of dyspnea.[38] However, this benefit was lost at 24 months after 1 year of active therapy. These data suggest that use and associated risk of cyclophospamide should be respected, and it is likely that a prolonged course of immunosuppression is needed. In a separate study that looked at the effects of intravenous cyclophosphamide on SSc-ILD, there was a nonstatistically significant improvement in FVC[66] after 6 months of intravenous cyclophosphamide followed by azathioprine.

Mycophenolate Mofetil

Uncontrolled case series and retrospective analysis showed that MMF (> 1g/day) may be helpful for ILD in SSc.[67,68] Additional prospective controlled studies are needed to provide guidance with the use of this medication in patients with SSc-ILD. By experience, use MMF as an alternative to cyclophosphamide or as a maintenance agent after initial induction therapy with cyclophosphamide is reasonable.

Azathioprine

Azathioprine was investigated as a maintenance agent in patients with SSc-ILD who were treated with 1 year of intravenous cyclophosphamide in a placebo-controlled randomized trial.[66] The results revealed no significant changes in FVC and DLCO, appearance on HRCT, and dyspnea scores between the two groups. Azathioprine is not recommended as a first-line induction agent.

Lung Transplantation

Lung transplantation is a viable alternative for SSc patients with ILD who were inadequately responsive to immunosuppressive therapy and meet the strict selection criteria. In a retrospective analysis of 47 SSc patients who underwent lung transplantation, the 1- and 3-year survival rates were 68% and 46%, respectively.[69] When compared with patients who underwent lung transplantation for other causes (e.g., idiopathic pulmonary fibrosis and idiopathic pulmonary hypertension), the patients with SSc had similar rates of mortality.[70] Lung transplantation needs to be carefully considered in SSc patients because of the common associated problem of gastrointestinal reflux disease. Our patient (Case 3) had no evidence of ILD on HRCT and PFT. The diagnosis of PAH was achieved by a screening echocardiogram and confirmatory right-sided heart catheterization.

References

1. LeRoy EC, Medsger Jr TA. Raynaud's phenomenon: a proposal for classification. Clin Exp Rheumatol 1992;10:485-8.
2. Wigley FM, Wise RA, Miller R, Needleman BW, Spence RJ. Anticentromere antibody as a predictor of digital ischemic loss in patients with systemic sclerosis. Arthritis Rheum 1992;35:688-93.
3. Boin F, Hummers LK. Scleroderma-like fibrosing disorders. Rheum Dis Clin North Am 2008;34:199-220; ix.
4. Allanore Y, Borderie D, Lemarechal H, Ekindjian OG, Kahan A. Acute and sustained effects of dihydropyridine-type calcium channel antagonists on oxidative stress in systemic sclerosis. Am J Med 2004;116:595-600.
5. Malamet R, Wise RA, Ettinger WH, Wigley FM. Nifedipine in the treatment of Raynaud's phenomenon. Evidence for inhibition of platelet activation. Am J Med 1985;78:602-8.
6. Thompson AE, Pope JE. Calcium channel blockers for primary Raynaud's phenomenon. A meta-analysis. Rheumatology (Oxford) 2005;44:145-50.
7. Fries R, Shariat K, von Wilmowsky H, Bohm M. Sildenafil in the treatment of Raynaud's phenomenon resistant to vasodilatory therapy. Circulation 2005;112:2980-5.
8. Gore J, Silver R. Oral sildenafil for the treatment of Raynaud's phenomenon and digital ulcers secondary to systemic sclerosis. Ann Rheum Dis 2005;64:1387.
9. Kumana CR, Cheung GT, Lau CS. Severe digital ischaemia treated with phosphodiesterase inhibitors. Ann Rheum Dis 2004;63:1522-4.
10. Gliddon AE, Dore CJ, Black CM, McHugh N, Moots R, Denton CP, et al. Prevention of vascular damage in scleroderma and autoimmune Raynaud's phenomenon: a multicenter, randomized, double-blind, placebo-controlled trial of the angiotensin-converting enzyme inhibitor quinapril. Arthritis Rheum 2007;56:3837-46.
11. Dziadzio M, Denton CP, Smith R, Howell K, Blann A, Bowers E, et al. Losartan therapy for Raynaud's phenomenon and scleroderma: clinical and biochemical findings in a fifteen-week, randomized, parallel-group, controlled trial. Arthritis Rheum 1999;42:2646-55.
12. Coleiro B, Marshall SE, Denton CP, Howell K, Blann A, Welsh KI, et al. Treatment of Raynaud's phenomenon with the selective serotonin reuptake inhibitor fluoxetine. Rheumatology (Oxford) 2001;40:1038-43.
13. Anderson ME, Moore TL, Hollis S, Jayson MI, King TA, Herrick AL. Digital vascular response to topical glyceryl trinitrate, as measured by laser Doppler imaging, in primary Raynaud's phenomenon and systemic sclerosis. Rheumatology (Oxford) 2002;41:324-8.
14. Arosio E, Montesi G, Zannoni M, Paluani F, Lechi A. Comparative efficacy of ketanserin and pentoxiphylline in treatment of Raynaud's phenomenon. Angiology 1989;40:633-8.
15. Rajagopalan S, Pfenninger D, Somers E, Kehrer C, Chakrabarti A, Mukherjee D, et al. Effects of cilostazol in patients with Raynaud's syndrome. Am J Cardiol 2003;92:1310-5.
16. Russell IJ, Lessard JA. Prazosin treatment of Raynaud's phenomenon: a double blind single crossover study. J Rheumatol 1985;12:94-8.
17. Wollersheim H, Thien T, Fennis J, van Elteren P, van 't Laar A. Double-blind, placebo-controlled study of prazosin in Raynaud's phenomenon. Clin Pharmacol Ther 1986;40:219-25.
18. Derk CT, Jimenez SA. Statins and the vasculopathy of systemic sclerosis. Potential therapeutic agents? Autoimmun Rev 2006;5:25-32.
19. Kuwana M, Kaburaki J, Okazaki Y, Yasuoka H, Kawakami Y, Ikeda Y. Increase in circulating endothelial precursors by atorvastatin in patients with systemic sclerosis. Arthritis Rheum 2006;54:1946-51.
20. Korn JH, Mayes M, Matucci Cerinic M, Rainisio M, Pope J, Hachulla E, et al. Digital ulcers in systemic sclerosis: Prevention by treatment with bosentan, an oral endothelin receptor antagonist. Arthritis Rheum 2004;50:3985-93.
21. Bogoch ER, Gross DK. Surgery of the hand in patients with systemic sclerosis: outcomes and considerations. J Rheumatol 2005;32:642-8.
22. Kotsis SV, Chung KC. A systematic review of the outcomes of digital sympathectomy for treatment of chronic digital ischemia. J Rheumatol 2003;30:1788-92.
23. Tomaino MM, Goitz RJ, Medsger TA. Surgery for ischemic pain and Raynaud's phenomenon in scleroderma: a description of treatment protocol and evaluation of results. Microsurgery 2001;21:75-9.
24. Sycha T, Graninger M, Auff E, Schnider P. Botulinum toxin in the treatment of Raynaud's phenomenon: A pilot study. Eur J Clin Invest 2004;34:312-3.
25. Van Beek AL, Lim PK, Gear AJ, Pritzker MR. Management of vasospastic disorders with botulinum toxin A. Plast Reconstr Surg 2007;119:217-26.
26. Belch JJ, Newman P, Drury JK, McKenzie F, Capell H, Leiberman P, et al. Intermittent epoprostenol (prostacyclin) infusion in patients with Raynaud's syndrome. A double-blind controlled trial. Lancet 1983;1:313-5.
27. Wigley FM, Wise RA, Seibold JR, McCloskey DA, Kujala G, Medsger Jr TA, et al. Intravenous iloprost infusion in patients with Raynaud phenomenon secondary to systemic sclerosis. A multicenter, placebo-controlled, double-blind study. Ann Intern Med 1994;120:199-206.
28. Dowd PM, Martin MF, Cooke ED, Bowcock SA, Jones R, Dieppe PA, et al. Treatment of Raynaud's phenomenon by intravenous infusion of prostacyclin (PGI2). Br J Dermatol 1982;106:81-9.
29. Mohrland JS, Porter JM, Smith EA, Belch J, Simms MH. A multiclinic, placebo-controlled, double-blind study of prostaglandin E1 in Raynaud's syndrome. Ann Rheum Dis 1985; 44:754-60.
30. Rosenbloom J, Jimenez SA. Molecular ablation of transforming growth factor beta signaling pathways by tyrosine kinase inhibition: the coming of a promising new era in the treatment of tissue fibrosis. Arthritis Rheum 2008;58:2219-24.
31. Vanthuyne M, Blockmans D, Westhovens R, Roufosse F, Cogan E, Coche E, et al. A pilot study of mycophenolate mofetil combined to intravenous methylprednisolone pulses and oral low-dose glucocorticoids in severe early systemic sclerosis. Clin Exp Rheumatol 2007;25:287-92.
32. DeMarco PJ, Weisman MH, Seibold JR, Furst DE, Wong WK, Hurwitz EL, et al. Predictors and outcomes of scleroderma renal crisis: the high-dose versus low-dose D-penicillamine in early diffuse systemic sclerosis trial. Arthritis Rheum 2002;46:2983-9.

33. Steen VD, Medsger Jr TA. Case-control study of corticosteroids and other drugs that either precipitate or protect from the development of scleroderma renal crisis. Arthritis Rheum 1998;41:1613-9.

34. Pope JE, Bellamy N, Seibold JR, Baron M, Ellman M, Carette S, et al. A randomized, controlled trial of methotrexate versus placebo in early diffuse scleroderma. Arthritis Rheum 2001;44:1351-8.

35. van den Hoogen FH, Boerbooms AM, Swaak AJ, Rasker JJ, van Lier HJ, van de Putte LB. Comparison of methotrexate with placebo in the treatment of systemic sclerosis: a 24 week randomized double-blind trial, followed by a 24 week observational trial. Br J Rheumatol 1996;35:364-72.

36. Stratton RJ, Wilson H, Black CM. Pilot study of anti-thymocyte globulin plus mycophenolate mofetil in recent-onset diffuse scleroderma. Rheumatology (Oxford) 2001;40:84-8.

37. Nihtyanova SI, Brough GM, Black CM, Denton CP. Mycophenolate mofetil in diffuse cutaneous systemic sclerosis--a retrospective analysis. Rheumatology (Oxford) 2007;46: 442-5.

38. Tashkin DP, Elashoff R, Clements PJ, Goldin J, Roth MD, Furst DE, et al. Cyclophosphamide versus placebo in scleroderma lung disease. N Engl J Med 2006;354:2655-66.

39. Griffiths B, Miles S, Moss H, Robertson R, Veale D, Emery P. Systemic sclerosis and interstitial lung disease: a pilot study using pulse intravenous methylprednisolone and cyclophosphamide to assess the effect on high resolution computed tomography scan and lung function. J Rheumatol 2002;29:2371-8.

40. Nash RA, McSweeney PA, Crofford LJ, Abidi M, Chen CS, Godwin JD, et al. High-dose immunosuppressive therapy and autologous hematopoietic cell transplantation for severe systemic sclerosis: long-term follow-up of the US multicenter pilot study. Blood 2007;110:1388-96.

41. Tehlirian CV, Hummers LK, White B, Brodsky RA, Wigley FM. High-dose cyclophosphamide without stem cell rescue in scleroderma. Ann Rheum Dis 2008;67:775-81.

42. Tyndall A, Furst DE. Adult stem cell treatment of scleroderma. Curr Opin Rheumatol 2007;19:604-10.

43. Levy Y, Amital H, Langevitz P, Nacci F, Righi A, Conforti L, et al. Intravenous immunoglobulin modulates cutaneous involvement and reduces skin fibrosis in systemic sclerosis: an open-label study. Arthritis Rheum 2004;50:1005-7.

44. Nacci F, Righi A, Conforti ML, Miniati I, Fiori G, Martinovic D, et al. Intravenous immunoglobulins improve the function and ameliorate joint involvement in systemic sclerosis: a pilot study. Ann Rheum Dis 2007;66:977-9.

45. Blum M, Wigley FM, Hummers LK. Scleromyxedema: a case series highlighting long-term outcomes of treatment with intravenous immunoglobulin (IVIG). Medicine (Baltimore) 2008;87:10-20.

46. Akhmetshina A, Dees C, Pileckyte M, Maurer B, Axmann R, Jüngel A, et al. Dual inhibition of c-abl and PDGF receptor signaling by dasatinib and nilotinib for the treatment of dermal fibrosis. FASEB J 2008;22:2214-22.

47. Bibi Y, Gottlieb AB. A potential role for imatinib and other small molecule tyrosine kinase inhibitors in the treatment of systemic and localized sclerosis. J Am Acad Dermatol 2008;59:654-8.

48. Pannu J, Asano Y, Nakerakanti S, Smith E, Jablonska A, Blaszczyk M, et al. Smad1 pathway is activated in systemic sclerosis fibroblasts and is targeted by imatinib mesylate. Arthritis Rheum 2008;58:2528-37.

49. Arcasoy SM, Christie JD, Ferrari VA, Sutton MS, Zisman DA, Blumenthal NP, et al. Echocardiographic assessment of pulmonary hypertension in patients with advanced lung disease. Am J Respir Crit Care Med 2003;167:735-40.

50. Hsu VM, Moreyra AE, Wilson AC, Shinnar M, Shindler DM, Wilson JE, et al. Assessment of pulmonary arterial hypertension in patients with systemic sclerosis: comparison of non-invasive tests with results of right-heart catheterization. J Rheumatol 2008;35:458-65.

51. Galie N, Ghofrani HA, Torbicki A, Barst RJ, Rubin LJ, Badesch D, et al. Sildenafil citrate therapy for pulmonary arterial hypertension. N Engl J Med 2005;353:2148-57.

52. Rubin LJ, Badesch DB, Barst RJ, Galie N, Black CM, Keogh A, et al. Bosentan therapy for pulmonary arterial hypertension. N Engl J Med 2002;346:896-903.

53. Denton CP, Humbert M, Rubin L, Black CM. Bosentan treatment for pulmonary arterial hypertension related to connective tissue disease: a subgroup analysis of the pivotal clinical trials and their open-label extensions. Ann Rheum Dis 2006;65:1336-40.

54. Williams MH, Das C, Handler CE, Akram MR, Davar J, Denton CP, et al. Systemic sclerosis associated pulmonary hypertension: Improved survival in the current era. Heart 2006;92:926-32.

55. Galie N, Rubin L, Hoeper M, Jansa A, Al-Hiti H, Meyer G, et al. Treatment of patients with mildly symptomatic pulmonary arterial hypertension with bosentan (EARLY study): a double-blind, randomised controlled trial. Lancet 2008;371:2093-100.

56. Barst RJA. Review of pulmonary arterial hypertension: role of ambrisentan. Vasc Health Risk Manag 2007;3:11-22.

57. Benza RL, Barst RJ, Galie N, Frost A, Girgis RE, Highland KB, et al. Sitaxsentan for the treatment of pulmonary arterial hypertension: a one year, prospective, open label, observation of outcome and survival. Chest 2008;134:775-82.

58. Badesch DB, Tapson VF, McGoon MD, Brundage BH, Rubin LJ, Wigley FM, et al. Continuous intravenous epoprostenol for pulmonary hypertension due to the scleroderma spectrum of disease. A randomized, controlled trial. Ann Intern Med 2000;132:425-34.

59. Olschewski H, Simonneau G, Galie N, Higenbottam T, Naeije R, Rubin LJ, et al. Inhaled iloprost for severe pulmonary hypertension. N Engl J Med 2002;347:322-9.

60. Simonneau G, Barst RJ, Galie N, Naeije R, Rich S, Bourqe RC, et al. Continuous subcutaneous infusion of treprostinil, a prostacyclin analogue, in patients with pulmonary arterial hypertension: a double-blind, randomized, placebo-controlled trial. Am J Respir Crit Care Med 2002;165:800-4.

61. Tapson VF, Gomberg-Maitland M, McLaughlin VV, Benza RL, Widlitz AC, Krichman A, et al. Safety and efficacy of IV treprostinil for pulmonary arterial hypertension: a prospective, multicenter, open-label, 12-week trial. Chest 2006;129: 683-8.

62. Altman RD, Medsger Jr TA, Bloch DA, Michel BA. Predictors of survival in systemic sclerosis (scleroderma). Arthritis Rheum 1991;34:403-13.

63. Steen VD, Medsger Jr TA. Severe organ involvement in systemic sclerosis with diffuse scleroderma. Arthritis Rheum 2000;43:2437-44.

64. White B. Interstitial lung disease in scleroderma. Rheum Dis Clin North Am 2003;29:371-90.

65. Mittoo S, Wigley FM, Wise R, Xiao H, Hummers L. Persistence of abnormal bronchoalveolar lavage findings after cyclophosphamide treatment in scleroderma patients with interstitial lung disease. Arthritis Rheum 2007;56:4195-202.

66. Hoyles RK, Ellis RW, Wellsbury J, Lees B, Newlands P, Goh NS, et al. A multicenter, prospective, randomized, double-blind, placebo-controlled trial of corticosteroids and intravenous cyclophosphamide followed by oral azathioprine for the treatment of pulmonary fibrosis in scleroderma. Arthritis Rheum 2006;54:3962-70.

67. Gerbino AJ, Goss CH, Molitor JA. Effect of mycophenolate mofetil on pulmonary function in scleroderma-associated interstitial lung disease. Chest 2008;133:455-60.

68. Liossis SN, Bounas A, Andonopoulos AP. Mycophenolate mofetil as first-line treatment improves clinically evident early scleroderma lung disease. Rheumatology (Oxford) 2006;45:1005-8.

69. Massad MG, Powell CR, Kpodonu J, Tshibaka C, Hanhan Z, Snow NJ, et al. Outcomes of lung transplantation in patients with scleroderma. World J Surg 2005;29:1510-5.

70. Schachna L, Medsger Jr TA, Dauber JH, et al. Lung transplantation in scleroderma compared with idiopathic pulmonary fibrosis and idiopathic pulmonary arterial hypertension. Arthritis Rheum 2006;54:3954-61.

Chapter 14

Targeted Treatment of the Idiopathic Inflammatory Myopathies

Maryam Dastmalchi and Helene Alexandersson

A 52-year-old woman presented with a 2-week history of progressive joint and muscle pain with stiffness in the upper arm and leg musculature. She had been exercising regularly for years and was in good physical shape. She also described a temperature of 38.2° C, Raynaud's phenomenon, symptoms of carpal tunnel syndrome, fatigue, palpitations, and shortness of breath. She was not taking any medications. On physical examination, no reduction of muscle strength was noted as measured by manual muscle test (MMT; explained later), but muscle endurance as measured by the functional index 2 (FI-2; explained later, see also Table 14-1 and reference 1) was reduced by 30% to 55% symmetrically in both the upper and lower extremity musculature and in the neck flexors. She was admitted to the hospital. On laboratory investigation, the thyroid stimulating hormone (TSH) level was moderately increased to 31 mE/L (0, 4–4, 7), T4 was

normal at 12 pmol/L (range 8–12 pmol/L), and T3 was reduced slightly at 3, 0 pmol/L (3, 5–5, 4). Serum creatine phophokinase (CK) levels were increased to 1932 IU/L. Electrophysiologic investigation revealed spontaneous activity in the biceps brachia, the deltoid, and the vastus lateralis muscles bilaterally. There were small light red skin eruptions overlying the knuckles and elbows. Chest x-ray examination and computed tomography (CT) examinations of the lungs revealed objective signs of interstitial lung disease (ILD) bilaterally, and enlargement of the heart including both the right and left chambers. There was no sign of pericarditis. Echocardiography revealed a small volume of pericardial fluid (3- to 5-mm layer). There were no signs of pulmonary hypertension, and there was no significant reduction of left ventricular function. Pulmonary function tests including vital capacity (VC) and total lung capacity (TLC) were reduced to

Table 14-1. *The Functional Index 2*

Tasks	Position	Pace (beats/min)	Maximal Number of Repetitions	Short Instruction
1. Shoulder flexion*	Sit on chair without back support	40	60	Raise the arm forward/upward
2. Shoulder abduction	Sit on chair without back support	40	60	Raise the arm to the side/upward
3. Head lift	Lay on a bench with horizontal head support without a pillow	40	60	Lift the head as much as possible
4. Hip flexion	Lay on back on a bench with straight legs	40	60	Lift one leg at the time (heel 40 cm from the bench)
5. Step test	Climb a 25 cm high stool	40	60	When climbing use the right leg, descending with the left.
6. Heel lift	Stand on both feet with balance support	80	120	Lift the heels as much as possible
7. Toe lifts	Stand on both feet with your hips and back against a wall	80	120	Lift the toes as much as possible

*Use a 1 kg weight cuff around the wrist.
Each task can be performed bilaterally or on the dominant side. Each task is scored as the number of correct performed repetitions giving a profile of muscle endurance impairment of the upper and lower extremities as well as the neck muscles. More detailed information, including pictures of all tasks, is included in an appendix in the original publication.[1]

less than 80% of the predicted values. Likewise, the single breath transfer factor for carbon monoxide (TLCO) was reduced to 50% of the predicted value. Electrocardiography (ECG) showed sinus tachycardia without any arrhythmia. There were no laboratory signs of infection. Antinuclear antibodies (ANAs) were absent; anti-Jo-1 antibodies were present by immunoblot analysis. A muscle biopsy was performed by the percutaneous conchotome method from the right vastus lateralis muscle.[2] Four small pieces of muscle tissue were obtained. The biopsy revealed scattered atrophic muscle fibers and signs of muscle fiber degeneration. Type II fiber atrophy was not present. Major histocompatibility complex-1 (MHC-1) was upregulated in a small number of predominately perifascicular fibers (Fig. 14-1). Some scattered CD 68 positive cells were also seen (macrophage marker). A diagnosis of Jo-1–positive dermatomyositis (DM) with heart and lung involvement was made. On further evaluation, including mammography, gynecologic examination, and CT of the abdomen, no sign of malignancy was found. The patient was started on small doses of levothyroxine replacement 4 days after admission. TSH normalized after 4 weeks of treatment with levothyroxine replacement. She was also given methylprednisolone 500 mg IV on 3 consecutive days and then oral prednisolone 50 mg (0.75 mg/kg). Concomitantly she received cyclophosphamide (CyX) pulses, 1000 mg monthly for 6 months. Tapering of prednisolone was started 6 weeks after diagnosis, initially in small decrements of 15% of the daily dosage per month. Six weeks after starting treatment (3 months after the onset of symptoms), muscle weakness had improved according to the FI-2, but the patient still had weakness of the neck flexors. Serum CK had steadily decreased and was now within the normal range (120 μ/L). At 3 months, there was

a further gradual improvement, and muscle function was almost normal as measured by the FI-2. Shortness of breath resolved completely after 4 months. Lung function tests were almost normalized, and a CT thorax showed almost complete regression of interstitial findings at 6 months. At the same time, echocardiography revealed regression of the previously noted cardiac enlargement. Muscle strength was completely normal at 6 months, serum CK had normalized, and a repeat muscle biopsy from the contralateral vastus lateralis muscle showed no inflammatory cell infiltrates and no MHC-1-positive fibers

After 6 months, the patient was on prednisolone 17.5 mg daily and continued tapering by 10% every 3 to 4 weeks. Additionally, she received methotrexate SC starting with 7.5 mg weekly, which was increased to 15 mg/week after 1 month. A carpal tunnel release was performed after 10 months, with resolution of the symptoms. One year after diagnosis, the patient was taking prednisolone 7.5 mg and MTX 15 mg weekly SC, as well as calcium and vitamin D supplementation and alendronic acid 70 mg weekly. She was going on daily walks with her dog for 1 hour and gradually increased to 2 hours. Already during the third week after diagnosis she had started doing home exercises in a myositis-specific training program, which entailed training five times weekly with increasing loads under supervision of a physical therapist (Fig. 14-2), and 1 year later she was still performing these exercises regularly.[3]

The differential diagnosis in this case was hypothyroidism versus DM. The patient had a discrete skin rash and she had symptoms such as fatigue that are common in both diagnoses. We considered the possibility that the patient's hypothyroidism might have caused the muscular symptoms. However, her hypothyroidism was of a mild degree, with T3 and T4 levels being almost normal, and clinical symptoms such as muscle weakness are uncommon in this situation. Patients with hypothyroidism may have changes on muscle biopsy such as type II fiber atrophy, which, however, was not present in this case. On the other hand, MMT did not reveal any muscle weakness, which made a diagnosis of myositis less probable. The FI-2 and muscle biopsy findings, and to a lesser extent the presence of anti-Jo-1 antibodies, elevation of CK level, Gottron's papules, and electrophysiologic changes contributed to a definitive diagnosis of DM in this case. This case illustrates the difficulty in diagnosing inflammatory myopathies if muscle weakness is minor. Pulse CyX therapy in combination with steroids may be an appropriate therapy alternative in some cases of severe polymyositis (PM)/DM. In this case, we chose CyX as second-line therapy because of lung and heart involvement. An important aspect of this case was the short delay between onsets of symptoms and initiation of treatment, which may have contributed to the complete resolution of symptoms. Another instructive aspect of this case is the fact that muscle function as measured by MMT was normal at disease onset, whereas FI-2 showed reduced muscle endurance.

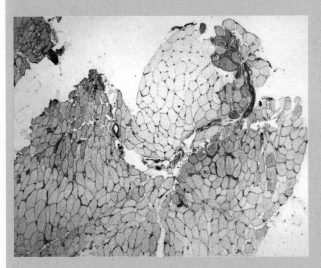

Figure 14-1. The biopsy revealed scattered atrophic muscle fibers and signs of muscle fiber degeneration. Type II fiber atrophy was not present. Major histocompatibility complex (MHC)-1 was upregulated in a small number of predominately perifascicular fibers. (Courtesy of Dr. Sevim Barbasso Helmers.)

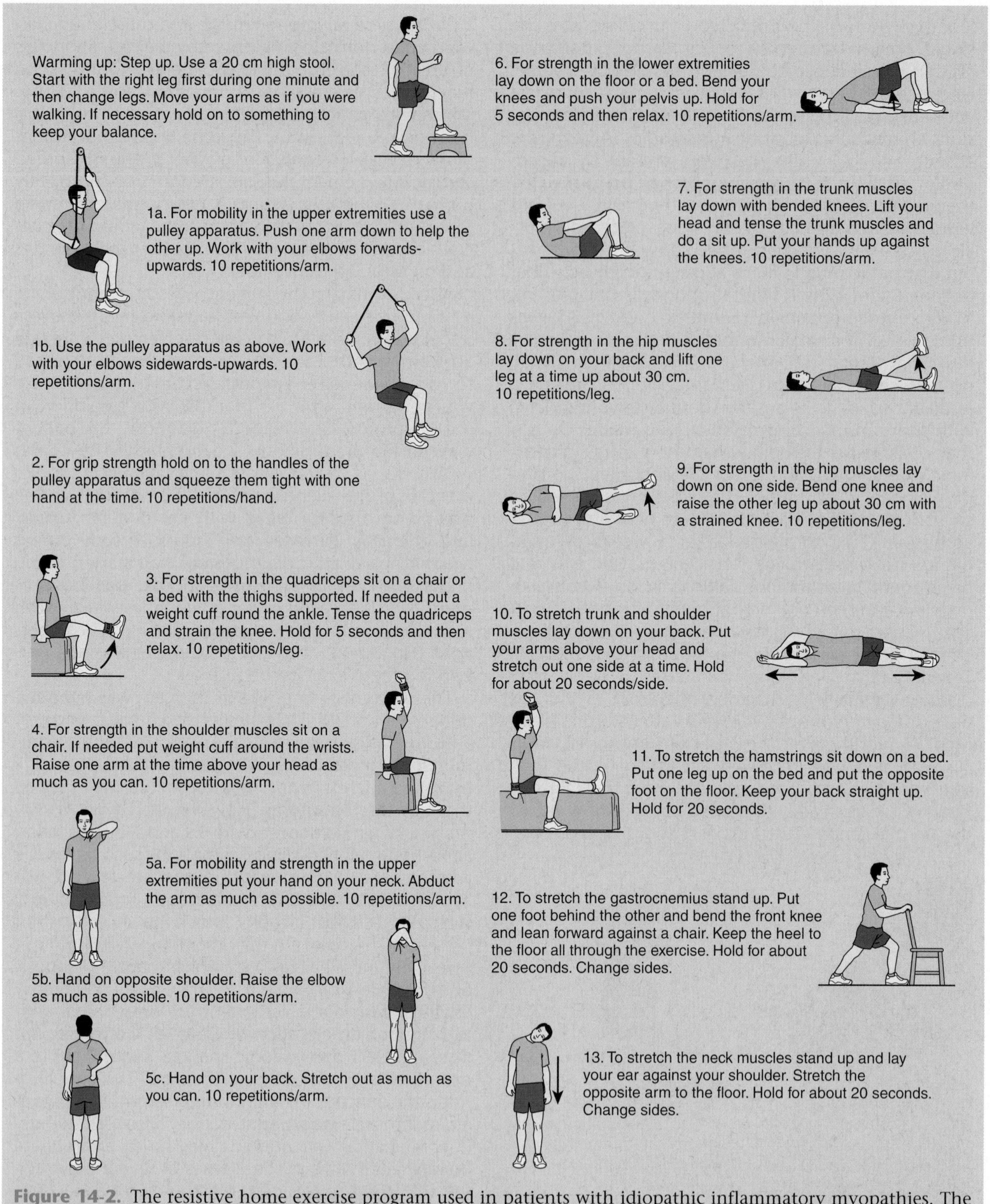

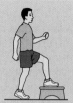

Warming up: Step up. Use a 20 cm high stool. Start with the right leg first during one minute and then change legs. Move your arms as if you were walking. If necessary hold on to something to keep your balance.

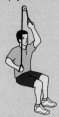

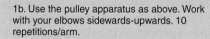

1a. For mobility in the upper extremities use a pulley apparatus. Push one arm down to help the other up. Work with your elbows forwards-upwards. 10 repetitions/arm.

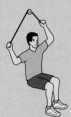

1b. Use the pulley apparatus as above. Work with your elbows sidewards-upwards. 10 repetitions/arm.

2. For grip strength hold on to the handles of the pulley apparatus and squeeze them tight with one hand at the time. 10 repetitions/hand.

3. For strength in the quadriceps sit on a chair or a bed with the thighs supported. If needed put a weight cuff round the ankle. Tense the quadriceps and strain the knee. Hold for 5 seconds and then relax. 10 repetitions/leg.

4. For strength in the shoulder muscles sit on a chair. If needed put weight cuff around the wrists. Raise one arm at the time above your head as much as you can. 10 repetitions/arm.

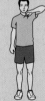

5a. For mobility and strength in the upper extremities put your hand on your neck. Abduct the arm as much as possible. 10 repetitions/arm.

5b. Hand on opposite shoulder. Raise the elbow as much as possible. 10 repetitions/arm.

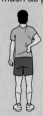

5c. Hand on your back. Stretch out as much as you can. 10 repetitions/arm.

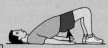

6. For strength in the lower extremities lay down on the floor or a bed. Bend your knees and push your pelvis up. Hold for 5 seconds and then relax. 10 repetitions/arm.

7. For strength in the trunk muscles lay down with bended knees. Lift your head and tense the trunk muscles and do a sit up. Put your hands up against the knees. 10 repetitions/arm.

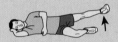

8. For strength in the hip muscles lay down on your back and lift one leg at a time up about 30 cm. 10 repetitions/leg.

9. For strength in the hip muscles lay down on one side. Bend one knee and raise the other leg up about 30 cm with a strained knee. 10 repetitions/leg.

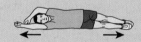

10. To stretch trunk and shoulder muscles lay down on your back. Put your arms above your head and stretch out one side at a time. Hold for about 20 seconds/side.

11. To stretch the hamstrings sit down on a bed. Put one leg up on the bed and put the opposite foot on the floor. Keep your back straight up. Hold for 20 seconds.

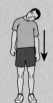

12. To stretch the gastrocnemius stand up. Put one foot behind the other and bend the front knee and lean forward against a chair. Keep the heel to the floor all through the exercise. Hold for about 20 seconds. Change sides.

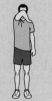

13. To stretch the neck muscles stand up and lay your ear against your shoulder. Stretch the opposite arm to the floor. Hold for about 20 seconds. Change sides.

Figure 14-2. The resistive home exercise program used in patients with idiopathic inflammatory myopathies. The patients performed 10 repetitions in one set per muscle group. (Modified from Alexanderson H. Exercise: An important component of treatment in the idiopathic inflammatory myopathies. Curr Rheumatol Rep 2005;7:115-24.)

INTRODUCTION

The idiopathic inflammatory myopathies (IIM) are systemic connective tissue diseases that are characterized by symmetric, proximal muscle weakness; decreased muscle endurance; and chronic inflammation in muscle tissue.[4,5] They can be subclassified into DM, PM, and inclusion body myositis (IBM) according to differences in clinical as well as histopathologic features.[4-6] DM may occur in both adults and children; in this chapter, however, we focus on the treatment of adult forms of myositis only. Myositis may exist as a disease entity on its own or may be linked to another inflammatory connective tissue disease such as systemic sclerosis or mixed connective tissue disease. Myositis may also be associated with a malignancy; this is particularly true for DM, whereas the association with PM is more controversial.[7] The IIMs are a somewhat heterogenous group of disorders, which is also reflected in their different responses to immunosuppressive therapies. Many studies have used Bohan and Peter criteria and the Griggs criteria for IBM to subgroup the patients.[8-10] Although these are the most frequently used diagnostic criteria, they have some limitations because even the subgroups PM or DM are not always homogeneous, with differences in response to treatment. Thus, there is a need for revised classification criteria to augment future studies of disease mechanisms.

Most patients with PM or DM present with subacute or slowly progressive proximal muscle weakness that is usually symmetric and represents a major source of disability for these patients.[3] They often experience difficulty raising the head when supine, lifting, carrying, climbing steps, dressing, and even walking on flat ground. Many patients need to use the handrail on stairways as a means of pulling themselves up. The patients also typically experience low muscle endurance, and their muscles are easily fatigued. As an example, they may be able to walk up one set of stairs, but then they cannot lift their legs any more and have to rest. The flexor muscles of the neck are affected more than the extensors. The musculature of the trunk can also be affected, which leads to difficulty in arising from supine positions. In contrast, the facial musculature is generally spared. Muscle pain is less common than muscle weakness and fatigue. Typically, the main discomfort arises after a workload and is often expressed by the patients as a sensation of "lactic acid in their legs."

IBM causes weakness and atrophy of distal and proximal muscles; involvement of quadriceps muscles and deep finger flexors are often clues to the diagnosis.[11] Patients often present with falls because their knees collapse due to quadriceps muscle weakness, or they have difficulty performing certain tasks such as turning keys owing to weakness of finger flexors. Neck flexors and extensors are frequently affected. Dysphagia occurs in up to 60% of patients with IBM, leading to choking episodes. Facial muscle weakness is not common, and extraocular muscles are not affected. Sensory function is usually normal.

The tendon reflexes, although preserved early in the disease, can diminish in the late stages as atrophy of major muscle groups becomes evident. Disease progression is slow but steady and resembles that of a muscular dystrophy. Most patients with IBM require an assistive device, such as a walker or wheelchair, within several years of onset.[12] IBM patients rarely have muscle pain.

The IIM are chronic disorders in most cases and up to two thirds of patients develop sustained functional impairment.[13,14] Several immunosuppressive treatments are available for the inflammatory myopathies, yet for many patients, recovery is incomplete.[15,16] Lifelong immunosuppressive therapy is often required, adverse side effects are common, and more effective therapies with fewer side effects are needed.[17]

EXTRAMUSCULAR MANIFESTATIONS

Extramuscular manifestations are common features in IIM. The most common extramuscular manifestations are from skin, affecting all with DM and some with PM. In both PM and in DM the lungs, joints, gastrointestinal (GI) channel, and heart may be affected, indicating that IIMs are systemic inflammatory diseases. They also frequently co-occur with other defined rheumatologic diseases such as systemic sclerosis, Sjögren's syndrome, and mixed connective tissue disease and less often with systemic lupus erythematosus (SLE) or rheumatoid arthritis. IBM is usually evident as an isolated muscle disease, although there are reports of an association with Sjögren's syndrome.[18]

PULMONARY DISEASE

Pulmonary complications constitute important clinical manifestations of DM or PM. The lungs may be involved either primarily with inflammation in the lung tissue, ILD, or as a complication of muscle weakness. Pulmonary involvement as a complication of PM or DM was primarily described by Hepper et al,[19] aspiration pneumonia, ventilatory insufficiency and interstitial pneumonia being the three most important types of associated lung involvement.[19] Interstitial pneumonia or ILD can be a serious complication of PM or DM. The reported prevalence of pulmonary involvement in PM or DM varies between 5% and 46% in cross-sectional studies, depending on whether clinical, radiologic, functional, or pathologic criteria have been used.[20,21] According to a recent reported prospective study, ILD is a common (65%) early manifestation in patients with PM or DM and is not always related to clinical symptoms.[22] The presence of ILD in patients with myositis affects the prognosis, with increased morbidity and mortality, and this often also has an influence on the choice of immunosuppressive treatment.

CUTANEOUS MANIFESTATIONS

Dermatologic manifestations usually precede the onset of muscle disease, and patients may experience significant cutaneous symptoms; however, studies of DM severity have historically focused with greater attention on the muscle disease.[8,9] The characteristic and possibly pathognomonic cutaneous features of DM are the heliotrope rash and Gottron's papules (Fig. 14-3). The heliotrope rash is composed of a violaceous erythematous rash with or without edema in a symmetric distribution involving the periorbital skin. Sometimes this sign is subtle and may involve only a mild discoloration along the eyelid margin. At other times, massive edema may develop. A heliotrope rash is rarely observed in patients with lupus erythematosus or scleroderma. Gottron's papules are present over bony prominences, particularly the metacarpophalangeal joints, the proximal interphalangeal joints, and the distal interphalangeal joints. They may also be found overlying the elbows, knees, and feet. These lesions consist of slightly elevated, violaceous papules and plaques. There may be a slight scale on some occasions. Within the lesions, there is often telangiectasia. These lesions may be clinically confused with lesions of SLE.

Skin calcinosis is a disabling complication, most commonly evident in children or young adults. Hard yellow nodules can arise over bony prominences. The deposits of calcium may erupt onto the skin surface and be the sites of secondary infection.

HEART INVOLVEMENT

Clinically manifest heart problems are relatively infrequent in patients with PM or DM. Subclinical cardiac involvement is more common and the frequency varies depending on the methods used. ECG changes are most common, and ECG abnormalities were observed in 32.5% to 72% of patients.[23,24] ECG abnormalities observed in PM and DM patients include atrial and ventricular arrhythmias, bundle branch block, AV blocks, high-grade heart block, prolongation of PR intervals, ventricular premature beats, left atrial abnormality, abnormal Q waves, as well as nonspecific ST-T wave changes. In the absence of controlled studies, it is still uncertain whether these manifestations are more frequent in the IIM than in an age- and gender-matched population.

GASTROINTESTINAL INVOLVEMENT

The most common GI symptom is dysphagia, caused by the weakness of the pharynx or esophagus and disordered esophageal motility. Esophageal dysfunction occurs in 15% to 50% of patients.

OTHER EXTRAMUSCULAR MANIFESTATIONS

Constitutional symptoms, such as fatigue and fever, often precede or accompany flares of disease and usually respond to glucocorticoids. Weight loss

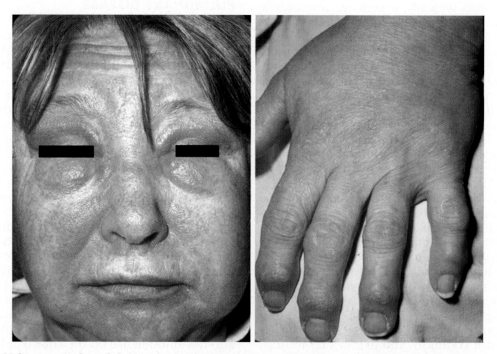

Figure 14-3. Heliotrope rash and Gottron's papules in a patient with severe dermatomyositis.

may relate to impaired swallowing. Raynaud's phenomenon is common and can often be managed by calcium channel blockers. Joint symptoms, which are nonerosive and involve both small and large joints, can improve by treatment with glucocorticoids.

TREATMENT

Pharmacologic Treatment

The treatment of the IIM is still largely empirical. Idiopathic inflammatory myopathies are rare diseases, and there are few randomized prospective clinical studies that have compared different methods of treatment (Table 14-2). Many studies of pharmacologic intervention have included a patient mix of acute and chronic disease. Spontaneous recovery from IIM has rarely been reported.[25] Patients with DM or PM respond to treatment differently than patients with IBM or myositis associated with another connective tissue disease. Assessment of therapeutic interventions is also limited owing to a lack of standardized methods for assessing IIM; this not only limits the ability of clinicians to evaluate therapeutic responses in individual patients, but also hinders interpretation of the few trials that have been conducted. During the past 30 years, there have been 24 prospective studies of treatments of adult myositis. Few of these were blinded and/or controlled trials (see Table 14-2). In addition to confirming the diagnosis and assessing extramuscular manifestations, defining disease activity by assessing changes in muscle strength is critical for managing the patient with IIM.

The primary aim for treatment of myositis is to improve muscle function. There are only a few treatment studies in which investigations of repeated muscle biopsies has been included as an outcome measure.[26-32] Thus, the molecular effect on muscle inflammation of most immunosuppressive drugs used today is largely unknown.

Investigations for Assessment of Treatment

Clinicians need to measure disease activity and to differentiate disease activity from chronic, irreversible changes that cause disability. The currently used diagnostic tools, muscle biopsy, elevation of serum enzyme activity, such as CK, and electrophysiologic investigation, have various limitations.[8,9] The most frequently used assessments for therapeutic responses are clinical evaluation of muscle strength and serum muscle enzyme activity.[13,22] Recently, magnetic resonance imaging (MRI) has been investigated as a possible tool for both diagnostic purposes and for assessment of disease activity.[33] Importantly, reduction of muscle function can be the result of both active muscle inflammation and of chronic changes, and therefore, any measurement of muscle function must be combined with assessments that reflect active muscle inflammation.[34]

The MMT has been used in trials to assess isometric muscle strength in myositis.[35-37] However, in patients with mild impairment, the MMT had limited reliability.[38] Another limitation of this measurement (and related ones) is that they measure strength, whereas patients with PM and DM often report impaired muscle endurance rather than, or in addition to, muscle weakness. The FI in myositis was the first functional impairment outcome measure developed specifically for patients with PM and DM.[39] The FI is based on repetitive movements involving selected muscle groups to capture decreased muscle endurance; it was validated as reliable regarding its ability to discriminate patients from healthy individuals. The FI is useful in assessing patients with moderate to severe impairment[3,40] but it has some ceiling and floor effects. A revised version, the FI-2, which also measures muscle endurance, has no ceiling or floor effects, and possesses satisfactory construct validity and interrater and intrarater reliability. It is not time consuming to administer, is well tolerated by patients with all stages of disease, and does not require any expensive equipment or formal training (see Table 14-1).[1] We recommend this measure for use in routine clinical care and clinical research. The disease-specific questionnaire Myositis Activities Profile (MAP) was developed in Sweden to assess limitations in activities of daily living and is valid for patients with PM and DM.[41] However, a possible limitation of a predefined questionnaire is that all questions might not be relevant for all patients. Therefore the MacMaster Toronto Arthritis Patient Preference Questionnaire (MACTAR), which was originally developed for arthritis patients, was validated for patients with PM and DM.[42] The MACTAR focuses on activities that are limited and important to improve for each individual and also contains questions about other aspects of health. The short form 36 (SF-36) is a generic questionnaire assessing quality of life that has been proven useful for myositis patients.[3,40,43]

Muscle Biopsy

Muscle biopsy is the gold standard for diagnosis of the IIM.[44] Obtaining a muscle specimen for histopathologic study is an important component of the diagnostic evaluation for most suspected myopathies. Histopathologic evaluation of muscle biopsies is also important to exclude other myopathies and to identify subsets of IIM. A muscle biopsy technique that allows for repeated biopsies is important to assess the effect of treatment at the tissue level. One such muscle biopsy technique is the percutaneous conchotome biopsy or the semiopen muscle biopsy.[2] This method has become widely used in Sweden and other Scandinavian countries, including our rheumatology clinic, during the past 20 years for both diagnostic and research purposes, but has received little attention outside Scandinavia. The percutaneous conchotome muscle biopsy technique gives a good size sample that allows for diagnostic evaluation and has a high

Table 14-2. *Prospective Treatment Studies in Adult Patients with Polymyositis, Dermatomyositis, and Inclusion Body Myositis*

Study	Design	Diagnosis	Number of Patients	Treatment	Effect of Therapy	Muscle Biopsy	Muscle Function Method
Bunch et al 1980[26]	Prospective, randomized, Double blind	PM/DM	16	Azathioprine/prednisolone versus placebo/prednisolone	Moderate, No difference between groups	Before/after	MMT
Bunch 1981[55]	Follow up after 3-year, uncontrolled	PM/DM	16	Azathioprine/prednisolone versus placebo/prednisolone	Study group require less pred	No	MMT
Cronin et al 1989[62]	Prospective open label	PM/DM/IBM	11	Monthly IV cyclophosphamide	No effect	No	MMT
Cherin et al 1991[67]	Prospective open label	PM/DM	20	Monthly IVIG	Good effect	No	MMT
Miller et al 1992[96]	Prospective, double-blind	PM/DM	42	Plasma exchange versus leukopheresis versus sham apheresis	No effect	No	MMT
Dalakas et al 1993[30]	Prospective, double-blind Placebo controlled, cross over	DM	15	Monthly IVIG	Good effect Prior study group	Before/after	MMT
Barohn et al 1995[32]	Prospective open label	IBM	8	Prednisolone	No effect	Yes	MMT
Leff et al 1993[97]	Prospective open label, cross over	IBM	11	Oral methotrexate/azathioprine versus biweekly methotrexate IV	No effect	No	MMT
Cherin et al 1995[98]	Prospective, open label	PM/DM	57	Plasma exchange	No effect	No	MMT
Villalba et al 1998[60]	Prospective randomized open label, cross over	PM/DM	30	Oral methotrexate/azathioprine versus biweekly intravenous methotrexate	Combination treatment prior	No	MMT
Adams et al 1999[99]	Prospective open label	PM/DM	16	Intravenous fludarabine	Moderate effect in subgroup	No	MMT
Oddis et al 1999[100]	Prospective, open label	IIM		Oral tacrolimus		No	MMT
Muscle study group 2001[101]	Prospective, randomized controlled	IBM	30	β INF	No effect No difference between groups	No	MMT, MVICT
Venkovsky et al 2000[66]	Prospective, randomized controlled	PM/DM	36	Cyclosporine A versus methotrexate	Methotrexate prior cyclosporine	No	MEFT

Table 14-2. *Prospective Treatment Studies in Adult Patients with Polymyositis, Dermatomyositis, and Inclusion Body Myositis—Cont'd*

Study	Design	Diagnosis	Number of Patients	Treatment	Effect of Therapy	Muscle Biopsy	Muscle Function Method
Danieli et al 2002[102]	Prospective, open label	PM/DM	20	Cyclosporine A/prednisolone versus cyclosporine A/prednisolone/IVIG/plasma exchange	Cyclosporine A/prednisolone/IVIG/prior plasma exchange no effect	No	MMT
Levine et al 2005[79]	Prospective open label pilot	DM	6	Rituximab	Good	Yes baseline	MMT
Badrising et al 2002[59]	Prospective randomized double-blind placebo-controlled	IBM	44	Methotrexate	No effect	No	MMT
Lindberg et al 2003[103]	Prospective, open label randomized	IBM	11	ATG versus methotrexate	ATG group prior	Before/after	MMT
Barohn et al, 2006[78]	Prospective open label pilot	IBM	9	Eternacept	No effect	No	MMT
Chung et al 2007[82]	Prospective open label	DM	8	Rituximab	Moderate	No	MMT
Mok et al 2007[80]	Prospective open label	PM	4	Rituximab	Moderate	No	MMT
Barbasso et al 2007[31]	Prospective open label	PM/DM, IBM	13	Monthly IVIG	No effect on myopathy	Before/after	FI
Hengstman et al 2008[73]	Prospective open label	PM/DM	6	Infliximab	No effect	No	MMT
Dastmalchi et al 2008[95]	Prospective open label pilot	PM/DM, IBM	13	Infliximab	No effect	Before/after	FI, MMT

ATG, anti-T-lymphocyte globulin; β INF, beta-interferon; DM, dermatomyositis; FI, functional index; IBM, inclusion body myositis; IIM, idiopathic inflammatory myopathies; IVIG, intravenous immune globulin; MEFT, muscle endurance functional testing; MMT, manual muscle testing; MVICT, maximum voluntary isometric contraction testing; PM, polymyositis.

yield in patients with myositis.[45] It is a simple procedure and is easy to learn and to perform, with a low complication rate and minimum discomfort for the patient.[2,46] The method can preferably be used as a diagnostic tool and repeated biopsies can help assess the effect of a given therapy for both clinical and research purposes. The percutaneous conchotome muscle biopsy technique is a sensitive method to simply and safely make diagnostic evaluations and to assess the effect of a given therapy on muscle tissue in patients with idiopathic inflammatory myopathies.[45,46] This semiopen biopsy technique can easily be performed by the rheumatologist in an outpatient clinic with a very low complication rate, and could be included as a tool for assessment of disease activity in clinical trials.[46] The problem with 'skip lesions' could be reduced by taking several biopsies from the same incision.[45] Another way to overcome this problem is to use MRI to select an appropriate site for muscle to be biopsied.[47] Further knowledge of disease pathogenesis and the effect of treatment at the molecular level could be obtained by performing repeated muscle biopsies and by correlating histologic findings with clinical outcome.

Various methods for sampling muscle tissue are available, and each has advantages and disadvantages. An open biopsy generally harvests the largest amount of tissue and can be performed on numerous muscles, but this technique is invasive and gives a large scar. Conversely, needle biopsy has become or is becoming the standard method of muscle biopsy at some institutions in North America, Europe, and elsewhere in the world.[48] Needle biopsy can be performed rapidly and is less invasive and less expensive, but the disadvantage is the smaller amounts of tissue per sample.

Glucocorticoids

The generally recommended treatment for DM and PM consists of glucocorticoids in high doses for the initial few months, with or without other immunosuppressive therapies.[4,50,51] Placebo-controlled trials of glucocorticoid treatment have never been performed, and therefore, the optimal initial dosage of glucocorticoids, as well as duration of treatment, is uncertain. In retrospective studies, improved muscle function was observed with an initial dose corresponding to prednisone 40 to 60 mg/day in 60% to 80% of the patients assessed by the MMT or by one of several muscle function scales.[8,9,13,52] It is notable that although a majority of patients improved, a complete recovery rate was reported in only 24% to 43%.

Lundberg and associates[53] examined muscle biopsies obtained from 10 patients with PM or DM before and after 12 to 24 weeks of treatment with prednisolone, 0.75 mg/kg/day. Strength improved in seven patients. Important changes were observed in the follow-up muscle biopsies, including a significant decrease in the expression of MHC-1 antigens on muscle cells. The major issue with the use of glucocorticoids to treat IIM is, of course, the development of significant side effects. Indeed, in studies of long-term outcomes of patients with IIM, steroid-induced side effects are major causes of disability.[54] In IBM, the results of several uncontrolled trials of glucocorticoids have shown stabilization or temporary improvement in muscle strength in some patients; however, these improvements are not usually maintained.[32] In a prospective trial of high-dose prednisolone for up to 12 months in eight patients with IBM muscle strength continued to deteriorate despite a fall in the serum CK concentrations, and repeat muscle biopsies showed an increase in the numbers of vacuolated and amyloid-containing fibers, despite a reduction in the numbers of T cells.[32] Thus, the bulk of the evidence does not support the use of glucocorticoids in most patients with IBM.

Immunosuppressive Agents

Although most patients with PM or DM respond, at least partially, to glucocorticoids, about 30% of patients do not respond at all.[13] Moreover, in a long-term follow-up study, a substantial number of patients developed increased disability with time owing to the side effects of glucocorticoid treatment.[17]

Several immunosuppressive agents have been reported both as steroid-sparing agents as well as being beneficial in patients who are steroid resistant, but few controlled therapeutic trials have been performed. Azathioprin (AZA) was reported to have a steroid-sparing effect as well as a favorable effect on clinical function compared with prednisone alone in a placebo-controlled trial.[26,55] However, treatment with AZA for 3 months did not have any impact on inflammation in the muscle as assessed by muscle biopsy (see Table 14-2).[26]

Retrospective studies, open prospective studies, and case reports have indicated a positive effect of MTX on muscle function in steroid-resistant patients with DM/PM,[56,57] but there have been no prospective controlled studies of this agent. The doses of MTX varied between 7.5 and 25 mg/week administered orally or IM, or up to 100 mg/week IV. In an additional open retrospective study, male patients with myositis with Jo-1 antibodies with incomplete clinical response to glucocorticoids were reported to have a more favorable clinical response to additional treatment with MTX compared with AZA.[58] In a randomized double-blind placebo-controlled study, 44 patients with IBM were treated with MTX. Quantitative muscle strength testing scores declined in both treatment groups but less so while on active treatment. This difference was not significant. There were no differences in MMT total scores, activity scale scores, and patients' own assessments after treatment. CK decreased significantly in the MTX group. The conclusion was that oral MTX did not slow the progression of muscle weakness.[59] In a prospective, randomized study, the combination of oral MTX with AZA was compared with high-dose intravenous MTX with leucovorin rescue. Both groups of patients with treatment-resistant PM/DM experienced modest improvements, but without a significant difference between the two treatments.[60]

The efficacy of CyX in IIM is unclear. In one open-label study, some patients were reported to benefit from daily oral CyX,[61] whereas IV pulse CyX was reported to be ineffective in another open study.[62]

There are a few reports of beneficial effects of cyclosporin A (CyA), mainly in treatment-resistant adult PM and DM cases.[63,64] In one open-label study of adult DM, CyA was reported to be beneficial as a first-line drug without corticosteroids.[65] Another controlled trial was conducted by Vencovsky and colleagues.[66] They investigated effectiveness and tolerance of treatment with CyA or MTX added to glucocorticoids in patients with severe, active PM and DM. Administration of MTX or CyA added to glucocorticoids was associated with clinical and laboratory improvement. Changes in CK and interleukin-1 receptor anatagonist (IL-1Ra) levels were not associated with parameters of clinical disease severity measured in this study. No patient recovered completely.

Intravenously administered high dosages of immunoglobulins (IVIG) are used in various autoimmune diseases, including the IIM. In a placebo-controlled trial, high-dose IVIG was beneficial in treatment-resistant DM patients, both regarding muscle function and muscle histopathology.[30] The therapeutic mechanisms of IVIG in DM are not known. Although the clinical effects were accompanied by decreased intercellular adhesion molecule 1 (ICAM-1) and MHC class I expression in repeat muscle biopsies, the number of patients that were subject to a repeat biopsy was small. The effect of IVIG in PM patients was less certain.[67] High doses of IVIG are usually well tolerated, but a drawback of high-dose IVIG treatment is the high cost. We performed an open, prospective trial in 13 treatment-resistant patients (six with PM, four with DM, two with IBM, and one adult person with juvenile-onset DM) who had signs of persistently active inflammatory disease.[31] The patients were treated with IVIG 2 g/kg 3 times at monthly intervals. Clinical evaluations as well as FI,[39] CK levels, and muscle biopsies were performed before treatment and after the third IVIG infusion in all subjects. Additional biopsies were taken 24 to 48 hours after the first infusion for molecular studies. Improved muscle function as measured by FI was recorded in three patients (one with PM, one with DM, and one with IBM), and CK levels decreased by more than 50% in five out of nine individuals with elevated levels, but median CK levels were not changed. Skin rash improved in three of four patients with DM. T cells, macrophages, MHC class I antigen on muscle fibers, IL-1, ICAM-1, and vascular cell adhesion molecule 1 (VCAM-1) expression and membranolytic attack complex (MAC)-deposits on capillaries were present to an equal degree in biopsies before and after IVIG treatment (Fig. 14-4). The relative frequency of muscle fiber type I and type II fibers was unchanged. High-grade muscle inflammation persisted after treatment in all patients. No correlation was seen between the clinical response and changes in proinflammatory molecules or fiber type characteristics. We concluded that the effects of IVIG treatment in IIM are limited.

Biologic Treatments

A few case reports have suggested beneficial effects of two different tumor necrosis factor (TNF) blockers in PM or DM.[34,68-72] A multicenter, prospective, open-label, controlled trial with infliximab combined with MTX in patients with recent-onset PM and DM was terminated prematurely because of a low inclusion rate and a high drop-out rate due to disease progression and the occurrence of infusion reactions.[73] The few patients who did reach the primary endpoint showed improvement in all aspects studied. We performed an open-label pilot study with infliximab in 13 patients with IIM. The patients received four infusions of infliximab combined with MTX or AZA. Muscle biopsies and MRI were performed at baseline and after four infusions. Clinical assessments included the disease activity core set proposed by The International Myositis Assessment and Clinical Studies Group (IMACS) including the MMT,[74,75] and serum levels of CK and lactate dehydrogenase (LD). Muscle impairment was also assessed by FI.[39] Clinical improvement was defined according to the proposal of IMACS as 20% improvement in three or more of the core set parameters and no more than two worsened by 25% (and not including MMT).[74-76] Worsening was defined by 30% reduction in any three of six variables of the IMACS core set disease activity measure.[77] Nine patients completed the study. Three patients discontinued due to adverse events and one due to a discovered malignancy. Three of the completers improved by 20% in three or more variables of the disease activity core set, four were unchanged and two worsened 30%. No patient improved in muscle strength by manual muscle test. At baseline, two completers had signs of muscle inflammation by MRI, and five at follow-up (Fig. 14-5). T lymphocytes, macrophages, cytokine expression, and MAC deposition in muscle biopsies were still evident after treatment. Type I interferon (IFN) activity was increased after treatment. Thus, anti-TNF treatment with infliximab was not effective in patients with myositis that was previously resistant to conventional immunosuppressive treatment. The clinical flares, signs of increased muscle inflammation on MRI scans, and the increase in type I IFN activity in the circulation and locally in muscle tissue suggest that infliximab could worsen muscle inflammation and that TNF blockade may not be appropriate for patients with treatment-resistant myositis. A pilot trial of the TNF-blocker etanercept in patients with IBM did not yield an improvement in composite muscle strength scores at 6 months, although there was a slight improvement in grip strength after 12 months of treatment.[78]

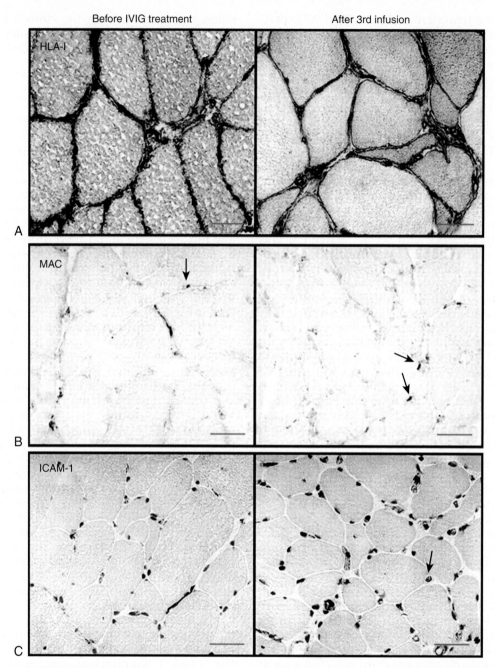

Before IVIG treatment   After 3rd infusion

HLA-I

MAC

A

B

ICAM-1

C

Figure 14-4. A, Major histocompatibility complex class I antigen expression on the muscle fiber membrane and sarco-plasma of the muscle fibers (*brown staining*) before intravenous immunoglobulin (IVIG) treatment remained unchanged in the repeat biopsies (patient 12, inclusion body myositis). **B,** Membranolytic attack complex (MAC) deposits in the capillaries (*arrows, brown staining*) before IVIG treatment remained unchanged in the repeat biopsies (patient 6, poly-myositis). **C,** Intercellular adhesion molecule-1 (ICAM-1) expression in capillaries (*arrow, red staining*) and inflammatory cells remained unchanged in the repeat biopsies (patient 9, dermatomyositis). Scale bar = 50 μm (original magnification ×250). (With permission from Helmers SB, Dastmalchi M, Alexanderson H, Nennesmo I, Esbjörnsson M, Lindvall B, et al. Limited effects of high-dose intravenous immunoglobulin (IVIG) treatment on molecular expression in muscle tissue of patients with inflammatory myopathies. Ann Rheum Dis 2007;66:1276-83.)

Rituximab, an anti-CD20 monoclonal anti-body that specifically depletes B-lineage lympho-cytes and has been approved for the treatment of B-cell lymphomas and rheumatoid arthritis, has also been studied in patients with PM and DM. A generally favorable effect has been reported in several uncontrolled trials. Thus, in an open-label uncontrolled trial of rituximab, seven patients with DM received four intravenous infusions of ritux-imab given at weekly intervals on days 1, 8, 15, and 22.[79] Muscle function, as measured by MMT, improved in all patients. Rituximab was well tol-erated in this small patient group. In another open trial, four adult patients with active PM were

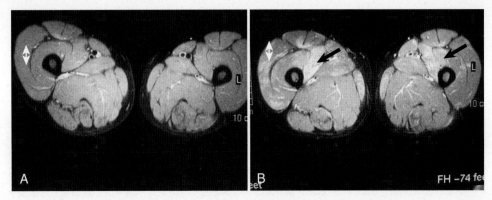

Figure 14-5. Magnetic resonance imaging scan of thigh muscles in a patient with polymyositis before **(A)** and after **(B)** infliximab treatment. New changes were seen after treatment visualized as increased signals (*arrows*). The sequences acquired were axial spin echo T1-weighted images, short tau inversion recovery (STIR) images, and spin echo T1-weighted images with fat suppression. (Reproduced with permission from Annals of Rheumatic Disease, the Eular Journal.)

included.[80] Although immunosuppressive agents were continued, rituximab (375 mg/m²) was given by intravenous infusion weekly for 4 consecutive weeks. Patients were followed every 4 weeks with serial assessment of muscle strength, serum muscle enzymes, physician's and patient's global impression of disease activity, disability, and quality-of-life scores. Significant improvement in the mean proximal muscle strength and reduction in CK levels in comparison to baseline were observed. Two patients had return of full muscle strength with significant drops in CK level. In another study, three patients with PM/DM received intravenous rituximab 1000 mg on days 0 and 14 on background prednisone plus MTX or AZA.[81] A normalization of CK levels was observed at 1 month postinfusion. Muscle strength improved in all three patients and returned to normal in two. The average daily prednisone dose decreased from 16.7 mg (range 10–20 mg) to 4 mg (range 0–7 mg) after treatment, and the MTX dose was tapered by 50% in 2 patients. The third patient eventually discontinued all additional therapies. A return of clinical symptoms with an elevated CK occurred in two patients at 6 and 10 months postinfusion, respectively; both patients were retreated with rituximab. The third patient remains disease free 12 months after initial treatment. Rituximab does not appear to be effective for dermatitis in patients with DM.[82]

Nonpharmacologic Therapy

Exercise

Historically patients with idiopathic inflammatory myopathies were discouraged from physical exercise due to fear of increased muscle inflammation. However, scientific evidence accumulating during the last 15 years supports the role of exercise as part of treatment in patients with adult inflammatory myopathies.

Most studies of exercise have evaluated safety and efficacy in patients with PM or DM. In a randomized, controlled exercise trial, patients with chronic, long-standing disease improved their aerobic capacity and muscle strength by 6-week cycling and step-up exercises on 65% of their maximal oxygen uptake compared with the control group without sustained increases in serum CK levels (Table 14-3).[37,84] A group of 10 patients with chronic long-standing PM or DM with stable disease activity and medication performed a resistance home exercise program resulting in improved muscle endurance and self-perceived health without signs of increased muscle inflammation assessed by muscle biopsies, MRI, or analysis of serum CK levels.[3] The 20-minute exercise program contained exercises against gravity or additional loads using weight cuffs for deltoids, neck flexors, quadriceps, hip flexors, abductors and extensors, and trunk muscles. The patients performed the home exercise program with additional 15-minute walks 5 days a week (see Fig. 14-2). A group of patients with active, recent-onset disease performed the same home exercise program without showing any signs of increased muscle inflammation, and having improved muscle function and quality of life.[40] Although this was an open-label study allowing concurrent tapering of the initial high-dose glucocorticoids treatment, the results clearly support the safety of exercise in early-onset disease. The same home exercise program was also studied in combination with creatine supplements in one of the largest randomized controlled double-blinded trials performed to date in the IIM. Thirty-seven patients with long-standing PM/DM were included and randomized into a creatine group and a control group.[85] All patients exercised 5 days a week for 5 months.[3] The creatine group improved significantly compared with the control group regarding physical capacity, muscle endurance, and muscle strength. The control group also improved significantly in muscle endurance. The creatine group showed an increased content of the phosphocreatine/β-nucleoside ratio compared with the control group. Similarly, dynamic exercise in combination with spa treatments was also

Table 14-3. *Exercise Studies in Adult Patients with Inflammatory Myopathies*

Study/Design	Patients (n)	Diagnosis	Disease Activity	Type of Exercise	Load/Intensity % of Max	Outcome Safety	Results Safety	Outcome Benefits	Results Benefits
Hicks et al Case report, 1993[36]	1	PM	Chronic	Isometric muscular	60	CPK	0	Isometric peak torque	+
Escalante et al Open study, 1993[35]	5	PM/DM	Active	Dynamic muscular	NR	CPK	0	Isometric peak torque	+
Spector et al Open study, 1997[90]	5	IBM	Chronic	Dynamic muscular	10–20 VRM	CPK Muscle biopsy	0 0	Isometric peak torque	0 +
Alexanderson et al Open study, 1999[3]	10	PM/DM	Chronic	Dynamic muscular	NR	CPK Mucle biopsy MRI	0	Muscle endurance (FI) Muscle fiber composition SF-36	+ + +
Wiesinger et al Randomized controlled, 1998[37]	14	PM/DM	Chronic	Aerobic	60	CPK	0	$VO2_{peak}$ Isometric peak torque	+ +
Wiesinger et al Controlled 1998[84]	13	PM/DM	Chronic	Aerobic	60	CPK	0	$VO2_{peak}$ Isometric peak torque Activity limitation (FASQ)	+ + +
Alexanderson et al Open study, 2000[40]	11	PM/DM	Active	Muscular dynamic	NR	CPK Muscle biopsy MRI	0 0 0	Muscle endurance (FI) SF-36	+ +
Heikkila et al Open study, 2001[86]	22	PM/DM/IBM	Chronic	Muscular dynamic	NR	CPK	0	Muscle endurance (FI) Activity limitation	+ 0
Varju et al Open study, 2003[87]	19	PM/DM	Chronic/ active	Muscular dynamic	NR	CPK	0	Isometric peak torque Forced vital capacity Activity limitation (HAQ)	+ + +
Arnardottir et al Open study, 2003[41]	7	IBM	Chronic	Muscular dynamic	NR	CPK Muscle biopsy	0 0	Isokinetic peak torque Muscle endurance (FI)	0 0

Table 14-3. *Exercise Studies in Adult Patients with Inflammatory Myopathies—Cont'd*

Study/Design	Patients (n)	Diagnosis	Disease Activity	Type of Exercise	Load/Intensity % of Max	Outcome Safety	Results Safety	Outcome Benefits	Results Benefits
Harris-Love et al Case report, 2005[104]	1	PM/IBM?	Chronic	Muscular dynamic	70	CPK Pain (VAS) ROM	0 0	Isometric peak torque	+
Chung et al Randomized, controlled double-blind study, 2007[85]	37	PM/DM	Chronic	Muscular dynamic	NR	CPK MRS Pain	0 + 0	Functional capacity (AFPT) Muscle endurance (FI) Muscle strength (MMT) Perceived health (NHP) Depression/anxiety	+ + + 0 0
Alexanderson et al Open study, repeated measures, 2007[88]	8	PM/DM	Chronic	Muscular dynamic	70	CPK Muscle biopsy Six-item core set	0 0 +(+)*	Muscle strength (10 VRM) Muscle endurance (FI-2) Activity limit (MAP) Participation restriction (VAS)	+ + 0(±)†

*Statistically significant improvement on group level as well as responders with decreased disease activity according to minimal clinically important criteria suggested by IMACS (ref);
†Unchanged group level with individual improvement and deterioration according to minimal clinically relevant criteria for improvement and deterioration according to Paulus et al (ref);
+, statistically significant improvement on group level; 0, unchanged group level; AFPT, aggregate functional performance time is a total score of measures; timed up and go, walking 15 feet, ascending descending 9 stair steps; DM, dermatomyosits; FASQ, Functional Assessment Screening Questionnaire; FI, Functional Index in myositis; HAQ, Stanford Health Assessment Questionnaire; IBM, inclusion body myositis; MAP, myositis activities profile; MMT, manual muscle test; NHP, Nottingham Health Profile; PM, polymyositis; ROM, range of motion; SF-36, short form 36-item questionnaire; VAS, visual analog scale; VO2_peak, maximal oxygen uptake; VRM, voluntary repetition maximum.

reported to be safe in patients with both active and chronic PM/DM.[86,87] Recently, an open repeated-measures design study reported improved muscle strength and endurance by an intensive resistance training program in a group of eight patients with long-standing PM/DM.[88] The patients exercised on a load of 10 voluntary repetitions maximum (VRM), allowing only 10 repetitions in each set, 3 days a week for 7 weeks. There were no signs of increased muscle inflammation assessed by muscle biopsies and serum CK levels. To the contrary, these patients had reduced extramuscular disease activity following the exercise program compared with baseline. Data were also analyzed individually according to responder criteria for disease activity[76] and disability.[89] Two patients were responders with reduced disease activity, and all patients were responders with at least 20% improved muscle strength and endurance.

Only two studies have focused on the effects of exercise in patients with IBM. One of these employed a resistance training program on a load of approximately five VRM and reported statistically significant improvements in all trained muscle groups. However, only minor changes with questionable clinical relevance was achieved in much affected muscle groups such as the quadriceps, whereas larger improvements were seen in less affected muscle groups such as the hamstrings and gluteus.[90] The other study employed the resistance home exercise program, but it did not detect any significant changes in muscle function.[91]

These few studies included a limited number of patients with PM or DM but they all came to the same conclusion: exercise is safe and beneficial. The role of exercise in patients with inclusion body myositis is more uncertain, although some data suggest that it is not harmful. There is an urgent need for larger randomized controlled trials, also including patients with IBM, to further increase knowledge of disease mechanisms causing disability, exercise effects, and what type of exercise program is most efficacious in patients with different types of IIM.

Approach to the Patient with Newly Diagnosed Idiopathic Inflammatory Myopathies

Based on the data reviewed earlier, we recommend a starting dose of prednisone (or equivalent) at 0.75 mg/kg/day as a single dose (Table 14-4). We would also advocate that the initial high dose of glucocorticoids is maintained for 4 to 12 weeks; this suggestion is based on the observation of a maximal improvement after a mean of 12 weeks.[13,24,92] Tapering of the glucocorticoid dosage should be guided by improved muscle function[4,5,50] and be conducted initially in small decrements of 15% to 20% of the daily dosage per month. Tapering of glucocorticoid could be started when close to normal muscle function has been achieved, regardless of elevated CK. We also recommend starting an immunosuppressive agent concomitantly with glucocorticoids. The most commonly used immunosuppressive in this setting are MTX or AZA regardless of whether the diagnosis is PM or DM (for IBM, see later). In patients with ILD or myocarditis, intravenous pulse methylprednisolone in combination with CyX may be instituted. CyX can be adminstered orally (2 mg/kg as a single dose) or alternatively intravenously at 1000 mg monthly for 3 to 6 months (Table 14-4 and Fig. 14-6).

To evaluate response to treatment, we propose a follow-up assessment post baseline at weeks 4, 12, 24, 36, and 52 weeks. Clinical assessments should include the disease activity core set proposed by IMACS, which includes the MMT,[74,75] serum levels of CK and LD, functional status measured by the Health Assessment Questionnaire, extramuscular disease activity measured by the myositis intention to treat index (MITAX), and the myositis disease activity assessment visual analog scale

Table 14-4. *Drugs Used in Inflammatory Myopathies, Dosage, and Side Effects*

Drug	Minimum Dosage	Maximum Dosage	Side Effects
Prednisolone	0.75 mg/kg day single dose	1 mg/kg day single dose	Muscle atrophy, osteoporosis, hypertension, diabetes
Methotrexate oral/SC	7.5 mg/week	25 mg/week	Liver toxicity, leukopenia
Azathioprine (AZA)	1 mg/kg twice a day	2.5 mg/kg twice a day	Liver toxicity, leukopenia
Methotrexate (MTX) IV	500 mg/m²	MTX 25 mg/week+ AZA 150 mg/day	Liver toxicity, leukopenia
Methotrexate + azathioprine	MTX 7.5 mg/week+ AZA 50 mg/day	2 mg/kg/day single dose MTX 25 mg/week	Liver toxicity, leukopenia
Cyclophosphamide oral	1 mg/kg/day single dose	2 g/kg every third month (maximum)	Leukopenia
Cyclophosphamide IV	500 mg monthly	1000 mg monthly	Leukopenia
IVIG	2 g/kg monthly (minimum)	5 mg/kg/day	Headache
Cyclosporin A	1 mg/kg/day	1000 mg IV	Hypertension
Rituximab	1000 mg IV		Allergic or infusion reactions, opportunistic infection

IV, intravenous; IVIG, intravenous globulin; SC, subcutaneous.

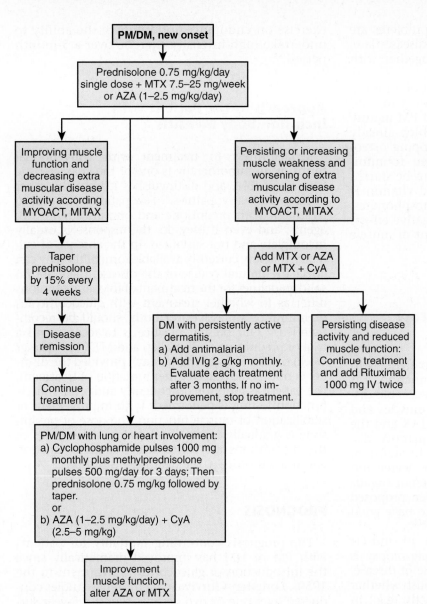

Figure 14-6. Proposed algorithm for treatment of new-onset polymyositis and dermatomyositis.

(MYOACT).[74,75] Additionally, our strong recommendation is to measure muscle function by the myositis functional index FI-2[1] at disease onset, 3, 9, and 12 months. Muscle biopsies should be performed at disease onset, and we recommend muscle biopsy at 6 months regardless of response to treatment. This recommendation may be appropriate for centers that use percutaneous conchotome biopsy or needle biopsy. The myositis damage index (MDI) is a comprehensive tool used to assess the extent and severity of damage developing in different organs and systems.[75] We propose scoring the MDI at a 6-month and 12-month visit, and then yearly. For defining clinical improvement and worsening, IMACS have proposed a tool that we recommend to follow, which is partly validated.[76,93] At the Karolinska University Hospital, active exercise is employed early, approximately 3 to 4 weeks after initiation of pharmacologic therapy when some clinical improvement has been noted. Usually the patient is started on the submaximal home exercise program (see Fig. 14-2)

5 days a week for 12 weeks under supervision of a physical therapist. Initial exercise load is decided according to the degree of muscle impairment as assessed by the FI-2. A second FI-2, along with the MAP is performed after 6 or 12 weeks.[41] Following improvements in muscle function the patient can continue with the home exercise program with increased loads, or begin supervised muscle training or aquatic training at approximately 50% of maximal load. When the patient has reached a stable, low disease activity, heavier muscle training at a load of 10 VRM, or aerobic exercise at 65% of maximal heart rate, can be employed 2 to 3 days a week. Patients with low disease activity and experienced in exercising can be referred to outpatient clinics or a gym of choice. The MACTAR can be helpful by identifying specific activities of daily living that are limited and important to the patient, and the exercise program and the goals that are set can be designed thereafter.[42] It is very important to perform regular follow-up at least once or twice a year and

to encourage patients to seek help if problems are encountered before that. In case of a disease flare, exercise loads need to be adjusted together with more frequent follow-up.

Osteoporosis is a frequent complication of long-standing glucocorticoid treatment and can lead to severe disability.[14] Because DM and PM mainly affect women in their middle age, which already may be at an increased risk of developing osteoporosis, much effort should be taken to minimize this risk. Preventive measures can be started concomitantly, including calcium and vitamin D substitution and treatment with bisphosphonates. Additionally, glucocorticoids have negative effects on muscles including the development of muscle atrophy.[52]

Approach to the Patient with Established Idiopathic Inflammatory Myopathies

When a physician is treating a patient with chronic IIM who has reduced muscle function, it is important to distinguish active and reversible disease from irreversible damage to the muscles and other organs. Two tools, known as MITAX and the MYOACT, have been developed to quantify disease activity in patients with IIM.[74,75] In addition, the MDI has been devised to assess the degree and severity of damage developing in different organs and systems. These measures have been proposed by the IMACS group and were found to have good face validity and to be comprehensive.[74,75]

Apart from accurate investigation of muscle function by MMT and FI-2, the muscle biopsy is an important tool in the chronic phase of disease. A repeat biopsy can be essential to establish whether the patient has been diagnosed correctly (e.g., in patients with IBM the initial biopsy can mimic PM histopathologically, and metabolic myopathies and drug-related myopathies have also sometimes resulted in incorrected diagnoses), and even more importantly, to determine if there is an ongoing inflammatory process, as evidenced by the presence of inflammatory cells, or by the expression of MHC-1. MRI investigation of affected muscles may also support the presence of active inflammation.

If these assessments support the presence of ongoing inflammation, then a renewed effort of controlling the inflammatory process with corticosteroids, immunosuppressives, IVIG, or even with experimental biologic treatments should be considered.

If, on the other hand, such investigations lead to the conclusion that the patient with chronic symptoms has inactive PM/DM, we propose a regimen of increased physical activity. Supervised physical training in combination with performing myositis home training for 3 to 6 months would be appropriate in these cases.[3] Creatine supplementation appears to increase the benefits of

exercise on endurance and improve the ability to undertake high-intensity exercise over a 5-month period.[85]

Approach to the Patient with Inclusion Body Myositis

Refractoriness to treatment with conventional forms of immunotherapy is one of the characteristic features of IBM, and distinguishes it from the other inflammatory myopathies.[83] Few patients respond to treatment with prednisone and immunosuppressive agents, and even if they do, the response is usually incomplete and not sustained. In the absence of evidence that any currently available form of therapy can affect the natural course of the disease, there are no solid guidelines for the treatment of IBM, and opinions differ as to whether treatment with glucocorticoids or immunosuppressives, or both, should be recommended.[83] Our present practice is to recommend a trial of prednisone (0.75 mg/kg) and MTX (10–25 mg/week) or AZA (1.5–2.5 mg/kg/day), provided the disorder is not too advanced. After initiation of treatment, the patient is monitored frequently and serial muscle function testing is performed. With improvement or stabilization of muscle function, the dose of prednisone is gradually tapered and maintenance doses of the medications are continued. If muscle function continues to worsen, the treatment is stopped.

PROGNOSIS

The prognosis concerning mortality for patients with PM or DM has improved dramatically since the introduction of glucocorticoid treatment in the 1950s. Long-term survival data from five studies conducted over one or two decades report a 5-year survival rate of 65% to 95% and a 10- to 15-year survival rate of 53% to 85%.[13,51,57] There seems to be no difference in survival rates between studies conducted during the past 20 to 30 years.

The remission rate varies between studies and with definitions of remission. Marie and coworkers[94] reported remission of DM or PM in 40% to 77% patients in France. Those who achieved remission were younger and had a tendency toward a shorter period of time between onset of symptoms and diagnosis.[94] Another study reported full remission in only 15% of patients.[15] Thus, despite improved survival with the introduction of glucocorticoid treatment, the majority of patients have persisting low muscle endurance and muscle weakness. It has remained common for patients to respond to treatment with partial improvement of muscle function but to be left with persistent reductions in muscle strength and endurance, despite the absence of classical signs of inflammation. Why these patients are still weak remains unknown. In this group of patients supervised training has a central role in improving muscle function.

CONCLUSION

In conclusion, the IIM are a group of muscle disorders where a considerable proportion of patients develop a chronic disability and reduced quality of life due to persistently decreased muscle function as well as to side effects of corticosteroid treatment. Until more controlled trials have been performed, we must mainly rely on uncontrolled studies when selecting treatments for patients with IIM. These studies support initial treatment with prednisone in starting doses of 0.75 mg/kg/day for approximately 4-12 weeks, with tapering doses according to muscle function thereafter. Because of the high corticosteroid doses that are required, the addition of a steroid-sparing immunosuppressive is usually indicated. Our findings suggest that the effects of IVIG treatment in IIM are limited, but a severe skin rash could be an indication for treatment with IVIG in patients with DM in whom other types of medication have failed or were not tolerated.

At this time, it seems appropriate to recommend combination therapy of glucocorticoids, immunosuppressives, and moderate exercise.[39,95] Whether active physical exercise could be introduced during an early stage of treatment to diminish the risk of persisting, chronic muscle weakness is still unclear and the optimal exercise program for patients with myositis still needs to be determined. Future recommendation may combine both strength and endurance training.

We expect that careful follow-up studies correlating clinical outcome with molecular findings in repeated muscle biopsies will achieve an increased knowledge concerning the pathogenesis as well as the effect of treatment at a molecular level. An improved understanding of the pathophysiologic changes in muscle tissue in patients with IIM is likely to lead to new therapeutic interventions and improved function in these patients.

References

1. Alexanderson H, Broman L, Tollback A, Josefson A, Lundberg IE, Stenstrom CH. Functional index-2: validity and reliability of a disease-specific measure of impairment in patients with polymyositis and dermatomyositis. Arthritis Rheum 2006;55:114-22.
2. Henriksson KG. [Muscle biopsy diagnosis in myopathies]. Scand J Rheumatol Suppl. 1979;30:135-43.
3. Alexanderson H, Stenstrom CH, Lundberg I. Safety of a home exercise programme in patients with polymyositis and dermatomyositis: a pilot study. Rheumatology (Oxford) 1999;38:608-11.
4. Dalakas MC. Polymyositis, dermatomyositis and inclusion-body myositis. N Engl J Med 1991;325:1487-98.
5. Plotz PH, Dalakas M, Leff RL, Love LA, Miller FW, Cronin ME. Current concepts in the idiopathic inflammatory myopathies: polymyositis, dermatomyositis, and related disorders. Ann Intern Med 1989;111:143-57.
6. Plotz PH, Rider LG, Targoff IN, Raben N, O'Hanlon TP, Miller FW. NIH conference. Myositis: immunologic contributions to understanding cause, pathogenesis, and therapy. Ann Intern Med 1995;122:715-24.
7. Dorph C, Lundberg IE. Idiopathic inflammatory myopathies—myositis. Best Pract Res 2002;16:817-32.
8. Bohan A, Peter JB. Polymyositis and dermatomyositis (second of two parts). N Engl J Med 1975;292:403-7.
9. Bohan A, Peter JB. Polymyositis and dermatomyositis (first of two parts). N Engl J Med 1975;292:344-7.
10. Griggs RC, Askanas V, DiMauro S, Engel A, Karpati G, Mendell JR, et al. Inclusion body myositis and myopathies. Ann Neurol 1995;38:705-13.
11. Sekul EA, Dalakas MC. Inclusion body myositis: new concepts. Semin Neurol 1993;13:256-63.
12. Peng A, Koffman BM, Malley JD, Dalakas MC. Disease progression in sporadic inclusion body myositis: observations in 78 patients. Neurology 2000;55:296-8.
13. Henriksson KG, Sandstedt P. Polymyositis—treatment and prognosis. A study of 107 patients. Acta Neurol Scand 1982;65:280-300.
14. Lundberg I, Nennesmo I, Hedfors E. A clinical, serological, and histopathological study of myositis patients with and without anti-RNP antibodies. Semin Arthritis Rheum 1992;22:127-38.
15. Adams EM, Plotz PH. The treatment of myositis. How to approach resistant disease. Rheum Dis Clin North Am 1995;21:179-202.
16. Lundberg I, Nyman U, Pettersson I, Hedfors E. Clinical manifestations and anti-(U1)snRNP antibodies: a prospective study of 29 anti-RNP antibody positive patients. Br J Rheumatol 1992;31:811-7.
17. Clarke AE, Bloch DA, Medsger Jr TA, Oddis CV. A longitudinal study of functional disability in a national cohort of patients with polymyositis/dermatomyositis. Arthritis Rheum 1995;38:1218-24.
18. Lindvall B, Bengtsson A, Ernerudh J, Eriksson P. Subclinical myositis is common in primary Sjogren's syndrome and is not related to muscle pain. J Rheumatol 2002;29:717-25.
19. Hepper NG, Ferguson RH, Howard Jr FM. Three types of pulmonary involvement in polymyositis. Med Clin North Am 1964;48:1031-42.
20. Frazier AR, Miller RD. Interstitial pneumonitis in association with polymyositis and dermatomyositis. Chest 1974;65:403-7.
21. Marie I, Hatron PY, Hachulla E, Wallaert B, Michon-Pasturel U, Devulder B. Pulmonary involvement in polymyositis and in dermatomyositis. J Rheumatol 1998;25:1336-43.
22. Bohan A, Peter JB, Bowman RL, Pearson CM. Computer-assisted analysis of 153 patients with polymyositis and dermatomyositis. Medicine 1977;56:255-86.
23. Fathi M, Dastmalchi M, Rasmussen E, Lundberg IE, Tornling G. Interstitial lung disease, a common manifestation of newly diagnosed polymyositis and dermatomyositis. Ann Rheum Dis 2004;63:297-301.
24. Taylor AJ, Wortham DC, Burge JR, Rogan KM. The heart in polymyositis: a prospective evaluation of 26 patients. Clin Cardiol 1993;16:802-8.
25. van de Vlekkert J, Hoogendijk JE, Frijns CJ, de Visser M. Spontaneous recovery of dermatomyositis and unspecified myositis in three adult patients. J Neurol Neurosurg Psychiatry 2008;79:729-30.
26. Bunch TW, Worthington JW, Combs JJ, Ilstrup DM, Engel AG. Azathioprine with prednisone for polymyositis. A controlled, clinical trial. Ann Intern Med 1980;92:365-9.
27. Dalakas MC, Koffman B, Fujii M, Spector S, Sivakumar K, Cupler E. A controlled study of intravenous immunoglobulin combined with prednisone in the treatment of IBM. Neurology 2001;56:323-7.
28. Dalakas MC. Intravenous immune globulin therapy for neurologic diseases. Ann Intern Med 1997;126:721-30.
29. Raju R, Dalakas MC. Gene expression profile in the muscles of patients with inflammatory myopathies: effect of therapy with IVIg and biological validation of clinically relevant genes. Brain 2005;128(Pt 8):1887-96.
30. Dalakas MC, Illa I, Dambrosia JM, Soueidan SA, Stein DP, Otero C, et al. A controlled trial of high-dose intravenous

immune globulin infusions as treatment for dermatomyositis. N Engl J Med 1993;329:1993-2000.

31. Barbasso Helmers S, Dastmalchi M, Alexanderson H, Nennesmo I, Esbjornsson M, Lindvall B, et al. Limited effects of high-dose intravenous immunoglobulin (IVIG) treatment on molecular expression in muscle tissue of patients with inflammatory myopathies. Ann Rheum Dis 2007;66:1276-83.

32. Barohn RJ, Amato AA, Sahenk Z, Kissel JT, Mendell JR. Inclusion body myositis: explanation for poor response to immunosuppressive therapy. Neurology 1995;45:1302-4.

33. Dion E, Cherin P. [Use of muscular MRI in inflammatory myopathies]. Rev Med Interne 2004;25:435-41.

34. Uthman I, El-Sayad J. Refractory polymyositis responding to infliximab. Rheumatology (Oxford) 2004;43:1198-9.

35. Escalante A, Miller L, Beardmore TD. Resistive exercise in the rehabilitation of polymyositis/dermatomyositis. J Rheumatol 1993;20:1340-4.

36. Hicks JE, Miller F, Plotz P, Chen TH, Gerber L. Isometric exercise increases strength and does not produce sustained creatinine phosphokinase increases in a patient with polymyositis. J Rheumatol 1993;20:1399-401.

37. Wiesinger GF, Quittan M, Aringer M, Seeber A, Volc-Platzer B, Smolen J, et al. Improvement of physical fitness and muscle strength in polymyositis/dermatomyositis patients by a training programme. Br J Rheumatol 1998;37:196-200.

38. Frese E, Brown M, Norton BJ. Clinical reliability of manual muscle testing. Middle trapezius and gluteus medius muscles. Phys Ther 1987;67:1072-6.

39. Josefson A, Romanus E, Carlsson J. A functional index in myositis. J Rheumatol 1996;23:1380-4.

40. Alexanderson H, Stenstrom CH, Jenner G, Lundberg I. The safety of a resistive home exercise program in patients with recent onset active polymyositis or dermatomyositis. Scand J Rheumatol 2000;29:295-301.

41. Alexanderson H, Lundberg IE, Stenstrom CH. Development of the myositis activities profile—validity and reliability of a self-administered questionnaire to assess activity limitations in patients with polymyositis/dermatomyositis. J Rheumatol 2002;29:2386-92.

42. Alemo-Munters L, Vollenhoven RV, Alexanderson H. Measurement properties of a Swedish MACTAR for patients with polymyositis and dermatomyositis. Arthritis Rheum 2006;1206:s503.

43. Sultan SM, Ioannou Y, Moss K, Isenberg DA. Outcome in patients with idiopathic inflammatory myositis: morbidity and mortality. Rheumatology (Oxford) 2002;41:22-6.

44. Engel A, Hohlfeld R, editors. Inflammatory myopathies: the polymyositis and dermatomyositis syndromes. New York: McGraw Hill Publishing; 2004.

45. Haddad MG, West RL, Treadwell EL, Fraser DD. Diagnosis of inflammatory myopathy by percutaneous needle biopsy with demonstration of the focal nature of myositis. Am J Clin Pathol 1994;101:661-4.

46. Dorph C, Nennesmo I, Lundberg IE. Percutaneous conchotome muscle biopsy. A useful diagnostic and assessment tool. J Rheumatol 2001;28:1591-9.

47. Pitt AM, Fleckenstein JL, Greenlee Jr RG, Burns DK, Bryan WW, Haller R. MRI-guided biopsy in inflammatory myopathy: initial results. Magn Reson Imaging 1993;11:1093-9.

48. Campellone JV, Lacomis D, Giuliani MJ, Oddis CV. Percutaneous needle muscle biopsy in the evaluation of patients with suspected inflammatory myopathy. Arthritis Rheum 1997;40:1886-91.

49. Adams EM, Chow CK, Premkumar A, Plotz PH. The idiopathic inflammatory myopathies: spectrum of MR imaging findings. Radiographics 1995;15:563-74.

50. Mastaglia FL, Phillips BA, Zilko P. Treatment of inflammatory myopathies. Muscle Nerve 1997;20:651-64.

51. Oddis CV. Therapy of inflammatory myopathy. Rheum Dis Clin North Am 1994;20:899-918.

52. Henriksson KG, Lindvall B. Polymyositis and dermatomyositis 1990—diagnosis, treatment and prognosis. Prog Neurobiol 1990;35:181-93.

53. Lundberg I, Kratz AK, Alexanderson H, Patarroyo M. Decreased expression of interleukin-1alpha, interleukin-1beta, and cell adhesion molecules in muscle tissue following corticosteroid treatment in patients with polymyositis and dermatomyositis. Arthritis Rheum 2000;43:336-48.

54. Ponyi A, Constantin T, Balogh Z, Szalai Z, Borgulya G, Molnar K, et al. Disease course, frequency of relapses and survival of 73 patients with juvenile or adult dermatomyositis. Clin Exp Rheumatol 2005;23:50-6.

55. Bunch TW. Prednisone and azathioprine for polymyositis: long-term followup. Arthritis Rheum 1981;24:45-8.

56. Malaviya AN, Many A, Schwartz RS. Treatment of dermatomyositis with methotrexate. Lancet 1968;2:485-8.

57. Metzger AL, Bohan A, Goldberg LS, Bluestone R, Pearson CM. Polymyositis and dermatomyositis: combined methotrexate and corticosteroid therapy. Ann Intern Med 1974;81:182-9.

58. Joffe MM, Love LA, Leff RL, Fraser DD, Targoff IN, Hicks JE, et al. Drug therapy of the idiopathic inflammatory myopathies: predictors of response to prednisone, azathioprine, and methotrexate and a comparison of their efficacy. Am J Med 1993;94:379-87.

59. Badrising UA, Maat-Schieman ML, Ferrari MD, Zwinderman AH, Wessels JA, Breedveld FC, et al. Comparison of weakness progression in inclusion body myositis during treatment with methotrexate or placebo. Ann Neurol 2002;51:369-72.

60. Villalba L, Hicks JE, Adams EM, Sherman JB, Gourley MF, Leff RL, et al. Treatment of refractory myositis: a randomized crossover study of two new cytotoxic regimens. Arthritis Rheum 1998;41:392-9.

61. Bombardieri S, Hughes GR, Neri R, Del Bravo P, Del Bono L. Cyclophosphamide in severe polymyositis. Lancet 1989;1:1138-9.

62. Cronin ME, Miller FW, Hicks JE, Dalakas M, Plotz PH. The failure of intravenous cyclophosphamide therapy in refractory idiopathic inflammatory myopathy. J Rheum 1989;16:1225-8.

63. Maeda K, Kimura R, Komuta K, Igarashi T. Cyclosporine treatment for polymyositis/dermatomyositis: is it possible to rescue the deteriorating cases with interstitial pneumonitis? Scand J Rheumatol 1997;26:24-9.

64. Saadeh C, Bridges W, Burwick F. Dermatomyositis: remission induced with combined oral cyclosporine and high-dose intravenous immune globulin. South Med J 1995;88:866-70.

65. Grau JM, Herrero C, Casademont J, Fernandez-Sola J, Urbano-Marquez A. Cyclosporine A as first choice therapy for dermatomyositis. J Rheumatol 1994;21:381-2.

66. Vencovsky J, Jarosova K, Machacek S, Studynkova J, Kafkova J, Bartunkova J, et al. Cyclosporine A versus methotrexate in the treatment of polymyositis and dermatomyositis. Scand J Rheumatol 2000;29:95-102.

67. Cherin P, Herson S, Wechsler B, Piette JC, Bletry O, Coutellier A, et al. Efficacy of intravenous gammaglobulin therapy in chronic refractory polymyositis and dermatomyositis: an open study with 20 adult patients. Am Journal Med 1991;91:162-8.

68. Hengstman GJ, van den Hoogen FH, Barrera P, Netea MG, Pieterse A, van de Putte LB, et al. Successful treatment of dermatomyositis and polymyositis with anti-tumor-necrosis-factor-alpha: preliminary observations. Eur Neurol 2003;50:10-5.

69. Hengstman GJ, van den Hoogen FH, van Engelen BG. Treatment of dermatomyositis and polymyositis with anti-tumor necrosis factor-alpha: long-term follow-up. Eur Neurol 2004;52:61-3.

70. Labioche I, Liozon E, Weschler B, Loustaud-Ratti V, Soria P, Vidal E. Refractory polymyositis responding to infliximab: extended follow-up. Rheumatology (Oxford) 2004;43:531-2.

71. Sprott H, Glatzel M, Michel BA. Treatment of myositis with etanercept (Enbrel), a recombinant human soluble fusion protein of TNF-alpha type II receptor and IgG1. Rheumatology (Oxford) 2004;43:524-6.

72. Efthimiou P, Schwartzman S, Kagen LJ. Possible role for tumour necrosis factor inhibitors in the treatment of resistant dermatomyositis and polymyositis: a retrospective study of eight patients. Ann Rheum Dis 2006;65:1233-6.

73. Hengstman GJ, De Bleecker JL, Feist E, Vissing J, Denton CP, Manoussakis MN, et al. Open-label trial of anti-TNF-alpha in dermato- and polymyositis treated concomitantly with methotrexate. Eur Neurol 2008;59:159-63.

74. Miller FW, Rider LG, Chung YL, Cooper R, Danko K, Farewell V, et al. Proposed preliminary core set measures for disease outcome assessment in adult and juvenile idiopathic inflammatory myopathies. Rheumatology (Oxford) 2001;40:1262-73.

75. Isenberg DA, Allen E, Farewell V, Ehrenstein MR, Hanna MG, Lundberg IE, et al. International consensus outcome measures for patients with idiopathic inflammatory myopathies. Development and initial validation of myositis activity and damage indices in patients with adult onset disease. Rheumatology (Oxford) 2004;43:49-54.

76. Rider LG, Giannini EH, Harris-Love M, Joe G, Isenberg D, Pilkington C, et al. Defining clinical improvement in adult and juvenile myositis. J Rheumatol 2003;30:603-17.

77. Oddis CV, Rider LG, Reed AM, Ruperto N, Brunner HI, Koneru B, et al. International consensus guidelines for trials of therapies in the idiopathic inflammatory myopathies. Arthritis Rheum 2005;52:2607-15.

78. Barohn RJ, Herbelin L, Kissel JT, King W, McVey AL, Saperstein DS, et al. Pilot trial of etanercept in the treatment of inclusion-body myositis. Neurology 2006;66(2 Suppl. 1):S123-4.

79. Levine TD. Rituximab in the treatment of dermatomyositis: an open-label pilot study. Arthritis Rheum 2005;52:601-7.

80. Mok CC, Ho LY, To CH. Rituximab for refractory polymyositis: an open-label prospective study. J Rheumatol 2007;34:1864-8.

81. Noss EH, Hausner-Sypek DL, Weinblatt ME. Rituximab as therapy for refractory polymyositis and dermatomyositis. J Rheumatol 2006;33:1021-6.

82. Chung L, Genovese MC, Fiorentino DF. A pilot trial of rituximab in the treatment of patients with dermatomyositis. Arch Dermatol 2007;143:763-7.

83. Oldfors A, Lindberg C. Inclusion body myositis. Curr Opin Neurol 1999;12:527-33.

84. Wiesinger GF, Quittan M, Graninger M, Seeber A, Ebenbichler G, Sturm B, et al. Benefit of 6 months long-term physical training in polymyositis/dermatomyositis patients. Br J Rheumatol 1998;37:1338-42.

85. Chung YL, Alexanderson H, Pipitone N, Morrison C, Dastmalchi M, Stahl-Hallengren C, et al. Creatine supplements in patients with idiopathic inflammatory myopathies who are clinically weak after conventional pharmacologic treatment: six-month, double-blind, randomized, placebo-controlled trial. Arthritis Rheum 2007;57:694-702.

86. Heikkila S, Viitanen JV, Kautiainen H, Kauppi M. Does improved spinal mobility correlate with functional changes in spondyloarthropathy after short term physical therapy? J Rheumatol 2000;27:2942-4.

87. Varju C, Petho E, Kutas R, Czirjak L. The effect of physical exercise following acute disease exacerbation in patients with dermato/polymyositis. Clin Rehabil 2003;17:83-7.

88. Alexanderson H, Dastmalchi M, Esbjornsson-Liljedahl M, Opava CH, Lundberg IE. Benefits of intensive resistance training in patients with chronic polymyositis or dermatomyositis. Arthritis Rheum 2007;57:768-77.

89. Paulus HE, Egger MJ, Ward JR, Williams HJ. Analysis of improvement in individual rheumatoid arthritis patients treated with disease-modifying antirheumatic drugs, based on the findings in patients treated with placebo. The Cooperative Systematic Studies of Rheumatic Diseases Group. Arthritis Rheum 1990;33:477-84.

90. Spector SA, Lemmer JT, Koffman BM, Fleisher TA, Feuerstein IM, Hurley BF, et al. Safety and efficacy of strength training in patients with sporadic inclusion body myositis. Muscle Nerve 1997;20:1242-8.

91. Arnardottir S, Alexanderson H, Lundberg IE, Borg K. Sporadic inclusion body myositis: pilot study on the effects of a home exercise program on muscle function, histopathology and inflammatory reaction. J Rehabil Med 2003;35:31-5.

92. Pearson CM. Patterns of polymyositis and their responses to treatment. Ann Intern Med 1963;59:827-38.

93. Oddis CV. Outcomes and disease activity measures for assessing treatments in the idiopathic inflammatory myopathies. Curr Rheumatol Rep 2005;7:87-93.

94. Marie I, Hachulla E, Hatron PY, Hellot MF, Levesque H, Devulder B, et al. Polymyositis and dermatomyositis: short term and long term outcome, and predictive factors of prognosis. J Rheumatol 2001;28:2230-7.

95. Dastmalchi M, Alexanderson H, Loell I, Stahlberg M, Borg K, Lundberg IE, et al. Effect of physical training on the proportion of slow-twitch type I muscle fibers, a novel non-immune-mediated mechanism for muscle impairment in polymyositis or dermatomyositis. Arthritis Rheum 2007;57:1303-10.

96. Miller FW, Leitman SF, Cronin ME, Hicks JE, Leff RL, Wesley R, et al. Controlled trial of plasma exchange and leukapheresis in polymyositis and dermatomyositis. N Engl J Med 1992;326:1380-1384.

97. Leff RL, Miller FW, Hicks J, Fraser DD, Plotz PH. The treatment of inclusion body myositis: a retrospective review and a randomized, prospective trial of immunosuppressive therapy. Medicine (Baltimore) 1993;72:225-235.

98. Cherin P, Auperin I, Bussel A, Pourrat J, Herson S. Plasma exchange in polymyositis and dermatomyositis: a multicenter study of 57 cases. Clin Exp Rheumatol 1995;13:270-271.

99. Adams EM, Pucino F, Yarboro C, Hicks JE, Thornton B, McGarvey C, et al. A pilot study: use of fludarabine for refractory dermatomyositis and polymyositis, and examination of endpoint measures. J Rheumatol 1999;26:352-360.

100. Oddis CV, Sciurba FC, Elmagd KA, Starzl TE. Tacrolimus in refractory polymyositis with interstitial lung disease. Lancet 1999;353:1762-1763.

101. Randomized pilot trial of betaINFla (Avonex) in patients with inclusion body myositis. Neurology 2001;57:1566-1570.

102. Danieli MG, Malcangi G, Palmieri C, Logullo F, Salvi A, Piani M, et al. Cyclosporin A and intravenous immunoglobulin treatment in polymyositis/dermatomyositis. Ann Rheum Dis 2002;61:37-41.

103. Lindberg C, Trysberg E, Tarkowski A, Oldfors A. Anti-T-lymphocyte globulin treatment in inclusion body myositis: a randomized pilot study. Neurology 2003;61:260-262.

104. Harris-Love MO. Safety and efficacy of submaximal eccentric strength training for a subject with polymyositis. Arthritis Rheum 2005;53:471-474.

POLYMYALGIA RHEUMATICA

CASE STUDY 1

A 72-year-old white woman requests urgent evaluation for increasing achiness of 6 weeks' duration.

Symptoms began shortly after a 3 day family reunion, during which time she "cooked and baked for 20 people." Initially attributed to overuse, symptoms have steadily worsened, unresponsive to ibuprofen in doses up to 1800 mg per day. Aching prominently involves the upper arms but has also recently affected the back of the neck and the posterior thighs. She awakens at night with pain, feels "like the tin man" on arising in the morning, and doesn't "loosen up" until 1:00 or 2:00 o'clock in the afternoon. She can no longer hook her bra in the back, and must be assisted with donning a blouse by her husband.

Past medical history includes hypercholesterolemia and hypertension. Her general health has been good. She has been on stable doses of atorvastain and hydrochlorthiazide for several years.

Musuculoskeletal examination is notable for limited abduction and internal rotation at both shoulders.

The erythrocyte sedimentation rate is 49 mm/hour, the C-reactive protein is 24.7 mg/L (normal 0–3).

Polymyalgia rheumatica is suspected, and prednisone 10 mg every morning, is started. She calls 1 week later, "50% better"; in another week, she reports that she is virtually symptom free with no nocturnal pain, minimal morning stiffness, and no functional limitations.

Diagnosis

Diagnostic criteria for polymyalgia rheumatica (PMR) have not been validated, although they are now under prospective evaluation by an international work group.[1] Previously formulated criteria for diagnosis[2-5] have been empirically derived, and include older age; recent onset of symptoms; prominent morning stiffness; proximally distributed symptoms; elevated acute phase reactants; and, in the Healey criteria,[3] the important stipulation of a brisk therapeutic response to low-dose corticosteroids (CS).

PMR is the quintessential systemic rheumatic disease of older adults: the mean age of onset is 73 years[5]; it occurs rarely in patients younger than the age of 50, if at all.

The onset of symptoms is recent and discrete, sometimes even precipitous—in contrast, for example, to the long duration of symptoms that is typical for the presentation of the patient with fibromyalgia. The requirement that symptoms be of more to 2 to 4 weeks in duration is intended to differentiate PMR from self-limited syndromes such as arthralgias and myalgias or viral etiologies. However, because the onset of symptoms in PMR may be abrupt, insistence on a disease duration of 1 month as a prerequisite for diagnosis may inappropriately delay efforts at treatment.

Morning stiffness is invariable in PMR. The gel phenomenon—stiffness with inactivity—is typically of notable intensity in PMR, and manifests as nocturnal pain, marked and prolonged morning stiffness (often resulting in the need for assistance with such activities of daily living as morning dressing), and stiffness with inactivity during the day.

Proximal achiness in PMR is symmetric, affecting the upper arms, posterior neck, and thighs. Achiness of the upper arms, with the complaint of difficulty raising the arms above the shoulders, is especially characteristic. Early in the disease, the lower extremities may be spared; accordingly, in an older adult, the new onset of symmetric aching of the upper arms should encourage consideration for a possible diagnosis of PMR. Physical examination may show limited range of motion about the shoulders and hips, especially the shoulders, owing to a pathophysiology that involves synovitis and bursitis.[6,7] The term "polymyalgia rheumatica," although embedded in the medical literature, is hence a misnomer. Range of motion may have returned to normal if the patient is examined later in the day. Muscle tenderness to palpation is a nonspecific sign of no clinical use. The motor examination, although sometimes problematic in the patient who is in significant pain, shows no weakness.

Elevations of the acute phase reactants are usual. The most familiar and most widely referenced of the acute phase reactants is the erythrocyte sedimentation rate (ESR), which, although sometimes elevated to triple figures, has a wide range in PMR. An increased ESR has generally been viewed as essential to the diagnosis; indeed, an ESR greater than 40 mm/h is specified in all proposed diagnostic criteria. But it is clear that PMR can present in the context of a "normal" ESR. The reported frequency of this occurrence varies considerably. Myklebust and Gran found ESRs less than 20 mm/h in only 2.3% of patients with PMR.[8] ESRs less than 40 mm/h have been reported in 7.3% to 22% of other series.[9-11] The spread among these percentages is difficult to reconcile, but clinical observation suggests that one important consideration is the length of time between when a patient develops symptoms and when he or she is seen and evaluated by a physician.

The well-known vagaries of the ESR (e.g., its susceptibility to variation with gender, age, anemia, and abnormal immunoglobulins) have played a role in an increased use of the C-reactive protein (CRP). Prospective head-to-head studies on the diagnostic value of the CRP versus the ESR in PMR, however, are remarkably few. However, growing clinical experience does suggest that the CRP may have superiority over the ESR for both the diagnosis of and follow-up of PMR. Practically, it is common to assess both acute phase reactants, and then to rely on the one that seems better to reflect the clinical activity of a given patient's disease.

Initial Treatment: The Therapeutic Trial of Low-Dose Corticosteroids

The prompt and virtually complete abolition of symptoms with low-dose CS may be the most striking clinical feature of PMR. Nonsteroidal anti-inflammatory drugs are not indicated because they are of minimal, if any, value for symptomatic management in this disease. Despite the indubitable benefit of CS for the treatment of PMR, controlled studies on the appropriate dose of this drug for initial management have not been done. Studies comparing various CS preparations (e.g., prednisone, prednisolone, and intramuscular methylprednisolone[12]) are similarly lacking. Doses between 10 and 20 mg of prednisone per day are normative.[13] Higher doses of CS of course are also effective, but they produce nonspecific symptomatic improvement in many musculoskeletal diseases, including those with local pathology, such as rotator cuff disease and osteoarthritis, whereas it is the exquisite symptomatic response to low-dose CS that has diagnostic value in the patient with possible PMR.

The response to low-dose CS may be immediate and seen after only a single dose, but it is common that a slightly longer period of time is required before a complete symptomatic response becomes fully manifest, especially in cases in which the inflammatory reaction is intense. In such cases, the use of divided doses of prednisone may be helpful.

Studies of serum interleukin 6 (IL-6) levels in PMR suggest a physiologic basis for this approach.[14] These levels are commonly elevated in PMR, often significantly so; they are promptly suppressed after a dose of CS, but within hours will begin to rebound. This rapid increase in IL-6 levels probably underlies the nocturnal recrudescence of aching and stiffness in the patient whose PMR remains active when under treatment with a single morning dose of CS.

The definition of remission in PMR has not been formalized; practically, however, if there has not been total or near-complete resolution of aching and stiffness after a 14- to 21-day trial of low-dose CS, the diagnosis of PMR should be strongly reconsidered and further diagnostic work-up undertaken. There are several approaches to the conduct of the diagnostic and therapeutic trial of CS, one of which could begin with prednisone 10 mg in a single morning dose. Because it is the immediate symptomatic response to CS that is of such diagnostic import, the patient in instructed to call in 1 week. If the therapeutic response is incomplete, the prednisone is split to 5 mg bid, and at the end of week 2, the patient is again told to call. If symptoms persist, the dose is increased to 10 mg in the morning and 5 mg at night. However, if there is not marked improvement by the end of week 3, further evaluation is advised. Very occasionally, if there is intense inflammation, a prednisone dose of more than 20 mg per day may be needed for initial treatment.

Differential Diagnosis

The differential diagnosis of diffuse achiness in an older adult includes other systemic rheumatic diseases, especially rheumatoid arthritis (RA). Distal symptoms and signs, however, may occur in PMR, and differentiation between PMR and RA with a polymyalgic presentation in an older adult can be difficult initially (see below, The Problem of Peripheral Synovitis). Pain may be part of the presentation of polymyositis or other myopathies, but such diseases manifest more often with weakness than with pain, without morning stiffness. Measurement of the serum creatine kinase (CK), which is always normal in PMR, will clarify the diagnosis.

Achiness may be among the nonspecific constitutional symptoms that can initially accompany various infections; fever, however, is rare in uncomplicated PMR and, if present, especially in the context of arthralgis and myalgias of recent onset, could indicate a diagnosis such as endocarditis and the need for blood cultures. Fever in true PMR raises concern for concurrent giant cell arteritis (GCA).

Diffuse pain may result from osseous disease, as in multiple myeloma. The possibility of widespread skeletal metastases must be borne in mind in the context of prior or even remote malignancy. Electrophoretic studies of the serum and urine and work-up for malignancy may be indicated. PMR is not a paraneoplastic syndrome, is not associated with an increased risk of cancer,[15] and does not require a malignancy work-up. That said, atypical features in the patient with suspected PMR, such as adenopathy or pulmonary infiltrates, must call the diagnosis into question. There appears to be an association of PMR with myelodysplastic syndromes, but in this unusual situation, PMR responds to low-dose CS in typically brisk fashion.[16]

Statin-related myopathy is commonly considered by both patient and physician in the differential diagnosis. The serum CK is elevated in patients with a bona fide statin myopathy; patients with statin-related myalgias and a normal CK are differentiated from PMR by the absence of a prominent gel phenomenon and the lack of symmetric and proximal localization of symptoms. Significantly symptomatic fibromyalgia is rather uncommon in older adults, and symptoms are generally of long duration, not of recent onset. Multifocal degenerative disease may generate an array of symptoms reminiscent of PMR. For example, rotator cuff disease is common in older adults, and if bilateral and accompanied by degenerative disc disease of the cervical spine or osteoarthritis at the hips, could suggest PMR. In this setting, morning stiffness is usually brief in duration, and acute phase reactants are not elevated. The stiffness that accompanies neurologic disease such as Parkinson's, can be distinguished from PMR by history and physical examination.

Although commonly included in the differential diagnosis, hypothyroidism rarely presents with symptoms that are confounded with PMR. Other conditions said to have the potential for diagnostic confusion with PMR have included calcium pyrophosphate dehydrate deposition disease,[17] purported late-onset spondyloarthropathy,[18] and malignancy,[19] but in clinical practice, such occurrences are also rare.

The Problem of Peripheral Synovitis

Distal symptoms and signs, which include carpal tunnel syndromes, peripheral arthritis, and distal swelling, occur in one half of patients with PMR.[20]

Carpal tunnel syndromes occur in as many as one of six patients with PMR and often remit with low-dose steroids.

A modest peripheral arthritis, which is never erosive, may affect the wrists, metacarpophalangeal joints, and knees, and responds with the same singular sensitivity to low-dose steroids as does the proximal symptomatology. Obviously, however, the presence of distal symptoms and signs could suggest a diagnosis of classic rheumatoid disease, which occasionally presents in older adults. The finding of peripheral arthritis in a patient with suspected PMR warrants measurement of rheumatoid factor or anticyclic citrullinated antibodies. The discovery of erosions, of course, indicates rheumatoid disease.

It is not unusual that overt polyarthritis of abrupt onset in an older adult is seronegative, thus confronting the clinician with the dilemma of distinguishing PMR from ostensible seronegative rheumatoid arthritis. Such patients have been described under the rubrics of late-onset rheumatoid arthritis[21] or elderly-onset rheumatoid arthritis,[22] but efforts to identify features that could distinguish at presentation among PMR, classic rheumatoid disease, or other entities have been largely unsuccessful. Practically, the distinction is made by vigilant follow-up, which may require 3 to 6 months before a clinical diagnosis can be firmly settled. The repeated appearance of overt peripheral synovitis during attempts to taper the prednisone dose to below 10 mg/day points to a diagnosis of rheumatoid disease rather than PMR.

Occasionally in older adults, prominent swelling over the dorsa of the hands and wrists presents explosively, which has been dubbed "RS3PE" (remitting symmetrical seronegative synovitis with peripheral edema) or the puffy edematous hand syndrome. This presentation is usually found in the setting of PMR. The syndrome, which may dominate proximal symptoms and also manifest as a relapse of PMR, responds to low-dose CS with characteristic briskness. Though sometimes construed as a unique entity, the puffy edematous hand syndrome (Fig. 15-1) seems most sensibly viewed as part of the spectrum of PMR.[23]

The Question of Giant Cell Arteritis

Clinically explicit, biopsy-proved GCA is customarily said to affect 15% of patients with PMR.[24] A recent prospective study reported GCA in 6% of 248 patients with PMR,[8] a figure that seems closer to clinical experience.

Evidence of arteritis has also been found on temporal artery (TA) biopsy in occasional PMR patients with no symptoms referable to GCA.[25] Evidence for the presence of subclinical GCA has also been found by recent imaging techniques. Using duplex ultrasonography, the halo sign

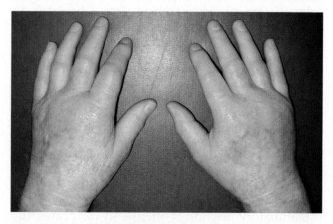

Figure 15-1. Puffy edematous hand syndrome in PMR.

(thought to represent edema of the vascular wall) or stenosis was seen in the temporal arteries of eight of 102 patients with PMR who were clinically asymptomatic for GCA, of whom four subsequently had TA biopsies positive for arteritis.[26] Using 18-fluorodeoxyglucose positron emission tomography (FDG-PET), an increased uptake in the subclavian arteries was noted in one third of 35 patients with PMR.[27] The prognostic and therapeutic significance of such subclinical arteritis is completely unknown.

TA biopsy is not routinely recommended in patients with PMR who have no clinical symptoms of GCA. Biopsy should be strongly considered if there are arteritic symptoms, especially new onset headache, jaw claudication, or amaurosis, or if fever is present. Biopsy should also be considered if physical examination demonstrates asymmetric blood pressures in the arms, vascular bruits by auscultation, or abnormalities of the temporal arteries to palpation. Similar consideration should be given to the occurrence of any of these symptoms and signs in the PMR patient already on treatment, because low-dose CS therapy is not a bulwark against the emergence of GCA.[28] Finally, it should be remembered that the clinical courses of PMR and GCA may not be synchronous, and that GCA may present in patients whose PMR is no longer active, and vice-versa.

Subsequent Treatment and Clinical Course

As is the case with the selection of the initial dose of CS for PMR, there are no evidence-based guidelines for the ensuing dosing of this drug, either for maintenance or as a taper. Whether CS treatment actually affects the natural history of PMR (i.e., whether it is remission inducing) is unknown; conceivably, it provides symptomatic management until the disease itself undergoes spontaneous remission. Accordingly, subsequent management of PMR is an exercise in empiricism, the goal of which is the identification of the lowest dose of CS that keeps the given patient comfortable and functional. Generally, after a patient has been asymptomatic for 1 month, dose reductions are initiated, every 2 to 4 weeks. Above 10 mg of prednisone per day, 2.5-mg decrements may be possible, but because symptoms in PMR are so steroid sensitive, the use of 1-mg decrement once the dose is below 10 mg/day is an effective strategy.

Some patients with PMR can be tapered smoothly and rather quickly off CS over a matter of mere months, but subsequent treatment is commonly punctuated by symptomatic relapses in up to 50% of cases,[29] necessitating upward adjustments in the dose of CS. Consequently, CS therapy can be prolonged. One recent study reported that a third of patients required CS treatment for more than 6 years,[30] whereas at another center, the median duration of some CS therapy for PMR was 37 months.[31] The data imply that there are two large subsets of PMR, one with milder disease, for which 1 to 2 years of treatment with CS suffices, and another with more protracted, relapsing disease, for which several years of such treatment is necessary. The potential length of treatment also implies that, when CS treatment is begun for PMR, the clinician must be prepared to commit to the care of an older adult for what can be an extended period of time with a medication that has an array of potential toxicities. Finally, in addition to relapses, the clinical course of PMR can also be marked by overt recurrences, that is, renewed activity of disease years after CS treatment has been stopped.[32]

Normalization of the ESR and CRP usually follows remission of symptoms in PMR. Increases in these tests may accompany relapses of symptoms, but not always, and a sizeable portion of symptomatic flares of PMR are not attended by such elevations, especially in the case of the ESR. Rises in the acute phase reactants in the absence of worsened symptoms, on the other hand, are not grounds for a reflexive escalation in the CS dose.

Ultimately, dose reductions of CS in PMR must be individualized. If, as often occurs, the CS taper cannot be uneventfully consummated, a minimum dose adequate for symptomatic relief is located. The frequency with which further dose reductions are attempted will vary, depending on the comfort level of the physician and patient with the given CS dose and the extent to which CS-related toxicities ensue. Because the CS dose is adjusted against the patient's symptoms, frequent assessment of the acute phase reactants seems of little practical use, unless a marked change in clinical status supervenes.

Toxicities of Corticosteroids

The toxicities of CS are well known and can occur even in the low doses used to treat PMR.

Axial bone loss can begin early in the course of CS treatment, for which aggressive prophylaxis with appropriate supplements of calcium and vitamin D is warranted in most patients, both women and men. Baseline bone mineral densitometry should be obtained. The value of bisphosphonates for reducing fracture risk due to CS use is well documented, and in clinical practice, the proactive deployment of such therapy has significantly decreased the incidence of fractures occurring during CS treatment for PMR.

An underacknowledged side effect of even low-dose CS in older adults is that of increased capillary fragility, which may result in widespread ecchymoses and in slowly healing superficial lacerations, a susceptibility exacerbated by concurrent treatment with aspirin, warfarin, or other anticoagulants. There is no treatment for this toxicity, aside from reduction in the CS dose.

The Difficult CS Taper

The taper of CS in PMR may be difficult for an assortment of reasons. PMR itself is prone to frequent relapses, as discussed earlier; the persistence of distal synovitis may prompt a revision of the operational diagnosis to rheumatoid disease; and CS-related toxicities may ensue. In addition, CS may produce capricious symptomatic improvement in a mixture of noninflammatory musculoskeletal conditions, such as osteoarthritis and rotator cuff disease. As CS are tapered, it is important to differentiate recrudescence of symptoms due to these local conditions from those arising from a true relapse of PMR, in order to avoid overtreatment.

Adjunctive Treatments for Polymyalgia Rheumatica

Although symptomatic treatment of PMR is invariably effective with the use of low-dose CS, such management in older adults may engender unacceptable toxicity, as has been discussed. Methotrexate (MTX) and tumor necrosis factor (TNF) alpha blockers have been explored as possible adjunctive treatments.

An earlier randomized control trial showed no benefit from the use of adjunctive MTX at a dose of 7.5 mg/week.[33] The more recent randomized control trial (RCT)[34] allocated 72 patients to treatment with prednisone alone vs prednisone and MTX at a dose of 10 mg/week. Prednisone was administered in an initial dose of 25 mg/week for 4 weeks, and then tapered by 2.5-mg decrements every 4 weeks, unless a flare (defined as increased symptoms of PMR and a rise in the ESR to greater than 30 or in the CRP to greater than 5 mg/L) prompted an increased dose. MTX was given for 48 weeks; patients were followed for 76 weeks. More patients treated in the MTX-treated group achieved the primary endpoint, discontinuation of CS ($P = 0.003$); they also had fewer flares and required a lower total cumulative CS dose.

The extent to which these conclusions can be generalized to practice is uncertain. The mean reduction in the prednisone dose in the MTX-treated group was little more than 1 mg/day; there were no differences in potential CS-related toxicities between the two groups; and the MTX dosing was low, by current standards.

The only RCT of TNF alpha blockade for the treatment of PMR involved infliximab (IFX).[35] In that study, 52 patients were randomized to treatment with prednisone alone versus prednisone and IFX, given at a dose of 3 mg/kg at weeks 0, 2, 6, 14, and 22. Prednisone was administered at an initial dose of 15 mg/day, and then tapered off by 16 weeks, unless a flare (defined as in the MTX study described above) required an increase in dose. Patients were followed for 52 weeks. The study was negative: there was no significant effect of IFX on any of the outcome variables, including numbers of relapse-free patients,

patients no longer taking prednisone, the number of flares, the duration of CS treatment, and cumulative CS dose.

A small, recent case series[36] described the use of etanercept, 25 mg twice weekly, in refractory PMR, defined as patients whose CS dose could not be reduced below 7.5 mg/day after 12 months of treatment, and who had relapsing symptoms of PMR and CS-related adverse events. In five of six patients the CS dose was decreased but not apparently stopped; whether CS-related toxicities were affected was not reported.

The routine use of methotrexate or TNF alpha blockade in the initial management of PMR is not recommended. Whether either of these medications is of value for the subsequent management of the PMR patient who develops CS-related toxicities is unclear. In practice, for patients with intolerable toxicities from even low-dose CS, MTX in contemporary doses of 15 to 25 mg/week seems to have a modestly steroid-sparing benefit, with the caveat that such doses have not been formally studied. The role of TNF alpha blockade at any point in a disease whose treatment involves only low-dose CS is uncertain, at best.

Conclusion

Low doses of CS are the foundation of treatment for PMR. Management should aim for the lowest dose of CS needed to maintain quality of life and functional status for the individual patient. Because of the extraordinary sensitivity of PMR to CS, use of 1-mg decrements for the taper of this drug is advantageous. Both patients and physicians should be aware of the frequency of relapses and of the potential need for long-term treatment.

GIANT CELL ARTERITIS

CASE STUDY 2

A 78-year-old woman is referred for emergency evaluation of sudden loss of vision in the left eye.

Two evenings previously, sudden and complete loss of vision in the left eye occurred. Thirty-six hours later, an ophthalmologist finds evidence for an acute ischemic optic neuropathy, prescribes 60 mg of prednisone, and requests emergency rheumatology consultation.

Two months previously, the left side of the head became tender to the touch, to an extent that the patient cancelled an appointment with her hairdresser for a permanent. She also experienced unilateral maxillary pain. Her primary care physician was consulted, who raised the possibility of sinusitis, for which a 2-week course of antibiotics was prescribed. Scalp pain receded, but was replaced with a low-grade, daily, occipital headache, somewhat improved with acetaminophen. Nine days ago, an "odd shape" appeared in the "left corner" of the eye for 10 minutes. She denies morning stiffness, jaw pain, fever, or weight loss.

There is a history of an anxiety disorder, paroxysmal atrial fibrillation, and osteoporosis, for which bisphosphonate therapy had been refused.

Medications include a beta blocker, aspirin 325 mg/day, and diazepam.

Physical examination shows an anxious patient, with no light perception in the left eye. Blood pressures are equal in the arms, 136/76 both arms. There are no vascular bruits or cardiac murmurs. TA pulsations are symmetric and nontender.

The ESR, obtained by the ophthalmologist earlier in the day, is 78.

Intravenous methylprednisone, 500 mg, is administered. The next day, unilateral TA biopsy is performed. Intravenous methylprednisolone is repeated that day and again the following morning. Histopathologic inspection of the TA shows a panarteritis, with disruption of the internal elastic lamina. Headache and facial pain resolve promptly, but visual loss in the left eye remains complete.

Diagnosis: Clinical Features

Like PMR, GCA is a disease of older adults: it rarely occurs in patients younger than 50 years of age, and 80% of the patients are older than 70 years of age.[37] Although any ethnic or racial group can be affected, the disease is unusual in blacks.[38]

The most frequent phenotype of GCA is that of so-called cranial arteritis, which presents as symptoms and signs referable to extracranial arteries, especially branches of the external carotid arteries. Headache in any location, whether it is temporal, frontal, parietal, or occipital, is common, affecting three quarters of patients. Jaw claudication occurs in slightly less than one-half of patients. Permanent visual loss, the most sinister complication of GCA, continues to be reported in 10% to 20% of patients (Table 15-1).[40-44] More than 90% of instances of vision loss are due to an anterior ischemic optic neuropathy, caused by occlusion of the posterior ciliary artery, which supplies the optic

nerve; most other cases of visual loss result from occlusion of the central retinal artery. Involvement of branches of the external carotid arteries can result in scalp tenderness, facial swelling, and pains in the tongue and throat.

Almost as common as headache in GCA are constitutional symptoms and signs, including anorexia, weight loss, malaise, sweats, and fevers. Fevers may be high-grade, exceeding 39° C,[45] and may account for one of six fevers of unknown origin in older adults.[46] In up to 10% of patients with GCA, systemic symptoms and signs dominate the clinical presentation, leading to evaluations for malignancy or infection. Also common in GCA are musculoskeletal symptoms and signs—not only PMR, which occurs in slightly under one-half of patients with GCA, but also distal findings, including peripheral arthritis, carpal tunnel syndromes, and distal extremity swelling with edema.[47]

Physical examination of the patient with suspected GCA should include careful palpation of the frontal and parietal branches of the superficial temporal arteries for tenderness, nodularity, enlargement, or decreased pulsation. Although these abnormalities are neither fully sensitive nor specific, they may be found in up to one half of patients with GCA. The self-evident converse should also be remembered: the temporal arteries are normal on palpation in at least one-half of patients.

Among laboratory data are anemia and thrombocytosis. Liver function tests may be elevated, most often the alkaline phosphatase, rarely more than twice normal.[48] The ESR is usually elevated, often significantly so, but neither high nor low values can be relied on to confirm or rule out a diagnosis of GCA. The medical literature and clinical experience are replete with biopsy-proved cases of GCA in patients whose ESRs were in a normal range or but modestly increased. In the Mayo Clinic series of 167 patients, 10.8% had ESRs less than 50, and 5.4% less than 40; the risk of visual loss in these patients was the same as patients with higher ESRs.[49] Ranges for the CRP in the initial diagnosis of GCA have not been studied.

Diagnosis: The Temporal Artery Biopsy

The definitive diagnosis of GCA is premised on histopathologic proof. Such proof is usually sought by biopsy of the most accessible of the cranial arteries, the TA. The procedure is simple, brief, and of little risk.

Some clinical features may argue for or against the diagnosis, but none is sufficiently specific or sensitive to be of conclusive diagnostic use to the clinician. The limitations of attempting a clinical diagnosis of GCA are suggested by the instructive meta-analysis assembled by Smetana and Shmerling[50] of 2680 positive and negative TA biopsies from 21 reports. The only symptoms that increased the likelihood of a positive TA biopsy were jaw claudication (likelihood ratio [LR] 4.2; 95% confidence interval [CI], 2.8–6.2)

Table 15-1. *Incidence of Permanent Visual Loss in Giant Cell Arteritis*

Study	Incidence (%)
Aiello (Mayo Clinic, 1993)[40a]	14.0
Font (Barcelona, Spain, 1997)[40]	15.75
Gonzalez-Gay (Northwestern Spain, 2000)[41]	14.9
Liozon (France, 2001)[42]	13.2
Nesher (Israel, 2004)[43]	18.3
Salvarani (Italy, 2005)[44]	19.1

and, interestingly, diplopia (LR 3.4; 95% CI, 1.3–8.6). The sensitivity, however, of these features was low: in biopsy-proved GCA, jaw claudication was present in only 34% (95% CI, 0.29–0.41) of cases, and diplopia in 9% (95% CI, 0.7–0.13). Conversely, the more prevalent clinical features of GCA (e.g., any headache, constitutional symptoms, and PMR) were not associated with increased LRs of a positive biopsy.

Palpation of the TA yielded more robust predictive information than most features of the history: "beaded," enlarged, or tender temporal arteries were all associated with increased LRs of 4.6 (95% CI, 1.1–18.4), 4.3 (95% CI, 2.1–8.9), and 2.6 (95% CI, 1.9–3.7). An ESR > 100 mm/h had a lesser predictive value for a positive biopsy (LR 1.9, 95% CI, 1.1–3.3) than findings on palpation of the temporal arteries, and the mean value of the ESR was not statistically different between biopsies that were positive and negative (Tables 15-2 and 15-3).

Thus, GCA is not a clinical diagnosis. But because the diagnostic stakes—loss of vision—are high, and because the treatment—high-dose CS—is rife with potential toxicities, TA biopsy should be performed in all patients with suspected GCA.

Histopathology of the Temporal Artery

A panarteritis with special predilection for the internal elastic lamina characterizes GCA. The cellular infiltrate includes T lymphocytes, macrophages, and

Table 15-3. *Sensitivity of Symptoms, Signs, and Laboratory Data in Suspected Giant Cell Arteritis*

Symptoms, Signs and Laboratory Data	Sensitivity (CI, 95%)
Symptoms	
Weight loss	0.43 (0.35–0.53)
Diplopia	0.09 (0.07–0.13)
Fever	0.42 (0.33–0.52)
Temporal headache	0.52 (0.36–0.67)
Any headache	0.76 (0.72–0.79)
Jaw claudication	0.34 (0.29–0.41)
Polymyalgia rheumatica	0.34 (0.28–0.41)
Unilateral vision loss	0.24 (0.14–0.36)
Signs	
Scalp tenderness	0.31 (0.20–0.44)
Beaded TA	0.16 (0.07–0.28)
Prominent/enlarged TA	0.47 (0.40–0.54)
Tender TA	0.41 (0.30–0.52)
Absent TA pulse	0.45 (0.26–0.66)
Laboratory Data	
ESR > 50 mm/h	0.83 (0.75–0.90)
ESR > 100 mm/h	0.39 (0.29–0.50)

CI, confidence interval; ESR, erythrocyte sedimentation rate; TA, temporal artery.
Adapted from Smetana GW, Shmerling RH. Does this patient have temporal arteritis? JAMA 2002;287:92-101.

giant cells, although the latter are not always identified. Fragmentation and duplication of the internal elastic lamina are common. Inflammation is variable and may be confined to the adentitia. Fibrinoid necrosis does not occur (Figs. 15-2 and 15-3).

The report of healed arteritis from a TA biopsy may be a cause of diagnostic consternation. This interpretation usually stems from the observation of focal duplication or disruption of the internal lamina of the artery without inflammation. The clinical significance of this finding is entirely unknown with respect to either prior or current disease activity. Whether to act on such a report is a venture in clinical judgment. In the absence of a compelling clinical scenario, treatment is probably not indicated.

Histopathologic stigmata of GCA may persist in the face of CS therapy for at least 2 weeks and probably longer.[51] Initiation of such therapy, pending biopsy and histopathologic interpretation, thus should not be postponed, if the clinical suspicion for GCA is high.

The Performance of the Temporal Artery Biopsy as a Diagnostic Test

The clinical value of the TA biopsy as a diagnostic test is bedeviled by concerns over its sensitivity. Because it is not fully sensitive, a negative biopsy still leaves the clinician to struggle with the peril of undetected disease and the attendant menace of sudden blindness. The problem with sensitivity has traditionally been ascribed to segmental involvement of the arterial wall by GCA, referred to as skip areas.[52] To improve the diagnostic sensitivity of the procedure, two canonical

Table 15-2. *Likelihood Ratios of Symptoms, Signs, and Laboratory Data in Suspected Giant Cell Arteritis*

Symptoms, Signs, and Laboratory Data	Positive LR (CI, 95%)	Negative LR (CI, 95%)
Symptoms		
Weight loss	1.3 (1.1–1.5)	0.89 (0.79–1.0)
Diplopia	3.4 (1.3–8.6)	0.95 (0.91–0.99)
Fever	1.2 (0.98–1.4)	0.92 (0.85–0.99)
Temporal headache	1.5 (0.76–3.0)	0.82 (0.64–1.0)
Any headache	1.2 (1.1–1.4)	0.7 (0.57–0.86)
Jaw claudication	4.2 (2.8–6.2)	0.72 (0.65–0.81)
Polymyalgia rheumatica	0.97 (0.76–1.2)	1.2 (1.0–1.3)
Unilateral vision loss	0.85 (0.58–1.2)	1.2 (1.0–1.3)
Signs		
Scalp tenderness	1.6 (1.2–2.1)	0.93 (0.86–1.0)
Beaded TA	4.6 (1.1–18.4)	0.93 (0.88–0.99)
Prominent or enlarged TA	4.3 (2.1–8.9)	0.67 (0.5–0.89)
Tender TA	2.6 (1.9–3.7)	0.82 (0.74–0.92)
Absent TA pulse	2.7 (0.55–13.4)	0.71 (0.36–1.3)
Laboratory Data		
ESR > 50	1.2 (1.0–1.4)	0.2 (0.08–0.51)
ESR > 100	1.9 (1.1–3.3)	0.8 (0.68–0.95)

CI, confidence interval; ESR, erythrocyte sedimentation rate; LR, likelihood ratio; TA, temporal artery.
Adapted from Smetana GW, Shmerling RH. Does this patient have temporal arteritis? JAMA 2002;287:92-101.

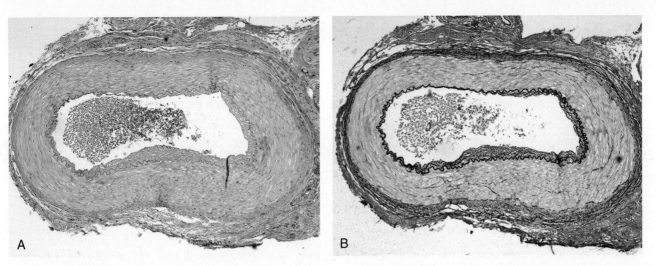

Figure 15-2. Histopathology, normal temporal artery. Hematoxylin and eosin stain (**A**) and elastin stain (**B**). (Courtesy of Dr. Robert F. Padera.)

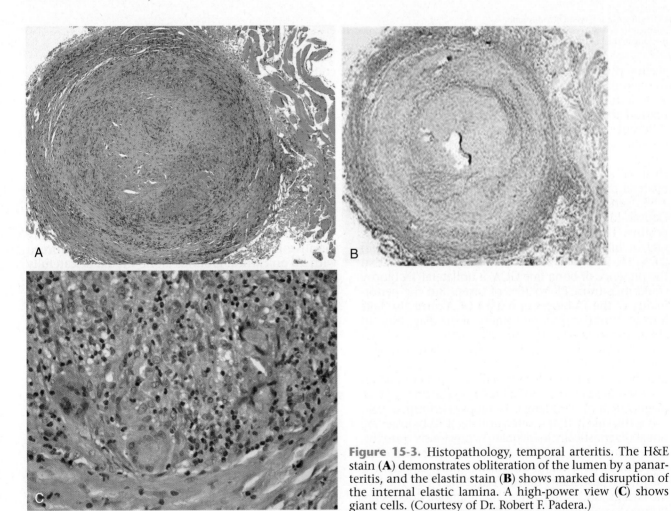

Figure 15-3. Histopathology, temporal arteritis. The H&E stain (**A**) demonstrates obliteration of the lumen by a panarteritis, and the elastin stain (**B**) shows marked disruption of the internal elastic lamina. A high-power view (**C**) shows giant cells. (Courtesy of Dr. Robert F. Padera.)

recommendations are often cited: acquire as long a specimen at biopsy as possible (minimum 2 cm), and perform bilateral TA biopsies.[39]

Recently, Mahr[53] has challenged the notion of the need for a long TA biopsy. In his large study of 1520 TA biopsy specimens, 15% of which had evi-dence of arteritis, biopsy length was investigated. Statistical analysis, based on piecewise logistic regres-sion, showed that the change point in the odds ratio for finding a positive TA biopsy occurred at a biopsy length of 0.5 cm (Table 15-4). Thus, biopsy lengths beyond 0.5 cm did not confer an increased diagnostic

Table 15-4. *Odds Ratio of Positive Temporal Artery Biopsy as a Function of Length of Biopsy*

	Diagnostic Sensitivity			
	All Giant Cell Arteritis		Giant Cell Arteritis with Giant Cells	
TAB Length	n/total n (%)	OR (95% CI)	n/total n (%)	OR (95% CI)
Class				
< 0.5 cm*	2/66 (3.0%)	1	2/66 (3.0%)	1
0.5–0.9 cm	56/381 (14.7%)	5.5 (1.3 to 23.2)	38/381 (10.0%)	3.5 (0.8 to 15.1)
1.0–1.4 cm	79/486 (16.3%)	6.2 (1.5 to 25.9)	61/486 (12.6%)	4.6 (1.1 to 19.2)
1.5–1.9 cm	45/290 (15.5%)	5.9 (1.4 to 24.9)	33/290 (11.4%)	4.1 (0.96 to 17.6)
2.0–2.4 cm	23/172 (13.4%)	4.9 (1.1 to 21.6)	19/172 (11.0%)	4.0 (0.9 to 17.6)
≥ 2.5 cm	18/125 (14.4%)	5.4 (1.2 to 24.0)	11/125 (8.8%)	3.1 (0.7 to 14.4)
Change Point				
< 0.5 cm*	2/66 (3.0%)	1	2/66 (3.0%)	1
≥ 0.5 cm	220/1454 (15.1%)	5.7 (1.4 to 23.6%)†	162/1454 (11.1%)	4.0 (0.97 to 16.5*)‡

*Reference values:
†*P* = 0.016.
‡*P* = 0.055.
CI, confidence interval; OR, odds ratio.
Adapted from Mahr A, Saba M, Kamboucher M, Polivka M, Baudrimont M, Brocheriou I, et al. Temporal artery biopsy for diagnosing giant cell arteritis: the longer, the better? Ann Rheum Dis 2006;65:826-8.

accuracy. (It should be noted biopsy lengths pertain to fixed pathology specimens, and that shrinkage of TA length between biopsy and histopathologic examination after fixation may be on the order of 20%.)

Recent reports have also suggested that the discordance between bilateral TA biopsies—that is, negative on one side, positive on the other—is low. Histopathologic findings were the same in 97% of 186 bilateral biopsies reported by Boyev and associates in 1999,[54] and in 99% of 91 bilateral biopsies reported by Danesh-Meyer and coworkers in 2000.[55] When only positive TA biopsies are considered, the discordance rate of bilateral biopsies ranges more widely—from 2.6%,[55] to 9.2%,[56] to 18.2%.[54] These data imply that, in the presence of bona fide GCA, a unilateral TA biopsy could miss from 1% to 10% of cases. But the performance of the TA biopsy as test for GCA must also take into account the prior probability of the diagnosis. In 2003, for instance, Hall and associates[57] found that only 1 of 88 patients with an initially negative biopsy who subsequently underwent a contralateral procedure had a positive biopsy, and that no patient had an adverse outcome (viz., visual loss), suggesting that, as diagnostic tool, a unilateral TA biopsy performed well.

It is thus likely that shorter, unilateral TA biopsies are not as diagnostically inadequate as previously thought. For example, the negative predictive value of such a biopsy may have major diagnostic utility, especially if the pretest probability of GCA is not high: e.g., the ethnic background is nonwhite; the temporal arteries are normal to palpation; or the ESR is less than 40.

If the clinical suspicion for GCA remains high despite a negative unilateral biopsy, contralateral biopsy should be pursued. It may be asked whether this sequential approach is warranted if a decision has already been made to go forward with treatment for a presumptive diagnosis of GCA, but the advantage to the clinician of a biopsy-confirmed diagnosis of GCA later in the course, should potential complications of the disease or its treatment ensue, is inestimable.

What if the biopsies are bilaterally negative? It can of course be concluded that GCA has been ruled out. Cranial GCA could still be present, although the possibility of this presentation has been significantly reduced, commensurate with the pretest probability of the diagnosis. Large vessel GCA, affecting the aorta or large arteries, cannot be excluded, because TA biopsies are positive in only one half of such patients, as discussed later (see Aneurysms of the Aorta, and Large Vessel Giant Cell Arteritis). In the face of bilaterally negative biopsies, however, the decision to proceed with CS on clinical grounds alone should be carefully weighed. An apparently favorable response to high-dose CS can be difficult to interpret with certainty: many symptoms may decrease, such as nonarteritic headaches, fatigue, and malaise, and the acute phase reactants often decline. Still, there will always be patients (e.g., those who have either undergone bilaterally negative biopsies or who have had a single negative biopsy and then refuse a contralateral biopsy) in whom the clinical imperative to undertake treatment cannot be ignored, and in whom management will be based on a diagnosis of biopsy-negative GCA.

Other Diagnostic Modalities: Imaging Procedures

Doppler ultrasonography of the temporal arteries has been recommended by some investigators as a noninvasive diagnostic tool for the diagnosis of GCA (Figs. 15-4 and 15-5).[58] The halo sign, a hypoechoic area around the artery, when combined with other ultrasonographic findings of stenosis and occlusion, has been reported to show a sensitivity of 88% for what was termed the "clinical diagnosis" of GCA and 95% for "positive findings on histologic examination".[59]

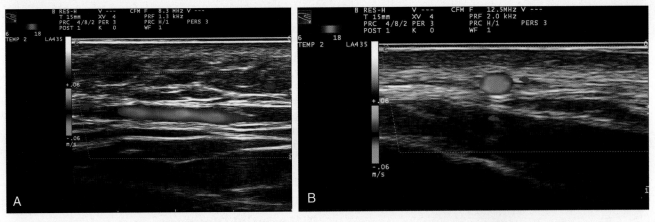

Figure 15-4. Color duplex ultrasonography of a normal temporal artery. Longitudinal (**A**) and transverse (**B**) views. (Courtesy of Dr. Wolfgang A. Schmidt).

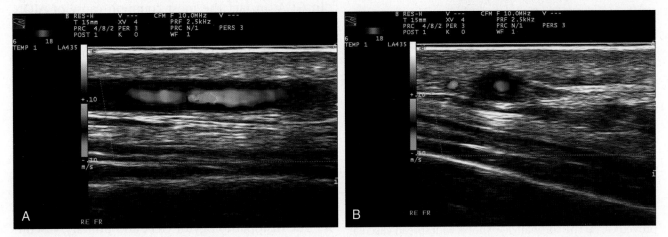

Figure 15-5. Color duplex ultrasonography, giant cell arteritis, temporal artery. Longitudinal (**A**) and transverse (**B**) views. Note hypoechoic swelling of the vessel wall. The longitudinal view also demonstrates turbulent flow suspicious for stenosis. (Courtesy of Dr. Wolfgang A. Schmidt.)

Other studies on the value of this technique for the diagnosis of GCA have been less favorable. A 2005 meta-analysis of studies of 2036 patients who had undergone diagnostic ultrasonography found that in biopsy-proved GCA, the combination of halo sign, stenosis, and occlusion had a sensitivity of 88% (95% CI, 74–95%) and a specificity of 78% (95% CI, 71–84%).[60] This analysis also noted that, if the pretest probability of GCA was low (less than 10%), a negative ultrasound examination virtually excluded the disease.

It is a truth universally acknowledged that, at present, ultrasonography is a highly operator-dependent procedure; as such, its use in the diagnosis of GCA remains controversial. Ultrasound of the TA—notwithstanding its virtues as a simple, inexpensive, risk-free technique—cannot now be recommended as a routine diagnostic surrogate for the TA biopsy.

FDG-PET of patients with GCA has demonstrated the remarkable extent of large artery involvement, particularly the subclavian arteries and the aorta. In one study of biopsy-proved GCA, three quarters of patients showed increased uptake in the subclavian arteries and one half showed increased uptake in the aorta (Figs. 15-6 and 15-7).[61] Whether such involvement predicts clinical outcome—the development of arterial stenoses or aneurysmal disease of the aorta—remains undetermined. Because their prognostic significance is unclear, findings on FDG-PET do not alter treatment strategies for GCA, and so this technique cannot be recommended for ordinary work-up. Because of the limited spatial resolution of FDG-PET, the TA itself cannot be visualized.

High-resolution, contrast-enhanced 3T magnetic resonance imaging (MRI) has also been studied.[62] Inflammation, identified on the basis of mural enhancement and thickening, can be detected in the extracranial arteries, including the temporal arteries.[62] A recent retrospective study reported that

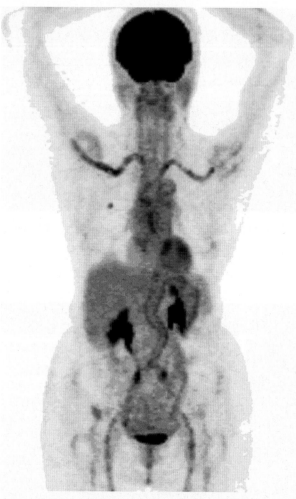

Figure 15-6. FDG PET scan of a patient with biopsy-proved GCA. The coronal view shows widespread vascular uptake, with increased avidity in the subclavian arteries bilaterally, thoracic and abdominal aorta, and femoral arteries.

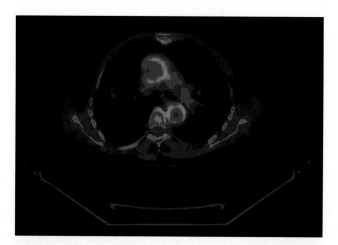

Figure 15-7. Fused image from FDG PET/CT scan of a patient with biopsy-proved GCA. An axial view shows increased avidity circumferentially in the wall of the ascending and descending aorta. Progressive aneurysmal dilation of the ascending aorta eventually led to the need for operative intervention; histopathology of the resected aortic root demonstrated active aortitis.

the sensitivity of high-resolution MRI and ultrasound, compared with TA biopsy, was the same (83% and 79%, respectively).[63] The technique of high-resolution MRI is in its infancy, and prospective, blinded studies in patients undergoing TA biopsies are lacking. The cost of both MRI and FDG-PET represents an obvious impediment to their widespread use.

At this time, the TA biopsy, notwithstanding its imperfect performance as diagnostic test, remains the proverbial gold standard for the definitive diagnosis of GCA.

Differential Diagnosis

Although anterior ischemic optic neuropathy (AION) due to arteritic occlusion of the posterior ciliary artery is the most frequent reason for vision loss in GCA, in fact the most common cause of AION in older adults is nonarteritic AION.[64] Diabetes mellitus, hypertension, and use of sildenafil are risk factors for nonarteritic AION, as is a small cup of the optic nerve head, but the basic cause is known. Affected patients are between the ages of 60 and 70 years of age and are rarely older. Loss of vision is characteristically first recognized when a patient awakens in the morning; the preceding days and weeks are uneventful, without noteworthy constitutional symptoms or premonitory visual symptoms. Acute phase reactants are normal. Involvement of the contralateral eye may occur in 12% to 19% of cases. Vision may improve with time, but there is no known treatment.

The histopathology of GCA and primary vasculitis of the central nervous system is similar, but the latter affects only intracranial arteries and is not associated with systemic symptoms and signs.

The TA may occasionally be involved by other systemic vaculitides, such as Wegener's granulomatosis or microscopic polyangiitis. Fibrinoid necrosis in the TA, which is not seen in GCA, should alert the pathologist and the clinician to the possibility of one of these diseases, which are further differentiated from GCA by their pulmonary or renal disease and the presence of antineutrophil cytoplasmic antibodies. Rarely, a TA biopsy will disclose amyloidosis, the clinical presentation of which may include jaw claudication and symptoms and signs referable to the shoulders.[65]

Initial Treatment: Corticosteroids

The effectiveness of CS in the treatment of GCA—above all as regards the prevention of permanent visual loss—has been ratified by decades of clinical experience. In an analysis of 245 patients with biopsy-proved GCA, all of whom were treated with CS, 34 patients (14%) had permanent visual loss. In 32 of 34 patients, loss of vision had already occurred before initiation of treatment with GC.[40a] In three of these 32 patients, there was further visual loss after treatment was started. Of the two instances of de novo visual loss that developed after beginning CS, one occurred in a patient who was 8 days into treatment with CS; the other, which occurred in a patient with a normal ESR 3 years after CS were begun and 1 year after they were discontinued, was in all likelihood unrelated to GCA. The ophthalmologists Hayreh and Zimmerman[66] described similar findings in 144 patients with biopsy-proved GCA. None of 53 patients without visual loss experienced deterioration of vision after beginning CS; of the 91 patients with visual loss at presentation, nine incurred additional deterioration of vision after beginning CS, all within 5 days of the start of treatment, in either the intially affected eye or the contralateral eye.

Permanent visual loss in GCA is not uncommon, occurring in 10% to 20% of cases; established visual loss is rarely reversible; established visual loss may occasionally progress after initiation of CS therapy; but in the overwhelming majority of patients with GCA and no visual loss at presentation, treatment with CS effectively abolishes the risk of subsequent loss of vision. Indeed, such is the efficacy of daily CS for the initial treatment of GCA that this drug is the yardstick against which any other therapy must be assessed.

Not codified, however, are the appropriate starting dose of CS, the speed of the taper of CS, and the necessary duration of treatment. Controlled studies on these important clinical issues do not exist, as is the case with the use of CS for the management of PMR. Given the unquestionable benefit of CS for the treatment of GCA, on the one hand, and the unquestionable potential toxicities of such treatment, on the other, optimal dosing of CS for the management of GCA poses a major challenge.

Earlier studies reported that smaller starting doses of CS (20–40 mg/day) were effective for the prevention of blindness. Ophthalmologists have typically promoted the use of substantially higher CS doses for initial management, no doubt as a consequence of their involvement with a population of cases of GCA in which visual loss has been threatened or already established. Because of the specter of blindness, current clinical practice usually opts for CS dose in the range of prednisone 40 to 60 mg/day, or 1 mg/kg, administered daily, although, as implied, such dosing is based on custom, not evidence. In the face of threatened visual loss (e.g., amaurosis fugax), high-dose intravenous methylprednisolone (500–1000 mg/day for 3 days) is traditionally tried, also without supportive evidence from controlled studies.

The upfront use of so-called pulse steroids (i.e., mega-doses of IV methylprednisolone) for the routine management of GCA has been proposed in one study.[67] Twenty-seven patients with biopsy-proved GCA were randomly allocated to treatment with either IV saline or IV methylprednisolone (15 mg/kg); both groups were also started on 40 mg of prednisone per day, which was then tapered according to a fixed schedule, unless relapse occurred, in which case the dose was adjusted upward. The duration of follow-up was 78 weeks. No blindness occurred in either group. A statistically significant percentage of patients who received pulse steroids attained a prednisone dose of 5 mg/day or less at 36, 52, and 78 weeks compared to patients treated with oral GC alone. However, the number of patients studied was small, and the lower cumulative dose of CS in the group treated with IV CS of oral CS held up only if the initial courses of IV methylprednisolone were not counted.

Could the initial dose of CS be varied? Could patients be stratified for their risks of blindness, and the CS dose be adjusted accordingly? Not surprisingly, most studies have flagged a history of prior transient visual loss (i.e., amaurosis fugax) as the strongest risk factor for subsequent permanent visual loss.[41-44] Curiously, a decreased risk of permanent visual loss has been noted in patients with a supposed strong inflammatory response, i.e. constitutional symptoms and signs, especially fever and weight loss, high ESR, and anemia.[41,43,44,68]

In any event, the use of stratification of risk to determine CS dosing is not now clinically useful in the individual patient, aside from the obvious point that symptoms of transient visual loss in suspected or proven GCA mandate immediate treatment with CS, either in the form of high-dose oral CS, or as is now common, with 3 days of high-dose intravenous CS.

Whatever the starting dose of CS, two points cannot be argued. First, if the clinical suspicion for GCA is high, CS treatment should begin promptly. Visual loss may occur with devastating swiftness, and may be irreversible; moreover, initiation of such treatment will not affect the interpretation of a TA biopsy even if several days are needed to orchestrate this procedure. Second, CS must be administered on a daily basis, as emphasized by Hunder and colleagues years ago.[69] The importance of daily CS use was recently underlined in the course of an investigation into the use of MTX for GCA.[70] In that study, an aggressive taper to alternate-day CS was associated with an alarming incidence of new visual loss.

A possible value for low-dose aspirin in the initial treatment of GCA has been suggested by two recent retrospective studies[71,72] and an enthusiastic editorial.[73] Patients with GCA who were taking antiplatelet therapy (mainly low-dose aspirin) at the time of diagnosis had significantly lowered odds ratios of so-called cranial ischemic complications—visual loss and strokes—during follow-up. Low-dose aspirin is now included in several recommendations for the initial treatment of GCA, but there are caveats. Whether antiplatelet therapy has a similar benefit in newly diagnosed patients with GCA to whose therapeutic regimen aspirin is then added is unproven. Thrombosis and embolism are not usually considered as figuring prominently in the pathophysiology of ischemia in GCA. And two newer studies have been unable to confirm a protective effect of low-dose aspirin against ischemic events in GCA.[74,75]

Therefore, the decision to add aspirin to the initial treatment with high-dose CS is not clear-cut. In a patient with no risk factors for bleeding, the risk of adding low-dose aspirin is probably low enough to support such use. But it should also be remembered that in an older adult, both high-dose CS as well as the concurrent administration CS and aspirin are among major risk factors for gastrointestinal bleeding, so that, if low-dose aspirin is used with high-dose CS, a proton pump inhibitor should be prophylactically prescribed.

In the initial management of GCA with high-dose CS, skin testing or other appropriate screening measures for tuberculosis should be up to date, as well as immunizations with flu vaccine and pneumococcal vaccine. Prophylaxis against *Pneumocystitis carinii* infection is not indicated, as infection with this organism is not increased in patients with GCA on high-dose GC alone.

Subsequent Treatment and Clinical Course

Deterioration of vision after the first week of CS is rare, and other symptoms and signs of GCA—headaches, scalp tenderness, fever, malaise, and others—recede quickly, usually within 1 or 2 weeks of beginning treatment. If such clinical improvement is not promptly forthcoming, especially in the case of biopsy-negative GCA, the diagnosis should be reassessed. Traditionally, the initial higher dose of CS, administered daily, is maintained for 2 to 4 weeks, at which time, a taper can be started. The recommendation of Hunder and Salvarani[24] that the dose then be reduced "each week or every two weeks by a maximum of 10% of the daily dose," although arbitrary, is grounded in common sense. With the important proviso that the clinical situation remain stable, it is reasonable to aim for a target dose of 40 mg of prednisone by 4 weeks, 20 mg/day by 12 weeks, and 5 to 10 mg/day by 26 weeks. The tempo of the taper is customarily slowed below prednisone 20 mg/day, because of what seems to be an increased frequency of symptomatic flares (e.g., recurring headache) at lower doses of CS. In many patients, CS treatment can then be terminated over the ensuing half year, after which true symptomatic flares of GCA are decidedly unusual.

What determines the speed at which the taper of CS can be safely pursued? Of primary clinical importance is an attentiveness to the recrudescence of symptoms and signs reminiscent of the patient's initial presentation. Accurate serologic gauges of disease activity would obviously be useful, and several have been proposed, including serum levels of IL-6.[76] Operationally, however, the clinician must work with the two venerable acute phase reactants, the ESR and the CRP.

Both the ESR and CRP usually decline to normal or near-normal values during the initial period of treatment; with higher-dose CS, the CRP declines more rapidly than the ESR. Observant follow-up may show that one or the other correlates better with the clinical assessment of disease activity, but in the management of GCA, both are often factored into decisions regarding the CS taper. The CRP, unlike the ESR, is not influenced by abnormalities of red blood cells and the serum immunoglobulins, not infrequent findings in older adults. Minor fluctuations in the acute phase reactants during the course of the taper are common and are not of themselves grounds for increased doses of CS, but if they rise significantly, the pace of the taper should be slowed or the CS dose modestly raised. Slavish titration of the CS dose against increases in the ESR or the CRP, without regard for the patient's clinical status, usually leads to overtreatment and CS-related toxicities.

The total duration of treatment with CS in reported series varies rather widely, but it is difficult to determine what figures in recommendations for routine CS use that is sustained beyond 1 or 2 years, apart from asymptomatic elevations of the acute phase reactants.

Clinical experience suggests that there is a tendency for CS use in GCA to be unduly prolonged at higher doses, and that in some instances, more morbidity ensues from the treatment of the disease than from the disease itself. It thus may be appropriate to consider aggressive monitoring of the acute phase reactants during the first 3 months of treatment, every 2 weeks, or before each reduction of the CS dose, if feasible. Whether such conscientious assessment would facilitate an expeditious and safe taper from initial high-dose prednisone to a dose in the range of 20 mg/day, or whether fewer side effects from CS, would ensue, is admittedly unproved.

Toxicities of CS

That older adults with GCA would be susceptible to the formidable toxicities attendant with the use of higher doses CS–diabetes mellitus, fracture, gastrointestinal bleeding, hypertension, infection, or posterior subcapsular cataract—is predictable.

Bone mineral densitometry should be obtained on all patients, both women and men, and all patients should receive supplemental calcium, 1000 to 1500 mg/day, and vitamin D, at least 800 units/day. Effective management of bone loss, which is mandatory, has been substantially facilitated by use of bisphosphonates. All patients with GCA on high-dose CS should be monitored regularly for possible deleterious effects of CS on blood pressure and glucose homeostasis.

Adjunctive Treatments for Giant Cell Arteritis

Despite the best efforts to use CS judiciously in the treatment of GCA, drug-related toxicities will occur, ranging from insulin-requiring diabetes mellitus and osteoporosis-related fragility fractures, which both physician and patient will agree are unacceptable, to weight gain or widespread capillary fragility, which the patient may view as equally, if not more, deplorable. In the hunt for a CS-sparing intervention, MTX and the TNF alpha blockers have been studied.

Discordant conclusions were reached in two RCTs of adjunctive MTX.

Jover and colleagues[77] treated 42 biopsy-proved GCA patients with prednisone and either MTX 10 mg/week or placebo. Prednisone was begun in a dose of 60 mg/day, tapered to 40 mg/day by 1 month, to 20 mg/day by 2 months, and then by 2.5-mg decrements every 2 weeks, unless relapse occurred, at which point prescribed dose adjustments were permitted. Relapse was defined as a recurrence of symptoms reversed by an increased prednisone dose; using this definition, the group treated with MTX compared with placebo had fewer relapses ($P = 0.018$). The MTX-treated group also had a lower cumulative CS dose ($P = 0.01$).

Hoffman and associates[70] treated 98 GCA patients, 83 of whom were biopsy-proved, with prednisone and either MTX 15 mg/week or placebo. Prednisone was begun in a dose of 1 mg/kg, maintained at that level for 4 weeks, tapered to 60 mg every other day by 3 months, and then tapered off by 6 months. Prescribed dose adjustments were again allowed if relapse occurred. Relapse was defined as an ESR greater than 40 and one feature of GCA (headache, fever, vision loss, other) not attributable to other conditions; using this definition, there was no statistically significant difference in relapses between the two groups. The cumulative CS dose was the same in both groups, as were CS-related toxicities.

In both studies, results may have been influenced by the dosing of MTX (10 to 15 mg/week), which, by current standards, is low. Possibly the conflicting conclusions (i.e., Jover found MTX to be CS sparing, Hoffman did not) were affected by the differing tapering regimens: Jover used daily doses of CS throughout, but Hoffman aimed to taper to alternate-day dose CS by 3 months. Ultimately, however, the differing verdicts of the two trials cannot be settled.

Mahr and associates[78] combined these two studies with another smaller RCT of 21 patients[79] to perform a careful meta-analysis on the use of adjunctive MTX in the treatment of GCA. He concluded that such use of MTX (e.g., in modest doses of 7.5–15 mg/week) reduced the risk of first and second relapse by 35% and 51%, respectively; decreased cumulative CS dose; and increased the probability of discontinuing CS entirely. On the other hand, and importantly, the meta-analysis found no reduction in CS-related toxicities with adjunctive MTX. The mean duration of follow-up was 55 weeks, which possibly was not long enough to detect such a reduction.

The MTX studies raise issues that complicate most efforts to identify adjunctive or alternative treatments for GCA. First, it is essential that, whatever the proposed regimen, visual loss be prevented, and any approach that cannot match the efficacy of monotherapy with appropriately administered CS for so doing does not merit further consideration. Second, the use of endpoints such as a decrease in clinical relapses, however defined, or a decrease in total CS dose, will be of no clinical consequence unless a beneficial effect on outcome can be demonstrated, viz., reduced CS-related toxicities. If there is no accompanying reduction in these toxicities, whether the risks inherent in adding a second drug will remain in doubt.

Adjunctive TNF alpha blockade for the treatment of GCA has been described in individual case reports, small series of cases, and one RCT. The RCT showed no benefit for adjunctive TNF alpha blockade compared with placebo in the treatment of newly diagnosed GCA.[80] In that study, 44 patients with GCA on treatment with GC for fewer than 4 weeks were randomized to concurrent treatment with placebo or infliximab, given at 5 mg/kg at 0, 2, and 6 weeks, and then every 8 weeks thereafter. Prednisone, in an initial dose of 40 to 60 mg/day, was tapered off by 6 months but could be adjusted for relapse, defined as an increased ESR from normal to 40 or more and one symptom or sign of GCA that could not be ascribed to other causes. Although planned for 52 weeks, the study was terminated at week 22 because there was no significant effect on either of the two primary outcome measures, the percentage of relapse-free patients and adverse events. Secondary outcome measures–time to first relapse, number of relapse-free patients when prednisone was tapered to 10 mg/day, and cumulative prednisone dose–were also no different in the groups treated with placebo compared with infliximab.

Attention should be paid to two case reports describing the emergence of GCA in the face of therapy with TNF alpha blockade. Both patients had seropositive rheumatoid arthritis, both were on active treatment for rheumatoid arthritis with MTX and TNF blockade (adalimumab or etanercept), and both evolved biopsy-proved GCA.[81,82] TNF alpha thus does not appear to play a major role in the initial pathogenesis of GCA.

Finally, it does appear that TNF alpha blockade is valuable for the management of some patients with Takayasu arteritis,[83] a systemic vasculitis that bears histopathologic similarities to GCA. The positive clinical experience with TNF alpha blockade in this arteritis, although not confirmed in controlled studies, suggests that a potential role for this therapy in the treatment of GCA could be further explored.

For adjunctive treatment of GCA, the benefits of MTX are at best modest, and at least at this time, those of TNF alpha blockade are uncertain. Neither adjunctive use of MTX nor TNF alpha blockade can therefore be recommended for initial or routine management. In a high-risk patient (e.g., one with potential or established CS-related toxicities, such as diabetes mellitus, significant hypertension, or osteoporosis with recurring fractures), the addition to CS therapy of MTX at doses of 20 to 25 mg/week could be considered. Efforts to identify a CS-sparing agent in the treatment for GCA that would result in a demonstrable reduction in CS-related toxicities remain important; identification of a treatment as efficacious as CS in the prevention of blindness but with lesser toxicities would be ideal.

Large Vessel Giant Cell Arteritis

Until recently the extent of "large-vessel GCA"–the term applied to GCA affecting the aorta and great vessels–has been underappreciated. In the Mayo Clinic's retrospective study of a population-based cohort of 168 cases of GCA, clinical large-vessel disease of any kind was found in one of four patents.[84] A high prevalence of subclinical large vessel involvement has also been shown with FDG-PET, as noted previously.[61]

Large Vessel Giant Cell Arteritis: Aneurysms of the Aorta

In an earlier study of the Mayo Clinic cohort by Hunder and associates, 16 of 96 patients were found to have aneurysms of the aorta, mainly in the ascending thoracic aorta.[84] Thoracic aorta aneurysms were 17.3 times more likely and abdominal aortic aneurysms 2.4 times more likely to occur in patients with GCA than in the general population. A later study from the Mayo Clinic reported aneurysmal disease of the aorta of 18% of 168 GCA patients.[85] Dissection occurred in one half of the 18 incident cases of aneurysm of the thoracic aorta.

Often these aneurysms were a late development in the course of GCA. In a descriptive study of aneurysms of the thoracic aorta in GCA, 8 of 41 patients were identified with aneurysms before or at the time of diagnosis of GCA, but in the remaining 33 patients

the median time between initial diagnosis of GCA and eventual diagnosis of aneurysm was 7 years.[86] Histopathologic evidence of active aortitis was seen in one half of the cases that came to surgery on post-mortem examination, thus implying two possible mechanisms for aneurysm formation–smoldering or recrudescent inflammation, on the one hand, or mechanical stress on an aorta structurally injured from initial inflammation, on the other (Fig. 15-8).

Although the incidence figures for aortic aneurysms in GCA reported from the Mayo Clinic may seem high, similar results have been published from 2 other centers.[87,88]

Data pertaining to risk factors for the clinical development of aneurysms are meager and conflicting. There is disagreement as to whether aneurysms are associated with traditional cardiovascular risk factors such as hypertension or hyperlipidemia, or with a strong or weak inflammatory response. The important issue as to whether sustained suppression of inflammation with CS affects the emergence of aneurysms has not been clarified.

Cost-effective screening strategies for aneurysms in GCA have not been vetted. An annual chest x-ray study is sensible. A more aggressive approach to screening has been proposed, beginning with annual transthoracic and abdominal ultrasound examinations.[89] Ultrasound, computed tomography (CT), and MRA are techniques of well-known sensitivity for detecting aneurysms or the aorta, but until there are prospective data confirming their diagnostic, therapeutic, and economic worth for routine screening of the GCA patient, clinical vigilance and the basic posteroanterior and lateral chest x-ray studies may have to suffice. If an aneurysm is suspected on plain films, CT of the chest should be obtained; if the aneurysm is documented, imaging of the entire vascular tree is warranted, usually with contrast MRI, and the clinician must then confront the issue of further management.

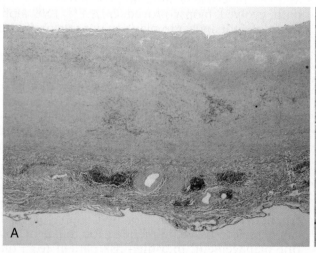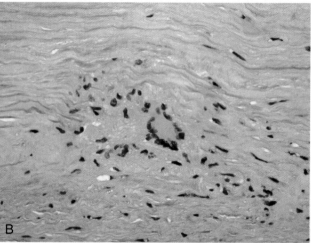

Figure 15-8. Histopathology, aorta. Aortitis in a patient with GCA. (**A**) The adventitia (bottom) is thickened and contains dense inflammatory infiltrates; the media also shows inflammatory infiltrates, and, on the left, an area of necrosis. (**B**) A high power view of the media shows an inflammatory infiltrate with a giant cell. (Courtesy of Dr. Robert F. Padera.)

Guidelines for the operative management of aortic aneurysms in GCA derive from recommendations for patients with aneurysms due to atherosclerosis. Surgery is recommended for aneurysms of ascending and descending thoracic aorta more than 5 and 6 cm in diameter, respectively, and for abdominal aortic aneurysms of more than 5.5 cm in diameter. In the management of lesser aneurysms, hypertension and other risk factors should be aggressively treated, and follow-up surveillance imaging is advised initially every 6 months. But two pivotal and related questions are difficult to answer: does the aneurysm contain active inflammation, and, if so, would treatment with CS prevent progression of the aneurysm?

The differentiation between damage and disease activity in large vessels is not easy. MRI with contrast can display luminal dimensions and wall thickening, but whether findings of mural edema or contrast enhancement with this technique correlate with the presence of ongoing inflammatory activity per se is less certain. This problem has been encountered with the use of MRI in the follow-up of patients with Takayasu arteritis, in which mural enhancement on post-contrast T1-sequences and mural edema on T2-sequences have related inconsistently to the subsequent evolution of overt vascular damage.[90] Similar uncertainties apply to the findings of increased uptake on FDG-PET. A recent study of MRI and FDG-PET, both performed in 25 patients with complicated GCA, could not correlate imaging abnormalities with CRP, ESR, or clinical findings.[91] The key question as to whether abnormal imaging of the vessel wall in GCA by MRA and FDG-PET reflects remodeling, inflammation, or both, remains unanswered. It is also a practical matter of no small importance that many insurers in the United States do not routinely cover FDG-PET for the diagnosis of vasculitis.

With this caution in mind, if there is an enlarging aneurysm, and if mural abnormalities are found on imaging studies in the face of elevated acute phase reactants, it is reasonable to resume or increase CS treatment, with the additional qualifications that a relationship between aortic inflammation and elevations of the acute phase reactants has never been proved, and that progression of an aneurysm may owe more to structural damage of the vessel wall than to ongoing inflammation. There is currently no evidence that MTX, TNF alpha blockers, or immunosuppressants are beneficial in this situation.

The unexpected finding of aortitis at the time of surgical repair of an aneurysm poses a comparably thorny problem. The typical scenario involves the discovery of aortitis by the pathologist on examination of a surgically excised aneurysm from a patient in whom systemic vasculitis was not suspected preoperatively. The differential diagnosis includes a variety of conditions that can usually be distinguished on clinical and pathologic grounds, including infections, such as syphilis and tuberculosis, and systemic rheumatic diseases, such as lupus, rheumatoid arthritis, and Takayasu arteritis. In an older adult, GCA often emerges as the leading diagnosis.

A prior history of symptoms and signs signalling PMR or GCA, or both, is sometimes obtained, sometimes not. The acute phase reactants cannot be relied on in the immediate post-operative period, so they should be measured after recovery from surgery, and the vascular tree should be completely imaged. In the absence of symptoms suggestive of PMR or GCA, the yield of a TA biopsy is likely to be low.

Once these data—history and physical examination, appropriate assessment of acute phase reactants, and vascular imaging—are collected, the matter of further treatment must be addressed. In patients in whom aortitis from a surgically repaired aneurysm appears to be clinically and radiologically localized to the ascending aorta, an argument could be made for conservative management, without pharmacologic intervention. In a series from the Mayo Clinic, only 1 of 19 such patients, treated without CS, developed a new aneurysm during a mean follow-up of almost 7 years.[92] In a similar series from the Cleveland Clinic, with a mean follow-up of 3.5 years, new aneurysms occurred in six of 25 patients treated without CS.[93] Of note, however, in the 11 patients from this latter series who did receive CS, no new aneurysms developed. Whether or not the plan of management includes CS, it is plain that attentive follow-up and imaging are essential.

The problem of aneurysms of the aorta in GCA–their prevention, appropriate surveillance for them, and their management—remains a work in progress. Notwithstanding these clinical uncertainties, the mortality of GCA patients with and without aortic aneurysms does not seem to be different.[94]

Large Vessel Giant Cell Arteritis: Involvement of the Great Vessels

Less common than aortic aneurysms is clinically diagnosed GCA of the great vessels, which was found in only 4% of the 168 GCA patients reported from the Mayo Clinic, most often at the subclavian and axillary arteries.[84] A much higher incidence of subclinical involvement of these arteries has been shown by ultrasound and FDG-PET scanning. Interestingly, the simultaneous occurrence of GCA of the aorta, manifested by aneurysm, and GCA of the great vessels, manifested by stenosis, is exceptional. Involvement of the femoral arteries is infrequent.

Subclavian/axillary GCA presents with claudication of the arms, i.e., heaviness or pain in the arms with use, better with cessation of activity. Blood pressure in the arms may be difficult to elicit or absent. Even in the absence of palpable arterial pulsations or blood pressures, overt consequences of arterial insufficiency, such as digital ulcerations or gangrene, are rare in GCA, by virtue of the usual development of an extensive collateral circulation.

The findings on angiography, which are typical for vasculitis in general and not unique to GCA, include smooth tapering of stenotic segments, both proximally and distally.[95] Involvement is nearly always bilateral, although not symmetric. If blood pressure in the arms cannot be obtained, formal dye angiography should be considered in order that central blood pressure can be assessed.

Some features distinguish subclavian/axillary GCA from other phenotypic presentations of GCA. In a study comparing 74 patients with angiographically proven subclavian/axillary GCA to 74 patients with biopsy-proved cranial GCA, PMR and constitutional symptoms were present with equal frequency in both groups, but headache occurred four times more commonly in the group with cranial GCA, and, as a not unexpected corollary, TA biopsy was negative in the 42% of patients with subclavian/axillary GCA.[96] In another study, the interval between the initial diagnosis of GCA and the detection of large-artery stenoses was 1.1 years, in contrast to the usually longer lag between initial diagnosis of GCA and the detection of aortic aneurysm.[84]

GCA presenting with large artery stenoses poses problems of management similar to those arising from the discovery of a GCA-related aortic aneurysm, and center on the question of how much of the clinical situation is due to irreversible structural damage as opposed to how much is due to ongoing inflammation. A careful history and physical examination, measurement of acute phase reactants, and vascular imaging are indicated, and may lead to a conclusion about the extent of active inflammation, but as is the case with the work-up of aortic aneurysm, such data may not be definitive. Although TA may be positive in only one half of cases, the finding of an active arteritis would justify a decision to proceed with an initial course of high-dose steroids. If the biopsy is negative, a trial of CS for treatment of claudication is still reasonable, though symptomatic improvement is unpredictable. Revascularization is rarely necessary; arterial stenting is occasionally necessary, but bypass procedures may be more durably successful.

Neurologic Involvement in Giant Cell Arteritis

Clinically significant neurologic involvement in GCA is unusual.

When strokes do occur, they usually result from involvement of the extradural internal carotid and vertebral arteries, more often the latter.[97] Accurate ascertainment of the prevalence of ischemic stroke in GCA is difficult because of the frequency of stroke in older patients in general; furthermore, whether a stroke occurring weeks or months after the diagnosis of GCA can be construed as an etiologically related event is unclear. Gonzalez-Gay and coworkers[98] reported stroke in 3% of 239 patients

with biopsy-proved GCA, all recorded within 30 days of the diagnosis. The actual prevalence of GCA in ischemic stroke as a whole is very low—only 0.15% of 4086 cases in the Lausanne Stroke Registry met histopathologic and radiologic criteria for the diagnosis of GCA.[99]

Involvement of the intracranial arteries by GCA is exceedingly rare: it was confirmed in all but two of 463 cases of clinically diagnosed central nervous system vasculitis reviewed by Salvarani and Hunder from the Mayo Clinic.[100] The rarity of this involvement has been attributed to the observation that these arteries lack an internal elastic lamina, a frequent site of histopatholgic changes in GCA. In this model, the proclivity for transient ischemic attacks and strokes in GCA to occur in the distribution of the vertebrobasilar circulation is explained by the preservation of an internal elastic lamina in the vertebral arteries for a few millimeters after they perforate the dura. The absence of vasa vasorum and key Toll-like receptors in intracranial arteries may also be important pathophysiologic considerations. When arteritis of the intracranial arteries due to GCA does occur, the course is poorly responsive to CS and often fatal.

Vestibular dysfunction and sensorineural hearing loss, although uncommon, can be part of the initial presentation of GCA and may reverse with CS treatment.[101]

Giant Cell Arteritis of the Breast and the Female Genital Tract

Exceptionally, GCA is found, usually by chance, on histopathologic examination of a surgically excised breast mass or organ of the female genital tract (ovary, fallopian tubes, or uterus). With GCA of the breast, evaluation for symptoms and signs pointing to PMR or GCA and assessment of the acute phase reactants are often unrevealing, surgical excision is usually curative, and CS treatment not indicated.[102] With involvement of the female genital tract, evidence for full-blown GCA, including positive TA biopsies, seems more frequent, which thus would mandate management with CS.[103]

Conclusion

No one regimen of CS use applies to the management of all cases of GCA, and as with PMR, treatment should be individualized. Visual loss after an initial course of higher dose, daily CS is rare. Subsequent treatment with higher doses of CS should not be unnecessarily protracted. It is possible that a concerted, careful effort at the subsequent taper of CS could decrease exposure to the drug and, accordingly, drug-related toxicities. Finally, a noninvasive marker that reliably reflects disease activity would be a great boon to the rational management of GCA.

Although the appropriate use of CS effectively abolishes visual loss from GCA, the incidence of this most serious of the complications of the disease has remained remarkably similar across case series reported from different countries over the years. One explanation for the persisting incidence of visual loss may be the lack of timely diagnosis, in turn impeding expeditious initiation of treatment. Continued efforts to educate clinicians in the recognition and diagnosis of GCA are also an important piece of the targeted treatment of this disease, the most common of the systemic vasculitides.

References

1. Dasgupta B, Salvarani C, Schirmer M, Crowson CS, Hutchings A, Matteson EL, and members of the American College of Rheumatology Work Group for Development of Classification Criteria for PMR. Developing classification criteria for polymyalgia rheumatica: comparison views from an expert panel and wider survey. J Rheumatol 2008;35:270-7.
2. Chuang TY, Hunder GG, Ilstrup DM, Kurland LT. Polymyalgia rheumatica. A 10-year epidemiologic and clinical study. Ann Int Med 1982;97:672-80.
3. Healey LA. Long-term follow-up of polymyalgia rheumatica: evidence for synovitis. Semin Arthritis Rheum 1984;13:322-8.
4. Bird HA, Esselinckx W, Dixon AS, Mowat AG, Wood PH. An evaluation of criteria for polymyalgia rheumatica. Ann Rheum Dis 1979;38:434-9.
5. Doran MF, Crowson CS, O'Fallon M, Hunder GG, Gabriel SE. Trends in the incidence of polymyalgia rheumatica over a 30 years period in Olmsted County, Minnesota, USA. J Rheumatol 2002;29:1694-7.
6. Cantini F, Salvarini C, Olivieri I, Niccoli L, Padula A, Macchioni L, et al. Shoulder ultrasonography in the diagnosis of polymyalgia rheumatica: a case-control study. J Rheumatol 2001;28:1049-55.
7. Cantini F, Niccoli L, Nannunu C, Padula A, Oliveiri I, Boiardi L, et al. Inflammatory changes of hip synovial structures in polymyalgia rheumatica. Clin Exp Rheumatol 2005;23:462-8.
8. Myklebust G, Gran JTA. Prospective study of 287 patients with polymyalgia rheumatic and temporal arteritis: clinical and laboratory manifestations at onset of disease and at the time of diagnosis. Br J Rheumatol 1996;35:1161-8.
9. Proven A, Gabriel SE, O'Fallon WM, Hunder GG. Polymyalgia rheumatica with low erythrocyte sedimentation rate at diagnosis. J Rheumatol 1999;26:1333-7.
10. Cantini F, Salvarani C, Olivieri I, Macchioni L, Ranzi A, Niccoli L, et al. Erythrocyte sedimentation rate and C-reactive protein in the evaluation of disease activity and severity in polymyalgia rheumatica: a prospective follow-up study. Semin Arthritis Rheum 2000;30:17-24.
11. Gonzalez-Gay MA, Rodriguez-Valerde V, Blanca R, Fernandez-Sueiro JL, Armona J, Figueroa M, et al. Polymyalgia rheumatica without significantly increased erythrocyte sedimentation rate. A more benign syndrome. Arch Intern Med 1997;157:317-20.
12. Dasgupta B, Dolan AL, Panati GS, Fernandes L. An initially double-blind controlled 96 week trial of depot methyl-prednisolone against oral prednisolone in the treatment of polymyalgia rheumatica. Br J Rheumatol 1998;37:189-95.
13. Salvarani C, Cantini F, Hunder GG. Polymyalgia rheumatica and giant cell arteritis. Lancet 2008;372:234-45.
14. Roche NE, Fulbright JW, Wagner AD, Hunder GG, Goronzy JJ, Weyand CM. Correlation of interleukin-6 production and disease activity in polymyalgia rheumatica and giant cell arteritis. Arthritis Rheum 1993;36:1286-94.
15. Myklebust G, Wilsgaard T, Jacobsen BK, Gran JT. No increased frequency of malignant neoplasms in polymyalgia and temporal arteritis. A prospective longitudinal study of 398 cases and matched population controls. J Rheumatol 2002;29:2143-7.
16. Espinosa G, Font J, Munoz-Rodriguez FJ, Cervera R, Ingelmo M. Myelodysplastic and myeloproliferative syndromes associated with giant cell arteritis and polymyalgia rheumatica: a coincidental coexistence or a causal relationship? Clin Rheumatol 2002;21:309-13.
17. Pego-Reigosa JM, Rodriguez-Rodriguez M, Hurtado-Hernandez Z, Gromaz-Martin J, Taboas-Rodriguez D, Millan-Cachinero C, et al. Calcium pyrophosphate deposition disease mimicking polymyalgia rheumatica: a prospective follow-up study of predictive factors for this condition in patients presenting with polymyalgia symptoms. Arthritis Rheum 2005;53:931-8.
18. Olivieri I, Garcia-Porrua C, Padula A, Cantini F, Salvarini C, Gonzalez-Gay MA. Late onset undifferentiated spondyloarthritis presenting with polymyalgia rheumatica features: description of 7 cases. Rheumatology Int 2007;27:927-33.
19. Niccoli L, Salvarani C, Baroncelli G, Padula A, Olivieri I, Cantini F. Renal cell carcinoma mimicking polymyalgia rheumatica. Clues for a correct diagnosis. Scand J Rheumatol 2002;31:103-6.
20. Salvarani S, Cantini F, Macchioni P, Olivieri I, Niccoli L, Padula A, et al. Distal musculoskeletal manifestations in polymyalgia rheumatica. Arthritis Rheum 1998;41:1221-6.
21. Pease CT, Haugeberg G, Morgan AW, Montague B, Hensor EMA, Bhakta BB. Diagnosing late onset rheumatoid arthritis, polymyalgia rheumatica, and temporal arteritis in patients presenting with polymyalgic symptoms. A prospective long-term evaluation. J Rheumatol 2005;32:1043-6.
22. Caporali R, Montecucco C, Epis O, Bobbio-Pallavicini F, Maio T, Cimmino MA. Presenting features of polymyalgia rheumatica (PMR) and rheumatoid arthritis with PMR-like onset: a prospective study. Ann Rheum Dis 2001;601:1021-4.
23. Salvarani C, Gabriel S, Hunder GG. Distal extremity swelling with pitting edema in polymyalgia rheumatica: report of nineteen cases. Arthritis Rheum 1996;26:517-21.
24. Salvarani C, Cantini F, Boiardi L, Hunder GG. Polymyalgia rheumatica and giant-cell arteritis. N Engl J Med 2002;347:261-70.
25. Gonzalez-Gay MA, Garcia-Porrua C, Amor-Dorado JC, Llora J. Giant cell arteritis without clinically evident vascular involvement in a defined population. Arthritis Rheum 2004;51:274-7.
26. Schmidt WA, Gromnica I. Incidence of temporal arteritis in patients with polymyalgia rheumatica: a prospective study using colour Doppler ultrasonography of the temporal arteries. Rheumatology 2002;41:46-52.
27. Blockmans D, De Ceuninck L, Vanderschueren S, Knockaert D, Mortelmans L, Bobbaers H. Repetitive 18-fluorodeoxy-glucose positron emission tomography in isolated polymyalgia rheumatica: a prospective study in 35 patients. Rheumatology 2007;46:672-7.
28. Hernandez-Rodriguez J, Font C, Garcia-Martinez A, Espigol-Frigole G, Sanmarti R, Canete JD, et al. Development of ischemic complications in patients with giant cell arteritis presenting with apparently isolated polymyalgia rheumatica: study of a series of 100 patients. Medicine (Baltimore) 2007;86:232-41.
29. Maradit Kremers H, Reinalda MS, Crowson CS, Zinsmeister AR, Hunder GG, Gabriel SE. Relapse in a population based cohort of patients with polymyalgia rheumatica. J Rheumatol 2005;32:65-73.
30. Cimmino MA, Salvarani C, Macchioni P, Gerli R, Bartoloni Bocci E, Montecucco C, et al. Long-term follow-up of polymyalgia rheumatica patients treated with methotrexate and steroids. Clin Exp Rheumatol 2008;26:395-400.
31. Ayoub WT, Franklin CM, Torretti D. Polymyalgia rheumatica. Duration of therapy and long-term outcome. Am J Med 1985;79:309-15.
32. Docken WP. Polymyalgia rheumatica can recur years after discontinuation of corticosteroid therapy. Clin Exp Rheumatol. 2009;27(suppl. 52):S25-7.

33. Ferraccioli G, Salaffi F, De Vita S, Casatta L, Bartoli E. Methotrexate in polymyalgia rheumatica: preliminary results of an open, randomized study. J Rheumatol 1996;23:624-8.

34. Caporali R, Cimmino MA, Ferraccioli G, Gerli R, Klersy C, Salvarani C, et al. Prednisone plus methotrexate for polymyalgia rheumatica: a randomized, double-blind, placebo-controlled trial. Ann Intern Med 2004;141:493-500.

35. Salvarani C, Macchioni P, Manzini C, Paolazzi G, Trotta A, Manganelli P, et al. Infliximab plus prednisone or placebo plus prednisone for the initial treatment of polymyalgia rheumatica: a randomized trial. Ann Intern Med 2007;146:631-9.

36. Catanoso MG, Macchioni P, Boiardi L, Pipitone N, Salvarani C. Treatment of refractory polymyalgia rheumatica with etanercept: An open pilot study. Arthritis Rheum 2007;57:1514-9.

37. Gonzalez-Gay MA, Barros S, Lopez-Diaz MJ, Garcia-Porrua C, Sanchez-Andrade A, Llorca J. Giant cell arteritis: disease patterns of clinical presentation in a series of 240 patients. Medicine (Baltimore) 2005;84:269-76.

38. Smith CA, Fidler WJ, Hall AJ. The epidemiology of giant cell arteritis. Report of a ten-year study in Shelby County, Tennessee. Arthritis Rheum 1983;26:1214-9.

39. Hall S, Persellin S, Lie JT, O'Brien PC, Kurland LT, Hunder GG. The therapeutic impact of temporal artery biopsy. Lancet 1983;2:1217-20.

40. Font C, Cid MC, Coll-Vinent B, Lopez-Soto A, Grau JM. Clinical features in patients with permanent visual loss due to biopsy-proven giant cell arteritis. Br J Rheumatol 1997;36:251-4.

40a. Aiello PD, Trautmann JC, McPhee TJ, Kunselman AR, Hunder GG. Visual prognosis in giant cell arteritis. Ophthalmology 1993;100:550-5.

41. Gonzalez-Gay MA, Garcia-Porrua C, Llorca J, Hajeer AH, Branas F, Dababneh A, et al. Visual manifestations of giant cell arteritis. Trends and clinical spectrum in 161 patients. Medicine (Baltimore) 2000;79:283-92.

42. Liozon E, Herrmann F, Ly K, Robert P, Loustand V, Soria P, et al. Risk factors of visual loss in giant cell (temporal arteritis): a prospective study of 174 patients. Am J Med 2001;111:211-7.

43. Nesher G, Berkun Y, Mates M, Baras M, Nesher R, Rubinow A, et al. Risk factors of cranial ischemic complications in giant cell arteritis. Medicine (Baltimore) 2004;83:114-22.

44. Salvarani C, Cimino L, Macchioni P, Consonni D, Cantini F, Bajocchi G, et al. Risk factors for visual loss in an Italian population-based cohort of patients with giant cell arteritis. Arthritis Rheum 2005;53:292-7.

45. Calamia KT, Hunder GG. Giant cell arteritis (temporal arteritis) presenting as fever of undetermined origin. Arthritis Rheum 1981;24:1414-8.

46. Knockaert DC, Vanneste LJ, Bobbaers HJ. Fever of unknown origin in elderly patients. J Am Geriatric Soc 1993;41:1187-92.

47. Salvarani C, Hunder GG. Musculoskeletal manifestations in a population-based cohort of patients with giant cell arteritis. Arthritis Rheum 1999;42:1259-66.

48. Gonzalez-Gay MA, Lopez-Diaz MJ, Barros S, Garcia-Porrua C, Sanchez-Andrade A, Paz-Carreira J, et al. Giant cell arteritis: laboratory tests at the time of diagnosis in a series of 240 patients. Medicine (Baltimore) 2005;84:277-90.

49. Salvarani C, Hunder GG. Giant cell arteritis with low erythrocyte sedimentation rate: frequency of occurrence in a population-based study. Arthritis Rheum 2001;45:140-5.

50. Smetana GW, Shmerling RH. Does this patient have temporal arteritis? JAMA 2002;287:92-101.

51. Achkar AA, Lie JT, Hunder GG, O'Fallon WM, Gabriel SE. How does previous corticosteroid treatment affect the biopsy findings in giant cell (temporal) arteritis? Ann Intern Med 1994;120:987-92.

52. Klein RG, Campbell RJ, Hunder GG. Skip areas in temporal arteritis. Mayo Clin Proc 1976;94:2072-7.

53. Mahr A, Saba M, Kamboucher M, Polivka M, Baudrimont M, Brocheriou I, et al. Temporal artery biopsy for diagnosing giant cell arteritis: the longer, the better? Ann Rheum Dis 2006;65:826-8.

54. Boyev LR, Miller NR, Green WR. Efficacy of unilateral versus bilateral temporal artery biopsies for the diagnosis of giant cell arteritis. Am J Ophthalmol 1999;128:211-9.

55. Danesh-Meyer HV, Savino PJ, Eagle RC, Kubis KC, Sergott RC. Low diagnostic yield with second biopsies in suspected giant cell arteritis. J Neuroophthalmol 2000;20:213-5.

56. Hayreh SS, Podhajsky PA, Raman R, Zimmerman B. Giant cell arteritis: validity and reliability of various diagnostic criteria. Am J Opthalmol 1997;123:285-96.

57. Hall JK, Volpe NJ, Galetta SL, Liu GT, Syed NA, Balcer LJ. The role of unilateral temporal artery biopsy. Ophthalmology 2003;110:543-8.

58. Schmidt WA, Kraft HE, Vorpahl K, Volker L, Gromnica-Ihle EJ. Color duplex ultrasonography in the diagnosis of temporal arteritis. N Engl J Med 1997;337:1336-42.

59. Schmidt WA, Gromnica-Ihle E. Duplex ultrasonography in temporal arteritis. Ann Int Med 2003;138:609.

60. Karassa FB, Matsagas MI, Schmidt WA, Ioannidis JP. Meta-analysis: test performance of ultrasonography for giant-cell arteritis. Ann Intern Med 2005;142:359-69.

61. Blockmans D, De Ceuninck L, Vanderschueren S, Knockaert D, Mortelmans L, Bobbaers H. Repetitive 18-flourodeoxy-glucose positron emission tomography in giant cell arteritis: a prospective study of 35 patients. Arthritis Rheum 2006;55:131-7.

62. Bley TA, Markl M, Schelp M, Uhl M, Frydrychowicz A, Vaith P, et al. Mural inflammatory hyperenhancement in MRI of giant cell (temporal) arteritis resolves under corticosteroid treatment. Rheumatology 2008;47:65-7.

63. Bley TA, Reinhard M, Hauenstein C, Markl M, Warnatz K, Hetzel A, et al. Comparison of duplex sonography and high-resolution magnetic resonance imaging in the diagnosis of giant cell (temporal) arteritis. Arthritis Rheum 2008;58:2574-8.

64. Mathews MK. Non-arteritic anterior ischemic optic neuropathy. Curr Opin Ophthalmol 2005;16:341-5.

65. Salvarani C, Gabriel SE, Gertz MA, Bjornsson J, Li CY, Hunder GG. Primary systemic amyloidosis presenting as giant cell arteritis and polymyalgia rheumatica. Arthritis Rheum 1994;17:1621-6.

66. Hayreh SS, Zimmerman B. Visual deterioration in giant cell arteritis patients while on high doses of corticosteroid therapy. Ophthalmology 2003;110:1204-15.

67. Mazlumzadeh M, Hunder GG, Easley KA, Calamia KT, Matteson EL, Griffing WL, et al. Treatment of giant cell arteritis using induction therapy with high-dose glucocorticoids: a double-blind, placebo-controlled, randomized prospective clinical trial. Arthritis Rheum 2006;54:3310-8.

68. Cid MC, Font C, Oristrell J, dela Sierra A, Coll-Vinent B, Lopez-Soto A, et al. Association between strong inflammatory response and low risk of developing visual loss and other cranial ischemic complications in giant cell (temporal) arteritis. Arthritis Rheum 1998;41:26-32.

69. Hunder GG, Sheps SG, Allen GL, Joyce JW. Daily and alternate-day corticosteroid regimens in treatment of giant cell arteritis: comparison in a prospective study. Ann Intern Med 1975;82:613-8.

70. Hoffman GS, Cid MC, Hellmann DB, Guillevin L, Stone JH, Schousboe J, et al. A multicenter, randomized, double-blind, placebo-controlled trial of adjuvant methotrexate treatment for giant cell arteritis. Arthritis Rheum 2002;46:1309-18.

71. Nesher G, Berkun Y, Mates M, Baras M, Rubinow A, Sonnenblick M. Low-dose aspirin and prevention of cranial ischemic complications in giant cell arteritis. Arthritis Rheum 2004;50:1332-7.

72. Lee MS, Smith SD, Galor A, Hoffman GS. Antiplatelet and anticoagulant therapy in patients with giant cell arteritis. Arthritis Rheum 2006;54:3306-9.

73. Hellman DB. Low-dose aspirin in the treatment of giant cell arteritis. Arthritis Rheum 2004;50:1026-7.

74. Narvaez J, Bernad B, Gomez-Vaquero C, Garcia-Gomez C, Roig-Vilaseca D, Juanola X, et al. Impact of antiplatelet therapy in the development of severe ischemic complications and in the outcome of patients with giant cell arteritis. Clin Exp Rheumatol 2008;26(Suppl. 49):S57-62.

75. Salvarani C, Della Bella C, Cimino L, Macchioni P, Formisano D, Bajocchi G, et al. Risk factors for severe cranial ischemic events in an Italian population based cohort of patients with giant cell arteritis. Rheumatology 2009;48:250-3.

76. Weyand CM, Fulbright JW, Hunder GG, Evans JM, Goronzy JJ. Treatment of giant cell arteritis: interleukin-6 as a biologic marker of disease activity. Arthritis Rheum 2000;43:1041-8.

77. Jover JA, Hernandez-Garcia C, Morado IC, Vargas E, Banares A, Fernandez-Gutierrez B. Combined treatment of giant-cell arteritis with methotrexate and prednisone. A randomized, double-blind, placebo-controlled trail. Ann Intern Med 2001;134:106-14.

78. Mahr AD, Jover JA, Speira RF, Hernandez-Garcia C, Fernandez-Gutierrez B, Lavalley MP, et al. Adjunctive methotrexate for treatment of giant cell arteritis: an individual patient data meta-analysis. Arthritis Rheum 2007;56:2789-97.

79. Spiera RF, Mitnick HJ, Kupersmith M, Richmond M, Spiera H, Peterson MG, et al. A prospective, double-blind, randomized placebo controlled trial of methotrexate in the treatment of giant cell arteritis (GCA). Clin Exp Rheumatol 2001;19:495-501.

80. Hoffman GS, Cinta-Cid M, Rendt-Zagar KE, Merkel PA, Weyand CM, Stone JH, et al. For the Infliximab-GCA study group. Infliximab for the maintenance of glucocorticoid-induced remission of giant cell arteritis: a randomized trial. Ann Intern Med 2007;146:621-30.

81. Seton M. Giant cell arteritis in a patient taking etanercept and methotrexate. J Rheumatol 2004;31:1467.

82. Leydet-Quilici H, Luc M, Armingeat T, Pham T, Lafforgue P. Giant cell arteritis during adalimumab treatment for rheumatoid arthritis. Joint Bone Spine 2007;74:303-4.

83. Molloy ES, Langford CA, Clark TM, Gota CE, Hoffman GS. Antitumour necrosis factor therapy in patients with refractory Takayasu arteritis; long-term follow-up. Ann Rheum Dis 2008;67:1567-9.

84. Evans JM, O'Fallon WM, Hunder GG. Increased incidence of aortic aneurysm and dissection in giant cell (temporal) arteritis: a population based study. Ann Intern Med 1995;122:502-7.

85. Nuenninghoff DM, Hunder GG, Christianson TJ, et al. Incidence and predictors of large-artery complication (aortic aneurysm, aortic dissection, and/or large-artery stenosis) in patients with giant cell arteritis: a population-based study over 50 years. Arthritis Rheum 2003;48:3522-31.

86. Evans JM, Bowles CA, Bjornsson J, Mullany CJ, Hunder GG. Thoracic aortic aneurysm and rupture in giant cell arteritis. A descriptive study of 41 cases. Arthritis Rheum 1994;37:1539-47.

87. Gonzalez-Gay MA, Garcia-Porrua C, Pineiro A, Pego-Reigosa R, Llorca J, Hunder GG. Aortic aneurysm and dissection in patients with biopsy-proven giant cell arteritis from northwestern Spain: a population-based study. Medicine (Baltimore) 2004;83:335-41.

88. Garcia-Martinez A, Hernandez-Rodriguez J, Arguis P, Paredes P, Segarra M, Lozano E, et al. Development of aortic aneurysm/dilation during the followup of patients with giant cell arteritis: a cross sectional screening of fifty-four prospectively followed patients. Arthritis Rheum 2008;59:422-30.

89. Bongartz T, Mateson EL. Large-vessel involvement in giant cell arteritis. Curr Opin Rheumatol 2006;18:10-7.

90. Tso E, Flamm SD, White RD, Schvartzman PR, Mascha E, Hoffman CS. Takayasu arteritis. Utility and limitations of magnetic resonance imaging in diagnosis and treatment. Arthritis Rheum 2002;46:1634-42.

91. Both M, Akmadi-Simab K, Reuter M, Dourvos O, Fritzer E, Ullrich S, et al. MRI and FDG-PET in the assessment of inflammatory aortic arch syndrome in complicated courses of giant cell arteritis. Ann Rheum Dis 2008;67:1030-3.

92. Miller DV, Isotalo PA, Weyand CM, Edwards WD, Aubry MC, Tazelaar HD. Surgical pathology of noninfectious ascending aortitis: a study of 45 cases with emphasis on an isolate variant. Am J Surg Pathol 2006;30:1150-8.

93. Rojo-Leyva F, Ratliff NB, Cosgrove DM, Hoffman GS. Study of 52 patients with idiopathic aortitis from a cohort of 1,204 surgical cases. Arthritis Rheum 2000;43:901-7.

94. Nuenninghoff DM, Hunder GG, Christianson TJH, McClelland RL, Matteson EL. Mortality of large-artery complication (aortic aneurysm, aortic dissection, and/or large-artery stenosis) in patients with giant cell arteritis: a population-based study over 50 years. Arthritis Rheum 2003;48:3532-7.

95. Stanson AW. Imaging findings in extracranial (giant cell) temporal arteritis. Clin Exp Rheumatol 2000;18(Suppl. 20):S43-8.

96. Brack A, Martinez-Taboada V, Stanson A, Goronzy JJ, Weyand CM. Disease pattern in cranial and large-vessel giant cell arteritis. Arthritis Rheum 1999;42:311-7.

97. Wilkinson IM, Russell RW. Arteries of the head and neck in giant cell arteritis: a pathological study to show the pattern of arterial involvement. Arch Neurol 1972;27:378-91.

98. Gonzalez-Gay MA, Blanco R, Rodriguez-Valerde V, Martinez-Taboada V, Delgado-Rodriguez M, Figueroa M, et al. Permanent visual loss and cerebrovascular accidents in giant cell arteritis: predictors and response to treatment. Arthritis Rheum 1998;41:1497-504.

99. Wiszniewska M, Devuyst G, Bogousslavsky J. Giant cell arteritis as a cause of first-ever stroke. Cerebrovasc Dis 2007;24:226-30.

100. Salvarani C, Giannini C, Miller DV, Hunder G. Giant cell arteritis: involvement of intracranial arteries. Arthritis Rheum 2006;55:985-9.

101. Amor-Dorado JC, Llorca J, Garcia-Porrua C, Costa C, Perez-Fernandez M, Gonzalez-Gay MA. Audiovestibular manifestations in giant cell arteritis: a prospective study. Medicine (Baltimore) 2003;82:13-26.

102. Hernandez-Rodriguez J, Tan CD, Molloy ES, Khasnis A, Rodriguez ER, Hoffman GS. Vasculitis involving the breast. A clinical and histopathologic analysis of 34 patients. Medicine (Baltimore) 2008;87:61-9.

103. Bajocchi G, Zamorani G, Cavazza A, Pipitone N, Versari A, Boiardi L, et al. Giant-cell arteritis of the female genital tract associated with occult temporal arteritis and FDGC-PET evidence of large-vessel vasculitis. Clin Exp Rheumatol 2007;25(Suppl. 44):S36-9.

CASE STUDY 1

A male patient was diagnosed at 48 years of age with Wegener's granulomatosis (WG) involving the sinuses, nose, and lungs. He was treated with daily cyclophosphamide and prednisolone for 1 year, after which the medication was tapered and discontinued. After being in remission for 48 months, he had a relapse involving the sinuses and the kidneys with a crescentic glomerulonephritis with a peak creatinine at 270 µg/L. He was once again treated with oral cyclophosphamide and prednisolone, and his creatinine normalized. After 5 months of treatment, he developed hematuria and elevated liver enzymes. Cystoscopy revealed cyclophosphamide-induced bladder injury. He was switched to azathioprine and did well for 2 years. He then had a relapse in the sinuses and lungs; azathioprine was discontinued, and he was treated with prednisolone and methotrexate (MTX). Subsequently, he has been on and off MTX for 6 years combined with low-dose prednisolone. He had some relapses in the sinuses, but reintroduction of MTX has always led to remission. He has residual sinus symptoms and a slighty elevated creatinine (150 µg/L) and his life has been complicated by diabetes mellitus and hypertension, but he is feeling generally well and is working full time.

Comments: This case illustrates the problems in treating patients with WG. The major problem is often not getting the patient into remission but to prevent relapse and organ damage without causing permanent adverse effects by the immunosuppressive treatment.

CASE STUDY 2

A woman born in 1967 with insulin-treated diabetes mellitus since 2000 was first admitted to a rheumatology unit in 1990 because of arthralgia and fatigue. She had a moderately elevated erythrocyte sedimentation rate (ESR), proteinuria 0.4 g/day, and antinuclear antibody (ANA) titer 1/100, and she was antineutrophil cytoplasmic antibody (ANCA) negative. On examination, she had no arthritis and no other pathologic findings. Her fatigue and arthralgia resolved spontaneously; she received no treatment and was followed by her family doctor. In 2006, she got increasingly tired, experienced a fever for 4 weeks, and was admitted. The laboratory studies included hemoglobulin, 94 g/L; ESR, 105 mm/h; creatinine, 158 µg/L. The examination also indicated that she had proteinuria and pulmonary infiltrate in the right underlobe. Her preliminary diagnosis was pneumonia, and she was treated with antibiotics.

However, her condition deteriorated with hemoptysis, increasing fever, and several additional pulmonary infiltrates. Repeat hemoglobulin was 75 g/L,

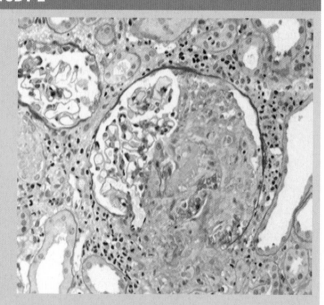

Figure 16-1. Crescentic glomerulonephritis; renal biopsy from patient in Case Study 2.

ESR 110 mm/h, serum creatinine 400 µg/L. The preliminary differential diagnosis included pneumonia, malignancy, and tuberculosis. Both a rheumatologist and a nephrologist were consulted, and further investigations were recommended including acute testing for ANCA, and antibodies against glomerular basal membrane (anti-GBM), and an acute kidney biopsy. She was positive for myeloperoxidase (MPO)-ANCA, and anti-GBM negative. Kidney biopsy showed a crescentic glomerulonephritis (Fig. 16-1). The diagnosis was microscopic polyangiitis (MPA).

She was treated with 10 pulses of cyclophosphamide 15 mg/kg IV plus prednisolone. She was in remission after 3 months of treatment, and after 6 months, the cyclophosphamide was discontinued and she was put on azathioprine as a remission maintenance therapy. After 2 years, she is doing well and still in remission. She has a stable serum creatinine at 150 µg/L and low-grade proteinuria, probably due to her diabetes.

Comments: This case illustrates the often difficult challenge of differentiating acute ANCA-associated vasculitis (AAV) from infection. In this case, the patient's acute condition was first diagnosed as pneumonia. However, resistance to antibiotic therapy, hemoptysis, and rising creatinine pointed to the diagnosis of MPA. Her positive MPO-ANCA and negative anti-GBM helped distinguish her condition from Goodpasture's syndrome.

INTRODUCTION

Vasculitis is defined as inflammation of the vessel walls. Vasculitis develops either primarily or secondarily to certain background conditions, such as malignancy, infections, and systemic rheumatic diseases. The primary systemic vasculitides cause inflammation of blood vessels resulting in occlusive, stenotic, or aneurismal change, leading to ischemic or hemorrhagic events. They are classified as small, medium, or large vessel vasculitis depending on the caliber of the vessels involved.[1] This chapter addresses the management of the adult spectrum of medium and small vessel vasculitides, which includes WG, MPA, Churg-Strauss syndrome (CSS), essential cryoglobulinemic vasculitis, polyarteritis nodosa (PAN) and Henoch-Schönlein purpura (Table 16-1).

Among the small vessel vasculitides, WG, MPA, and CSS are distinct from classic PAN and have common characteristics: the affected vessels are arterioles, capillaries, and venules; the most common organs affected are the kidney and lungs; and they involve ANCAs as the common pathogenesis.[2] Therefore, MPA, WG, and CSS are called ANCA-associated vasculitides. The frequency of ANCA positivity differs from one vasculitis to another: ANCAs are present in more than 80% of WG patients, around 75% of patients with MPA, and only 40% of those with CSS.[3-6]

OVERALL ASPECTS ON THE MANAGEMENT OF MEDIUM AND SMALL VESSEL VASCULITIS, INCLUDING THE DISEASES ASSOCIATED WITH ANTINUCLEAR ANTIBODIES

A primary vasculitis may be life-threatening, and therefore, rapid and correct management is mandatory for the survival of the patient. Therefore, patients with primary small and medium vessel vasculitides should be managed at centers of expertise. The rarity of primary systemic vasculitis makes it hard to maintain expertise in their management.[7-10] Expert guidance is needed to differentiate damage from disease activity and to consider differential diagnoses. Patients with vasculitis may require interventions by specialists with a deep knowledge of vasculitis, such as specialized radiography,[11,12] renal transplantation,[13] or therapeutic injection of a subglottic stenosis.[14,15] Vasculitis may relapse years after remission, even in previously unaffected organ systems.[16,17] Patients may also develop complications from the treatment many years after discontinuation.[18]

ANCA testing should be performed by indirect immunofluorescence to detect the characteristic labeling: cytoplasmic or perinuclear. All serum samples positive for ANCA by immunofluorescence should be tested for reactivity to proteinase 3 (PR3) and MPO.[19] A positive test for cytoplasmic ANCA targeted to PR3, or perinuclear ANCA against MPO has a high sensitivity and specificity for the diagnosis of ANCA-associated vasculitis.[20,21] PR3-ANCA occur in 75% to 90% of patients with WG, whereas 5% to 20% of patients with WG have MPO-ANCA.[22] MPO-ANCAs are seen in 50% to 80% of patients with MPA, with 10% to 20% having PR3-ANCA. ANCA is also found in up to 40% of patients with CSS when anti-MPO ANCA are seen predominantly. Patients with isolated granulomatous disease of the upper or lower respiratory tract may not have a positive ANCA. Therefore, the absence of a positive test does not rule out a diagnosis.[23,24]

The initial observation that ANCA levels were higher in those with active disease gave rise to hope that ANCA could be a biomarker for disease activity. However, in a prospective study of 156 patients, only a weak association with disease activity was demonstrated; decreases in PR3-ANCA during remission induction treatment were not associated with a shorter time to sustained remission; and increases in PR3-ANCA levels were not associated with relapse in the following year.[25] Therefore, serial ANCA levels should not be used to monitor disease activity or guide decisions concerning immunosuppressive treatment in ANCA-associated vasculitis.

Table 16-1. *Names and Definitions Adopted by the Chapel Hill Consensus Conference on The Nomenclature of Medium-Sized Vessel Vasculitides and Small Vessel Vasculitides*

Condition	Signs and Symptoms
Medium-Sized Vessel Vasculitides	
Polyarteritis nodosa	Necrotizing inflammation of medium-sized or small arteries without glomerulonephritis or vasculitis in arterioles, capillaries and venules.
Kawasaki disease	Arteritis involving large, medium-sized, and small arteries, and associated with mucocutaneous lymph node syndrome. Coronary arteries are often involved. Aorta and veins can be involved. Usually occurs in children
Small Vessel Vasculitides	
Wegener's granulomatosis	Granulomatous inflammation involving the respiratory tract, and necrotizing vasculitis affecting small to medium-sized vessels (e.g., capillaries, venules, arterioles, and arteries). Necrotizing glomerulonephritis is common. Strongly associated with antineutrophil cytoplasm (ANCA)
Churg-Strauss syndrome	Eosinophil-rich and granulomatous inflammation involving the respiratory tract, and necrotizing vasculitis affecting small- to medium-sized vessels, associated with asthma and eosinophilia. Strongly associated with antineutrophil cytoplasm autoantibodies (ANCAs).
Microscopic polyangiitis	Necrotizing vasculitis, with few or no immune deposits, affecting small vessels (i.e., capillaries, venules and/or arterioles). Necrotizing glomerulonephritis is common. Strongly associated with antineutrophil cytoplasm autoantibodies. Pulmonary capillaritis often occurs.
Henoch-Schönlein purpura	Vasculitis with IgA-dominant immune deposits, affecting small-vessels (i.e., capillaries, venules and/or arterioles). Typically involves skin, gut, and glomeruli, and is associated with arthralgias and arthritis.
Cryoglobulin-associated vasculitis	Vasculitis with cryoglobulin immune deposits, affecting small vessels (i.e., capillaries, venules and/or arterioles), associated with cryoglobulin in serum. Skin and glomeruli are often involved
Cutaneous leukocytoclastic angiitis	Isolated cutaneous leukocytoclastic angiitis without systemic vasculitis or glomerulonephritis.

Biopsy is highly recommended because it can strongly support a diagnosis of vasculitis. Histopathologic evidence of vessel wall inflammation is the gold standard for the diagnosis of vasculitis. The diagnostic yield of biopsies showing either vasculitis (glomerulonephritis in a kidney biopsy) or granuloma is more than 90%,[24,26,27] but the yield of the biopsy may vary due to the organ sampled, the skill of the operator, and the sampling method used.[26-30] A biopsy may be especially helpful in patients with negative ANCA test.[26] Biopsies are also important to rule out other diagnoses. The site of the biopsy must be determined by individual assessment. In renal involvement, repeated biopsies may be of value to follow up treatment results, disease relapse, and chronic damage.

CLINICAL ASSESSMENT AND EVALUATION OF VASCULITIS AND DISEASE SCORING

In several complex rheumatic diseases, measurement of disease activity is becoming increasingly important. Patients with rheumatoid arthritis,

systemic lupus erythematosus (SLE) and vasculitis are expected to live for many years, having frequent episodes of relapse, accumulation of damage, and drug toxicity. In this context, indices of clinical disease assessment have become necessary because of the failure of serologic markers to provide accurate information for selecting appropriate treatments. Multiorgan involvement is very common in primary systemic vasculitis. Therefore, it is important to have a structured clinical assessment conducted in all patients with a suspicion of vasculitis. In vasculitis, the Birmingham Vasculitis Activity Score (BVAS)[31,32] (Tables 16-2 and 16-3) has been adopted to assess disease activity, whereas the Vasculitis Damage Index (VDI)[33] (Table 16-4) provides information on disease damage. BVAS and VDI have become internationally recognized assessment tools, allowing comparison of studies from different continents and effective collaboration in multicenter studies. Clinical trials using these tools have provided a firm evidence base for treatment decisions in vasculitis. The first version of the BVAS was published in 1994.[31] Since then, the list of clinical features has been revised by the European Vasculitis Study Group (EUVAS).[32] The BVAS is divided into nine organ-based systems,

Table 16-2. *Vasculitis Activity Score 2003*

Center _____ Assessor _____ Paper case _____

Patient Initials / No _____ Assessment number _____ Date _____ *BVAS 2003 Study*

VASCULITIS ACTIVITY SCORE 2003

○ Tick box only if abnormality represents active disease (use the Vasculitis Damage Index [VDI] to score items of damage). If there are no abnormalities in a system, please tick the "None" box

□ If all the abnormalities recorded represent smouldering/low grade/grumbling disease, and there are no new/worse features, please remember to tick the box at the bottom right corner

	None	Active disease		None	Active disease
1. General	○		**6. Cardiovascular**	○	
Myalgia		○	Loss of pulses		○
Arthralgia or arthritis		○	Valvular heart disease		○
Fever ≥ 38.0 °C		○	Pericarditis		○
Weight Loss ≥ 2 kg		○	Ischemic cardiac pain		○
			Cardiomyopathy		○
2. Cutaneous	○		Congestive cardiac failure		○
Infarct		○			
Purpura		○	**7. Abdominal**	○	
Ulcer		○	Peritonitis		○
Gangrene		○	Bloody diarrhea		○
Other skin vasculitis		○	Ischemic abdominal pain		○
3. Mucous Membranes/Eyes	○		**8. Renal**	○	
Mouth ulcers/granulomata		○	Hypertension		○
Genital ulcers		○	Proteinuria >1+		○
Adnexal inflammation		○	Hematuria ≥10 rbc/hpf		○
Signigicant proptosis		○	Creatinine 125-249 μmol/l		○
Red eye (Epi)scleritis		○	Creatinine 250-499 μmol/l		○
Red eye conjunctivitis/ blepharitis/keratitis		○	Creatinine ≥ 500 μmol/l		○
Blurred vision		○	Rise in creatinine > 30% or creatinine clearance fall > 25%		○
Sudden visual loss		○			
Uveitis		○	**9. Nervous system**	○	
Retinal vasculitis/retinal vessel thrombosis/retinal exudates/retinal hemorrhages		○	Headache		○
			Meningitis		○
			Organic confusion		○
4. EHT	○		Seizures (not hypertensive)		○
Bloody nasal discharge/nasal crusts/ulcers and/or granulomata		○	Stroke		○
			Cord lesion		○
Paranasal sinus involvement		○	Cranial nerve palsy		○
Subglottic stenosis		○	Sensory peripheral neuropathy		○
Conductive hearing loss		○	Motor mononeuritis multiplex		○
Sensorineural hearing loss		○	**10. Other**	○	
5. Chest	○				○
Wheeze		○			○
Nodules or cavities		○			○
Pleural effusion/pleurisy		○			○
Infiltrate		○	**Persistent Disease Only:**		
Endobronchial involvement		○	Tick here if all the above abnormalities are due to low grade grumbling disease and not due to new/worse disease		☐
Massive hemoptysis/alveolar hemorrhage		○			
Respiratory failure		○			

BVAS 2003 15/04/04

Modified from Luqmani RA, Bacon PA, Moots RJ, Janssen BA, Pall A, Emery P, et al. Birmingham Vasculitis Activity Score (BVAS) in systemic necrotizing vasculitis. QJ Med 1994;87:671-8.

Table 16-3. *Glossary and Scoring Birmingham Vasculitis Activity Score (BVAS) 2003*

Glossary and scoring for BVAS 2003. GENERAL RULE: disease features are scored only when they are due to active vasculitis, after excluding other causes (e.g., infection, hypertension, etc.). If the feature is due to active disease, it is scored in the boxes. It is essential to apply these principles to each item below. Scores have been weighted according to the severity which each symptom or sign is thought to represent. Tick "Persistent Disease" box if all the abnormalities are due to active (but not new or worse) vasculitis. If any of the abnormalities are due to new/worse disease, DO NOT tick the "Persistent Disease" box. For some features, further information (from specialist opinion on further tests) is required if abnormality is newly present or worse. Remember that in most instances, you will be able to complete the whole record when you see the patient. However, you may need further information before entering some items. Please leave these items blank, until the information is available, and then fill them in. For example, If the patient has new onset of stridor, you would usually ask an ENT colleague to investigate this further to determine whether or not it is due to active Wegener's granulomatosis.		BVAS persistent	BVAS new/worse
1. General	**Maximum scores**	2	3
Myalgia	Pain in the muscles	1	1
Arthralgia or arthritis	Pain in the joints or joint inflammation	1	1
Fever at 38.0 °C	Documented oral/axillary temperature elevation. Rectal temps are 0.5 °C higher	2	2
Weight loss	At least 2 kg loss of body weight (not fluid) having occurred since last assessment or in the 4 weeks not as a consequence of dieting	2	2
2. Cutaneous	**Maximum scores**	3	6
Infarct	Area of tissue necrosis or splinter hemorrhages	1	2
Purpura	Petechiae (small red spots), palpable purpura, or ecchymoses (large plaques) in skin or oozing (in the absence of trauma) in the mucous membranes.	1	2
Ulcer	Open sore in a skin surface.	1	4
Gangrene	Extensive tissue necrosis (e.g., digit)	2	6
Other skin vasculitis	Livedo reticularis, subcutaneous nodules, erythema nodosum, etc.	1	2
3. Mucous membranes/eyes	**Maximum scores**	3	6
Mouth ulcers/granulomata	Aphthous stomatitis, deep ulcers and/or "Strawberry" gingival hyperplasia, excluding lupus erythematosus, and infection	1	2
Genital ulcers	Ulcers localized in the genitalia or perineum, excluding infections.	1	1
Adnexal inflammation	Salivary (diffuse, tender swelling unrelated to meals) or lacrimal gland inflammation. Exclude other causes (infection). Specialist opinion preferably required.	2	4
Significant proptosis	Protrusion of the eyeball due to significant amounts of inflammation in the orbit; if unilateral, there should be a difference of 2 mm between one eye and the other. This may be associated with diplopia due to infiltration of extra-ocular muscles. Developing myopia (measured on best visual acuity, see later) can also be a manifestation of proptosis	2	4
Red eye (Epi)scleritis	Inflammation of the sclerae (specialist opinion usually required). Can be heralded by photophobia.	1	2
Red eye conjunctivitis	Inflammation of the conjunctivae (exclude infectious causes and excluding uveitis as cause of red eye, also exclude conjunctivitis sicca which should not be scored as this is not a feature of active vasculitis): (specialist opinion not usually required).	1	1
Blepharitis	Inflammation of eyelids. Exclude other causes (trauma, infection). Usually no specialist opinion is required		
Keratitis	Inflammation of central or peripheral cornea as evaluated by specialist		
Blurred vision	Altered measurement of best visual acuity from previous or baseline, requiring specialist opinion for further evaluation.	2	3
Sudden visual loss	Sudden loss of vision requiring ophthalmological assessment.		6
Uveitis	Inflammation of the uvea (iris, ciliary body, choroid) confirmed by ophthalmologist.	2	6

Continued

Table 16-3. *Glossary and Scoring Birmingham Vasculitis Activity Score (BVAS) 2003—Cont'd*

		BVAS persistent	BVAS new/worse
Retinal vasculitis	Retinal vessel sheathing on examination by specialist or confirmed by retinal fluoroscein angiography	2	6
Retinal vessel thrombosis	Arterial or venous retinal blood vessel occlusion		
Retinal exudates	Any area of soft retinal exudates (exclude hard exudates) seen on ophthalmoscopic examination.		
Retinal hemorrhages	Any area retinal hemorrhage seen on ophthalmoscopic examination.		
4. ENT	**Maximum scores**	3	6
Bloody nasal discharge/ nasal crusts/ulcers and/ or granulomata	Bloody, mucopurulent, nasal secretion, light or dark brown crusts frequently obstructing the nose, nasal ulcers and/or granulomatous lesions observed by rhinoscopy	3	6
Paranasal sinus involvement	Tenderness or pain over paranasal sinuses usually with pathologic imaging (CT, MR, x-ray, ultrasound)	1	2
Subglottic stenosis	Stridor and hoarseness due to inflammation and narrowing of the subglottic area observed by laryngoscopy	3	6
Conductive hearing loss	Hearing loss due to middle ear involvement confirmed by otoscopy and/ or tuning fork examination and/or audiometry	1	3
Sensorineural hearing loss	Hearing loss due to auditory nerve or cochlear damage confirmed by audiometry	2	6
5. Chest	**Maximum scores**	3	6
Wheeze	Wheeze on clinical examination	1	2
Nodules or cavities	New lesions, detected by CXR		3
Pleural effusion/pleurisy	Pleural pain and/or friction rub on clinical assessment or new onset of radiologically confirmed pleural effusion. Other causes (e.g., infection, malignancy) should be excluded	2	4
Infiltrate	Detected by CXR or CT scan. Other causes (infection) should be excluded	2	4
Endobronchial involvement	Endobronchial pseudotumor or ulcerative lesions. Other causes such as infection or malignancy should be excluded. NB: smooth stenotic lesions to be included in VDI; subglottic lesions to be recorded in the ENT section.	2	4
Massive hemoptysis/ alveolar hemorrhage	Major pulmonary bleeding, with shifting pulmonary infiltrates; other causes of bleeding should be excluded if possible	4	6
Respiratory failure	Dyspnea which is sufficiently severe as to require artificial verification	4	6
6. Cardiovascular	**Maximum scores**	3	6
Loss of pulses	Loss of pulses in any vessel detected clinically; this may include loss of pulses leading to threatened loss of limb	1	4
Valvular heart disease	Significant valve abnormalities in the aortic mitral or pulmonary valves detected clinically or echocardiographically.	2	4
Pericarditis	Pericardial pain and/or friction rub on clinical assessment.	1	3
Ischemic cardiac pain	Typical clinical history of cardiac pain leading to myocardial infarction or angina. Consider the possibility of more common causes (e.g., atherosclerosis)	2	4
Cardiomyopathy	Significant impairment of cardiac function due to poor ventricular wall motion confirmed on echocardiography	3	6
7. Abdominal	**Maximum scores**	4	9
Peritonism	Acute abdominal pain with peritonism/peritonitis due to perforation/ infarction of small bowel, appendix or gallbladder, etc., or acute pancreatitis confirmed by radiology/surgery/elevated amylase	3	9
Bloody diarrhea	Of recent onset; inflammatory bowel disease and infectious causes excluded.	3	9
Ischemic abdominal pain	Severe abdominal pain with typical features of ischemia confirmed by imaging or at surgery, with typical appearances of aneursyms or abnormal vasculature characteristic of vasculitis.	2	6

		BVAS persistent	BVAS new/worse
8. Renal	**Maximum scores**	6	12
Hypertension	Diastolic BP>95, accelerated or not, with or without retinal changes.	1	4
Proteinuria	>1+ on urinalysis; >0.2 g/24 hours infection should be excluded.	2	4
Hematuria	10 or more RBC per hpf (high power field), excluding urinary infection and urinary uthlasis (stone)	3	6
Creatinine 125-249	Serum creatinine values 125-249 µmol/l at first assessment only.	2	4
Creatinine 250-499	Serum creatinine values 250-499 µmol/l at first assessment only.	3	6
Creatinine ≥ 500	Serum creatinine values 500 µmol/l or greater at first assessment only.	4	8
Rise in creatinine > 30% or creatinine clearance fall > 25%	Significant deterioration in renal function attributable to active vasculitis.		6
9. Nervous system	**Maximum scores**	6	9
Headache	New, unaccustomed & persistent headache	1	1
Meningitis	Severe headache with neck stiffness ascribed to inflammatory meningitis after excluding infection/bleeding	1	3
Organic confusion	Impaired orientation, memory or other intellectual function in the absence of metabolic, psychiatric, pharmacological or toxic causes.	1	3
Seizures (not hypertensive)	Paroxysmal electrical discharges in the brain & producing characteristic physical changes including tonic & clonic movements & certain behavioral changes.	3	9
Stroke	Cerebrovascular accident resulting in focal neurological signs such as paresis, wetness, etc. A stroke due to other causes (e.g., atherosclerosis) should be considered & appropriate neurological advice is recommended	3	9
Cord lesion	Transverse myelitis with lower extremity wetness or sensory loss (usually with a detectable sensory level) with loss of sphincter control (rectal & urinary bladder).	3	9
Cranial nerve palsy	Facial nerve palsy, recurrent nerve palsy, oculomotor nerve palsy, etc. excluding sensorineural hearing loss and ophthalmic symptoms due to inflammation	3	6
Sensory peripheral neuropathy	Sensory neuropathy resulting in glove and/or stocking distribution of sensory loss. Other causes should be excluded (e.g., idiopathic, metabolic, vitamin deficiencies, infectious, toxic, hereditary).	3	6
Motor mononeuritis multiplex	Simultaneous neuritis of single or many peripheral nerves, only scored if motor involvement. Other causes should be excluded (diabetes, sarcoidosis, carcinoma, amyloidosis).	3	9
10. Other	Other feature of active vasculitis-please describe		

with each section including symptoms and signs that are typical of that particular organ involvement in systemic vasculitis. Altogether, 66 clinical features are included. The clinician only scores features believed to be due to active vasculitis. Each item is given a numeric value according to its clinical relevance. The different organ systems are also weighted according to clinical relevance by applying maximal scores for each system. For example, ear-nose-throat (ENT) has a maximal score of 6, whereas the renal system has 12. The latest version of BVAS is called BVAS 2003.[32,34] A glossary of terms was also developed for the BVAS and published along with the new version of the assessment tool[34] (see Table 16-3), emphasizing the importance of scoring an item only if it is due to active vasculitis, based on clinical judgment.

Damage caused by vasculitis or its treatment may prove more troublesome to the patient than disease activity and is highly unlikely to respond to immunosuppressive treatment. In a longitudinal WG cohort from the National Institutes of Health, 86% of patients had permanent damage as a consequence of the disease itself and 42% had treatment-related

Table 16-4. *Vasculitis Damage Index (VDI)*

This is for recording organ damage that has occurred in patients *since the onset of vasculitis*
Patients often have co-morbidity before they develop vasculitis, **which must not be scored**
Record features of active disease using the Birmingham Vasculitis Activity Score (BVAS)
A new patient should *usually have a VDI score of zero*, unless:
(a) they have had vasculitis for more than three months of onset of disease, **and**
(b) the damage has developed or become worse since the onset of vasculitis

	No	Yes
1. Musculoskeletal		
None	☐	
Significant muscle atrophy or weakness		○
Deforming/erosive arthritis		○
Osteoporosis/vertebral collapse		○
Avascular necrosis		○
Osteomyelitis		○
2. Skin/Mucous membranes		
None	☐	
Alopecia		○
Cutaneous ulcers		○
Mouth ulcers		○
3. Ocular		
None	☐	
Cataract		○
Retinal change		○
Optic atrophy		○
Visual impairment/diplopia		○
Blindness in one eye		○
Blindness in second eye		○
Orbital wall destruction		○
4. ENT		
None	☐	
Hearing loss		○
Nasal blockage/chronic discharge/crusting		○
Nasal bridge collapse/septal perforation		○
Chronic sinusitis/radiological damage		○
Subglottic stenosis (no surgery)		○
Subglottic stenosis (with surgery)		○
5. Pulmonary		
None	☐	
Pulmonary hypertention		○
Pulmonary fibrosis		○
Pulmonary infarction		○
Pleural fibrosis		○
Chronic asthma		○
Chronic breathlessness		○
Impaired lung function		○
6. Cardiovascular		
None	☐	
Angina angioplasty		○
Myocardial infarction		○
Subsequent myocardial infarction		○
Cardiomyopathy		○
Valvular disease		○
Pericarditis ≥3 mths or pericardectomy		○
Diastolic BP ≥95 or requiring antihypertensives		○

Name
Trial Number
Date
Center

	No	Yes
7. Peripheral vascular disease		
None	☐	
Absent pulses in one limb		○
2nd episode of absent pulses in one limb		○
Major vessel stenosis		○
Claudication >3 mths		○
Minor tissue loss		○
Major tissue loss		○
Subsequent major tissue loss		○
Complicated venous thrombosis		○
8. Gastrointestinal		
None	☐	
Gut infarction/resection		○
Mesenteric insufficiency/pancreatitis		○
Chronic peritonitis		○
Esophageal stricture/surgery		○
9. Renal		
None	☐	
Estimated/measured GFR ≤ 50%		○
Proteinuria ≥ 0.5 g/24 hr		○
End stage renal disease		○
10. Neuropsychiatric		
None	☐	
Cognitive impairment		○
Major psychosis		○
Seizures		○
Cerebrovascular accident		○
2nd cerebrovascular accident		○
Cranial nerve lesion		○
Peripheral neuropathy		○
Transverse myelitis		○
11. Other		
None	☐	
Gonadal failure		○
Marrow failure		○
Diabetes		○
Chemical cystitis		○
Malignancy		○
Other		○

Total VDI Score. Record the number of positive items (1 point for each). The VDI score can either increase or remain the same over time. Remember to carry forward any previous items of damage.

☐

VDI Modified from Exley AR, Bacon PA, Luqmani RA, Kitas GD, Gordon C, Savage CO, et al. Development and initial validation of the Vasculitis Damage Index for the standardized clinical assessment of damage in the systemic vasculitides. Arthritis Rheum 1997;40:371-80.

morbidity. This damage included, for example, end-stage renal disease, chronic pulmonary dysfunction, saddle-nose deformities, blindness, and death.[16] VDI is composed of 64 items of damage grouped into 11 organ systems and records items of change, due to vasculitis, treatment, or unrelated, that have occurred since the onset of vasculitis. Completion of the form provides a numeric score. The VDI was first published in 1997[33] and is constructed to be a cumulative index; therefore, the VDI score can never decrease over time. A comprehensive overview of the clinical evaluation of vasculitis and the development of the BVAS 2003 and the VDI was published in 2007.[35]

Training is an essential part of these assessment tools. Because of this, a training manual is provided by the EUVA, along with a practical guide.

A helpful tool for evaluating prognosis is the five-factor score (FFS). It is a prognostic score developed by the French vasculitis study group and has been proven accurately to predict survival for patients with PAN, MPA, and CSS.[36,3] The FFS is based on five clinical items, with the presence of each accorded one point for a maximum score of 5: renal insufficiency, proteinuria, central nervous system involvement, cardiomyopathy, and severe gastrointestinal involvement. For PAN, MPA, and CSS, 5-year survival rates were 88% when FFS was 0; 74% when FFS equaled 1; and 54% when FFS 2 or more.[36]

It is very important during treatment of vasculitis to critically assess the effect of given therapy, disease activity, disease progress and to notice adverse events (for example, infections due to immunomodulation, drug-induced pneumonitis, or bladder toxicity). Urinalysis should be performed on each patient at each visit to screen for renal relapse or response, infection, and bladder toxicity in patients treated with cyclophosphamide.[18,38,39] It is important to monitor a full blood count and liver enzymes at regular intervals to screen for drug toxicity, along with inflammatory markers and renal function parameters at 1- to 3-month intervals in order to monitor disease evaluation and treatment response.[40,41] A declining renal function may necessitate drug alteration or dose adjustment of the immunosuppressive agent. A drastic fall in white cell count or a slowly progressive leukopenia may require discontinuation or reduction of the immunomodulation.

It is important to categorize the ANCA-associated vasculitides by different levels of severity to arrive at treatment decisions. Treating physicians need to be aware of the fact that patients with different levels of disease severity respond to different treatment strategies, which has been demonstrated by clinical trials conducted by the EUVAS.[40,42-44] It may be appropriate to treat a patient with early systemic or local AAV with methotrexate, but the same patient will need cyclophosphamide if he or she develops a more generalized disease or a life-threatening disease manifestation.[42,43,45] The EUVAS disease categorization of AAV is shown in Table 16-5.[46]

Table 16-5. *The European Vasculitis Study Group (EUVAS) Disease Categorization of Antinuclear Cytoplasmic Antibody–Associated Vasculitis*

Category	Definition
Localized	Upper or lower respiratory tract disease without any other systemic involvement or constitutional symptoms
Early systemic	Any, without organ-threatening or life-threatening disease
Generalized	Renal or other organ-threatening disease, serum creatinine < 500 µmol/L (5.6 mg/dL)
Severe	Renal or other vital organ failure, serum creatinine > 500 µmol/L (5.6 mg/dL)
Refractory	Progressive disease unresponsive to glucocorticoids and cyclophosphamide

PHARMACOLOGIC TREATMENT

The treatment of systemic vasculitis has to be individualized depending on the distribution and level of severity of the disease. The treatment strategy consists of two steps:
1. Remission induction.
2. Remission maintenance.

A current overall therapeutic approach is presented in Table 16-6.[47] The European League Against Rheumatism (EULAR) has developed recommendations for the management of small and medium vessel vasculitis.[46]

The Role of High Dose Glucocorticoids in Remission-Induction Therapy

Clinical trials and cohort studies conducted in the vasculitides have generally employed glucocorticoid therapy in combination with immunosuppressive medications. It is recommended to start prednisolone at 1 mg/kg/day, as has been done in recent clinical trials.[40,42,48] The initial high dose should be maintained for approximately 1 month, and it is not recommended to reduce the dose to less than

Table 16-6. *Therapeutic Approaches to ANCA Associated Vasculitis*

Induction	Maintenance	Indication
Cyclophosphamide + glucocorticoids	Azathioprine	Severe disease
Cyclophosphamide + glucocorticoids	Methotrexate	Severe disease
Cyclophosphamide + glucocorticoids	Mycophenolate mofetil	Severe disease
Methotrexate + glucocorticoids	Methotrexate	Non-severe disease

15 mg/day for the first 12 weeks.[49,50] Intravenous pulse methylprednisolone can be used in addition to oral prednisolone as part of remission induction therapy when a rapid effect is wanted.[51,52]

Induction of Remission in Non–Organ-Threatening or Non–Life-Threatening Disease Antinuclear Cytoplasmic Antibody–Associated Vasculitis

Methotrexate (20–25 mg/week) in combination with prednisolone (1 mg/kg/day initially, max 80 mg/day) can be used as an alternative to cyclophosphamide in patients with less severe disease and in whom renal function is normal.[17,42,45,48,53-57] Methotrexate should be started at a dose of 15 mg/week and increased to 20 to 25 mg/week over the next 1 to 2 months until remission has been reached and then for another 3 months. A proposed schedule is given in Table 16-7.[42] In the randomized controlled NORAM trial, it was shown that this regimen is equal to cyclophosphamide plus glucocorticoids in its capacity to induce remission.[42] Sometimes it may take longer time to induce remission with methotrexate compared with cyclophosphamide in patients

with pulmonary involvement. Patients with methotrexate should receive folic acid supplementation.

Some cases of CSS can be treated with glucocorticoids alone.

Induction of Remission in Generalized Primary Small and Medium Vessel Vasculitis

For remission-induction in patients with generalized primary small and medium vessel vasculitis, a combination of cyclophosphamide (intravenous or oral) and glucocorticoids is the therapy of choice. Continuous oral cyclophosphamide at 2 mg/kg/day (maximum 200 mg/day) plus prednisolone 1 mg/kg/day (max 80 mg/day) has been used for remission induction in ANCA-associated vasculitis since the 1970s. Proposed treatment schedules are given in Tables 16-8 and 16-9.[16] A meta-analysis of three randomized controlled trials concluded that pulsed monthly cyclophosphamide was more likely to induce remission than continuous oral therapy, and with a lower risk of side effects, but that it may be associated with a higher risk of relapse.[51,58-61] However, it must be taken into consideration that the trials were not readily comparable because of

Table 16-7. *Proposed Protocol for Remission Induction with Methotrexate in Patients Between 18 and 70 Years of Age*

Time from Start of Therapy	Prednisone or Prednisolone*	Methotrexate (mg/week)
0	1 mg/kg/day	15
1 week	0.75 mg/kg/day	15
2 weeks	0.5 mg/kg/day	17.5
4 weeks	0.4 mg/kg/day	20
6 weeks	0.33 mg/kg/day	22.5
8 weeks	0.28 mg/kg/day	25
10 weeks	0.25 mg/kg/day	25
3 months	15 mg daily	25
4 months	12.5 mg daily	25
5 months	10 mg daily	25
6 months	10 mg daily	25
12 months	7.5 mg daily	22.5
15 months	5 mg daily	22.5
18 months	2.5 mg daily	20
21 months	0	15
24 months	0	12.5
30 months	0	7.5
36 months	0	0

*Max dosage prednisolone 80 mg/day.

Table 16-8. *Proposed Protocol for Remission Induction with Oral Continuous Cyclophosphamide in Patients Between 18 and 70 Years*†

Time for Start of Therapy	Prednisolone (mg/kg/day)‡	Cyclophosphamide (mg/kg/day)	Azathioprine (mg/kg/day)
0	1	2.0	0
1 week	0.75	2.0	0
2 weeks	0.5	2.0	0
4 weeks	0.4	2.0	0
6 weeks	0.33	2.0	0
8 weeks	0.28	2.0	0
10 weeks	0.25	2.0	0
3 months	15 mg/day	2.0	0
4 months	12.5 mg/day	1.5	0
5 months	10 mg/day	0	2.0
6 months	10 mg/day	0	2.0
12 months	7.5 mg/day	0	2.0
15 months	5 mg/day	0	2.0
18 months	2.5 mg/day	0	1.5
21 months	0	0	1.5
24 months	0	0	1.0
30 months	0	0	0

*Patients between 60 and 70 years of age: Reduce cyclophosphamide and azathioprine with 50 mg/day.
†Max dosage for cyclophosphamide and azathioprine 200 mg daily.
‡Max dosage prednisolone 80 mg/daily.

Table 16-9. *Proposed Protocol for Remission Induction with Oral Continuous Cyclophosphamide in Patients Older than 70 Years*

Time for Start of Therapy	Prednisolone (mg/kg/day)	Cyclophosphamide (mg/kg/day)	Azathioprine (mg/kg/day)
0	0.75	1.5	0
1 week	0.5	1.5	0
2 weeks	0.4	1.5	0
4 weeks	0.2	1.5	0
6 weeks	15 mg/day	1.5	0
8 weeks	12.5 mg/day	1.0	0
3 months	10 mg/day	1.0	0
4 months	10 mg/day	1.0	0
5 months	7.5 mg/day	0	1.5
12 months	5 mg/day	0	1.5
18 months	5 mg/day	0	1
24 months	0	0	0.5
30 months	0	0	0

different therapeutic regimes. The CYCLOPS trial (daily oral vs pulse cyclophosphamide during induction therapy for generalized vasculitis) was designed and tested by the EUVAS group to analyze a treatment regimen of intravenous cyclophosphamide at a dose of 15 mg/kg (max 1.2 g) every 2 weeks for the first three pulses, followed by infusions every 3 weeks for the next three to six pulses (summarized in Table 16-10).[49,60,62-64] The results of this large randomized controlled trial suggest that pulse and continuous oral cyclophosphamide were equally effective in achieving remission and that pulse therapy had a dramatically lower rate of side effects.[63] In clinical trials, dose adjustments of pulsed cyclophosphamide were made for age and renal function (Table 16-11).[63,64] For continuous oral cyclophosphamide, the dose should be reduced for age (see proposed protocol in Table 16-9).

In patients with CSS and PAN, the combination of cyclophosphamide and glucocorticoids achieves better control of disease compared with monotherapy with glucocorticoids alone, whereas the long-term survival rate seems to remain unchanged.[65] In a prospective, randomized trial in 62 patients, the

Table 16-10. *Proposed Protocol for Remission Induction with Pulse Cyclophosphamide for Patients Between 18 and 60 Years of Age*

Time for Start of Therapy	Prednisolone (mg/kg/day)*	Pulse no	Cyclophosphamide (mg/kg/pulse)†	Azathioprine (mg/kg/day)‡§
0	1	1	15 mg/kg IV	0
1 week	0.75	0	0	0
2 weeks	0.5	2	15 mg/kg IV	0
4 weeks	0.4	3	15 mg/kg IV	0
7 weeks	0.33	4	15 mg/kg IV or oral	0
10 weeks	0.25	5	15 mg/kg IV or oral	0
13 weeks	15 mg/day	6	15 mg/kg IV or oral	0
16 weeks	12.5 mg/day	7	15 mg/kg IV or oral	0
19 weeks	12.5 mg/day	8	15 mg/kg IV or oral	0
22 weeks	10 mg/day	9	15 mg/kg IV or oral	0
26 weeks	10 mg/day	10	15 mg/kg IV or oral	0
28 weeks	10 mg/day	0	0	2.0
9 months	7.5 mg/day	0	0	2.0
12 months	5 mg/day	0	0	1.5
15 months	2.5 mg/day	0	0	1.5
18 months	0	0	0	1.5
24 months	0	0	0	1.0
30 months	0	0	0	0

*Max dosage prednisolone 80 mg/day.
†Max dosage cyclophosphamide 1200 mg/pulse.
‡Max dosage azathioprine 200 mg/day.
§Patients between 60 and 70 years of age: reduce azathioprine with 50 mg/day.

Table 16-11. *Dose Modification of Pulsed Cyclophosphamide as Used in the CYCLOPS Trial**

Age (years)	Creatinine (µmol/L)	
	< 300 (mg/kg/pulse)	300–500 (mg/kg/pulse)
<60	15	12.5
60-70	12.5	10
>70	10	7.5

*Pulsed cyclophosphamide dose reductions for renal function and age.

combination therapy produced sustained remission of greater then 18 months among a majority of the patients.[66]

Pulsed intravenous cyclophosphamide has been used in CSS and PAN with equal efficacy and a lower incidence of adverse events when compared with daily oral cyclophosphamide.[67,68] The intravenous route may achieve a more rapid clinical response than oral cyclophosphamide, and this may be particularly important for patients with active disease. When combined with glucocorticoids, intravenous cyclophosphamide should not exceed 12 pulses.[69]

In patients with rapidly progressive severe renal disease, plasma exchange is recommended to improve renal survival.[46] There is also evidence for improved renal survival in patients with severe renal disease (serum creatinine > 500 µl/L) when plasma exchange is used as an adjuvant to daily oral cyclophosphamide and prednisolone.[43] It is not known whether it benefits patients with less severe renal disease.[70,71] The effect of plasma exchange on extrarenal manifestations has not been studied in a convincing manner.

Cyclophosphamide metabolites are toxic to the urethelium and can therefore cause hemorrhagic cystitis in the short term and malignancy in the long term.[18,38,39] Patients should be encouraged to drink plenty of fluids, or be given intravenous fluids on the day of the infusion to dilute metabolites in the urine. Patients given intravenous cyclophosphamide should also be given oral or intravenous 2-mercaptoethanesulfonate sodium (Mesna, Baxter, Chicago, IL), which binds to acrolein, a toxic metabolite of cyclophosphamide, making it nontoxic.[17] Mesna also reduces the toxic acrolein urine products by retarding the degradation of 4-hydroxymetabolites and may also be beneficial in patients receiving continuous oral cyclophosphamide.[16,17,72] Antiemetic therapy should routinely be administered with intravenous cyclophosphamide. Monitoring for cyclophosphamide-related side effects should include regular monitoring of blood and liver function tests.

Prophylaxis against *Pneumocystis jiroveci* (formerly *Pneumocystis carinii*) should be given to all patients being treated with cyclophosphamide using trimethoprim/sulphamethoxazole 400/80 mg daily or on alternate days, unless contraindicated.[73-75]

Remission-Maintenance Therapy

For many years, long-term cyclophosphamide therapy has been used to maintain remission in patients with AAV.[16] However, the toxicity of long-term cyclophosphamide makes it an undesirable option.[18,38,39] Azathioprine (2 mg/kg/day) is safer than cyclophosphamide but is as effective at 18 months in preventing relapse.[40,76] Methotrexate (20–25 mg weekly) has also been effectively used for maintenance therapy after remission induction with cyclophosphamide, if the serum creatinine is less than 130 µmol/L.[77,78] Leflunomide (20–30 mg/day) may also be effective.[79] Mycophenolate mofetil (MMF) has been tested for maintenance therapy in 14 patients with WG; the results were encouraging but its ability to prevent relapses remains to be proven.[80] The EUVAS group is currently evaluating MMF for maintenance treatment with a regimen using pulse or oral cyclophosphamide for induction (6 months), followed by randomization to azathioprine versus MMF to maintain remission (3 years); results from this trial have not yet been published.

The addition of trimethoprim/sulphamethoxazole (800/160 mg twice daily) to standard remission maintenance therapy can reduce the risk of relapse in WG[81]; however, trimethoprim/sulphamethoxazole monotherapy may not be effective for maintenance of remission.[82] Because chronic nasal carriage of *Staphylococcus aureus* is associated with a higher relapse rate[83] in patient with nasal involvement, treatment with the topical antibiotic mupirocin could also be considered as an additional therapy.

The glucocorticoid dose should be tapered to a maintenance dose of 10 mg/day or less prednisolone (or equivalent) during remission.[40] After 6 to 18 months, this dose can be gradually reduced further, depending on the patient's response to treatment, and with the aim of discontinuing glucocorticoid therapy, if possible.

At present, there is ample evidence for recommending a combination of low-dose glucocorticoid therapy plus azathioprine (see Tables 16-8 to 16-10) for remission-maintenance.

The optimal duration of maintenance therapy remains uncertain. It is likely that relapse occurs more frequently in patients who are off treatment, but prolonging therapy must be balanced against the potential for relapses that still can occur on medication, drug toxicity, and the ability of some patients to come off treatment. For newly diagnosed patients who do not have significant organ damage, treatment should be continued for at least 2 years in the absence of toxicity, after which time the physician can consider tapering the dose toward discontinuation. In patients who have relapsed or who have had severe permanent organ damage, treatment for a longer duration may become necessary.

Alternative Immunomodulatory Therapy in Patients Refractory to Maximal Doses of Standard Therapy

Patients who do not achieve remission or relapse on maximal doses of standard therapy should be considered for alternative immunomodulatory therapy. Because of their efficacy, safety and good tolerance, intravenous immunoglobulins should be considered in this group of patients. In small prospective open studies, complete to partial responses were observed in 45% and 75%, respectively, of the patients given IVIG alone or in combination with other immunosuppressants or glucocorticoids.[84-86] One placebo-controlled trial in patients with relapsed AAV demonstrated better outcomes in vasculitis patients treated with IVIG.[84] The study evaluated the efficacy of a single cycle of IVIG (0.4 g/kg/day for 5 days) in patients with persistent disease activity despite conventional therapy. After 1 year, responses were seen in 14 out of 17 patients in the single IVIG versus 6 out of 17 in the placebo group. Recently, a prospective open multicenter trial in French patients with relapsed AAV was conducted. The patients received a monthly infusion of IVIG for 6 months in addition to conventional treatment.[87] Complete remission was obtained in 13 (59%) of the 22 patients, without any serious adverse events. It is important before treatment with IVIG to measure serum immunoglobulins because a pre-existing hypergammaglobulinemia may become aggravated, leading to a hyperviscosity state; and patients with selective IgA deficiency may develop an anaphylactic reaction on receiving IVIG.

For patients with progressive disease in spite of optimal therapy, alternative options may also include biologic agents such as rituximab, infliximab, etanercept, antithymocyte globulin, or conventional immunosuppressants such as MMF and 15-deoxyspergualin.[44,88-96]

The anti-TNF monoclonal antibody infliximab (Remicade, Johnson & Johnson, Horsham, PA) or the soluble TNF receptor-Ig construct etanercept (Enbrel, Immunex Corporation, Thousand Oaks, CA) have been studied in the treatment of AAV. In an open, uncontrolled, prospective trial, infliximab in combination with conventional therapy led to clinical remission in 88% (28/32) of patients with acute or persistently active AAV after a mean of 6.4 weeks.[90] Serious infections and death were reported in seven and two patients, respectively, whereas five patients had a relapse at a mean of 27 weeks.

Etanercept has been studied in patients with AAV in conjuction with conventional therapy to reduce the relapse rate. In combination with cyclophosphamide, or methotrexate in limited disease, etanercept did not confer any advantage for relapse prevention compared with cyclophosphamide or methotrexate alone.[48] Moreover, six cases of cancer were diagnosed during this trial, all in the etanercept arm, raising a concern about the rarely used combination of etanercept with alkylating agents; three more cancers were diagnosed later, two of them in the placebo arm.[48]

Antithymocyte globulin polyclonal antibody preparations have also been tested in AAV. In one study, 13 out of 15 patients with extremely refractory WG had a good primary response but it was not sustained in seven of them.[97]

In five open-label trials of the B-cell depleting monoclonal antibody rituximab (Rituxan, Genentech, San Francisco, CA; Mabthera, Roche, Nutley, NJ) in refractory or relapsing AAV, 42 of 46 (91%) patients achieved remission within 6 months.[92-96] In the largest case series of rituximab use for AAV patients published to date, 15 patients with refractory or relapsing AAV received 4 weekly infusions of 375 mg/m^2 rituximab.[98] B-cell depletion was achieved in all patients and partial or complete remission was seen in 14 of 15 patients with a significant decline in BVAS compared with baseline. However, some differences were noted in time to and extent of the therapeutic responses for constitutional and "vasculitic" manifestations of the disease as compared with granulomatous lesions, such as lung nodules in WG or orbital pseudotumors, with the latter regressing more slowly, sometimes 4 to 6 months after the first rituximab administration.[96] The potential benefit of rituximab in treating disease manifestations that are typically not improved by standard immunosuppressive regimens such as subglottic stenosis and retrobulbar granulomas has also been addressed. In a small study, 8 patients (5 with retrobulbar and 1 with pulmonary/sinus granulomas and 2 with subglottic stenosis) who had not responded to conventional immunosuppression and anti-TNF antibody therapy, were treated with four weekly infusions of rituximab. Improvement of the disease manifestations was observed in the patient with pulmonary/sinus granuloma and in one of the patients with subglottic stenosis, but in none of the patients with retrobulbar disease.[99] Further studies of rituximab in patients with AAV are needed to better understand its effectiveness and its long-term usefulness, a randomized double-blind trial (RAVE) is currently underway to compare rituximab with cyclophosphamide for remission induction of severe active WG.

A pilot study using MMF in relapsing or resistant AAV indicated that MMF may provide effective treatment for systemic small vessel AAV.[100] In a recently published single-center nonblinded clinical trial, the clinical efficacies of MMF and intermittent cyclophosphamide pulse therapy as induction treatment in patients with AAV and moderate renal involvement (serum creatinine < 500 μmol/L) were compared.[101] Fourteen of 18 patients (77.8%) in the MMF group and 8 of 17 patients (47.1%) receiving cyclophosphamide had a complete remission and 44.4% respectively, 15.4% recovered renal function. This suggests that MMF may effectively ameliorate disease activity and considerably improve renal function in patients with AAV.

The presence of activated T lymphocytes in WG lesions has raised the question as to whether interference with T-cell costimulation could modulate disease. Currently, a pilot study is ongoing investigating the T-cell costimulation-blocker abatacept (Orencia, Bristol Meyers Squibb, Princeton, NJ) in mild relapsing WG. There has been no published experience with abatacept in AAV so far.

The modulation of cytokine profiles by interferon-α may be an alternative in refractory CSS and has been reported to be effective in CSS patients in whom disease was refractory to glucocorticoids and cyclophosphamide.[102]

Treatment of Mixed Essential Cryoglobulinemic Vasculitis

No clinical trials have been performed for the treatment of essential (hepatitis C negative) cryoglobulinemic vasculitis. Therefore, the recommendation is that this disease should be treated in the same way as the other small vessel diseases discussed earlier, with immunomodulatory agents and glucocorticoids. Patients with rapidly progressive severe renal disease should also be treated with plasma exchange.

Rituximab may be of benefit but has mainly been used in patients with hepatitis C–associated cryoglobulinemic vasculitis.[103,104]

The use of interferon-α to induce remission in hepatitis C–associated cryoglobulinemia is well documented.[105-109] However, combination therapy with ribavirin and interferon-α may be more effective than interferon-α alone.[110,111]

Treatment of Hepatitis B–Associated Polyarteritis Nodosa

High-dose glucocorticoid therapy tapered over 2 weeks, followed by antiviral agents accompanied by plasma exchange has been shown to achieve a high rate of remission induction in hepatitis B–associated PAN.[112] Rituximab may be used in refractory cases.[103]

Treatment of Henoch-Schönlein Purpura

In mild cases of Henoch-Schönlein purpura, no specific therapy or only glucocorticoids in low doses is needed. Patients with glomerulonephritis should be treated with an immunosuppressive regimen, including high-dose glucocorticoids and another immunosuppressive agent such as cyclophosphamide, azathioprine, or MMF, depending on disease severity.[113]

References

1. Jennette JC, Falk RJ, Andrassy K, Bacon PA, Churg J, Gross WL, et al. Nomenclature of systemic vasculitides. Proposal of an international consensus conference. Arthritis Rheum 1994;37:187-92.
2. Ozaki S. ANCA-associated vasculitis: diagnostic and therapeutic strategy. Allergol Int 2007;56:87-96.
3. Kallenberg CG, Brouwer E, Weening JJ, Tervaert JW. Anti-neutrophil cytoplasmatic antibodies: current diagnostic and pathophysiological potential. Kidney Int 1994;46:1-15.
4. Guillevin L, Durand-Gasselin B, Cevallos R, Gayraud M, Lhote F, Callard P, et al. Microscopic polyangiitis: clinical and laboratory findings in eighty-five patients. Arthritis Rheum 1999;42:421-30.
5. Sinico RA, Di Toma L, Maggiore U, Bottero P, Radice A, Tosconi C, et al. Prevalence and clinical significance of antineutrophil cytoplasmatic antibodies in Churg-Strauss syndrome. Arthritis Rheum 2005;52:2926-35.
6. Sable-Fourtassou R, Cohen P, Mahr A, Pagnoux C, Mouthon L, Jayne D, et al. Antineutrophil cytoplasmatic antibodies and the Churg-Strauss syndrome. Ann Intern Med 2005;143:632-8.
7. Koldingsnes W, Nossent H. Epidemiology of Wegener's granulomatosis in northern Norway. Arthritis Rheum 2000;43:2481-7.
8. Reinhold-Keller E, Herlyn K, Wagner-Bastmeyer R, Gross WL. Stable incidence of primary systemic vasculitides over five years: results from the German vasculitis register. Arthritis Rheum 2005;53:93-9.
9. Carruthers DM, Watts RA, Symmons DP, Scott DG. Wegener's granulomatosis—increased incidence or increased recognition? Br J Rheumatol 1996;35:142-5.
10. Pettersson EE, Sundelin B, Heigl Z. Incidence and outcome of pauciimmune necrotizing and crescentic glomerulonephritis in adults. Clin Nephrol 1995;43:141-9.
11. Reuter M, Schnabel A, Wesner F, Tetzlaff K, Risheng Y, Gross WL, et al. Pulmonary Wegener's granulomatosis: correlation between high-resolution CT findings and clinical scoring of disease activity. Chest 1998;114:500-6.
12. Lohrmann C, Uhl M, Warnatz K, Kotter E, Ghanem N, Langer M. Sinonasal computed tomography in patients with Wegener's granulomatosis. J Comput Assist Tomogr 2006;30:122-5.
13. Elmedhem A, Adu D, Savage CO. Relapse rate and outcome of ANCAassociated small vessel vasculitis after transplantation. Nephrol Dial Transplant 2003;18:1001-4.
14. Hoffman GS, Thomas-Golbanov CK, Chan J, Akst LM, Eliachar I. Treatment of subglottic stenosis, due to Wegener's granulomatosis, with intralesional corticosteroids and dilation. J Rheumatol 2003;30:1017-21.
15. Langford CA, Sneller MC, Hallahan CW, Hoffman GS, Kammerer WA, Talar-Williams C, et al. Clinical features and therapeutic management of subglottic stenosis in patients with Wegener's granulomatosis. Arthritis Rheum 1996;39:1754-60.
16. Hoffman GS, Kerr GS, Leavitt RY, Hallahan CW, Lebovics RS, Travis WD, et al. Wegener granulomatosis: an analysis of 158 patients. Ann Intern Med 1992;116:488-98.
17. Reinhold-Keller E, Beuge N, Latza U, de Groot K, Rudert H, Nolle B, et al. An interdisciplinary approach to the care of patients with Wegener's granulomatosis: long-term outcome in 155 patients. Arthritis Rheum 2000;43:1021-32.
18. Talar-Williams C, Hijazi YM, Walther MM, Linehan WM, Hallahan CW, Lubensky I, et al. Cyclophosphamide-induced cystitis and bladder cancer in patients with Wegener granulomatosis. Ann Intern Med 1996;124:477-84.
19. Savige J, Gillis D, Benson E, Davies D, Esnault V, Falk RJ, et al. International Consensus Statement on Testing and Reporting of Antineutrophil Cytoplasmic Antibodies (ANCA). Am J Clin Pathol 1999;111:507-13.
20. Hagen EC, Daha MR, Hermans J, Andrassy K, Csernok E, Gaskin G, et al. Diagnostic value of standardized assays for anti-neutrophil cytoplasmic antibodies in idiopathic systemic vasculitis. EC/BCR Project for ANCA Assay Standardization. Kidney Int 1998;5:743-53.

21. Choi HK, Liu S, Merkel PA, Colditz GA, Niles JL. Diagnostic performance of antineutrophil cytoplasmic antibody tests for idiopathic vasculitides: metaanalysis with a focus on antimyeloperoxidase antibodies. J Rheumatol 2001;28: 1584-90.

22. Bosch X, Guilabert A, Font J. Antineutrophil cytoplasmatic antibodies. Lancet 2006;368:404-18.

23. Finkielman JD, Lee AS, Hummel AM, Viss MA, Jacob GL, Homburger HA, et al. ANCA are detectable in nearly all patients with active severe Wegener's granulomatosis. Am J Med 2007;120(643):e9-14.

24. Stone JH. Limited versus severe Wegener's granulomatosis: baseline data on patients in the Wegener's granulomatosis etanercept trial. Arthritis Rheum 2003;48:2299-309.

25. Finkielman JD, Merkel PA, Schroeder D, Hoffman GS, Spiera R, St. Clair EW, et al. Antiproteinase 3 antineutrophil cytoplasmatic antibodies and disease activity in Wegener granulomatosis. Ann Intern Med 2007;147:611-9.

26. Jennings CR, Jones NS, Dugar J, Powell RJ, Lowe J. Wegener's granulomatosis—a review of diagnosis and treatment in 53 subjects. Rhinology 1998;36:188-91.

27. Cadoni G, Prelajade D, Campobasso E, Calo L, Agostino S, Manna R, et al. Wegener's granulomatosis: a challenging disease for otorhinolaryngologists. Acta Otolaryngol 2005;125:1105-10.

28. Schnabel A, Holl-Ulrich K, Dalhoff K, Reuter M, Gross WL. Efficacy of transbronchial biopsy in pulmonary vasculitides. Eur Respir J 1997;10:2738-43.

29. Maguchi S, Fukuda S, Takizawa M. Histological findings in biopsies from patients with cytoplasmic-antineutrophil cytoplasmic antibody (cANCA)-positive Wegener's granulomatosis. Auris Nasus Larynx 2001;28(Suppl.):S53-8.

30. Aasarod K, Bostad L, Hammerstrom J, Jorstad S, Iversen BM. Renal histopathology and clinical course in 94 patients with Wegener's granulomatosis. Nephrol Dial Transplant 2001;16:953-60.

31. Luqmani RA, Bacon PA, Moots RJ, Janssen BA, Pall A, Emery P, et al. Birmingham Vasculitis Activity Score (BVAS) in systemic necrotizing vasculitis. Q J Med 1994;87:671-8.

32. Luqmani RA, Exley AR, Kitas GD, Bacon PA. Disease assessment and management of the vasculitides. Baillieres Clin Rheumatol 1997;11:423-46.

33. Exley RA, Bacon PA, Luqmani RA, Kitas GD, Carruthers DM, Moots R. Examination of disease severity in systemic vasculitis from the novel perspective of damage using the vasculitis damage index (VDI). Br J Rheumatol 1998;37:57-63.

34. Luqmani RA. Evaluation of vasculitis disease activity in Europe. Eur J Intern Med 2001;12:401-2.

35. Flossman O, Bacon PA, de Groot K, Jayne D, Rasmussen N, Seo P, et al. Development of comprehensive disease assessment in systemic vasculitis. Ann Rheum Dis 2007;66: 283-92.

36. Guillevin L, Lhote F, Gayraud M, Cohen P, Jarrousse B, Lortholary O, et al. Prognostic factors in polyarteritis nodosa and Churg-Strauss syndrome. A prospective study in 342 patients. Medicine (Baltimore) 1996;75:17-28.

37. Gayraud M, Guillevin L, le Tounglin P, Cohen P, Lhote F, Casasuss P, et al. Long term follow up of polyarteritis nodosa, microscopic polyangiitis and Churg-Strauss syndrome, analysis of four prospective trials including 278 patients. Arthritis Rheum 2001;44:666-75.

38. Stillwell TJ, Benson Jr RC, DeRemee RA, McDonald TJ, Weiland LH. Cyclophosphamide-induced bladder toxicity in Wegener's granulomatosis. Arthritis Rheum 1988;31: 465-70.

39. Knight A, Askling J, Granath F, Sparen P, Ekbom A. Urinary bladder cancer in Wegener's granulomatosis: risks and relation to cyclophosphamide. Ann Rheum Dis 2004;63: 1307-11.

40. Jayne D, Rasmussen N, Andrassy K, Bacon P, Tervaert JW, Dadoniene J, et al. A randomized trial of maintenance therapy for vasculitis associated with antineutrophil cytoplasmic autoantibodies. N Engl J Med 2003;349:36-44.

41. Chakravarty K, McDonald H, Pullar T, Taggart A, Chalmers R, Oliver S, et al. BSR & BHPR guideline for disease-modifying anti-rheumatic drug (DMARD) therapy in consultation with the British Association of Dermatologists. Rheumatology (Oxford) 2008;47:924-5.

42. De Groot K, Rasmussen N, Bacon PA, Tervaert JW, Feighery C, Gregorini G, et al. Randomized trial of cyclophosphamide versus methotrexate for induction of remission in early systemic antineutrophil cytoplasmic antibody-associated vasculitis. Arthritis Rheum 2005;52:2461-9.

43. Jayne DR, Gaskin G, Rasmussen N, Abramowicz D, Ferrario F, Guillevin L, et al. Randomized trial of plasma exchange or high-dosage methylprednisolone as adjunctive therapy for severe renal vasculitis. J Am Soc Nephrol 2007;18:2180-8.

44. Schmitt WH, Hagen EC, Neumann I, Nowack R, Flores-Suarez LF, van der Woude FJ. Treatment of refractory Wegener's granulomatosis with antithymocyte globulin (ATG): an open study in 15 patients. Kidney Int 2004;65:1440-8.

45. Hoffman GS, Leavitt RY, Kerr GS, Fauci AS. The treatment of Wegener's granulomatosis with glucocorticoids and methotrexate. Arthritis Rheum 1992;35:1322-9.

46. Mukthyar C, Guillevin L, Cid M, Dasgupta B, de Groot K, Gross W, et al. EULAR recommendations for the management of primary small and medium vessel vasculitis. Ann Rheum Dis 2009;68:310-7.

47. Molloy ES, Langford CA. Advances in the treatment of small vessel vasculitis. Rheum Dis Clin North Am 2006;32: 157-72.

48. Wegeners Granulomatosis Etanercept Trial group. Etanercept plus standard therapy for Wegener's granulomatosis. N Engl J Med 2005;352:351-61.

49. Jayne DR, Rasmussen N. Treatment of antineutrophil cytoplasm autoantibody-associated systemic vasculitis: initiatives of the European Community Systemic Vasculitis Clinical Trials Study Group. Mayo Clin Proc 1997;72: 737-47.

50. Koldingsnes W, Nossent JC. Baseline features and initial treatment as predictors of remission and relapse in Wegener's granulomatosis. J Rheumatol 2003;30:80-8.

51. Guillevin L, Cordier JF, Lhote F, Cohen P, Jarrousse B, Royer I, et al. A prospective, multicenter, randomized trial comparing steroids and pulse cyclophosphamide versus steroids and oral cyclophosphamide in the treatment of generalized Wegener's granulomatosis. Arthritis Rheum 1997;40: 2187-98.

52. Guillevin L, Cohen P, Mahr A, Arène JP, Mouthon L, Puèchal X, et al. Treatment of polyareteritis nodosa and microscopic polyangiitis with poor prognosis factors: a prospective trial compairing glucocorticoids and six or twelve cyclophopshamide pulses in sixty-five patients. Arthritis Rheum 2003;49:93-100.

53. Sneller MC, Hoffman GS, Talar-Williams C, Kerr GS, Hallahan CW, Fauci AS. An analysis of forty-two Wegener's granulomatosis patients treated with methotrexate and prednisone. Arthritis Rheum 1995;38:608-13.

54. Stone JH, Tun W, Hellman DB. Treatment of non-life threatening Wegener's granulomatosis with methotrexate and daily prednisone as the initial therapy of choice. J Rheumatol 1999;26:1134-9.

55. Langford CA, Talar-Williams C, Sneller MC. Use of methotrexate and glucocorticoids in the treatment of Wegener's granulomatosis. Long-term renal outcome in patients with glomerulonephritis. Arthritis Rheum 2000;43:1836-40.

56. de Groot K, Muhler M, Reinhold-Keller E, Paulsen J, Gross WL. Induction of remission in Wegener's granulomatosis with low dose methotrexate. J Rheumatol 1998;25:492-5.

57. Metzler C, Hellmich B, Gause A, Gross WL, de Groot K. Churg Strauss syndrome—successful induction of remission with methotrexate and unexpected high cardiac and pulmonary relapse ratio during maintenance treatment. Clin Exp Rheumatol 2004;22(Suppl. 36):S52-61.

58. de Groot K, Adu D, Savage CO. The value of pulse cyclophosphamide in ANCA-associated vasculitis: meta-analysis and critical review. Nephrol Dial Transplant 2001;16: 2018-27.

59. Haubitz M, Frei U, Rother U, Brunkhorst R, Koch KM. Cyclophosphamide pulse therapy in Wegener's granulomatosis. Nephrol Dial Transplant 1991;6:531-5.

60. Adu D, Pall A, Luqmani RA, Richards NT, Howie AJ, Emery P, et al. Controlled trial of pulse versus continuous prednisolone and cyclophosphamide in the treatment of systemic vasculitis. QJM 1997;90:401-9.

61. de Groot K, Schmidt DK, Arlt AC, Gross WL, Reinhold-Keller E. Standardized neurologic evaluations of 128 patients with Wegener granulomatosis. Arch Neurol 2001;58:1215-21.

62. Rihova Z, Jancova E, Merta M, Zabka J, Rysava R, Bartunkova J, et al. Daily oral versus pulse intravenous cyclophosphamide in the therapy of ANCA associated vasculitis—preliminary single center experience. Prague Med Rep 2004;105:64-8.

63. de Groot K, Harper L, Jayne D, Suarez L, Gregorini G, Gross W, et al. Pulse versus daily oral cyclophosphamide for induction of remission in ANCA-associated vasculitis. Ann Intern Med 2009;150:670-80.

64. Haubitz M, Bohnenstengel F, Brunkhorst R, Schwab M, Hofmann U, Busse D. Cyclophosphamide pharmacokinetics and dose requirements in patients with renal insufficiency. Kidney Int 2002;61:1495-501.

65. Guillevin L, Jarrousse B, Lok C, Lhote F, Jais JP, Le Thi Huong Du D, et al. Longterm followup after treatment of polyarteritis nodosa and Churg-Strauss angiitis with comparison of steroids, plasma exchange and cyclophosphamide to steroids and plasma exchange. A prospective randomized trial of 71 patients. The Cooperative Study Group for Polyarteritis Nodosa. J Rheumatol 1991;18:567-74.

66. Guillevin L, Lhote F, Cohen P, Jarrousse B, Lortholary O, Genereau T, et al. Corticosteroids plus pulse cyclophosphamide and plasma exchanges versus corticosteroids plus pulse cyclophosphamide alone in the treatment of polyarteritis nodosa and Churg-Strauss syndrome patients with factors predicting poor prognosis. A prospective, randomized trial in sixty-two patients. Arthritis Rheum 1995;38:1638-45.

67. Cohen P, Pagnoux C, Mahr A, Arene JP, Mouthon L, Le Guern V, et al. Churg-Strauss syndrome with poor-prognosis factors: A prospective multicenter trial comparing glucocorticoids and six or twelve cyclophosphamide pulses in forty-eight patients. Arthritis Rheum 2007;57:686-93.

68. Gayraud M, Guillevin L, Cohen P, Lhote F, Cacoub P, Deblois P, et al. Treatment of good-prognosis polyarteritis nodosa and Churg-Strauss syndrome: comparison of steroids and oral or pulse cyclophosphamide in 25 patients. French Cooperative Study Group for Vasculitides. Br J Rheumatol 1997;36:1290-7.

69. Guillevin L, Pagnoux C. Therapeutic strategies for systemic necrotizing vasculitides. Allergology Int 2007;56:105-11.

70. Allen A, Pusey C, Gaskin G. Outcome of renal replacement therapy in antineutrophil cytoplasmic antibody-associated systemic vasculitis. J Am Soc Nephrol 1998;9:1258-63.

71. Guillevin L, Fain O, Lhote F, Jarrousse B, Le Thi Huong D, Bussel A, et al. Lack of superiority of steroids plus plasma exchange to steroids alone in the treatment of polyarteritis nodosa and Churg-Strauss syndrome. A prospective, randomized trial in 78 patients. Arthritis Rheum 1992;35:208-15.

72. Hellmich B, Kausch I, Doehn C, Jocham D, Holl-Ulrich K, Gross WL. Urinary bladder cancer in Wegener's granulomatosis: is it more than cyclophosphamide? Ann Rheum Dis 2004;63:1183-5.

73. Chung JB, Armstrong K, Schwartz JS, Albert D. Cost-effectiveness of prophylaxis against Pneumocystis carinii pneumonia in patients with Wegener's granulomatosis undergoing immunosuppressive therapy. Arthritis Rheum 2000;43:1841-8.

74. Ognibene FP, Shelhamer JH, Hoffman GS, Kerr GS, Reda D, Fauci AS, et al. Pneumocystis carinii pneumonia: a major complication of immunosuppressive therapy in patients with Wegener's granulomatosis. Am J Respir Crit Care Med 1995;151:795-9.

75. Jarrousse B, Guillevin L, Bindi P, Hachulla E, Leclerc P, Gilson B, et al. Increased risk of Pneumocystis carinii pneumonia in patients with Wegener's granulomatosis. Clin Exp Rheumatol 1993;11:615-21.

76. Slot MC, Tervaert JW, Boomsma MM, Stegeman CA. Positive classic antineutrophil cytoplasmic antibody (C-ANCA) titer at switch to azathioprine therapy associated with relapse in proteinase 3-related vasculitis. Arthritis Rheum 2004;51:269-73.

77. Langford CA, Talar-Williams C, Barron KS, Sneller MC. Use of a cyclophosphamide-induction methotrexate-maintenance regimen for the treatment of Wegener's granulomatosis: extended follow-up and rate of relapse. Am J Med 2003;114:463-9.

78. Reinhold-Keller E, Fink CO, Herlyn K, Gross WL, De Groot K. High rate of renal relapse in 71 patients with Wegener's granulomatosis under maintenance of remission with low-dose methotrexate. Arthritis Rheum 2002;47:326-32.

79. Metzler C, Miehle N, Manger K, Iking-Konert C, de Groot K, Hellmich B, et al. Elevated relapse rate under oral methotrexate versus leflunomide for maintenance of remission in Wegener's granulomatosis. Rheumatology (Oxford) 2007;46:1087-91.

80. Langford CA, Talar-Williams C, Sneller MC. Mycophenolate mofetil for remission maintenance in the treatment of Wegener's granulomatosis. Arthritis Rheum 2004;51:278-83.

81. Stegeman CA, Tervaert JW, de Jong PE, Kallenberg CG. Trimethoprimsulfamethoxazole(co-trimoxazole) for the prevention of relapses of Wegener's granulomatosis. Dutch Co-Trimoxazole Wegener Study Group. N Engl J Med 1996;335:16-20.

82. Reinhold-Keller E, De Groot K, Rudert H, Nolle B, Heller M, Gross WL. Response to trimethoprim/sulfamethoxazole in Wegener's granulomatosis depends on the phase of disease. QJM 1996;89:15-23.

83. Stegeman CA, Tervaert JW, Sluiter WJ, Manson WL, de Jong PE, Kallenberg CG. Association of chronic nasal carriage of Staphylococcus aureus and higher relapse rates in Wegener granulomatosis. Ann Intern Med 1994;120:12-7.

84. Jayne DR, Chapel H, Adu D, Misbah S, O'Donoghue D, Scott D, et al. Intravenous immunoglobulin for ANCA-associated systemic vasculitis with persistent disease activity. Q J Med 2000;93:433-9.

85. Jayne DR, Lockwood CM. Intravenous immunoglobulins as sole therapy for systemic vasculitis. Br J Rheumatol 1996;35:1150-3.

86. Levy Y, Uziel Y, Zandman GG, Amital H, Sherer Y, Langevitz P, et al. Intravenous immunoglobulins in peripheral neuropathy associated with vasculitis. Ann Rheum Dis 2003;62:1221-3.

87. Martinez V, Cohen P, Pagnoux C, Vinzio S, Mahr A, Mouthon L, et al. Intravenous immunoglobulins for relapses of ANCA-associated systemic vasculitides: final analysis of a prospective, open and multicenter trial. Arthritis Rheum 2008;58:308-17.

88. Koukoulaki M, Jayne DR. Mycophenolate mofetil in antineutrophil cytoplasm antibodies-associated systemic vasculitis. Nephron Clin Pract 2006;102:100-7.

89. Birck R, Warnatz K, Lorenz HM, Choi M, Haubitz M, Grunke M, et al. 15-Deoxyspergualin in patients with refractory ANCA-associated systemic vasculitis: a six-month open-label trial to evaluate safety and efficacy. J Am Soc Nephrol 2003;14:440-7.

90. Booth A, Harper L, Hammad T, Bacon P, Griffith M, Levy J, et al. Prospective study of TNFalpha blockade with infliximab in anti-neutrophil cytoplasmic antibody-associated systemic vasculitis. J Am Soc Nephrol 2004;15:717-21.

91. Stassen PM, Cohen Tervaert JW, Stegeman CA. Induction of remission in active anti-neutrophil cytoplasmic antibody-associated vasculitis with mycophenolate mofetil in patients who cannot be treated with cyclophosphamide. Ann Rheum Dis 2007;66:798-802.

92. Keogh KA, Wylam ME, Stone JH, Specks U. Induction of remission by B lymphocyte depletion in eleven patients with refractory antineutrophil cytoplasmic antibody-associated vasculitis. Arthritis Rheum 2005;52:262-8.

93. Keogh KA, Ytterberg SR, Fervenza FC, Carlson KA, Schroeder DR, Specks U. Rituximab for refractory Wegener's granulomatosis: report of a prospective, open-label pilot trial. Am J Respir Crit Care Med 2006;173:180-7.

94. Stasi R, Stipa E, Del Poeta G, Amadori S, Newland AC, Provan D. Longterm observation of patients with anti-neutrophil cytoplasmic antibody-associated vasculitis treated with rituximab. Rheumatology (Oxford) 2006;45:1432-6.

95. Brihaye B, Aouba A, Pagnoux C, Cohen P, Lacassin F, Guillevin L. Adjunction of rituximab to steroids and immunosuppressants for refractory/relapsing Wegener's granulomatosis: a study on 8 patients. Clin Exp Rheumatol 2007;25(Suppl. 4):S23-7.

96. Eriksson P. Nine patients with anti-neutrophil cytoplasmic antibodypositive vasculitis successfully treated with rituximab. J Intern Med 2005;257:540-8.

97. Schmitt WH, Hagen EC, Neumann I, Nowack R, Flores-Suarez LF, van der Woude FJ. Treatment of refractory Wegener's granulomatosis with antithymocyte globulin (ATG): an open study in 15 patients. Kidney Int 2004;65:1440-8.

98. Lovric S, Erdbruegger U, Kümpers P, Woywodt A, Koenecke C, Wedemeyer H, et al. Rituximab as rescue therapy in anti-neutrophil cytoplasmatic antibody-associated vasculitis: single centre experience with 15 patients. Nephrol Dial Transplant 2009;24:179-85.

99. Aries PM, Hellmich B, Voswinkel J, Both M, Nölle B, Holl-Ulrich K, et al. Lack of efficacy of rituximab in Wegener's granulomatosis with refractory granulomatous manifestations. Ann Rheum Dis 2006;65:853-8.

100. Joy MS, Hogan SL, Jennette JC, Falk RJ, Nachman PH. A pilot study using mycophenolate mofetil in relapsing or resistant ANCA small vessel vasculitis. Nephrol Dial Transplant 2005;20:2725-32.

101. Hu W, Liu C, Xie H, Chen H, Liu Z, Li L. Mycophenolate mofetil versus cyclophosphamide for inducing remission of ANCA vasculitis with moderate renal involvement. Nephrol Dial Transplant 2008;23:1307-12.

102. Tatsis E, Schnabel A, Gross WL. Interferon-α treatment of four patients with the Churg-Strauss syndrome. Ann Intern Med 1998;129:370-4.

103. Zaja F, De Vita S, Mazzaro C, Sacco S, Damiani D, De Marchi G, et al. Efficacy and safety of rituximab in type II mixed cryoglobulinemia. Blood 2003;101:3827-34.

104. De Vita S, Quartuccio L, Fabris M. Rituximab in mixed cryoglobulinemia: increased experience and perspectives. Dig Liver Dis 2007;39(Suppl. 1):122-8.

105. Misiani R, Bellavita P, Fenili D, Vicari O, Marchesi D, Sironi PL, et al. Interferon alfa-2a therapy in cryoglobulinemia associated with hepatitis C virus. N Engl J Med 1994;330:751-6.

106. Mazzaro C, Colle R, Baracetti S, Nascimben F, Zorat F, Pozzato G. Effectiveness of leukocyte interferon in patients affected by HCV-positive mixed cryoglobulinemia resistant to recombinant alpha-interferon. Clin Exp Rheumatol 2002;20:27-34.

107. Adinolfi LE, Utili R, Zampino R, Ragone E, Mormone G, Ruggiero G. Effects of long-term course of alpha-interferon in patients with chronic hepatitis C associated to mixed cryoglobulinaemia. Eur J Gastroenterol Hepatol 1997;9:1067-72.

108. Mazzaro C, Carniello GS, Colle R, Doretto P, Mazzi G, Crovatto M, et al. Interferon therapy in HCV-positive mixed cryoglobulinaemia: viral and host factors contributing to efficacy of the therapy. Ital J Gastroenterol Hepatol 1997;29:343-50.

109. Cohen P, Nguyen QT, Deny P, Ferriere F, Roulot D, Lortholary O, et al. Treatment of mixed cryoglobulinemia with recombinant interferon alpha and adjuvant therapies. A prospective study on 20 patients. Ann Med Interne (Paris) 1996;147:81-6.

110. Saadoun D, Resche-Rigon M, Thibault V, Piette JC, Cacoub P. Antiviral therapy for hepatitis C virus–associated mixed cryoglobulinemia vasculitis: a long-term followup study. Arthritis Rheum 2006;54:3696-706.

111. Mazzaro C, Zorat F, Comar C, Nascimben F, Bianchini D, Baracetti S, et al. Interferon plus ribavirin in patients with hepatitis C virus positive mixed cryoglobulinemia resistant to interferon. J Rheumatol 2003;30:1775-81.

112. Guillevin L, Mahr A, Callard P, Godmer P, Pagnoux C, Leray E, et al. Hepatitis B virus-associated polyarteritis nodosa: clinical characteristics, outcome, and impact of treatment in 115 patients. Medicine (Baltimore) 2005;84:13-22.

113. Flynn JT, Smoyer WE, Bunchman TE, Kershaw DB, Sedman AB. Treatment of Henoch-Schonlein purpura glomerulonephritis in children with high-dose corticosteroids plus oral cyclophosphamide. Am J Nephrol 2001;21:128-33.

Chapter 17

Management of CNS Vasculitis and Takayasu's Arteritis

Richard Keating

CENTRAL NERVOUS SYSTEM VASCULITIS

CASE STUDY 1

A 34-year-old woman is admitted to the intensive care unit (ICU) following presentation to the emergency department with slurred speech, right-sided arm and leg weakness, severe headache, and mental status changes. Screening computed tomography (CT) scan in the emergency department showed several subacute ischemic infarctions in a widespread distribution. Initial laboratories were remarkable for an erythrocyte sedimentation rate (ESR) of 40 mm/h and a negative antinuclear antibody (ANA) test. You are asked by the ICU attending to evaluate the patient for possible central nervous system (CNS) vasculitis.

Introductory Comments

A request to "rule out CNS vasculitis" is often met with a feeling of anxiety. The consulting rheumatologist knows that this is a rare disease, and it is difficult to make the diagnosis with certainty. CNS vasculitis is probably the least commonly encountered form of vasculitis seen by a rheumatologist. The consultant is caught between the fear of missing a serious diagnosis and withholding needed therapy, and just as easily making the diagnosis inappropriately in the setting of a condition that mimics vasculitis and treating the patient too aggressively, with the potential to cause serious iatrogenic harm. There is no gold standard test to lead to the diagnosis, and clinical judgment and experience are of paramount importance. The rheumatologist should never feel alone in the evaluation of a patient with possible CNS vasculitis and should readily obtain the assistance and counsel from colleagues in neurology, vascular medicine, infectious diseases and imaging consultants, among others. To meet the challenge of offering the patient the optimum outcome in this difficult disease requires a team approach.

Several early points need to be covered before we try to address the question of whether our patient has CNS vasculitis. Importantly, CNS vasculitis is not one disease entity but a broad term that is imprecisely applied by too many physicians. Under the banner of CNS vasculitis are myriad vascular based abnormalities that may affect the CNS but do not reflect a true necrotizing vasculitis in etiology.

Our understanding of vasculitis of the CNS over the past decade has grown deeper. Described first almost 50 years ago, CNS vasculitis was considered a fatal disease.[1] As recently as 1988, only 46 cases had been described.[2] The advent of contrast angiography has probably contributed to the increase in diagnosis of CNS vasculitis since the 1970s, but making this diagnosis based solely on angiographic findings is tenuous. Newer imaging modalities have contributed to a far greater sensitivity in identifying CNS ischemia, but the modalities to identify true vascular inflammation as the etiology for that ischemia has not improved concurrently.[3] Simply put, we are far better at identifying ischemia and damage to the brain than we are at identifying its exact etiology.

Our understanding of CNS vasculitis is fraught with many problems. There are no controlled trials that have addressed best practices for either the diagnosis or treatment of CNS vasculitis. There is a paucity of long-term follow-up data on patients diagnosed with CNS vasculitis. We lack an animal study model. Also, there is no classification criteria widely accepted within the rheumatology community for categorizing and reporting on CNS vasculitis. Regardless, a condition originally viewed as inexorably devastating without aggressive treatment is now viewed in a far more nuanced way with an appreciation that CNS vasculopathy has a spectrum of involvement and outcomes.

Definitions and Clinical Subsets

CNS vasculitis has been variously titled, over the past many years, as isolated angiitis of the CNS, primary CNS vasculitis, or primary vasculitis of the CNS (Table 17-1). The currently accepted classification of CNS vasculitis, while still in evolution, can be

Table 17-1. *Definitions*

Primary angiitis of the central nervous system (PACNS) is vasculitis limited to the CNS (brain, spinal cord, and meninges). Either contrast angiography or pathologic confirmation is employed to make this diagnosis. Should a biopsy be obtained, its results can then be used to further clarify PACNS as either *"Granulomatous Angiitis of the CNS (GACNS)"* or *"Non-Granulomatous angiitis of the CNS (NGACNS)."*[1]

PACNS can be further classified based on the type of study used to make the diagnosis as either *"Histologically Defined Angiitis of the CNS (HDACNS)"* or *"Angiographically Defined Angiopathy of the CNS (ADACNS)."*[2]

Secondary vasculitis of the central nervous system (SVCNS) is the nosology used to describe those patients with a systemic disease, often a systemic vasculitis or diffuse connective tissue disease, that has features referable to the CNS. SLE with CNS involvement would be a good example.

Reversible cerebral vasoconstriction syndromes (RCVS) is a vasospastic variant of CNS vascular disease.[3] This condition is defined by its reversible nature. This condition has at various times been called isolated benign cerebral vasculitis, benign acute cerebral angiopathy, CNS pseudovasculitis, migraine angiitis, and others. Most recently, it has been titled *Benign Angiopathy of the central nervous system (BACNS)*, which emphasized its better prognosis.[4] RCVS is the current preferred name, reinforcing the concept of vascular process reversibility.

[1] Younger DS, Calabrese LH, Hays AP. Granulomatous angiitis of the nervous system. Neurol Clin 1997;15:821.
[2] Woolfenden AR, Tong DC, Marks MP, Ali AO, Albers GW. Angiographically defined primary angiitis of the CNS. Is it really benign? Neurology 1998;51:183-8.
[3] Calabrese LH, Dodick DW, Schwedt TJ, Singhal AB. Narrative review: Reversible cerebral vasoconstriction syndromes. Ann Intern Med 2007;146:34-45.
[4] Calabrese L, Gragg LA, Furlan AJ: Benign angiopathy: A distinct subset of angiographically defined primary angiitis of the central nervous system. J Rheumatol 1993;20:2046.

broadly approached and divided along the following schema, which has helped bring some order to a heterogeneous set of terms and conditions:

Primary angiitis of the central nervous system (PACNS) is, by definition, limited to the CNS (brain, spinal cord, and meninges). Either contrast angiography or pathologic confirmation is employed to make this diagnosis. Should a biopsy be obtained, its results can then be used to further clarify PACNS as either *granulomatous angiitis of the CNS* (GACNS) or non-granulomatous angiitis, sometimes referred to as *atypical PACNS*.[4] One group has proposed a classification based on the type of study used to make the diagnosis with two subsets defined as "histologically defined angiitis of the CNS" (HDACNS) or "angiographically defined angiopathy of the CNS" (ADACNS).[5] PACNS is a rare disease, with an incidence estimated at 2.4 cases per 1,000,000 person years.[6]

Secondary vasculitis of the central nervous system (SVCNS) is the term applied in the nosology of CNS vasculitis to describe those patients with a systemic disease, often a systemic vasculitis or diffuse connective tissue disease, that has features referable to the CNS. Systemic lupus erythematosus (SLE) with CNS involvement would be a good example.

Reversible Cerebral Vasoconstriction Syndromes (RCVS) is another variant of the condition. This more recent addition to the nomenclature came from the realization that there are a subset of patients with a vasospastic variant of CNS vascular disease.[7] The terminology in this condition has evolved as its reversible nature has become more central to our understanding of its course and prognosis. This condition has at various times been called isolated benign cerebral vasculitis, benign acute cerebral angiopathy, CNS pseudovasculitis, migraine angiitis, and others. Most recently, it was titled benign

angiopathy of the central nervous system (BACNS), which emphasized its better prognosis.[8] RCVS is the current preferred name, enforcing the concept of reversibility in the vascular anomaly.

The implication of an RCVS diagnosis is that the course of disease should be more benign by virtue of reversible vasospasm and that this reversibility portends a far better prognosis. The modifier 'benign' has been called into question though as some with this diagnosis do suffer significant and additive morbidity.[5]

A difficulty at the time of presentation and initial diagnosis of CNS vasculitis lies in the dilemma that one cannot be certain that the clinical course is going to be one of vasospastic reversibility (RCVS) or progressive disease from necrotizing vasculitis (PACNS). The consulting rheumatologist must marshal all of his or her skills to evaluate and classify the patient quickly and correctly.

Differential Diagnosis

A large list of CNS vasculitis mimics, as well as consideration that CNS vasculitis might be a component of a larger, more systemic vasculitis, needs to be considered when evaluating a patient for CNS vasculitis (Table 17-2). A thorough history and physical examination will go far in addressing each of the possible diagnoses.

An immunocompromised state raises the risk for an opportunistic infectious process. Patients with underlying autoimmune diseases on aggressive immunosuppression regimens are especially problematic. The rheumatologist needs to consider the possibility that the underlying disease is the reason for new CNS manifestations (such as CNS lymphoma) as well as the possibility that the

Table 17-2. *Differential Diagnosis of Central Nervous System Vasculopathy*

Secondary vasculitis of the CNS (SVCNS):
  Polyarteritis nodosa
  Allergic granulomatosis (Churg-Strauss syndrome)
  Hypersensitivity vasculitis
  Wegener's granulomatosis
  Takayasu's arteritis
  Behçet's disease
  Lymphomatoid granulomatosis
  Cogan's syndrome
  Vasculitis from a diffuse connective tissue
    disease (SLE, MCTD)

Infection:
  Bacterial (endocarditis, meningitis, tuberculosis,
    spirochetal)
  Viral (herpes, HIV, hepatitis C)
  Fungal (aspergillus, histoplasmosis)

Neoplasm:
  Carcinomatous meningitis
  Glioma
  Malignant angioendotheliomatosis
  Multiple myeloma
  Angioimmunoproliferative disorders
  CNS lymphoma

Drugs:
  Amphetamine
  Ephedrine
  Cocaine
  Ergotamine
  Phenylpropanolamine
  Heroin

Heritable Disorders:
  Cerebral autosomal dominant arteriopathy with
    subcortical infarcts and leukoencephalopathy (CADASIL)

Vasospastic disorders:
  Postpartum angiopathy
  Eclampsia
  Pheochromocytoma
  Subarachnoid hemorrhage
  Migraine
  Dissection
  Hypertension associated
  Exertional headaches

Other "mimics":
  Fibromuscular dysplasia
  Amyloid
  Moyamoya disease
  Thrombotic thrombocytopenic purpura
  Sickle cell anemia
  Neurofibromatosis
  Atherosclerosis
  Myxoma embolism
  Paraprotein
  Cholesterol embolism
  Pregnancy and post-partum vasculopathy
  Demyelinating disease
  Sarcoidosis
  Embolic processes
  Eale's disease
  Acute posterior placoid pigment epitheliopathy
    and cerebral vasculitis
  Hypercoagulable states/antiphospholipid syndrome
  Radicular vasculopathy
  Traumatic dissection

CNS, central nervous system; HIV, human immunodeficiency virus; MCTD, mixed connective tissue disease; SLE, systemic lupus erythematosus.
From Calabrese LH, Duna GF. Vasculitis of the central nervous system. In: Weisman MH, Weinblatt ME, Louie JS, editors. Treatment of the Rheumatic Diseases. Philadelphia: W.B. Saunders; 2001; pp 345-52; and Calabrese LH, Furlan AJ, Gragg LA, Ropos TJ. Primary angiitis of the central nervous system: diagnostic criteria and clinical approach. Cleveland Clinic J Med 1992;59:293-306.

immunosuppression created with medications has allowed for an opportunistic infection.

Infectious angiitis can mimic PACNS and a high degree of suspicion for an infectious process should be maintained. Some of the infectious causes of angiitis include human immunodeficiency virus (HIV), hepatitis C, herpes zoster (HZV), histoplasmosis, Lyme disease, and syphilis. Fungal infections have a predilection for the base of the brain. Often these patients are immunosuppressed or ill from comorbid conditions. The need for consultation with an infectious disease specialist can't be overemphasized.

Drug use can mimic CNS vasculitis and is often an inciting agent for RCVS, although the clinical picture can mimic PACNS. Careful history taking, often from family members, should concentrate on recent ingestion of cocaine, amphetamines, and ephedrine containing products (marketed for rapid weight loss). Urine toxicologic screening is recommended.

Attention should be paid to the age of the patient as drug abuse is more common in the younger age groups, whereas atherosclerosis, cerebral amyloid, and neoplasm are more common in the older population. Cerebral amyloid angiopathy should be in the differential diagnosis for an older patient with cerebral hemorrhages. The amyloid is usually found in the vessels in the leptomeninges and cortex with sparing of white matter.

A curious entity to consider in the setting of possible CNS vasculitis is after varicella zoster virus (VZV) contralateral hemiplegia. Approximately 1 to 4 weeks following a VZV infection as in herpes zoster ophthalmicus or trigeminal nerve involvement, a patient may develop a syndrome of contralateral hemiplegia. The current understanding of this curious clinical presentation is that a vasculitis involves the ipsilateral carotid artery or its middle cerebral artery branch.[9] If in doubt, and a VZV-associated process is being considered, consultation with an infectious diseases expert and therapy for HZV should be considered.

Diagnostic Evaluation

Symptoms and Signs

The most common symptom of PACNS is *headache,* which becomes more chronic. Most patients diagnosed with CNS vasculitis have been ill for an extended period of time, often measured in months. Headache might then be followed by *encephalopathy,* and finally, *multiple infarcts* develop. Other neurologic features reported include stroke, seizure, hemorrhage, cranial neuropathies, cerebellar dysfunction, a mass lesion, spinal cord involvement, and cauda equina syndrome.[10,11]

There is usually a delay in diagnosis from weeks to months as neurologic involvement increases. Although imaging may show multiple strokes, a key point is that the strokes are often of varying age, suggesting an ongoing process with repeated showering of infarcts. Generally, new neurologic events occur. Fever and weight loss are not requisite findings, nor do they preclude CNS vasculitis. Curiously, most cases of biopsy-proven PACNS occur in men.

A "thunderclap headache" characterized by an abrupt onset with evolution to maximal pain measured in minutes is more likely to herald the presentation of RCVS than of PACNS, which has a more indolent cephalgia presentation. There may be self-limited resolution and then recurrence of the headache before presentation and final diagnosis. This headache and clinical picture of RCVS is more common in women than men. The headache will then be followed by other neurologic signs and symptoms. RCVS may be spontaneous or secondary to ingested vasoactive substances, or as a finding in the postpartum period.[12] Again, particular attention should be paid to the possibility of the patient using cannabis, decongestants, weight-loss supplements, and selective serotonin reuptake inhibitors (SSRIs) (Table 17-3).

Laboratory Evaluation

Laboratory evaluation is, unfortunately, nonspecific in CNS vasculitis. There is no diagnostic serologic test for PACNS. Many patients are systemically ill, and this is reflected in an anemia of chronic disease, elevated acute phase reactants, and other nonspecific laboratory values reflecting an inflammatory condition. The laboratory is employed more to evaluate for the mimics of PACNS than to confirm the diagnosis of PACNS. A basic evaluation should include an evaluation for autoimmune disease, a hypercoaguable state (to include antiphospholipid antibodies), HIV, syphilis, blood cultures for bacteria, fungi, and mycobacteria.

Cerebrospinal fluid (CSF) analysis is usually abnormal in PACNS. The typical CSF fluid finding in PACNS is an elevated CSF protein with a CSF lymphocytosis.

The typical CSF fluid finding in RCVS is more bland, with a few cells but near normal, if not

Table 17-3. *Precipitating Factors and Conditions Associated with Reversible Cerebral Vasoconstriction Syndromes*

Pregnancy and Puerperium
- Early puerperium
- Late pregnancy
- Eclampsia
- Preeclampsia
- Delayed postpartum eclampsia

Catecholamine-Secreting Tumor
- Pheochromocytoma
- Bronchial carcinoid tumor

Exogenous Exposures
- Drugs
  - Cannabis
  - Cocaine
  - "Ecstasy"
  - Amphetamine derivatives
  - Lysergic acid diethylamine
- Medications
  - SSRIs
  - Ergotamine tartrate
  - Methergine
  - Bromocriptine
  - Lisuride
  - Sumatriptan
  - Isometheptine
  - Tacrolimus
  - Cyclophosphamide
  - Interferon alpha
  - Nasal decongestants
  - Phenylpropanolamine
  - Pseudoephedrine
  - Ephedrine
- Red blood cell transfusion
- IVIG
- Alcohol
- Miscellaneous
  - Hypercalcemia
  - Porphyria
  - Head trauma
  - Spinal subdural hematoma
  - Postcarotid endarterectomy

IVIG, intravenous immunoglobulin; SSRIs, selective serotonin reuptake inhibitors.
From Ducros A, Boubobza M, Porcher R, Sarov M, Valade D, Boussser MG. The clinical and radiological spectrum of reversible cerebral vasoconstriction syndrome. A prospective series of 67 patients. Brain 2007;130:3091-101; and Calabrese LH, Dodick DW, Schwedt TJ, Singhal AB. Narrative review: reversible cerebral vasoconstriction syndromes. Ann Intern Med 2007;146:34-44.

normal, protein. In approximately 50% of cases of RCVS, the CSF analysis is entirely normal. It usually resembles the analyses obtained in chronic meningitis.

Imaging Studies

Brain magnetic resonance imaging (MRI) study has supplanted brain CT as the imaging modality of choice for CNS vasculitis. It offers unparalleled sensitivity for detecting abnormalities. MRI is abnormal in more than 90% of cases.[13] Specificity, however, is still wanting. The usual PACNS MRI findings include multiple, bilateral lesions that are usually infarcts or nonspecific signal change. Typical locations for lesions include the subcortical white matter, deep gray matter, deep white matter, and cortex. Although a normal brain MRI has a strong negative predictive value for PACNS, pathologic diagnosis has been made when the imaging study was unremarkable.[14] Prominence of the meninges on gadolinium-enhanced MRI may be a finding in PACNS. MRI angiography (MRA) may well be abnormal but does not guarantee the level of clarity needed for the size blood vessel usually affected in PACNS, and so a transfemoral contrast angiogram is often required.

Most patients with CNS vasculitis are diagnosed now with contrast angiography. Traditional contrast angiography in CNS vasculitis would be expected to demonstrate classic "beading" of small vessels with alternating constrictions, ectasia, and dilatation. Microaneurysms are far less common than in polyarteritis nodosa. Commonly affected vessels include the small branches of the middle anterior arteries or the posterior cerebral arteries. Unless affected by atherosclerotic vascular disease, the more proximal and larger vessels are not affected by PACNS. The finding of atherosclerotic changes in the carotid siphon or other vessels should raise concern if the angiogram is then interpreted as showing vasculitis. It needs to be remembered that vasculitis is a dynamic, pathophysiologic process, and a contrast angiogram is no more than an imaging modality of intraluminal architecture and many processes other than vasculitis can result in a similar imaging result. It really cannot be stressed enough that even when an angiogram is "positive," the careful clinician must maintain a healthy level of skepticism and consider alternative explanations to vasculitis for the angiographic findings. Many patients will still have another explanation for the luminal findings.[14] Even a well-performed contrast angiogram lacks specificity for CNS vasculitis.[3]

An abnormal angiogram then, while important to the diagnosis of CNS vasculitis, can be misleading because multiple conditions may lead to a similar picture. The radiologist's report that an angiogram is *consistent with vasculitis* must be interpreted with caution and a circumspect approach taken by the treating rheumatologist. The angiographic findings in PACNS and RVCS may well be indistinguishable in the acute setting with no pathognomonic angiographic feature for necrotizing CNS vasculitis. A follow-up angiogram after several months of treatment is sometimes necessary to confirm that the initial findings represented a reversible process (RVCS) versus a necrotizing process (PACNS).

Just as a positive angiogram can lead to early diagnostic closure, a normal angiogram may not rule out vasculitis. GACNS, confirmed histologically, can sometimes result in a normal angiogram because the size of the affected vessels may be below the resolution of the imaging study. Most patients with a so-called positive angiogram have some condition other than GACNS.[3,4,13]

Pathologic Evaluation

Biopsy of the leptomeninges/underlying cortex is the definitive method for confirming the diagnosis of PACNS. Some would argue that this procedure should be pursued before committing a patient to high-dose corticosteroids and cyclophosphamide with their attendant side effects.[15] The procedure is subject to sampling bias with the possibility for a false-negative finding. It is recommended that the biopsy be taken from the nondominant temporal lobe.[16] It should be appreciated that there is the potential for morbidity from the procedure itself although it is low (2% in one study).[17] The risk of biopsy needs to be put into context when one considers the risk of empiric treatment with a cytotoxic agent or agents for a prolonged time period for a condition that does not have histologic confirmation. It is important to remember that angiography alone lacks specificity.

The pathology of PACNS is an inflammatory process centered about smaller veins and arterioles and is more prominent in the leptomeninges than in the deeper cortex. As noted previously, the infiltrate may be either granulomatous or nongranulomatous. A patchy distribution of involvement leads to sampling error.[18]

Brain biopsy has a sensitivity for PACNS of approximately 80%.[19]

In summary, a biopsy in conjunction with an angiogram is preferred in making the diagnosis of PACNS. The need for both studies is necessitated by the reality that an angiogram alone is too nonspecific. The added information obtained with biopsy supports a decision to give aggressive immunosuppression. Biopsy material should be submitted for staining for infectious etiologies in addition to routine histology.

In reality, obtaining a biopsy is not always feasible. In a clinical scenario that supports the diagnosis of RCVS, one could consider a delayed biopsy if treatment with corticosteroids and a calcium channel blocker for a predetermined time period does not result in clinical improvement.

Diagnostic Evaluation Summary

Making the definitive diagnosis of CNS vasculitis can clearly be challenging. A high index of suspicion must drive the evaluation because there is no single serologic test or imaging modality result that will confirm the diagnosis for the consulting rheumatologist with absolute certainty. The concept of benign disease (usually vasospasm) at one end of the spectrum and a truly inflammatory vasculitis at the opposite pole underpins our current understanding of CNS vasculitis. Finding the point on this spectrum that defines the individual patient is difficult and requires careful clinical judgment. A meticulous history and physical examination is of paramount importance. Interviewing family members is necessary to ascertain whether vasoactive drugs have been ingested. Over-the-counter supplements and illegal drug use must be addressed.

A variety of diagnostic tests are then employed in approaching the CNS vasculitis evaluation, and it is worth remembering that the majority of patients who are evaluated for CNS vasculitis are eventually diagnosed with another condition. An echocardiogram to evaluate for an embolic etiology to CNS findings is usually obtained. Electroencephalography, CT, and MRI imaging, and CSF analysis typically follow, both to evaluate for the mimics (see Differential Diagnosis) of vasculitis as well as to pursue the diagnoses of PACNS or RCVS. A totally normal MRI and CSF analysis strongly argues against PACNS, and when both studies are normal, they offer a high negative predictive value for vasculitis.

However, if these tests are abnormal and a high index of suspicion remains for vasculitis, then they should be followed by contrast angiography and then, finally, a leptomeningeal/cortical brain biopsy. It is natural to want to avoid an invasive procedure such as leptomeningeal biopsy and to depend on an angiogram report for diagnostic confirmation, but the predictive value of an angiogram is low and the consulting rheumatologist may well need to pursue tissue diagnosis. A diagnosis based solely on angiography is more tenuous than one based on histopathologic results. RCVS is a more likely diagnosis when only contrast angiography is used to make the diagnosis.

A follow-up contrast angiogram in 6 to 12 weeks is the confirmatory test for the diagnosis of RCVS. A failure to show angiographic resolution should raise the suspicion that something other than vasospasm is causing the patient's clinical picture.

Diagnostic Criteria—Primary Angiitis of the Central Nervous System

The currently employed classification scheme originated with Calabrese and Mallek in their 1988 review and is a useful guide to diagnosis of PACNS.[20]
1. A history or clinical finding of an acquired neurologic deficit that remained unexplained after a thorough initial basic evaluation.
2. Either classic (high-probability) angiographic evidence or histopathologic demonstration of angiitis within the CNS.
3. No evidence of systemic vasculitis or any other condition to which the angiographic or pathologic features could be secondary.

Although no readily agreed-upon diagnostic criteria are accepted, a *definite* diagnosis of PACNS could be given with a compelling set of symptoms and signs including headache, additive neurologic deficits, a lack of an alternative explanation or diagnosis, supporting imaging studies, and a histologic sample demonstrating vasculitis.

Diagnostic Criteria—Reversible Cerebral Vasoconstriction Syndromes

RCVS or reversible cerebral vasoconstrictive syndrome is probably more common than is realized. Although this group of conditions does have a better prognosis than PACNS or SVCNS, it is easy for a patient to be misdiagnosed with PACNS with resultant unnecessarily aggressive treatment. Five elements have been proposed for the diagnosis of reversible cerebral vasoconstrictive syndrome[7]:
1. Presence of multifocal segmental cerebral artery vasoconstriction documented by direct or indirect angiography (transfemoral angiograpy, computerized tomographic angiography [CTA], magnetic resonance angiography [MRA])
2. No evidence of aneursymal, subarachnoid hemorrhage (which is often observed after a stroke)
3. CSF analysis shows normal or near-normal results (e.g., protein level < 80 mg/dL, leukocytes < 10 mm^3, normal glucose level)
4. Severe, acute headaches, with or without additional neurologic signs or symptoms
5. Reversibility of angiographic abnormalities within 12 weeks after onset.

Treatment

There are no placebo-controlled, large scale, randomized trials performed that have defined the best approach to therapy for either PACNS or RCVS. This reflects the diagnostic uncertainty and low incidence of both PACNS and RCVS. Often, therapy is begun when one is not even certain which of these conditions is the correct diagnosis. Clinical judgment drives the treatment plan for all form of CNS vasculopathy. Continuous reevaluation of the diagnosis and assessment of response to therapy will allow for a measured change in treatment as time progresses.

Primary Angiitis of the Central Nervous System

Experience has shown that corticosteroids are first-line agents for PACNS, and most rheumatologists would favor 3 days of 1000 mg of methylprednisolone daily before transitioning to a regimen of 1 mg/kg/day of prednisone. The prednisone dose should be continued until clinical improvement is noted and inflammatory markers, if present, are improved. This is likely to take a month or more. A slow taper follows, if response is forthcoming, over the ensuing many months.

The addition of cyclophosphamide or other therapies should be considered on an individual basis for PACNS. Cyclophosphamide in combination with corticosteroids has a record of success dating back to the early 1980s, when a report on four patients with what was then called isolated angiitis of the central nervous system was published.[21] Combination therapy was thus established as a standard of care, and it is generally accepted that true PACNS should be treated with more than corticosteroids alone. Aggressive therapy with the combination of corticosteroids and cyclophosphamide is generally advocated when the patient has a heavy disease burden along with a compelling diagnostic evaluation. If the patient can take oral medications, cyclophosphamide is dosed at 2 mg/kg/day starting along with corticosteroids. Some will delay, adding cyclophosphamide to see if monotherapy with corticosteroids results in prompt improvement, thereby trying to avoid cyclophosphamide. However, the threshold for adding cyclophosphamide for a firm diagnosis of PACNS is low. Prophylactic therapy for *Pneumocystis jiroveci* is recommended when cyclophosphamide is combined with corticosteroids. The duration of treatment and the tapering schedule for the corticosteroid/cyclophosphamide combination is empiric, but modeling the treatment on a Wegener's granulomatosis regimen seems reasonable. Disease severity warranting the institution of cyclophosphamide may result in a treatment course extending to 2 years after clinical improvement.

Reversible Cerebral Vasoconstriction Syndromes

RCVS, especially if induced by a drug or other removable cause, does not necessarily require immunosuppression. In the setting of a firm diagnosis of RCVS, some advocate treatment with a calcium channel blocker either alone or combined with a faster tapering course of prednisone than would be used in PACNS. Frustratingly, the presentation of RCVS is often clouded by a less-than-clear diagnosis and so an initial course of corticosteroids is a prudent treatment. If response is forthcoming and the clinical picture becomes more consistent with a reversible angiopathy, then the initial corticosteroid dosing may be followed by a quick taper over approximately 3 months.[19,22] Avoidance of all sympathomimetic drugs is mandatory.[23] As a more developed understanding of RCVS has evolved, so has its treatment. A shorter during of corticosteroid therapy in combination with calcium channel blockers has become accepted. Calcium channel blockers are often continued long term.

A follow-up angiogram in 12 weeks would, if pursued, confirm the reversible nature of RCVS and offer significant prognostic data. Also, a lack of reversibility on angiogram would lend support to a diagnosis of PACNS and suggest the need for a longer and perhaps more intensive course of treatment.

At first presentation, when the rheumatologist is uncertain if the patient has PACNS or RCVS, clinical judgment should dictate just how aggressively to treat the patient. A fulminant presentation would warrant combined therapy with corticosteroids and cyclophosphamide, whereas a presentation consistent with RCVS (female, thunderclap headache, normal CSF) could be approached with corticosteroids and/or calcium channel blockers as the mainstay of therapy.

Prognosis

A retrospective study of a cohort of 101 patients with PACNS followed at Mayo Clinic was reported and indicated that four presentation manifestations were associated with an increased mortality rate. These features included focal neurologic deficits, cognitive impairment, cerebral infarction, and large vessel involvement. Treatment was continued for 12 to 18 months. Relapse occurred in 21 of the 101 patients, but those affected still had a similar outcome to those without relapse.[24]

RCVS is not without potential morbidity. Cortical subarachnoid hemorrhage, intracerebral hemorrhage, seizure, and reversible posterior leukoencephalopathy have all been seen early in the course, usually in the first week of symptoms. In the second week, cerebral infarction and transient ischemic attack (TIA) may be seen. Still, the prognosis for RCVS is believed to be far better than that for PACNS. No relapse was seen in at least one study of 67 patients with RCVS, who were followed for a mean of 16 months.[12] Sixteen patients with RCVS were followed for a mean of almost 3 years with excellent recovery, although one patient did have some form of relapse after therapy was tapered. No death occurred in this sample.[25]

Summary

PACNS is a rare disease but one with an increased rate of mortality and morbidity if not recognized and treated early. Angiography and biopsy are key elements in the diagnostic approach and are complimentary. Early recognition and treatment are necessary to impact on its significant morbidity and mortality rates. High-dose corticosteroids, usually in combination with cyclophosphamide, are mainstays of treatment.[6]

RCVS is characterized by its reversibility, usually over the course of several months. Headache is a heralding presentation. It has a number of exogenous triggers including drugs, pregnancy, or in the puerperium. CSF analysis is usually normal as are autoimmune serologies. A contrast angiogram usually shows segmental cerebral arterial vasoconstriction, which reverses by 12 weeks. Treatment is empirical but may include only observation with removal of an identified, inciting agent or some combination of calcium channel blockers and possible high-dose corticosteroids for a limited period of time. Most patients do well (Table 17-4).[7]

Case Presentation Follow-Up

Our 34-year-old woman underwent an extensive evaluation to include normal or negative laboratories including antinuclear cytoplasmic antibodies (ANCAs), rapid plasma regain (RPR), blood cultures, hypercoagulability evaluation, and infectious disease work-up. She had a normal echocardiogram. CSF analysis revealed normal protein, glucose, and cell analysis. An angiogram documented multiple segmental areas of cerebral artery vasoconstriction

Table 17-4. *Summary of Critical Elements for the Diagnosis of Reversible Cerebral Vasoconstriction Syndromes*

1. Transfemoral angiography or indirect CTA or MRA documenting multifocal segmental cerebral artery vasoconstriction
2. No evidence for aneurysmal subarachnoid hemorrhage
3. Normal or near-normal cerebrospinal fluid analysis
   • Protein level < 80 mg/dL
   • Leukocytes < 10 mm³
   • Normal glucose level
4. Severe, acute headaches, with or without additional neurologic signs or symptoms
5. Reversibility of angiographic abnormalities within 12 weeks after onset. If death occurs before the follow-up studies are completed, autopsy rules out conditions such as vasculitis, intracranial atherosclerosis, and aneurysmal subarachnoid hemorrhage, which can also manifest with headache and stroke

CTA, computed tomography angiography; MRA, magnetic resonance angiography.
From Calabrese LH, Dodick DW, Schwedt TJ, Singhal AB. Narrative review: reversible cerebral vasoconstriction syndromes. Ann Intern Med 2007;146:34-44.

with areas of stenosis and beading. She was started on high-dose corticosteroids during the initial evaluation. As she slowly improved, the history was elicited from family members that she had been ingesting a commercial, weight loss supplement containing pseudoephedrine and that the severe headache which brought her to the emergency department was of sudden onset. The corticosteroids were weaned over the course of several weeks and replaced by a calcium channel blocker. A repeat angiogram 12 weeks later, after discontinuation of all nonprescribed medications, showed normalization of the previously seen stenoses and beading. She was diagnosed with RCVS (Table 17-5).

Table 17-5. *Infectious Etiologies of Central Nervous System Vasculitis*

1. Viruses
   • HIV
   • CMV
   • VZV
   • Others
2. Syphilis
3. *Borrelia burgdorferi*
4. Bartonella
5. *Mycobacterium tuberculosis*
6. Fungi
   • Aspergillus
   • Coccidioides
   • Others
7. Bacteria (multiple)
8. Rickettsiae
   • Rocky Mountain spotted fever
   • Typhus
   • Others

CMV, cytomegalovirus; HIV, human immunodeficiency virus; VZV, varicella zoster virus.
From Calabrese LH, Duna GF, Lie JT. Vasculitis in the central nervous system. Arthritis Rheum 1997;40:1189-201.

TAKAYASU'S ARTERITIS

CASE STUDY 2

A 33-year-old woman presented with slurred speech and left upper extremity weakness for 10 to 15 minutes. These symptoms resolved but recurred 2 weeks later. She was evaluated by a neurologist who obtained an MRI of her brain that was unremarkable. However, he also heard a bruit at the right common carotid artery and ordered a cerebral angiogram. This study documented an aneurysm in the right brachiocephalic artery and a near-occlusion of the right internal carotid artery, as well as a near-occlusion of the right vertebral artery. She was referred to rheumatology for further evaluation.

Introductory Comments

An uncommon disease, Takayasu's Arteritis (TA) or "pulseless disease" is named for a Japanese ophthalmologist who reported the case of a 21-year-old woman with sudden visual loss and a vascular anomaly about the optic disc.[26]

TA is an inflammatory vascular disease that generally affects the aorta, its main branches, and the pulmonary arteries. It results in a granulomatous panarteritis of the aorta and its major branches. TA is historically associated with young Asian women. This is probably a reflection of Takayasu's report emanating from Asia. However, we know there were many preceding reports of an unnamed condition involving the larger vessels in younger women worldwide characterized by aneurysms and stenoses.

TA affects all ethnic groups and is found worldwide, although it does affect women more than men. TA shares many clinical features with giant cell arteritis (GCA) with its predilection for large vessel vascular trees. An inciting event in a susceptible host initiates an inflammatory process in the vessel wall with resultant damage that progresses to a final stage with either stenosis or aneurysmal dilatation.

The initial systemic phase of the disease is often accompanied by malaise, fatigue, fever (including FUO), night sweats, weight loss, and arthalgias/myalgias although these systemic features may be absent and the patient seemingly starts the disease with vascular inflammation in isolation. Relapse is common, even with treatment. In one large series, 45% of patients studied experienced at least one disease relapse and a full 23% never achieved a remission. TA has the potential for significant morbidity.[27]

Definitions and Clinical Subsets

Table 17-6 provides the American College of Rheumatology (ACR) Classification Criteria for TA. Of particular note, the 1990 criteria set an age of

Table 17-6. *1990 Criteria for the Classification of Takayasu's Arteritis**

1. Age at disease onset < 40 years
   Development of symptoms or findings related to Takayasu arteritis at age 40 years
2. Claudication of extremities
   Development and worsening of fatigue and discomfort in muscles of 1 or more extremity while in use, especially the upper extremities
3. Decreased brachial artery pulse
   Decreased pulsation of 1 or both brachial arteries
4. BP difference > 10 mm Hg
   Difference of > 10 mm Hg in systolic blood pressure between arms
5. Bruit over subclavian arteries or aorta
   Bruit audible on auscultation over 1 or both subclavian arteries or abdominal aorta
6. Arteriogram abnormality
   Arteriographic narrowing or occlusion of the entire aorta, its primary branches, or large arteries in the proximal upper or lower extremities, not due to arteriosclerosis, fibromuscular dysplasia, or similar causes; changes usually focal or segmental

* For purposes of classification, a patient shall be said to have Takayasu's arteritis if at least three of these six criteria are present. The presence of any three or more criteria yields a sensitivity of 90.5% and a specificity of 97.8%.
BP, blood pressure (systolic; difference between arms).
From Arend WP, Michel BA, Bloch DA, Hunder GG, Calabrese LH, Edworthy SM, et al. The American College of Rheumatology 1990 criteria for the classification of Takayasu's arteritis. Arthritis Rheum 1990;33:1129-34.

onset younger than 40 years. In reality, the age of the population at risk does not always fit this cut-off. Some patients do develop this disease after the age of 40 years, and it should always be considered in the differential diagnosis of a large vessel vasculitis. This is especially true when approaching a patient with an FUO. A patient with early, nonocclusive vascular inflammation may also fail to meet criteria until the disease progresses to a symptomatic stage.

Differential Diagnosis and Diagnostic Criteria

Figure 17-1 offers a graphic depiction of how vessel size correlates with the various forms of vasculitis. There are several rheumatologic diseases that can affect the aorta but these conditions are not usually confused with TA by virtue of their associated signs and symptoms. One rheumatologic disease, GCA, deserves special comment. Because TA often first presents after the age of 40 years, there is an overlap in the clinical features of TA and GCA. Clues to differentiating between these two forms of vasculitis include the following features:
1. TA more frequently has involvement of the aortic branches than does GCA.
2. TA has a far greater female preponderance than does GCA.
3. TA may have pulmonary vessel involvement, whereas GCA usually does not.

Diagnostic Evaluation

Symptoms and Signs
A large cohort of patients with TA collected internationally documented that there is a clear predilection for upper extremity arterial involvement as compared to lower extremity involvement. However, lower extremity or even visceral vessel involvement may be seen in almost one half of patients who have TA.[28] The aorta and left subclavian artery are the most frequently affected vessels. Other arterial vessels commonly affected include the carotid and renal.[27]

Disease-associated morbidity may include hypertension, aortic valvular disease resulting in aortic insufficiency, myocardial infarction, aneurysmal rupture, heart failure, visual disturbances,

Figure 17-1. Depiction of how vessel size correlates with the various forms of vasculitis.

CLASSIFICATION OF THE VASCULITIDES

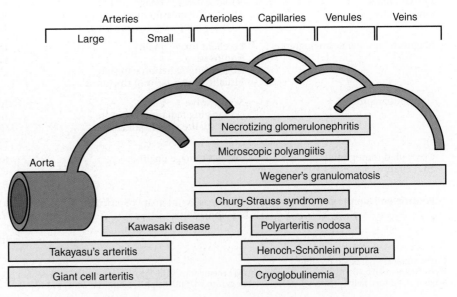

cerebrovascular disease, diminished pulses or discordant upper extremity blood pressure measurement, bruits, carotidynia, and vascular claudication.[27] Coronary heart disease may occur with both coronary aneurysms as well as stenosis.[29] Involvement of the pulmonary arteries can result in hemoptysis, chest pain, cough, and dsypnea. Obviously, the affected vessel or vessels will dictate the individual patient's signs and symptoms.

Fatigue, malaise, fever, arthralgias, myalgias, night sweats, and weight loss may accompany the vascular inflammation phase of disease. These nonspecific features might not even suggest TA to the uninitiated, especially if they occur prior to a more classic "vascular insufficiency" period of symptoms such as claudication. In the absence of claudication or a vascular event, the diagnosis may remain elusive for years because TA is not often considered in the differential diagnosis of such nonspecific symptoms. One important lesson is that TA should always be considered in the FUO patient's diagnostic evaluation. TA is a diagnosis that often follows years of low-grade vascular inflammation. Only the astute clinician's consideration of this diagnosis will initiate the sequence of events that results in its proper diagnosis.

Absent or discordant pulses should raise the specter of TA (as well as GCA and Buerger's disease). Attention on physical examination then should be directed to searching for discordant pulses or blood pressure readings, vascular tenderness, or bruits. Skin involvement, albeit rare, does occur in TA as both nodular and ulcerative lesions. Myocarditis is also an unusual presenting manifestation. Erythema nodosum can rarely be a presenting feature.

Laboratory Evaluation

The usual but nonspecific laboratory findings seen in many inflammatory disorders are seen in TA as well. Elevation of the ESR and C-reactive protein (CRP), an anemia of chronic inflammation, a polyclonal gammopathy, leukocytosis, and thrombocytosis may be evident. There is no specific diagnostic laboratory test for TA. Autoantibodies are typically absent, and complement levels are normal. On occasion, the entire laboratory evaluation for a patient with active TA is completely *normal*. It remains difficult to accurately gauge disease activity in TA simply by laboratory measure. Cohort series of patients with established TA have shown that the ESR is not an accurate reflector of disease activity. Biopsy material from large vessels may very well show active vasculitis in the setting of a normal ESR.[27]

Imaging Studies

The advent of advanced, noninvasive vascular imaging has opened a new window on TA diagnosis and management. Different imaging modalities provide different types of information. Diagnosis is made earlier and modalities to follow disease response or progression are now widely available, although none is without its limitations. Contrast angiography, MR angiography, CT angiography, and high-resolution Doppler ultrasound all play roles in diagnosis and management. Positron emission tomography (PET) is starting to play a role as well. Table 17-7 provides a comparison of these various imaging techniques in TA, with both advantages and disadvantages listed. Importantly, MRA does not produce ionizing radiation.

Table 17-7. *Comparison of Imaging Techniques in Takayasu's Arteritis*

Technique	Advantages	Disadvantages
Conventional angiography	"Gold standard" image quality Allows CAP measurement Allows angioplasty at same time	Invasive Radiation exposure Does not visualize vessel wall thickness
Magnectic resonance angiography	Excellent image quality Noninvasive No ionizing radiation exposure Visualizes vascular wall thickness	Image quality not "gold standard" Cannot use in patients with pacemaker CAP measurement not posssible
Ultrasonography	Noninvasive No ionizing radiation exposure Can visualize vessel wall edema	Image quality not "gold standard" Image quality affected by obesity Operator dependent CAP measurement not possible
Computed tomography angiography	Excellent image quality	Ionizing radiation exposure CAP measurement not possible Intravenous contrast agent required
Positron emission tomography	Can measure intensity of vascular inflammation	Ionizing radiation exposure Vascular anatomy not well seen CAP measurement not possible Intravenous contrast agent required

CAP, Central arterial blood pressure.
From Hellman DH. Giant cell arteritis, polymyalgia rheumatica, and Takayasu's arteritis. In: Firestein GS, Budd RC, Harris ED Jr, McInnes IB, Ruddy S, Sergent JS, editors. Kelly's Textbook of Rheumatology, 8th ed. Philadelphia: Saunders; 2008; p. 1409-28.

Vascular wall thickening can be visualized with MRA even before the development of stenoses or aneurysms. These modalities may suggest early, endovascular inflammation. MRA with "edema weighting" can show vessel wall edema, although the positive predictive value of seeing such edema is uncertain. Edema may be an early sign in inflammation, or it may be a feature of post-inflammatory vascular remodeling. Some patients with obvious edema do not progress to vascular stenosis in the absence of treatment. Regardless, MRA with its ability to image large portions of the great vessels and its capacity to better define the vascular wall is a major tool in diagnosis and monitoring of the vascular tree.[30]

Doppler ultrasound imaging is still being evaluated for applicability in monitoring TA. Its use is probably optimal in the common carotid artery and vertebral arteries, but it is of limited applicability in defining flow in the proximal subclavian and distal internal carotid arteries.

Vascular luminal anatomy and mapping can be obtained with conventional contrast angiography and also offer the advantage of central pressure monitoring and coronary artery imaging. Angiography defines luminal irregularities and has the ability to map occlusions, aneurysms, and stenoses in the vascular tree and is still considered the gold standard for investigating TA. It is, of course, invasive and is unable to ascribe a finding of stenosis to active inflammation versus scarring and fibrosis. Lesions frequently are located at the origin of the primary branches of the aorta. Luminal narrowing or irregularity may proceed to stenoses or aneurysms, and often one sees a characteristic mix of stenoses and aneurysms alternating with segments of normal vessel. Contrast angiography is often obtained when surgical intervention is planned. Its disadvantage is its invasive nature and difficulty in using the same modality over time to monitor disease activity.

The consultant rheumatologist is all too often left in the uncomfortable position of trying to discern just where the patient is along the spectrum from reversible inflammation at one pole through to irreversible scarring at the other extreme. Although we are in a better position to "know the anatomy" of TA we are still far too often hampered by not knowing whether the anatomic abnormality visualized is caused by active or past inflammation.

New, noninvasive imaging studies might hold promise for TA disease diagnosis and monitoring if it can identify intravascular inflammation and differentiate active vasculitis from post-inflammatory changes. 18F-FDG PET has shown some promise in evaluating TA patients when coregistered with enhanced CT scanning. This interesting imaging modality was found in a study of 14 TA patients (11 in the active, inflammatory stage and three in the inactive stage) to have a sensitivity of 91% and specificity of 89%. This technique nicely showed aorta, aortic branches, and pulmonary artery inflammation. 18-FDG-PET is expensive, results in significant radiation exposure, and is often limited in both availability and access. In an older patient, it can be difficult to differentiate vascular inflammation from TA from that of atherosclerosis.[31,32]

Pathologic Evaluation

TA is characterized by adventitial thickening and cellular infiltration of the tunica media along with destruction of elastin and vascular smooth muscle. Myofibroblast proliferation results in intimal hyperplasia which is then followed by fibrosis of the tunica media and intima with eventual stenosis. Aneurysm formation ensues when local destruction of the media predominates.

On occasion, the diagnostic possibility of TA is only first entertained when a pathologic specimen from a large vessel is interpreted by the pathologist as showing granulomatous inflammation. A vessel may be biopsied during a "routine" vascular revascularization procedure for claudication and the pathologic finding returns as a surprise to both the pathologist and surgeon. Asymptomatic inflammation in the vessel wall may be followed by stenosis or aneurysms.[27] One series that reviewed 1204 aortic surgical specimens accrued over 20 years at one institution found unexpected aortitis in 52 of the patients, whereas only one of the 52 had features of a systemic illness at the time of surgery. Sixteen of the 52 had had a history of vasculitis or other systemic disease that was not believed to be active at the time of surgery. New aneurysms were noted in six of 25 patients who were not treated with glucocorticoids followed for 41 months and in zero of 11 patients who were treated with glucocorticoids and followed for 35.5 months. One could argue then that the pathologic finding of an unexpected vasculitis does not necessarily warrant immunosuppression, although it certainly warrants careful and continued observation.

Diagnostic Evaluation and Management Summary

The difficult truth in caring for a patient with TA is that there is no single test that consistently and accurately reflects disease activity. Up to one third of those with clinically active disease had a normal ESR in one series, and conversely, a little more than half of the patients with TA had an elevated ESR in the setting of disease quiescence.[27]

Many TA patients are essentially asymptomatic at diagnosis, with an incidental bruit on physical examination leading to a revealing evaluation of the larger vascular tree involvement. The ESR may be normal in the face of active vasculitis, luminal irregularity on contrast angiography might represent vasculitis or post-inflammatory scarring, systemic symptoms may be absent in the setting of active vasculitis, and new vascular ischemic deficits might be the result of progressive vascular occlusion from scarring and not from a reversible vasculitis. Not all vascular insufficiency symptoms are due to active inflammation. All of a clinician's diagnostic skills are taxed in diagnosing and caring for a TA patient.

Treatment

TA disease treatment is largely empiric, with no controlled trials performed that definitively answer the question of best therapy. Treatment choices have to be predicated on the assumption that TA is a chronic disease and one that can be expected to have periods of both activity and quiescence. Therefore, the treatment should be tailored to disease activity. Treatment may be directed at some point in time to addressing inflammation and at other times to addressing fixed vascular lesions. It is important to keep in mind that the treatment of TA is one that will necessarily change as the disease evolves. Almost all responses to therapy is temporary, and relapse is, unfortunately, an expected development.

Attention must be given to blood pressure control and the possibility of evolving renovascular disease. Bilateral blood pressure measurement should be a standard of care in examining TA patients so as to identify evolving subclavian lesions. Listening for bruits and pulse checks at each visit is part of the standard of care for the TA population.

Treatment of hypertension with an angiotensin converting enzyme inhibitor or an angiotensin II receptor antagonist is preferred in light of the increased risk for renovascular hypertension in TA. Caution in initiating these agents must be applied to first ensure that there is not bilateral renal artery stenosis.

Increased attention to cardiovascular risk reduction is also important with the recognition of accelerated atherogenesis, which seems intrinsic to all inflammatory disorders. Discontinuation of smoking is paramount. Lipid reduction should be addressed as well, and the pleiotropic effects of statins to modulate endovascular function makes them an attractive cotreatment in TA. Finally, many have a low threshold for instituting low-dose aspirin as an adjunctive cardiovascular protective therapy.

Glucocorticoids

Glucocorticoids have always been and still are a mainstay of treatment for TA. Active disease should be treated with 0.5 to 1.0 mg/kg per day of prednisone. The correct dose and time course of treatment is rather empiric as there are a lack of comparative studies evaluating different treatment regimens in TA. Regardless, features of TA that might warrant high-dose prednisone would include fever, elevation of acute phase reactants, acute vascular claudication symptoms, critical organ ischemia, and typical angiographic lesions. Remission can be induced in more than half of patients treated with corticosteroids. Treatment is given for 4 to 12 weeks before

a slow taper is instituted. Unfortunately, many do relapse.[27] A pragmatic initial approach to a new patient with TA might include using glucocorticoids in the acute setting until a response is noted or additional imaging reveals a fixed lesion that appears unresponsive to immunosuppressive therapy. Most patients with TA seem to need 5 to 10 mg/day of prednisone chronically to prevent a flare.

Additional immunosuppressive therapy is employed when a steroid taper results in disease flare or when one is unable to lower the steroid to a "tolerable" dose. No one agent has been shown, to date, to have superiority over another for treating TA. The choice of additional therapy following corticosteroids or concomitant with corticosteroids must be individualized and take into consideration comorbidities, patient preference, and physician comfort with the individual agents.

Methotrexate

Methotexate (MTX) is often used to supplement or even to try and supplant corticosteroids. One treatment study in TA started patients on MTX orally at 0.3 mg/kg (not to exceed 15 mg) weekly and increased the dose every 1 to 2 weeks to a maximal 25 mg weekly in conjunction with prednisone at a standard dose of 1 mg/kg/day. The prednisone was then tapered after the first month to an every other day dosing plan after 3 to 6 months. If the disease appeared to be controlled after 6 months of MTX, then the MTX was continued for another 6 months while a further prednisone taper was offered. After the prednisone was weaned, the MTX was finally tapered. This regimen resulted in an 81% remission rate at 1 year in the 16 patients treated, and 25% of these patients went on to a medication free remission of up to 1 year. Unfortunately, as is all too common with TA, the remissions did not hold and more than half had a relapse. Fortunately, half of these patients saw "disease capture" and a second remission when treated with the same regimen.[33] MTX, to many rheumatologists, is the preferred agent for combined initial therapy with corticosteroids in the treatment of TA and has taken on the role as the first choice therapy in combination with corticosteroids.

Cyclophosphamide

Cyclophosphamide use in TA is less well studied in TA than its use in other forms of systemic vasculitis. Its use was more popular before the widespread application of MTX, and much of our understanding of its use in TA is modeled on its use in Wegener's granulomatosis. Its attendant side effects have also lessened enthusiasm for its use. Regardless, cyclophosphamide is still prescribed for life-threatening disease or after a failure of corticosteroids/MTX to control disease activity. A small series of patients were treated with cyclophosphamide at 2 mg/kg/day, and it was continued for 1 year following remission before tapering off, a regimen similar to that used in Wegener's granulomatosis. The group given cyclophosphamide all had active disease despite three months of glucocorticoid therapy and all seven treated responded as measured by ability to lower the corticosteroid dose. Vascular lesion progression was halted in four.[34] If cyclophosphamide is used, it is now given usually for only 3 to 6 months before transitioning to MTX or azathioprine (AZA). Some favor an initial intravenous pulse of cyclophosphamide (750 mg/m[2]), followed by a second infusion 2 weeks later and then monthly for 6 months.[35] Most would favor using MTX in conjunction with prednisone first and reach for cyclophosphamide only if the MTX/prednisone combination proves ineffective or is not tolerated or if the MTX did not allow for prednisone weaning.

Azathioprine and Mycophenolate Mofetil

AZA and mycophenolate mofetil (MMF) have been used for patients with TA, but the published data on their efficacy is still somewhat scanty. AZA was employed in a study of 15 patients with TA in conjunction with prednisone. AZA (2 mg/kg/day) was given with prednisolone at 1 mg/kg/day in newly diagnosed patients with TA, and the prednisolone was then tapered to 5 to 10 mg per day over 12 weeks if there was a positive clinical response. A slower taper was used if disease activity continued. Prednisolone was continued for 1 year at a maintenance dose of 5 to 10 mg per day. All responded well, and all had angiograms at 1 year that showed no new lesions. AZA can certainly be considered a viable alternative then to MTX in the treatment of TA.[36] A report of three patients treated with MMF at 2 g/day suggested efficacy and allowed tapering of corticosteroids to a very low level, in one case to complete removal. Two of the three patients had previous treatment with several immunosuppressive regimens, and the third had only been treated with corticosteroids.[37] Although there is limited experience with AZA and MMF use in TA, they both may well play a role as steroid-sparing agents.

Tumor Necrosis Factor Inhibitors

Tumor necrosis factor (TNF) inhibitors have been studied now in TA as well. Because TA is a granulomatous vasculitis and TNF-α plays a central role in granuloma formation, it makes intuitive sense that a TNF inhibitor might offer disease control. A pilot study of 15 patients with relapsing TA demonstrated improvement in 14 who were treated with either etanercept or infliximab, and 10 patients saw a prolonged and complete remission that lasted from 1 to 3.3 years in the absence of corticosteroids.[38] A follow-up study with additional patients from the same center (Cleveland Clinic) also showed an ability to lower the corticosteroid dose in refractory TA patients following initiation of infliximab or etanercept. Twenty patients were treated with infliximab, nine were treated with etanercept, and four patients received both. Before starting the TNF inhibitor, all of the patients were unable to achieve remission despite corticosteroids and additional

immunosuppressive drugs.[39,40] Clearly, TNF inhibition is a promising avenue of therapy in TA and well worth considering in the individual patient. They would appear to offer remission or at least significant improvement in disease management. Stopping the TNF inhibitor did result in disease recurrence, not surprisingly. The disappointing results in other granulomatous vasculitis disease states treated with anti-TNF therapies does raise caution in too readily embracing this therapy.

A recent case report raises some very intriguing possibilities for additional biologic therapy of TA. Interleukin-6 (IL-6) expression is increased in the aortic tissue of patients with TA, and tocilizumab is a humanized IL-6 receptor antibody. A 20-year-old woman with refractory active TA complicated by ulcerative colitis received treatment with tocilizumab. Both the TA and the ulcerative colitis improved, and the patient was able to wean her previously high-dose corticosteroid regimen to 7.5 mg/day of prednisolone.[41]

Abatacept, a CTLA4-Ig antibody approved for use in rheumatoid arthritis, which acts as a T-cell costimulator inhibitor, is to be evaluated in an National Institutes of Health (NIH) study as a treatment for both GCA and TA. Enrollment for this study has yet to begin.

Surgical Treatment

TA often requires surgical intervention, usually to address fixed, stenotic lesions or aneurysms. Hemodynamically significant lesions may necessitate revascularization. Cervicocranial occlusions with the incipient risk for a cerebrovascular accident, coronary artery disease, aortic regurgitation, coarctation of the aorta, limb-threatening claudication, renal artery stenosis, or progressive aneurismal dilatation may all need intervention. The diagnosis of TA is often first made only when the patient has progressed to the point of a vascular occlusion or aneurysm necessitating repair.

Modern revascularization procedures, which include percutaneous transluminal angioplasty and bypass grafting, have benefited many patients with TA. A vascular surgeon experienced in the care of TA patients is integral to optimal care, as is a vascular radiologist. Timing of vascular procedures is critical, because revascularization during periods of active vasculitis will result in poorer results.[42] Not every stenosis requires a procedure because collateralization is expected over time. Immediate revascularization should be considered if a stenosis is causing significant symptoms or vascular flow compromise or a dissection seems imminent.

Angioplasty and vascular stenting were initially thought to be very promising treatments for the vascular occlusions induced by TA. Unfortunately, the NIH cohort of TA patients who underwent angioplasty did not demonstrate significant long-term benefit. The initial success rate was only 56%, and almost half had subsequent restenosis, aneurysm formation, or other complication.[27] A cohort of patients who underwent the angioplasty procedures at the Cleveland Clinic, half of whom had stents employed, showed a very high restenosis rate.[28] Although angioplasty can open an occluded vessel and provide immediate improvement to an ischemic region, the long-term benefit from these procedures is less than clear. Stents impregnated with immunosuppressive or antiproliferative medications to abrogate restenosis have not been studied in large series of patients with TA.

Arterial bypass and reconstruction probably provides better long-term vessel patency than angioplasty or stenting, but it, too, suffers from a high restenosis rate, usually in the range of 20% to 30%. Anastomotic aneurysms are a potential risk.[44] Similar restenosis rates were reported after long-term follow-up in the NIH series (50 bypass procedures were performed in 23 patients). Interestingly, there was a lesser restenosis rate in those who received autologous grafts.[27]

Timing is critical in any procedure. Active disease is probably best treated medically, and surgical results are better when inflammation is controlled. The difficulty is in knowing just where a patient is in the phase of TA activity: the inflammatory phase versus the scarring phase.

Prognosis

Although TA can be self-limited or even have a uniphasic course with resolution after one course of treatment, this is the exception. Most patients with TA have a propensity to recurring exacerbations and to accrue new lesions over time.[27,28] Disability is very common among those affected by TA. The NIH cohort showed some form of functional disability in 74% of those diagnosed, with 47% fully disabled.[27] Large series of patients with TA and long periods of follow-up are few so that the true natural history of this disease is not entirely clear.

The overall survival rate in two North American series of patients was promising. A Mayo Clinic series of 32 patients followed over a 13-year period had a survival rate of 94%.[44] An NIH cohort of 60 patients had two deaths during their study period. One of these two committed suicide, and one died suddenly after 9 years of disease while the disease was in remission.[27] Mortality data would suggest that heart failure is the leading cause of death from TA.[45,46]

Summary

TA is a large vessel vasculitis of uncertain etiology that results in a chronic disease, marked by periods of activity and quiescence, with a progressive toll in morbidity and disability. Close cooperative care with a vascular surgeon and radiologist who understand the nuances of TA is essential to optimizing outcome and management. Disease activity is not reflected well by standard laboratory tests, so clinical assessment based on history, physical examination, and imaging plays an even larger role in patient management.

Case Presentation Follow-Up

Our patient presented with a very abnormal angiogram report. On further questioning, she did note right upper extremity pain with exertion or even when walking briskly. She would experience almost immediate relief when she stopped the activity or stopped walking. A thorough physical examination revealed a blood pressure of 136/83 in the left arm and 120/70 in the right arm, and a diminished radial pulse on the right. Bruits were heard over both carotid regions and both subclavian regions. Screening laboratories returned with an ESR of 27 mm/h, a normal CRP, and a negative ANA test.

An MRA showed ascending aorta dilatation, intimal thickening, a right brachiocephalic aneurysm, significant stenosis of the proximal left common carotid artery, right subclavian stenosis, and irregularity of the distal vertebral arteries bilaterally. The right vertebral artery, previously described as occluded, was now apparently patent. A diagnosis of Takayasu's arteritis was made. The patient was started on prednisone at 1 mg/kg/day and methotrexate at 15 mg po weekly, along with 1 mg/day of folic acid. The initial plan was to repeat the MRA in 6 weeks and assess for any response in her occlusions.

References

1. Cravioto M, Feigin I. Non-infectious granulomatous angiitis with a predilection for the central nervous system. Neurology 1959;9:599-609.
2. Calabrese LH, Mallek JA. Primary angiitis of the central nervous system: Report of eight new cases, review of the literature and proposal for diagnostic criteria. Medicine (Baltimore) 1988;67:20.
3. Duna G, Calabrese L. Limitations in the diagnostic modalities in the diagnosis of primary angiitis of the central nervous system (PACNS). J Rheumatol 1995;22:662-7.
4. Younger DS, Calabrese LH, Hays AP. Granulomatous angiitis of the nervous system. Neurol Clin 1997;15:821.
5. Woolfenden AR, Tong DC, Marks MP, Ali AO, Albers GW. Angiographically defined primary angiitis of the CNS. Is it really benign? Neurology 1998;51:183-8.
6. Salvarani C, Brown RD, Calamia KT, Christianson TJH, et al. Primary central nervous system vasculitis: analysis of 101 patients. Ann Neurol 2007;62:442-51.
7. Calabrese LH, Dodick DW, Schwedt TJ, Singhal AB. Narrative review: Reversible cerebral vasoconstriction syndromes. Ann Intern Med 2007;146:34-45.
8. Calabrese L, Gragg LA, Furlan AJ: Benign angiopathy: A distinct subset of angiographically defined primary angiitis of the central nervous system. J Rheumatol 1993;20:2046.
9. MacKenzie RA, Forbes GS, Karnes WE. Angiographic findings in herpes zoster arteritis. Ann Neurol 1981;10:458.

10. Calabrese LH, Furlan AJ, Gragg LA, Ropos TJ. Primary angiitis of the central nervous system: Diagnostic criteria and clinical approach. Cleve Clin J Med 1992;59:293-306.

11. Duna GF, George T, Rybicki L, Calabrese LH. Primary angiitis of the central nervous system: an analysis of unusual presentations (abstract). Arthritis Rheum 1995;38(Suppl. 9):S340.

12. Ducros A, Boubobza M, Porcher R, Sarov M, Valade D, Boussser MG. The clinical and radiological spectrum of reversible cerebral vasoconstriction syndrome. A prospective series of 67 patients. Brain 2007;130:3091-101.

13. Chu C, Gray L, Goldstein L, Hulette CM. Diagnosis of intracranial vasculitis: A multidisciplinary approach. J Neuropathol Exp Neurol 1998;57:30-8.

14. Vanderzant C, Bomberg M, MacGuire A, McCune J. Isolated small-vessel angiitis of the central nervous system. Arch Neurol 1988;45:683-7.

15. Moore PM. Vasculitis of the central nervous system. Semin Neurol 1994;14:307-12.

16. Moore P. Diagnosis and management of isolated angiitis of the central nervous system. Neurology 1989;39:167-73.

17. Whitely RJ, Cobbs G, Alford CA. Diseases that mimic herpes simplex encephalitis: diagnosis, presentation, outcome. JAMA 1989;262:234-9.

18. Sigal LH. The neurologic presentation of vasculitic and rheumatologic syndromes: a review. Medicine 1987;66:157-80.

19. Calabrese LH, Duna GF, Lie JT. Vasculitis in the central nervous system. Arthritis Rheum 1997;40:1189-201.

20. Calabrese LH, Mallek JA: Primary angiitis of the central nervous system: report of eight new cases, review of the literature and proposal for diagnostic criteria. Medicine (Baltimore) 1988;67:20.

21. Cupps TR, Moore PM, Fauci AS: Isolated angiitis of the central nervous system. Am J Med 1983;74:97.

22. Calbrese LH: Vasculitis of the central nervous system. Rheum Dis Clin North Am 1995;21:1059.

23. Calabrese LH, Duna GT: Drug induced vasculitis. Curr Opin Rheumatol 1996;8:34.

24. Salvarani C, Brown RD, Calamia KT, Christianson TJH, Weigand SD, Miller DV, et al. Primary central nervous system vasculitis: analysis of 101 patients. Ann Neurol 2007;62:442-51.

25. Hajj-Ali RA, Furlan A, Abou-Chebel A, Calabrese LH. Benign angiopathy of the central nervous system: cohort of 16 patients with clinical course and long-term followup. Arthritis Care Res 2002;47:662-9.

26. Takayasu M. A case with peculiar changes of the retinal central vessels. Acta Societatis Ophthalmological Japonicae 1908;12:554-5.

27. Kerr GS, Hallahan CW, Giordano J, Leavitt RY, Fauci AS, Rottem M, et al. Takayasu's arteritis. Ann Intern Med 1994;120:919.

28. Maksimowicz-McKinnon K, Clark TM, Hoffman GS. Limitations of therapy and a guarded prognosis in an American cohort of Takayasu arteritis patients. Arthritis Rheum 2007;56:1000-9.

29. Endo M, Tomizawa Y, Nishida H, Aomi S, Nakazawa M, Tsurumi Y, et al. Angiographic findings and surgical treatment of coronary artery involvement in Takayasu arteritis. J Thorac Cardiovasc Surg 2003;125:570.

30. Tso E, Flamm SD, White RD, Schvartzman PR, Mascha E, Hoffma GS. Takayasu arteritis: Utility and limitations of magnetic resonance imaging in diagnosis and treatment. Arthritis Rheum 2002;46:1634-42.

31. Blockmans D, Stroobants S, Maes A, Mortelmans L. Positron emission tomography in giant cell arteritiis and polymyalgia rheumatica: evidence for inflammation of the aortic arch. Am J Med 2000;108:246-9.

32. Kobayashi Y, Ishii K, Oda K, Nariai T, Tanaka Y, Ishiwata K, et al. Aortic wall inflammation due to Takayasu arteritis imaged with 18F-FDG PET coregistered with enhanced CT. J Nucl Med 2005;46:917-22.

33. Hoffman GS, Leavitt RY, Kerr GS, Rottem M, Sneller MC, Fauci AS. Treatment of glucocorticoid-resistant or relapsing Takayasu's arteritis with methotrexate. Arthritis Rheum 1994;37:578.

34. Shelhamer JH, Volkman DJ, Parillo JE, Lawley TJ, Johnston MR, Fauci AS. Takayasu's arteritis and its therapy. Ann Intern Med 1985;103:121.

35. Andrews J, Mason JC. Takayasu's arteritis - recent advances in imaging offer promise. Rheumatology 2007;46:6-15.

36. Valsakumar AK, Valappil UC, Jorapur V, Garg N, Nityanand S, Sinha N. Role of immunosuppressive therapy on clinical, immunological, and angiographic outcome in active Takayasu's arteritis. J Rheumatol 2003;30:1793-8.

37. Daina E, Schieppati A, Remuzzi G. Mycophenolate mofetil for the treatment of Takayasu arteritis: report of three cases. Ann Intern Med 1999;130:422-6.

38. Hoffman GS, Merkel PA, Brasington RD, Lenschow DJ, Liang P. Anti-tumor necrosis factor therapy in patients with difficult to treat Takayasu arteritis. Arthritis Rheum 2004;50:2296-304.

39. Molloy ES, Langford CA, Clark TM. Durable remission in patients with refractory Takayasu's arteritis treated with infliximab and etanercept. Arthritis Rheum 2006;54:4093.

40. Molloy ES, Langford CA, Clark TM, Gota CE, Hoffman GS. Anti-tumour necrosis factor therapy in patients with refractory Takayasu arteritis: Long term follow-up. Ann Rheum Dis 2008;67:1567-9.

41. Nishimoto N, Nakahara H, Yoshio-Hoshino N, Mima T. Successful treatment of a patient with Takayasu arteritis using a humanized anti-interleukin-6 receptor antibody. Arthritis Rheum 2008;58:1197-200.

42. Fields C, Bower T, Cooper L, Hoskin T, Noel AA, Panneton JM, et al. Takayasu's arteritis: operative results and the influence of disease activitiy. J Vasc Surg 2006;43:64-71.

43. Miyata T, Sato O, Koyama H, Shigematsu H, Tada Y. Long-term survival after surgical treatment of patients with Takayasu's arteritis. Circulation 2003;108:1474-80.

44. Hall S, Barr W, Lie JT, Stanson AW, Kazmier FJ, Hunder GG. Takayasu's arteritis: a study of 32 North American patients. Medicine 1985;64:89.

45. Lupi-Herrera E, Sanchez-Torres G, Marcushamer J, Mispireta J, Horwitz S, Vela JE. Takayasu's arteritis: clinical study of 107 cases. Am Heart J 1977;93:94-103.

46. Subramanyan R, Joy J, Balakrishnan K. Natural history of aortoarteritis (Takayasu's disease). Circulation 1989;80:429-37.

Chapter 18

Management of Sarcoidosis, Behçet's Disease, and Other Rare Rheumatic Diseases

Karla L. Miller and Grant W. Cannon

SARCOIDOSIS

Introduction

Sarcoidosis is a multisystem inflammatory disease of uncertain etiology associated with the accumulation of noncaseating granulomas in clinically involved tissues and, occasionally, in asymptomatic tissues.[1,2] This disease has been reported worldwide in all sexes, ages, and ethnic groups, and the disease manifestations have been widely depicted in the literature since it was initially described in 1877.

Epidemiology

The incidence of sarcoidosis varies considerably worldwide, with the highest annual incidence reported in patients of northern European and African-American ancestry.[3,4] It typically develops before the age of 50 years, and incidence peaks between the ages of 20 to 39.[4] Females are affected more commonly than males worldwide.

Possible Etiologies

The precise etiology and pathogenesis of sarcoidosis is still unknown, although our knowledge of immunopathogenic mechanisms has advanced in the last decade. Current evidence would suggest that there is not a single etiology for this condition and that there are multiple causes of sarcoidosis accounting for the variety of clinical features that characterize the disease.[2] A variety of agents have been implicated as the inciting antigen in sarcoidosis. Environmental and occupational exposures such as inorganic particles, mold, insecticides, pollens, metalworking, and firefighting have been reported in association with sarcoidosis.[5-7] Both mycobacterial and propionibacterial DNA and RNA have been detected by polymerase chain reaction (PCR) techniques in lymph nodes affected by sarcoidosis, although no causal relationship has been established.[8] The variety in reported environmental triggers suggests that sarcoidosis may be the result of exaggerated immune responses to more than one antigen.

Genetic Features

Genetic contributions to the development of sarcoidosis have been suspected on the basis of several reports of multiple family members being affected with the disease.[9-11] Both human leukocyte antigen (HLA) class I and II antigens have been associated with risk of developing sarcoidosis in various studies, including HLA-A1, B8, and DR3 in whites. Some haplotypes appear to predispose to a specific clinical presentation, disease chronicity, or disease severity. For example, HLA-DR3 and DQ2 are associated with an acute Lofgren's presentation and a good prognosis, but HLA-B5 appears to be associated with chronic disease.[12] Other genes have been implicated in sarcoidosis susceptibility via genome wide linkage and association studies, such as butyrophilin-like 2 gene and annexin A11.[13] Based on the available genetic data and the variability in clinical manifestations, it is doubtful that a single gene defect alone is the cause of sarcoidosis.

Pathogenesis

Sarcoidosis is characterized histologically by the formation of noncaseating epithelioid granulomas. Sarcoid granulomas are dense collections of macrophages and epithelioid cells encircled by lymphocytes, and later by fibroblasts and collagen. Granulomas generally serve to protect the surrounding tissue by confining the inciting pathogen or trigger, thereby containing the inflammatory response. Granuloma formation involves a series of steps, of which the hallmark is the activation of antigen-specific T helper 1 (Th1) lymphocytes via interaction of naïve CD4+ T cells with antigen-presenting cells bearing HLA class II molecules.[14,15] These Th1 cells secrete the cytokines interleukin-2 (IL-2) and interferon-γ (IFN-γ). Further proliferation and differentiation of T lymphocytes is stimulated by IL-2, in addition to IL-15 and tumor necrosis factor-α (TNF-α) released from macrophages. IFN-γ amplifies the local cellular immune response and is essential to granuloma formation. TNF-α appears to play an important role in perpetuation of the inflammatory response and maintenance of granulomas.

Most sarcoidal granulomas resolve spontaneously, but some persist or lead to fibrosis. It is still unclear what determines the eventual outcome of the granulomas in sarcoidosis, but a shift to cytokines produced by Th2 lymphocytes (IL-4, IL-10, and IL-13) may be key to the development of fibrosis in some patients.[14,15]

Clinical Manifestations and Diagnosis

Sarcoidosis involves the lung most frequently, but up to 30% of patients develop extrapulmonary manifestations.[16] Constitutional symptoms such as fatigue, malaise, fever, and anorexia may also be present, particularly in the elderly.[17] Abnormalities due to sarcoidosis can be seen in any organ, but most clinical disease involves hilar lymphadenopathy, pulmonary disease, skin or eye manifestations, or a combination of these findings.

Pulmonary

Respiratory involvement occurs in 95% of patients, and ranges in presentation from asymptomatic hilar lymphadenopathy to interstitial lung disease with alveolitis.[18] Endobronchial involvement exists in 40% to 70% of patients and is more common in the later stages. These lesions can progress to cause clinically significant airway stenosis infrequently. The sinuses, pharynx, and larynx can also be affected by sarcoidal granulomas. Dry cough, dyspnea, and chest pain are common presenting symptoms, and hemoptysis is generally rare, but when present may indicate aspergillus infection of a cavitary lesion. The stage of pulmonary involvement is based on the chest radiograph, which provides an anatomic guide to lung involvement, but does not indicate disease chronicity. Stage 0 is normal, and stage 1 consists only of bilateral hilar adenopathy. Stage 2 is defined by adenopathy with concurrent pulmonary infiltrates, stage 3 by pulmonary infiltrates only, and stage 4 by reticular opacities or fibrosis with volume loss. Pulmonary function tests can indicate restriction or diffusion capacity abnormalities, but do not correlate with change radiographic staging.[19] High-resolution computed tomography (HRCT) of the lungs can be helpful, particularly in the setting of respiratory symptoms and a normal chest radiograph.[20] Bronchoalveolar lavage (BAL) characteristically shows an elevated CD4/CD8 T cell ratio, but chronic and extrapulmonary disease are associated with increased levels of CD8+ T cells and neutrophils.[21] However, BAL alone cannot establish the diagnosis of sarcoidosis, and transbronchial biopsies of both the upper and lower lobes increase the diagnostic yield.

Dermatologic

Cutaneous manifestations of sarcoid are seen in up to 20% to 30% of patients, and are often present at the time of diagnosis.[22] A wide range of skin lesions have been reported with sarcoidosis, and the most common of these is a maculopapular skin eruption involving the face, neck, and back. Sarcoid nodules tend to occur over the extensor surfaces of the extremities and on the torso. Some subcutaneous nodules remit spontaneously. Plaque-like sarcoidal skin lesions tend to be associated with chronic disease. Lupus pernio refers to an indurated, violaceous, plaque-like eruption that most frequently occurs on the nose, cheeks, chin, and forehead. This manifestation tends to affect black women more commonly and is associated with upper respiratory disease, pulmonary fibrosis, and bony involvement. Erythema nodosum is a panniculitis that most frequently affects women, commonly appearing in the lower extremities below the knees, and tends to be the only sarcoidal lesion associated with pain. It is a component of Lofgren's syndrome (erythema nodosum, hilar adenopathy, and migratory polyarthritis), and is associated with an acute presentation that generally resolves spontaneously. Biopsies of sarcoidal skin lesions are helpful in establishing the diagnosis, except in the case of erythema nodosum, which is nonspecific and associated with other inflammatory conditions.

Ophthalmologic

Eye involvement occurs in 25% to 80% of patients, and most commonly presents as an acute anterior uveitis with blurred vision and photophobia.[23] Other eye manifestations include posterior uveitis, retinal vasculitis, optic neuritis, keratoconjunctivitis, lacrimal gland enlargement, and conjunctival nodules. Posterior uveitis is frequently accompanied by central nervous system involvement. Because ocular involvement in sarcoidosis can be asymptomatic and lead to visual loss if untreated, a baseline slit-lamp and fundoscopic examination should be performed as a part of the initial evaluation.[23]

Cardiac

The granulomatous inflammation of sarcoidosis can infiltrate multiple areas of the heart including the ventricular septum and conduction system, leading to cardiomyopathy, arrhythmias, complete heart block, and sudden death. Papillary muscle involvement and pericardial effusions have also been documented. It does not generally cause valvular disease. Symptomatic involvement occurs in 5% of patients with sarcoidosis, but some studies have demonstrated that it may be more prevalent at autopsy (20% to 67%).[24] Cardiac magnetic resonance imaging (MRI) with gadolinium and positron emission tomography (PET) scanning can be useful in the diagnosis of cardiac sarcoidosis. However, the diagnostic yield of the endomyocardial biopsy in sarcoidosis is characteristically low, owing to the irregular distribution of granulomas in cardiac tissue.[25]

Neurologic

Only 5% to 10% of all patients with sarcoidosis present with neurologic symptoms, but up to 25% have central nervous system (CNS) involvement at autopsy.[26] It can occur alone or in combination with pulmonary and/or other extrapulmonary manifestations. Most CNS manifestations are due to granulomatous infiltration of the basal meningeal tissues or nearby structures, and include mass lesions, lymphocytic meningitis, hypothalamic hypopituitarism, central diabetes insipidus, hydrocephalus, seizures, psychosis, cognitive dysfunction and cranial nerve palsies. The most common neurologic presentation is a unilateral facial nerve palsy. MRI with gadolinium is the best imaging modality in the evaluation of sarcoidosis involving the brain, spinal cord, or meninges. Cerebral spinal fluid (CSF) may demonstrate multiple abnormalities, including elevated protein, low glucose, lymphocytic pleocytosis, oligoclonal bands, elevated opening pressure, and elevated angiotensin-converting enzyme (ACE) level. Brain biopsies are invasive and generally of low diagnostic yield, so other more accessible biopsy sites are preferred whenever possible.

Musculoskeletal

Involvement of the musculoskeletal system can occur in up to 10% of patients with sarcoidosis including the joints, muscle, and bone. Arthralgias are the most common musculoskeletal symptom (70%). Acute arthritis can present alone or as a part of Lofgren's syndrome, which is characterized by hilar adenopathy, acute polyarthritis, and erythema nodosum. This type of arthritis usually involves the ankles or knees, is self-limiting, and tends to resolve within 2 years. Close to a third of these patients may progress to a more chronic type of arthritis. Several types of chronic joint involvement have been reported including dactylitis, non-deforming arthritis, Jaccoud-type arthropathy, joint swelling due to a sarcoidal bone lesion, and chronic joint effusions. Myositis due to sarcoid has been reported both as an acute presentation, and also as a more insidious disease. Electromyography (EMG) can reveal a myopathic pattern, and open surgical biopsies may reveal granulomatous inflammation. Plain radiographs of joints are frequently normal except for soft tissue swelling. Cystic phalangeal lesions can occur but do not seem to correlate with the arthritis or symptoms. Sclerotic bone lesions of the axial skeleton have also been reported, but are of unclear clinical consequence. Arthrocentesis of an affected joint typically yields minimal, mildly inflammatory synovial fluid with a predominance of lymphocytes. Arthroscopic synovial biopsies can reveal typical noncaseating granulomas, but closed needle biopsies are of little diagnostic value.[27] Overall, the diagnosis of musculoskeletal involvement in sarcoidosis can be challenging, unless more commonly involved organ systems are concurrently affected. Therefore, it is important to fully evaluate the chest, skin, and eyes of a patient in whom musculoskeletal sarcoidosis is suspected.

Other

Painless peripheral lymphadenopathy is not uncommon in acute and chronic sarcoidosis. Parotid glands, thyroid, liver, and spleen can be infiltrated in patients with known sarcoidosis. Gastrointestinal granulomatous ulcerations and pancreatic involvement have been reported, but are rare manifestations.[28] Increased intestinal absorption of calcium can occur due to overproduction of 1, 25-hydroxyvitamin D as it is converted by sarcoidal macrophages from the less active metabolite 25-hydroxyvitamin D. This can lead to hypercalciuria, hypercalcemia, nephrocalcinosis, and nephrolithiasis.[29] Fortunately, renal failure due to granulomatous infiltration is rare.

CASE STUDY 1 LOFGREN'S SYNDROME

A 44-year-old woman presents to the rheumatology clinic with a 2-week history of large, painful red "lumps" that developed over her legs below the knees. She also notes progressive pain, redness, and swelling involving her left ankle over the last week, which has caused her to walk with a limp. She denies any high fever, dyspnea, cough, or chest pain, but reports malaise, muscle aches, and generalized fatigue. Her examination is notable for normal vital signs, lung, and cardiac exam. There are four large erythematous subcutaneous nodules over the lower extremities below the knees that are tender to palpation. The left ankle examination reveals a moderate effusion associated with mild erythema and warmth. There is mild discomfort with range of motion. Laboratory studies include a normal complete blood count (CBC) with differential. A comprehensive metabolic panel demonstrated a normal rheumatoid factor, anti-CCP antibody serum uric acid and a slightly elevated calcium of 10.5 mg/dL. Erythrocyte sedimentation rate (ESR) of 38 mm/h, and a C-reactive protein (CRP) of 2.0 mg/dL were noted. An attempted arthrocentesis of the left ankle did not yield any synovial fluid. Radiograph of the left ankle was normal except for diffuse soft tissue swelling, and chest radiograph revealed bilateral hilar lymphadenopathy but was otherwise normal. The patient was diagnosed with acute sarcoidosis presenting as Lofgren's syndrome based on her clinical presentation, and no further diagnostic work-up was pursued. Naproxen 500 mg twice daily was started due to the painful arthritis involving her left ankle, and her symptoms were significantly improved 1 week later. She reported resolution of her skin lesions and joint swelling after 4 weeks, and remained asymptomatic at her 1-year follow-up visit.

Discussion of Case Study 1

Patients who present with a classic Lofgren's triad of erythema nodosum, arthritis, and bilateral hilar lymphadenopathy may not need a biopsy, so long as there is no alternative explanation for the symptoms and they resolve promptly without complication. Fever is a common occurrence in Lofgren's syndrome but is not always present. Tissue biopsy should be pursued whenever possible if a reasonably accessible lesion is present, such as lymph nodes, dermatologic lesions, cutaneous nodules, and enlarged parotid or lacrimal glands. Biopsy of erythema nodosum in sarcoidosis is not recommended because it will show a nonspecific panniculitis rather than granulomas.[30] Nonsteroidal anti-inflammatory drugs (NSAIDs) are the first line of treatment for arthralgias and mild arthritis, and glucocorticoids are generally reserved for organ dysfunction or progressive disease that does not respond to NSAIDs. It is important to recognize that this presentation of sarcoidosis is typically self-limiting and associated with a benign prognosis.

CASE STUDY 2 PULMONARY SARCOIDOSIS

A 50-year-old man is referred to rheumatology clinic 10 months after being diagnosed with stage III pulmonary sarcoidosis and bilateral anterior uveitis. His primary complaints have been dyspnea and fatigue, and uveitis was found incidentally on his baseline ophthalmologic exam. He was initially started on prednisone 60 mg daily, but has been unable to wean below 20 mg without experiencing recurrent dyspnea. Transbronchial biopsies at the time of diagnosis were consistent with granulomatous inflammation, and bacterial and fungal cultures were negative. Pulmonary function tests showed mild restricton with a reduced diffusion capacity, and his oxygen saturations decreased to 86% with ambulation. He is currently on 30 mg of prednisone daily and his oxygen saturations are maintaining at 89% to 91% with ambulation. He has only mild dyspnea on exertion. His exam is notable for moon facies and central obesity, and his blood pressure is 146/88. His lung examination reveals few basilar rales, but is otherwise unremarkable. Methotrexate is initiated at 7.5 mg once weekly, and up titrated over 6 weeks to 15 mg weekly. He tolerates the methotrexate well and is able to wean down to 10 mg of prednisone daily over the following 6 months and repeat pulmonary studies are stable. His follow-up eye examinations are without evidence of recurrent uveitis.

Discussion of Case Study 2

This case illustrates the need for additional immunosuppressive therapy, particularly in the setting of a high corticosteroid requirement and evidence of medication toxicity. Although many patients with sarcoidosis undergo spontaneous remission, less than 30% of patients with stage III pulmonary disease undergo remission.[2] Oral corticosteroids are the first-line treatment for symptomatic or progressive stage II and III lung disease. Randomized, controlled data assessing the use of additional immunosuppressive therapy in sarcoidosis is limited, and primarily based on small studies and case reports.[31] In a patient who experiences significant glucocorticoid side effects, develops progressive disease despite adequate dosing glucocorticoids, or is unable to taper to less than 15 mg daily, alternative or additional immunosuppressive therapy should be considered. One randomized, controlled trial compared methotrexate to placebo in patients being treated with corticosteroids, and found that it was effective as a steroid-sparing agent.[32] However, there were no differences between the groups in terms of pulmonary measures. Other alternative cytotoxic agents that can be considered in this setting include azathioprine and cyclophosphamide.

CASES

Treatment

The goal of therapy in sarcoidosis is to suppress the inflammatory response, reduce granuloma burden, and prevent irreversible damage from disease progression. Corticosteroids are the most commonly used agents for control of symptoms and disabling systemic involvement, due to their potent effects on the inflammatory response. However, it is important to note that there have been no well-controlled trials documenting improvement in long-term outcomes with this therapy. Because the majority of patients with sarcoidosis are not disabled by the disease, the decision to start corticosteroid therapy should involve careful consideration of prognostic signs, risks, and benefits. The optimal dose of corticosteroid is the lowest dose necessary to adequately control symptoms and disease progression in patients in whom this therapy is indicated.

Therapy with corticosteroids is indicated in pulmonary sarcoidosis when there are progressive symptoms, worsening radiographic changes, or deterioration in lung function. In extrapulmonary sarcoidosis, the threshold for treatment of neurologic, cardiac, ocular, and renal involvement is lower because the complications are more serious in nature. Other indications for corticosteroids include severe constitutional symptoms, hepatic insufficiency, neuropathy, upper airway involvement, and disfiguring skin disease. Use of additional immunosuppressive therapy in the treatment of sarcoidosis is generally reserved for those who do not respond adequately to corticosteroids, develop intolerable side effects, or are unable to wean to lower doses of corticosteroids without disease recurrence.

Pulmonary

The following symptoms are indications for treatment of pulmonary sarcoidosis:

1. Progressive dyspnea, cough, chest pain, or hemoptysis
2. A fall in total lung capacity of at least 10 percent, forced vital capacity of 15%, or in diffusing capacity of 20%
3. Worsening interstitial opacities, cavities, fibrosis, honeycombing, or signs of new pulmonary hypertension on imaging

Corticosteroids are generally started at 0.5 to 1 mg/kg ideal body weight, and the patient is reevaluated at 4 to 6 weeks. The dose is then tapered by 5 to 10 mg every 4 to 8 weeks down to a goal of half of the starting dose. The dose should be tapered until achieving an acceptable maintenance dose, preferably to doses no greater than 10 to 15 mg daily. A total course of treatment of 1 year is recommended, but a slightly longer course may be required if exacerbations of disease are frequent and require periods of higher corticosteroid dosing.[30]

Adverse glucocorticoid effects, progression of disease despite adequate dosing, and inability to wean to lower doses of medication, are among the primary reasons for considering additional immunosuppressive therapy. As noted in the discussion of Case 2, methotrexate is most commonly used as a steroid-sparing agent in this setting based on a randomized, controlled trial demonstrating efficacy when used for this purpose.[32] However, successful use of other therapies such as azathioprine, leflunomide, cyclophosphamide, cyclosporine, and infliximab has been reported in small trials and case reports.

Ophthalmologic

Anterior uveitis can generally be treated with topical cycloplegics (e.g., scopolamine or atropine), and topical steroids (e.g., prednisolone acetate). Oral steroids may be used in severe or recalcitrant cases. Granulomatous infiltration of the lacrimal glands and surrounding structures or panuveitis require oral corticosteroids or periocular subtenon steroid injections every 3 to 4 weeks. Optic neuritis is always treated with systemic corticosteroid therapy. Successful treatment of chronic uveitis has been reported with other immunosuppressive therapies such as methotrexate, azathioprine, and infliximab.[33]

Dermatologic

Limited, nondisfiguring skin lesions of sarcoidosis, such as small plaques and papules, may be treated with topical or intralesional corticosteroids. Erythema nodosum is usually self-limited, and, therefore, requires no specific treatment. Lupus pernio and larger plaques can lead to permanent scarring and therefore need more aggressive therapies such as systemic corticosteroids, methotrexate, and antimalarials. There are anecdotal reports of successful treatment with cyclosporine, chlorambucil, retinoids, photochemotherapy (PUVA), minocycline, and thalidomide.[34]

Cardiac

Because cardiac sarcoidosis can be associated with high morbidity and mortality rates, treatment is usually aggressive. Ventricular arrhythmias and cardiomyopathy should be treated early and with high doses of prednisone of 60 mg per day or greater.[35] Tapering of prednisone to lower doses of 10 to 15 mg over 6 months is recommended. Other immunosuppressive agents such as cyclophosphamide, methotrexate, azathioprine, and chlorambucil have been used with limited success in refractory cases. In patients with recurrent ventricular arrhythmias, implantable defibrillators have been used.[36]

Neurologic

Randomized, controlled data addressing the treatment of neurosarcoidosis are lacking, but recommendations are made on consensus that these patients should be treated with corticosteroids. Severity of disease coupled with initial response to therapy dictate dose and duration of treatment. Prednisone is typically started at doses of 60 to 80 mg per day and then tapered according to the severity of the underlying neurologic disease.[37] As in cardiac sarcoidosis, other immunosuppressive agents such as methotrexate, antimalarials, azathioprine, cyclophosphamide, cyclosporine, and infliximab have been used with some success in treatment of refractory cases of neurosarcoidosis.[37-39] Cranial or spinal irradiation has also been used in refractory cases, usually in addition to immunosuppressive therapy.[40]

Musculoskeletal

Lofgren's arthritis or periarthritis does not usually require treatment beyond NSAIDs, because it tends to be self-limiting. If NSAIDs at maximum doses do not provide adequate relief, colchicine, hydroxychloroquine, or moderate doses of glucocorticoids can be used. In refractory cases or in chronic arthritis requiring higher doses of steroids, weekly low-dose methotrexate can be effective.[41] Sarcoidosis involving the bone generally responds inadequately to treatment with corticosteroids. Acute sarcoidal myositis responds much better to corticosteroid therapy than chronic muscle disease overall.

Renal and Hypercalcemia

Treatment of hypercalcemia and hypercalciuria is indicated if there is significant concern for nephrolithiasis, nephrocalcinosis, or worsening renal insufficiency. These conditions respond very well to moderate doses of oral prednisone, but there is evidence suggesting that agents such as chloroquine and ketoconazole can achieve a more prolonged response on calcium levels.[42]

Refractory Disease and Future Therapy

Because TNF-α appears to play a key role in the formation of granulomas, this cytokine would appear to be a reasonable target for inhibition in the treatment of sarcoidosis and other granulomatous diseases.[43] Use of thalidomide and pentoxifylline in the treatment of sarcoidosis has been proposed on this basis, but further studies are necessary. Infliximab, a chimeric anti-TNF-α monoclonal antibody, has demonstrated some benefit in the treatment of refractory pulmonary and extrapulmonary sarcoidosis.[43-45] However, TNF-α blockade using the dimeric fusion protein etanercept has not yielded the same results, although efficacy is similar between the two drugs in the treatment of rheumatoid arthritis. This suggests that simple neutralization of TNF-α, despite its role in granuloma formation and maintenance, is not sufficient in producing a sustained remission. A better understanding of the immunopathogenesis of sarcoidosis is necessary in the development of targeted treatments addressing this complicated disease.

BEHÇET'S DISEASE

Introduction

Behçet's disease (BD) is a chronic inflammatory disease whose most prominent feature is recurrent oral apthae. This disease is best characterized as a multisystem vasculitis, and it is associated with multiple systemic manifestations including mucocutaneous lesions, ocular disease, cutaneous lesions, neurologic disease, vascular disease, and arthritis. BD is unique among the systemic vasculitides in its propensity to involve a variety of blood vessels including small, medium, and large arteries, as well as the venous circulation.

Epidemiology

BD is most common in Turkey and along the ancient silk road, which courses from eastern Asia to the Mediterranean.[46] The prevalence of this disease ranges from 13.5 to 20 per 100,000 in Japan, China, Korea, Iran, Iraq, and Saudi Arabia, and from 1:15,000 to 1:500,000 in Northern American and Northern European countries.[46] The disease typically presents between the ages of 20 to 40 years, affecting men more commonly in the Mediterranean, and women more commonly in Northern Europe.[47,47a]

Etiology and Genetic Features

The etiopathogenesis of BD is yet unknown, but as is the case with many systemic inflammatory diseases, it is likely multifactorial with a prominent genetic component. Because most cases of BD are sporadic, the genetic features of the disease do not reflect a mendelian inheritance pattern. Certain HLAs, particularly HLA-B51, have been associated with increased risk of disease development and severity among various ethnic groups.[47,48] HLA-B52, B57, B27, and B15 have also been reported variably in association with BD, however one study found less than 20% HLA-B contribution among patients with BD.[49] Other non-HLA genes may also help determine susceptibility to disease. Genetic polymorphisms of the intercellular adhesion molecule (ICAM)-1 gene, endothelial nitric oxide synthetase gene, TNF genes, and vascular endothelial growth factor (VEGF) gene have been shown to play a role in disease susceptibility.[50-53]

A dysregulated and exaggerated Th1 immune response is thought to be the predominant feature in BD pathogenesis, but some studies have shown evidence for Th2 contribution as well. It is likely that the pathogenesis of this disease involves a mixture of both pathways.[54,55] Although no causal environmental trigger has been proven in BD, the many possible etiologic factors form a broad spectrum ranging from infectious agents to pollution. Heat shock proteins (HSPs), which are produced by many cells in response to stress, demonstrate substantial sequence homology between bacteria and humans. These shared epitopes may be targeted by the immune system by way of molecular mimicry, and this could play a role in the initiation of BD.[56] Other infectious agents such as *Streptococcus saguis*, *Staphylococcus aureus*, herpes simplex virus-1, and Prevotella species have been implicated as potential triggers of disease.[57,58]

Endothelial dysfunction is a prominent feature of BD, and activation of blood vessel endothelium in BD mediates vascular inflammation and thrombosis.[59-61] Elevated serum nitric oxide levels, homocysteine, antiendothelial antibodies, and vascular endothelial growth factor have been documented in patients with BD, and may play significant roles in the induction and perpetuation of vascular injury.[59,62-64]

Clinical Manifestations

Recurrent and painful mucocutaneous ulcers are the hallmark feature of BD, and the other clinical manifestations vary depending on the patient and the population. Men are more commonly and more seriously affected in the Middle East and Mediterranean, whereas women are more commonly affected in Japan, Korea, and Northern Europe.[47,65] Ocular, vascular, and central nervous system involvement are associated with the greatest morbidity and mortality.

Oral Ulcerations

The oral ulcers of BD are similar in appearance and histology to the common oral ulcer and ulcer associated with recurrent aphthous stomatitis. However, they are generally more extensive, and frequently multiple ulcers occur simultaneously. Healing generally occurs over 1 to 3 weeks. They may become less frequent with disease chronicity.

Urogenital Ulcerations

Genital lesions that appear similar to the oral apthae of BD occur in approximately 75% of patients with this syndrome. They are generally found on the scrotum in men and on the vulva in women. Scar formation occurs commonly with these lesions, but they tend to recur less frequently than the oral lesions. Salpingitis, epididymitis, and other pelvic inflammatory conditions have been reported in association with BD.[66]

Dermatologic Lesions

A variety of cutaneous lesions are seen in association with BD. These may include acneiform lesions, papulovesicular lesions, erythema nodosum, nodules, superficial thrombophlebitis, pyoderma gangrenosum–like ulcerations, and palpable purpura. The acneiform lesions of BD are difficult to distinguish from ordinary acne and may be more common in those patients with arthritis.[58,67]

The pathergy reaction refers to a hyperreactivity of the skin to local injury in the form of an erythematous papule or pustule. A lesion greater than 5 mm typically develops 24-48 hours after needle prick. This reaction is very specific to BD, however it is reported much more commonly in Turkey and Japan, than in Northern Europe or the United States.

Ocular Disease

Eye involvement is reported in 25% to 75% of patients with BD, and is usually less severe in North American populations, resulting in a lower incidence of blindness.[68] Uveitis is the most common type of eye involvement in BD. It is usually chronic, bilateral, and episodic, often involving the entire uveal tract. Hypopyon is an anterior uveitis with severe inflammation in the anterior chamber that is primarily seen in patients with BD. It is associated with a poor prognosis owing to its association with retinal vasculitis.[69] Posterior uveitis, optic neuritis, retinal vasculitis, and vascular occlusion can rapidly progress to irreversible visual impairment if left untreated. Neovascularization, cataracts, glaucoma, and occasionally conjunctival ulceration can also be seen in patients with BD.[70] Conjunctivitis, scleritis, sicca syndrome, and isolated anterior uveitis are rare.

Arthritis

Joint involvement occurs in 50% of patients and typically presents as a nonerosive, asymmetric, and nondeforming oligoarthritis. Medium and large joints are more commonly affected than smaller ones, and synovial fluid is inflammatory.[71] The arthritis often occurs during times of disease exacerbation and resolves over 1 to 3 weeks.

Neurologic Disease

Neurologic involvement is observed in less than 15% of patients with BD.[72] It occurs more commonly in men than women. The most frequent type of involvement is focal parenchymal lesions, which have a severe prognosis. The lesions can be located in the brain stem, spinal cord, corticospinal tract, periventricular white matter, and basal ganglia. The first signs of clinical involvement may be personality change, psychosis, dementia, parasthesias, focal weakness, and sphincter disturbances. Nonparenchymal involvement is typically in the form of arterial or venous thrombosis. Peripheral neuropathy is uncommon.[73]

Vascular Disease

BD is unique in its ability to involve blood vessels of all sizes in both the arterial and venous circulation. Venous disease occurs more frequently than arterial, and is often an early feature of BD. Although superficial and deep vein thromboses are the most common types of venous involvement, other venous obstructive lesions such as dural sinus thrombosis, Budd-Chiari syndrome, and superior or inferior vena cava occlusion can also occur. Small vessel vasculitis is the typical arterial involvement, although medium and large vessel disease also occur resulting in significant morbidity and mortality. Among the larger arteries, the carotid, pulmonary, aortic, iliac, femoral, and popliteal arteries are most frequently involved. Pulmonary artery aneurysms occur more commonly in BD than in any other vasculitis and are a leading cause of death.[74] It typically presents with recurrent episodes of hemoptysis, and should be distinguished from pulmonary embolus because anticoagulation could result in a worse outcome. Involvement of the cerebral, renal, and coronary vessels is unusual.[69]

Cardiac Involvement

Cardiac disease resulting in clinical symptoms is rare in BD. Pericarditis, myocarditis, coronary vasculitis, valvular lesions, and atrial or ventricular septal aneurysms have been reported sporadically.[75] BD does not appear to be associated with accelerated coronary atherosclerosis, as occurs in other autoimmune diseases such as systemic lupus erythematosus and rheumatoid arthritis.[76]

Gastrointestinal Involvement

Discrete gastrointestinal ulcerations occur in some patients and may lead to intestinal perforation. They are typically observed in the terminal ileum but can also be found in the cecum and ascending colon.[77] Abdominal pain, nausea, diarrhea, and anorexia may be among the initial symptoms. Distinguishing the gastrointestinal involvement of BD from inflammatory bowel disease can be difficult, because oral apthae can occur in both entities.

Other

Constitutional symptoms such as fever, malaise, and fatigue are not uncommon in BD. Glomerulonephritis, hematuria, proteinuria, and mild renal insufficiency can be seen in BD, but is rare. Secondary (AA) amyloidosis can develop in long-standing BD, and usually presents with nephritic syndrome.[78] Voiding abnormalities and erectile dysfunction may occur due to neuropathy or vascular disease.[79] One study suggested an association between BD and myelodysplasia.[80]

Diagnosis

BD is diagnosed based primarily on clinical findings because there are no laboratory tests or serologies specific to the diagnosis. Laboratory testing during active disease typically reveals elevated markers of inflammation such as CRP and the erythrocyte sedimentation rate, but these findings are nonspecific. The current international classification criteria require the presence of recurrent oral apthae occurring three times in 1 year, plus two of the following[81]:
- Recurrent genital apthae
- Eye lesions observed by an ophthalmologist
- Skin lesions characteristic of BD

- Positive pathergy test (papule 2 mm or greater developing 24 to 48 hours after oblique insertion of a 20- to 25-gauge needle 5 mm into the skin, performed on the forearm)

These criteria are thought to be of higher sensitivity and specificity than previous criteria, but it is important to note that their primary function is in defining the disease for the purposes of clinical and basic research.[82] The use of these criteria in the individual patient may be of limited use, making the diagnosis of BD fairly challenging in some instances.

Treatment

Management of BD is focused on treating the inflammatory attacks, thereby limiting tissue damage and minimizing recurrences in order to decrease the overall disease burden. Treatment is dictated by the type of organ involved and by disease severity within that organ. Typically multiple organ systems are involved in BD, and treatment is then guided by disease severity in the most critical organ. Mucocutaneous disease is common to most patients, but the highest morbidity and mortality rates are

---

CASE STUDY 3

A 46-year-old white woman presents to the rheumatology clinic reporting a 5-year history of recurrent oral ulcers, history of vaginal ulcers confirmed by her gynecologist, episodic nodules on her legs below the knees, intermittent pustular rashes, and chronic diarrhea that is occasionally bloody. She has been evaluated by multiple specialists in the community including a rheumatologist about 3 years ago. She underwent angiography of her abdominal vessels at that time that showed no evidence of vasculitis or aneurysms. A dermatologist evaluated her lesions and diagnosed erythema nodosum. A pathergy test was performed and resulted in a 5 mm pustular lesion 48 hours later. She has been treated intermittently with corticosteroids for likely BD for the last 3 years, and is currently taking prednisone 15 mg daily. She has been hospitalized on two occasions owing to abdominal pain, diarrhea, and dehydration. During these hospitalizations her laboratory tests demonstrated marked elevations in ESR and CRP, as well as a mild anemia. Blood and stool cultures have always been negative. A colonoscopy 3 years ago revealed ulcerations at the cecum and ascending colon and was believed to be consistent with possible Crohn's disease. Her genital ulcerations and erythema nodosum have subsided while on chronic prednisone, and her diarrhea is significantly improved as well. She has had significant difficulty weaning below 15 to 20 mg of prednisone due to recurrence in diarrhea. Colchicine therapy was poorly tolerated due to worsening diarrhea. Azathioprine was added 2 years ago

as a steroid-sparing therapy which has allowed her to taper to her current dose of prednisone. Her examination at the time of evaluation was notable for moderate central obesity, abdominal striae, and one small oral ulcer. She is very concerned about her inability to wean to lower corticosteroids, particularly because she has developed multiple cataracts, glaucoma, obesity, and mild diabetes as a result. After discussing treatment options for BD, she decides to proceed with infliximab and is loaded at a dose of 5 mg/kg, and maintained every 8 weeks without adverse effects. She continues on azathioprine. After 6 months, she is weaned to 5 mg of prednisone daily, and her diarrhea is markedly improved and stable. Her oral ulcers have also decreased in frequency substantially.

Discussion of Case Study 3
The clinical presentation of this patient meets the current classification criteria for BD. Because diagnostic laboratory or imaging studies for this disease do not exist, the diagnosis is often delayed and multiple specialists are necessary in the evaluation of the patient. As described later, treatment is generally directed at the manifestation causing the most morbidity, or associated with the highest mortality. This patient had persistant bowel involvement and evidence of steroid toxicity, which directed her therapy. Infliximab has been used successfully to treat gastrointestinal complications of BD as described later, and would be a reasonable addition because the current first-line therapy is not providing adequate disease control.

due to ocular, large vessel, and neurologic involvement. Patients with severe manifestations require timely and effective treatment of inflammation in order to prevent irreversible tissue damage.

The literature addressing treatment of BD comes primarily from case reports and small case series, with few randomized, controlled trials (RCTs) assessing efficacy of treatments. This has resulted in a limited ability to compare trials and pool data, thus hindering the data collection necessary for improvements in the management of BD.[83] Since 1998, there have been small advances in the literature addressing BD treatment, particularly in evaluating colchicine for mucocutaneous disease, and the anti-TNF-α therapies. Treatment of BD is discussed within the context of minor and major disease manifestations.

Minor Disease Manifestations

Manifestations in this category include mucocutaneous disease, arthritis, and various skin lesions, which interfere with patient quality of life but do not substantially compromise organ function. Topical sucralfate as a mouthwash was shown to reduce pain and healing time of oral ulcers in BD.[84] Colchicine has been used widely to treat many symptoms of BD, and has been shown to be effective in the treatment of genital ulcers, erythema nodosum, and arthritis in a 2-year controlled trial.[85] Acneiform skin disease can also be treated with colchicine. Thalidomide is also effective in treating oral and genital apthae, and acneiform lesions, but symptoms recur on discontinuation and side effects limit long-term use.[86] However, erythema nodosum in BD is distinct from its presence in other entities in that it frequently represents a medium vessel vasculitis and occasionally undergoes ulceration.[87] Glucocorticoid or azathioprine therapy may be more effective for erythema nodosum in this setting if the initial response to colchicine is unfavorable. Additionally, it is important to note that pyoderma gangrenosum in the patient with BD is often complicated by the pathergy reaction. As a result, débridement of these lesions in BD can cause local expansion of the lesion rather than healing. Prompt immunosuppressive therapy should also be considered in this scenario.

Major Disease Manifestations

Ocular, neurologic, and large vessel involvement are the primary disease manifestations that can result in significant organ dysfunction and even death. Anterior uveitis is generally treated with mydriatic agents to prevent formation of synechiae, but some cases may require topical or oral glucocorticoids. Posterior uveitis, focal brain lesions, encephalitis, and medium-vessel cerebral vasculitis are all treated similarly due to their potentially devastating consequences. Large vessel disease requires a combination of immunosuppressive therapy, and occasionally surgical grafting. High dose glucocorticoid therapy helps reduce the acute inflammatory features of severe disease, but additional immunosuppressive agents are usually necessary to prevent disease relapse while tapering. Prednisone 1 mg/kg or intravenous methylprednisolone 1 mg/day for three days are typically used as initial therapy in organ-threatening disease.[88] Infliximab, cyclophosphamide, cyclosporine, and azathioprine have all been employed in the treatment of serious complications of BD, but evidence-based data on efficacy are limited. Choice of treatment should primarily be based on the safety profile of the drug in the individual patient. Infliximab dosed at 5 mg/kg has exhibited rapid control of resistant uveitis, but treatment must continue indefinitely due to disease relapses.[89] It has also been used successfully in the treatment of neuro-BD manifestations and gastrointestinal involvement.[88,90] Azathioprine use in BD may lead to a more favorable long-term outcome if it is employed early in the disease course.[91] Cyclophosphamide is used in combination with high-dose steroids in severe complications such as pulmonary aneurysms and CNS disease.[74] Cyclosporine has primarily been evaluated in the treatment of severe ocular disease, and is not generally used in treating CNS disease owing to its potential for neurotoxicity.[92] Venous thrombosis is treated with standard anticoagulation regimens. The role of primary anticoagulation with aspirin or warfarin is yet unknown, but control of the systemic inflammation in BD should be the primary goal in preventing thrombotic events.

Identification of underlying pathogenetic mechanisms will be critical to better understanding BD and should help direct therapeutic modalities. More multidisciplinary and long-term trials assessing treatment efficacy and relapse prevention are needed in order to develop better management plans for this complicated disease.

References

1. Cox CE, Davis-Allen A, Judson MA. Sarcoidosis. Med Clin North Am 2005;89:817-28.
2. Newman LS, Rose CS, Maier LA. Sarcoidosis. N Engl J Med 1997;336:1224-34.
3. Pietinalho A, Hiraga Y, Hosoda Y, Lofroos AB, Yamaguchi M, Selroos O. The frequency of sarcoidosis in Finland and Hokkaido, Japan. A comparative epidemiological study. Sarcoidosis 1995;12:61-7.
4. Rybicki BA, Major M, Popovich J, Jr., Maliarik MJ, Iannuzzi MC. Racial differences in sarcoidosis incidence: a 5-year study in a health maintenance organization. Am J Epidemiol 1997;145:234-41.
5. Izbicki G, Chavko R, Banauch GI, Weiden MD, Berger KI, Aldrich TK, et al. World Trade Center sarcoid-like granulomatous pulmonary disease in New York City Fire Department rescue workers. Chest 2007;131:1414-23.
6. Moller DR, Chen ES. What causes sarcoidosis? Curr Opin Pulm Med 2002;8:429-34.
7. Newman LS, Rose CS, Bresnitz EA, Rossman MD, Barnard J, Frederick M, et al. A case control etiologic study of sarcoidosis: environmental and occupational risk factors. Am J Respir Crit Care Med 2004;170:1324-30.
8. Eishi Y, Suga M, Ishige I, Kobayashi D, Yamada T, Takemura T, et al. Quantitative analysis of mycobacterial and propionibacterial DNA in lymph nodes of Japanese and European patients with sarcoidosis. J Clin Microbiol 2002;40:198-204.

9. Rybicki BA, Harrington D, Major M, Simoff M, Popovich J, Jr., Maliarik M, et al. Heterogeneity of familial risk in sarcoidosis. Genet Epidemiol 1996;13:23-33.

10. Rybicki BA, Iannuzzi MC, Frederick MM, Thompson BW, Rossman MD, Bresnitz EA. Familial aggregation of sarcoidosis. A case-control etiologic study of sarcoidosis (ACCESS). Am J Respir Crit Care Med 2001;164:2085-91.

11. Rybicki BA, Kirkey KL, Major M, Maliarik MJ, Popovich J, Jr., Chase GA, et al. Familial risk ratio of sarcoidosis in African-American sibs and parents. Am J Epidemiol 2001;153:188-93.

12. Visser H, Vos K, Zanelli E, Verduyn W, Schreuder GM, Speyer I, et al. Sarcoid arthritis: clinical characteristics, diagnostic aspects, and risk factors. Ann Rheum Dis 2002;61:499-504.

13. Grunewald J. Genetics of sarcoidosis. Curr Opin Pulm Med 2008;14:434-9.

14. Agostini C, Basso U, Semenzato G. Cells and molecules involved in the development of sarcoid granuloma. J Clin Immunol 1998;18(3):184-92.

15. Conron M, Du Bois RM. Immunological mechanisms in sarcoidosis. Clin Exp Allergy 2001;31:543-54.

16. Rizzato G, Palmieri G, Agrati AM, Zanussi C. The organ-specific extrapulmonary presentation of sarcoidosis: a frequent occurrence but a challenge to an early diagnosis. A 3-year-long prospective observational study. Sarcoidosis Vasc Diffuse Lung Dis 2004;21:119-26.

17. Chevalet P, Clement R, Rodat O, Moreau A, Brisseau JM, Clarke JP. Sarcoidosis diagnosed in elderly subjects: retrospective study of 30 cases. Chest 2004;126:1423-30.

18. Baughman RP. Pulmonary sarcoidosis. Clin Chest Med 2004;25:521-30, vi.

19. Judson MA, Baughman RP, Thompson BW, Teirstein AS, Terrin ML, Rossman MD. Two year prognosis of sarcoidosis: the ACCESS experience. Sarcoidosis Vasc Diffuse Lung Dis 2003;20:204-11.

20. Nishimura K, Itoh H, Kitaichi M, Nagai S, Izumi T. Pulmonary sarcoidosis: correlation of CT and histopathologic findings. Radiology 1993;189:105-9.

21. Poulter LW, Rossi GA, Bjermer L, Costabel U, Israel-Biet D, Klech H, et al. The value of bronchoalveolar lavage in the diagnosis and prognosis of sarcoidosis. Eur Respir J 1990;3:943-4.

22. Roberts SD, Mirowski GW, Wilkes D, Kwo PY, Knox KS. Sarcoidosis. Part II: extrapulmonary and systemic manifestations. J Am Acad Dermatol 2004;51:628-30.

23. Bonfioli AA, Orefice F. Sarcoidosis. Semin Ophthalmol 2005;20:177-82.

24. Chapelon-Abric C, de Zuttere D, Duhaut P, Veyssier P, Wechsler B, Huong DL, et al. Cardiac sarcoidosis: a retrospective study of 41 cases. Medicine (Baltimore) 2004;83(6):315-34.

25. Uemura A, Morimoto S, Hiramitsu S, Kato Y, Ito T, Hishida H. Histologic diagnostic rate of cardiac sarcoidosis: evaluation of endomyocardial biopsies. Am Heart J 1999; 138(2 Pt 1):299-302.

26. Scott TF, Yandora K, Valeri A, Chieffe C, Schramke C. Aggressive therapy for neurosarcoidosis: long-term follow-up of 48 treated patients. Arch Neurol 2007;64:691-6.

27. Pettersson T. Rheumatic features of sarcoidosis. Curr Opin Rheumatol 1998;10:73-8.

28. Sprague R, Harper P, McClain S, Trainer T, Beeken W. Disseminated gastrointestinal sarcoidosis. Case report and review of the literature. Gastroenterology 1984;87:421-5.

29. Berliner AR, Haas M, Choi MJ. Sarcoidosis: the nephrologist's perspective. Am J Kidney Dis 2006;48:856-70.

30. Statement on Sarcoidosis. Joint Statement of the American Thoracic Society (ATS), the European Respiratory Society (ERS) and the World Association of Sarcoidosis and Other Granulomatous Disorders (WASOG) adopted by the ATS Board of Directors and by the ERS Executive Committee, February 1999. Am J Respir Crit Care Med 1999;160: 736-55.

31. Paramothayan S, Lasserson TJ, Walters EH. Immunosuppressive and cytotoxic therapy for pulmonary sarcoidosis. Cochrane Database Syst Rev 2006;3:CD003536.

32. Baughman RP, Winget DB, Lower EE. Methotrexate is steroid sparing in acute sarcoidosis: results of a double blind, randomized trial. Sarcoidosis Vasc Diffuse Lung Dis 2000;17:60-6.

33. Rothova A. Ocular involvement in sarcoidosis. Br J Ophthalmol 2000;84:110-6.

34. English JC, 3rd, Patel PJ, Greer KE. Sarcoidosis. J Am Acad Dermatol 2001;44:725-43.

35. Reuhl J, Schneider M, Sievert H, Lutz FU, Zieger G. Myocardial sarcoidosis as a rare cause of sudden cardiac death. Forensic Sci Int 1997;89:145-53.

36. Winters SL, Cohen M, Greenberg S, Stein B, Curwin J, Pe E, et al. Sustained ventricular tachycardia associated with sarcoidosis: assessment of the underlying cardiac anatomy and the prospective utility of programmed ventricular stimulation, drug therapy and an implantable antitachycardia device. J Am Coll Cardiol 1991;18:937-43.

37. Gullapalli D, Phillips LH, 2nd. Neurologic manifestations of sarcoidosis. Neurol Clin 2002;20:59-83, vi.

38. Carter JD, Valeriano J, Vasey FB, Bognar B. Refractory neurosarcoidosis: a dramatic response to infliximab. Am J Med 2004;117:277-9.

39. Sharma OP. Effectiveness of chloroquine and hydroxychloroquine in treating selected patients with sarcoidosis with neurological involvement. Arch Neurol 1998;55(9):248-54.

40. Menninger MD, Amdur RJ, Marcus RB, Jr. Role of radiotherapy in the treatment of neurosarcoidosis. Am J Clin Oncol 2003;26:e115-8.

41. Kaye O, Palazzo E, Grossin M, Bourgeois P, Kahn MF, Malaise MG. Low-dose methotrexate: an effective corticosteroid-sparing agent in the musculoskeletal manifestations of sarcoidosis. Br J Rheumatol 1995;34:642-4.

42. Sharma OP. Vitamin D, calcium, and sarcoidosis. Chest 1996;109:535-9.

43. Baughman RP, Iannuzzi M. Tumour necrosis factor in sarcoidosis and its potential for targeted therapy. BioDrugs 2003;17:425-31.

44. Baughman RP, Drent M, Kavuru M, Judson MA, Costabel U, du Bois R, et al. Infliximab therapy in patients with chronic sarcoidosis and pulmonary involvement. Am J Respir Crit Care Med 2006;174:795-802.

45. Denys BG, Bogaerts Y, Coenegrachts KL, De Vriese AS. Steroid-resistant sarcoidosis: is antagonism of TNF-alpha the answer? Clin Sci (Lond) 2007;112:281-9.

46. Yurdakul S, Hamuryudan V, Yazici H. Behcet syndrome. Curr Opin Rheumatol 2004;16:38-42.

47. Sakane T, Takeno M, Suzuki N, Inaba G, Behcet's disease. N Engl J Med 1999;341:1284-91.

47a. O'Duffy JD. Behcet's disease. Curr Opin Rheumatol 1994;6:39-43.

48. Kotter I, Gunaydin I, Stubiger N, Yazici H, Fresko I, Zouboulis CC, et al. Comparative analysis of the association of HLA-B*51 suballeles with Behcet's disease in patients of German and Turkish origin. Tissue Antigens 2001;58:166-70.

49. Gul A, Hajeer AH, Worthington J, Barrett JH, Ollier WE, Silman AJ. Evidence for linkage of the HLA-B locus in Behcet's disease, obtained using the transmission disequilibrium test. Arthritis Rheum 2001;44:239-40.

50. Ahmad T, Wallace GR, James T, Neville M, Bunce M, Mulcahy-Hawes K, et al. Mapping the HLA association in Behcet's disease: a role for tumor necrosis factor polymorphisms? Arthritis Rheum 2003;48:807-13.

51. Chmaisse HN, Fakhoury HA, Salti N, Makki RF. The ICAM-1 469 T/C gene polymorphism but not 241 G/A is associated with Behcets disease in the Lebanese population. Saudi Med J 2006;27:604-7.

52. Salvarani C, Boiardi L, Casali B, Olivieri I, Cantini F, Salvi F, et al. Vascular endothelial growth factor gene polymorphisms in Behcet's disease. J Rheumatol 2004;31:1785-9.

53. Salvarani C, Boiardi L, Casali B, Olivieri I, Ciancio G, Cantini F, et al. Endothelial nitric oxide synthase gene polymorphisms in Behcet's disease. J Rheumatol 2002;29:535-40.

54. Hamzaoui K, Hamzaoui A, Guemira F, Bessioud M, Hamza M, Ayed K. Cytokine profile in Behcet's disease patients. Relationship with disease activity. Scand J Rheumatol 2002;31:205-10.

55. Raziuddin S, al-Dalaan A, Bahabri S, Siraj AK, al-Sedairy S. Divergent cytokine production profile in Behcet's disease. Altered Th1/Th2 cell cytokine pattern. J Rheumatol 1998;25:329-33.

56. Direskeneli H, Hasan A, Shinnick T, Mizushima R, van der Zee R, Fortune F, et al. Recognition of B-cell epitopes of the 65 kda HSP in Behcet's disease. Scand J Immunol 1996;43:464-71.

57. Direskeneli H. Behcet's disease: infectious aetiology, new autoantigens, and HLA-B51. Ann Rheum Dis 2001;60:996-1002.

58. Hatemi G, Bahar H, Uysal S, Mat C, Gogus F, Masatlioglu S, et al. The pustular skin lesions in Behcet's syndrome are not sterile. Ann Rheum Dis 2004;63:1450-2.

59. Direskeneli H, Keser G, D'Cruz D, Khamastha MA, Akoglu T, Yazici H, et al. Anti-endothelial cell antibodies, endothelial proliferation and von Willebrand factor antigen in Behcet's disease. Clin Rheumatol 1995;14:55-61.

60. Kayikcioglu M, Aksu K, Hasdemir C, Keser G, Turgan N, Kultursay H, et al. Endothelial functions in Behcet's disease. Rheumatol Int 2006;26:304-8.

61. Triolo G, Accardo-Palumbo A, Carbone MC, Ferrante A, Giardina E. Enhancement of endothelial cell E-selectin expression by sera from patients with active Behcet's disease: moderate correlation with anti-endothelial cell antibodies and serum myeloperoxidase levels. Clin Immunol 1999;91:330-7.

62. Cekmen M, Evereklioglu C, Er H, Inaloz HS, Doganay S, Turkoz Y, et al. Vascular endothelial growth factor levels are increased and associated with disease activity in patients with Behcet's syndrome. Int J Dermatol 2003;42:870-5.

63. Evereklioglu C, Turkoz Y, Er H, Inaloz HS, Ozbek E, Cekmen M. Increased nitric oxide production in patients with Behcet's disease: is it a new activity marker? J Am Acad Dermatol 2002;46:50-4.

64. Ozdemir R, Barutcu I, Sezgin AT, Acikgoz N, Ermis N, Esen AM, et al. Vascular endothelial function and plasma homocysteine levels in Behcet's disease. Am J Cardiol 2004;94:522-5.

65. Zouboulis CC, Vaiopoulos G, Marcomichelakis N, Palimeris G, Markidou I, Thouas B, et al. Onset signs, clinical course, prognosis, treatment and outcome of adult patients with Adamantiades-Behcet's disease in Greece. Clin Exp Rheumatol 2003;21(Suppl. 30):S19-26.

66. Kaklamani VG, Vaiopoulos G, Markomichelakis N, Kaklamanis P. Recurrent epididymo-orchitis in patients with Behcet's disease. J Urol 2000;163:487-9.

67. Diri E, Mat C, Hamuryudan V, Yurdakul S, Hizli N, Yazci H. Papulopustular skin lesions are seen more frequently in patients with Behcet's syndrome who have arthritis: a controlled and masked study. Ann Rheum Dis 2001;60:1074-6.

68. Nussenblatt RB. Uveitis in Behcet's disease. Int Rev Immunol 1997;14:67-79.

69. Seyahi E, Melikoglu M, Yazic H. Clinical features and diagnosis of Behcet's syndrome. Int J Adv Rheumatol 2007;5:8-13.

70. Zamir E, Bodaghi B, Tugal-Tutkun I, See RF, Charlotte F, Wang RC, et al. Conjunctival ulcers in Behcet's disease. Ophthalmology 2003;110:1137-41.

71. Kim HA, Choi KW, Song YW. Arthropathy in Behcet's disease. Scand J Rheumatol 1997;26:125-9.

72. Akman-Demir G, Serdaroglu P, Tasci B. Clinical patterns of neurological involvement in Behcet's disease: evaluation of 200 patients. The Neuro-Behcet Study Group. Brain 1999;122(Pt 11):2171-82.

73. Atasoy HT, Tunc TO, Unal AE, Emre U, Koca R, Esturk E, et al. Peripheral nervous system involvement in patients with Behcet disease. Neurologist 2007;13:225-30.

74. Hamuryudan V, Er T, Seyahi E, Akman C, Tuzun H, Fresko I, et al. Pulmonary artery aneurysms in Behcet syndrome. Am J Med 2004;117:867-70.

75. Gurgun C, Ercan E, Ceyhan C, Yavuzgil O, Zoghi M, Aksu K, et al. Cardiovascular involvement in Behcet's disease. Jpn Heart J 2002;43:389-98.

76. Kural-Seyahi E, Fresko I, Seyahi N, Ozyazgan Y, Mat C, Hamuryudan V, et al. The long-term mortality and morbidity of Behcet syndrome: a 2-decade outcome survey of 387 patients followed at a dedicated center. Medicine (Baltimore) 2003;82:60-76.

77. Korman U, Cantasdemir M, Kurugoglu S, Mihmanli I, Soylu N, Hamuryudan V, et al. Enterolysis findings of intestinal Behcet disease: a comparative study with Crohn disease. Abdom Imaging 2003;28:308-12.

78. Melikoglu M, Altiparmak MR, Fresko I, Tunc R, Yurdakal S, Hamuryudan V, et al. A reappraisal of amyloidosis in Behcet's syndrome. Rheumatology (Oxford) 2001;40:212-5.

79. Erdogru T, Kocak T, Serdaroglu P, Kadioglu A, Tellaloglu S. Evaluation and therapeutic approaches of voiding and erectile dysfunction in neurological Behcet's syndrome. J Urol 1999;62:147-53.

80. Tada Y, Koarada S, Haruta Y, Mitamura M, Ohta A, Nagasawa K. The association of Behcet's disease with myelodysplastic syndrome in Japan: a review of the literature. Clin Exp Rheumatol 2006;24(Suppl. 42):S115-9.

81. International Study Group for Behcet's Disease. Criteria for diagnosis of Behcet's disease. Lancet 1990;335:1078-80.

82. Ferraz MB, Walter SD, Heymann R, Atra E. Sensitivity and specificity of different diagnostic criteria for Behcet's disease according to the latent class approach. Br J Rheumatol 1995;34:932-5.

83. Saenz A, Ausejo M, Shea B, Wells G, Welch V, Tugwell P. Pharmacotherapy for Behcet's syndrome. Cochrane Database Syst Rev 2000;CD001084.

84. Alpsoy E, Er H, Durusoy C, Yilmaz E. The use of sucralfate suspension in the treatment of oral and genital ulceration of Behcet disease: a randomized, placebo-controlled, double-blind study. Arch Dermatol 1999;135:529-32.

85. Yurdakul S, Mat C, Tuzun Y, Ozyazgan Y, Hamuryudan V, Uysal O, et al. A double-blind trial of colchicine in Behcet's syndrome. Arthritis Rheum 2001;44:2686-92.

86. Hamuryudan V, Mat C, Saip S, Ozyazgan Y, Siva A, Yurdakul S, et al. Thalidomide in the treatment of the mucocutaneous lesions of the Behcet syndrome. A randomized, double-blind, placebo-controlled trial. Ann Intern Med 1998;128:443-50.

87. Kim B, LeBoit PE. Histopathologic features of erythema nodosum–like lesions in Behcet disease: a comparison with erythema nodosum focusing on the role of vasculitis. Am J Dermatopathol 2000;22:379-90.

88. Pipitone N, Olivieri I, Cantini F, Triolo G, Salvarani C. New approaches in the treatment of Adamantiades-Behcet's disease. Curr Opin Rheumatol 2006;18:3-9.

89. Sfikakis PP, Kaklamanis PH, Elezoglou A, Katsilambros N, Theodossiadis PG, Papaefthimiou S, et al. Infliximab for recurrent, sight-threatening ocular inflammation in Adamantiades-Behcet disease. Ann Intern Med 2004;140:404-6.

90. Travis SP, Czajkowski M, McGovern DP, Watson RG, Bell AL. Treatment of intestinal Behcet's syndrome with chimeric tumour necrosis factor alpha antibody. Gut 2001;49:725-8.

91. Hamuryudan V, Ozyazgan Y, Hizli N, Mat C, Yurdakul S, Tuzun Y, et al. Azathioprine in Behcet's syndrome: effects on long-term prognosis. Arthritis Rheum 1997;40:769-74.

92. Sajjadi H, Soheilian M, Ahmadieh H, Hassanein K, Parvin M, Azarmina M, et al. Low dose cyclosporin-A therapy in Behcet's disease. J Ocul Pharmacol 1994;10:553-60.

Management of the Connective Tissue Diseases of Childhood

Dawn M. Wahezi and Norman T. Ilowite

Rheumatic diseases in childhood, although biologically similar to those in adults, represent a unique class of disorders that often possess distinctive differences in clinical manifestations, therapeutic goals, and overall prognostic implications. The relative rarity of many of these diseases, accompanied with the ethical challenges of studying children, often limits adequate scientific research and clinical trials. Thus, management in children is often based largely on adult-based literature, retrospective reviews, case series, and anecdotal evidence, although some randomized studies have been performed. The purpose of this chapter is to describe, in detail, therapies for connective tissue diseases that are very unique in childhood (juvenile dermatomyositis [JDM], Kawasaki's disease [KD], Henoch-Schönlein purpura [HSP], neonatal lupus, and linear scleroderma), while emphasizing variations in management of children with inflammatory diseases generally more prevalent in adults (systemic lupus erythematosus [SLE], antiphospholipid syndrome, Wegener's granulomatosus [WG], and polyarteritis nodosa [PAN]).

JUVENILE DERMATOMYOSITIS

JDM, the most common inflammatory myopathy of childhood, is a rare multisystemic autoimmune vasculopathy, primarily characterized by proximal muscle weakness and pathognomonic skin rashes (Fig. 19-1). It affects approximately 3.2 million children in the United States per year, with the average onset at 7 years old.[1] Other organ systems, particularly gastrointestinal, pulmonary, and cardiac may also be involved. Calcinosis of the cutaneous and subcutaneous tissues, muscles, tendons and ligaments, a rare complication in adult dermatomyositis, occurs in approximately 20% to 40% of children, particularly those in whom there is a delay to diagnosis or inadequate control of active disease inflammation. Children with extensive calcinosis may suffer from significant long-term disability; therefore, aggressive treatment regimens are often aimed at prevention of this outcome.

CASE STUDY 1

A 4-year-old girl with no significant past medical history presents with erythematous, scaly papules on her hands, elbows, knees and ankles bilaterally. According to her mother, the rash had been present for 3 months, with minimal improvement after using various topical treatments prescribed by her primary doctor. Recently, the patient has had decreased activity, refusing to rise up from a seated position on the floor or to climb up onto the couch. Her mother states that her symptoms have progressed, and the child prefers to "lie down in bed all day long." She denies any dysphonia, dysphagia, or choking episodes. The patient has been afebrile and tolerating feeds without issue. Physical examination reveals an uncomfortable child, lying still in bed. Skin examination reveals a heliotrope discoloration of bilateral eyelids with mild periorbital edema and Gottron's papules over her elbows, knees, dorsal proximal interphalangeal (PIP) joints, and metacarpophalangeal (MCP) joints bilaterally. Nailbed capillaroscopy reveals mild dilation and tortuosity of the vessels. The patient has significant proximal muscle weakness bilaterally, including a mild head lag and Trendelenberg gait. Initial laboratory evaluation reveals a creatine phophokinase (CPK) of 11,782, aldolase of 168, lactate dehydrogenase (LDH) of 1402, and aspartate aminotransferase (AST) of 1064.

Differential Diagnosis

The differential diagnosis of JDM differs greatly from inflammatory myositis seen in adults. Children very rarely have polymyositis, focal myositis, inclusion body myositis, eosinophilic myositis, or dermatomyositis associated with malignancy. More commonly, etiologies to consider are postinfectious myositis, primary neuromuscular myopathies, and inflammatory myopathies associated with other connective tissue diseases including scleroderma and mixed connective tissue disease. Acute, transient, postinfectious myositis may follow various infections including viruses, particularly influenza A/B,

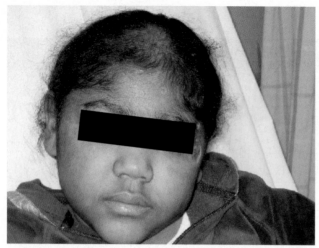

Figure 19-1. Alopecia and heliotrope discoloration, with vasculitic infarcts and ulceration, in an 8-year-old girl with juvenile dermatomyositis.

coxsackievirus B and varicella; or bacterial infections such as staphylococcal or streptococcal bacteremia. These illnesses are typically preceded by fever, symptoms of upper respiratory infection (URI), nausea, vomiting and headache. Myalgias in viral myositis are more commonly found in the proximal calf and may result in transient elevations of muscle specific enzymes. Similarly, myositis secondary to bacterial infections, are typically transient; however, complications with localized abscess formation may occur. In contrast, primary neuromuscular myopathies, such as Duchenne's muscular dystrophy, often lack constitutional symptoms and muscle tenderness. Instead, they are often characterized by marked elevation of serum CPK levels, slowly progressive proximal muscle weakness, and hypertrophy of distal

muscles, particularly the calves. Suspicion for these disorders should be elevated in cases of younger children with an absence of characteristic skin changes, loss of developmental milestones, and a positive family history. Electromyographic findings or muscle biopsy pathology are often necessary for diagnostic purposes. Finally, children with connective tissue diseases such as SLE, scleroderma, and mixed connective tissue disease may have skin and muscle involvement that may initially appear similar to those seen in JDM, however, additional organ manifestations and serologic laboratory evaluations should provide further definitive diagnostic information. Overall, the presence of the characteristic rash, proximal muscle weakness, and elevated muscle enzymes is often sufficient to make the diagnosis; however, in certain cases muscle histopathology not only aids in diagnosis but also may provide evidence of prognostic features, including perifascicular myopathy, obvious capillary loss, central nucleation of myofibers, necrosis, and fibrosis (Fig. 19-2).[2] Reports suggest that the pathogenesis of vasculopathy seen in JDM may be secondary to an imbalance between angiostatic and angiogenic chemokines within muscle, resulting in significantly higher levels of interferon-induced angiostatic chemokines, which often parallels the degree of vasculopathy.[3]

Treatment

Historically, outcomes in JDM varied dramatically; with one third of patients spontaneously recovering, one third developing moderate to severe disability, and the final third eventually succumbing to the illness. In the 1970s, with the introduction of corticosteroids as the mainstay of treatment in JDM, functional outcomes and mortality have

Figure 19-2. Muscle biopsy in a patient with juvenile dermatomyositis revealing capillary loss, variable myofiber atrophy, infarct and central nuclei. (From Miles L, Bove KE, Lovell D, Wargula JC, Bukulmez H, Shao M, et al. Predictability of the clinical course of juvenile dermatomyositis based on initial muscle biopsy: a retrospective study of 72 patients. Arthritis Care Res 2007;57:1183-91.)

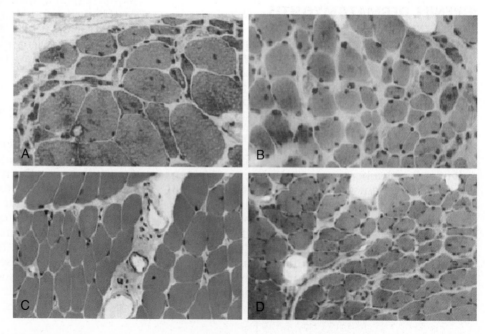

significantly improved. Owing to the lack of randomized, controlled clinical trials, management depends primarily on information from retrospective reviews, observational data, and clinical experience. In an emergent setting, adequacy of ventilatory effort, swallowing ability, and risk of aspiration must be rapidly assessed and aggressively treated. Over time, goals of therapy should be aimed at suppression of both clinical and laboratory signs of immunoinflammatory response, preservation of muscle strength and function, and prevention of long-term complications, including calcinosis, lipodystrophy and functional disability.

Assessment of treatment efficacy is often measured in terms of frequent assessments of muscle strength and function, as well as improvement in serum concentrations of muscle enzymes. Collaborative study groups have standardized and validated clinical disease activity scales including the Childhood Myositis Assessment Scale (CMAS) as a tool to assess adequate clinical response to treatment.[4-6] In addition, muscle enzymes are frequently monitored; however, individual enzyme levels do not always correlate with disease activity. In particular, creatine kinase may be the poorest predictor of disease exacerbation, whereas LDH and AST, although less specific, more often mirror disease activity.[7] The measurement of immunologic and endothelial activation markers, including von Willebrand's factor antigen, neopterin, mononuclear cell subsets, cytokines, and adhesion molecules may also have a role in the assessment of disease activity; however there is not yet general acceptance of these latter biomarkers.[8,9] Changes seen in magnetic resonance imaging (MRI) scans, particularly short tau inversion recovery or fat-suppressed T2-weighted images, may be a more sensitive, quantitative assessment of initial muscle inflammation and subsequent recovery following treatment (Fig. 19-3).[10,11] Changes in dermatologic manifestations seem to correlate moderately with changes in measures of muscle inflammation;

however, skin improvement is unpredictable and therefore should not guide therapeutic decisions.[5]

Corticosteroids

Early and adequate treatment with high-dose oral corticosteroids has been widely accepted as a critical component in the management of JDM. Typically, patients receive prednisone (up to 2 mg/kg/day divided into two to three doses) for 2 months, with close monitoring for resolution of both clinical and laboratory manifestations. With an adequate response evident, corticosteroids are then slowly tapered over a 2-year period.[12] Several studies also suggest that aggressive initial management with intravenous (IV) pulse corticosteroids may result in a more favorable outcome.[13-16] The proposed rationale is to gain rapid control of inflammation, preventing both acute and chronic complications, and in the long-term, minimizing chronic corticosteroid use and associated toxicity. In addition, early aggressive management may induce earlier disease remission and greatly decrease hospitalizations.[17] Further justification suggests that a likely gastrointestinal vasculopathy in active JDM may impair oral corticosteroid absorption therefore impairing efficacy.[18] In contrast, data reported in a retrospective, propensity score analysis did not support any significant difference in efficacy outcomes between standard therapy with oral prednisone and aggressive management with IV corticosteroids.[19]

Despite significant improvements in prognosis of JDM, calcinosis remains a considerable source of long-term morbidity (Figs. 19-4 and 19-5). It appears that calcinosis is significantly correlated with a longer time to diagnosis and overall longer active disease duration.[13] Retrospective data and observational studies are somewhat inconsistent; however, the majority indicate that early treatment with IV methylprednisolone (30 mg/kg), followed by high-dose oral corticosteroids may be associated with a more rapid normalization of muscle

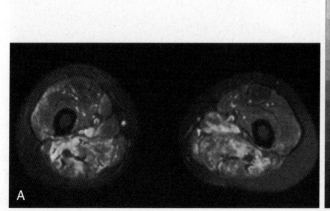
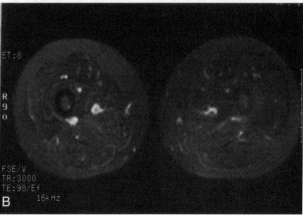

Figure 19-3. A, Fat-suppressed T2-weighted magnetic resonance imaging (MRI) scan before initiation of therapy in a 7-year-old patient with juvenile dermatomyositis. Hyperintense signal can be noted predominantly in the hamstrings bilaterally, as well as the quadriceps muscles. **B,** Follow up T2-weighted MRI in the same patient after treatment with corticosteroids and methotrexate showing attenuation of abnormal signal.

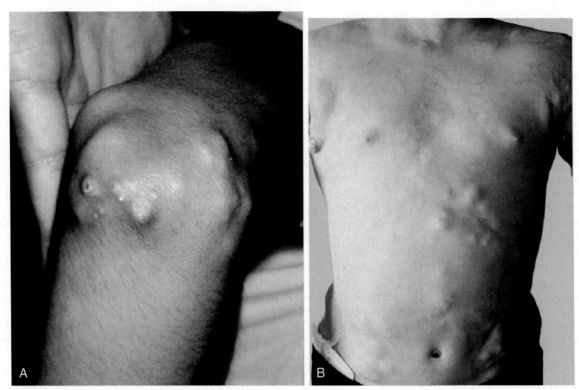

Figure 19-4. **A,** Calcinosis circumscripta—superficial plaques of dystrophic calcium deposition in subcutaneous tissue in a patient with juvenile dermatomyositis. **B,** Tumoral calcinosis (i.e., calcinosis universalis)–nodular calcium deposits into deeper tissue layers. (Courtesy of Dr. Lisa G. Rider, MD, NIH.)

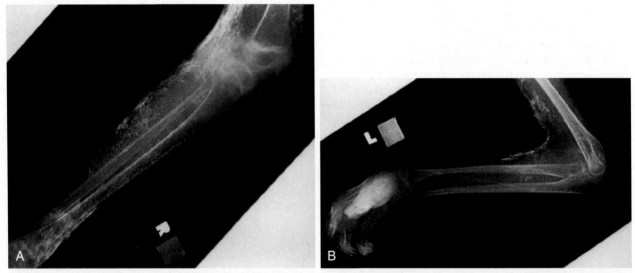

Figure 19-5. **A,** Radiographic evidence of planar calcinosis in the arm of a patient with juvenile dermatomyositis. **B,** Further delineation of interfascial deposition of calcium in the same patient.

enzymes, earlier clinical remission, and therefore, decreased incidence of calcinosis.[13,14,20] Similarly, some studies propose that intermittent IV methylprednisolone pulses given on a weekly to monthly basis many induce remission more rapidly.[13,21] Retrospective reviews, in which a reduction of calcinosis was not significantly associated with initial management with IV methylprednisolone, noted

the likelihood of higher disease severity in these patients and, therefore, the increased risk of long-term complications.[19,22]

Despite the enormous benefits gained from corticosteroids, long-term use is often associated with undesirable steroid toxicity. Among others, side effects that may limit therapy include significant osteopenia, osteoporosis, avascular necrosis of bone, compression fractures, Cushing's syndrome, growth retardation, and steroid myopathy. Subsequent management and the institution of additional immunosuppressant medications often aim to reduce corticosteroid dose while maintaining adequate disease control. The addition of calcium and vitamin D appears to be beneficial in the reduction of bone loss; however, they may be insufficient in the management of severe osteoporosis. In contrast, calcitonin and bisphosphonates have been shown to be effective in the treatment of adults with osteoporosis; however, use in children is limited due to unknown long-term effects on growing bone.[23,24] At present, there is an increasing body of evidence that bisphosphonates are relatively safe in the treatment of osteoporosis in children with rheumatic and metabolic bone disease.[24]

Hydroxychloroquine

Based primarily on anecdotal evidence, hydroxychloroquine (6 mg/kg/day) has been recommended as a steroid-sparing agent, particularly in patients with prominent dermatologic manifestations.[25,26] In general, hydroxychloroquine is considered a safe, well-tolerated medication. Side effects may include gastrointestinal intolerance, headache, lightheadedness, and skin hyperpigmentation. Rarely, retinal toxicity may occur; therefore, all children should have routine ophthalmologic monitoring assessing for changes in visual acuity, visual fields, color vision, and retinal changes.[27]

Methotrexate

Second-line medications, including immunosuppressive agents, are typically considered as adjunctive therapy in cases of steroid resistance, steroid dependence or unacceptable steroid toxicity. Of all the immunosuppressive drugs, methotrexate (MTX) is widely used as the preferred agent for refractory JDM (0.35–2 mg/kg/week; max dose = 50 mg). More recently, MTX has also been recommended as a component of initial therapy to additionally improve clinical outcome.[21,28] Experience from the use of low-dose MTX in other pediatric rheumatologic diseases has proven its safety and limited long-term toxicity.[29] Several small, uncontrolled, retrospective studies have also shown efficacy of MTX in JDM, demonstrating decreased disease activity, decreased calcinosis, as well as a more rapid discontinuation of corticosteroids and therefore decreased steroid toxicity.[13,21,28,30] Initially, MTX is often administered orally, with a change to subcutaneous administration should gastrointestinal side effects evolve.[28] In cases of suspected gastrointestinal vasculopathy with potentially impaired absorption, some authors may propose an earlier change to parenteral administration due to greater bioavailability. Overall, MTX is generally well tolerated, with typical side effects including gastrointestinal intolerance, risk of infection and hepatotoxicity.[29] Although potentially a concern, these effects are often transient and resolve with discontinuation of the drug.[21,28] In cases of

persistent gastrointestinal intolerance, leucovorin (5 mg given 24 hours following the weekly dose of MTX) may be given to reduce potential toxicity.

Cytotoxic Agents

In addition to MTX, other immunosuppressive agents used in refractory JDM include azathioprine (AZA), cyclophosphamide (CYC), cyclosporine, and mycophenolate mofetil (MMF). Of these agents, the greatest amount of published evidence available for the use of these agents in JDM is for cyclosporine therapy (3–5 mg/kg/day); however these data are primarily based on case reports and retrospective reviews.[31,32] These reports generally reveal favorable outcomes; however, the benefits must be weighed against the risks of side effects, particularly renal impairment, hypertension, and hepatotoxicity. Although few studies exist, some authors suggest AZA (1–3 mg/kg/day) may be as efficacious and a potentially safe steroid-sparing agent should MTX fail.[4,33] Similarly, CYC (1 mg/kg/day oral or 0.5–1 g/m²/month IV) is seen as a potentially effective medication with minimal evidence of serious toxicity in short-term use, however mixed results have been seen in adult dermatomyositis.[34] Potential side effects of CYC include alopecia, cytopenias, bladder toxicity, gastrointestinal intolerance, and infertility. In addition, there have been some recent reports suggesting the benefits of MMF with generally few side effects.[35]

Intravenous Immunoglobulin

Intravenous immunoglobulin (IVIG) has been shown to be a safe and effective treatment in adults with dermatomyositis. Potential mechanisms of action of IVIG in autoimmune and inflammatory disorders are not fully understood, but data suggest that they involve modulation of expression and/or function of Fc receptors, increased activity of complement or proinflammatory cytokines, idiotype/anti-idiotype interactions, and effects of T, B, and dendritic cells.[36] In a small, double-blinded, placebo-controlled trial, IVIG was shown to result in significant improvement in muscle strength, neuromuscular symptoms and histologic findings on muscle biopsy.[37] In children, however, there are no controlled clinical trials, evidence is therefore based on retrospective reviews and anecdotal reports.[38–40] These reports concluded that IVIG (1–2 g/kg/month) is beneficial in reducing clinical manifestations and sparing corticosteroid toxicity in cases of severe, refractory JDM. It appears that repeated treatments may be necessary for long-term benefits due to a tendency for relapse after the cessation of IVIG.[37,40] Administration of IVIG to immunoglobulin A (IgA)–deficient patients may result in anaphylaxis; therefore, IgA levels should be routinely measured before administration, or as soon as possible if immediate use is indicated. In addition, reports suggest that children, particularly those with autoimmune disorders, may have increased incidence of side effects including fever, nausea, and vomiting. This may be related to concentrations of IgA more than 15 µg/mL; therefore, preparations with lower concentrations of IgA are preferred (Gammagard, Baxter, Deerfield, IL; 2.2 µg/mL).[41] Other potential side effects include headache and aseptic meningitis.

Biologic Agents

Tumor necrosis factor-α (TNF-α) has been identified in high levels in patients with JDM, particularly in those with a prolonged disease course or complicated by calcinosis.[42] The use of TNF-α inhibitors, particularly infliximab (6–10 mg/kg via infusions every 4–8 weeks) and etanercept (0.8 mg/kg; max 50 mg/week), appear to show promising results in severe, refractory JDM. Few small clinical trials have been published suggesting clinical benefits, including improved muscle weakness, joint range of motion, and regression of calcinosis.[43,44] Similarly, rituximab, a monoclonal antibody to B cells, may have clinical benefits; however, clinical trials are still underway.[45,46] In very severe cases of JDM that are recalcitrant to other therapies, plasmapheresis may also be considered.[47]

Supportive Measures

In addition to the therapies listed earlier, supportive measures including skin care for ulcerations, nutritional assessments for risk of aspiration and malnutrition, psychological support and education, and physical therapy are essential in the management of patients with JDM. Despite active inflammation, physical therapy should be initiated at the time of diagnosis with passive range-of-motion exercises to prevent decreased range of motion. Once acute inflammation has subsided; active, muscle-strengthening exercises should be gradually introduced to minimize muscle atrophy and contractures.

One of the major aims of treatment in JDM is to avoid long-term complications, including calcinosis and lipodystrophy (Fig. 19-6). Once these complications develop, there are no treatments that have proven to be consistently effective. Case reports and anecdotal evidence suggest that therapies including colchicine, warfarin, bisphosphonates, probenecid, diltiazem, and aluminum hydroxide may offer variable responses in the management of calcinosis.[48] The authors have had some success with treatment with colchicine, especially when superficial calcinosis lesions cause ulceration and crystal-induced cellulitis. It should also be noted that calcinosis is often complicated by concurrent infection, and appropriate antibiotic administration can be critical. In addition, there is generalized consensus that early aggressive control of active disease inflammation; using corticosteroids, MTX, IVIG, and cytotoxic agents have a preventative role in the formation and progression of calcinosis. In some cases, calcinosis may spontaneously regress; however, depending on location, in rare cases surgical excision may

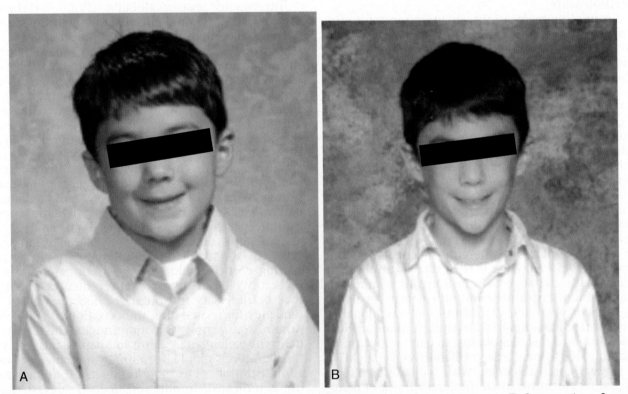

Figure 19-6. A, Six-year-old boy who was ultimately diagnosed with juvenile dermatomyositis. **B,** Same patient, 2 years later (age 8) showing significant facial lipodystrophy. Note absence of subcutaneous fat in the malar areas. Similar loss of fat was present in the extremities.

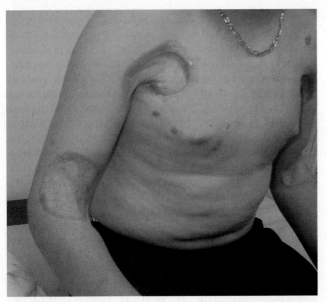

Figure 19-7. Skin grafting after excision of large tumoral calcinosis lesions in the axillae and antecubital fossae of an adolescent boy with juvenile dermatomyositis.

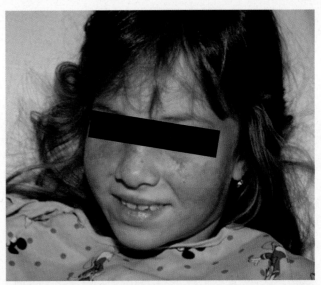

Figure 19-8. Malar rash in a 9-year-old girl with juvenile systemic lupus erythematosus.

be required (Fig. 19-7). In addition, careful monitoring must be performed in the prevention of serious infections potentially associated with calcinosis and ulceration.

SYSTEMIC LUPUS ERYTHEMATOSUS

SLE is a chronic, autoimmune disease often characterized by the presence of widespread inflammation, multiorgan system involvement and an episodic course of disease flare and remission. For the most part, clinical features of pediatric SLE are similar to those in adult-onset SLE; therefore, for the purposes of this chapter, we focus on features unique to childhood disease and highlight differences in presentation, treatment, and prognosis between the two groups. Of all patients diagnosed with SLE, it is estimated that approximately 15% to 20% have disease onset in childhood, with the highest proportion in adolescence, female gender, positive family history and those of Native American, black, and Hispanic descent. Constitutional symptoms including unexplained fever, malaise, weight loss, rash and arthritis/arthralgias are the most common manifestations of SLE in children and adolescents (Figs. 19-8 and 19-9). In addition, many children may have evidence of hematologic, neurologic, or cardiopulmonary involvement on presentation; renal disease, however, remains a major cause of morbidity and mortality, with more than 75% of children having some form of clinically evident nephritis.

Children with SLE are often reported to have a more aggressive clinical course with more significant internal organ involvement than adult-onset disease.[49,50] Despite this, with medical advances in treatment and monitoring, the overall long-term

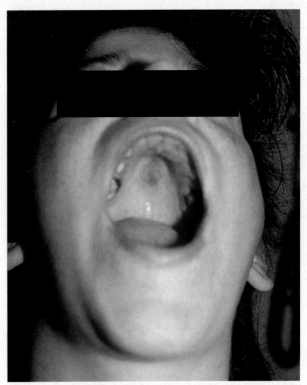

Figure 19-9. Classic palatal ulceration in an adolescent female with juvenile systemic lupus erythematosus.

prognosis has greatly improved over the years. Satisfactory outcome in children currently depends on an estimated 50- to 60-year survival time, resulting in a prolonged duration of potential disease burden and treatment-related morbidity. Assessments of disease activity and nonreversible damage that were developed for adults have been validated in children and include the SLE Disease Activity Index (SLEDAI), the Systemic Lupus Activity Measure

(SLAM), the British Isles Lupus Assessment Group Activity Index (BILAG), and the Systemic Lupus International Clinics Damage Index (SLICC). Specific limitations, however, exist with regard to use in children including the variation in the definition of and significance given to the presence of renal involvement, the lack of clearly defined cognitive impairment (including behavioral changes and school failure), and the significance of prolonged corticosteroid therapy both on overall prognosis and long-term morbidity (including musculoskeletal and neurocognitive growth and development).[49,51]

CASE STUDY 2

A 16-year-old girl, with no significant past medical history, presents with a history of prolonged fever of unknown etiology, fatigue, malaise, and a 10-pound weight loss over the last three weeks. She notes mild pain in her fingers bilaterally, and has noticed progressive difficulty writing in her morning classes at school. In addition, she has experienced a decline in school performance, which she attributes to her fatigue, recurrent school absences, and "not being able to focus and remember things as I used to." Review of systems reveals recent hair loss and daily headaches. Physical exam reveals a thin female with prominent frontal alopecia. Head, eye, ear, nose, and throat (HEENT) examination reveals mild malar erythema, normal fundoscopic exam and enlarged cervical lymphadenopathy bilaterally. Musculoskeletal examination reveals tenderness, swelling, and erythema of the PIP joints bilaterally, as well as bilateral knee effusions. Laboratory evaluation reveals anemia, mild lymphopenia, highly elevated erythrocyte sedimentation rate (ESR) and a normal CRP. Urinalysis reveals proteinuria with a urine protein/urine creatinine elevated to 1.2. Further evaluation reveals an antinuclear antibody level of 1:320 speckled, increased anti-dsDNA, increased anti-SSa (Ro), and reduced levels of C3 and C4.

Differential Diagnosis

The differential diagnosis of SLE is extensive and highly variable based on clinical presentation. Among the vast differential diagnosis, the presence of nonspecific, constitutional symptoms including fever, malaise, and weight loss, often compel physicians to exclude other chronic and potentially life-threatening diagnoses including malignancy (particularly leukemia and lymphoma), infectious disease (such as human immunodeficiency virus [HIV], tuberculosis, Epstein-Barr virus [EBV], cytomegalovirus [CMV]), primary immunodeficiency, endocrinopathies (such as hypo/hyperthyroidism) and other rheumatologic disorders.

Treatment

Owing to the potential for more severe disease, major organ involvement, longer disease burden, and morbidity of chronic corticosteroid use in pediatric SLE many physicians would support a more aggressive approach at the onset of disease and an earlier introduction of steroid toxicity–sparing agents. Challenges of management specific to adolescents with SLE include issues of defiance, noncompliance with therapy, fear of corticosteroid impact on body image, and impact of disease manifestations and frequent hospital visits on school performance.

General supportive treatment measures include establishing a multidisciplinary approach to care, providing psychosocial support, avoidance of unnecessary limitations on activity, and optimizing each individual's childhood experience. Dietary counseling as well as supplementation with vitamins including calcium, vitamin D, and folic acid are important adjuvants to therapy, aiding in reduction of complications such as excessive weight gain, osteoporosis and atherosclerosis. In addition, all patients with SLE are advised to use sunscreen (SPF 30 or greater) with ultraviolet A and ultraviolet B protection year round, both indoors and outdoors, to prevent disease exacerbation. Finally, pneumococcal and meningococcal vaccination is highly recommended secondary to an increased incidence of functional asplenia among children with lupus.

Nonsteroidal Anti-Inflammatory Drugs

Nonsteroidal anti-inflammatory drugs (NSAIDs) are primarily used in pediatric SLE for fever and mild musculoskeletal manifestations, including arthritis, myalgias, and arthralgias.[52] Aspirin (ASA), another potential therapeutic option in these scenarios, is less commonly used in children due to the potential for hepatotoxicity and Reye's syndrome. Toxicity from NSAIDs is limited; however, risks most often include gastritis, decreased glomerular filtration rate, and rarely aseptic meningitis. Pseudoporphyria has also been described in children using naproxen.[53]

Antimalarials

Hydroxychloroquine (6 mg/kg/day, max 400 mg/day) is routinely used at the onset of disease in children and adolescents with SLE to reduce symptoms of fatigue, mucocutaneous manifestations, and alopecia, as well as a steroid toxicity–sparing agent. Efficacy of antimalarials in SLE has been demonstrated in clinically stable adults, with removal of the drug, resulting in increased incidence of disease activity. Although typically well tolerated, the primary concern in the use of hydroxychloroquine is the rare incidence of retinal toxicity; therefore, yearly ophthalmologic monitoring is indicated.

Corticosteroids

The introduction of corticosteroids as the mainstay of treatment has greatly improved the prognosis in children with SLE, allowing for a more rapid control of acute manifestations and increased overall life expectancy.[54-56] Depending on initial presentation, high-dose oral corticosteroids (prednisone 1–2 mg/kg/day, divided into two doses to maximize antiinflammatory effects) are often initiated, particularly in cases of major organ involvement including renal, central nervous system (CNS), pulmonary and hematologic manifestations. In cases of severe CNS or renal involvement, IV methylprednisolone (30 mg/kg/day for 3 consecutive days) may be indicated to achieve a more rapid resolution of symptoms.[57,58] In addition, intermittent monthly doses of intravenous methylprednisolone may aid in the long-term management of these patients while decreasing overall corticosteroid use and associated toxicity.

Although many children will respond to treatment with corticosteroids, complications often arise with prolonged use, including adrenal suppression, hypertension, hyperglycemia, cataracts, avascular necrosis, myopathy, CNS disturbances, immunosuppression, and dislipoproteinemia.[59] Among the most concerning toxicities in children is the risk of significant osteopenia, osteoporosis, and growth retardation. In addition, alterations in emotional liability and physical appearance due to cushingoid facies, obesity, hirsuitism, and acne, may have significant impact on adolescent psychosocial well-being. Therefore, early introduction of a slow, gradual taper of corticosteroids while maintaining adequate disease control is critical. Steroid toxicity–sparing strategies may also include consolidation to a single morning dose initially and eventual reduction to alternate-day therapy.

Immunosuppressive Agents

The addition of an immunosuppressive or cytotoxic agent is often indicated in cases of proliferative glomerulonephritis, CNS involvement (Fig. 19-10), and pulmonary hemorrhage; as well as with evidence of steroid dependence or unacceptable steroid toxicity. Common immunosuppressive agents currently used in pediatric SLE are CYC, AZA, cyclosporine, MMF, and MTX.

CYC has been considered the adjunctive therapy of choice for the most severe manifestations of SLE, particularly severe proliferative lupus nephritis and CNS disease, often resulting in reduced disease activity, preservation of renal and neurological function and overall reduction in corticosteroid dose.[60-62] Although there have been no randomized, controlled trials in children, several case series and comparative studies have similarly reported efficacy and superiority over AZA or prednisone alone.[58,63-66] Significant toxicity limits use in less severe cases, and caution must be taken in monitoring for bone marrow suppression, infection, alopecia, nausea, vomiting, and hemorrhagic cystitis. The incidence of alopecia, a potentially distressing complication

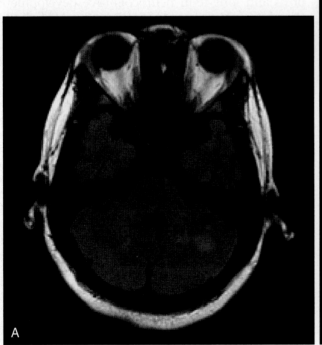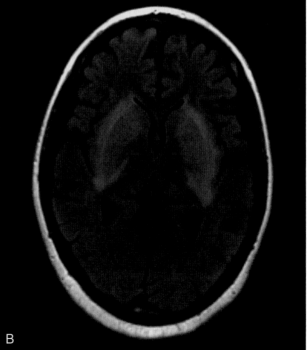

Figure 19-10. **A,** Magnetic resonance imaging scan with increased signal abnormality in the left cerebellar white matter in a 14-year-old patient with systemic lupus erythematosus and focal dysmetria. **B,** Evidence of bilateral signal abnormality in the basal ganglia of the same patient.

in adolescents, may be reduced with the use of scalp-cooling techniques including cryogel packs, cold air circulation, and specialized caps with liquid coolant circulation.[67] Long-term risks including secondary malignancy may be higher than that in adults; whereas permanent gonadal damage has been reported to be lower in the pediatric population. Although data are limited in children, semen cryopreservation and gonadotropin-releaseing hormone (GnRH)–analogs may provide additional protection in adolescents receiving CYC.[68] Typically IV CYC (0.5–1 g/m²/month), given in an induction phase of seven monthly doses, followed by a maintenance phase of one dose every 3 months for 2 years, is preferred over oral CYC to reduce overall cumulative toxicity.[65]

In cases of mild to moderate organ involvement other, less toxic, immunosuppressive agents may be necessary to obtain better disease control and reduced corticosteroid dosing. AZA (1–2 mg/kg/day, max 150 mg/day), has been used most frequently in pediatric SLE as an effective steroid-sparing agent with limited toxicity, including potential hematologic and gastrointestinal side effects.[69] Controversy exists regarding efficacy in proliferative SLE nephritis; however, some reports suggest sustained disease remission with decreased long-term toxicity when used as maintenance therapy following CYC induction.[62,70,71] Similarly, cyclosporine (3–5 mg/kg/day) may be an effective therapy in steroid-resistant or steroid-dependent children with SLE; however, its role in severe lupus nephritis is still undetermined.[72,73] Potential for hypertension and nephrotoxicity with cyclosporine may further limit use in these cases.[74] Recent experience with MMF (1–3 g/day) in pediatric SLE has shown promising results, particularly in cases of class V membranous glomerulonephritis and as maintenance therapy following CYC induction in cases of proliferative glomerulonephritis.[71,75,76] Further reports suggest that MMF may be as effective as CYC with significantly less toxicity in adults with proliferative lupus nephritis; however, long-term data regarding risks and benefits, and use in pediatric SLE are still to be determined.[76-78] Finally, the use of MTX has been suggested in the management of persistent arthritis and skin disease; however, sole use may be insufficient to control disease flare in cases of major organ system involvement.[69,79,80]

Biologic Agents

Many biologic agents are currently being evaluated in adults with refractory SLE; however, data in pediatrics remain limited. Rituximab, an anti-CD20 monoclonal antibody (375–500 mg/m²/dose IV for two doses given 2 weeks apart) may be effective in treatment of severe autoimmune cytopenia and potentially as an adjunct to therapy in refractory nephritis.[81-86] Interpretation of this data is difficult owing to the use of other immunosuppressive agents simultaneously with rituximab. Other agents, such as IVIG, B-cell modulators (LJP 394), anti-interleukin 10 monoclonal antibodies, and therapies targeted against CD-40/CD-40 ligand and CTLA4-Ig are currently being investigated.[87,88]

Other Considerations

Children with SLE often show signs of dyslipoproteinemia, with evidence of elevated triglycerides and decreased high-density lipoproteins (HDLs), which may predispose them to early atherosclerosis and early cardiovascular sequelae.[89,90] Therefore, routine screening is indicated, with early intervention with diet and exercise if levels are abnormal. In some cases. pharmacologic intervention with statins and bile acid sequestrants may be necessary. In addition, hydroxychloroquine may have some beneficial lipid-lowering effects.[91]

ANTIPHOSPHOLIPID ANTIBODY SYNDROME

Antiphospholipid antibody syndrome (APLS) is characterized by the presence of antiphospholipid antibodies in association with clinical signs of hypercoagulability, including arterial/venous thrombosis, pulmonary embolism, and stroke. Children with APLS are more likely to exhibit clinical manifestations including migraine, chorea, epilepsy, thrombocytopenia and hemolytic anemia. In addition, there is evidence that maternal antiphospholipid antibodies can cross the placenta and may have a partial role in the pathogenesis of neonatal thrombosis and long-term neurocognitive development; therefore, infants born to mothers with APLS should be closely monitored with routine neurodevelopmental monitoring.[92,93]

There are limited data on management of pediatric APLS; therefore, recommendations are made primarily based on adult-based literature and algorithms.[94] In general, therapeutic options of anticoagulation are chosen largely based on the presence of prior arterial or venous thrombosis. Children with serologic evidence of antiphospholipid antibodies who are asymptomatic typically do not require treatment. Antibodies must be confirmed on at least two occasions due to the incidence of transient, inconsequential elevations in antiphospholipid antibodies with many bacterial and viral infections in childhood, such as mycoplasma, parvovirus, cytomegalovirus, varicella zoster, HIV, staphylococcus, and streptococcus. Prophylactic treatment with low-dose ASA is typically not indicated in asymptomatic children, and caution must be taken owing to the risk of Reye's syndrome.[95] Similar to adults with APLS, the presence of arterial or venous thrombosis is an indication for anticoagulation with either low-molecular-weight heparin (LMWH) (starting at 1 mg/kg/dose every 12 hours) or coumadin (starting at 0.1–0.2 mg/kg/day;

therapeutic International Normalized Ratio [INR] of 2–3). In cases of major organ thrombosis, arterial thrombosis, recurrent thrombosis, or recurrent fetal loss, long-term anticoagulation with a higher therapeutic target (INR 3–4) may be indicated.[96,97] In addition, data are limited on the safety of anticoagulation in children; however, several reports have demonstrated that LMWH appears to be safe and efficacious in both the treatment and prophylaxis of thromboembolism in children.[98-100]

NEONATAL LUPUS ERYTHEMATOSUS

Neonatal lupus erythematosus (NLE) is a rare syndrome caused by the transplacental passage of autoantibodies directed against Ro and La proteins, most commonly resulting in cardiac, dermatologic, hematologic, and hepatic manifestations. Although mothers with positive autoantibodies are at risk, only 1% to 3% of infants will actually develop the syndrome. The most severe complication associated with NLE is the development of complete congenital heart block, which occurs in 15% to 30% of infants with NLE. Cardiac manifestations are thought to be secondary to direct attack on fetal cardiocytes with prolonged inflammation and eventual fibrosis (Fig. 19-11). Once scarring has developed, cardiac effects are essentially irreversible and mortality may occur in up to 30% of infants. Early detection with serial echocardiograms is critical, and interven-tion with fluorinated steroids (oral dexamethasone 4 mg/day) with or without IVIG may be beneficial in reducing early inflammation.[101-104] In addition, persistent fetal bradycardia in utero may require the use of sympathomimetics or inotropic agents.[105,106] Infants born with symptomatic congenital heart block require permanent pacemaker insertion shortly after delivery, whereas those who are asymptomatic may be cautiously monitored. Owing to the high incidence of morbidity and mortality in these patients, pacemaker placement is often required before the end of childhood.[107] Other manifestations of NLE including discoid skin lesions, occurring primarily on the face, scalp, and neck (Fig. 19-12); cytopenias and hepatic inflammation are reversible and typically resolve spontaneously. Occasionally, topical corticosteroids may be used to hasten the resolution of the dermatologic manifestations.

CHILDHOOD VASCULITIC SYNDROMES

Kawasaki Disease

KD, one of the most common vasculitides of childhood, is a febrile systemic vasculitis, characterized by inflammation in small and medium sized vessels. Typically, KD occurs in children younger than 5 years old, with an increased incidence in persons of Asian descent. Diagnostic

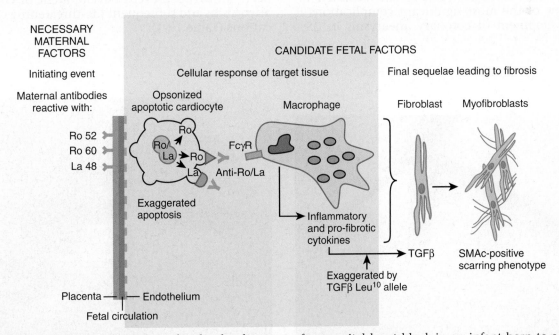

Figure 19-11. Proposed pathogenesis for the development of congenital heart block in an infant born to a mother with anti-Ro and anti-La antibodies. (Redrawn from Clancy RM, Buyon JP. Autoimmune-associated congenital heart block: dissecting the cascade from immunologic insult to relentless fibrosis. Anat Rec A Discov Mol Cell Evol Biol 2004;280:1027-35.)

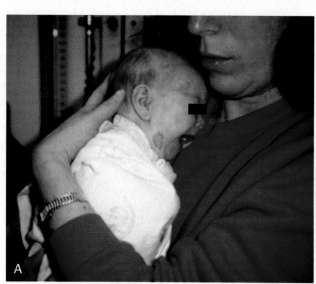

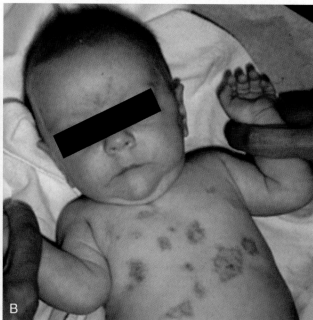

Figure 19-12. A, Classic discoid skin lesions in a 2-week-old infant with neonatal lupus erythematosus, noted predominantly on the face and scalp. **B,** Evidence of the rash on the trunk of the same infant.

criteria require fever for more than 5 days' duration, plus four of the following: bilateral conjunctival injection, oral mucous membrane changes (injection, fissured lips and/or strawberry tongue), peripheral extremity changes (erythema, swelling or desquamation), polymorphous rash, and cervical lymphadenopathy greater than 1.5 cm (Figs. 19-13 and 19-14). Although typically a self-limited illness, one of the most significant complications is the development of coronary aneurysms in 25%

of untreated patients, making KD one of the most common causes of acquired heart disease in children in the developed world. Demonstration of coronary artery aneurysms in children whose febrile illness did not fulfill diagnostic criteria has led to the concept of incomplete or atypical KD. Proper diagnosis of these patients is critical, because treatment has been shown to prevent development of coronary aneurysms and subsequent life-threatening complications (Table 19-1).

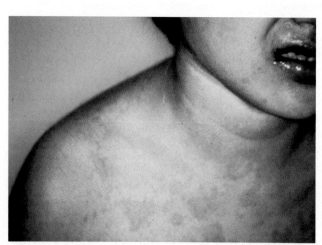

Figure 19-13. Erythematous, fissured lips (cheilosis) and polymorphous exanthem in a child with Kawasaki's disease.

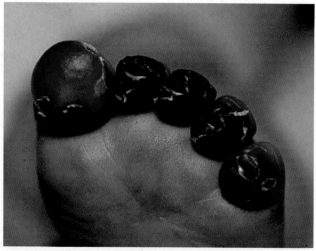

Figure 19-14. Desquamation and vasculitic infarcts in the foot of a patient with Kawasaki's disease. (Courtesy of Dr. Robert Sundel.)

CASE STUDY 3

A 2-year-old boy presents with a fever for 6 days. According to the mother, the patient has been very cranky. She notes mild rhinorrhea at the onset of symptoms, followed by the development of conjunctival erythema, cracked lips and an erythematous diaper rash. On physical examination, the patient is irritable, but nontoxic in appearance. Skin examination reveals an erythematous, macular rash in the perineal region with early signs of desquamation. HEENT exam reveals bilateral, nonexudative conjunctivitis with limbic sparing, dry lips and a strawberry tongue. The remainder of the physical examination is benign. Laboratory evaluation reveals significantly elevated ESR and CRP levels. In addition, the patient has normochromic, normocytic anemia, elevated liver transaminases and sterile pyuria on urinalysis. Based on the algorithm set forth by the American Heart Association (see Fig. 19-15), the patient met criteria for atypical KD. He was subsequently treated and underwent echocardiogram for further evaluation.

Table 19-1. *Clinical Features of Kawasaki's Disease*

Fever persisting for 5 days or more
Presence of at least four principal clinical features
   Bilateral conjunctival injection without exudate
   Polymorphous exanthem
   Cervical lymphadenopathy (at least one node greater
     than 1.5 cm)
   Oropharyngeal changes including erythema, dry/fissured
     lips, strawberry tongue, injected pharyngeal mucosa
   Changes in extremities including erythema and/or
     edema of the hands and feet (acute) and periungal
     peeling of fingers (subacute)
Exclusion of other disease processes

Differential Diagnosis

The differential diagnosis of KD, at the onset of disease, includes a wide spectrum of illnesses commonly associated with fever and mucocutaneous manifestations. The differential diagnosis includes, but is not limited to, viral infections, toxin-mediated illnesses, immune reactions and other rheumatologic diseases. Viral illnesses, including measles, EBV, and adenovirus may have similar mucocutaneous manifestations; however, these illnesses generally lack extremity and cardiac involvement. In contrast, toxin-mediated illnesses, particularly group A streptococcal infections such as scarlet fever and toxic shock syndrome, may have significant signs of inflammation and major organ involvement. These illnesses, however, often lack the ocular and articular involvement seen in KD. Other infections, such as Rocky Mountain spotted fever, differ due to a predominance of headaches and gastrointestinal complaints. Finally, immune reactions such as Stevens-Johnson syndrome, serum sickness, and rheumatologic diseases including systemic-onset

juvenile idiopathic arthritis, can mimic KD; however, subtle differences are seen in ocular and mucosal manifestations.

Treatment

KD is an acute, self-limited illness, which often resolves spontaneously in less than 2 weeks without therapy. However, persistent vascular inflammation may result in the development of coronary artery aneurysms with the potential to cause severe complications and significant long-term morbidity and mortality. In general, goals of therapy include control of acute inflammation, resolution of symptoms and prevention of long-term sequelae. The American Academy of Pediatrics and the American Heart Association currently recommend that first-line therapy of KD should include high-dose ASA and IVIG given within the first 10 days of illness.[108] In cases of suspected incomplete KD, algorithms developed by consensus, have been proposed to aid in clinical management (Fig. 19-15).[108]

Several scoring systems have been established to identify children at highest risk of developing coronary artery abnormalities. Common presenting features in potentially high-risk patients include age younger than 1 year old, male gender, elevated white blood cell count, elevated acute phase reactants, decreased hematocrit, and decreased albumin.[109] In certain regions of Japan, these factors have been used to stratify which patients should receive treatment with IVIG. However, owing to the significant implications of inadequate treatment, all patients diagnosed with KD should be treated with IVIG and ASA, and to use laboratory markers, as well as echocardiogram findings, to determine subsequent management. Finally, there is currently growing evidence that circulating endothelial cells and endothelial microparticles, as detected by markers including E-selectin and CD-105, are significantly elevated in active childhood systemic vasculitis, particularly in patients with KD and coronary artery abnormalities as compared with children with inactive vasculitis, febrile illnesses and healthy controls.[110,111] In addition, significant reduction in E-selectin and CD-104 were better predictors of response than ESR and CRP further suggesting potential use as a clinical biomarker.[110]

Aspirin

ASA was the first medication used in KD owing to its anti-inflammatory and antiplatelet properties. During the acute phase of illness, high-dose ASA (80 to 100 mg/kg/day divided into four doses) has important anti-inflammatory effects; however it does not seem to effect the development of coronary aneurysms.[112,113] In vitro data suggest that high dose ASA may be prothrombotic; therefore, once the patient has been afebrile for 48 to 72 hours, ASA is reduced to antithrombotic doses (3–5 mg/kg/day), which is then maintained for a minimum of 6 to 8 weeks until platelet counts normalize and echocardiogram findings remain clear of any evidence of coronary

EVALUATION OF SUSPECTED INCOMPLETE KAWASAKI DISEASE (KD)[1]

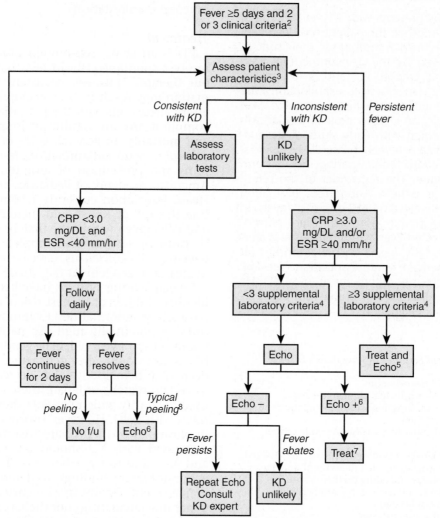

Figure 19-15. Proposed algorithm for diagnosis and management of incomplete Kawasaki's disease. (1) This algorithm represents the informed opinion of the expert committee. (2) Infants 6 months old on day 7 of fever without other explanation should undergo laboratory testing +/– echocardiogram. (3) Characteristics suggesting disease other than KD include exudative conjunctivitis, exudative pharyngitis, discrete intraoral lesions, bullous or vesicular rash, or generalized adenopathy. (4) Supplemental laboratory criteria: albumin 3.0 g/dL, anemia for age, elevation of alanine aminotransferase, platelets after 7 days 450,000/mm^3, white blood cell count 15,000/mm^3, and urine 10 white blood cells/high-power field. (5) Can treat before echocardiogram. (6) Echocardiogram is considered positive for purposes of this algorithm if any of 3 conditions are met: z score of LAD or RCA 2.5, coronary arteries meet Japanese Ministry of Health criteria for aneurysms, or 3 other suggestive features exist, including perivascular brightness, lack of tapering, decreased LV function, mitral regurgitation, pericardial effusion, or z scores in LAD or RCA of 2–2.5. (7) If the echocardiogram is positive, treatment should be given to children within 10 days of fever onset and those beyond day 10 with clinical and laboratory signs (CRP, ESR) of ongoing inflammation. (8) Typical peeling begins under nail bed of fingers and then toes. (Adapted from Newburger JW, Takahashi M, Gerber MA, Gewitz MH, Tani LY, Burns JC, et al. Diagnosis, treatment and long-term management of Kawasaki disease: A statement for health professionals from the committee on rheumatic fever, endocarditis, and Kawasaki disease, council on cardiovascular disease in the young, American Heart Association. Circulation 2004;110:2747–71.)

changes. The risks of ASA include transient hearing loss and chemical hepatitis. In addition, Reye's syndrome, a rare, but potentially fatal disease consisting of hepatitis and severe encephalopathy, may occur in children who contract the influenza virus while taking ASA; therefore, all children, who are undergoing long-term ASA therapy should receive annual influenza vaccinations.

Intravenous Immunoglobulin

The beneficial effects of IVIG in the prevention of coronary artery abnormalities in KD have been well established since the early 1980s.[114,115] Initially, doses were divided over four consecutive days, however, studies later indicated that a single, large dose (2 g/kg over 10–12 hours) resulted in significantly more rapid resolution of clinical and laboratory manifestations of inflammation, decreased incidence of coronary artery complications and decreased hospital length of stay.[113,116,117] IVIG is most effective in the reduction of coronary abnormalities when given within 10 days of the onset of fever; however, it is also recommended to treat once the diagnosis is made even after 10 days of illness have elapsed if there continues to be evidence of active inflammation. Owing to the requirement of fever for 5 days as part of diagnostic criteria, most authors accept that there is little benefit in treating patients with IVIG before day 5, showing no significant reduction in the development of coronary aneurysms.[118,119] In addition, some studies even suggest that early treatment may result in a greater requirement for additional IVIG.[118] Approximately 10% to 30% of children treated with IVIG are refractory to primary treatment. In cases of prolonged or recrudesced fever, most experts recommend repeat treatment with a second and potentially a third dose of IVIG (2 g/kg).[108,120]

Corticosteroids

Despite adequate initial treatment with high dose IVIG, 5% of children with KD develop subsequent coronary aneurysms; 1% developing giant aneurysms. Patients who appear refractory to additional doses of IVIG may benefit from treatment with corticosteroids (either IV pulse methylprednisolone [30 mg/kg/day for 3 days] or conventional doses of oral prednisone). Although clearly beneficial in other forms of vasculitis, corticosteroid use in KD has previously been considered contraindicated, with potential concerns for worsening incidence of coronary artery abnormalities.[121,122] Further analysis, however, has revealed that these studies were deeply flawed. At present, most studies support a potential role for corticosteroids in the management of KD, revealing more rapid resolution of fever, improvement in laboratory markers, shorter length of hospitalization, and no significant difference in coronary artery abnormalities as compared with IVIG and ASA alone.[123-126] Other recent studies report reduced incidence of coronary aneurysms in patients treated with corticosteroids.[127-129] Although there has been little demonstrated long-term risk regarding the use of corticosteroids, several studies have noted an increased incidence of transient dilation of coronary arteries during pulse therapy.[122,130,131] Therefore, in general, corticosteroids are currently not recommended as routine initial treatment of KD and should be reserved for use in refractory KD.

Other Therapeutic Approaches

Other therapies that are of proven or theoretical benefit in other forms of vasculitis have been tried in KD, including pentoxifylline, CYC, cyclosporine, infliximab and plasmapheresis. Pentoxyfylline, an effective vasodilator and inhibitor of platelet aggregation, may have similar effects as ASA when given in conjunction with IVIG.[132] In addition, anti-TNF agents (such as infliximab), cytotoxic agents, and plasmapheresis may also have a role in patients resistant to treatment with IVIG and corticosteroids.[133-135] Finally, patients who exhibit significant coronary artery enlargement may require antiplatelet agents including abciximab, clopidogrel and dipyridamole; or antithrombotic medications including heparin and warfarin to aid in long-term prevention of coronary thrombosis.

Henoch-Schönlein Purpura

HSP, one of the most common vasculitides in children, is a leukocytoclastic small vessel vasculitis, most frequently occurring in children ages 3 to 15 years old. Although the exact etiology is unknown, the universal deposition of IgA suggests that the vasculitis is an IgA-mediated immune response to infections, including β-hemolytic streptococci and upper respiratory tract infections. It is characterized by the presence of nonthrombocytopenic palpable purpura (Fig. 19-16), arthritis/arthralgia, abdominal pain, genitourinary involvement, and renal disease (Table 19-2).

In the majority of patients, HSP is self-limited without significant sequelae. Typically, short-term morbidity is related to arthritis, genitourinary symptoms, and gastrointestinal manifestations; including intussusception (typically ileoileal), bowel infarction or perforation. Long-term complications are primarily a consequence of renal involvement, with approximately one third of patients developing nephritis and less than 10% eventually developing chronic renal disease.[136,137]

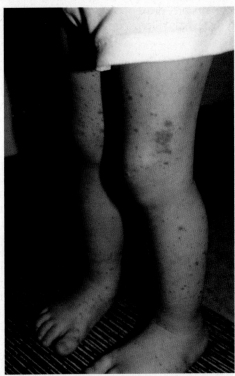

Figure 19-16. Classic palpable purpura on the lower extremities in a child with Henoch-Schönlein purpura.

Table 19-2. *Henoch-Schönlein Purpura*

Presence of two or more of the following:
   Age younger than 20 years old at the onset of first
      symptoms
   Palpable purpura (not related to thrombocytopenia)
   Bowel angina: diffuse abdominal pain, worse after meals,
      may be associated with bloody diarrhea
   Histopathology revealing granulocytes in the walls of
      arterioles and venules

CASE STUDY 4

A 4-year-old boy with no significant past medical history, presents with an erythematous, nonblanching, purpuric rash on his lower extremities and buttocks, worsening over the past 5 days. According to his mother, he has been complaining of pain in his right knee and bilateral ankles for 2 days before presentation. She has noticed swelling in his ankles and states that he has been ambulating with a limp. In addition, she notes complaints of vague, intermittent, generalized abdominal pain and a low-grade fever. His mother denies the presence of any diarrhea, melena, dysuria, or hematuria. Physical examination reveals a well appearing male in no apparent distress. Skin examination reveals scalp edema and palpable purpura on his lower extremities and buttocks bilaterally. Abdominal examination is benign, revealing no tenderness or palpable masses. Musculoskeletal examination reveals pain and periarticular swelling of his right knee and bilateral ankles. There is no erythema, warmth, or limited range of motion on examination. Scrotal swelling and tenderness to palpation are present. Stool guaiac is negative. Urinalysis reveals microscopic hematuria.

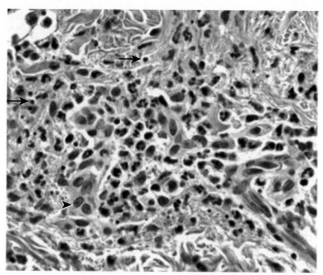

Figure 19-17. Skin biopsy revealing leukocytoclastic vasculitis in a boy with Henoch-Schönlein purpura. Neutrophilic infiltration with endothelial swelling can be seen (*arrows*). (Adapted from Zaidi M, Singh N, Kamran M. Acute onset of hematuria and proteinuria with multiorgan involvement of the heart, liver, pancreas, kidneys and skin in a patient with Henoch-Schonlein purpura. Kidney Int 2008;72:503-8.)

Differential Diagnosis

The differential diagnosis of HSP varies based on clinical presentation, particularly in cases in which arthritis, gastrointestinal, or renal manifestations precede the appearance of purpura (Fig. 19-17). Purpuric rashes must be distinguished from those associated with disease states including idiopathic thrombocytopenic purpura, hemolytic uremic syndrome, septicemia, coagulopathies, malignancy, SLE, and other forms of vasculitis. Laboratory evaluations including platelets, coagulation studies, serum complement levels, and autoimmune markers help to differentiate these etiologies. Acute hemorrhagic edema of infancy (AHEI) is a self-limited, leukocytoclastic vasculitis, presenting as a purpuric rash in infants younger than 2 years old. Histologically, it appears similar to HSP, with occasional demonstration of perivascular IgA deposition; however, involvement of other organ systems, including the kidneys and gastrointestinal tract, is uncommon. AHEI has been thought to be along a clinical spectrum of HSP, because younger patients with HSP may present with minimal gastrointestinal and renal involvement. Other causes of purpura associated with arthritis may include parvovirus infection, hepatitis, mixed cryoglobulinemia, hypersensitivity vasculitis, and underlying rheumatic diseases such as SLE and dermatomyositis. In addition, patients with IgA nephropathy, poststreptococcal glomerulonephritis, and Berger's disease may present with similar immunologic and histopathologic findings on renal biopsy, however, extrarenal manifestations suggest HSP.

Treatment

Typically, two thirds of patients follow a self-limited course with complete resolution in 4 to 6 weeks. In general, treatment goals should be focused on acute pain management, mitigating short-term gastrointestinal and urogenital morbidity, and prevention of chronic renal disease. Review of the literature reveals no universally accepted practice guidelines and few significant therapeutic trials. Thus, current management of HSP is based on retrospective reviews, limited prospective evidence and primarily anecdotal experience.

Supportive Care

For the majority of patients, HSP is managed with supportive care and pain management alone. In general, supportive care includes maintenance of adequate hydration, nutrition, and electrolyte balance. In addition, surveillance for signs of gastrointestinal involvement (including intussusception or hemorrhage) and potential testicular torsion is essential. Patients with significant renal disease may require hospitalization and anti-hypertensive medications.

Nonsteroidal Anti-Inflammatory Drugs

Pain management includes the use of nonsteroidal anti-inflammatory drugs (NSAIDs) to help control significant joint and abdominal pain (ex. naproxen 10–15 mg/kg/day divided in two doses). There are currently no randomized, controlled studies regarding the use of NSAIDs; however, there is generalized consensus that anti-inflammatory medications are effective. In these cases, caution must be taken to rule out evidence of gastrointestinal bleed or glomerulonephritis because these conditions may be exacerbated by the use of NSAIDs.

Corticosteroids

In more severe cases, the use of corticosteroids may help facilitate a more rapid resolution of symptoms (prednisone 1–2 mg/kg/day for 1–2 weeks, followed by a taper). However, the use of steroids is controversial, with variable evidence regarding the benefits of administration.

Use of steroids in the treatment of severe arthritis and significant abdominal pain has been advocated in several studies of HSP; demonstrating decreased severity and a more rapid resolution of symptoms.[138-143] Although conflicting data exist, further support has been demonstrated through case reports indicating that the use of corticosteroids, including IV methylprednisolone, further reduces gastrointestinal complications including hemorrhage and intussusception.[136,144,145] Similarly, prednisone has also been advocated in the management of orchitis, potentially preventing surgical intervention.[146,147]

The studies regarding the role of steroids in the prevention of renal disease are less conclusive. Several small, retrospective studies provide conflicting evidence regarding the reduction of renal progression with early use of prednisone.[141,142,146,148,149] Two prospective, randomized, controlled studies examining the use of steroids early in the course of HSP have been performed. Both studies concluded that prednisone did not prevent the development of renal symptoms, however, in the latter trial, prednisone was shown to be effective in resolving established nephritis more rapidly.[139,150] Similarly, in a systematic, meta-analysis review of the literature, early corticosteroid administration significantly reduced the odds of developing persistent renal disease.[140] In cases of significant renal manifestations, evidence suggests the use of IV methylprednisolone, cyclosporine, AZA, CYC, IVIG, anticoagulation, and plasma exchange may have a role in the management of HSP nephritis.[137,151-153]

In general, steroids should be considered for severe arthritis, gastrointestinal disease, or orchitis. Milder symptoms including cutaneous manifestations, mild abdominal pain, and mild arthritis are adequately managed with supportive care. The use of routine steroids for the prevention of renal complications is not adequately supported; however, there may be a role for corticosteroids in the long-term management of renal disease. In addition, there is sufficient evidence that initial presentation of renal disease in HSP is highly indicative of long-term prognosis.[153] Therefore, patients with initial evidence of heavy proteinuria, hematuria, or renal insufficiency should be referred for renal biopsy. Evidence predictive of a poor outcome, including fibrous crescents in greater than 50% of glomeruli, necessitates the institution of aggressive empiric therapy.

Wegener's Granulomatosis

WG is a necrotizing, granulomatous vasculitis, typically characterized by involvement of upper and lower respiratory tracts and pauci-immune glomerulonephritis. Although uncommon in children, the initial presentation often includes constitutional symptoms, nasopharyngeal inflammation, sinusitis, cough, chest pain, hemoptysis, myalgias, and arthralgias. Childhood-onset disease differs from that in adults in that there often is a female predominance, with a significantly higher prevalence of upper respiratory tract manifestations, including subglottic stenosis and nasal deformity (Fig. 19-18).[154-157] Renal disease complicates the course in more than 60% of children and is often rapidly progressive. In cases of spared renal involvement, the term local or limited WG may be employed. Diagnostic criteria include a positive anti neutrophil cytoplasmic antigen (ANCA), specifically in a cytoplasmic pattern directed against proteinase-3 (PR3). Tissue biopsy of lung, skin, or kidney often provides additional confirmation revealing granulomas, neutrophilic vasculitis and necrosis.

Differential Diagnosis

The differential diagnosis of WG primarily includes other forms of granulomatous disease. History and laboratory evaluation aid in distinguishing other etiologies including fungal, mycobacterium and helminth infections; as well as immunodeficiencies, such as chronic granulomatous disease. Similarly, other vasculitides may present with granulomatous vasculitis, including Churg-Strauss syndrome, primary angiitis of the CNS, and lymphomatoid granulomatosis. Finally, other forms of pulmonary-renal syndromes should be excluded including Goodpasture's syndrome, microscopic polyangiitis, PAN, SLE, and mixed connective tissue disease.

Treatment

Before the introduction of a standard therapeutic protocol, WG was considered highly fatal. Current management, based primarily on adult-onset WG literature, includes a combination of corticosteroids and cytotoxic agents and has led to disease remission in 70% to 90% of patients. Although highly efficacious, concerns have arisen regarding unacceptable drug toxicity during the maintenance phase of therapy, resulting in the addition of potentially less toxic agents into treatment regimens. Despite adequate management, frequent relapses may occur, often coinciding with corticosteroid tapering. Some evidence suggests that acute increases in ANCA titers

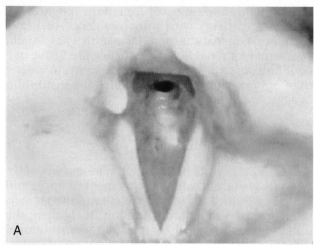

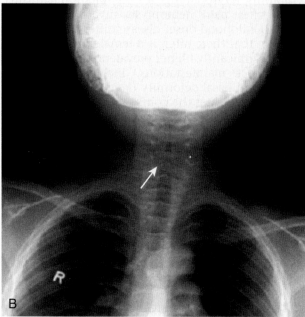

Figure 19-18. Subglottic stenosis in a 13-year-old boy with Wegener's granulomatosus as shown by bronchoscopy (**A**) and x-ray study (**B**). (Adapted from Lee HK, Cho HY, Cheong HI, Choi Y, Ha IS. A case of Wegener's granulomatosis with multi-organ involvement in childhood. J Korean Soc Pediatr Nephrol 2007;11:118-25.)

may indicate disease relapse; however, this is less evident in pediatric literature and clinical correlation is essential.[155,158,159]

Induction

The standard treatment of choice for induction of therapy in WG is similar to that in adults and includes high-dose oral prednisone (1–2 mg/kg/day divided into two to three doses) in combination with oral CYC (2 mg/kg/day) for a total of 4 weeks duration.[154,160,161] In critically ill patients, IV methylprednisolone (30 mg/kg/day for 1–3 days) or plasmapheresis should be considered.[156,162] Owing to the significant toxicity and risk of infection associated with oral CYC, several studies have examined the potential benefits of IV pulse CYC as an alternative approach to decrease overall cumulative toxicity.[155,163,164]

Maintenance

Approximately half of the patients with pediatric WG will experience one or more relapses after induction therapy. Traditional standard maintenance therapy includes oral prednisone (1 mg/kg/day) tapered gradually to an alternate-day dose and oral CYC (2 mg/kg/day) tapered after 1 year of complete remission.[154,164]

Alternative approaches to maintenance therapy, including MTX, AZA, MMF, cyclosporine, rituximab, and etanercept, have been considered in adult WG; however, pediatric data are limited. Low-dose MTX (0.3–1 mg/kg PO or SC weekly) has been demonstrated in both adults and children to maintain similar rates of remission as compared with oral CYC with significantly decreased toxicity.[165-168] Rates of relapse may be increased in patients with severe disease; therefore, MTX may be more appropriate in cases of milder or limited WG.[155,169] Similarly, the use of AZA in childhood WG has been demonstrated to maintain disease remission while allowing for reduction in corticosteroid dose; this is in contrast to cyclosporine, which has had variable success in sustaining disease control.[156,161] Agents including MMF, rituximab, and etanercept are currently being studied for refractory disease in adult-onset WG literature with inconclusive benefits and require further review.[170-173]

Increased risk of respiratory tract infections may be associated with triggered relapses in patients with WG. Based on this notion, studies have demonstrated the use of trimethoprim/sulfamethoxazole (TMP/SMZ) to reduce incidence of relapses.[174,175] TMP/SMZ, however, is not effective as a primary maintenance therapy; therefore, these drugs should be reserved for use as an adjunctive measure.[166]

Additional Therapeutic Measures

Children with WG are more likely to have limited or localized disease, primarily involving the upper respiratory passages. As a result, nasal deformities and subglottic stenosis are more frequent complications. In these patients, immunosuppression and cytotoxic agents may not be sufficient. Surgical intervention, including intratracheal dilation and corticosteroid injections may be necessary.[154,165]

Polyarteritis Nodosa

PAN is a rare, systemic, necrotizing vasculitis, affecting primarily small and medium-sized muscular arteries, often resulting in characteristic aneurysm formation. PAN is uncommon in childhood, with the highest frequency occurring in the fifth and sixth decades of life. Clinical manifestations vary depending on pattern of vascular involvement, with common clinical manifestations including fever, weight loss, arthritis and arthralgia, abdominal pain, myalgias, cutaneous abnormalities, renal disease, hypertension, and neurologic abnormalities (Table 19-3).[176] In some series, PAN has been

Table 19-3. *Proposed Criteria for Polyarteritis Nodosa in Childhood**

Major criteria
  Renal involvement
  Musculoskeletal findings
Minor criteria
  Cutaneous findings
  Gastrointestinal involvement
  Peripheral neuropathy
  Central nervous system disease
  Cardiac involvement
  Lung involvement
  Constitutional symptoms
  Acute phase reactants
  Presence of hepatitis B surface antigen

*The presence of at least five criteria, including at least one major criterion is highly suggestive of the diagnosis.

preceded by infections including group A streptococcus, parvovirus, and cytomegalovirus, suggesting that infection is a potential inciting event. Although, hepatitis B and C infections are often linked with PAN in adults, these associations are less frequently described in children. Cutaneous polyarteritis (CPA), thought to be along a similar spectrum of disease as PAN, may also result in a panarteritis. CPA, however, is primarily restricted to skin, musculoskeletal, and peripheral neurologic abnormalities, resulting in a favorable prognosis and therefore is better classified as a distinct entity.

Differential Diagnosis

Differential diagnosis of PAN varies from that in adults and primarily includes infections, such as bacterial endocarditis and chronic viral infections; and other vasculitides, such as WG, microscopic polyangiitis, and sarcoidosis. Histopathologic features often help differentiate the condition, revealing nongranulomatous, necrotizing arteritis with fibrinoid necrosis in small to medium sized vessels particularly at sites of bifurcation. In addition, angiographic demonstration of vascular beading and aneurysm formation in renal, celiac and mesenteric vessels is characteristic of PAN.

Treatment

Management of PAN in childhood is primarily based on adult literature and retrospective data. Reported prognosis and outcome varies by study; however, in general, children have better renal outcome, improved survival, and lower relapse rates, as compared with adults.[177] Corticosteroid therapy is an integral part of therapy for the majority of children with PAN. Depending on initial presentation, oral prednisone (1–2 mg/kg/day) is typically given, followed by a slow taper.[178-180] In cases of severe CNS, renal, and gastrointestinal involvement, IV methylprednisone (30 mg/kg/day for 3 days) should be considered.[181] In addition, immunosuppressant therapy including CYC or AZA, have been shown to be beneficial in both adults and children with life-threatening disease.[177,179,182,183] In cases with a

demonstrated streptococcal or hepatitis B infection, treatment with penicillin or antiviral medications has been advocated.[184,185] Finally, other agents, such as IV immunoglobulin have been reported to be successful in some cases of relapsing PAN.[186,187]

Localized Scleroderma

Scleroderma, characterized by excessive accumulation of collagen and fibrosis in tissue, is subdivided into three categories: diffuse cutaneous systemic scleroderma, limited cutaneous systemic scleroderma, and localized scleroderma. Systemic forms of scleroderma are rare in childhood, with management primarily based on adult-supported literature. Therefore, for the purposes of this chapter, we focus on localized forms of scleroderma, with manifestations primarily confined to skin and subcutaneous tissue.

Localized scleroderma can be broadly divided into three major types: linear scleroderma, morphea and generalized morphea. Briefly, linear scleroderma, the most common type of scleroderma in children, is characterized by linear streaks of indurated tissue. In contrast, morphea, typically round or oral plaques, is subcategorized by depth of subdermal involvement and defined as generalized when individual plaques become confluent or affect three or more anatomic sites. Although the exact etiology is unknown, the pathogenesis is thought to be secondary to activation of immunologic factors, vascular endothelium and fibroblasts, resulting in excessive collagen synthesis and fibrosis. Several studies have investigated the role of autoimmunity, demonstrating variably increased autoantibodies [including antinuclear antibodies, antihistone antibodies, anti–single-stranded DNA antibodies, and rheumatoid factor], cell surface markers, cytokines and soluble cytokine receptors [including interleukin-2 receptor].[188-193] Actively progressing disease may be suggested by elevations in rheumatoid factor, ESR, eosinophils, or immunoglobulins, and clinically by the presence of erythema, warmth, and edema surrounding the sclerodermatous plaque.

Differential Diagnosis

Various dermatologic conditions may mimic localized scleroderma. Although not always necessary for diagnosis, biopsy and histologic evaluation may reveal inflammatory infiltrate with subsequent increases in collagen and fibroblasts and eventual sclerosis. More importantly, localized scleroderma must be distinguished from systemic scleroderma, typically by the presence of focal, more distal, cutaneous manifestations and the lack of findings including Raynaud's phenomenon, cardiopulmonary, gastrointestinal, renal, and CNS involvement. However, recent evidence suggests that extracutaneous manifestations may occur in a selected group of children with localized scleroderma, particularly articular, neurologic, vascular and ophthalmologic manifestations; therefore, careful evaluation and monitoring are essential.[194] In addition, autoantibodies often found in adults with systemic scleroderma, including anti-topoisomerase I (Scl-70) and anticentromere antibodies, are rarely seen in local disease.

Treatment

Localized scleroderma is typically a self-limited disease, with spontaneous remission occurring in approximately 3 to 5 years. However, significant morbidity may occur in cases of extensive involvement of the face (en coup de sabre or Parry-Romberg syndrome) or limb involvement (Fig. 19-19). Potential complications include significant facial disfigurement/atrophy, ambylopia, uveitis, seizures, joint contractures, significant atrophy/growth retardation of the affected limb and neurovascular consequences (Fig. 19-20). Therefore, in cases of active disease, topical or systemic therapy should be considered. Owing to the lack of reliable, standardized assessments of disease activity, therapeutic recommendations have been based primarily on anecdotal evidence, case series, and retrospective reviews. Several outcome measures have been used with variable success, including the Localized Scleroderma Severity Index (LoSSI), computerized skin score (CSS), visual analog scale (VAS), thermography, ultrasound, and MRI.

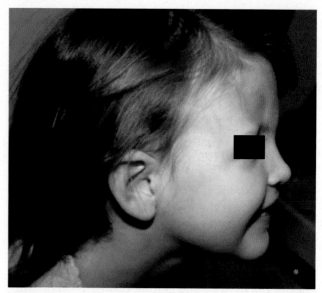

Figure 19-19. En coup de sabre affecting the right forehead in a young girl with localized scleroderma.

Owing to the wide spectrum of clinical disease and associated morbidity, treatment options vary based on the depth of subdermal involvement, anatomic location, presence of irreversible structural deformity, and the potential involvement of extracutaneous features. In cases of isolated, superficial plaques of morphea, systemic treatment is generally

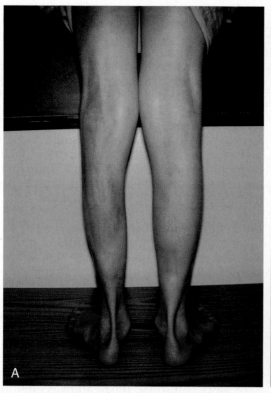

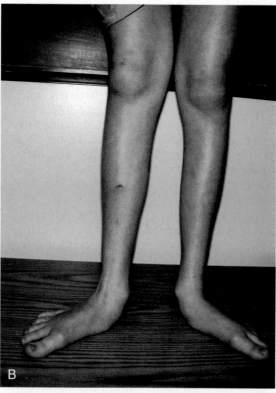

Figure 19-20. A, Linear scleroderma extending over the left knee joint, resulting deformity and significant muscular atrophy. **B,** Further evidence of muscle wasting can be seen with involvement of the entire left lower extremity. (**A** and **B** Courtesy of Ronald Laxer.)

unwarranted. Therapy typically includes topical agents, such as corticosteroids and synthetic vitamin D_3 analogs, including calcipotriene. Although potentially effective, corticosteroids may result in local atrophy and telangiectasias; whereas topical calcipotriene binds vitamin D receptors, altering immunoregulation, fibroblast proliferation, and collagen synthesis, and may result in improved sclerodermatous lesions without signs of toxicity.[195] Similarly, oral calcitriol has been used in cases of systemic sclerosis and extensive morphea with some success; however, a recent double-blind, placebo-controlled trial revealed little benefit.[196-198] In addition, several studies using ultraviolet A phototherapy (UVA) and psoralen plus ultraviolet A photochemotherapy (PUVA) have demonstrated significant reduction in skin sclerosis with improvement in elasticity of plaques.[199-202] Furthermore, phototherapy used in conjunction with vitamin D_3 analog ointment, calcipotriol, may be additionally effective.[203]

In cases of linear scleroderma and deep morphea, in which potential disfigurement or disability may occur, treatment with immunosuppressive agents should be considered. Current literature supports the use of combined oral or IV corticosteroid therapy (oral prednisone 1 mg/kg/day or IV methylprednisolone 30 mg/kg/day for 3 days/month) with MTX (PO or SC, 0.3–1 mg/kg/week, max dose 25 mg/dose).[204-207] Using various forms of assessment, combined systemic corticosteroids and MTX appear to be a well tolerated, effective approach to reducing the progression of active lesions while improving skin appearance, thickness and induration. In addition, some studies have proposed a benefit of initial pulse IV methylprednisolone (given 3 days/month for 3–6 months) as an inducing agent to reduce overall clinical corticosteroid toxicity.[204,205] One potential obstacle to this regimen is the relatively high rate of relapse which may occur upon cessation of therapy; therefore a continuation of maintenance therapy with a gradual reduction of corticosteroid dose is recommended.[205] Other agents that have been used with variable success include D-penicillamine, antimalarials, cyclosporine, and bosentan.[208-212] Finally, patients with severe disfigurement or disability may benefit from surgical intervention; however, caution should be taken to undergo reconstruction once there is no longer evidence of active disease.

References

1. Mendez EP, Lipton R, Ramsey-Goldman R, Roettcher P, Bowyer S, Dyer A, et al. for the NIAMS Juvenile DM Registry Physician Referral Group. US incidence of juvenile dermatomyositis, 1995–1998: results from the National Institute of Arthritis and Musculoskeletal and Skin Diseases Registry. Arthritis Rheum 2003;49:300-5.
2. Miles L, Bove KE, Lovell D, Wargula JC, Bukulmez H, Shao M, et al. Predictability of the clinical course of juvenile dermatomyositis based on initial muscle biopsy: a retrospective study of 72 patients. Arthritis Rheum 2007;15:1183-91.
3. Fall N, Bove K, Stringer K, Lovell DJ, Brunner HI, Weiss J, et al. Association between lack of angiogenic response in muscle tissue and high expression of angiostatic ELR-negative CXC chemokines in patients with juvenile dermatomyositis. Arthritis Rheum 2005;52:3175-80.
4. Feldman BM, Rider LG, Reed AM, Pachman LM. Juvenile dermatomyositis and other idiopathic inflammatory myopathies of childhood. Lancet 2008;371:2201-12.
5. Huber AM, Feldman BM, Rennebohm RM, Hicks JE, Lindsley CB, Perez MD, et al. Validation and clinical significance of the childhood myositis assessment scale for assessment of muscle function in the juvenile inflammatory myopathies. Arthritis Rheum 2004;50:1595-603.
6. Rider LG, Giannini EH, Brunner HI, Ruperto N, James-Newton L, Reed AM, et al. International consensus on preliminary definitions of improvement in adult and juvenile myositis. Arthritis Rheum 2004;50:2281-90.
7. Guzman J, Petty RE, Malleson PN. Monitoring disease activity in juvenile dermatomyositis: the role of von Willebrand factor and muscle enzymes. J Rheumatol 1994;21:739-43.
8. Baechler EC, Bauer JW, Slattery CA, Ortmann WA, Espe KJ, Novitzke J, et al. An interferon signature in the peripheral blood of dermatomyositis patients is associated with disease activity. Mol Med 2007;13:59-68.
9. Pachman LM. An update on juvenile dermatomyositis. Curr Opin Rheumatol 1995;7:437-41.
10. Maillard SM, Jones R, Owens C, Pilkington C, Woo P, Wedderburn LR, et al. Quantitative assessment of MRI T2 relaxation time of thigh muscles in juvenile dermatomyositis. Rheumatology 2004;43:603-8.
11. Hernandez RJ, Sullivan DB, Chenevert TL, Keim DR. MR imaging in children with dermatomyositis: musculoskeletal findings and correlation with clinical and laboratory findings. AJR Am J Roentgenol 1993;161:359-66.
12. Bowyer SL, Blane CE, Sullivan DB, Cassidy JT. Childhood dermatomyositis: factors predicting functional outcome and development of dystrophic calcification. J Pediatr 1983;103:882-8.
13. Fisler RE, Liang MG, Fuhlbrigge RC, Yalcindag A, Sundel RP. Aggressive management of juvenile dermatomyositis results in improved outcome and decreased incidence of calcinosis. J Am Acad Dermatol 2002;47:505-11.
14. Pachman LM. Inflammatory myopathy in children. Rheum Dis Clin North Am 1994;20:919-42.
15. Callen AM, Pachman LM, Hayford J, Chung A, Ramsey-Goldman R. Intermittent high-dose intravenous methylprednisone (IV pulse) therapy prevents calcinosis and shortens disease course in juvenile dermatomyositis. Arthritis Rheum 1994;37(Suppl. 6):R10.
16. Huang JL. Long-term prognosis of patients with juvenile dermatomyositis initially treated with intravenous methylprednisolone pulse therapy. Clin Exp Rheumatol 1999;17:621-4.
17. Klein-Gitelman MS, Waters T, Pachman LM. The economic impact of intermittent high-dose intravenous versus oral corticosteroid treatment of juvenile dermatomyositis. Arthritis Care Res 2000;13:360-8.
18. Rouster-Stevens KA, Gursahaney A, Ngai K-L, Daru JA, Pachman LM. Pharmacokinetic study of oral prednisolone compared with intravenous methyl-prednisolone in patients with juvenile dermatomyositis. Arthritis Rheum 2008;58:222-6.
19. Seshadri R, Feldman B, Ilowite N, Cawkwell G, Pachman L. The role of aggressive corticosteroid therapy in patients with juvenile dermatomyositis. A propensity score analysis 2008;59:989-95.
20. Laxer RM, Stein LD, Petty RE. Intravenous pulse methyl prednisolone treatment of juvenile dermatomyositis. Arthritis Rheum 1987;30:328-34.
21. Al-Mayouf S, Al-Mazyed A, Bahabri S. Efficacy of early treatment of severe juvenile dermatomyositis with intravenous methylprednisolone and methotrexate. Clin Rheumatol 2000;19:138-41.
22. Huber AM, Lang B, LeBlanc CM, Birdi N, Bolaria RK, Malleson P, et al. Medium- and long-term functional outcomes in a multicenter cohort of children with juvenile dermatomyositis. Arthritis Rheum 2000;43:541-9.

23. Milojevic DS, Ilowite NT. Treatment of rheumatic diseases in children: special considerations. Rheum Dis Clin N Am 2002;28:461-82.

24. Cimaz R. Osteoporosis in childhood rheumatic diseases: prevention and therapy. Best Pract Res Clin Rheumatol 2002;16:397-409.

25. Olsen NY, Lindsley CB. Adjunctive use of hydroxychloroquine in childhood dermatomyositis. J Rheumatol 1989;16:1545-7.

26. Woo TY, Callen JP, Voorhees JJ, Bickers DR, Hanno R, Hawkins C, et al. Cutaneous lesions of dermatomyositis are improved by hydroxychloroquine. J Am Acad Dermatol 1984;10:592-600.

27. Marmor MF, Carr RE, Easterbrook M, Farjo AA, Mieler WF. Recommendations on screening for chloroquine and hydroxychloroquine retinopathy: a report by the American Academy of Ophthalmology. Ophthalmology 2002;109:1377-82.

28. Ramanan AV, Campbell-Webster N, Ota S, Parker S, Tran D, Tyrrell PN, et al. The effectiveness of treating juvenile dermatomyositis with methotrexate and aggressively tapered corticosteroids. Arthritis Rheum 2005;52:3570-78.

29. Singsen BH, Goldbach-Mansky R. Methotrexate in the treatment of juvenile rheumatoid arthritis and other pediatric rheumatoid and nonrheumatic disorders. Rheum Dis Clin North Am 1997;23:811-40.

30. Miller LC, Sisson BA, Tucker LB, DeNardo BA, Schaller JG. Methotrexate treatment of recalcitrant childhood dermatomyositis. Arthritis Rheum 1992;35:1143-9.

31. Kobayashi I, Yamada M, Takahashi Y, Kawamura N, Okano M, Sakiyama Y, et al. Interstitial lung disease associated with juvenile dermatomyositis: clinical features and efficacy of cyclosporine A. Rheumatology (Oxf) 2003;42:371-4.

32. Heckmatt J, Hasson N, Sunders C, Thompson N, Peters AM, Cambridge G, et al. Cyclosporine in juvenile dermatomyositis. Lancet 1989;1:1063-6.

33. Ponyi A, Constantin T, Balogh Z, Szalai Z, Borgulya G, Molnar K, et al. Disease course, frequency of relapses and survival of 73 patients with juvenile or adult dermatomyositis. Clin Exp Rheumatol 2005;23:50-6.

34. Riley P, Maillard SM, Wedderburn LR, Woo P, Murray KJ, Pilkington CA. Intravenous cyclophosphamide pulse therapy in juvenile dermatomyositis. A review of efficacy and safety. Rheumatology 2004;43:491-6.

35. Edge JC, Outland JD, Dempsey JR, Callen JP. Mycophenolate mofetil as an effective corticosteroid-sparing therapy for recalcitrant dermatomyositis. Arch Dermatol 2006;142:65-9.

36. Negi V, Elluru S, Siberil S, Graff-Dubois S, Mouthon L, Kazatchkine MD, et al. Intravenous immunoglobulin: an update on the clinical use and mechanisms of action. J Clin Immunol 2007;27:233-45.

37. Dalakas MC, Illa I, Dambrosia JM, Soueidan SA, Stein DP, Otero C, et al. A controlled trial of high-dose intravenous immune globulin infusions as treatment of dermatomyositis. N Engl J Med 1993;329:1993-2000.

38. Al-Mayouf SM, Laxer RM, Schneider R, Silverman ED, Feldman BM. Intravenous immunoglobulin therapy for juvenile dermatomyositis: efficacy and safety. J Rheumatol 2000;27:2498-503.

39. Sansome A, Dubowitz V. Intravenous immunoglobulin in juvenile dermatomyositis-four year review of nine cases. Arch Dis Child 1995;72:25-8.

40. Lang BA, Laxer RM, Murphy G, Silverman ED, Roifman CM. Treatment of dermatomyositis with intravenous gammaglobulin. Am J Med 1991;91:169-72.

41. Manlhiot C, Tyrell PN, Liang L. Safety of intravenous immunoglobulin in the treatment of juenile dermatomyositis: adverse reactions are associated with immunoglobulin A content. Pediatrics 2008;121:e626-30.

42. Pachman LM, Liotta-Davis MR, Hong DK, Kinsella TR, Mendez EP, Kinder JM, et al. TNFalpha-308A allele in juvenile dermatomyositis: association with increased production of tumor necrosis factor alpha, disease duration and pathologic calcifications. Arthritis Rheum 2000;43:2368-77.

43. Miller ML, Smith RL, Abbott KA, et al. Use of etanercept in chronic juvenile dermatomyositis (JDM). Arthritis Rheum 2002;46:S306.

44. Riley P, McCann LJ, Maillard SM, Woo P, Murray KJ, Pilkingtion CA. Effectiveness of infliximab in the treatment of refractory juvenile dermatomyositis with calcinosis. Rheumatology (Oxford) 2008;47:877-80.

45. Levine TD. A pilot study of rituximab therapy for refractory dermatomyositis. Arthritis Rheum 2002;46:S488.

46. Cooper MA, Willingham DL, Brown DE, French AR, Shih FF, White AJ. Rituximab for the treatment of juvenile dermatomyositis; a report of four pediatric patients. Arthritis Rheum 2007;56:3107-11.

47. Dau PC, Bennington JL. Plasmapheresis in childhood dermatomyositis. J Pediatr 1981;98:237-40.

48. Boulman N, Slobodin G, Rozenbaum M, Rosner I. Calcinosis in rheumatic diseases. Semin Arthritis Rheum 2005;35:202-3.

49. Brunner HI, Silverman ED, To T, Bombardier C, Feldman BM. Risk factors for damage in childhood-onset systemic lupus erythematosus. Arthritis Rheum 2002;46:436-44.

50. Jimenez S, Cervera R, Font J, Ingelmo M. The epidemiology of systemic lupus erythematosus. Clin Rev Allergy Immunol 2003;25:3-12.

51. Brunner HI, Feldman BM, Bombardier C, Silverman ED. Sensitivity of the Systemic Lupus Erythematosus Disease Activity Index, British Isles Lupus Assessment Group Index and Systemic Lupus Activity Measure in the evaluation of clinical change in childhood-onset systemic lupus erythematosus. Arthritis Rheum 1999;42:1354-60.

52. Ostensen M, Villliger PM. Non-steroidal anti-inflammatory drugs in systemic lupus erythematosus. Lupus 2001;10:135-9.

53. Levy ML, Barron KS, Eichenfield A, Honig PJ. Naproxen induced pseudoporphyria: a distinctive photodermatitis. J Pediatr 1990;117:660-4.

54. Glidden RS, Mantzouranis EC, Borel Y. Systemic lupus erythematosus in childhood: clinical manifestations and improved survival in fifty-five patients. Clin Immunol Immunopathol 1983;29:196-210.

55. Walravens P, Chase HP. The prognosis of childhood systemic lupus erythematosus. Am J Dis Child 1976;130:929-33.

56. Chatham WW, Kimberly RP. Treatment of lupus with corticosteroids. Lupus 2002;10:140-7.

57. Barron KS, Person DA, Brewer EJ, Beale MG, Robson AM. Pulse methylprednisolone therapy in diffuse proliferative lupus nephritis. J Pediatr 1982;101:137-41.

58. Benseler SM, Silverman ED. Neuropsychiatric involvement in pediatric systemic lupus erythematosus. Lupus 2007;16:564-71.

59. Ilowite NT. Premature atherosclerosis in systemic lupus erythematosus. J Rheumatol Suppl 2000;58:15-9.

60. Takada K, Illei GG, Boumpas DT. Cyclophosphamide for the treatment of systemic lupus erythematosus. Lupus 2001;10:154-61.

61. Boumpas DT, Austin HA 3rd, Vaughn EM, Klippel JH, Steinberg AD, Yarboro CH, et al. Controlled trial of pulse methylprednisolone versus two regimens of pulse cyclophosphamide in severe lupus nephritis. Lancet 1992;340:741-5.

62. Steinberg AD, Decker JL. A double-blind controlled trial comparing cyclophosphamide, azathioprine and placebo in the treatment of glomerulonephritis. Arthritis Rheum 1974;17:923-37.

63. Baca V, Lavalle C, Garcia R, Catalan T, Sauceda JM, Sanchez G, et al. Favorable response to intravenous methylprednisolone and cyclophosphamide in children with severe neuropsychiatric lupus. J Rheumatol 1999;26:432-9.

64. Yancey CL, Doughty RA, Athreya BH. Central nervous system involvement in childhood systemic lupus erythematosus. Arthritis Rheum 1981;24:1389-95.

65. Lehman TJA, Onel K. Intermittent intravenous cyclophosphamide arrests progression of the renal chronicity index in childhood systemic lupus erythematosus. J Pediatr 2000;136:243-7.

66. Lehman TJ. A practical guide to systemic lupus erythematosus. Pediatr Clin North Am 1995;42:1223-38.

67. Massey CS. A multicentre study to determine the efficacy and patient acceptability of the Paxman scalp cooler to prevent hair loss in patients receiving chemotherapy. Eur J Oncol Nurs 2004;8:121-30.

68. Silva CAA, Brunner HI. Gonadal functioning and preservation of reproductive fitness with juvenile systemic lupus erythematosus. Lupus 2007;16:593-9.

69. Silverman E. What's new in the treatment of pediatric SLE. J Rheumatol 1996;23:1657-60.

70. Tucker LB. Controversies and advances in the management of systemic lupus erythematosus in children and adolescents. Best Pract Res Clin Rheumatol 2002;16:471-80.

71. Contreras G, Pardo V, Leclercq B, Lenz O, Tozman E, O'Nan P, et al. Sequential therapies for proliferative lupus nephritis. N Engl J Med 2004;350:971-80.

72. Feutren G, Querin S, Noel LH, Chatenoud L, Beaurain G, Tron F, et al. Effects of cyclosporine in severe systemic lupus erythematosus. J Pediatr 1987;111:1063-8.

73. Fu LW, Yang LY, Chem WP, Lin CY. Clinical efficacy of cyclosporine A (Neoral) in the treatment of pediatric lupus nephritis with heavy proteinuria. Br J Rheumatol 1998;37:217-21.

74. Griffiths B, Emery P. The treatment of lupus with cyclosporine A. Lupus 2001;10:165-70.

75. Buratti S, Szer IS, Spencer CH, Bartosh S, Reiff A. Mycophenolate mofetil treatment of severe renal disease in paediatric onset systemic lupus erythematosus. J Rheumatol 2001;28:2103-8.

76. Lau KK, Ault BH, Jones DP, Butani L. Induction therapy for pediatric focal proliferative lupus nephritis: cyclophosphamide versus mycophenolate mofetil. J Pediatr Health Care 2008;22:282-8.

77. Ginzler EM, Dooley MA, Aranow C, Kim MY, Buyon J, Merrill JT, et al. Mycophenolate mofetil or intravenous cyclophosphamide for lupus nephritis. N Engl J Med 2005;353:2219-28.

78. Chan TM, Li FK, Tang CS, Wong RW, Fang GX, Ji YL, et al. Efficacy of mycophenolate mofetil in patients with diffuse proliferative lupus nephritis. N Engl J Med 2000;343:1156-62.

79. Abud-Mendoza C, Sturbaum AK, Vazquez-Compean R, Gonzalez-Amaro R. Methotrexate in childhood systemic lupus erythematosus. J Rheumatol 1993;20:731-3.

80. Ravelli A, Ballardini G, Viola S, Villa I, Ruperto N, Martini A. Methotrexate therapy in refractory pediatric onset systemic lupus erythematosus. J Rheumatol 1998;25:572-5.

81. Willems M, Haddad MD, Niaudet P, Kone-Paut I, Bensman A, Cochat P, et al. Rituximab therapy for childhood-onset systemic lupus erythematosus. J Pediatr 2006;148:623-7.

82. Marks SD, Patey S, Brogan PA, Hasson N, Pilkington C, Woo P, et al. B lymphocyte depletion therapy in children with refractory systemic lupus erythematosus. Arthritis Rheum 2005;52:3168-74.

83. El-Hallack M, Binstadt BA, Leichtner AM, Bennett CM, Neufeld EJ, Fuhlbrigge RC, et al. Clinical effects and safety of rituximab for treatment of refractory pediatric autoimmune diseases. J Pediatr 2007;150:376-82.

84. Podolskaya A, Stadermann M, Pilkington C, Marks SD, Tullus K. B cell depletion therapy for 19 patients with refractory systemic lupus erythematosus. Arch Dis Child 2008;93:401-6.

85. Nwobi O, Abitbol CL, Chandar J. Rituximab therapy for juvenile-onset systemic lupus erythematosus. Pediatr Nephrol 2008;23:413-9.

86. Huggins JL, Brunner HI. Targeting B cells in the treatment of childhood-onset systemic lupus erythematosus. J Pediatr 2006;148:571-3.

87. Rauova L, Lukac J, Levy Y, Rovensky J, Shoenfeld Y. High-dose intravenous immunoglobulins for lupus nephritis-a salvage immunomodulation. Lupus 2001;10:209-13.

88. MacDermott EJ, Adams A, Lehman TJA. Systemic lupus erythematosus in children: current and emerging therapies. Lupus 2007;16:677-83.

89. Tyrrell PN, Beyene J, Benseler SM, Sarkissian T, Silverman ED. Predictors of lipid abnormalities in children with new-onset systemic lupus erythematosus. J Rheumatol 2007;10:2112-9.

90. Ilowite NT, Cooperman N, Leicht T, Kwong T, Jacobson MS. Effects of dietary modifications and fish oil supplementation on dyslipoproteinemia in pediatric systemic lupus erythematosus. J Rheumatol 1995;22:1347-51.

91. Ardoin SR, Sandborg C, Schanberg LE. Management of dyslipidemia in children and adolescents with systemic lupus erythematosus. Lupus 2007;16:618-26.

92. Boffa MC, Lachassine E. Infant perinatal thrombosis and antiphospholipid antibodies: a review. Lupus 2007;16:634-41.

93. Nacinovich R, Galli J, Bomba M, Filippini E, Parrinello G, Nuzzo M, et al. Neuropsychological development of children born to patients with antiphospholipid syndrome. Arthritis Rheum 2008;59:345-51.

94. Lim W, Crowther MA, Eikelboom JW. Management of antiphospholipid antibody syndrome: a systematic review. JAMA 2006;295:1050-7.

95. Ravelli A, Martini A. Antiphospholipid antibody syndrome in pediatric patients. Rheum Dis Clin North Am 1997;23:657-76.

96. Avcin T. Antiphospholipid syndrome in children. Curr Opin Rheumatol 2008;20:595-600.

97. Kamat AV, D'Cruz DP, Hunt BJ. Managing antiphospholipid antibodies and antiphospholipid syndrome in children. Haematologica 2006;91:1674-80.

98. Dix D, Andrew M, Marzinotto V, Charpentier K, Bridge S, Monagle P, et al. The use of low-molecular-weight heparin in pediatric patients: a prospective cohort study. J Pediatr 2000;136:439-45.

99. Burak CR, Bowen MD, Barron TF. The use of enoxaparin in children with acute, nonhemorrhagic stroke. Pediatr Neurol 2003;29:295-8.

100. Punzalan RC, Hillery CA, Montgomery RR, Scott CA, Gill JC. Low-molecular-weight heparin in thrombotic disease in children and adolescents. J Pediatr Hematol Oncol 2000;22:137-42.

101. Buyon JP, Rupel A, Clancy RM. Neonatal lupus syndromes. Lupus 2004;13:705-12.

102. Saleeb S, Copel J, Friedman D, Buyon JP. Comparison of treatment with fluorinated glucocorticoids to the natural history of autoantibody-associated congenital heart block: retrospective review of the research registry for neonatal lupus. Arthritis Rheum 1999;42:2335-45.

103. Bierman FZ, Baxi L, Jaffe I, Driscoll J. Fetal hydrops and congenital complete heart block: response to maternal steroid. J Pediatr 1988;112:646-8.

104. Wong JP, Kwek KY, Tan JY, Yeo GS. Fetal congenital complete heart block: prophylaxis with intravenous immunoglobulin and treatment with dexamethasone. Aust N Z J Obstet Gynecol 2001;41:339-41.

105. Groves AM, Allan LD, Rosenthal E. Therapeutic trial of sympathomimetics in three cases of complete heart block in the fetus. Circulation 1995;92:3394-6.

106. Minassian VA, Jazayeri A. Favorable outcome in a pregnancy with complete fetal heart block and severe bradycardia. Obstet Gynecol 2002;100:1087-9.

107. Eronen M, Siren MK, Ekblad H, Tikanoja T, Julkunen H, Paavilainen T. Short and long-term outcome of children with congenital complete heart block diagnosed in utero or as a newborn. Pediatrics 2000;106:86-9.

108. Newburger JW, Takahashi M, Gerber MA, Gewitz MH, Tani LY, Burns JC, et al. Diagnosis, treatment and long-term management of Kawasaki disease: a statement for health professionals from the committee on Rheumatic Fever, Endocarditis and Kawasaki disease, council on cardiovascular disease in the young, American Heart Association. Circulation 2004;110:2747-71.

109. Harada K. Intravenous gamma-globulin treatment in Kawasaki disease. Acta Paediatr Jpn 1991;33:805-10.

110. Brogan PA, Shah V, Brachet C, Harnden A, Mant D, Klein N, et al. Endothelial and platelet microparticles in vasculitis of the young. Arthritis Rheum 2004;50:927-36.

111. Nakatani K, Takeshita S, Tsujimoto H, Kawamura Y, Tokutomi T, Sekine I. Circulating endothelial cells in Kawasaki disease. Clin Exp Immunol 2003;131:536-40.

112. Durongpisitkul K, Gururaj VJ, Park JM, Martin CF. The prevention of efficacy of aspirin and immunoglobulin treatment. Pediatrics 1995;96:1057-61.

113. Terai M, Shulman ST. Prevalence of coronary artery abnormalities in Kawasaki disease is highly dependent on gamma globulin dose but independent of salicylate dose. J Pediatr 1997;131:888-93.

114. Furusho K, Kamiya T, Nakano H, Kiyosawa N, Shinomiya K, Hayashiedera T, et al. High-dose intravenous gammaglobulin for Kawasaki disease. Lancet 1984;2:1055-8.

115. Newburger JW, Takahashi M, Burns JC, Beiser AS, Chung KJ, Duffy CE, et al. The treatment of Kawasaki syndrome with intravenous gamma globulin. N Engl J Med 1986;315:341-7.

116. Newburger JW, Takahashi M, Beiser AS, Burns JC, Bastian J, Chung KJ, et al. A single intravenous infusion of gamma globulin as compared with four infusions in the treatment of acute Kawasaki syndrome. N Engl J Med 1991;324:1633-9.

117. Sato N, Sugimura T, Akagi T, Yamakawa R, Hashino K, Eto G, et al. Selective high dose gamma-globulin treatment in Kawasaki disease: assessment of clinical aspects and cost effectiveness. Pediatr Int 1999;41:1-7.

118. Muta H, Ishii M, Kimiyasu E, Furui J, Sugahara Y, Akagi T, et al. Early intravenous gamma-globulin treatment for Kawasaki disease: the nationwide surveys in Japan. J Pediatr 2004;144:496-9.

119. Yanagawa H, Nakamura Y, Sakata K, Yashiro M. Use of intravenous gamma globulin for Kawasaki disease: effects on cardiac sequelae. Pediatr Cardiol 1997;18:19-23.

120. Sundel RP, Burns JC, Baker A, Beiser AS, Newburger JW. Gamma globulin re-treatment in Kawasaki disease. J Pediatr 1993;123:657-9.

121. Kato H, Koike S, Yokoyama T. Kawasaki disease: effect of treatment on coronary artery involvement. Pediatrics 1979;63:175-9.

122. Han RK, Silverman ED, Newman A, McCrindle BW. Management and outcome of persistent or recurrent fever after initial intravenous gamma globulin therapy in acute Kawasaki disease. Arch Pediatr Adolesc Med 2000;154:694-9.

123. Sundel RP, Baker AL, Fulton DR, Newburger JW. Corticosteroids in the initial treatment of Kawasaki disease: report of a randomized trial. J Pediatr 2003;142:611-6.

124. Wright DA, Newburger JW, Baker A, Sundel RP. Treatment of immune globulin-resistant Kawasaki disease with pulsed doses of corticosteroids. J Pediatr 1996;128:146-9.

125. Nonaka Z, Maekawa K, Okabe T, Eto Y, Kubo M. Randomized controlled study of intravenous prednisolone and agamma globulin treatment in 100 cases with Kawasaki disease. Kawasaki Disease. In: Firth International Kawasaki disease symposium. Philadelphia: Elsevier Science; 1994.

126. Newburger JW. Treatment of Kawasaki disease: corticosteroids revisited. J Pediatr 1999;135:411-3.

127. Shinohara M, Sone K, Tomomasa T, Morikawa A. Corticosteroids in the treatment of the acute phase of Kawasaki disease. J Pediatr 1999;135:465-9.

128. Wooditch AC, Aronoff SC. Effect of initial corticosteroid therapy on coronary artery aneurysm formation in Kawaski disease: a meta-analysis of 862 children. Pediatrics 2005;116:989-95.

129. Inoue Y, Okada Y, Shinohara M, Kobayashi T, Tomomasa T, Takeuchi K, et al. A multicenter prospective randomized trial of corticosteroids in primary therapy for Kawasaki disease: clinical course and coronary artery outcome. J Pediatr 2006;149:336-41.

130. Hashino K, Ishii M, Iemura M, Akagi T, Kato H. Re-treatment for immune globulin-resistant Kawasaki disease: a comparative study of additional immune globulin and steroid pulse therapy. Pediatr Int 2001;43:211-7.

131. Furukawa T, Kishiro M, Akimoto K, Nagata S, Shimizu T, Yamashiro Y. Effects of steroid pulse therapy on immunoglobulin-resistant Kawasaki disease. Arch Dis Child 2008;93:142-6.

132. Furukawa S, Matsubara T, Umezawa Y, Motohashi T, Ino T, Yabuta K. Pentoxifylline and intravenous gamma globulin combination therapy for acute Kawasaki disease. Eur J Pediatr 1994;153:663-7.

133. Weiss JE, Eberhard BA, Chowdhury D, Gottlieb BS. Infliximab as a novel therapy for refractory Kawasaki disease. J Rheumatol 2004;31:808-10.

134. Wallace CA, French JW, Kahn SJ, Sherry DD. Initial intravenous gamma-globulin treatment failure in Kawasaki disease. Pediatrics 2000;105:E78.

135. Raman V, Kim J, Sharkey A, Chatila T. Response of refractory Kawasaki disease to pulse steroid and cyclosporin A therapy. Pediatr Infect Dis J 2001;20:635-7.

136. Szer IS. Gastrointestinal and renal involvement in vasculitis: management strategies in Henoch-Schönlein purpura. Cleveland Clin J Med 1999;66:312-7.

137. Scharer K, Krmar R, Querfeld U, Ruder H, Waldherr R, Schaefer F. Clinical outcome of Schonlein-Henoch purpura nephritis in children. Pediatr Nephrol 1999;13:816-23.

138. Saulsbury FT. Henoch-Schonlein purpura in children. Report of 100 patients and review of the literature. Medicine 1999;78:395-409.

139. Ronkainen J, Koskimies O, Ala-Houhala M, Antikainen M, Merenmies J, Rajantie J, et al. Early prednisone therapy in Henoch-Schonlein purpura: a randomized, double blind, placebo-controlled trial. J Pediatr 2006;149:241-7.

140. Weiss PF, Feinstein JA, Luan X, Burnham JM, Feudtner C. Effects of corticosteroid on Henoch-Schonlein purpura: a systematic review. Pediatrics 2007;120:1079-87.

141. Buchanec J, Galanda V, Belakova S, Minarik M, Zibolen M. Incidence of renal complications in Schonlein-Honch purpura syndrome in dependence of an early administration of steroids. Int Urol Nephrol 1988;20:409-12.

142. Saulsbury FT. Corticosteroid therapy does not prevent nephritis in Henoch-Schonlein purpura. Pediatr Nephrol 1993;7:69-71.

143. Szer IS. Henoch-Schonlein purpura: when and how to treat. J Rheumatol 1996;23:1661-5.

144. Rosenblum N, Winter H, Harland S. Steroid effects on the course of abdominal pain in children with Henoch-Schonlein purpura. Pediatrics 1987;79:1018-21.

145. Wang L, Huang FC, Ko SF, Cheng MT. Successful treatment of mesenteric vasculitis caused by Henoch-Schonlein purpura with methylprednisolone pulse therapy. Clin Rheumatol 2003;22:140-2.

146. Mollica F, Li Volti S, Garozzo R, Russo G. Effectiveness of early prednisone therapy in preventing the development of nephropathy in anaphylactoid purpura. Eur J Pediatr 1992;151:140-4.

147. Rigante D, Canelli M, Federico G, Bartolozzi F, Porri MG, Stabile A. Predictive factors of renal involvement or relapsing disease in children with Henoch-Schonlein purpura. Rheumatol Int 2005;25:45-8.

148. Temmel AFP, Emminger W, Schroth B, Zaunschirm HA, Gadner H. Early prednisone therapy and nephropathy in anaphylactoid purpura. Eur J Pediatr 1993;152:782-3.

149. Kaku Y, Nohara K, Honda S. Renal involvement in Henoch-Schonlein purpura: a multivariate analysis of prognostic factors. Kidney Int 1998;53:1755-9.

150. Huber AM, King J, McLaine P, Klassen T, Pothos M. A randomized, placebo-controlled trial of prednisone in early Henoch-Schonlein purpura. BMC Med 2004;2:7.

150. Iijinma K, Ito-Kariya S, Nakamura H, Yoshikawa N. Multiple combined therapy for severe Henoch-Schonlein nephritis in children. Pediatr Nephrol 1998;12:244-8.

151. Flynn JT, Smoyer WE, Bunchman TE, Kershaw DB, Sedman AB. Treatment of Henoch-Schonlein purpura glomerulonephritis in children with high dose corticosteroids plus oral cyclophosphamide. Am J Nephrol 2001;21:128-33.

153. Tarshish P, Bernstein J, Edelmann CM. Henoch-scholein purpura nephritis: course of disease and efficacy of cyclophosphamide. Pediatr Nephrol 2004;19:51-6.

154. Rottem M, Fauci AS, Hallahan CW, Kerr GS, Lebovics R, Leavitt RY, et al. Wegener's granulomatosis in children and adolescents: clinical presentation and outcome. J Pediatr 1993;122:26-31.

155. Akikusa JD, Schneider R, Harvey EA, Hebert D, Thorner PS, Laxer RM, et al. Clinical features and outcomes of pediatric Wegener's granulomatosis. Arthritis Rheum 2007;57:837-44.

156. Belostotsky VM, Shah V, Dillon MJ. Clinical features in 17 paediatric patients with Wegener granulomatosus. Pediatr Nephrol 2002;17:754-61.

157. Halstead LA, Karmody CS, Wolff SM. Presentation of Wegener's granulomatosus in young patients. Otolaryngol Head Neck Surg 1986;94:368-71.

158. Lurati-Ruiz F, Spertini F. Predictive value of antineutrophil cytoplasmic antibodies in small-vessel vasculitis. J Rheumatol 2005;32:2167-72.

159. Girard T, Mahr A, Noel LH, Cordier JF, Lesavre P, Andre MH, et al. Are antineutrophil cytoplasmic antibodies a marker predictive of relapse in Wegener's granulomatosis? Rheumatology (Oxford) 2001;40:147-51.

160. Moorthy AV, Cheswney RW, Segar WE, Groshong T. Wegener's granulomatosis in childhood: prolonged survival following cytotoxic therapy. J Pediatr 1977;91:616-8.

161. Stegmayr BG, Gothefors L, Malmer B, Muller Wiefel DE, Nilsson K, Sundelin B. Wegener's granulomatosus in children and young adults: a case study in ten patients. Pediatr Nephrol 2000;14:208-13.

162. Harrison HL, Linshaw MA, Lindsley CB, Cuppage FE. Bolus corticosteroids and cyclophosphamide for initial treatment of Wegener's granulomatosis. JAMA 1980;89:403-10.

163. De Groot K, Adu D, Savage CO. EUVAS (European Vasculitis Study Group). The value of pulse cyclophosphamide in ANCA-associated vasculitis: metanalysis and critical review. Nephrol Dial Transplant 2001;16:2018-27.

164. Guillevin L, Cordier JF, Lhote F, Cohen P, Jarrousse B, Royer I, et al. A prospective randomized trial comparing steroids with pulse cyclophosphamide versus steroids and oral cyclophosphamide in the treatment of generalized Wegener's granulomatosis. Arthritis Rheum 1997;40:2187-98.

165. Langford CA, Talar-Williams C, Barron KS, Sneller MC. A staged approach to the treatment of Wegener's granulomatosis: induction of remission with glucocorticoids and daily cyclophosphamide switching to methotrexate for remission maintenance. Arthritis Rheum 1999;42:2666-73.

166. De Groot K, Reinhold-Keller E, Tatsis E, Paulsen J, Heller M, Nolle B, et al. Therapy for the maintenance of remission in sixty-five patients with generalized Wegener's granulomatosis. Arthritis Rheum 1996;39:2052-61.

167. Hoffman GS, Leavitt RY, Kerr GS, Fauci AS. Treatment of Wegener's granulomatosis with glucocorticoids and methotrexate. Arthritis Rheum 1992;35:1322-9.

168. Gottlieb BS, Miller LC, Ilowite NT. Methotrexate treatment of Wegener's granulomatosis in children. J Pediatr 1996;129:604-7.

169. Langford CA, Talar-Williams C, Barron KS, Sneller MC. Use of a cyclophosphamide-induction methotrexate-maintenance regimen for the treatment of Wegener's granulomatosis: extended follow-up and rate of relapse. Am J Med 2003;114:463-9.

170. Langford CA, Talar-Williams C. Mycophenolate mofetil for remission maintenance in the treatment of Wegener's granulomatosis. Arthritis Rheum 2004;51:278-83.

171. Specks U, Fervenza FC, McDonald TJ, Hogan MC. Response of Wegener's granulomatosis to anti-CD20 chimeric monoclonal antibody therapy. Arthritis Rheum 2001;44:2836-40.

172. Keogh KA, Wylam ME, Stone JH, Specks U. Induction of remission by B lymphocyte depletion in eleven patients with refractory antineutrophil cytoplasmic antibody-associated vasculitis. Arthritis Rheum 2005;52:262-8.

173. Wegener's Granulomatosis Etanercept Trial (WGET) Research Group. Etanercept plus standard therapy for Wegener's granulomatosis. N Engl J Med 2005;352:351-61.

174. DeRemee RA. The treatment of Wegener's granulomatosis with trimethoprim/sulfamethoxazole: illusion or vision? Arthritis Rheum 1988;31:1068-74.

175. Weir A, Lipman M, Congleton J. Co-trimoxazole in Wegener's granulomatosis. N Engl J Med 1996;335:1769-70.

176. Ozen S, Besbas N, Saatci U, Bakkaloglu A. Diagnostic criteria for polyarteritis nodosa in childhood. J Pediatr 1992;120:206-9.

177. Ozen S, Anton J, Arisoy N, Bakkaloglu A, Besbas N, Brogan P, et al. Juvenile polyarteritis: results of a multicenter survey of 110 children. J Pediatr 2004;145:517-22.

178. Sundel R, Szer I. Vasculitis in childhood. Rheum Dis Clin N Am 2002;28:625-54.

179. Besbas N, Ozen S, Saatci U, Topaloglu R, Tinaztepe K, Bakkaloglu A. Renal involvement in polyarteritis nodosa: evaluation of 26 Turkish children. Pediatr Nephrol 2000;14:325-7.

180. Maeda M, Kobayashi M, Okamoto S, Fuse T, Matsuyama T, Watanabe N, et al. Clinical observation of 14 cases of childhood PAN in Japan. Acta Paediatr Jpn 1997;39:277-9.

181. Blau EB, Morris RF, Yunis EJ. Polyarteritis nodosa in older children. Pediatrics 1977;60:227.

182. Guillevin L, Jarrousse B, Lok C, Lhote F, Jais JP, Le Thi Huong Du D, et al. Long-term followup after treatment of polyarteritis nodosa and Churg-Strauss angiitis with comparison of steroids, plasma exchange and cyclophosphamide to steroids and plasma exchange. A prospective randomized trial of 71 patients. J Rheumatol 1991;18:489-90.

183. Fauci AS, Katz P, Haynes BF, Wolff SM. Cyclophosphamide therapy of severe systemic necrotizing vasculitis. N Engl J Med 1979;301:235-8.

184. Till SH, Amos RS. Long-term follow-up of juvenile-onset cutaneous polyarteritis nodosa associated with streptococcal infection. Br J Rheumatol 1997;36:909-11.

185. Guillevin L, Lhote F, Jarrousse B, Fain O. Treatment of polyarteritis nodosa and Churg-Strauss syndrome. A meta-analysis of 3 prospective controlled trials including 182 patients over 12 years. Ann Med Intern 1992;143:405-16.

186. Gedalia A, Correa H, Kaiser M, Sorensen R. Case report: steroid sparing effect of intravenous gamma globulin in a child with necrotizing vasculitis. Am J Med Sci 1995;309:226-8.

187. Albornoz MA, Benedetto AV, Korman M, McFall S, Tourtellotte CD, Myers AR. Relapsing cutaneous polyarteritis nodosa associated with streptococcal infections. Int J Dermtol 1998;37:664-6.

188. Zulian F, Athreya BH, Laxer R, Nelson AM, Feitosa de Oliveira SK, Punaro MG, et al. Juvenile localized scleroderma: clinical and epidemiological features in 750 children. An international study. Rheumatology 2006;45:614-20.

189. Takehara K, Moroi Y, Nakabayashi Y, Ishibashi Y. Antinuclear antibodies in localized scleroderma. Arthritis Rheum 1983;26:612-6.

190. Rosenberg AM, Uziel Y, Krafchik BR, Hauta SA, Prokopchuk PA, Silverman ED, et al. Antinuclear antibodies in children with localized scleroderma. J Rheumatol 1995;22:2337-43.

191. Hanson V, Drexler E, Kornreich H. Rheumatoid factor (anti-gamma-globulins) in children with focal scleroderma. Pediatrics 1974;53:945-7.

192. Uziel Y, Krafchik BR, Feldman B, Silverman ED, Rubin LA, Laxer RM. Serum levels of soluble interleukin-2 receptor. A marker of disease activity in localized scleroderma. Arthritis Rheum 1994;37:898-901.

193. Nelson AM, Laxer RM. Localized sclerodermas. In: Cassidy JT, Petty RE, Laxer RM, Lindsley CB, editors. Textbook of Pediatric Rheumatology. 5th ed. Philadelphia, Elsevier; 2005; p. 472-81.

194. Zulian F, Vallongo C, Woo P, Russo R, Ruperto N, Harper J, et al. Localized scleroderma in childhood is not just a skin disease. Arthritis Rheum 2005;52:2873-81.

195. Cunningham BB, Landells ID, Langman C, Sailer DE, Paller AS. Topical calcipotriene for morphea/linear scleroderma. J Am Acad Dermatol 1998;39:211-5.

196. Hulshof MM, Pavel S, Breedveld FC, Dijkmans BA, Vermeer BJ. Oral calcitriol as a new therapeutic modality for generalized morphea. Arch Dermatol 1994;130:1290-3.

197. Humbert PG, Dupond JL, Rochefort A, Vasselet R, Lucas A, Laurent R, et al. Localized scleroderma-response to 1,25-dihydroxyvitamin D3. Clin Exp Dermatol 1990;15:396-8.

198. Hulshof MM, Bouwes Bavinck J, Bergman W, Masclee AA, Heickendorff L, Breedveld FC, et al. Double-blind, placebo-controlled study of oral calcitriol for the treatment of localized and systemic scleroderma. Am Acad Dermatol 2000;43:1017-23.

199. Stege H, Berneburg M, Humke S, Klammer M, Grewe M, Grether-Beck S, et al. High-dose UVA1 radiation therapy for localized scleroderma. J Am Acad Dermatol 1997;36:938-44.

200. Kerscher M, Dirschka T, Volkenandt M. Treatment of localized scleroderma by UVA1 phototherapy. Lancet 1995;28:1166.

201. Pasic A, Ceovic R, Lipozencic J, Husar K, Susic SM, Skerlev M, et al. Phototherapy in pediatric patients. Pediatr Dermatol 2003;20:71-7.

202. Breuckmann F, Gambichler T, Altmeyer P, Kreuter A. UVA/UVA1 phototherapy and PUVA photochemotherapy in connective tissue diseases and related disorders: a research based review. BMC Dermtology 2004;4:11.

203. Kreuter A, Gambichler T, Avermaete A, Jansen T, Hoffman A, Hoffman K, et al. Combined treatment with calcipotriol ointment and low-dose ultraviolet A1 phototherapy in childhood morphea. Pediatr Dermatol 2001;18:241-5.

204. Uziel Y, Feldman BM, Krafchik BR, Yeung RS, Laxer RM. Methotrexate and corticosteroid therapy for pediatric localized scleroderma. J Pediatr 2000;136:91-5.

205. Weibel L, Sampaio MC, Visentin MT, Howell KJ, Woo P, Harper JI. Evaluation of methotrexate and corticosteroids for the treatment of localized scleroderma (morphea) in children. Br J Dermatol 2006;155:1013-20.

206. Fitch PG, Retting P, Burnham JM, Finkel TH, Yan AC, Akin E, et al. Treatment of pediatric localized scleroderma with methotrexate. J Rheumatol 2006;33:609-14.

207. Kreuter A, Gambichler T, Breuckmann F, Rotterdam S, Freitag M, Stuecker M, et al. Pulsed high dose corticosteroids combined with low dose methotrexate in severe localized scleroderma. Arch Dermatol 2005;141:847-52.

208. Falanga V, Medsger TA. D-penicillamine in the treatment of localized scleroderma. Arch Dermatol 1990;126:609.

209. Krafchik BR. Localized cutaneous scleroderma. Semin Dermatol 1992;11:65–72.

210. Weiss JS. Antimalarial medications in dermatology: a review. Dermatol Clin 1991;9:377-85.

211. Peter RU, Ruzicka T, Eckert F. Low-dose cyclosporine A in the treatment of disabling morphea. Arch Dermatol 1991;127:1420-1.

212. Roldan R, Morote G, Castro MDC, Miranda MD, Moreno JC, Collantes E. Efficacy of bosentan in treatment of unresponsive cutaneous ulceration in disabling pansclerotic morphea in children. J Rheumatol 2006;33:2538-40.

Chapter 20

Septic Arthritis

Matija Tomšič, Sonja Praprotnik, James S. Louie, and John Townes

ORGANISMS RESPONSIBLE FOR SEPTIC ARTHRITIS

HOST FACTORS IMPORTANT IN SEPTIC ARTHRITIS

DIAGNOSTIC WORK-UP OF THE PATIENTS WITH SUSPECTED INFECTIOUS ARTHRITIS

THERAPY OF SEPTIC ARTHRITIS

The best practices for the management of infectious agent arthritis change rapidly, due to the development of new antibiotic drugs, and emerging research surrounding antibiotic resistance. Therefore, in order to ensure best patient care, the editors decided to update this chapter on an ongoing basis, and publish it in its entirety on www.expertconsult.com.

INTRODUCTION

Lyme disease, first recognized in 1976 because of an epidemic of oligoarthritis in children in Lyme, CT, is now the most common vector borne illness in both North America and Europe.[1,2] The causative organism, *Borrelia burgdorferi*, was isolated from the tick vector, *Ixodes scapularis*, in 1982[3] and from patients in 1983.[4,5] Erythema migrans (EM), a characteristic rash seen in the majority of cases, was reported in Sweden in 1909.[6] The neurologic manifestations of Lyme disease, particularly peripheral neuropathy in association with meningitis, were described in Europe in the 1940s.[7] Although Lyme disease in North America is almost always caused by *B. burgdorferi*, related species in Europe and Asia, *Borrelia afzelli* and *Borrelia garinii*, cause somewhat different clinical illnesses.[8] Ticks capable of transmitting Lyme disease are part of the *Ixodes ricinus* complex, including *I. scapularis* in the northeastern and north central United States, *I. pacificus* in the western states, *I. ricinus* in Europe and *Ixodes persulcatus* in Asia.[9]

In the United States, about 20,000 cases of Lyme disease are reported to the Centers for Disease Control and Prevention (CDC) annually (Fig. 21-1).[10,11] Most cases occur in the coastal northeastern states (Massachusetts to Virginia), the Midwest (Minnesota and Wisconsin), and the western states (California, Oregon and parts of Nevada) (Fig. 21-2).[12,13] Lyme disease is underreported to health authorities, so the actual number of cases in the United States may be five- to 10-fold higher than the number of reported cases.[14,15] In association with a rapidly increasing incidence, there has been geographic expansion and widespread media interest, often sensationalizing Lyme disease.

Lyme disease has characteristic clinical features, and once the disease is established, confirmatory diagnostic tests. For the rheumatologist, Lyme arthritis can be recognized in the same way that gout or rheumatoid arthritis are diagnosed clinically, but confusion exists in the identification of Lyme disease, and it is often overdiagnosed and overtreated.[16-19] In considering targeted therapies for Lyme disease, a well-grounded understanding of clinical manifestations will solve many treatment problems.

Lyme disease can be divided into stages[20,21]:
1. Early localized infection.
2. Early disseminated infection.
3. Late Lyme disease.

Because Lyme disease is a tick-borne spirochetal infection, the earliest manifestations of the disease occur primarily during the late spring and early summer (Fig. 21-3),[22] when nymphal ixodes ticks are active (Fig. 21-4).[23] Early Lyme disease begins after an incubation period of days to several weeks following exposure to *B. burgdorferi*.[24] Late disease occurs weeks to years later. Lyme arthritis, a late manifestation, often begins in the fall or early winter, 3 to 6 months after initial infection.

Overlap can occur between stages. The pattern of illness has changed somewhat since Lyme disease was described thirty years ago, primarily because the disease is more often recognized and treated at onset and such treatment is almost always curative.[25] For this reason, fewer patients progress to early disseminated infection or to Lyme arthritis. For the same reason, Lyme arthritis patients are less likely to report antecedent EM. Recognition of EM leads to treatment, preventing progression of disease. Still, the concept of early and late disease is useful in recognizing patterns of illness. In considering whether a patient has Lyme disease, the clinician needs to understand how progression can occur and to approach the diagnosis based on suspicion of a specific stage of the illness.

EARLY DISEASE

Early Localized Infection

Early infection is most frequently recognized because of the EM rash seen in perhaps 80% of patients at the onset of Lyme disease.[21,26] In early localized disease, spirochetal infection is confined to the skin. *B. burgdorferi* can be successfully cultured from EM lesions more frequently than from other sites later in the disease.[27] There may be mild fever, malaise, and arthralgias, but other significant manifestations will be lacking. EM is an expanding erythematous rash, often with a well-demarcated

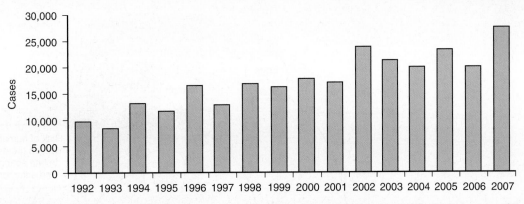

Figure 21-1. Reported cases of Lyme disease by year, 1992–2007—United States. In 2007, 27,444 cases of Lyme disease were reported, yielding a national average of 9.1 cases per 100,000 persons. In the 10 states where Lyme disease is most common, the average was 34.7 cases per 100,000 persons. (Adapted from Center for Disease Control and Prevention. Reported cases of Lyme disease by year—United States, 1992-2007. Accessed online October 4, 2008, at: http://www.cdc.gov/ncidod/dvbid/lyme/resourse/Lyme07Cases.pdf.)

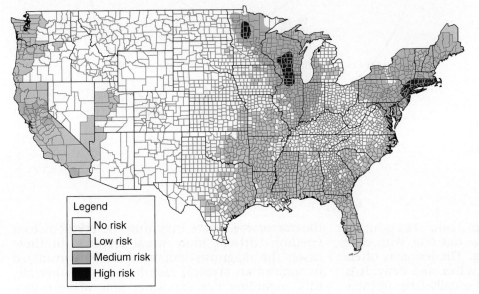

Legend
- No risk
- Low risk
- Medium risk
- High risk

Figure 21-2. Lyme disease risk—United States. (Adapted from http://www.aldf.com/usmap.shtml.)

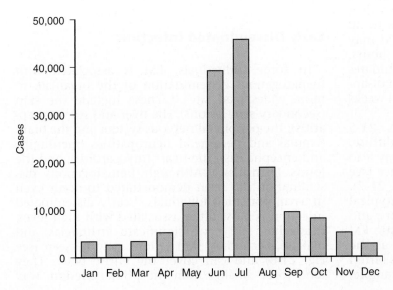

Figure 21-3. Reported cases of Lyme disease by month of illness onset, 1992–2004—United States. Patients with Lyme disease are most likely to have illness onset in June, July, or August and less likely to have illness onset from December through March. (Adapted from http://www.cdc.gov/ncidod/dvbid/lyme/resources/ld_rptmtho-fill_04.pdf.)

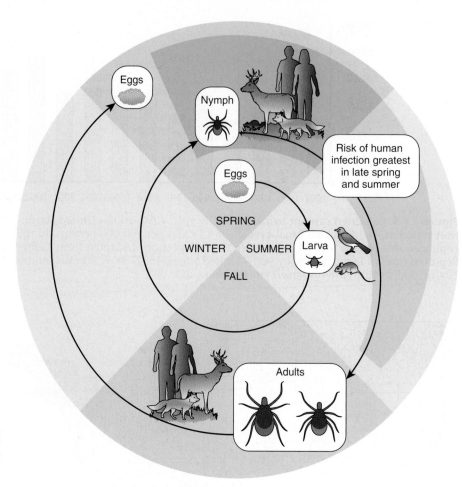

Figure 21-4. Life cycle of *Ixodes scapularis*. (Adapted from http://www.cdc.gov/ncidod/dvbid/lyme/ld_transmission.htm.)

outer border (Figs. 21-5 through 21-8).[28] The primary lesion occurs at the site of the tick bite, with centrifically expanding erythema. The lesion is often raised, sometimes indurated, warm, and itchy. It is not often painful. The rash is usually large (greater than 5 cm), and its size will usually distinguish EM from smaller, noninfectious, irritant skin reactions that occur at the bite site in many individuals. EM most typically develops 7 to 10 days after a deer tick bite, with a range of a few days to up to 30 days, but rarely occurs beyond this time. EM may expand within days or sometimes within hours. Appropriate antibiotic therapy promptly eliminates the rash and, even in untreated patients, EM disappears without scarring several days to several weeks after onset.[26,28]

Patterns of EM are recognized (see Figs. 21-5 through 21-7),[28] the most common being a diffuse, homogeneous rash (see Fig. 21-5). There may also be central clearing or a bull's eye appearance (see Fig. 21-6). Vesiculation may occur (see Fig. 21-7). But beyond these patterns, EM may have atypical features, may be transient, lasting only hours, and does not occur in all patients. Characteristic EM rashes are observed on flat surfaces, such as the chest or in the groin, but if an individual is bitten on a contoured or irregular surface, for example,

the ear or toe, there may only be erythematous swelling without more usual features. In these cases, the diagnosis will need to be considered in spite of an atypical rash because of other factors, including tick exposure, time of year, geographic risk of infection, and if present, laboratory confirmation.

Early Disseminated Infection

In some individuals, EM is associated with hematogenous dissemination of the organism to more widespread sites.[29] These include the skin (secondary skin lesions), the liver and spleen (hepatitis), the peripheral nervous system and the brain (cranial and peripheral neuropathies, meningitis and encephalitis), the heart (myocarditis), and the joints (arthritis).[21] Although hematogenous dissemination has been demonstrated to occur even in asymptomatic individuals,[29] early disseminated infection is most often associated with high fever, headaches, stiff neck, significant arthralgias, and malaise. Secondary skin lesions may be seen (see Fig. 21-8) and can cover the entire body. They tend to be smaller than the primary lesion, wax

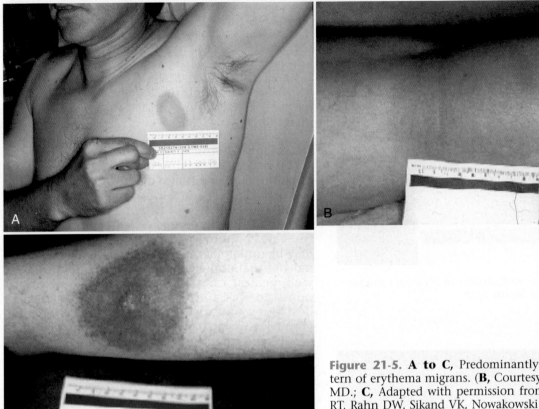

Figure 21-5. **A to C,** Predominantly homogeneous pattern of erythema migrans. (**B,** Courtesy of Robert P. Smith, MD.; **C,** Adapted with permission from Smith RP, Schoen RT, Rahn DW, Sikand VK, Nowakowski L, Parenti DL, et al. Clinical characteristics and treatment outcome of early Lyme disease in patients with microbiologically confirmed erythema migrans. Ann Intern Med 2002;136:421-8.)

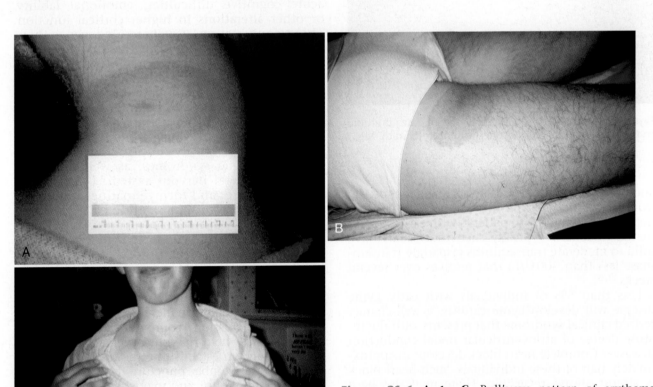

Figure 21-6. **A to C,** Bull's-eye pattern of erythema migrans. (**A,** Adapted with permission from Smith RP, Schoen RT, Rahn DW, Sikand VK, Nowakowski L, Parenti DL, et al. Clinical characteristics and treatment outcome of early Lyme disease in patients with microbiologically confirmed erythema migrans. Ann Intern Med 2002;136:421–8; **C,** Courtesy of Robert P. Smith, MD.)

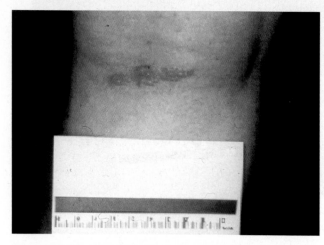

Figure 21-7. Central vesiculation of erythema migrans. (Courtesy of Robert P. Smith, MD.)

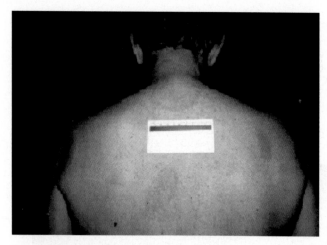

Figure 21-8. Early disseminated Lyme disease: multiple erythema migrans lesions. (Courtesy of Robert P. Smith, MD.)

and wane over time, and resolve independently from the primary lesion. Lyme disease causes mild hepatitis in about 5% of patients with early disseminated infection. Typically such individuals have mild to moderate transaminitis (aspartate transaminase less than 400 U/L) that resolves over several weeks.[21,29]

Less than 5% of individuals with early Lyme disease will develop Lyme carditis, a well-characterized clinical syndrome that presents with fluctuating degree of atrioventricular nodal conduction disease.[21] Complete heart block develops in approximately half of these individuals. Such heart block is almost always reversible. There may also be a mild acute myocarditis, but involvement of the heart valves does not occur, nor are there other cardiac arrhythmias such as atrial fibrillation or distal conduction system disease. Lyme carditis has been

suggested as a cause of chronic cardiomyopathy in Europe,[30] but there have been no well-documented cases in the United States.[31] One elderly patient coinfected with both the *B. burgdorferi* and *Babesia microtii* died from cardiac complications of infection.[32]

Neurologic Disease

The neurologic manifestations of Lyme disease present the most difficult diagnostic problems, but the neurologic features of early Lyme disease are often characteristic.[21,33] Patients may have disease of the peripheral nervous system; cranial neuropathies are common, particularly facial palsy, which may be unilateral or bilateral. There may be external ophthalmoplegia, and patients may initially seek medical care for diplopia. These manifestations can wax and wane, occur with other manifestations of early disseminated infection, and may be associated with meningitis or, less commonly, encephalitis. Many patients with early neurologic infection have headache, fever, and stiff neck. A significant percentage of these are found to have Lyme meningitis with a mild to moderate lymphocytic pleocytosis, elevated cerebral spinal fluid (CSF) protein levels and an increased CSF index (ratio of CSF to serum *B. burgdorferi* antibody titers greater than 1). Rare patients have a pattern consistent with meningoencephalitis and have acute cognitive difficulties, emotional lability, or other alterations in higher cortical function. These manifestations usually resolve even without antibiotic treatment, but untreated patients with Lyme meningoencephalitis may take months to recover.[34]

A distinction is made between early and late stage neurologic disease, although this may be a continuum. Late Lyme disease can occasionally affect the central nervous system (CNS). Patients may have cognitive dysfunction, such as memory loss, fatigue syndromes, as well as disease of the peripheral nervous system. Upper motor neuron disease and demyelinating syndromes have been reported, but causation has not been established.[35]

Patients with late neurologic Lyme disease usually have an antecedent history of earlier manifestations, such as EM, cranial nerve palsies or oligoarticular arthritis, and this is helpful in diagnosis.[35] Diagnostic imaging tests of the CNS, such as brain magnetic resonance imaging or brain single-photon emission computerized tomography scanning, may help rule out other conditions, but are not useful in establishing the diagnosis of CNS Lyme disease. Lumbar puncture testing, as in early disease, is important and may show mild lymphocytic pleocytosis, increased CSF protein, and an elevated CSF index (ratio of CSF to serum *B. burgdorferi* antibodies by enzyme-linked immunosorbent assay [ELISA] greater than 1).[35]

LATE DISEASE

Lyme Arthritis

Lyme disease was recognized in the United States in patients with Lyme arthritis, a late manifestation of the disease.[1] Affected individuals are often active outdoors in locations endemic for Lyme disease and typically have a characteristic pattern of arthritis.[36] In the past, most patients also had antecedent EM, but this is now less likely because recognition of EM leads to curative treatment. Such treated individuals will not develop further disease manifestations, including Lyme arthritis. On the other hand, if early Lyme disease is not treated, 60% of these individuals will subsequently develop Lyme arthritis, often 3 to 6 months after disease exposure (Fig. 21-9).[36] Some patients develop migratory arthralgias without frank arthritis, but most develop monoarthritis or, less frequently, an asymmetric oligoarthritis arthritis, usually including the knee (Fig. 21-10). Lyme arthritis usually affects fewer than five joints, typically large joints (Fig. 21-11).[36]

Lyme arthritis tends to occur in intermittent attacks lasting from several days to several weeks, although in about 10% of untreated patients, joint swelling lasts for more than a year and can be considered chronic.[36] Large joint effusions are common in the knees and elsewhere, and often recur after aspiration. Popliteal cysts occur and can rupture if tense synovial effusions are allowed to persist. The arthritis is often not painful and usually resolves with surprisingly little joint dysfunction, although chronic, unremitting arthritis sometimes causes permanent joint destruction.[36]

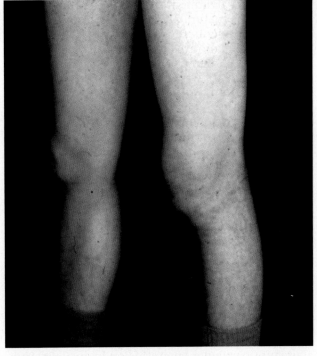

Figure 21-10. Lyme disease: monoarthritis of the knee. (Courtesy of Allen C. Steere, MD.)

Although Lyme arthritis is an infection, there are only two reports of successful cultivation of *B. burgdorferi* from synovial fluid.[37,38] However, *B. burgdorferi* DNA is detectable in synovial fluid by polymerase chain reaction (PCR) in most untreated Lyme arthritis patients[39] and synovial fluid PCR testing is usually

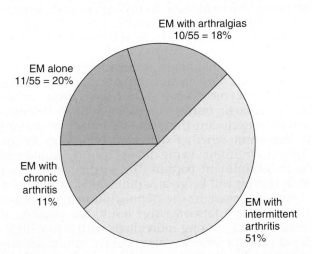

Figure 21-9. Frequency of joint involvement in 55 Lyme disease patients. (Adapted with permission from Steere AC, Schoen RT, Taylor E. The clinical evolution of Lyme arthritis. Ann Intern Med 1987;107:725–31.)

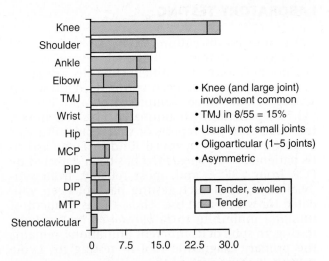

Figure 21-11. Lyme arthritis: distribution of joints affected. (Adapted with permission from Steere AC, Schoen RT, Taylor E. The clinical evolution of Lyme arthritis. Ann Intern Med 1987;107:725–31.)

negative after treatment. Antibiotic therapy clearly improves the natural history of Lyme arthritis,[40] but not all patients respond immediately. It often requires several months for arthritis to resolve, even with successful therapy.

It is unclear why Lyme arthritis responds promptly to antibiotic therapy in some patients but not others. There is evidence that in some patients, persistent Lyme arthritis results from postinfectious, immune reactivity, rather than persistent infection.[41] There may both bacterial[42] and host determinants of arthritis propensity, severity and antibiotic responsiveness.[43,44] Clinically, patients with Lyme arthritis can be divided into two groups: *antibiotic responsive* (successful antibiotic treatment in less than three months) and *antibiotic refractory* (treatment requires more than three months).[45] It is not possible to prospectively identify which patients will be antibiotic refractory, but as discussed later, these patients may require nonantibiotic therapies to achieve resolution of arthritis.

Although Lyme arthritis is an infectious, inflammatory arthritis, its frequent presentation as an acute monoarticular knee effusion in an active individual is often confused with a mechanical internal derangement. Compared with other forms of bacterial arthritis, Lyme arthritis is only occasionally associated with fever or significant constitutional symptoms and is usually less painful. Lyme arthritis shares some clinical features with spondyloarthropathy, but not with most cases of rheumatoid arthritis, because it is not polyarticular or symmetric. There is no convincing evidence that Lyme disease causes osteoarthritis or an osteoarthritic predisposition.

LABORATORY TESTING

It is possible to culture B. burgdorferi from EM skin biopsy specimens,[27] but such testing is usually not necessary or routinely clinically available. B. burgdorferi has also been cultured, in a research setting, from blood samples from 93 of 213 (43.7%) patients with untreated EM.[29] As noted, there are only two reports of successful culture of B. burgdorferi from synovial fluid in Lyme arthritis patients.[37,38] B. burgdorferi has been detected by PCR from CSF[46,47] and, most reliably, from synovial fluid,[39] but such testing has not been validated for widespread use. Thus, the assessment of humoral immunity to B. burgdorferi by serologic testing, in spite of its inherent limitations, remains the primary diagnostic tool in testing for Lyme disease. Because such testing relies on the patient's immune response, which can take up to 4 weeks to develop, a significant minority of patients with early localized infection will be seronegative for B. burgdorferi antibodies by ELISA at the onset of illness.[48] Because the goal of treatment at this

stage is not only to shorten the duration of EM but also prevent late stage manifestations of disease, it is appropriate to treat such individuals with antibiotics based on clinical suspicion, even in the absence of serologic confirmation. These patients will not only have complete recovery but may never make a detectable serologic response against B. burgdorferi.

As B. burgdorferi infection becomes more established, however, most patients with early disseminated Lyme disease will have B. burgdorferi–specific antibodies by ELISA, and virtually all patients with late stage Lyme disease will have such seroreactivity.[25,49] Criteria have been established to determine positive tests for B. burgdorferi by ELISA and Western blot (WB).[50] According to validated standards, established by the CDC/Association of State and Territorial Public Health Laboratory directors, the criteria for immunoglobulin G (IgG) reactivity require the presence of five or more significant bands.[51] These criteria were developed to maximize sensitivity and specificity in the diagnosis of all stages of Lyme disease. Patients with Lyme arthritis usually widely exceed this WB IgG reactivity and often have IgM reactivity as well (Table 21-1).

Lyme disease test results must be interpreted in the clinical context of the patient's history. Not only are negative serologic responses often seen during the first several weeks of infection but persistent positive responses are seen in many patients for months after successful antibiotic therapy for early Lyme disease. Among individuals with Lyme arthritis, the immune response against B. burgdorferi is even more robust. For this reason, most patients with Lyme arthritis remain seropositive for years after successful antibiotic therapy. Such seropositivity, in the absence of other evidence for infection, is not an indication for retreatment and may confer protective immunity. In my experience, patients with a history of Lyme arthritis are unlikely, for a period of several years, to be reinfected with Lyme disease.

For the rheumatologist, evaluating patients with chronic musculoskeletal complaints and questions about late Lyme disease ("Do I have Lyme arthritis?"), serologic testing is a useful adjunct in establishing or excluding the diagnosis, but it is important to determine whether signs and symptoms fit the clinical syndrome. Lyme disease testing should not be indiscriminant because the predictive value of such testing will be greatly diminished if the prevalence of disease in the population being tested is low. Although false-negative results are possible at disease onset, among individuals with a low likelihood of Lyme disease, false-positive results are the bigger problem. At the present time, hundreds of thousands of Lyme disease serologies are being performed to find hundreds of cases. As a result, the predictive value of Lyme disease serologies has been diminished, and false-positive tests are a common clinical problem.[52]

Table 21-1. *Lyme Disease Western Blot Results*

Test Name	Result		Reference
Lyme Disease IgG and IgM, WB			
Lyme Disease (IgG), WB	**POSITIVE**	**ABN**	NEGATIVE
18 kD (IgG) band	**REACTIVE**	**ABN**	
23 kD (IgG) band	**REACTIVE**	**ABN**	
28 kD (IgG) band	**REACTIVE**	**ABN**	
30 kD (IgG) band	**REACTIVE**	**ABN**	
39 kD (IgG) band	**REACTIVE**	**ABN**	
41 kD (IgG) band	**REACTIVE**	**ABN**	
45 kD (IgG) band	**REACTIVE**	**ABN**	
58 kD (IgG) band	**REACTIVE**	**ABN**	
66 kD (IgG) band	**REACTIVE**	**ABN**	
93 kD (IgG) band	**REACTIVE**	**ABN**	

NOTE: IgG Western Blot strips which have 5 (or more) of the 10 significant bands are considered positive for specific antibody to *B. burgdorferi*. The diagnosis of Lyme disease must include careful clinical evaluation and should not be based only on detection of antibodies to *B. burgdorferi*. A negative western blot interpretation does not exclude the possibility of infection with *B. burgdorferi*. (From Dressler F, Whalen JA, Reinhardt BN, Steere AC. Western blotting in the serodiagnosis of Lyme disease. J Infect Dis 1993;167:392–400 and the Recommendations of the Second Conference of Lyme Disease, Dearborn, Michigan, 1994.)

Lyme Disease (IgM), WB	**POSITIVE**	**ABN**	NEGATIVE
23 kD (IgM) band	**REACTIVE**	**ABN**	
39 kD (IgM) band	NON-REACTIVE		
41 kD (IgM) band	**REACTIVE**	**ABN**	

NOTE: IgM Western Blot strips which have a minimum of 2 of the 3 significant bands are considered positive for specific antibody to *B. burgdorferi*. The diagnosis of Lyme disease must include careful clinical evaluation and should not be based only on detection of antibodies to *B. burgdorferi*. A negative western blot interpretation does not exclude the possibility of infection with *B. burgdorferi*. (From Dressler F, Whalen JA, Reinhardt BN, Steere AC. Western blotting in the serodiagnosis of Lyme disease. J Infect Dis 1993; 167:392–400 and the Recommendations of the Second Conference of Lyme Disease, Dearborn, Michigan, 1994.)

The State of CT asks us to remind all physicians to report all cases of Lyme disease. Please call them at 860–509–7994 for reporting forms.

Courtesy of Quest Diagnostics.

CASE PRESENTATIONS

CASE STUDY 1 Early Localized Infection

A 56-year-old construction foreman was turkey hunting in Orange, CT, in May. To hunt turkey, he sat on the ground in the woods for several hours. Following this, he noted a minimally engorged deer tick in the right groin. He believed that he had been bitten one and a half hours before he removed the tick. Two days later he developed an erythematous rash in the right groin that was 3 inches in diameter. He otherwise felt well but suspected Lyme disease and visited his primary care physician. He was diagnosed with EM and given doxycycline 100-mg two pills in one dose. He was told to return if he developed any new symptoms. Over 4 days the rash resolved, but 2 weeks later, he developed fever, achiness, and headache. He was seen again by his primary doctor and given doxycycline 50 mg bid to be taken for 21 days.

By day 8 of this therapy, he was improved but still had significant fatigue and was unable to function full time at the construction job site. His employer suggested that he get a second opinion about treatment.

A second physician evaluated him in mid June. On examination, the skin was clear. The right groin revealed a bite site, but no rash. There was no significant inguinal lymphadenopathy. The remainder of the examination was unremarkable. The past medical history was one of generally good health. The patient reported having had three previous episodes of EM, 3 years, 5 years, and 8 years previously. Each of these was treated with antibiotic therapy with prompt resolution of illness.

The patient was given doxycycline 100 mg PO bid for an additional 10 days. At the completion of this treatment, his energy had returned to normal and he was entirely asymptomatic 1 month later in follow-up.

Discussion of Case 1

Lyme disease risk is a function of the time of year, geographic exposure, and vocational or recreational activities that increase the likelihood of deer tick bites. This individual, a turkey hunter, spent prolonged periods sitting on the ground during hunting season in the late spring in Connecticut. Perhaps it is not surprising that this was his fourth EM episode.[53] When Lyme disease is recognized and treated at the onset, most patients develop little protective immunity, become seronegative within weeks or months, and may develop the illness again if re-exposed.

This patient was aware of a deer tick bite and removed the tick, by his estimate, one and a half hours after exposure. He saved the tick. It was not engorged. In spite of this, he developed EM. This is not typical. Generally, the duration of tick attachment predicts the likelihood of disease development. The transmission of *B. burgdorferi* from the mid gut of *I. scapularis* to a host is relatively inefficient. In experimental animal models[54] and in humans,[55] 24 to 48 hours of tick attachment is required for infection to become reliably established. Therefore, prompt tick removal is one protective strategy to prevent Lyme disease. This patient noted the tick bite and the EM rash in the groin. Warm, moist sites such as the groin

or the axilla are common locations for tick bites (see Fig. 21-5A). It is also common for an individual engaging in high-risk activity, such as turkey hunting, to sustain multiple bites, and it is conceivable that the patient was unaware of the actual tick bite that caused this infection.

The patient recognized that he had early Lyme disease. He presented to his primary care physician, who confirmed this diagnosis based on his risk for Lyme disease and the typical appearance of the EM rash. However, the physician prescribed only two doxycycline 100 mg pills. This is an acceptable strategy to prevent Lyme disease in asymptomatic individuals with engorged deer tick bites.[56] Another appropriate strategy is simply to tell the patient to watch for signs and symptoms of Lyme disease and withhold any treatment,[57] but it is not an appropriate treatment of early Lyme disease. EM indicates that a localized skin infection is already present. In this patient, single dose doxycycline was insufficient to eradicate infection, and he went on, over several weeks, to have further symptoms of early Lyme disease. When seen in follow-up, the patient's physician again correctly recognized the persistence of Lyme disease but gave less than a full dose of doxycycline therapy. The patient improved but had persistent fatigue that prevented him from returning to work. He felt better after doxycycline was increased to 100 mg bid. Full-dose doxycycline was continued for 10 days. As expected, he was cured of the illness and did well.

CASE STUDY 2 Early Disseminated Infection

A 21-year-old man developed headache and vomiting in August. There was no history of tick bites, but several days previously, when he first became ill, the patient had noted a "spot" on his chest that "looked like a hive" and lasted for 36 hours. Because of headache and vomiting, he was taken to a hospital emergency room, where an ear infection was suspected. The past medical history was noteworthy in that shortly after birth, he had been given a diphtheria/pertussis/tetanus vaccination and developed a postvaccination encephalopathy resulting in some persistent cognitive impairment. He also had juvenile-onset diabetes mellitus requiring insulin treatment.

In the emergency room, the patient was given cefdinir (Omnicef, Abbott Laboratories, North Chicago, IL), a first-generation cephalosporin, and seemed to improve somewhat over the next several days. One week later, however, he complained of severe back pain, recurrent headache, nausea and vomiting. He returned to the emergency room. A Lyme disease screening ELISA was positive, and a WB IgM test showed 23, 39, 41 reactive bands. He was given doxycycline 100 mg bid.

Over the next week, he felt somewhat better but not well. He still had headaches and vomiting. He was taken to another hospital. A lumbar puncture

was performed. The CSF opening pressure was normal, but there was a CSF lymphocytic pleocytosis (98 nucleated cells/mm^3, predominantly lymphocytes and 3 red cells/mm^3) and CSF protein was elevated at 131 mg/dL. Early disseminated Lyme disease with meningitis was diagnosed. He was hospitalized and given ceftriaxone (Rocephin, Roche Laboratories, Nutley, NJ) 2 g daily. Within 48 hours he felt much improved. This therapy was continued as an outpatient for a total duration of three weeks. The patient subsequently remained well.

Discussion of Case Study 2

Often the diagnosis of early Lyme disease is made easily from the clinical features of illness-geographic risk, time of year, history of a deer tick bite, characteristic EM appearance, and associated clinical symptoms, but sometimes it is not so easy. This patient illustrates several challenges in the diagnosis of early Lyme disease; most individuals with Lyme disease are not aware of a deer tick bite. Not all EM lesions have a typical appearance, and many are transient. An ear infection as a CNS cause for nausea and vomiting was considered initially in this patient, but Lyme disease was not. His pre-existing neurologic condition may also have hampered communication.

Early Lyme disease is readily cured with appropriate antibiotic therapy,[58] but some antibiotics, including the first-generation cephalosporin given initially to this patient (also sulfa drugs and quinolones) are ineffective in treating Lyme disease.[59] Several studies demonstrate that both doxycycline, which was eventually given, and amoxicillin successfully cure 95% of patients with early disease.[60,61] Unfortunately for this patient, treatment failures in early Lyme disease occasionally occur in individuals with unrecognized meningitis. Once meningitis was confirmed, the patient responded promptly to a parenteral third-generation cephalosporin (ceftriaxone). In some studies, oral doxycycline therapy has been found to be as effective as ceftriaxone in early Lyme disease with meningitis,[62] but based on my experience with this and similar patients, I treat Lyme meningitis, at least initially, with parenteral ceftriaxone or penicillin. It might have been possible to switch this patient from ceftriaxone to oral doxycycline after several days of parenteral therapy, but both the patient and his family were wary of any further potential for inadequate treatment.

Sometimes patients have rashes for which differentiation between EM and cellulitis is difficult. As in this patient, EM will not respond to a first-generation cephalosporin, and doxycycline may sometimes be inadequate for cellulitis. In these patients, amoxicillin/clavulanate (Augmentin, GlaxoSmithKline, Philadelphia, PA) may be a good alternative.

CASE STUDY 3 Lyme Arthritis

In early December, a 51-year-old man developed left shoulder and left elbow pain that resolved within 48 hours. This was followed by right knee swelling, which also lasted only a day. He then developed a left knee effusion. An orthopedic surgeon aspirated 70 mL from the left knee on December 13 and reaspirated 70 mL on December 14 (Table 21-2). He administered doxycycline, cephalexin, and indomethacin and referred the patient to a rheumatologist on December 15. Aside from left knee pain and swelling, the patient felt well. He denied fever, psoriasis, diarrhea, or antecedent EM. He worked as a United States Treasury Special Agent and conducted extensive weapons training in the field for other agents in Rhode Island. There was a history of deer tick bites.

On examination the patient was afebrile. There were no rashes. There was limitation of motion in the left knee due to a large effusion. Other joints were normal except for unilateral edema of the left ankle. Laboratory testing included a WBC 7300 cell/mcL, hematocrit 42.2%, erythrocyte sedimentation rate 67 mm/hr and CRP 8.6 mg/dL (normal less than 0.8). The uric acid was 4.4 mg/dL. The rheumatoid factor was 21 IU/mL (normal less than 14). Lyme disease testing showed ELISA 5.9 (normal less than 1), WB positive (see Table 21-1).

The rheumatologist diagnosed Lyme arthritis. Doxycycline 100 mg bid was continued for 30 days. A large left knee synovial effusion persisted and recurred in spite of repeated aspiration (see Table 21-2). *B. burgdorferi* PCR testing demonstrated reactivity during the first 3 weeks of antibiotic therapy but not subsequently. Doxycycline was given for a total of 60 days. In spite of this, there was persistent pain, stiffness, and a recurrent synovial effusion. On February 20, the patient was given ceftriaxone 2 g daily for 28 days. After 10 days, the left knee synovial effusion had not recurred for the first time and the patient had minimal pain. Ten days after completing ceftriaxone therapy, he reported resolution of left knee arthritis, but mild stiffness of the right knee. Examination showed an unremarkable left knee but a moderate right knee effusion with limitation of flexion. Recurrent Lyme arthritis in the right knee was diagnosed. He was treated with doxycycline 100 mg PO bid for 30 days. By day 7, he reported that both his knees were normal. He remained well in long-term follow-up.

Table 21-2. *Synovial Fluid Analysis of the Left Knee*

Date	Volume (cc)	WBC	Lyme Disease PCR	Routine Culture
12/13/05	70	37,000	–	Negative
12/14/05	85	18,250	–	–
12/15/05	75	14,300	Detected	–
01/05/06	38	17,200	Detected	–
01/25/06	24	14,300	Not detected	–
02/07/06	54	25,200	Not detected	–
02/17/06	70	18,250	–	–

–, data not available; PCR, polymerase chain reaction; WBC, white blood cell count.

Discussion of Case Study 3

Because EM is more frequently recognized and treated, Lyme arthritis patients are less likely than in the past to present to rheumatologists with antecedent EM. In this patient, Lyme arthritis was suggested by an asymmetric oligoarthritis with marked knee swelling. The diagnosis was also supported by the geographic location, the patient's occupation, and the onset in the early winter several months after potential exposure to Lyme disease. As is almost universal in patients with Lyme arthritis, serologic testing in this case revealed markedly positive antibody responses against *B. burgdorferi*.[49,50] As expected, the peripheral white blood cell count was not significantly elevated, but synovial fluid white blood cell counts showed an inflammatory response. The ESR and CRP were somewhat elevated. As in this patient, false-positive rheumatoid factor (or antinuclear antibodies) are occasionally seen.[63]

In individuals with the mildest involvement, Lyme arthritis is self-limited, lasting days or weeks, even in the absence of antibiotic therapy. Because such attacks of arthritis, if untreated, can recur,[36] antibiotic therapy should be given to prevent future recurrences in untreated patients even if an attack has already resolved. In other patients, Lyme arthritis is more persistent and untreated attacks can last for months, or even longer.

At present, most patients are treated initially with oral doxycycline or amoxicillin.[40] The majority of patients respond within 1 to 3 months and can be considered *antibiotic sensitive*.[45] A minority of patients with Lyme arthritis treated with antibiotics for up to 3 months will not immediately respond and are *antibiotic refractory*. Differences in susceptibility to treatment reflect either persistent infection or a postinfectious, immune-mediated inflammatory reaction,[45] but for individual patients, it is generally not possible to prospectively predict response to treatment. In any case, even difficult-to-treat patients usually have gradual resolution of Lyme arthritis over time.[36] As in this patient, I typically treat when necessary for up to 60 days with oral antibiotic therapy. In the minority of patients who do not respond, I then treat with ceftriaxone 2 g daily for 30 days. Along the way, an expectant approach may be appropriate, and courses of antibiotic therapy may be spaced between periods of no treatment, because improvement may occur even in the absence of antibiotics. Some studies suggest that 14 days of parenteral antibiotic therapy may be as effective as 30 days with less risk of adverse effects,[64] but I continue to treat most patients who require parenteral antibiotics for 30 days.

In this patient, 60 days of oral antibiotic therapy failed to resolve left knee arthritis. He continued to develop large, recurrent knee effusions and was unable to work. When he was subsequently given ceftriaxone, he promptly improved, but then had recurrence of arthritis in the contralateral knee. What should be done at that point? In my experience, most, but not all, patients with Lyme disease monoarthritis, successfully treated with antibiotic therapy, do not have subsequent recurrences in other joints. When they do, as in this patient, the recurrences are often milder and less protracted than the original episode of arthritis. It was for this reason that I used additional doxycycline therapy to treat the patient's subsequent attack of arthritis. This attack resolved promptly with only oral antibiotic therapy.

What should be done for patients with Lyme arthritis who do not respond to 60 days of oral antibiotic therapy, followed by a month of parenteral antibiotic therapy? As infection persists, the spirochete generates an expanding range of host immune responses.[49] From a clinical perspective, this explains the multiple reactive bands seen on WB testing.[50] There is, however, a diminishing return to continuing antibiotic treatment.[40] It may be that in these individuals, the arthritis becomes less an infectious process and more a postinfectious, inflammatory reactive arthritis.

In antibiotic-refractory patients, several strategies are possible. Over the long run (measured in weeks and months), the natural history of Lyme arthritis even in these refractory individuals is one of gradual resolution[36] and an expectant approach may be part of their treatment. Beyond this, two strategies have been used most extensively to treat refractory Lyme arthritis. The first is arthroscopic synovectomy for Lyme arthritis of the knee.[65] Among 20 patients with Lyme arthritis of the knee refractory to multiple courses of oral and intravenous antibiotic therapy, arthroscopic synovectomy successfully treated 80%. Presumably, the mechanism of arthroscopic synovectomy is debulking of the inflamed/infected synovium. Unlike synovectomies for other inflammatory rheumatic diseases, the long-term natural history of the arthroscopic synovectomy in Lyme arthritis is not one of recurrent inflammatory arthritis.

A second approach to refractory Lyme arthritis has been to use disease-modifying antirheumatic drugs.[45] Such treatment should be considered only after extensive antibiotic therapy because there is concern that immunosuppressive therapy might retard resolution of infection. Although there is some experience with more potent agents, interest has centered mostly on hydroxychloroquine because of its limited immunosuppressive potential. Patients are typically treated for 6 months. The results to date suggest a possible benefit when compared with a historical control group, but the small number of patients treated has not demonstrated a statistically significant improvement.[45] Careful patient selection has not been associated with reports of adverse outcomes. More experience is needed.

Beyond antibiotic therapy in the management of Lyme arthritis, there is a place for adjunctive measures. During the acute phase of arthritis in which recurrent effusions are common, partial non-weight bearing and nonsteroidal anti-inflammatory drugs help limit joint swelling and protect against complications such as popliteal cyst rupture. In some patients, such as in this case, recurrent aspiration of the inflamed joint is also necessary to relieve pressure on a tensely swollen joint. It is possible, but unproven, that such recurrent drainage enhances the resolution arthritis. I avoid corticosteroid injections in patients with Lyme arthritis,

because limited information has associated this with delayed cure.[66] Joint effusions often come back when aspirated but, as in this patient, the first evidence of successful treatment may be that the drained effusion does not recur.

CASE STUDY 4 Lyme Disease and Rheumatoid Arthritis

A 64-year-old woman reported a 10-year history of generalized stiffness in her fingers, followed several years later by stiffness in her feet. These symptoms were not severe. She tore an anterior cruciate ligament at age 60 years and had ongoing knee stiffness. Two months before her visit to a rheumatologist, the patient abruptly developed pain in the neck and in both shoulders. Initially, she attributed this pain to disturbed sleep because her symptoms were worse in the morning, but she then developed increased pain in her shoulder, hips, and right elbow, with swelling of the right hand. Because of these symptoms, she visited her primary care physician. His testing included a positive rheumatoid factor (patient = 19 IU, normal less than 14), positive antinuclear antibody (patient = 1:320 homogeneous) and positive Lyme disease ELISA (patient = 1.52, normal less than 0.9). Her physician treated her with doxycycline and referred her to a rheumatologist. The past medical history included a bull's eye rash in 1996 diagnosed as Lyme disease for which the patient was given doxycycline for 2 weeks.

On examination, there was no psoriasis. The joint examination revealed mild synovitis of the second and third metacarpophalangeal joints bilaterally, somewhat limited flexion and extension of the elbows, and pain with abduction of both shoulders. There was some pain with abduction and external rotation of the hips.

The rheumatologist diagnosed rheumatoid arthritis based on the patient's history of a symmetric inflammatory arthritis associated with morning stiffness. The patient was told that she did not have Lyme disease or systemic lupus erythematosus.

Discussion of Case Study 4
In rheumatology, laboratory testing needs to be an adjunct to a well-formulated clinical suspicion. This patient described a symmetric polyarthritis affecting both large and small joints associated with morning stiffness. Her examination showed a proliferative synovitis in the small joints of her hands. These findings are expected in rheumatoid arthritis. They do not suggest Lyme arthritis. Her laboratory testing showed a positive rheumatoid factor consistent with the diagnosis of rheumatoid arthritis. She also had a low positive antinuclear antibody, seen in many patients with rheumatoid arthritis, and a low positive Lyme disease ELISA. Her positive Lyme disease serology may reflect previous exposure to B. burgdorferi (she had a bull's eye rash in 1996), or the positive Lyme disease serology may simply be a false-positive result. Polyclonal B cell activation in rheumatoid arthritis or other chronic inflammatory conditions increases the likelihood of a false positive Lyme disease serology.[49]

For patients with recent-onset inflammatory arthritis, Lyme arthritis may be a more appealing diagnosis than rheumatoid arthritis, because antibiotic therapy in Lyme disease is curative, but current treatment in rheumatoid arthritis is not. Patients with inflammatory arthritis who live in Lyme disease endemic locations (and some such patients living in nonendemic locations) may seek the diagnosis of Lyme disease. However, the rheumatologist needs to recognize the clinical differences between Lyme disease and rheumatoid arthritis, recognize the limitations of laboratory testing in both these diseases, and counsel patients accurately.

CASE STUDY 5 Lyme Disease, Chronic Lyme Disease, and Fibromyalgia

A 52-year-old woman from southeastern Connecticut noted a tick bite on the right inner thigh in June. Shortly after this, she traveled to Tennessee for vacation. She noted an expanding erythematous rash around the bite site and suspected that she had Lyme disease. Initially, she felt well. Because she was on vacation and was concerned that "physicians in Tennessee might not understand Lyme disease," she did not seek medical attention. Over 2 weeks, she developed increasing headache, achiness, and flu-like symptoms. She returned to Connecticut and saw her primary care physician, who diagnosed her as having Lyme disease and treated her for 2 weeks with doxycycline. She then felt well.

In September, the patient noted recurrent achiness, fatigue, and headaches. She suspected a recurrence of Lyme disease. Repeat Lyme disease ELISA in October was positive (patient = 3.08; normal less than 0.9). WB testing showed IgM positive (23 and 41 kd bands) and IgG negative. She was given a month of doxycycline therapy. She felt somewhat better.

Early in the following year she returned to her physician with fatigue, widespread musculoskeletal pain and concern that she had chronic Lyme disease. A Lyme disease serology was obtained and was again positive (ELISA = 1.53; Western blot IgM positive, IgG negative, as before). She was given doxycycline again for 1 month, but her symptoms did not improve. She was referred to a rheumatologist.

The patient was perimenopausal. She reported disturbed sleep more than 1 year. Her past medical history included hypertension and lumbar disc surgery. She worked as an administrator. On examination there was mild obesity. The skin was clear. The joint examination was without synovitis except mild osteoarthritic changes of the DIP joints in both hands.

The rheumatologist diagnosed "history of Lyme disease, treated," and fibromyalgia based on her history of disturbed sleep, fatigue, and widespread musculoskeletal pain. She was given amitriptyline 25 mg at bedtime, and a regular exercise program was recommended. When seen in follow-up 6 months later, she reported that she was relieved not to have chronic Lyme disease and her symptoms were somewhat improved.

Discussion of Case Study 5

Most patients treated for Lyme disease, whether early or late stage, do not develop chronic symptoms.[67] But Lyme disease is overdiagnosed, overtreated,[16–19] and sometimes misdiagnosed based on common, nonspecific symptoms that have other causes, even in patients who have no supportive features of Lyme disease. When given the diagnosis of Lyme disease for symptoms such as fatigue and widespread musculoskeletal pain, such patients will have no benefit or only a transient placebo-associated improvement from antibiotic therapy for a disease that they do not have.

Some individuals, such as this patient, have a well-documented antecedent history of Lyme disease but no longer have active infection. These patients frequently have persistently positive Lyme disease serologies even after curative antibiotic therapy. If they are given antibiotics for nonspecific flu-like symptoms or fatigue syndromes, they often experience a transient placebo-associated benefit. As in this case, that benefit typically diminishes over time, and the patient and the treating physician come to recognize that they are pursuing a therapeutic dead end.

Depression and associated somatoform disorders are common. Rheumatologists focus on musculoskeletal symptoms in patients with somatoform disorders and currently consider such individuals as having "fibromyalgia." Such a label may or may not be useful, but it does acknowledge the presence of a common problem. Some patients with somatoform symptoms who are, in fact, depressed resist the diagnosis of depression and seek the diagnosis of Lyme disease.[19] They also seek "Lyme literate" physicians who will give them this diagnosis.[68] But most patients simply want answers and are open to an honest understanding of their problem. These patients present the rheumatologist with a gratifying opportunity to reduce anxiety about chronic Lyme disease, which they do not have and to give them treatment more likely to relieve their symptoms.

LYME DISEASE TREATMENT

The Infectious Disease Society of America[25] and others[69] have recently reviewed evidence-based recommendations for the prevention and treatment of Lyme disease (Table 21-3).

Prevention

Unfortunately, preventive strategies have had limited impact on Lyme disease. In the northeastern United States, agriculture has waned, reforestation has occurred, and deer populations have increased exponentially in the absence of significant predators or hunting pressure.[8] In geographically isolated regions, such as the barrier islands off Massachusetts, it has been demonstrated that reductions in deer populations can decrease the prevalence of Lyme disease.[70] It is unlikely that such strategies will be employed over larger geographic areas.

Thus, currently available preventive measures rely on individual protection. The individual risk of Lyme disease can be somewhat predicted because the geographic risk of Lyme disease exposure is well characterized (see Fig. 21-2) and vocational and recreational activities are also important predictors of risk. For individuals at high risk for exposure, a

case-controlled study demonstrated that protective clothing was 40% effective and routine use of tick repellents on skin or clothing was 20% effective in preventing Lyme disease.[71] Other routinely recommended personal protective strategies, including checking one's body for ticks or spraying property with acaracides were not effective.[71] However, the transmission of Lyme disease from an infected tick to an individual requires tick attachment for up to 48 hours.[54,55] Therefore, in persons at risk, tick checks and prompt tick removal would seem prudent. A Lyme disease vaccine (Lymerix), consisting of a recombinant outer surface protein (Osp A) in adjuvant was available for persons between the ages of 15 and 70 who lived in or visited high risk areas and have frequent or prolonged exposure to *I. scapularis*,[72] but this vaccine has been withdrawn from commercial use.

It is controversial whether asymptomatic individuals should be given prophylactic antibiotic treatment after deer tick bites (see Table 21-3).[56,57] Although *B. burgdorferi* infection rates in *Ixodes* ticks from endemic areas can be high (between 5% and 50%),[73] the likelihood of acquiring Lyme disease after a deer tick bite in an endemic area is much lower, perhaps 1%,[57] presumably because of the prolonged duration of attachment to an individual required for transmission of infection.[54,55] Prophylactic antibiotic

Table 21-3. *Treatment of Lyme Disease**

Disorder	Drug‡	Usual Adult Dosage (range)†	Pediatric Dosage‡
Tick Bite			
	Doxycycline§,¶ and/or observation	200 mg PO bid × 1 dose	>8 y: 4 mg/kg × 1 dose
Erythema Migrans	Doxycycline¶ or	100 mg PO bid x 14 days (10–21)	>8 y: 1–2 mg/kg bid
	Amoxicillin	250–500 mg PO tid × 14 days (14–21)	25–50 mg/kg/day tid
	Ceftriazone axetil	500 mg PO bid x 14 days (14–21)	30 mg/kg/day bid
Neurologic Disease			
Facial nerve palsy	Doxycycline¶ or	100 mg PO bid × 14 days (14–21)	>8 y: 1–2 mg/kg bid
	Amoxicillin	250–500 mg PO tid 14 days (14–21)	25–50 mg/kg/day divided bid
More serious disease¶	Ceftriaxone††	2 g q24 h IV × 14 days (10–28)	50–75 mg/kg/day
Cardiac Disease			
Mild (first-degree AV block, PR <300 msec)	Doxycycline¶ or	100 mg PO bid × 14 days (14–21)	>8 y: 1–2 mg/kg bid
More serious disease††	Amoxicillin	250–500 mg PO tid × 14 days (14–21)	25–50 mg/kg/day tid
	Ceftraxone**	2 g q24 h IV × 14 days (14–21)	50–75 mg/kg/day
Arthritis‡‡			
Arthritis without neurologic disease	Doxycycline¶ or	100 mg PO bid × 14 days (14–21)	>8 y: 1–2 mg/kg bid
	Amoxicillin	400 mg PO tid 28 days	25–50 mg/kg/day
Persistent or recurrent§§	Ceftriaxone**	2 g q24 h IV × 14 days (14–28)	50–75 mg/kg/day

*Regardless of the clinical manifestation of Lyme disease, complete response to treatment may be delayed beyond the treatment duration. Relapse may occur with all of these regimens; patients who relapse may need a second course of treatment. Many repeat courses of therapy or excessively prolonged treatment is not recommended.

†Based on severity and/or response.

‡Should not exceed adult dosage. Duration of therapy is the same as in adult patients.

§Prophylaxis with doxycycline can be considered when: 1) the attached tick can be reliably identified as an adult or nymphal. *I.scapularis* tick that is estimated to have been attached for >36 hours based on the degree of engorgement of the tick with blood or on certainty about the time of exposure to the tick; b) prophylaxis can be started within 72 hours of the time that the tick was removed; c) the local rate of infection of these ticks with *B. burgdorferi* is >20%; and d) doxycycline is not contraindicated. For individuals who do not fulfill these criteria, observation is recommended.

¶Should generally not be used for children <8 years old or for pregnant or lactating women. Gastrointestinal toxicity and photosensitivity are common adverse effects.

¶Available data in European neuroborreliosis indicated that doxycycline and ceftriaxone are equally effective in Lyme meningitis. Data are lacking on the efficacy of doxycycline in Lyme encephalitis or Lyme encephalopathy. In the absence of brain or spinal cord involvement, doxycycline may be considered an acceptable treatment option if the illness is not severe.

**Intravenous cefotaxime 2 g q8 h is an acceptable alternative; the dose in pediatric patients is 150 to 200 mg/kg/day in 3 to 4 divided doses (max 6 g/day).

††Includes hospitalized patients with first-degree AV block with symptoms, or with a PR interval >200 milliseconds, or second- or third-degree AV block.

‡‡In late disease, the response to treatment may be delayed for several weeks or months.

§§Patients with mild persistent or recurrent arthritis may be treated with a second course of oral antibiotics.

Modified with permission from Treatment of Lyme disease. Med Lett Drugs Ther 2007;49:49-51 with permission.

treatment has a small risk of adverse affects, and in controlled clinical trials, such treatment has not been shown to confirm a major benefit.[57] In one study, however, administration of a single 200-mg dose of doxycycline after a deer tick bite reduced the incidence of EM from 3.2% in the control population to 0.4% in the treated group.[56]

Early Disease Treatment

For early stage disease (local and disseminated), the goal of antibiotic therapy is to shorten the duration of EM and associated symptoms and to prevent the development of late-stage illness. Most patients with EM can be cured with oral antibiotic therapy. Lyme carditis and early neurologic Lyme disease may require parenteral antibiotic therapy (see Table 21-3 and Case Study 2).

For EM, the drug of choice for adults (except pregnant women) and for children with permanent dentition, is doxycycline, 100 mg orally twice daily for 14 to 21 days or amoxicillin, 250 to 500 mg orally three times daily for 14 to 21 days (for children with permanent dentition, doxycycline, 1 to 2 mg/kg bid or amoxicillin, 25 to 50 mg/d divided tid).

The range in treatment duration suggested reflects variable severity of disease at onset. I treat most patients with mild illness for 2 weeks. Because the severity of disease at onset predicts for the risk of late disease manifestations in inadequately treated patients, I use 3 weeks of antibiotics for individuals with more than mild illness. Some studies suggest that a shorter duration is adequate.[74] Both doxycycline and amoxicillin are effective, but an advantage of doxycycline may be better CNS penetration. Also, doxycycline is effective against *Anaplasma phagocytophilum* (previously referred to as *Ehrlichia phagocytophila*), the causative organism of human granulocytic anaplasmosis, and some patients with Lyme disease may be coinfected with this tick-transmitted organism. But for most cases of Lyme disease, amoxicillin is just as effective as doxycycline for early Lyme disease and should be used in young children and pregnant women. For patients who cannot be treated with doxycycline or amoxicillin, cefuroxine axetil (Ceftin, GlaxoSmithKline, Philadelphia, PA) is an alternative.[61] Azithromycin, clarithromycin, or erythromycin are less effective. Maternal-to-fetal transmission of *B. burgdorferi* occurs rarely, if at all. Therefore, it is recommended that pregnant women receive standard therapy, although doxycycline should be avoided in pregnant women. First-generation cephalosporins, such as cephalexin (Keflex, Middlebrook Pharmaceuticals, Inc., Westlake, TX) are ineffective for Lyme disease (see Case Study 2).[59]

Treatment of Neurologic Manifestations

For patients with mild neurologic disease, such as facial palsy alone, oral doxycycline may be adequate therapy. For most patients with neurologic involvement, however, intravenous ceftriaxone (Rocephin) given for 2 to 4 weeks is recommended.[75] Cefotaxime (Claforen, Sanofi-Aventis, Bridgewater, NJ) or penicillin G are alternatives. The signs and symptoms of acute neuroborreliosis usually resolve within weeks, and relapses are unlikely after a 4-week course of parenteral antibiotic therapy.[75]

Treatment of Cardiac Disease

Patients with first-degree heart block and a PR interval of less than 0.3 seconds may be treated orally like other individuals with EM. For patients with higher grade atrioventricular nodal block and a PR interval of greater than 0.3 seconds, parenteral antibiotic therapy as listed in Table 21-3 and cardiac monitoring are recommended. Because Lyme carditis resolves without conduction system damage, a permanent pacemaker, even in patients with transient complete heart block, can almost always be avoided.[25,69]

Treatment of Lyme Arthritis

Several oral regimens are successful in treating Lyme arthritis in approximately 75% of patients and can, thus, avoid the morbidity and expensive intravenous antibiotic therapy. In adults, these antibiotics include doxycycline 100 mg orally twice daily for 30 days to 60 days and amoxicillin 500 mg three times a day for 30 to 60 days.[25,40,69] In patients who do not respond to oral antibiotic therapy, the intravenous regimens described in Case Study 3 and Table 21-3 (ceftriaxone and penicillin) are an alternative.[25,69] Despite either oral or intravenous antibiotic therapy, about 10% of patients in the United States have persistent joint inflammation for months, or even several years, after antibiotic therapy.[45] These patients may benefit from anti-inflammatory agents, arthroscopic synovectomy,[65] and occasionally hydroxychloroquine[45] as described in Case Study 3.

Management of Chronic Lyme Disease

Early Lyme disease is common and underreported.[14,15] Late Lyme disease, excluding Lyme arthritis, is rare, overdiagnosed, and overtreated.[16–19] Some patients are diagnosed as having "chronic Lyme disease" who, in fact, have never had this disorder. Some have a well-documented antecedent history of Lyme disease, treated according to standard regimens, but continue to have subjective symptoms, such as musculoskeletal pain, neurocognitive difficulties, or fatigue syndromes (see Case Study 5). Some advocates of "chronic Lyme disease" make this diagnosis and recommend treatment in the absence of any well-defined clinical criteria or validated laboratory studies. Not uncommonly, these patients have other medical conditions, such as rheumatoid arthritis, multiple sclerosis, fibromyalgia or, most frequently, depression.[19] There is no evidence that they will benefit from long-term antibiotic therapy, either intravenous or oral.[76] Long-term antibiotic therapy for patients given the diagnosis of chronic Lyme disease has been associated with adverse events,[19] including biliary complications[77] and death.[78] Supportive care, reassurance, and in many instances, treatment of the underlying disease, including depression, are more likely to be helpful.

References

1. Steere AC, Malawista SE, Syndman DR, Shope RE, Andiman WA, Ross MR, et al. Lyme arthritis: An epidemic of oligoarticular arthritis in children and adults in three Connecticut communities. Arthritis Rheum 1977;20:7-17.
2. Dennis DT, Hayes EB. Epidemiology of Lyme Borreliosis. In: Kahl O, Gray JS, Lane RS, Stanek G, editors. Lyme borreliosis: biology, epidemiology and control. Oxford, UK: CABI Publishing; 2002. p. 251-80.

3. Burgdorfer W, Barbour AG, Hayes SF, Benach JL, Grunwaldt E, Davis JP, et al. Lyme disease—a tick-borne spirochetosis? Science 1982;216:1317-9.

4. Steere AC, Grodzicki RL, Kornblatt AN, Craft JE, Barbour AG, Burgdorfer W, et al. The spirochetal etiology of Lyme disease. N Engl J Med 1983;308:733-40.

5. Benach JL, Bosler EM, Hanrahan JP, Coleman JL, Habicht GS, Bast TF, et al. Spirochetes isolated from the blood of two patients with Lyme disease. N Engl J Med 1983;308:740-2.

6. Afzelius A. Erythema chronicum migrans. Acta Dermatol Venerol (Stockh) 1921;2:120-5.

7. Bannworth A. Zur Klinik und Pathogenese der "chronischen lymphocytaren Meningitis". Arch Psychiatr Nervenkt 1944;117:161-85.

8. Steere AC, Coburn J, Glickstein L. The emergence of Lyme disease. J Clin Invest 2004;113:1093-101.

9. Lane RS, Piesman J, Burgdorferi W. Lyme borreliosis: relation of its causative agent to its vectors and hosts in North America and Europe. Annu Rev Entomol 1991;36:587-609.

10. Jajosky RA, Hall PA, Adams DA, Dawkins FJ, Sharp P, Anderson WA, et al. Centers for Disease Control and Prevention. Summary of notifiable diseases—United States, 2004. MMWR Morb Mortal Wkly Rep 2006;53:1-79.

11. Center for Disease Control and Prevention. Reported cases of Lyme disease by year—United States, 1992-2007. Available at: http://www.cdc.gov/ncdod/dvbid/lyme/resourse/Lyme07 Cases.pdf [Accessed online October 4, 2008].

12. Orloski KA, Hayes EB, Campbell GL, Dennis DT. Surveillance for Lyme disease United States 1992-1998, MMWR Morb Mortal Wkly Rep 2000;49:1-11.

13. American Lyme Disease Foundation. U.S. Maps and Statistics-Lyme disease risk. Available at: http://www.aldf.com/usmap.shtml [Accessed online October 4, 2008].

14. Meek JI, Roberts CL, Smith EV, Cartter ML. Underreporting of Lyme disease by Connecticut physicians, 1992. J Public Health Manage Practice 1996;2:61-5.

15. Coyle BS, Strickland GT, Liang YY, Pena C, McCarter R, Israel E, et al. The public health impact of Lyme disease in Maryland. J Infect Dis 1996;173:1260-2.

16. Sigal LH. Summary of the first 100 patients seen at a Lyme disease referral center. Am J Med 1990;88:577-81.

17. Steere AC, Taylor E, McHugh GL, Logigian E. The overdiagnosis of Lyme disease. JAMA 1993;269:1812-6.

18. Feder HM, Hunt MS. Pitfalls in the diagnosis and treatment of Lyme disease in children. JAMA 1995;274:66-8.

19. Reid MC, Schoen RT, Evans J, Rosenberg JC, Horwitz RI. The consequences of overdiganosis and overtreatment of Lyme disease: an observational study. Ann Intern Med 1998;128:354-62.

20. Asbrink E, Hovmark A. Early and late cutaneous manifestations of Ixodes-borne borreliosis (erythema migrans borreliosis, Lyme borreliosis). Ann N Y Acad Sci 1988;539:4-15.

21. Steere AC. Lyme disease. N Engl J Med 1989;321:586-96.

22. Centers for Disease Control and Prevention. Reported cases of Lyme disease by Month of Illness Onset United States, 1992-2004. Available at: http://www.cdc.gov/ncidod/dvbid/lyme/resourses/ld_rptmthofill_04.pdf. [Accessed online October 4, 2008].

23. Centers for Disease Control and Prevention. Life cycle of black-legged ticks. Available at: http://www.cdc.gov/ncidod/dvbid/lyme/ld_transmission.htm. [Accessed online October 4, 2008].

24. Steere AC. Lyme disease. N Engl J Med 2001;345:115-25.

25. Wormser GP, Dattwyler RJ, Shapiro ED, Halperin JJ, Steere AC, Klempner MS, et al. The clinical assessment, treatment and prevention of Lyme disease, human granulocytic anaplasmosis, and babesiosis: clinical practice guidelines by the Infectious Diseases Society of America. Clin Infect Dis 2006;43:1089-134.

26. Steere AC, Bartenhagen NH, Craft JE, Hutchinson GJ, Newman JH, Rahn DW, et al. The early clinical manifestations of Lyme disease. Ann Intern Med 1983;99:76-82.

27. Berger BW, Kaplan MH, Rothenberg IR, Barbour AG. Isolation and characterization of the Lyme disease spirochete from the skin of patients with erythema chronicum migrans. J Am Acad Dermatol 1985;13:444-9.

28. Smith RP, Schoen RT, Rahn DW, Sikand VK, Nowakowski L, Parenti DL, et al. Clinical characteristics and treatment outcome of early Lyme disease in patients with microbiologically confirmed erythema migrans. Ann Intern Med 2002;136:421-8.

29. Wormser GP, McKenna D, Carlin J, Nadelman RB, Cavaliere LF, Holmgren D, et al. Brief communication: hematogenous dissemination in early Lyme disease. Ann Intern Med 2005;142:751-5.

30. Stanek G, Klein J, Bittner R, Glogar D. Isolation of Borrelia burgdorferi from the myocardium of a patient with long-standing cardiomyopathy. N Engl J Med 1990;322:249-52.

31. Sonnesyn SW, Diehl SC, Johnson RC, Kubo SH, Goodman JL. A prospective study of the seroprevalance of Borrelia burgdorferi infection in patients with severe heart failure. Am J Cardiol 1995;76:97-100.

32. Marcus LC, Steere AC, Duray PH, Anderson AE, Mahoney EB. Fatal pancarditis in a patient with coexistent Lyme disease and babesiosis: demonstration of spirochetes in the myocardium. Ann Intern Med 1985;103:374-6.

33. Pachner AR, Steere AC. The triad of neurologic manifestations of Lyme disease: Meningitis, cranial neuritis, and radiculoneuritis. Neurology 1985;35:47-53.

34. Steere AC, Pachner AR, Malawista SE. Neurologic abnormalities of Lyme disease: Successful treatment with high-dose intravenous penicillin. Ann Intern Med 1983;99:767-72.

35. Logigian EL, Kaplan RF, Steere AC. Chronic neurologic manifestation of Lyme disease. N Engl J Med 1990;323:1438-44.

36. Steere AC, Schoen RT, Taylor E. The clinical evolution of Lyme arthritis. Ann Intern Med 1987;107:725-31.

37. Syndman DR, Schenkein DP, Berardi VP, Lastavica CC, Pariser KM. Borrelia Burgdorferi in joint fluid in chronic Lyme arthritis. Ann Intern Med 1986;104:798-800.

38. Schmidli J, Hunziker T, Moesli P, Schaad UB. Cultivation of Borrelia Burgdorferi from joint fluid three months after treatment of facial palsy due to Lyme borreliosis. J Infect Dis 1988;158:905-6.

39. Nocton JJ, Dressler F, Rutledge BJ, Rys PN, Persing DH, Steere AC, et al. Detection of Borrelia burgdorferi DNA by polymerase chain reaction in synovial fluid in Lyme arthritis. N Engl J Med 1994;330:229-34.

40. Steere AC, Levin RE, Molloy PJ, Kalish RA, Abraham JH 3rd, Liu NY, et al. Treatment of Lyme arthritis. Arthritis Rheum 1994;37:878-88.

41. Steere AC, Glickstein L. Elucidation of Lyme arthritis. Nature Rev Immunol 2004;4:143-52.

42. Pal U, Wang P, Bao F, Yang X, Samanta S, Schoen R, et al. Borrelia burgdorferi basic membrane proteins A and B participate in the genesis of Lyme arthritis. J Exp Med 2008;205:133-41.

43. Kannain P, McHugh G, Johnson BJ, Bacon RM, Glickstein LJ, Steere AC, et al. Antibody responses to Borrelia burgdorferi in patients with antibiotic-refractory antibiotics responsive or non-antibiotic treated Lyme arthritis. Arthritis Rheum 2007;56:4216-25.

44. Shin JJ, Glickstein LJ, Steere AC. High levels of inflammatory chemokines and cytokines in joint fluid and synovial tissue throughout the course of antibiotic-refractory Lyme arthritis. Arthritis Rheum 2007;56:1325-35.

45. Steere AC, Angelis SM. Therapy for Lyme arthritis: strategies for the treatment of antibiotic-refractory arthritis. Arthritis Rheum 2006;54:3079-86.

46. Lebech AM, Hansen K, Rutledge BJ, Kolbert CP, Rys PN, Persing DH. Diagnostic detection and direct genotyping of Borrelia burgdorferi by polymerase chain reaction in cerebrospinal fluid in patients with Lyme neuroborreliosis. Mol Diagn 1998;3:131-41.

47. Nocton JJ, Bloom BJ, Rutledge BJ, Persing DH, Logigian EL, Schmid CH, et al. Detection of Borrelia burgdorferi DNA by polymerase chain reaction in cerebrospinal fluid in Lyme neuroborreliosis. J Infect Dis 1996;174:623-7.

48. Shrestha M, Grodzicki R, Steere AC. Diagnosing early Lyme disease. Am J Med 1985;78:235-40.

49. Craft JE, Grodzicki RL, Steere AC. The antibody response in Lyme disease: evaluation of diagnostic tests. J Infect Dis 1984;149:789-95.

50. Dressler F, Whalen JA, Reinhardt BN, Steere AC. Western blotting in the serodiagnosis of Lyme disease. J Infect Dis 1993;167:392-400.

51. Second International Conference on serologic diagnosis of Lyme disease. Recommendations for test performance and interpretation. MMWR Morb Mortal Wkly Rep 1995;44: 590-1.

52. Kaslow RA. Current perspective on Lyme borreliosis. JAMA 1992;267:1381-3.

53. Krause PJ, Foley DT, Burke GS, Christianson D, Closter L, Spielman A, et al. Reinfection and relapse in early Lyme disease. Am J Trop Med Hyg 2006;75:1090-4.

54. Piesman J, Maupin GO, Campos EG, Happ CM. Duration of adult female *Ixodes dammini* attachment and transmission of *Borrelia burgdorferi* with a description of a needle aspiration isolation method. J Infect Dis 1991;163:891-7.

55. Piesman J. Dynamics of *Borrelia burgdorferi* transmission by nymphal *Ixodes dammini* ticks. J Infect Dis 1993;167: 1082-5.

56. Nadelman RB, Nowakowski J, Fish D, Falco RC, Freeman K, McKenna D, et al. Single dose doxycycline prophylaxis for prevention of Lyme disease after an *Ixodes scapularis* tick bite. N Engl J Med 2001;345:79-84.

57. Shapiro ED, Gerber MA, Holabird NB, Berg AT, Feder HM Jr, Bell GL, et al. A controlled trial of antimicrobial prophylaxis for Lyme disease after deer-tick bites. N Engl J Med 1992;327:1769-73.

58. Wormser GP. Early Lyme disease. N Engl J Med 2006;354: 2794-801.

59. Nowakowski J, McKenna D, Nadelman RB, Cooper D, Bittker S, Holmgren D, et al. Failure of treatment with cephalexin for Lyme disease. Arch Fam Med 2000;9:563-7.

60. Dattwyler RJ, Volkman DJ, Conaty SM, Platkin SP, Luft BJ. Amoxycillin plus probenecid versus doxycycline for treatment of erythema migrans borreliosis. Lancet 1990;336: 1404-6.

61. Nadelman RB, Luger SW, Frank E, Wisniewski M, Collins JJ, Wormser GP. Comparison of cefuroxime axetil and doxycycline in the treatment of early Lyme disease. Ann Intern Med 1992;117:273-80.

62. Dattwyler RJ, Luft BJ, Kunkel MJ, Finkel MF, Wormser GP, Rush TJ, et al. Ceftriaxone compared with doxycycline for the treatment of acute disseminated Lyme disease. N Engl J Med 1997;337:289-94.

63. Axford JS, Rees DH, Mageed RA, Wordsworth P, Alavi A, Steere AC. Increased IgA rheumatoid factor and V(H)1 associated cross reactive idiotype expression in patients with Lyme arthritis and neuroborreliosis. Ann Rheum Dis 1999;58: 757-61.

64. Dattwyler RS, Wormser GP, Rush TJ, Finkel MF, Schoen RT, Grunwaldt E, et al. A comparison of two treatment regimens of ceftriaxone in late Lyme disease. Wien Klin Wochenschr 2005;117:393-7.

65. Schoen RT, Aversa JM, Rahn DW, Steere AC. Treatment of refractory chronic Lyme arthritis with arthroscopic synovectomy. Arthritis Rheum 1991;34:1056-60.

66. Dattwyler RJ, Halperin JJ, Volkman DJ, Luft BJ. Treatment of late Lyme borreliosis - randomized comparison of ceftriaxone and penicillin. Lancet 1988;1:1191-4.

67. Feder Jr HM, Johnson BJ, O'Connell S, Shapiro ED, Steere AC, Wormser GP, et al. A critical reappraisal of "chronic Lyme disease". N Engl J Med 2007;357:1422-30.

68. Tonks A. Lyme wars. BMJ 2007;375:910-2.

69. Treatment of Lyme disease. Med Lett Drugs Ther 2007;49: 49-51.

70. Wilson ML, Telford III SR, Peisman J, Spielman A. Reduced abundance of immature *Ixodes dammini* (Acari: Ixodiae) following elimination of deer. J Med Entomol 1988;25:224-8.

71. Vazquez M, Muehlenbein C, Cartter M, Hayes EB, Ertel S, Shapiro ED. Effectiveness of personal protective measures to prevent Lyme disease. Emerg Infect Dis [serial on the Internet]. Available at: http://www.cdc.gov/EID/content/14/2/210.htm; 2008 Feb. [Accessed online October 4, 2008].

72. Steere AC, Sikand VK, Meurice F, Parenti DL, Fikrig E, Schoen RT, et al. Vaccination against Lyme disease with recombinant *Borrelia burgdorferi* outer-surface lipoprotein A with adjuvant. N Engl J Med 1998;339:209-15.

73. American Lyme Disease Foundation. Available at: http://www. aldf.com/about.shtml [Accessed online October 4, 2008].

74. Wormser GP, Ramanathan R, Nowakowski J, McKenna D, Holmgren D, Visintainer P, et al. Duration of antibiotic therapy for early Lyme disease: A randomized, double blind, placebo-controlled trial. Ann Intern Med 2003;238:697-704.

75. Halperin JJ, Shapiro EN, Logigian E, Belman AL, Dotevall L, Wormser GP, et al. Practice parameter: Treatment of nervous system Lyme disease (an evidence-based review). Neurology 2007;69:91-102.

76. Klempner MS, Hu LT, Evans J, Schmid CH, Johnson GM, Trevino RP, et al. Two controlled trials of antibiotic treatments in patients with persistent symptoms and a history of Lyme disease. N Engl J Med 2001;345:85-92.

77. Ettestad PJ, Campbell GL, Weibel SF, Genese CA, Spitalmy KC, Marchetti CM, et al. Biliary complications in the treatment of unsubstantiated Lyme disease. J Infect Dis 1995;171: 356-61.

78. Patel R, Grogg KL, Edwards WD, Wright AJ, Schwenk NM. Death from inappropriate therapy for Lyme disease. Clin Infect Dis 2000;31:1107-9.

Chapter 22

Gout and Crystal Deposition Disease

Brian F. Mandell

A 66-year-old man is seen in consultation for acute foot pain 3 days following partial colectomy with reanastomosis for diverticulitis. There had been no surgical complications. He recalled no similar episodes of foot pain. A year earlier, he had experienced knee pain and swelling, for which he took over-the-counter ibuprofen following dancing at his daughter's wedding. The patient's past medical history included a myocardial infarction several years ago without adverse sequelae, hyperlipidemia, hypertension, type 2 diabetes, and a nephrectomy for renal cell carcinoma 10 years earlier. Medications at home included aspirin, atorvastatin, glyburide, hydrochlorthiazide, and enalapril. All of these medications except enalapril are still being held since his diet is being advanced to full liquids following surgery. He is receiving unfractionated heparin 5000 U every 8 hours. His oral temperature is 100.8° F; other vitals include a heart rate of 86 and blood pressure of 146/92. His examination is remarkable for a clean surgical wound and nontender abdomen. Lungs are clear and there is a soft systolic ejection quality murmur (also noted on admission). There is trace pitting edema of both pretibial areas. The left foot is warmer than the right, with tenderness of the midfoot when it is squeezed, and there is marked swelling and warmth around the medial malleolus with extreme pain to any motion of the ankle. There are normal pulses and no embolic lesions. Laboratory studies, obtained before the consultation are notable for a white blood cell count of 10,200, with 84% neutrophils, glucose of 174, normal electrolytes, creatinine 1.8, serum urate of 6.8, and an ESR of 54.

Discussion of Differential Diagnosis

The patient has acute arthritis of the ankle and probably midfoot in the perioperative setting. On a statistical basis, this is most likely a result of crystal-induced inflammation, probably due to monosodium urate (gout). Because the rates of morbidity and mortality (11%) associated with bacterial infectious arthritis are high, infection should be directly excluded as a cause of the arthritis, particularly in the postoperative patient who has several potential portals of infection. In several retrospective studies, delay in diagnosis and

appropriate treatment of infectious arthritis has been shown to be associated with an increased likelihood of permanent joint dysfunction.

Among 100 consecutive patients with acute monoarticular arthritis in the hospital and emergency room setting, 80% was due to microcrystalline disease (Mandell BF, unpublished information). Other potential etiologies, such as psoriasis, enteropathic, and spondylitis, are relatively uncommon and generally occur in patients with known underlying disease (e.g., psoriasis, inflammatory bowel disease, and ankylosing spondylitis). The immediate distinction in this patient must be made between crystal-induced and infectious arthritis. This distinction cannot be reliably made on clinical grounds. The presence or absence of fever, elevated peripheral white blood cell count, or elevated acute phase reactants will not distinguish crystal-induced from septic arthritis. This has been shown in several published studies,[1] and in the postoperative setting, there are additional reasons for the vital signs and laboratory studies to be abnormal. Radiographs are of little assistance in determining the etiology of acute peripheral joint arthritis, and obtaining these studies often delays the appropriate evaluation.

The serum urate level is generally higher than the saturation point of 6.7 mg/dL at the time of an acute attack of gout, but this is not always the case. Also, patients with infectious arthritis or acute arthritis of other etiologies may also have hyperuricemia because it is so common in the general population. Additionally, an acute *decrease* in the serum urate level due to the initiation of a hypouricemic drug[2] or acute intravenous hydration is a well recognized and frequent initiator of acute gouty arthritis. Thus, measurement of the serum urate level is not a sensitive or specific test to determine the etiology of acute arthritis and should not be relied on to distinguish between crystal-induced and infectious arthritis.

The test of choice in determining the etiology for acute monoarticular arthritis is synovial fluid analysis, with culture being the gold standard to diagnose bacterial infection[3] and polarized microscopy the test of choice for crystal-induced arthritis. Anticoagulation, in this case heparin, should not be a deterrent to synovial fluid aspiration. Gram staining of the fluid to demonstrate the presence of bacteria is notoriously insensitive[4] and fraught with the additional problem of false-positive results due to misinterpretation. Higher synovial white blood cell counts (>50,000 cells per mm[3]) are more frequently associated with infection than with crystals, but there is too much overlap to use the total white blood cell count or percentage of neutrophils to make this distinction with confidence.[5] The patient with inflammatory fluid and the absence of observed crystals should generally be treated as if he or she has septic arthritis until the cultures return clearly negative. The finding of crystals in the fluid confirms the diagnosis of gout (monosodium urate) or pseudogout (calcium pyrophosphate) but does not exclude the relatively uncommon[6] coexistence of infection and crystal disease. Thus, it is reasonable to send fluid for culture even if crystals have been observed in the fluid, especially if the suspicion for infection is particularly high (i.e., in the setting of recently documented or suspected bacterial infection elsewhere in the patient or if intra-articular corticosteroid therapy is planned).

The role of polymerase chain reaction and other molecular tests to confirm the diagnosis of septic arthritis has yet to be fully defined. Synovial fluid glucose or lactate levels are not routinely useful. Crystals, although present, may occasionally not be observed on the initial evaluation; thus, subsequent aspirated fluid samples should be re-examined for the presence of crystals. The fluid can be centrifuged in a conical test tube, and the pellet evaluated for the presence of crystals. This may increase the sensitivity of the crystal analysis. Alizarin stain may be used to facilitate the recognition of calcium-containing crystals. However, this stain is not universally available, and should be filtered before use because it tends to precipitate. If necessary, synovial fluids can be stored in the absence of anticoagulant and examined at a later point in time when a more experienced observer is available.

In the described patient, monosodium urate crystals were observed in the fluid aspirated from his ankle. The midfoot tenderness also had suggested gout as the likely diagnosis, because this is one of very few anatomic areas affected by gout but generally not by infection in the acute setting. Culture of the fluid was negative. He was treated with 1.0 mg of intravenous colchicine (a therapy no longer available in many regions due to safety concerns). He had a rapid response over 24 hours, with normalization of his temperature and relief of most of his pain, avoiding the less specific antipyretic and the gastric and renal effects of nonsteroidal anti-inflammatory drugs (NSAIDs) and the hyperglycemic and (theoretical) wound healing effects of corticosteroids. Appropriately dosed intravenous colchicine does not cause nausea or diarrhea.

It is worth noting the multiple risk factors for coronary artery disease (CAD) that this patient exhibited. This is not unusual in patients with gout.

CASE STUDY 2   Polyarticular Gout

A 59-year-old woman was seen in the office for evaluation and treatment of chronic polyarticular arthritis. The arthritis has been present for several years, and her daily function has deteriorated since going on hemodialysis for chronic kidney disease (CKD) due to biopsy-documented damage from hypertension and diabetes. The arthritis affected her peripheral interphalangeal (PIP) joints more than the metacarpophalangeal (MCP) joints of both hands, both wrists, ankles, and knees. She had chronic olecranon bursitis. She had a positive antinuclear antibody (ANA) test (homogenous), antimicrosomal antibodies, and rheumatoid factor in the past. She had no detectable hepatitis B or C antibodies before receiving the hepatitis B vaccine last year. She had experienced minimal response to methotrexate a few years previously, with reduced swelling and stiffness of the hands, but still had experienced arthritis flares requiring steroid therapy with "dose packs." The methotrexate was stopped as the renal function worsened. Over the past year, there had been fewer flares, but increased pain and stiffness of the involved joints. Medications included folic acid, multivitamins, a baby aspirin, furosemide, hydralazine, metoprolol, enalapril, insulins, thyroid replacement, and pravastatin. Examination was notable for heart rate of 66 with blood pressure of 142/88. The above-mentioned joints had cool proliferative synovium with a generally symmetric distribution. There was slight bilateral, cool, and nontender olecranon bursal distention; the left bursa contained several small nodules. The skin was dry, there was no psoriasis, and the left thumb pad had a nontender intradermal nodule (shown in Fig. 22-1). Hand radiographs from 2 years previously reported osteoarthritis of the finger PIP and distal interphalangeal (DIP) joints, normal joint spaces of the MCP and intercarpal joints, several carpal bone cysts, but no erosions.

Discussion of Differential Diagnosis

This patient was referred for management of seropositive rheumatoid arthritis (RA) and osteoarthritis; she had experienced a less than ideal response to methotrexate, and now was experiencing greater difficulties in performing daily activities due to joint stiffness. The presence of diabetes and CKD complicated the choice of medications.

The symmetrical polyarthritis is consistent with rheumatoid disease, as is the positive rheumatoid factor in the past. A positive ANA can be found in patients with RA as well as in those with autoimmune thyroid disease. The radiographs were consistent with

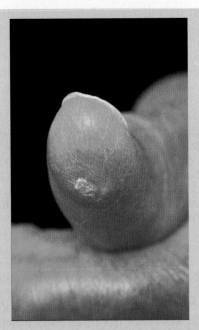

Figure 22-1. Intradermal urate deposit (tophus).

osteoarthritis but did not exclude the coexistence of RA or an alternative inflammatory arthritis affecting the wrists. The lack of a complete response to methotrexate does not exclude the diagnosis of RA. Chronic hepatitis C, which can cause a "pseudorheumatoid" polyarthritis without erosions, was excluded by the absence of viral antibodies. There was nothing in the history or on examination to suggest psoriatic, enteropathic, or spondylitis-associated peripheral arthritis (these entities often, although not always, cause a fairly more asymmetric arthritis). The time course and examination did not suggest bacterial infection. The clinical wrist involvement, in the absence of a history of wrist trauma, made the diagnosis of generalized osteoarthritis affecting the wrists unlikely. The arthropathy preceded the dialysis; hence, dialysis-associated amyloidosis was not tenable.

Although no calcinosis was seen on radiographs, the diagnoses of chronic pseudogout and hemochromatosis were considered. However, the olecranon nodules (thought to be tophi) and the thumb lesion, a characteristic intradermal deposit of urate, strongly suggested

that the arthritis was due to chronic progressive gout with likely coexistent osteoarthritis. On careful questioning, most patients with chronic gout, or their family members, will recall a history of intermittent flares at the outset of the arthritis. As in this case, occasional patients with chronic established disease have symptoms and findings of chronic swelling and discomfort which can mimic rheumatoid or psoriatic (more asymmetric) arthritis. The diagnosis of gout was confirmed by aspiration of a few drops of fluid from the olecranon bursa demonstrating monosodium urate crystals.

Retrospective studies suggest that the frequency of gout flares may decrease with the development of end stage renal disease,[7] perhaps due to decreased inflammatory cell reactivity to the crystals. But as in this patient, symptoms from chronic proliferative gouty synovitis may not abate. The serum urate level was between 9 and 10 mg/dL on two occasions. Because renal transplantation was being considered and it was believed that the use of calcineurin antagonist therapy would likely accelerate the gouty arthritis, it was believed that it was imperative to initiate hypouricemic therapy.

She was started on celecoxib prophylactically to reduce the likelihood of a gout flare with the introduction of hypouricemic therapy. A cyclooxygenase-2 (COX-2) selective NSAID was chosen because of its slightly decreased gastrointestinal (GI) bleeding risk and lack of antiplatelet effect compared with a nonselective NSAID in a patient taking (cardioprotective) aspirin and likely having kidney failure–associated platelet dysfunction. Because the patient was already on dialysis, there was no concern over worsening the renal function with celecoxib. Low-dose allopurinol (50 mg) was subsequently added and increased to a dose that decreased the serum urate to less than 6.0 mg/dL. The patient was monitored for systemic hypersensitivity reaction or rash as the dose of allopurinol was increased. It has been suggested by some (but not all) authors that the risk of hypersensitivity reactions is higher in patients with renal dysfunction.[8] It should be noted that the promulgated guidelines for allopurinol dosing in patients with renal insufficiency have not been rigorously validated[9] and, if adhered to, will result in suboptimal control of serum urate levels in a significant majority of patients.

TREATMENT OF THE ACUTE ATTACK

The acute gout attack is a dramatic inflammatory response to urate crystals. In addition to being membranolytic, recent studies have elucidated a mechanism by which crystals trigger inflammatory cells to release interleukin 1 (IL-1) via a toll-like receptor (Fig. 22-2), which then activates a polymeric protein complex in the cytoplasm (inflammasome). The inflammasome generates active IL-1 beta, which then triggers and amplifies the local and systemic inflammatory response to crystals. The primary role of IL-1 can be demonstrated by the ability of

IL-1 antagonists to block animal responses to urate crystals and it has been used to successfully treat human gout. Downstream from the effect of IL-1, other inflammatory mediators are released including prostaglandins, leukotrienes, and interleukin 8.

Acute attacks of gout are generally responsive to high doses of several different anti-inflammatory therapies. The clinical choice of therapeutic agents is generally dependent on the risk of side effects in a given patient based on his or her comorbidities and concomitant medications, as well as the personal preferences of the prescribing physician (and patient). It has been

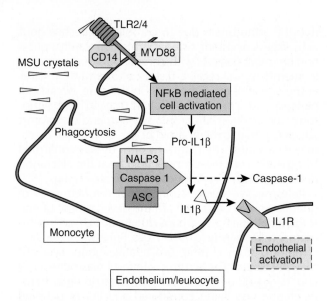

Figure 22-2. Uric acid crystals activate mononuclear cells to release interleukin 1 via toll-like receptor and the NALP3 inflammasome. (From So A. Uric acid crystals activate mononuclear cells to release interleukin 1 via toll like receptor and the NALP3 inflammasome. Arth Res Therapy 2008;10:221-7.)

suggested that the earlier an attack is treated, the easier it is to treat. Some authors have described their experience with having patients abort an incipient attack if low doses of oral colchicine or an NSAID are taken at the first twinge of joint pain that can be recognized by the patient as gout. Once established, an attack may need to be treated for a longer period of time until it completely resolves and does not recur when the treatment is discontinued. In one retrospective review of 90 hospitalized patients treated with intravenous colchicine, the duration of symptoms before therapy did not influence the response (Khurana, PS and Mandell, BF presented at the Soc Gen Int Med annual meeting, 1999), but there is little other information to refute the common concept that the longer an attack persists, the harder it is to quickly get it to resolve. Agents that are effective in treating the acute gout attack include virtually all NSAIDs (aspirin is generally not used for this) including some COX-2 selective ones, corticosteroids (oral, parenteral and intra-articular), and colchicine (oral and previously intravenous). Narcotics blunt some of the pain but will not resolve the attack, and some clinicians (including myself) believe that they are not as effective as the anti-inflammatory medications in relieving the pain. Recently, there have been a few case reports on the efficacy of specific biologic therapies including anti-tumor necrosis factor (TNF) and anti-IL1 agents. These are briefly discussed later in this chapter.

There have been few controlled trials studying acute gout; even fewer have included a placebo (or narcotic) arm. The historic approach to the treatment of gout attacks with repeated hourly (or bihourly) doses of oral colchicine was demonstrated to be more effective than placebo within 24 hours.[10] However, virtually all patients suffered GI side effects with this regimen, and most clinicians avoid this approach. Using just a few

oral colchicine pills (one taken hourly) at the first onset of an attack can be effective, without GI side effects, according to some authors (and patients). Intravenous colchicine was safe and effective in several retrospective studies (one published in full form[11]) totaling approximately 250 patients. Despite some benefits of using low dose intravenous (IV) administration (limited GI side effects with appropriate dosing; no effect on bleeding; no general antipyretic effect; no leukocytosis, which can cause diagnostic confusion; and no effect on glucose levels or renal function); the multiple published case reports of morbidity and deaths attributed to IV colchicine use (many with therapeutic overdose) have led to removal of this formulation from the marketplace.

NSAIDs have been a popular choice for treating acute gout attacks. Indomethacin has had a time-honored role as the gold standard therapy. It is believed to be quickly absorbed and rapidly effective. But given its proclivity to cause headache and confusion in the elderly, as well as gastric bleeding, and its potency in adversely affecting renal function, it has slowly and partially been replaced in general use by other NSAIDs. In a controlled double-blind comparison between indomethacin (50 mg every 8 hours) and the COX-2 selective NSAID etoricoxib (120 mg), significant pain relief was achieved with both agents by 4 hours after the first dose.[12] Naproxen (500 mg twice daily) was shown in a different controlled trial as equivalent in efficacy to prednisolone (35 mg once daily).[13] Pain was reduced to 50% of baseline with both agents by approximately 48 hours. NSAID therapy should be continued for several days after complete resolution of the attack to avoid resumption of the inflammation and pain. The well-accepted efficacy of NSAIDs in treating acute gout is tempered by the frequent presence of comorbidities in gouty patients, which often make the use of high-dose NSAIDs less than ideal. The demography of patients with gout includes a high prevalence of hypertension, renal insufficiency, metabolic syndrome, coronary disease and alcohol use. Owing to this situation and the increased awareness of the gastric toxicity of NSAIDs, many clinicians now use corticosteroids as first-line therapy for acute attacks of gout, particularly in hospitalized patients.

For years, there was a dearth of data supporting what clinicians already knew, that steroids effectively can treat the acute gout attack.[13] Textbooks stated that use of corticosteroids was associated with "rebound" attacks of gout on discontinuation. My own interpretation of this hackneyed caveat is that steroid therapy was frequently used for too short of a period of time, and if therapy (steroids or NSAIDs) of an attack of gout is stopped too soon, the attack is not resolved and symptoms resume. In 1990, a small experience was reviewed that documented the efficacy and lack of rebound attacks with steroid therapy.[14] There is still no uniformly accepted dose, and many clinicians use some permutation of a scheme that involves initial treatment with approximately 40 mg daily of prednisone or the equivalent until symptoms resolve and then slowly taper the steroid over another 7 days.

Adrenocorticotropic hormone is also effective,[15] with animal models suggesting that its mechanisms of action include a direct peripheral anti-inflammatory effect as well as eliciting cortisol release from the adrenal gland. A single dose is generally not sufficient for the reasons noted earlier, and it is expensive therapy. Intra-articular steroid is effective, assuming the joint is accessible to injection. But, even though some animal studies and a study in pediatric patients with septic arthritis[16] suggest that systemic steroids are not harmful, and may be beneficial when provided with appropriate antibiotics, there remains a strong theoretical concern with injecting a deposit formulation of steroid into an infected joint because once injected, it cannot be removed. The difficulties in rapidly and reliably distinguishing infection from crystal-induced arthritis were discussed earlier. Thus, I have some reluctance to use intra-articular steroids to treat gout attacks if there is any increased concern over the possibility of co-existent infection.

TREATMENT OF HYPERURICEMIA

A biologic prerequisite for the development of gouty arthritis is a persistent serum urate level above 6.7 mg/dL, the concentration at which urate begins to crystallize in connective tissue. By maintaining the urate below this level, urate deposits will dissolve, pass into the serum, and be excreted into urine. Based on the pathophysiology alone, it thus makes sense to treat everyone who has experienced a gout attack with hypouricemic medication in order to prevent future attacks or progression to chronic polyarticular gout, as in Case Study 2 earlier. However, most patients with gout do not progress to severe disease, and some patients only have rare repeated attacks over years and do not wish to take on the cost and even minimal risk of taking a medication for the rest of their life. It is impossible to predict with certainty at the time of the first attack the disease course in a given patient, although repeated attacks at a young age, the presence of a transplanted organ with cyclosporine therapy, and early formation of tophi or erosions presage a more difficult course. Controlled interventional studies have not been conducted to compare the different approaches of early hypouricemic therapy versus treating the inflammatory episodes without addressing the hyperuricemia in terms of patient quality of life, medical and social costs and function. Authors have advocated, without hard data, initiating hypouricemic therapy following a defined number of gouty attacks (sometimes two or three) or the presence of visible or radiographic tophi. The first suggestion seems overly arbitrary. I favor instead to use the following points when discussing this treatment decision with patients: How disruptive will attacks of gout be if they continue to occur (does the patient travel a lot)? Are there relative contraindications to the use of medications needed to treat acute attacks (renal insufficiency, peptic ulcer disease, diabetes, etc.)? Is it likely that the attack frequency will increase over time (presence of tophi, attacks began at a young age or are increasing in frequency, the likely need for medication that may increase urate levels further). Multiple studies and clinical experience have shown that the maintenance of low serum urate (< 6.0 mg/dL) reduces the frequency of gout attacks as patients are followed over a long period of time.

When making the decision to institute hypouricemic therapy for the purpose of controlling the progression of gouty arthritis and ultimately eliminate attacks of gout, it is critical that both physician and patient recognize that these goals can be reached only after many months of therapy as the total urate burden in the body is reduced. It is also critical to recognize (and inform the patient) that if the urate level is abruptly reduced for any reason, including with medication, that there is a significant risk of inducing an attack of gout within the first several months of therapy. There is a suggestion that the more the urate is lowered, the greater the chance of inducing an attack.[17] Hence, it is reasonable practice to use a prophylactic anti-inflammatory therapy such as low dose oral colchicine or an NSAID for the initial months of hypouricemic therapy. The presence of renal insufficiency can complicate the decision regarding prophylaxis, requiring a decrease in the colchicine dose to below the often-used dose of 0.6 mg twice daily and avoidance of NSAIDs entirely. In patients with severe gout, the likelihood of an attack may be as high as 40% over the 8 weeks following the start of hypouricemic therapy, even with prophylaxis.

It has been recognized for more than 100 years that hyperuricemia, as defined by a level greater than population normal (which is higher than the biologically relevant level of 6.7 mg/dL at which urate is saturated in biologic fluids), is associated with a number of other conditions. Hyperuricemia was strongly linked as a causative agent of gout, Lesch-Nyhan syndrome, tumor lysis syndrome, and uric acid nephrolithiasis. Hyperuricemia has also been associated with CKD, CAD, hypertension, and components of the metabolic syndrome including diabetes. However, several analyses of the epidemiologic data led authors to conclude that the urate was more likely a consequence than a cause of these latter conditions, and the general teaching for the past few decades had been that hyperuricemia is "benign" and does not in and of itself require treatment.

Re-examination of this association in large observational and retrospective studies, other than the Framingham database, has led to a growing opinion that hyperuricemia may be a proximate cause of cardiovascular disease, and not simply an innocent bystander or epiphenomenon.[18,19] Serum urate has even been suggested as an independent predictor of all-cause as well as cardiovascular mortality.[20] Stronger evidence for a direct role of urate in the development of hypertension and cardiovascular disease comes from the rat model of mild hyperuricemia developed by Johnson and colleagues.[21] Moderate acute hyperuricemia induced by inhibition of endogenous uricase in rats induces reversible hypertension in the absence of crystal deposition or acute renal injury. If left untreated, the hyperuricemia induces microvascular disease and a salt-sensitive hypertension that no longer can be reversed by normalization of the hyperuricemia. If this pathophysiology is mimicked in humans, it could explain why patients with long-standing hypertension and hyperuricemia do not normalize their blood pressure with treatment of the hyperuricemia.

In an attempt to mimic the timing of hypouricemic therapy in the animal studies, Feig and colleagues[22] followed up on observations that hyperuricemia in adolescents and young adults predicts the future development of hypertension and in a placebo-controlled crossover design trial treated adolescents with new-onset primary hypertension and hyperuricemia with allopurinol. Treatment with allopurinol, but not placebo, reversibly and significantly lowered the blood pressure. Some, but not all, interventional studies in patients with chronic kidney disease have shown that administering allopurinol can slow the progression of kidney dysfunction.[23,24]

In a parallel body of data, there is growing recognition that high-fructose intake, as is common in the United States, predisposes to glucose intolerance, weight gain, and the complete metabolic syndrome.[25] It has been proposed that this contributes to the obesity epidemic in young Americans, and may also contribute to the rising prevalence of hyperuricemia and gout. Experimental data in rats have been published supporting the hypothesis that fructose contributes to the development of all of these outcomes via an increase in serum urate levels.[26] Conclusive data in humans, however, have not yet been published.

Inhibition of xanthine oxidase with allopurinol has been the most used, best tolerated, and most effective hypouricemic therapy in the United States. It has been shown to be effective in "inefficient renal excretors" of uric acid (probably > 90% of hyperuricemic patients), as well as "hyperproducers." If allopurinol is used, there is no necessity in obtaining a 24-hour urinary uric acid excretion before starting therapy. However, in very young patients, in patients with a striking family history of gout, or in those patients likely to be provided a uricosuric agent to lower their serum urate, two 24-hour urine uric acid excretion tests should be performed. Some authors have recommended in the absence of nephrolithiasis that a spot urine uric acid/creatinine excretion should be measured, and if it is low, then a 24-hour excretion does not need to be evaluated. (Simkin, P letter to editor Arth Rheum 49:735, 2003). This is a reasonable approach, although one not yet prospectively validated.

In the United States, probenecid is the generally used uricosuric agent, but in general, most clinicians prefer to start with allopurinol because it is easier to take (once daily), does not require extra water intake, works in the setting of renal insufficiency (see comments regarding use of allopurinol in the setting of renal insufficiency), and tends to be more effective. The angiotensin receptor blocker losartan is unique in its probenecid-like uricosuric effect but is generally less effective than full-dose probenecid. It can be used in conjunction with allopurinol and is a reasonable adjunct therapy in the hypertensive hyperuricemic patient. Uricosurics should be avoided in patients excreting more than 1 g of uric acid daily and those with a history of nephrolithiasis because increasing uric acid excretion in these patients may increase the chance of further stone formation. Outside of the United States, some countries have access to benzbromarone, a uricosuric with greater efficacy than probenecid. However there have been difficulties with hepatotoxicity.

Allopurinol is generally well tolerated. It should be started at a low dose, perhaps at one half of a 100 mg tablet once daily to avoid a rapid fall in the urate level, which seems more likely to induce a gouty attack. Perhaps 8% experience a rash, and a small percentage of those patients develop Stevens-Johnson syndrome or a systemic hypersensitivity reaction, which can be serious and life threatening. Hence, any rash, fever or elevations in transaminases in a patient taking allopurinol must be taken seriously. It has been suggested that severe hypersensitivity reactions are more common in patients with renal insufficiency. However, it is not certain that adjusting the dose of allopurinol in patients with CKD reduces the risk of adverse reactions. Patients with mild skin reactions can be desensitized to allopurinol,[28] but a new xanthine oxidase inhibitor (febuxostat) was approved by the FDA and this will make desensitization unnecessary for these relatively few patients. Studies with febuxostat suggest a daily dose of 80 or 120 mg has an equal if not greater hypouricemic effect than 300 mg allopurinol.

Once hypouricemic therapy is initiated as part of a total program to lower the serum urate, reduce the total body uric acid load, and reduce the frequency of gout attacks, it is generally a life-long therapy. The urate level should be checked a few weeks after each change in dose until the target level is achieved, and then approximately every 6 months. The target urate level should be approximately 6.0 mg/dL to maintain the urate level below its saturation point of 6.7 mg/dL. Over time, urate crystals will disappear from the synovial fluid and presumably from the synovial tissue.[29]

Although the current trend of thought in 2009 is moving toward the concept that hyperuricemia is deleterious and a primary mediator of several aspects of cardiovascular disease morbidity and mortality, there are as yet no data of sufficient strength in humans to warrant a paradigm shift toward routinely treating asymptomatic hyperuricemia. There are also conceptually conflicting data that suggest urate can be biologically beneficial to endothelial function[27] and that elevated urate levels perhaps act as a circulating antioxidant.[30] Although these data need to be addressed, I believe that the weight of information supports trying to avoid hyperuricemia and that controlled interventional trials are warranted to guide our clinical decision making. In the meantime, as I counsel patients on ways to limit cardiovascular risk and limit progression of CKD, I note the growing amount of information on the adverse effects of hyperuricemia. I also am particularly attentive to treating the comorbid, potentially unrecognized, cardiovascular risk in patients who have known gouty arthritis.

TREATMENT OF INTERCRITICAL GOUT

Gouty arthritis, for most untreated patients, is characterized by intermittent flares separated by periods of time ("intercritical-gout") when there are no joint symptoms. Over time, these intercritical periods may become shorter as the flare frequency increases. However, this time course is notoriously difficult to predict for most patients. In a few patients, chronic gout develops, as in Case Study 2. If attacks are few, intercritical periods very long and the attacks are easy to treat then it is a reasonable strategy for many patients to simply treat the attacks as they arise. It must be remembered, however, that with this approach the uric acid burden in the body is likely increasing, and tophi, joint damage, or an increase in attack frequency may occur (as may other complications of hyperuricemia—see earlier discussion). Clinician and patient must be vigilant for evidence of tophi deposition or worsening joint symptoms.

Lowering the serum urate will, over time, lengthen periods of intercritical gout as it decreases the frequency of attacks. But, this may not be apparent for close to a year. Gout flare frequency may also be decreased by chronic suppressive anti-inflammatory therapy, independent of urate lowering therapy. NSAIDs or prednisone would likely decrease attack frequency (never tested in a formal way in a large study), but the side effects of chronic therapy with these agents in gouty patients would likely be fraught with side effects. Low-dose colchicine (0.6 mg tablets once or twice daily) is generally well tolerated as a chronic therapy, and can decrease the frequency of gout flares, but without lowering the uric acid burden in the body. Loose stools and occasionally intolerable diarrhea may necessitate reduction in dose or discontinuation of therapy.

A toxicity of concern in patients on long-term low-dose colchicine prophylactic therapy is some combination of a vacuolar myopathy and axonal neuropathy.[31] It may be painful and associated with weakness, pain, and reduced deep tendon reflexes as well as elevated CPK values. It is reversible over weeks to months if it is recognized and

the drug is stopped. It is more common in patients with a reduced glomerular filtration rate (GFR), but can also occur suddenly due to the addition of drugs that influence colchicine metabolism or intracellular distribution (macrolide antibiotics, most statins, cyclosporine and some calcium channel blockers).

A long-term comparative study between the strategies of urate-lowering versus long-term suppressive therapy has never been undertaken. Experience has informed us that patients with tophacious or severe recurrent gout do better with hypouricemic therapy plus prophylactic anti-inflammatory therapy in an effort to reduce attacks and reduce uric acid burden, including visible tophi. However, in the middle-aged to older patient with their first flare, or in older healthy patients with a few intermittent attacks, the ideal strategic approach must be empiric and based on discussion between patient and physician.

TREATMENT CONSIDERATIONS IN SPECIAL PATIENT GROUPS

There are several special patient groups that warrant specific comment because of unique aspects of their presentation or difficulties in therapeutic management. Gout is generally thought of as a disease of men. There is a striking male predominance, but women do get gout. I have a sense that it is underrecognized by primary care physicians. Women develop gout later in life, generally after menopause, when their serum urate levels increase to a range comparable to males. The postmenopausal increase in urate is due to the loss of estrogen, and estrogen (in animal studies) suppresses the transporter responsible for uric acid reabsorption in the proximal tubule.[32] Perhaps due to late recognition, women more commonly have tophi and multiple joint involvement at the time of initial diagnosis of gout than men. Additionally, there seems to be frequent involvement of the finger DIP joints. Red, tender Heberden's nodes from gout can be misdiagnosed as acute inflammatory osteoarthritis.[33] As discussed earlier, once the correct diagnosis is made, treatment is based on the patient's comorbidities and the clinician's estimated likelihood that the disease will progress or cause significant morbidity.

Patients who have received solid organ transplants and are prescribed a calcineurin antagonist, particularly cyclosporine, to prevent rejection are especially prone to develop rapidly progressive tophacious gout. The exact mechanisms by which cyclosporine exacerbates gout and hyperuricemia is not totally clear, but the rapidity of tophi formation and polyarticular joint involvement suggest something more than just a reduction in the GFR, or altered tubular handling of uric acid with resultant hyperuricemia. Diuretics, which are frequently required in heart and kidney transplant patients, exacerbate the hyperuricemia and gout. Because xanthine oxidase metabolizes azathioprine, allopurinol (or febuxostat) must be used with extreme caution and lowered azathioprine doses must be used when the patient is receiving azathioprine. Because of the background immunosuppression, the risk for infection is always present, and joints should be aspirated rather than assuming the etiology of an acute arthritis is gout. Gout usually starts within 5 years of the transplant,[34] if there is no prior history of gout. Patients with hyperuricemia at the time of transplantation are at greater risk to develop gout following the transplant. Management is complicated by the many drug interactions and the likelihood of some degree of renal impairment. Gout may be manifest primarily in tendons or as an enthesitis. If possible, in patients with known gout who are expecting a transplant, I try to reduce their serum urate before transplantation. Discussion with the transplant team is of value because antirejection regimens avoiding azathioprine can be utilized if the continued use of allopurinol is desired.

Gout occurs frequently following surgery, generally in patients who have a prior history of gout attacks (often not asked about on admission to the hospital). The likely reasons for postoperative flares include fluid shifts that alter the serum urate level and may favor new crystal formation in the joint fluid, as well as new medications that may elicit increases or decreases in serum urate. Additionally, allopurinol and prophylactic anti-inflammatory medications are often held before surgeries when the patient is not eating. The average time following surgery before an attack of gout is about 4 days,[35] and multiple joints are frequently involved. Treatment is complicated by the many potential drug interactions. Postoperative gout (or pseudogout) can be a vexing cause of postoperative fever, especially in the intubated or otherwise noncommunicating patient.

The patient with CKD and gout was discussed above (see Case Study 2), but a few points are worth reiterating. It was observed that the frequency of allopurinol hypersensitivity reactions seemed to be increased in patients with renal insufficiency. Because allopurinol's key active metabolite oxypurinol is cleared by the kidney, it was proposed that allopurinol dosing be adjusted based on the estimated GFR.[36] However the data to support that these "guidelines" reduce the frequency of hypersensitivity reactions are scant, and there are data refuting this premise.[8] Treating hyperuricemia with a uricosuric drug is not likely to be effective in the setting of a reduced GFR. A nonpurine inhibitor of xanthine oxidase (febuxostat), which is not cleared by the kidney, has been approved by the FDA. There are only limited data available on its use in patients with severe CKD. NSAIDs are relatively contraindicated in the setting of severe kidney disease, although once the patient is on dialysis, these agents can be used (some form of gastric protection should be considered). Use of colchicine in the setting of CKD or end-stage renal disease (ESRD) is potentially dangerous, and full-dose treatment of an acute attack or chronic full-dose prophylactic dosing should be avoided because there is a high risk for colchicine toxicity.

The patient with severe tophacious gout and a history of allopurinol intolerance had posed a special set of problems because there was not another extremely efficacious hypouricemic agent. If the intolerance was a mild skin reaction, desensitization therapy may be effective.[37] However, if the intolerance was demonstrated as GI symptoms, severe rash, or a systemic hypersensitivity reaction, there was no satisfactory treatment. Probenecid or other uricosurics are often not extremely effective, and even with a severe low purine diet, they are not likely to lower the serum urate sufficiently. Febuxostat may provide the alternative to this small group of patients, but information on the tolerance of this drug by patients who had an allopurinol systemic hypersensitivity reaction is still limited. We have utilized the drug successfully in 8 such patients.

EXPERIMENTAL APPROACHES AND DRUGS IN DEVELOPMENT FOR GOUT

Gout is generally not an extremely difficult condition to treat, even with currently available agents. The major problems seem to be related to patient compliance and physician education regarding the treatment of this disease. As noted earlier, there are certain groups of patients with gout who pose special management problems with our current available drugs.

There are specific situations in which the drugs used to treat the acute attack (i.e., NSAIDs, corticosteroids, and colchicine) are relatively strongly contraindicated or even ineffective. Based on current knowledge of the mediators of the acute gouty attack, several investigators have published their experiences using targeted biological therapy to treat the acute attack. Antagonizing IL-1 with anakinra,[37] as expected from the data on crystal activation of IL-1 via the inflammasome discussed earlier, or TNF-α[38] has been successful. There are a number of published and unpublished anecdotal successes in difficult or refractory gout patients using these currently available agents. Despite the very significant expense, these may be extremely useful drugs in highly selected patients. One personal caveat to these successes, I have cared for three patients on chronic anti-TNF therapy for nongouty diseases (two with etanercept and one with adalimumab) who have experienced continued intermittent attacks of gout (two patients) and pseudogout. An additional problematic issue with the use of these targeted therapies is that they are likely contraindicated in the setting of infection, a situation when an alternative to corticosteroids would be of real value.

Humans lack a functional (enzyme) uricase, which degrades urate into the more soluble allantoin. Raspuricase is a preparation of uricase available for clinical use in the treatment of the tumor lysis syndrome, and it has been used anecdotally to try to dissolve tophi and reduce the total body burden of uric acid in order to prevent further attacks of gout. It is antigenic, however, and cannot be used on a long-term basis. In an effort to limit the antigenicity and allergic potential, pegylated uricase has been developed and has been utilized in clinical trials in patients with severe tophaceous gout and allopurinol intolerance.[39] It has been effective when infused every 2 or 4 weeks at lowering the serum urate and dramatically dissolving tophi. A plenary report at the annual 2008 scientific meeting of the American College of Rheumatology included data describing the efficacy, but also raised some concerns regarding potential cardiac toxicity. At the present time, it has not been resolved whether this is a significant issue of concern.[40]

PSEUDOGOUT (CALCIUM PYROPHOSPHATE DEPOSITION DISEASE)

Other naturally occurring crystals can elicit an acute or chronic arthritis. Calcium pyrophosphate deposition disease (CPPD) can result in an acute inflammatory arthritis that is clinically indistinguishable from gout; hence, the term "pseudogout." The biochemical inflammatory cascade may be similar to that triggered by monosodium urate,[41,42] and the acute inflammatory response may respond to the same anti-inflammatory agents, including colchicine and an IL-1 antagonist.[43] The joint distribution and demographics are somewhat different in patients with CPPD as compared with those with gout. More women get CPPD, and the wrists (knees and MCPs) are far more common than the first metatarsophalangeal (MTP) joint. Patients with CPPD only extremely rarely get visible/palpable crystal masses or radiographically visible erosive tophi. Instead, they frequently get calcification of cartilaginous structures, including the menisci and fibrocartilage. It should be noted that this "chondrocalcinosis" can be seen radiographically in patients who have had no clinical inflammatory arthritis, and in this case, the condition requires no therapy. Multiple bone cysts may be prominent findings on radiographs, initially in the absence of joint space narrowing. A myriad of metabolic and other disorders have been associated with CPPD, but the association may be tenuous with many. However, hyperparathyroidism is an important consideration, particularly because pseudogout attacks are strikingly common immediately following curative parathyroid surgery. Distinguishing CPPD from gout is important; although the acute attacks can be treated similarly, the chronic disease management is different because patients with CPPD do not need their serum urate levels lowered. The serum urate level should not be used to distinguish CPPD from gout because patients with pseudogout may have hyperuricemia for unrelated reasons. There are fewer reported studies, but many (not all) patients with chronic, recurrent pseudogout respond to prophylactic therapy with colchicine and/or NSAIDs.

References

1. Margaretten ME, Kohlwes J, Moore D, Bent S. Does this adult patient have septic arthritis? JAMA 2007;297:1478-88.
2. Logan JA, Morrison E, McGill PE. Serum uric acid in acute gout. Ann Rheum Dis 2007;56:696-7.
3. Coakley G, Mathews C, Field M, Jones A, Kingsley G, Walker D, et al. On behalf of the British Society for Rheumatology Standards, Guidelines and Audit Working Group. BSR & BHPR, BOA, RCGP and BSAC guidelines for management of the hot swollen joint in adults. Rheumatology 2006;45:1039-41.
4. Pascual E, Jovani V. Synovial fluid analysis. Best Pract Res Clin Rheumatol 2005;19:371-86.
5. Coutlakis P, Roberts WN, Wise C. Another look at synovial fluid leukocytosis and infection. J Clin Rheumatol 2002;8:67-71.
6. Shah K, Spear J, Nathanson LA, McCauley J, Edlow JA. Does the presence of crystal arthritis rule out septic arthritis? J Emerg Med 2007;32:23-6.
7. Ohno I, Ichida K, Okabe H, Hikita M, Uetake D, Kimura H, et al. Frequency of gouty arthritis in patients with end-stage renal disease in Japan. Intern Med 2005;44:706-9.
8. Dalbeth N, Stamp L. Allopurinol dosing in renal impairment: Walking the tightrope between adequate urate lowering and adverse events. Semin Dial 2007;20:391-5.
9. Perez-Ruiz F, Calabozo M, Pijoan JI, Herrero-Beites AM, Ruibal A. Effect of urate-lowering therapy on the velocity of size reduction of tophi in chronic gout. Arthritis Rheum 2002;47:356-60.
10. Ahern MJ, Reid C, Gordon TP, McCredie M, et al. Does colchicine work? The results of the first controlled study in acute gout. Aust NZ J Med 1987;17:301-4.
11. Maldonado MA, Salzman A, Varga J. Intravenous colchicine use in crystal-induced arthropathies: a retrospective analysis of hospitalized patients. Clin Exp Rheumatol 1997;15:487-92.
12. Schumacher HR, Boice JA, Daikh DI, Mukhopadhyay S, Malmstrom K, Ng J, et al. Randomized double blind trial of etoricoxib and indomethacin in treatment of acute gouty arthritis. BMJ 2002;324:1488-92.
13. Janssens HJ, Jannssen M, van de Lisdonk EH, van Riel PL, van Weel C. Use of oral prednisolone or naproxen for the treatment of gout arthritis: a double-blind, randomised equivalence trial. Lancet 2008;371:1854-60.
14. Groff GD, Franck WA, Raddatz DA. Systemic steroid therapy for acute gout: a clinical trial and review of the literature. Semin Arthritis Rheum 1990;9:329-36.
15. Siegel LB, Alloway JA, Nashel DJ. Comparison of adrenocorticotropic hormone and triamcinolone, acetonide in the treatment of acute gouty arthritis. J Rheumatol 1994;21:1325-7.
16. Odio CM, Ramirez T, Arias G, Abdelnour A, Hidalgo I, Herrera ML, et al. Double blind, randomized, placebo-controlled study of dexamethasone therapy for hematogenous septic arthritis in children. Pediatr Infect Dis J 2003;22:883-8.
17. Schumacher HR, Becker MA, Wortmann RL, MacDonald PA, Hunt B, Streit J, et al. Effects of febuxostat versus allopurinol and placebo in reducing serum urate in subjects with hyperuricemia and gout: a 28-week, phase III, randomized, double-blind, parallel-group trial. Arthritis Rheum 2008;59:1540-8.

18. Feig DI, Kang D, Johnson R. Uric acid and cardiovascular risk. N Engl J Med 2008;359:1811-21.
19. Alderman MH. Podagra, uric acid, and cardiovascular disease. Circulation 2007;116:880-3.
20. Ioachimescu AG, Brennan DM, Hoar BM, Hazen SL, Hoogwerf B. Serum uric acid is an independent predictor of all-cause mortality in patients at high risk of cardiovascular disease. Arthritis Rheum 2008;58:623-30.
21. Mazzali M, Hughes J, Kim YG, Jefferson JA, Kang DH, Gordon KL, et al. Elevated uric acid increases blood pressure in the rat by a novel crystal-independent mechanism. Hypertension 2001;38:1101-6.
22. Feig DI, Soletsky B, Johnson RJ. Effect of allopurinol on blood pressure of adolescents with newly diagnosed essential hypertension: a randomized trial. JAMA 2008;300:8.
23. Siu Y, Leung K, Tong MK, Kwan T. Use of allopurinol in slowing the progression of renal disease through its ability to lower serum uric acid level. Am J Kidney Dis 2006;47:51-9.
24. Mene P, Punzo G. Uric acid: bystander or culprit in hypertension and progressive renal disease? J Hypertension 2008; 26:2085-92.
25. Nakagawa T, Hu H, Zharikov S, Tuttle KR, Short RA, Glushakova O, et al. A causal role for uric acid in fructose-induced metabolic syndrome. Am J Physiol Renal 2006;290:F625-31.
26. Johnson RJ, Segal MS, Sautin Y, Nakagawa T. Potential role of sugar (fructose) in the epidemic of hypertension, obesity and the metabolic syndrome, diabetes, kidney disease, and cardiovascular disease. Am J Clin Nutr 2007;86:899-906.
27. Waring WS, McKnight JA, Webb DJ, Maxwell S. Uric acid restores endothelial function in patients with type 1 diabetes and regular smokers. Diabetes 2006;55:3127-32.
28. Fam AG, Dunne SM, Iazetta J, Paton TW. Efficacy and safety of desensitization to allopurinol following cutaneous reactions. Arthritis Rheum 2001;44:231-8.
29. Waring WS, Convery A, Mishra V, Shenkin A, Webb DJ, Maxwell SRJ. Uric acid reduces exercise-induced oxidative stress in healthy adults. Clin Sci 2003;105:425-30.
30. Pascual E, Sivera F. The time required for disappearance of urate crystals from synovial fluid after successful hypouricemic treatment relates to the duration of gout. Ann Rheum Dis 2007;66:1056-8.
31. Kuncl RW, Duncan G, Watson D, Alderson K, Rogawski MA, Peper M. Colchicine myopathy and neuropathy. N Engl J Med 1987;316:1562-8.
32. Hediger MA, Johnson RJ, Miyazi H, Endou H. Molecular physiology of urate transport. Physiology 2005;20:125-33.
33. Meyers D, Monteagudo C. Gout in women. Clin Exp Rheum 1985;3:105-9.
34. Stamp L, Ha L, Searle M, O'Donnell J, Frampton C, Chapman P. Gout in renal transplant recipients. Nephrology 2006;11:367-71.
35. Kang EH, Lee EY, Lee YJ, Song YW, Lee EB. Clinical features and risk factors of postsurgical gout. Ann Rheum Dis 2008;67:1271-5.
36. Hande KR, Noone RM, Stone WJ. Severe allopurinol toxicity: descriptions and guidelines for prevention in patients with renal insufficiency. Am J Med 1984;76:47-56.
37. McGonagle D, Tan AL, Shankaranarayana S, Madden J, Emery P, McDermott MF. Management of treatment resistant inflammation of acute on chronic tophaceous gout with anakinra. Ann Rheum Dis 2007;66:1683-4.
38. Tausche AK, Richter K, Grässler A, Hänsel S, Roch B, Schröder HE. Severe gouty arthritis refractory to anti-inflammatory drugs: treatment with anti-tumour necrosis factor as a new therapeutic option. Ann Rheum Dis 2004;63:1351-2.
39. Sundy JS, Becker MA, Baraf SB, Barkhuizen A, Moreland LW, Huang W, et al. Reduction of plasma urate levels following treatment with multiple doses of pegloticase in patients with treatment failure gout: results of a phase II randomized study. Arthritis Rheum 2008;58:2882-91.
40. Sundy JS, Baraf HS, Becker MA, Barkhuizen A, Moreland LW, Huang W, et al. Efficacy and safety of Intravenous (IV) Pegloticase (PGL) in subjects with Treatment Failure Gout (TFG): Phase 3 results from GOUT1 and GOUT2. Arthritis Rheum 2008;58:S400.
41. So A. Uric acid crystals activate mononuclear cells to release interleukin 1 via toll like receptor and the NALP3 inflammasome. Arth Res Therapy 2008;10:221-7.
42. Martinon F, Pétrilli V, Mayor A, Tardivel A, Tschoop J. Gout-associated uric acid crystals activate the NALP3 inflammasome. Nature 2006;440:237-41.
43. McGonagle D, Tan AL, Madden J, Emery P, McDermott MF. Successful treatment of resistant pseudogout with anakinra. Arthritis Rheum 2008;58:631-3.

Section IV Management of the Degenerative Rheumatic Diseases

Chapter 23

Management of Osteoarthritis: Pharmacotherapy

Mathilde Michon, Jérémie Sellam, and Francis Berenbaum

INTRODUCTION

Osteoarthritis (OA) is the most common chronic joint disorder and is characterized by a degradative and repair process of cartilage and subchondral bone associated with synovial inflammation that may be triggered by a variety of biochemical as well as mechanical insults. OA should not be considered as a degenerative cartilage disease anymore but as a dynamic process including destruction and repair, as well as inflammation.

Pharmacologic therapies include oral (systemic) agents, topical agents, dietary supplements, and intra-articular (IA) therapies. All of these therapies have, to some degree, a symptomatic effect, and belong to the symptom-modifying osteoarthritis drug (SMOAD) family. Some of them may also have a beneficial effect on the structural damage and could be considered disease-modifying osteoarthritis drug (DMOAD). A better understanding of OA pathogenesis is bringing new opportunities for novel targeted therapies, some of which are already under clinical investigation.

The primary outcome measures recommended by Outcome Measures in Rheumatology Clinical Trials (OMERACT) for clinical trials of OA comprise four core domains: pain, physical function, patient global assessment, physician global assessment and, for studies of at least 1 year in duration, joint imaging.[1] For the study of DMOADs, primary endpoints should include joint space narrowing, pain, and physical function (Table 23-1).[2]

ANALGESICS

Acetaminophen (Paracetamol)

Acetaminophen (also known as paracetamol) is a simple analgesic that has both analgesic and antipyretic actions.

As a treatment for symptoms of OA, acetaminophen at up to 4 g/day is widely recommended as first-line therapy, for example, by the European League Against Rheumatism (EULAR),[3,4] the American College of Rheumatology (ACR),[5] and the Osteoarthritis Research Society International (OARSI).[6]

Symptomatic Efficacy

The description of efficacy and safety of acetaminophen for the treatment of OA has been well updated in a recent meta-analysis.[7] Acetaminophen was given at a dosage of 2600 to 4000 mg/day in the patient's knee or hip OA. Most of the studies lasted around 6 weeks and reported a superiority of acetaminophen compared with placebo. A pooled analysis of five trials demonstrated a statistically significant reduction in pain compared with placebo (pain decreased by 4 points on a scale of 0–100 in the acetaminophen group compared with placebo). The clinical significance of such a low effect remains debatable. No beneficial effect was observed on physical function.

Comparing acetaminophen with nonselective nonsteroidal anti-inflammatory drugs (NSAIDs) (ibuprofen, diclofenac, naproxen, and others) or selective cyclooxygenase-2 (COX-2) inhibitors (celecoxib, rofecoxib, and others), acetaminophen was less effective than NSAIDs in terms of pain reduction (pain decreased by 6 points on a scale of 0 to 100 in people who took NSAIDs compared with acetaminophen), improvement in global assessments (patient and investigator), stiffness and improvement in some parameters of functional status such as the Western Ontario and McMaster Universities (WOMAC) function scale, but not in the 50-foot walk time, nor in the Health Assessment Questionnaire (HAQ) or the Lequesne's algofunctional index.

Safety

In people taking NSAIDs, gastrointestinal (GI) discomfort occurred more frequently than in those taking acetaminophen (relative risk [RR], 1.47; 95% confidence interval [CI], 1.08-2.00) or a COX-2-selective NSAID.[7]

In this meta-analysis, no conclusion could be drawn concerning the serious adverse events, including serious GI, renal, and cardiovascular safety, because of the small number of participants and the relatively short period of time in most studies (6 days to 2 years).[7]

García Rodríguez and associates[8] reviewed the data on the risk of upper GI complications associated with NSAIDs or acetaminophen, and provided evidence that high-dose acetaminophen may not be as safe as previously thought. Surprisingly, in two

Table 23-1. *Clinicians Guide to Anti-Inflammatory Therapy*

Type of Risk	No or Low GI Risk	NSAID GI Risk
No CV risk (without aspirin)	NS-NSAID (cost consideration)	Coxib or NS-NSAID + PPI or Coxib + PPI for patients with previous GI bleeding
CV risk (with aspirin)	Naproxen* Addition of PPI if GI risk warrants gastroprotection	Add PPI irrespective of NSAID Coxib + PPI for those with previous gastrointestinal bleeding

*NS or selective (low-dose) NSAID without established aspirin interaction if naproxen is ineffective.
CV, cardiovascular; GI, gastrointestinal; (NS) NSAID, (nonselective) nonsteroidal anti-inflammatory drug; PPI, proton pump inhibitor.
From Lin J, Zhang W, Jones A, Doherty M. Efficacy of topical non-steroidal anti-inflammatory drugs in the treatment of osteoarthritis: meta-analysis of randomised controlled trials. BMJ 2004;329:324.

long-term studies, acetaminophen was associated with an increased risk for serious upper GI complications, with a clear dose-effect relationship. There was also evidence of a very strong interaction between the use of acetaminophen at doses of 2000 mg/day or more and NSAIDs (RR, 16.6; 95% CI, 11-24.9). However, a bias due to channeling cannot be ruled out in such an epidemiologic study. Hepatic toxicity was also reported in patients taking high doses (4 g/day) in particular when associated with alcohol consumption. Finally, recent data suggest that high-dose acetaminophen could induce hypertension, although the explanation remains unclear.

Conclusion

Acetaminophen is considered a safe treatment of OA, but the effect-size (improvement expressed as the fraction of the standard deviation) is modest (0.21; 95% CI, 0.02-0.41).[6] NSAIDs have a higher effect size than acetaminophen for pain relief (effect size 0.32; 95% CI, 0.24-0.39) but a less favorable safety profile. The choice of treatment for each patient ultimately depends on both effectiveness and safety profile in addition to availability, cost, and patient acceptance. According to the recommendation by EULAR, ACR, and OARSI, acetaminophen remains the first line oral analgesic in the management of OA. Additional randomized controlled trials (RCTs) are necessary to better identify the patients with OA who are more likely to benefit from acetaminophen.

Opioids

Opioids are potent analgesics targeting the opioid receptors. Biologic studies have shown that opioid receptors are present in inflamed OA synovial tissue.

Symptomatic Efficacy

In a systematic literature analysis of RCTs, Avouac and colleagues[9] found that opioids significantly decrease pain intensity but have small benefits on function compared with placebo in patients with OA. In two meta-analyses, Cepeda and coworkers[10,11] sought to determine the effect of oral tramadol (mean daily dose: 200 mg, during 1 week to 3 months) in patients with symptomatic hip or knee OA. The placebo-controlled studies indicated that participants who received tramadol had less pain (-8.5 units on a 0 to 100 scale; 95% CI, -12.0 to -5.0) than patients who received placebo. The reduction in the WOMAC index was 8.5% larger in the tramadol group than the placebo group. In the three placebo-controlled studies that followed participants for more than eight weeks, tramadol was more effective than placebo concerning pain intensity and patient global assessment. Thus, pooled results suggest that in people with OA, tramadol may decrease pain, improve overall well-being, slightly decrease stiffness and slightly improve function more than placebo.

In knee OA, no difference has been shown between tramadol (200 mg/day) and placebo among nonresponders to naproxen; in contrast, patients responding to naproxen had a significant improvement with tramadol and were able to reduce their dosage of the NSAID.[12]

Safety

According to Cepeda and associates,[10,11] participants who received tramadol had 2.27 times the risk of developing minor adverse events and 2.6 times the risk of developing major adverse events, compared with participants receiving placebo (minor adverse events: 39% versus 18% and major adverse events: 21% versus 8% respectively). The most common adverse events were nausea, vomiting, dizziness, constipation, somnolence, tiredness, and headache. There was no report of any life-threatening event. No comparison in terms of adverse events with other opioid drugs used in OA has been performed to date. Adverse events, although reversible and not life-threatening, may lead to discontinuation of the drug and could limit the use of tramadol.

Conclusion

Therefore, for patients suffering from severe pain or for which other analgesics/NSAIDs are contraindicated, opioids may be a reasonable alternative but should be monitored closely.[6]

NONSTEROIDAL ANTI-INFLAMMATORY DRUGS

NSAIDs decrease inflammation and pain by inhibiting the enzyme cyclooxygenase (COX) and thereby reducing prostaglandin production, COX-1, found in most normal tissues including the GI tract, kidneys, and platelets, is considered a housekeeping enzyme that regulates the production of prostaglandins and thromboxane A_2 for several physiologic functions such as protection of gut mucosal integrity, vascular vasoconstriction, and platelet activation; COX-2, found particularly in the kidney, brain, bone and reproductive organs, is upregulated substantially in any tissue with inflammation or injury and is a key mediator of inflammation, explaining its role in arthritis pain. NSAIDs differ in their ability to inhibit COX-1 and COX-2: nonselective NSAIDs inhibit COX-1 and COX-2, whereas coxibs inhibit selectively COX-2.

Nonselective Nonsteroidal Anti-inflammatory Drugs

Symptomatic Efficacy

Several trials have compared nonselective NSAIDs with acetaminophen for hip and knee OA.[13-16] All studies except one[13] have found nonselective NSAIDs to be superior to acetaminophen.

In the Ibuprofen, Paracetamol Study in Osteoarthritis (IPSO) study, the analgesic efficacy of ibuprofen 400 mg as a single dose and as multiple doses (1200 mg/day) was compared with that of acetaminophen either as a single dose of 1000 mg or as multiple doses (3000 mg/day) in patients with knee or hip OA.[16] Over 2 weeks, pain intensity, stiffness, and functional disability decreased significantly more in the ibuprofen than in the acetaminophen group.

Pincus and colleagues[14] found significantly higher levels of improvement for diclofenac plus misoprostol than for acetaminophen over 6 weeks. This superiority of diclofenac plus misoprostol was observed especially in patients with more severe OA, whereas patients with mild OA had similar improvements with both therapeutic options. Melo Gomes and coworkers[17] found that the efficacy of diclofenac/misoprostol in treating the signs and symptoms of OA was at least comparable to that of piroxicam or naproxen.

Safety

Gastrointestinal Disorders

In a meta-analysis of dyspepsia and NSAIDs, Ofman and associates[18] found that dyspeptic symptoms occur in 4.8% of patients receiving NSAIDs compared with 2.3% receiving placebo and that they are the most common reason for cessation of therapy. Dyspeptic symptoms are dose-dependent but are a poor predictor of peptic ulcers: of those investigated for dyspepsia, 50% have a normal endoscopy, 15% gastro-esophageal reflux disease, 25% peptic ulcers,

and 2% malignancies.[19] Endoscopic abnormalities are more likely in patients older than 45 years of age. Serious events such as perforation or bleeding from upper GI ulcers occur in 2% of NSAID users,[20] but are usually not preceded by symptoms. The link between ulcers on endoscopy and these complications needs to be investigated further. It has been shown that prostaglandin analogues (misoprostol 800 µg/day), proton pump inhibitors (PPIs), and double-dose H2-receptor antagonists are effective at preventing chronic NSAID-related endoscopic gastric and duodenal ulcers (misoprostol: RR, 0.17; 95% CI, 0.11-0.24, PPIs: RR, 0.40; 95% CI, 0.32-0.51, H2-receptor antagonists: RR, 0.44; 95% CI, 0.26-0.74).[21]

NSAIDs may also cause lower intestinal side effects, such as ulcers, bleeding, inflammation and scarring in the small intestine and colon: lower intestinal events account for nearly 40% of the serious GI events in a population of patients with rheumatoid arthritis (RA) treated with naproxen.[22]

Predictors of serious toxicity are

- Age 65 years or older: the risk rises for each decade after age 50, with an RR for those between age 50 and 60 years of 1.8 (compared with those younger than 50), and an RR of 9.2 for those older than the age of 80 years.[23]
- People with a past history of peptic ulcer disease: for example, the RR for serious toxicity using naproxen in such patients is 13.5.[24,25]
- People also taking anticoagulants: RRs exceed 6.0.[26,27]
- People also using corticosteroids: RRs vary between 2 and 6.[26,28]
- People using NSAIDs for prolonged periods.[24]

Cardiovascular Effects

Singh and coworkers[29] reviewed the published evidence and assessed the risk of acute myocardial infarction with nonselective NSAIDs. Nonselective NSAIDs as a class were associated with an increased risk for acute myocardial infarction (RR, 1.19; 95% CI, 1.08-1.31). Similar results were found for diclofenac (RR, 1.38; 95% CI, 1.22-1.57) and ibuprofen (RR, 1.11; 95% CI, 1.06-1.17) but not for naproxen (RR, 0.99; 95% CI, 0.88-1.11). Increases in blood pressure, which can be seen with any NSAID, may be one explanation for these increases in cardiovascular risk.

Renal Effects

Prostaglandins control renal blood flow, glomerular filtration rate, and salt and water excretion by the kidney. NSAIDs may cause sodium retention, hyporeninemic hypoaldosteronism, prerenal azotemia, acute interstitial nephritis, and nephritic syndrome. Acute renal dysfunction has been reported with NSAIDs.[30,31] Moreover, many of the nonselective NSAIDs have been implicated as causing chronic renal failure with RRs ranging from 2 to 8.[32,33]

Thus, special vigilance is needed in patients treated with antihypertensive drugs, those at risk for renal diseases such as diabetes, and in the elderly.

Other Adverse Effects

Other adverse effects including skin rashes, allergic reactions, mouth ulcers, headaches, tinnitus, exacerbation of asthma, and aggravation of inflammatory bowel disease have been described.

Selective Cyclooxygenase-2 Inhibitors (Coxibs)

Symptomatic Efficacy

In order to assess the effectiveness of COX-2–selective NSAIDs for the management of OA and RA, Chen and colleagues[34] undertook a meta-analysis of RCTs for each COX-2 selective NSAID compared with placebo and nonselective NSAIDs. The coxibs were found to be similar to nonselective NSAIDs for the symptomatic relief of OA.[34]

Safety

Gastrointestinal Disorders

Compared with non-selective NSAIDs, COX-2 selective NSAIDs (celecoxib, rofecoxib, and lumiracoxib) were found to be associated with significantly fewer clinical upper GI events, the reduction being around 50%. Although coxibs offer protection against serious upper GI events, the amount of evidence for this protective effect may vary across individual drugs.[34] Moreover, no difference has been demonstrated when a coxib is compared with a classic NSAID plus PPI.[35] Importantly, in patients at high GI risk, such as patients with previous ulcer bleeding induced by nonselective NSAIDs, neither celecoxib nor diclofenac plus omeprazole adequately prevents ulcer recurrence[36]: in this population, celecoxib plus a PPI is more effective than celecoxib alone for the prevention of recurrent ulcer bleeding.[37]

Recent studies have shown that coxibs might have the additional advantage of a lower risk for GI complications, which cannot be achieved by other strategies. (Currently available gastroprotective therapies such as PPI do not protect the lower GI tract.) A post hoc analysis of serious lower GI clinical events in a prospective, double-blind trial in RA patients randomly assigned to naproxen 500 mg twice daily or rofecoxib 50 mg daily, found a rate of serious lower GI events (serious bleeding, perforation, obstruction, ulceration, or diverticulitis) per 100 patient-years of 0.41 for rofecoxib and 0.89 for naproxen (RR, 0.46; 95% CI, 0.22-0.93; $P = 0.032$). Serious lower GI events were 54% lower with the use of the selective COX-2 inhibitor rofecoxib.[38] A more recent systematic review identified studies of NSAID or coxibs that reported on lower GI integrity (e.g., permeability), visualization (e.g., erosions, ulcers), and clinical events. Coxibs had significantly fewer harmful effects than nonselective NSAIDs in three of four integrity studies, one endoscopic study (RR for mucosal breaks: 0.3), and two randomized studies (RR for lower GI clinical events: 0.5; hematochezia: 0.4).[39] Nevertheless, these data have not

been confirmed in a recent prospective trial assessing lower GI clinical events in patients with OA or RA randomly treated with the COX-2–selective inhibitor etoricoxib (60 or 90 mg daily) versus the nonselective NSAID diclofenac (150 mg daily): no statistically significant decrease in lower GI clinical events was seen in this study. The risk of a lower GI clinical event with NSAID use seemed to be constant over time, and the major risk factors were a prior lower GI event and older age.[40] More trials are warranted to more precisely estimate the effects of nonselective NSAIDs and coxibs on the lower GI tract.

The concept of CSULGIEs (Clinically Significant Upper and/or Lower GI Events) as the first and only available composite endpoint designed to evaluate the entire GI tract, may help physicians to consider the entire GI tract when choosing NSAIDs and protective therapies.

Two trials comparing celecoxib with a nonselective NSAID using CSULGIEs as a primary endpoint are in progress. The study outcomes will provide important information on the entire GI safety of these two commonly used therapies.

Cardiovascular Effects

There is still a debate on a specific cardiovascular risk of coxibs compared with classic NSAIDs. A coxib-induced imbalance between PGI_2 secretion in endothelial cells and thromboxane A_2 (TXA_2) platelet synthesis could explain why COX-2 inhibitors may increase the risk of CV events. In a meta-analysis of the incidence of serious vascular events in RCTs, coxibs were associated with a 42% relative increase in the incidence of serious vascular events compared with placebo, corresponding mainly to an excess of myocardial infarctions. There was no significant heterogeneity among the different coxibs. However, the incidence of serious vascular events was similar between a coxib and nonselective NSAID except naproxen.[41]

Renal Effects

Concerning renal events, significant heterogeneity of renal effects across agents is observed suggesting that there is no class effect. Celecoxib is associated with a lower risk of both renal dysfunction (RR, 0.61; 95% CI, 0.40-0.94) and hypertension (RR, 0.83; 95% CI, 0.71-0.97) compared with NSAID controls.[42]

Other Adverse Effects

COX-2 inhibitors share most of the side effects seen with the classical NSAIDs. Recently, lumiracoxib has been withdrawn because of its hepatotoxicity.

Conclusion

The choice between a classic NSAID and a coxib depends on the patient's history and comorbidities.[43] In any case, COX-2–selective and classic NSAIDs should be used at the lowest effective dose for the shortest possible duration of treatment. However, it is not rare that chronic use of the highest dose is necessary to achieve the clinical goals. Further trials assessing the relative efficacy of COX-2–selective NSAIDs versus combination of nonselective NSAIDs and gastroprotective agents in people at standard risk and those at a higher risk are needed.

Topical Nonsteroidal Anti-inflammatory Drugs and Capsaicin

In a meta-analysis of RCTs of short duration (less than 4 weeks), topical NSAIDs were found to be superior to placebo in relieving OA pain and stiffness and improving function in the first 2 weeks of treatment only.[44] Effect sizes for pain at weeks 1 and 2 were modest at 0.41 (95% CI, 0.16-0.66) and 0.40 (95% CI, 0.15-0.65), respectively. However, topical NSAIDs were inferior to oral NSAIDs in the first week of treatment and associated with local side effects such as rash, itch, or burning. These results were in contradiction with those of a meta-analysis of long-term studies of topical NSAIDs in knee OA that found a pooled effect of topical NSAIDs at 4 weeks or beyond superior to placebo/vehicle in pain relief (mean effect size –0.28; 95% CI, –0.42 to –0.14), suggesting that topical NSAIDs are effective for pain relief in knee OA for a longer duration.[45]

Topical capsaicin cream contains a lipophilic alkaloid extracted from chili peppers. Its efficacy in knee or hand OA is supported by a meta-analysis of RCTs: capsaicin cream was better than placebo in providing pain relief in OA (odds ratio [OR], 4.36; 95% CI, 2.77–6.88). However, complete blinding was impossible because of the initial discomfort associated with topical capsaicin (local burning, stinging or erythema).[46]

SYMPTOMATIC SLOW-ACTING DRUGS IN OSTEOARTHRITIS

Glucosamine

Glucosamine is a natural precursor of the cartilage extracellular matrix component glycosaminoglycan. It has been widely promulgated as a remedy for OA on the basis that it might provide a substrate for matrix synthesis and repair. There are no dietary sources of glucosamine, and commercially available glucosamine is derived from shellfish. As a nutritional supplement, it is available in three forms: glucosamine hydrochloride (GH), glucosamine sulfate (GS), and N-acetyl-glucosamine.

The mechanisms of action for glucosamine in OA are poorly understood. In vitro studies have shown that adding GS to human chondrocytes results in increased proteoglycan synthesis.[47,48] Antiarthritic effects of glucosamine are presumed to result from the provision of glucosamine as a substrate for articular cartilage glycosaminoglycan synthesis, stimulating the production of cartilaginous matrix. In addition, anti-inflammatory properties have been proposed.[49]

The recommended dose of glucosamine in OA is 1250 mg/day.

Symptomatic Efficacy

The efficacy of glucosamine has been described in a meta-analysis according to the Cochrane guidelines.[50] Comparing GS or GH versus placebo, glucosamine was significantly superior to placebo in decreasing pain (on a scale of 0 to 100, glucosamine achieved a 13-point greater improvement than placebo) and in improving the Lequesne's Index (with a difference in the change from baseline between glucosamine and placebo of 2.3 units on the Lequesne scale). In contrast, there was no statistical difference between glucosamine and placebo for the WOMAC total score nor for its different subscales (pain, stiffness, function).

In a randomized trial, glucosamine (1500 mg/day), chondroitin sulfate (1200 mg/day), and the combination of both all failed to show a benefit on pain in a group of patients with OA of the knee, but post-hoc analyses suggested that the combination of glucosamine and chondroitin sulfate may be effective in the subgroup of patients with moderate-to-severe knee pain.[51]

Structural Efficacy

Three meta-analyses suggested the ability of GS to delay structural progression in knee OA. In Poolsup and associates,[52] the risk of disease progression was reduced by 54% (pooled RR, 0.46; 95% CI, 0.28-0.73; $P = 0.0011$). The number needed to treat was nine (95% CI, 6-20). Similar results were described by Richy and colleagues,[53] who showed significant efficacy of glucosamine on joint space narrowing with an effect size of 0.41 (95% CI, 0.21-0.60; $P < 0.001$), which corresponds to a low to medium effect. These results were corroborated by those reported by the Cochrane Collaboration.[50] It is noteworthy that these results are based on the assessment of joint space narrowing on x-ray studies. Because several biases are known to interfere with this measure (level of pain, positioning, and others), the clinical consequence of the reported differences remains questionable. Moreover, data on the long-term use of glucosamine in knee OA are sparse. One trial in radiographic knee OA (Kellgren-Lawrence grade 2 or grade 3 changes and joint space width of at least 2 mm at baseline) compared the structural efficacy of glucosamine 500 mg three times daily, chondroitin sulfate 400 mg three times daily, the combination of glucosamine and chondroitin sulfate, celecoxib 200 mg daily, or placebo over 24 months. At 2 years, no treatment achieved a predefined threshold of clinically important difference in the loss of joint space width as compared with placebo.[54] Further long-term trials and trials evaluating different forms of glucosamine are warranted before the widespread use of this agent for the prevention of structural progression could be recommended.

Safety

Long-term treatment with glucosamine is well tolerated. The number of reported adverse effects was not significantly different between glucosamine and placebo.[50,52] The most common problems reported to be associated with glucosamine were generally transient and considered mild to moderate, including abdominal pain, dyspepsia, diarrhea, increased blood pressure, fatigue, and rash.

Chondroitin sulfate

Chondroitin is a highly hydrophilic polysaccharide macromolecule. Its hydrocolloid properties confer much of the compressive resistance of cartilage. Proposed mechanisms of action of chondroitin sulfate include restoration of the extracellular matrix of the cartilage, prevention of further cartilage degradation,[55] and/or a role in overcoming a dietary deficiency of sulfur-containing amino acids that are essential building blocks for cartilage extracellular matrix molecules.[56] The recommended dose of chondroitin in OA is 1000 to 1200 mg/day.

Symptomatic Efficacy

A recent meta-analysis examined data on symptomatic and structural efficacy and safety of chondroitin in knee or hip OA, versus placebo or no treatment.[57] The analysis revealed a high degree of heterogeneity among the trials. Large-scale, methodologically sound trials indicated that the symptomatic benefit is minimal, with an effect size of –0.03 (95% CI, –0.13 to –0.07) corresponding to a difference of 0.6 mm on a 100-mm VAS. These results differ from a previous meta-analysis in knee or hip OA,[58] in which the aggregate effect size was 0.78 (95% CI, 0.60-0.95). When only high-quality or large trials were considered, this effect size was substantially lower, suggesting that quality issues and publication biases may have played a critical role. The effect sizes were relatively consistent for pain and functional outcomes.

In the recent RCT referred to earlier,[51] which compared glucosamine (1500 mg daily), chondroitin sulfate (1200 mg daily), glucosamine plus chondroitin sulfate, celecoxib (200 mg daily), and placebo for 24 weeks in patients with knee OA, it was shown that the response to chondroitin sulfate, either alone or in combination with glucosamine, was not significantly higher than the response to placebo.

Structural Efficacy

Differences in changes between chondroitin and placebo groups revealed a small effect in favor of chondroitin: 0.16 mm on minimum joint space width (95% CI, 0.08-0.24) and 0.23 mm on mean joint space width (95% CI, 0.09-0.37), that corresponds to small effect sizes (e.g., 0.12 and 0.18, respectively).[57] These effects are small, and their clinical significance is uncertain. Moreover, there was no evidence for structural efficacy of chondroitin versus placebo in radiographic knee OA in a 24-months study.[54]

Safety

The RR for any adverse event with chondroitin sulfate does not differ from that of placebo.[57]

Diacerein

Several studies (both in vitro and in animal models) suggest that the active diacetyl derivative of diacerein, rhein, may inhibit interleukin-1 (IL-1) production and the secretion of metalloproteinases without affecting the synthesis of prostaglandins.[59-61] Diacerein has also been implicated in the regulation of transforming growth factor (TGF) beta-1 and beta-2 in articular chondrocytes.[62] The recommended dose of diacerein in OA is 100 mg/day.

Symptomatic Efficacy

Rintelen and coworkers[63] performed a systematic meta-analysis of RCTs with diacerein for knee and/or hip OA to provide an evidence-based assessment of its symptomatic efficacy. Diacerein was significantly superior to placebo during the active treatment phase (reducing pain, changes in functional impairment, global efficacy rating by patients), and comparable to standard treatments (mostly NSAIDs). However, diacerein, but not NSAIDs, showed a carryover effect, persisting up to 3 months after treatment, with a significant analgesic-sparing effect during the follow-up period. A meta-analysis performed by Fidelix and colleagues[64] reviewed RCTs in order to confirm the effectiveness and safety of diacerein. When compared with placebo, pain on a VAS (0–100 mm) showed a statistically significant difference in favor of diacerein. However, a subgroup analysis according to the localization (knee or hip OA) showed an absence of efficacy. There was no improvement in the Lequesne's index, either in the group as a whole or in the subgroup analyses. Concerning total hip replacement, no evidence of a benefit was found. When comparing diacerein with NSAIDs, no significant difference was found in terms of pain on VAS, WOMAC function, or analgesic intake. Nevertheless, the studies were heterogeneous, evaluated different joints (knee or hip) for a short period (mean of 2.5 months), and the results were expressed with very large confident intervals. One 8-week study in hip OA, comparing diacerein plus NSAID with placebo showed better results in the former group in reducing pain and improving function (Lequesne's index).[64] Diacerein was compared with other symptomatic slow-acting drugs in osteoarthritis such as NRD 101 (a new hyaluronic acid [HA] high-molecular-weight polysaccharide) in knee OA for 1 year or harpadol in knee or hip OA for 4 months. In separate subgroup analyses, there was no difference between the groups in the following outcomes: pain (VAS 0–100 mm), Lequesne's index, global efficacy patient assessment, painful days in the previous month and radiographic progression.[64]

Structural Efficacy

In the 3-year controlled ECHODIAH trial including 507 patients suffering from painful OA of the hip, diacerein was compared with placebo. Structural progression was evaluated radiographically, and defined as the time to a 0.5-mm loss of joint space width. Using a life table approach, progression was significantly less frequent, and average time-to-progression significantly longer, in the diacerein group.[65]

Safety

Tolerability assessments revealed a statistically significant inferiority of diacerein versus placebo.[63,64] Diacerein is an anthraquinonic derivative; therefore, diarrhea was the most frequent adverse event (from 39% to 42% of patients treated by diacerein). The severity of diarrhea was mild to moderate, occurred within the first 2 weeks of the treatment, and resolved on continuing treatment. In most patients, this did not result in treatment interruption. The second most prevalent side effect is discoloration of the urine, which has no clinical consequences but may interfere with the blinding design in clinical trials. Finally, allergic events affecting the skin (pruritus, rash) are not rare.

Avocado-Soybean Unsaponifiables

It has recently been shown that avocado-soybean unsaponifiables (ASUs) can counteract stress-activated signaling pathways in chondrocytes.[66] The recommended dose in OA is 300 mg/day (100 mg avocado oil and 200 mg soybean oil).

Symptomatic Efficacy

The symptomatic efficacy of ASU in hip or knee OA has been evaluated in a meta-analysis of RCTs.[67] The average trial duration was 6 months. Both pain reduction and the Lequesne index favored ASU (effect size 0.39; 95% CI, 0.01-0.76; $P = 0.04$, and 0.45; 95% CI, 0.21-0.70; $P = 0.0003$, respectively), but results were heterogeneous between trials. The number of responders following ASU compared with placebo (OR, 2.19; $P = 0.007$) corresponded to a number needed to treat 6 (4–21) patients. Meta-analysis data support better chances of success in patients with knee OA than in those with hip OA.

Structural Efficacy

One randomized, double-blind, placebo-controlled pilot trial failed to demonstrate a structural effect of ASU in 108 patients suffering from hip OA (Kellgren-Lawrence grade 1 to 3).[68] However, in a post hoc analysis, ASU significantly reduced the progression of joint space loss as compared with placebo in the subgroup of patients with advanced joint space narrowing, suggesting that ASU could have a structural effect. Confirmation in a larger placebo-controlled study is required.

Safety

ASU is generally well tolerated. Occasional regurgitations with unpleasant taste can be avoided by taking the pill in the middle of a meal. Allergic reactions are rare. Hepatic disorders can occur but remain exceptional.

S-adenosylmethionine

S-adenosylmethionine (SAMe) is a dietary supplement now available in the United States. SAMe is proposed as an antidepressant, a medication for cholestasis and liver disorders, a treatment for migraines, and a therapy for fibromyalgia or OA. In OA, its mechanism of action remains controversial.

The efficacy of SAMe has been assessed in a meta-analysis of RCTs versus placebo or NSAIDs.[69] When compared with placebo, SAMe was more effective in reducing functional limitation (effect size 0.31; 95% CI, 0.099-0.520), but not in reducing pain, but data were based on only two studies. SAMe appeared to be as effective as NSAIDs in reducing pain (effect size 0.12; 95% CI, –0.029 to 0.273) and in improving functional limitation (effect size 0.025; 95% CI, –0.127 to 0.176) without the adverse effects often associated with NSAID therapies.

INTRA-ARTICULAR THERAPIES

Intra-articular Corticosteroids

Intra-articular (IA) corticosteroid injection for hip or knee OA should be considered particularly when patients have moderate to severe pain despite oral analgesic/anti-inflammatory agents, especially in patients with effusion or other signs of local inflammation.[3,5,6]

Six products are available: betamethasone (5 mg prednisone = 0.75 mg betamethasone), cortivazol (5 mg prednisone = 0.3 mg cortivazol), methylprednisolone (5 mg prednisone = 4 mg methylprednisolone), prednisolone acetate (5 mg prednisone = 5 mg prednisolone), triamcinolone hexacetonide (5 mg prednisone = 4 mg triamcinolone), and triamcinolone acetonide (5 mg prednisone = 4 mg triamcinolone).

Symptomatic Efficacy

In a recent Cochrane review,[70] IA corticosteroid was more effective than IA placebo for pain reduction up to 3 weeks post-injection. At 4 to 24 weeks post injection, no significant effect on pain was observed. Data on function were sparse, and no short- and long-term differences were detected. For patient global assessment, studies consistently showed lack of effect longer than 1 week postinjection. Therefore, it appears that the beneficial effects of IA corticosteroids are rapid in onset but may be relatively short lived (approximately 1 to 3 weeks). Comparisons of different IA corticosteroids against each other showed that triamcinolone hexacetonide was superior to betamethasone in terms of the number of patients reporting pain reduction up to 4 weeks postinjection (RR, 2.00; 95% CI, 1.10-3.63). No difference was detected between hydrocortisone tertiary-butylacetate and hydrocortisone acetate. None of the trials comparing one corticosteroid against another showed any statistically significant differences for the global assessment.[70]

For hip OA, Flanagan and coworkers[71] prospectively compared triamcinolone, bupivacaine, and saline in patients awaiting hip replacement. The three agents did not reliably give long-term benefit, but some short-term relief was obtained. Comparisons of IA corticosteroid (cortivazol or triamcinolone acetonide) and arthroscopic joint lavage showed no differences in any of the efficacy outcome measures (pain, function, global assessment).[70] In a recent meta-analysis, joint lavage in knee OA provided no benefit at 3 months in pain or function compared with placebo. Combination of lavage and IA steroid injection is not more effective than lavage alone.[72]

Safety

In the Cochrane review,[70] placebo comparisons did not show any statistically significant differences in the total number of withdrawals, in the number of patients reporting post injection flares or in the number of patients reporting local discomfort. Concerning corticosteroid versus joint lavage plus IA placebo, no statistically significant differences were detected in the total withdrawals overall, in the number of withdrawals due to lack of efficacy, or in the number of patients reporting local discomfort. Comparisons of different IA corticosteroids against each other did not show statistically significant differences for the number of patients reporting local pain after injection.

Although complications of IA corticosteroids remain rare, the physician should be aware of them to weigh the benefits and risks of these treatments. The following adverse effects have been reported: post injection flare, crystal-induced synovitis, tissue atrophy, fat necrosis, calcification, sepsis, and hematoma. Rarely, the systemic diffusion of the IA corticosteroid may result in hyperglycemia or hypertension.

Conclusion

IA corticosteroids are effective for the short-term symptomatic treatment of knee and hip OA. Their onset of action is fast, with effects on pain detectable at 1 week postinjection and lasting for 2 to 3 weeks. Some patients experience more dramatic and prolonged symptom relief than others: clinical predictors of good response should be further investigated, in particular those associated with inflammation and structural damage.

Hyaluronic Acid

Viscosupplementation is based on the physiologic importance of HA in synovial joints. To date, the long-term effect of viscosupplementation is not well understood. It may be based on a sequence of events that restores the trans-synovial flow and subsequently the metabolic and rheologic homeostasis of the joint.

Several different formulations of viscosupplements (hyaluronan and hylan) are available and differ in their molecular weights and in their source. This difference is thought to be of some importance with respect to the volume/amount and number of injections, the residue time in the joint and the biologic effects. In fact, injected HA is cleared from the osteoarthritic joint in less than 1 day.[73] To increase average molecular weight and half-life in the joint, HAs have been modified to form hylan, chemically cross-linked HA molecules with average molecular weights up to 23.10^6 Daltons, resulting in prolonged half-lives (e.g., 1.5–9 days).[74]

Symptomatic Efficacy

The pooled analyses reveal that viscosupplementation may be an effective treatment for knee OA, superior to placebo with respect to pain, function, and patient global assessment.[75]

When comparing HA products with placebo or IA corticosteroids, the dynamics of the response are such that a statistically significant effect on pain and function 1 to 4 weeks postinjection is not always achieved, but becomes evident and clinically important by the 5th to 13th week after injection, with an improvement from 28% to 54% for pain and from 9% to 32% for function. This suggests a later onset but a more durable response to HA treatment.[75]

Importantly, there are considerable differences between HA products in terms of their effects in time and on various outcomes in OA, and therefore, the clinical effects compared with placebo may be moderate to large depending on the product, the variable studied, and the time point at which it is measured. However, there are few randomized head-to-head comparisons of different viscosupplements, and prescribers should be cautious in drawing conclusions regarding the relative value of different products.[75]

A recent randomized double-blind trial in patients with painful knee OA showed that HA 2 mL or distention with physiological saline 20 mL did not significantly reduce pain compared with physiologic saline placebo 2 mL.[76] It has been suggested that higher viscosity and longer IA half-life could lead to better effectiveness. To determine whether high-molecular-weight hylan, or standard HA differ in their effectiveness and safety, Reichenbach and associates[77] performed a systematic review and meta-analysis of RCTs comparing these products in knee OA. They found no robust evidence for a clinically relevant benefit of hylan compared with HA. The pooled effect size was small (effect size 0.27; 95% CI, 0.55-0.01), favoring hylan, but between-trial heterogeneity was high.

The symptomatic effect of HA has also been assessed in other OA sites. Concerning hip OA, Qvistgaard and coworkers[78] showed some clinical improvement (effect size 0.6; 95% CI, 0.1-1.1; P = 0.021 compared to saline) at 3 months. Tikiz and colleagues[79] found a significant clinical improvement from baseline during a 6-month follow-up period with a lower molecular weight hyaluronan or with a higher molecular weight viscosupplement, but without a significant difference between the higher and lower molecular weight compounds. A few studies aimed to assess the effects of HA in trapezometacarpal joint osteoarthritis. Studies comparing hylan versus corticosteroid or placebo,[80] sodium hyaluronate versus triamcinolone acetonide,[81] or hyaluronate versus methylprednisolone[82] showed a delayed (1 month) but long-lasting (up to 6 months) effect of HA on pain, grip strength and fine hand function, whereas corticosteroids had earlier but more short-lived efficacy. HA has also been tested in ankle OA, and provided sustained relief of pain and improvement of function compared with saline placebo injection.[83,84]

Structural Efficacy

A structural effect of local hyaluronan injections in knee OA was suggested in an ex vivo study coming from a randomized open-label clinical trial comparing IA injections of hyaluronan or of methylprednisolone acetate.[85] Both treatment strategies modified a number of structural variables of the synovial membrane of the osteoarthritic human knee toward the appearance of that of normal synovium. These data were supported in a histomorphometric study on cartilage samples taken from osteoarthritic human knees before and 6 months after IA injections of hyaluronan or methylprednisolone acetate.[86] Six months after hyaluronan treatment, a significant reconstitution of the superficial layer was observed, with an improvement in chondrocyte density and territorial matrix appearance. Results obtained with hyaluronan were significantly superior to those with methylprednisolone and provided further evidence of a potential structure-modifying activity of hyaluronan in OA. However, these products have not yet proved to be DMOADs in OA patients.

Safety

Except for a high incidence of injection site pain, the safety profile of HA seems acceptable.[75] These occasional local reactions tend to be transient, resolving either spontaneously or with simple intervention. A meta-analysis revealed that patients treated with hylan were approximately twice as likely as patients treated with HA to experience local adverse events. The pooled RRs for hylan were of 1.91 (95% CI, 1.04-3.49) for local adverse events (ranging from pain, swelling, or warmth to severe inflammatory reactions of the treated knee), 2.04 (95% CI, 1.18-3.53) for flares and 2.40 (95% CI, 1.21-4.76) for joint effusions.[77]

NEW PERSPECTIVES

Bone-Targeted Therapies

Subchondral bone is now considered as one of the actors involved in the pathophysiology of OA. Based on these recent discoveries, trials with bone-targeted therapies have been published and others are ongoing (Table 21-2).

Table 23-2. *Drugs Under Investigation in Humans*

Class	Name	Goal	Route of Administration
Bone-targeted	Alendronate	DMOAD	Oral
	Strontium ranelate	DMOAD	Oral
	Calcitonin	DMOAD	Oral
	Vitamin D	DMOAD	Oral
Biologic agents	IL-1 inhibitors	DMOAD and/or SMOAD	IA
	TNF inhibitors	DMOAD and/or SMOAD	Subcutaneous, IA?
	NGF inhibitors	SMOAD	Infusion
	FGF-18	DMOAD	IA
NSAID derived	Naproxcinod	SMOAD	Oral
	Licofelone	SMOAD	Oral
MMP inhibitors	Doxycycline	DMOAD	Oral
TRPV1 agonist	Capsaicin	SMOAD	Infusion

DMOAD, disease-modifying osteoarthritis drug; FGF-18, fibroblast growth factor-18; IA, intra-articular; IL-1, interleukin 1; MMP, matrix metalloproteinase; NGF, nerve growth factor; NSAID, nonsteroidal anti-inflammatory agent; SMOAD, symptom-modifying osteoarthritis drug; TNF, tumor necrosis factor; TRPV1, transient receptor potential vanilloid receptor.

Bisphosphonates

Because bisphosphonates could have a chondro-protective effect, reducing the incidence and progression of osteophytes in animal models and modifying osteoblast function in vitro, this therapeutic class has been tested in OA with interesting results. Risedronate may be responsible for less subchondral bone attrition and less bone marrow edema–like change by magnetic resonance imaging (MRI), and also decreases the level of markers of cartilage degradation. Unfortunately, no clinically relevant effect was observed with this treatment.[87] Alendronate use was associated with decreased spinal osteophyte formation and less progression of disc space narrowing in spinal OA.[88] Etidronate has shown some beneficial effect on OA pain.[89] In conclusion, the theoretical chondroprotective effect of biphosphonates gives a rationale to test them in OA, but before wide-spread use in clinical practice can be recommended, further trials are needed to determine if there is a clinically relevant benefit.

Strontium Ranelate

Strontium ranelate is a new drug indicated for the treatment of postmenopausal osteoporosis, which has been proven to be effective in the reduction of vertebral and hip fractures. According to in vitro studies showing an effect of strontium ranelate on extracellular cartilage matrix synthesis and an enhancement of insulin-like growth factor activity on proteoglycan synthesis, a potential effect on OA of this drug has to be considered. According to a post hoc analysis of two RCTs in women with osteoporosis and prevalent spinal OA, strontium ranelate reduces the radiographic progression of spinal OA and decreased back pain related to OA (studied in patients with no prevalent vertebral fracture during the study).[90] A randomized controlled trial in knee OA is ongoing.

Oral Salmon Calcitonin

Oral salmon calcitonin, available as a therapeutic agent in metabolic bone diseases for more than 30 years, could be potentially effective in the treatment of OA. Recently, a phase II clinical trial in knee OA has shown an improvement in functional disability and a decrease in levels of biomarkers reflecting cartilage loss.[91] A phase III clinical trial is currently performed to further investigate the effect of this therapy in knee OA (ClinicalTrials.gov Identifier: NCT00704847).

Vitamin D

Vitamin D may play a role in OA progression because vitamin D deficiency is associated with incidence and progression of OA.[92,93] However, the ben-efit of vitamin D supplementation in OA patients with vitamin D deficiency needs to be investigated.

Biologic Agents

Interleukin-1

Interleukin 1 (IL-1) plays a pivotal role in the pathogenesis of OA, and therefore, local injection of the IL-1 receptor antagonist (IL-1Ra) has recently been studied in knee OA with some minimal effects in a few patients.[94] This treatment option needs further investigation.

Tumor Necrosis Factor

TNF is another cytokine involved in the inflammatory component of OA and has proved to be an effective therapeutic target in RA. An open-pilot study of TNF inhibition (adalimumab) in the erosive/inflammatory subgroup of hand OA has been performed but the results were disappointing.[95] However, an RCT evaluating adalimumab is currently conducted in symptomatic hand OA (ClinicalTrials.gov Identifier: NCT00597623).

Nerve Growth Factor

Nerve growth factor (NGF) is a key mediator involved in peripheral pain. Recently, a humanized (NGF)–neutralizing monoclonal antibody (tanezumab, formerly known as RN624) has been proposed as a good candidate for the treatment of chronic pain. In a recently reported phase II trial, a large beneficial effect on pain of IV tanezumab once every 8 weeks was seen in severe knee OA patients, as assessed by the OMERACT-OARSI responder index and the WOMAC physical function, pain, and stiffness scores.[96] Because of unacceptable neurologic side effects seen in this trial with the highest doses, a phase III clinical trial with lower dosages is scheduled in 2009.

Fibroblast Growth Factor-18

Fibroblast growth factor-18 is one of the growth factors involved in matrix stabilization and cartilage repair.[97] Studies of repeated IA injections of this mediator are being considered in knee OA.

New Drugs Derived from Nonsteroidal Anti-inflammatory Drugs
Nitric Oxide Nonsteroidal Anti-inflammatory Drugs

Given the efficacy, safety, and tolerability issues associated with NSAIDs, the development of new agents to manage the pain associated with arthritis but without the cardiovascular and GI adverse events remains a priority. Cyclooxygenase-inhibiting nitric oxide–donating drugs (CINODs) may offer one alternative. These drugs are synthesized by linking a nitric oxide moiety to an NSAID via an ester linkage. They have been shown in laboratory and early clinical studies to be efficacious in the treatment of pain and inflammation, and they may help to reduce NSAID-induced gastric damage. Naproxcinod was shown to induce significantly less gastric damage than the parent compound naproxen, while exhibiting equivalent analgesic and anti-inflammatory activities in an animal model.[98] Furthermore, clinical studies have demonstrated a trend toward lower blood pressure in patients receiving naproxcinod as compared with naproxen.[99] More research will help to determine whether CINODs have a better benefit-risk profile than classical NSAIDs and than coxibs in OA.[100]

Licofelone

Licofelone is a molecule with anti-COX and anti-lipoxygenase activities. Pilot studies have shown interesting results in terms of efficacy and safety in OA but a large RCT is needed in order to compare its profile with the other NSAIDs.[101]

Matrix Metalloproteinase Inhibitors

Doxycycline has been tested in OA based on its anti-matrix metalloproteinase (MMP) activity demonstrated in vitro. Unfortunately, the results were disappointing.[102] Other MMP inhibitors have also been studied, but unacceptable musculoskeletal side effects occurred.[103] However, recent basic discoveries in the field of MMP biology has lead to novel targets, which are now being tested in humans.

Transient Receptor Potential Vanilloid Receptor Inhibitors

Transient receptor potential vanilloid receptor (TRPV1) belongs to the transient receptor potential vanilloid subfamily that is involved in nociception. Topical capsaicin, an agonist of TRPV1, is commonly used in some countries for the symptomatic treatment of OA. An injectable preparation of capsaicin (ALGRX-4975) is in development for long-lasting pain relief (phase II and III clinical trials are ongoing).[104]

CONCLUSIONS

Although many potential targets for a disease-modifying drug are now considered in OA, we must admit today that the pharmacologic approach relies only on treating the symptoms. Many international recommendations have recently been published to help doctors in their choice among the different available therapeutic agents. However, these recommendations have been based on analyses of trials that compare groups of patients. Although such comparisons are important, the implementation of these recommendations should always take into account the individual patient profiles we encounter in the clinic. Each prescription should be tailor made and should rely on an individual evaluation of the benefit-to-risk ratio for each drug.

References

1. Bellamy N, Kirwan J, Boers M, Brooks P, Strand V, Tugwell P, et al. Recommendations for a core set of outcome measures for future phase III clinical trials in knee, hip, and hand osteoarthritis. Consensus development at OMERACT III. J Rheumatol 1997;24:799-802.
2. Abadie E, Ethgen D, Avouac B, Bouvenot G, Branco J, Bruyere O, et al. Group for the Respect of Excellence and Ethics in Science. Recommendations for the use of new methods to assess the efficacy of disease-modifying drugs in the treatment of osteoarthritis. Osteoarthritis Cartilage 2004;12:263-8.
3. Jordan KM, Arden NK, Doherty M, Bannwarth B, Bijlsma JW, Dieppe P, et al. Standing Committee for International Clinical Studies Including Therapeutic Trials ESCISIT. EULAR Recommendations 2003: an evidence based approach to the management of knee osteoarthritis: Report of a Task Force of the Standing Committee for International Clinical Studies Including Therapeutic Trials (ESCISIT). Ann Rheum Dis 2003;62:1145-55.
4. Zhang W, Doherty M, Arden N, Bannwarth B, Bijlsma J, Gunther KP, et al. EULAR Standing Committee for International Clinical Studies Including Therapeutics (ESCISIT). EULAR evidence based recommendations for the management of hip osteoarthritis: report of a task force of the EULAR Standing Committee for International Clinical Studies Including Therapeutics (ESCISIT). Ann Rheum Dis 2005;64:669-81.
5. American College of Rheumatology Subcommittee on Osteoarthritis Guidelines. Recommendations for the medical management of osteoarthritis of the hip and knee: 2000 update. Arthritis Rheum 2000;43:1905-15.
6. Zhang W, Moskowitz RW, Nuki G, Abramson S, Altman RD, Arden N, et al. OARSI recommendations for the management of hip and knee osteoarthritis, Part II: OARSI evidence-based, expert consensus guidelines. Osteoarthritis Cartilage 2008;16:137-62.
7. Towheed TE, Maxwell L, Judd MG, Catton M, Hochberg MC, Wells G. Acetaminophen for osteoarthritis. Cochrane Database Syst Rev 2006;(1):CD004257.
8. García Rodríguez LA, Hernández-Díaz S. Relative risk of upper gastrointestinal complications among users of acetaminophen and nonsteroidal anti-inflammatory drugs. Epidemiology 2001;12:570-6.
9. Avouac J, Gossec L, Dougados M. Efficacy and safety of opioids for osteoarthritis: a meta-analysis of randomized controlled trials. Osteoarthritis Cartilage 2007;15:957-65.
10. Cepeda MS, Camargo F, Zea C, Valencia L. Tramadol for osteoarthritis: a systematic review and metaanalysis. J Rheumatol 2007;34:543-55.
11. Cepeda MS, Camargo F, Zea C, Valencia L. Tramadol for osteoarthritis. Cochrane Database Syst Rev 2006;19(3):CD005522.
12. Schnitzer TJ, Kamin M, Olson WH. Tramadol allows reduction of naproxen dose among patients with naproxen-responsive osteoarthritis pain: a randomized, double-blind, placebo-controlled study. Arthritis Rheum 1999;42:1370-7.
13. Bradley JD, Brandt KD, Katz BP, Kalasinski LA, Ryan SI. Comparison of an antiinflammatory dose of ibuprofen, an analgesic dose of ibuprofen, and acetaminophen in the treatment of patients with osteoarthritis of the knee. N Engl J Med 1991;325:87-91.
14. Pincus T, Koch GG, Sokka T, Lefkowith J, Wolfe F, Jordan JM, et al. A randomized, double-blind, crossover clinical trial of diclofenac plus misoprostol versus acetaminophen in patients with osteoarthritis of the hip or knee. Arthritis Rheum 2001;44:1587-98.
15. Case JP, Baliunas AJ, Block JA. Lack of efficacy of acetaminophen in treating symptomatic knee osteoarthritis: a randomized, double-blind, placebo-controlled comparison trial with diclofenac sodium. Arch Intern Med 2003;163:169-78.

16. Boureau F, Schneid H, Zeghari N, Wall R, Bourgeois P. The IPSO study: ibuprofen, paracetamol study in osteoarthritis. A randomised comparative clinical study comparing the efficacy and safety of ibuprofen and paracetamol analgesic treatment of osteoarthritis of the knee or hip. Ann Rheum Dis 2004;63:1028-34.

17. Melo Gomes JA, Roth SH, Zeeh J, Bruyn GA, Woods EM, Geis GS. Double-blind comparison of efficacy and gastroduodenal safety of diclofenac/misoprostol, piroxicam, and naproxen in the treatment of osteoarthritis. Ann Rheum Dis 1993;52:881-5.

18. Ofman JJ, Maclean CH, Straus WL, Morton SC, Berger ML, Roth EA, et al. Meta-analysis of dyspepsia and nonsteroidal antiinflammatory drugs. Arthritis Rheum 2003;49:508-18.

19. Williams B, Luckas M, Ellingham JH, Dain A, Wicks AC. Do young patients with dyspepsia need investigation? Lancet 1988;2:1349-51.

20. Tramèr MR, Moore RA, Reynolds DJ, McQuay HJ. Quantitative estimation of rare adverse events which follow a biological progression: a new model applied to chronic NSAID use. Pain 2000;85:169-82.

21. Rostom A, Dube C, Wells G, Tugwell P, Welch V, Jolicoeur E, et al. Prevention of NSAID-induced gastroduodenal ulcers. Cochrane Database Syst Rev 2002;(4):CD002296.

22. Laine L, Connors LG, Reicin A, Hawkey CJ, Burgos-Vargas R, Schnitzer TJ, et al. Serious lower gastrointestinal clinical events with nonselective NSAID or coxib use. Gastroenterology 2003;124:288-92.

23. Hernández-Díaz S, Rodríguez LA. Association between nonsteroidal anti-inflammatory drugs and upper gastrointestinal tract bleeding/perforation: an overview of epidemiologic studies published in the 1990s. Arch Intern Med 2000;160:2093-9.

24. MacDonald TM, Morant SV, Robinson GC, Shield MJ, McGilchrist MM, Murray FE, et al. Association of upper gastrointestinal toxicity of non-steroidal anti-inflammatory drugs with continued exposure: cohort study. BMJ 1997;315:1333-7.

25. Fries JF, Bruce B. Rates of serious gastrointestinal events from low dose use of acetylsalicylic acid, acetaminophen, and ibuprofen in patients with osteoarthritis and rheumatoid arthritis. J Rheumatol 2003;30:2226-33.

26. García Rodríguez LA, Jick H. Risk of upper gastrointestinal bleeding and perforation associated with individual nonsteroidal anti-inflammatory drugs. Lancet 1994;343:769-72 [Erratum in: Lancet 1994;343:1048].

27. Shorr RI, Ray WA, Daugherty JR, Griffin MR. Concurrent use of nonsteroidal anti-inflammatory drugs and oral anticoagulants places elderly persons at high risk for hemorrhagic peptic ulcer disease. Arch Intern Med 1993;153:1665-70.

28. Laine L, Bombardier C, Hawkey CJ, Davis B, Shapiro D, Brett C, et al. Stratifying the risk of NSAID-related upper gastrointestinal clinical events: results of a double-blind outcomes study in patients with rheumatoid arthritis. Gastroenterology 2002;123:1006-12.

29. Singh G, Wu O, Langhorne P, Madhok R. Risk of acute myocardial infarction with nonselective non-steroidal anti-inflammatory drugs: a meta-analysis. Arthritis Res Ther 2006;8:R153.

30. Griffin MR, Yared A, Ray WA. Nonsteroidal antiinflammatory drugs and acute renal failure in elderly persons. Am J Epidemiol 2000;151:488-96.

31. Pérez Gutthann S, García Rodríguez LA, Raiford DS, Duque Oliart A, Ris Romeu J. Nonsteroidal anti-inflammatory drugs and the risk of hospitalization for acute renal failure. Arch Intern Med 1996;156:2433-9.

32. Perneger TV, Whelton PK, Klag MJ. Risk of kidney failure associated with the use of acetaminophen, aspirin, and nonsteroidal antiinflammatory drugs. N Engl J Med 1994;331:1675-9.

33. Sandler DP, Burr FR, Weinberg CR. Nonsteroidal anti-inflammatory drugs and the risk for chronic renal disease. Ann Intern Med 1991;115:165-72.

34. Chen YF, Jobanputra P, Barton P, Bryan S, Fry-Smith A, Harris G, et al. Cyclooxygenase-2 selective non-steroidal anti-inflammatory drugs (etodolac, meloxicam, celecoxib, rofecoxib, etoricoxib, valdecoxib and lumiracoxib) for osteoarthritis and rheumatoid arthritis: a systematic review and economic evaluation. Health Technol Assess 2008;12:1-278, iii.

35. Chan FK, Hung LC, Suen BY, Wu JC, Lee KC, Leung VK, et al. Celecoxib versus diclofenac and omeprazole in reducing the risk of recurrent ulcer bleeding in patients with arthritis. N Engl J Med 2002;347:2104-10.

36. Chan FK, Hung LC, Suen BY, Wong VW, Hui AJ, Wu JC, et al. Celecoxib versus diclofenac plus omeprazole in high-risk arthritis patients: results of a randomized double-blind trial. Gastroenterology 2004;127:1038-43.

37. Chan FK, Wong VW, Suen BY, Wu JC, Ching JY, Hung LC, et al. Combination of a cyclo-oxygenase-2 inhibitor and a proton-pump inhibitor for prevention of recurrent ulcer bleeding in patients at very high risk: a double-blind, randomised trial. Lancet 2007;369:1621-6.

38. Laine L, Connors LG, Reicin A, Hawkey CJ, Burgos-Vargas R, Schnitzer TJ, et al. Serious lower gastrointestinal clinical events with nonselective NSAID or coxib use. Gastroenterology 2003;124:288-92.

39. Laine L, Smith R, Min K, Chen C, Dubois RW. Systematic review: the lower gastrointestinal adverse effects of nonsteroidal anti-inflammatory drugs. Aliment Pharmacol Ther 2006;24:751-67.

40. Laine L, Curtis SP, Langman M, Jensen DM, Cryer B, Kaur A, et al. Lower gastrointestinal events in a double-blind trial of the cyclo-oxygenase-2 selective inhibitor etoricoxib and the traditional nonsteroidal anti-inflammatory drug diclofenac. Gastroenterology 2008;135:1517-25.

41. Kearney PM, Baigent C, Godwin J, Halls H, Emberson JR, Patrono C. Do selective cyclo-oxygenase-2 inhibitors and traditional non-steroidal anti-inflammatory drugs increase the risk of atherothrombosis? Meta-analysis of randomised trials. BMJ 2006;332:1302-8.

42. Zhang J, Ding EL, Song Y. Adverse effects of cyclooxygenase 2 inhibitors on renal and arrhythmia events: meta-analysis of randomized trials. JAMA 2006;296:1619-32.

43. Jones R, Rubin G, Berenbaum F, Scheiman J. Gastrointestinal and cardiovascular risks of nonsteroidal anti-inflammatory drugs. Am J Med 2008;121:464-74.

44. Lin J, Zhang W, Jones A, Doherty M. Efficacy of topical non-steroidal anti-inflammatory drugs in the treatment of osteoarthritis: meta-analysis of randomised controlled trials. BMJ 2004;329:324.

45. Biswal S, Medhi B, Pandhi P. Longterm efficacy of topical nonsteroidal antiinflammatory drugs in knee osteoarthritis: metaanalysis of randomized placebo controlled clinical trials. J Rheumatol 2006;33:1841-4.

46. Zhang WY, Li Wan Po A. The effectiveness of topically applied capsaicin. A meta-analysis. Eur J Clin Pharmacol 1994;46:517-22.

47. Bassleer C, Rovati L, Franchimont P. Stimulation of proteoglycan production by glucosamine sulfate in chondrocytes isolated from human osteoarthritic articular cartilage in vitro. Osteoarthritis Cartilage 1998;6:427-34.

48. Bassleer C, Henrotin Y, Franchimont P. In-vitro evaluation of drugs proposed as chondroprotective agents. Int J Tissue React 1992;14:231-41.

49. Hungerford MW, Valaik D. Chondroprotective agents: glucosamine and chondroitin. Foot Ankle Clin 2003; 8:201-19.

50. Towheed TE, Maxwell L, Anastassiades TP, Shea B, Houpt J, Robinson V, et al. Glucosamine therapy for treating osteoarthritis. Cochrane Database Syst Rev 2005;(2):CD002946.

51. Clegg DO, Reda DJ, Harris CL, Klein MA, O'Dell JR, Hooper MM, et al. Glucosamine, chondroitin sulfate, and the two in combination for painful knee osteoarthritis. N Engl J Med 2006;354:795-808.

52. Poolsup N, Suthisisang C, Channark P, Kittikulsuth W. Glucosamine long-term treatment and the progression of knee osteoarthritis: systematic review of randomized controlled trials. Ann Pharmacother 2005;39:1080-7.

53. Richy F, Bruyere O, Ethgen O, Cucherat M, Henrotin Y, Reginster JY. Structural and symptomatic efficacy of glucosamine and chondroitin in knee osteoarthritis: a comprehensive meta-analysis. Arch Intern Med 2003;163:1514-22.

54. Sawitzke AD, Shi H, Finco MF, Dunlop DD, Bingham 3rd CO, Harris CL, et al. The effect of glucosamine and/or chondroitin sulfate on the progression of knee osteoarthritis: a report from the glucosamine/chondroitin arthritis intervention trial. Arthritis Rheum 2008;58:3183-91.

55. Johnson KA, Hulse DA, Hart RC, Kochevar D, Chu Q. Effects of an orally administered mixture of chondroitin sulfate, glucosamine hydrochloride and manganese ascorbate on synovial fluid chondroitin sulfate 3B3 and 7D4 epitope in a canine cruciate ligament transection model of osteoarthritis. Osteoarthritis Cartilage 2001;9:14-21.

56. Cordoba F, Nimni ME. Chondroitin sulfate and other sulfate containing chondroprotective agents may exhibit their effects by overcoming a deficiency of sulfur amino acids. Osteoarthritis Cartilage 2003;11:228-30.

57. Reichenbach S, Sterchi R, Scherer M, Trelle S, Bürgi E, Bürgi U, et al. Meta-analysis: chondroitin for osteoarthritis of the knee or hip. Ann Intern Med 2007;146:580-90.

58. McAlindon TE, LaValley MP, Gulin JP, Felson DT. Glucosamine and chondroitin for treatment of osteoarthritis: a systematic quality assessment and meta-analysis. JAMA 2000;283:1469-75.

59. Boittin M, Rédini F, Loyau G, Pujol JP. Effect of diacerhein (ART 50) on the matrix synthesis and collagenase secretion by cultured joint chondrocytes in rabbits. Rev Rhum Ed Fr 1993;60(6):68S-76S.

60. Moore AR, Greenslade KJ, Alam CA, Willoughby DA. Effects of diacerhein on cytokine determinations in a model of cartilage degradation induced by granuloma in mice. Rev Prat 1997;47(17 Suppl.):S24-6.

61. Pelletier JP, Mineau F, Fernandes JC, Duval N, Martel-Pelletier J. Diacerhein and rhein reduce the interleukin 1beta stimulated inducible nitric oxide synthesis level and activity while stimulating cyclooxygenase-2 synthesis in human osteoarthritic chondrocytes. J Rheumatol 1998;25:2417-24.

62. Felisaz N, Boumediene K, Ghayor C, Herrouin JF, Bogdanowicz P, Galerra P, et al. Stimulating effect of diacerein on TGF-beta1 and beta2 expression in articular chondrocytes cultured with and without interleukin-1. Osteoarthritis Cartilage 1999;7:255-64.

63. Rintelen B, Neumann K, Leeb BF. A meta-analysis of controlled clinical studies with diacerein in the treatment of osteoarthritis. Arch Intern Med 2006;166:1899-906 [Erratum in: Arch Intern Med 2007;167:444].

64. Fidelix TS, Soares BG, Trevisani VF. Diacerein for osteoarthritis. Cochrane Database Syst Rev 2006;(1):CD005117.

65. Dougados M, Nguyen M, Berdah L, Maziéres B, Vignon E, Lequesne M. ECHODIAH Investigators Study Group. Evaluation of the structure-modifying effects of diacerein in hip osteoarthritis: ECHODIAH, a three-year, placebo-controlled trial. Evaluation of the Chondromodulating Effect of Diacerein in OA of the Hip. Arthritis Rheum 2001;44:2539-47.

66. Gabay O, Gosset M, Levy A, Salvat C, Sanchez C, Pigenet A, et al. Stress-induced signaling pathways in hyalin chondrocytes: inhibition by avocado-soybean unsaponifiables (ASU). Osteoarthritis Cartilage 2008;16:373-84.

67. Christensen R, Bartels EM, Astrup A, Bliddal H. Symptomatic efficacy of avocado-soybean unsaponifiables (ASU) in osteoarthritis (OA) patients: a meta-analysis of randomized controlled trials. Osteoarthritis Cartilage 2008;16:399-408.

68. Lequesne M, Maheu E, Cadet C, Dreiser RL. Structural effect of avocado/soybean unsaponifiables on joint space loss in osteoarthritis of the hip. Arthritis Rheum 2002;47:50-8.

69. Soeken KL, Lee WL, Bausell RB, Agelli M, Berman BM. Safety and efficacy of S-adenosylmethionine (same) for osteoarthritis. J Fam Pract 2002;51:425-30.

70. Bellamy N, Campbell J, Robinson V, Gee T, Bourne R, Wells G. Intraarticular corticosteroid for treatment of osteoarthritis of the knee. Cochrane Database Syst Rev 2006;(2):CD005328.

71. Flanagan J, Casale FF, Thomas TL, Desai KB. Intra-articular injection for pain relief in patients awaiting hip replacement. Ann R Coll Surg Engl 1988;70:156-7.

72. Avouac J, Bardin T, Richette P. Effects of joint lavage in patients with osteoarthritis of the knee: meta-analysis of randomized controlled trials. Arthritis Rheum 2008;58:S485.

73. Fiorentini R. Proceedings of the United States Food and Drug Administration Advisory Panel on Orthopaedic and Rehabilitation Devices. Fairfax (VA): CASET Associates; 1996.

74. Berkowitz D. Proceedings of the United States Food and Drug Administration Advisory Panel on Orthopaedic and Rehabilitation Devices. Fairfax (VA): CASET Associates; 1996.

75. Bellamy N, Campbell J, Robinson V, Gee T, Bourne R, Wells G. Viscosupplementation for the treatment of osteoarthritis of the knee. Cochrane Database Syst Rev 2006;(2):CD005321.

76. Lundsgaard C, Dufour N, Fallentin E, Winkel P, Gluud C. Intra-articular sodium hyaluronate 2 ml versus physiological saline 20 ml versus physiological saline 2 ml for painful knee osteoarthritis: a randomized clinical trial. Scand J Rheumatol 2008;37:142-50.

77. Reichenbach S, Blank S, Rutjes AW, Shang A, King EA, Dieppe PA, et al. Hylan versus hyaluronic acid for osteoarthritis of the knee: a systematic review and meta-analysis. Arthritis Rheum 2007;57:1410-8.

78. Qvistgaard E, Christensen R, Torp-Pedersen S, Bliddal H. Intra-articular treatment of hip osteoarthritis: a randomized trial of hyaluronic acid, corticosteroid, and isotonic saline. Osteoarthritis Cartilage 2006;14:163-70.

79. Tikiz C, Unlü Z, Sener A, Efe M, Tüzün C. Comparison of the efficacy of lower and higher molecular weight viscosupplementation in the treatment of hip osteoarthritis. Clin Rheumatol 2005;24:244-50.

80. Heyworth BE, Lee JH, Kim PD, Lipton CB, Strauch RJ, Rosenwasser MP. Hylan versus corticosteroid versus placebo for treatment of basal joint arthritis: a prospective, randomized, double-blinded clinical trial. J Hand Surg [Am] 2008;33:40-8.

81. Fuchs S, Mönikes R, Wohlmeiner A, Heyse T. Intra-articular hyaluronic acid compared with corticoid injections for the treatment of rhizarthrosis. Osteoarthritis Cartilage 2006;14:82-8.

82. Stahl S, Karsh-Zafrir I, Ratzon N, Rosenberg N. Comparison of intraarticular injection of depot corticosteroid and hyaluronic acid for treatment of degenerative trapeziometacarpal joints. J Clin Rheumatol 2005;11:299-302.

83. Cohen MM, Altman RD, Hollstrom R, Hollstrom C, Sun C, Gipson B. Safety and efficacy of intra-articular sodium hyaluronate (Hyalgan) in a randomized, double-blind study for osteoarthritis of the ankle. Foot Ankle Int 2008;29:657-63.

84. Salk RS, Chang TJ, D'Costa WF, Soomekh DJ, Grogan KA. Sodium hyaluronate in the treatment of osteoarthritis of the ankle: a controlled, randomized, double-blind pilot study. J Bone Joint Surg Am 2006;88:295-302.

85. Pasquali Ronchetti I, Guerra D, Taparelli F, Boraldi F, Bergamini G, Mori G, et al. Morphological analysis of knee synovial membrane biopsies from a randomized controlled clinical study comparing the effects of sodium hyaluronate (Hyalgan) and methylprednisolone acetate (Depomedrol) in osteoarthritis. Rheumatology (Oxford) 2001;40:158-69.

86. Guidolin DD, Ronchetti IP, Lini E, Guerra D, Frizziero L. Morphological analysis of articular cartilage biopsies from a randomized, clinical study comparing the effects of 500-730 kda sodium hyaluronate (Hyalgan) and methylprednisolone acetate on primary osteoarthritis of the knee. Osteoarthritis Cartilage 2001;9:371-81.

87. Bingham 3rd CO, Buckland-Wright JC, Garnero P, Cohen SB, Dougados M, Adami S, et al. Risedronate decreases biochemical markers of cartilage degradation but does not decrease symptoms or slow radiographic progression in patients with medial compartment osteoarthritis of the knee: results of the two-year multinational knee osteoarthritis structural arthritis study. Arthritis Rheum 2006;54:3494-507.

88. Neogi T, Nevitt MC, Ensrud KE, Bauer D, Felson DT. The effect of alendronate on progression of spinal osteophytes and disc-space narrowing. Ann Rheum Dis 2008;67:1427-30.

89. Fujita T, Fujii Y, Okada SF, Miyauchi A, Takagi Y. Analgesic effect of etidronate on degenerative joint disease. J Bone Miner Metab 2001;19:251-6.

90. Bruyere O, Delferriere D, Roux C, Wark JD, Spector T, Devogelaer JP, et al. Effects of strontium ranelate on spinal osteoarthritis progression. Ann Rheum Dis 2008;67:335-9.

91. Manicourt DH, Azria M, Mindeholm L, Thonar EJ, Devogelaer JP. Oral salmon calcitonin reduces Lequesne's algofunctional index scores and decreases urinary and serum levels of biomarkers of joint metabolism in knee osteoarthritis. Arthritis Rheum 2006;54:3205-11.

92. Chaganti RK, Parimi N, Dam T, Cawthon P, Nevitt M, Lane N. The association of serum vitamin D with prevalent radiographic hip osteoarthritis in older men. Arthritis Rheum 2008;58(Suppl.):S676.

93. Kinjo M. Serum 25OH vitamin D level and symptomatic knee osteoarthritis: Analysis in a population-based U.S. sample Kinjo M. Arthritis Rheum 2008;58(Suppl.):S239.

94. Chevalier X, Giraudeau B, Conrozier T, Marliere J, Kiefer P, Goupille P. Safety study of intraarticular injection of interleukin 1 receptor antagonist in patients with painful knee osteoarthritis: a multicenter study. J Rheumatol 2005;32:1317-23.

95. Magnano MD, Chakravarty EF, Broudy C, Chung L, Kelman A, Hillygus J, et al. A pilot study of tumor necrosis factor inhibition in erosive/inflammatory osteoarthritis of the hands. J Rheumatol 2007;34:1323-7.

96. Lane NE, Schnitzer TJ, Smith MD, Brown MT. Tanezumab relieves moderate to severe pain due to osteoarthritis of the knee: A Phase 2 Trial. Arthritis Rheum 2008;58(Suppl.):S896.

97. Moore EE, Bendele AM, Thompson DL, Littau A, Waggie KS, Reardon B, et al. Fibroblast growth factor-18 stimulates chondrogenesis and cartilage repair in a rat model of injury-induced osteoarthritis. Osteoarthritis Cartilage 2005;13:623-31.

98. Mizoguchi H, Hase S, Tanaka A, Takeuchi K. Lack of small intestinal ulcerogenecity of nitric oxide-releasing indomethacin, NCX-530, in rats. Aliment Pharmacol Ther 2001;15:257-67.

99. Schnitzer TJ, Kivitz A, Rankin B, Fisher C, Marker H, Frayssinet H, et al. Comparison of naproxcinod to naproxen and placebo: results of a 13-week phase 3 pivotal trial in patients with osteoarthritis of the knee with particular focus on blood pressure effects. Ann Rheum Dis 2008;67(Suppl. II):394.

100. Berenbaum F. New horizons and perspectives in the treatment of osteoarthritis. Arthritis Res Ther 2008;10(Suppl. 2):S1.

101. Kulkarni SK, Singh VP. Licofelone: the answer to unmet needs in osteoarthritis therapy? Curr Rheumatol Rep 2008;10:43-8.

102. Brandt KD, Mazzuca SA, Katz BP, Lane KA, Buckwalter KA, Yocum DE, et al. Effects of doxycycline on progression of osteoarthritis: results of a randomized, placebo-controlled, double-blind trial. Arthritis Rheum 2005;52:2015-25.

103. Krzeski P, Buckland-Wright C, Bálint G, Cline GA, Stoner K, Lyon R, et al. Development of musculoskeletal toxicity without clear benefit after administration of PG 116800, a matrix metalloproteinase inhibitor, to patients with knee osteoarthritis: a randomized, 12 month, double-blind, placebo-controlled study. Arthritis Res Ther 2007;9:R109.

104. Remadevi R, Szallisi A. Adlea (ALGRX-4975), an injectable capsaicin (TRPV1 receptor agonist) formulation for long-lasting pain relief. IDrugs 2008;11:120-32.

Chapter 24

Osteoporosis

Marc C. Hochberg

Osteoporosis has been defined as a systemic skeletal disorder characterized by compromised bone strength predisposing to an increased risk of fracture.[1] Bone strength is determined by many factors, including bone mass. Bone mass is estimated in clinical practice by the measurement of area bone mineral density (BMD), the quantity of mineral (grams of calcium) divided by the area of the bone, using the technique of dual x-ray absorptiometry (DXA). There is a strong nonlinear relationship between BMD and the risk of fracture, such that for every decrease in one standard deviation below the age-adjusted mean for total hip BMD, the risk of hip fracture increases by a factor of greater than two.[2] The World Health Organization (WHO) defined osteoporosis in white women as a BMD measured at the femoral neck of 2.5 or more standard deviations below the mean of young white women aged 20 to 39 years.[3] This definition has been generalized to nonwhite women and men, with the recommendation that normative data for young persons should be sex specific.[4]

The most important osteoporotic fractures, from the standpoint of both incidence and consequences, are vertebral and hip fractures.[5,6] Systematic reviews and meta-analyses of placebo-controlled randomized clinical trials (RCTs) have demonstrated that treatment of postmenopausal women with either prevalent vertebral fractures or low BMD (femoral neck or total hip BMD T-score of –2.0 or below) can reduce the risk of vertebral and nonvertebral, including hip fractures.[7-9] Similarly, treatment of men with low BMD and adults receiving chronic oral glucocorticoid therapy has been shown to increase BMD and reduce the risk of vertebral fractures.[8,9]

This chapter reviews recommendations for identifying persons who should undergo measurement of BMD, persons with low BMD who should receive treatment to reduce their risk of fracture, and the therapies available in the United States for those individuals. Drugs not approved for treatment of osteoporosis in the United States, such as strontium ranelate,[10] human parathyroid hormone 1-84,[11] and tibolone[12] are not discussed. Furthermore, surgical management of fractures, including the use of kyphoplasty and vertebroplasty for management of back pain due to vertebral fractures, are not covered; the reader is referred to a recent chapter on this topic.[13]

WHO SHOULD HAVE BMD MEASURED?

The most widely recognized guidelines in the United States are those of the National Osteoporosis Foundation (NOF) that were updated in 2008 (Table 24-1).[14] The NOF currently recommends that all postmenopausal women and men age 50 and older should be evaluated for osteoporosis risk in order to determine the need for BMD testing. The NOF recommends that BMD be measured using DXA in (1) all postmenopausal women aged 65 and older and men age 70 and older, regardless of risk factors; (2) younger postmenopausal women and men age 50 to 69 about whom there is concern based on their risk factor profile; (3) women in the menopausal transition if there is a specific risk factor associated with increased fracture risk such as low body weight, prior low-trauma fracture or use of high-risk medications; (4) adults who have a fracture after age 50; (5) adults with a condition (Table 24-2) or taking a medication

---

Table 24-1. *Indications for Measurement of Bone Mineral Density*

Women age 65 and older, and men age 70 and older, regardless of clinical risk factors

Younger postmenopausal women and men age 50 to 69 years with risk factors for fracture

Women in the menopausal transition with risk factors for fracture, such as low body weight, prior low-trauma fracture, or use of high-risk medication

Adults who have a low-trauma fracture after age 50

Adults with a condition (e.g., rheumatoid arthritis) or taking a medication (e.g., glucocorticoids in a daily dose ≥ 5 mg prednisone or equivalent for three months or longer) associated with low bone mass or bone loss

Anyone being considered for pharmacologic therapy for osteoporosis

Anyone being treated for osteoporosis, to monitor treatment effect

Anyone not receiving therapy in whom evidence of bone loss would lead to treatment

From Clinician's Guide to Prevention and Treatment of Osteoporosis, National Osteoporosis Foundation, Washington, D.C., 2008; and 2007 ISCD Official Positions (accessed at www.iscd.org on October 13, 2008).

Table 24-2. *Conditions Associated with Low Bone Mineral Density or Bone Loss*

Genetic Disorders
Cystic fibrosis
Homocystinuria
Osteogenesis imperfecta
Ehlers-Danlos syndrome
Hypophosphatasia
Glycogen storage disease
Gaucher's disease
Porphyria
Idiopathic hypercalciuria
Hemochromatosis
Marfan's syndrome
Riley-Day syndrome
Menkes' steely hair syndrome

Hypogonadal States
Anorexia nervosa
Hyperprolactinemia
Turner's syndrome
Panhypopituitarism
Athletic amenorrhea
Klinefelter's syndrome
Ovarian failure
Androgen insensitivity

Endocrine Disorders
Acromegaly
Cushing's syndrome
Adrenal insufficiency
Thyrotoxicosis
Hyperparathyroidism
Diabetes mellitus, type I

Gastrointestinal Diseases
Gastrectomy
Malabsorption

Primary biliary cirrhosis
Celiac disease
Inflammatory bowel disease

Hematologic Disorders
Hemophilia
Multiple myeloma
Systemic mastocytosis
Thalassemia
Sickle cell disease
Leukemias and lymphomas

Rheumatic Diseases
Ankylosing spondylitis
Lupus
Rheumatoid arthritis

Miscellaneous
Alcoholism
Emphysema
Multiple sclerosis
Amyloidosis
Epilepsy
End-stage renal disease
Depression
Scoliosis
Post-transplant bone disease
Immobilization
Sarcoidosis
Muscular dystrophy
Metabolic acidosis
Heart failure

Modified from Department of Health and Human Services. Bone health and osteoporosis: a report of the Surgeon General. Rockville, MD: Department of Health and Human Services; 2004.

Table 24-3. *Medications Associated with Secondary Osteoporosis or Accelerated Rate of Decline in Bone Mass*

Anticoagulants
Anticonvulsants
Antidepressants
Aromatase inhibitors
Cancer chemotherapeutic drugs
Cyclosporine A and tacrolimus
Depo-medroxyprogesterone
Glucocorticoids
Gonadotropin-releasing hormone agonists
Lithium
Proton-pump inhibitors
Thyroxine

Updated from Department of Health and Human Services. Bone health and osteoporosis: a report of the Surgeon General. Rockville, MD: Department of Health and Human Services; 2004.

(Table 24-3) associated with low bone mass or bone loss; (6) anyone being considered for pharmacologic therapy for osteoporosis; (7) anyone being treated for osteoporosis, to monitor treatment effect; and (8) anyone not receiving therapy in whom evidence of bone loss would lead to treatment.

The evidence that links universal testing of women aged 65 and older with a reduced rate of fractures is derived from two studies.[15,16] LaCroix and colleagues randomized more than 9000 women aged 60 to 80 years who were not taking hormone therapy or other osteoporosis medications to one of three groups: universal testing (n = 1986), testing based on results of the SCORE questionnaire[17] (n = 1940), and testing based on results of a 17-item questionnaire adapted from known risk factors for hip fracture (n = 5342).[15] During a mean follow-up of 33 months, the rate of osteoporotic fractures was 74.11, 99.44, and 91.77 per 1000 woman-years, respectively ($P < 0.05$ comparing the universal screening group with the other two groups). The rate of hip fractures was also lower in the universal screening group, but differences were not statistically significant (8.54, 9.04, and 13.31 per 1000 woman-years, respectively). These results were supported by an analysis of data from the Cardiovascular Health Study.[16] In this observational cohort study, 1378 participants enrolled in the Sacramento County (California) and Allegheny County (Pennsylvania) sites completed measurement of BMD at the hip, whereas 1685 participants enrolled in the Washington County (Maryland) and Forsyth County (North Carolina) sites received usual care; the mean age of participants was 76 years, the majority were women and more than 80% were white. The incidence of hip fractures over a mean follow-up of 4.9 years was 4.8 and 8.2 per 1000 person-years in the screened group and usual care group, respectively: adjusted relative risk (RR) = 0.64 (95% confidence interval [CI], 0.41–0.99). There was no evidence of a statistical interaction between screening and sex, age group or race; however, there were only four hip fractures in the 532 black participants. Hence, these two studies support the recommendations for universal BMD testing in older women.

WHO SHOULD BE TREATED TO REDUCE FRACTURE RISK?

Solomon and colleagues performed a systematic review of the English-language literature using MEDLINE and HealthStar for the period between January 1992 and December 2003 to identify osteoporosis treatment guidelines.[18] They identified 18 unique guidelines; 17 provided recommendations for postmenopausal women, and 13 provided recommendations for men. There was considerable heterogeneity in the recommendations, however.

Delmas and colleagues, in outlining the position of the International Osteoporosis Foundation (IOF), concluded that treatment of postmenopausal women with established osteoporosis is always cost effective and that additional scenarios exist when treatment is cost effective.[19] These additional scenarios depend upon crossing an "intervention threshold," where the future morbidity from osteoporotic fractures, largely derived from the risk and costs of hip fracture, exceeds the costs of interventions that have been shown to reduce the risk of these fractures. Additional risk factors that contribute to the estimate of this risk, independent of BMD, were identified through a series of meta-analyses conducted by Professor John Kanis and colleagues under the auspices of the WHO; these risk factors include age, sex, prior history of fragility fracture, parental history of hip fracture, current smoking, use of systemic glucocorticoids, alcohol intake in excess of 3 units per day, and presence of rheumatoid arthritis (Table 24-4).[20-27] An algorithm named the WHO Fracture Risk Assessment Tool (FRAX) was developed to allow calculation of the person-specific 10-year risk for both a major osteoporotic fracture (hip, shoulder, wrist and clinical vertebral combined) and a hip fracture alone[28]; FRAX can be accessed at www.shef.ac.uk/FRAX/index.htm (Fig. 24-1). If BMD has not been measured, the person's weight and height can be substituted in the calculation. Some caveats need to be recognized by providers who are going to use FRAX in their practices: (1) it is not intended for use in persons younger than 50 years of age; (2) it applies only to previously untreated patients; (3) lumbar spine BMD cannot be substituted for either femoral neck or total hip BMD (hence, it cannot be used in persons with bilateral total hip arthroplasties); and (4) before entry into the computer algorithm, the patient's BMD T-score must be converted to an

Table 24-4. *Clinical Risk Factors Included in WHO Fracture Risk Assessment Model (FRAX)*

Current age
Sex
Weight
Height
History of previous spontaneous or low-trauma fracture, including radiographic vertebral fracture without symptoms
Parental history of hip fracture
Current smoking
Use of glucocorticoids for more than 3 months at a dose of prednisolone of 5 mg daily or more (or equivalent doses of other glucocorticoids)
Alcohol intake of 3 or more units per day
Rheumatoid arthritis
Other causes of secondary osteoporosis

WHO, World Health Organization.
From FRAX: WHO Fracture Risk Assessment Tool (accessed at www.shef.ac.uk/FRAX/index.htm on October 13, 2008).

appropriate T-score using the "FRAX Patch," which is available on the NOF's website ("www.nof.org/frax_patch.htm").

The NOF suggests, based on cost-effectiveness modeling, that postmenopausal women and men age 50 and older should be considered for treatment if (1) they have either a hip or vertebral fracture; (2) they have osteoporosis based on a BMD T-score of –2.5 or below at the femoral neck or lumbar spine; or (3) they have low BMD (T-score between –1.0 and –2.5 at the femoral neck or lumbar spine) with a 10-year risk of a hip or a major osteoporotic fracture of 3% or 20% or greater, respectively (Table 24-5).[29,30] Note that glucocorticoid use is included among the factors considered in estimating the 10-year fracture risk; hence, the FRAX model is applicable to patients being considered for treatment of glucocorticoid-induced osteoporosis. An algorithm developed by the author summarizing the approach to BMD testing and the use of BMD in making decisions about whom to treat based on the NOF recommendations is shown in Figure 24-2.

TREATMENT TO REDUCE FRACTURE RISK

The management of the individual patient with osteoporosis requires a combination of nonpharmacologic and pharmacologic modalities.[31] Before instituting pharmacologic therapies, however, all patients should be evaluated for secondary causes of osteoporosis and, if identified, these conditions should be treated appropriately. A set of routine laboratory tests that are useful to identify common causes of secondary osteoporosis includes a complete blood count and differential, erythrocyte sedimentation rate, routine chemistry profile, 25-hydroxyvitamin vitamin D level (see later), thyroid-stimulating hormone, if the patient is receiving thyroid hormone supplementation and

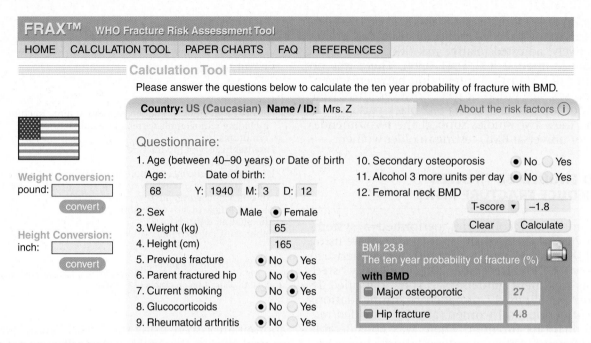

Figure 24-1. WHO Fracture Risk Assessment Tool (FRAX) completed for a postmenopausal woman age 68 years. The patient has a weight of 65 kg and height of 165 cm, a history of hip fracture in a parent, and is a current smoker. She has not had a prior fracture, taken oral glucocorticoids, been diagnosed with rheumatoid arthritis, or consumed three or more units of alcohol per day. Her femoral neck BMD T-score is –1.8. Her 10-year risk of a major osteoporotic fracture is 27% and a hip fracture is 4.8%. Based on the National Osteoporosis Foundation recommendations, she should be treated to reduce her fracture risk.

Table 24-5. *Indications for Treatment of Osteoporosis*

A vertebral or hip fracture
Bone mineral density T-score of –2.5 or below at the
   femoral neck or lumbar spine
Low bone mass and a 10-year probability of major
   osteoporotic fracture of 20% or higher
Low bone mass and a 10-year probability of hip fracture
   of 3% or higher

From Clinician's Guide to Prevention and Treatment of Osteoporosis. Washington, DC: National Osteoporosis Foundation; 2008.

---

a 24-hour urine for measurement of calcium excretion; other tests can be ordered if any of the above are abnormal (Table 24-6).[32] In addition, serum testosterone levels should be measured in all men.

Nonpharmacologic Modalities

Key components of the nonpharmacologic treatment program are patient education, adequate nutrition, particularly protein, calcium and vitamin D intake, muscle strengthening and balance exercises to prevent falls, smoking cessation, and avoidance or limitation of alcohol intake.

Patient Education

Several studies have demonstrated an association between adherence and persistence with oral bisphosphonates and fracture risk reduction[33]; hence, use of educational materials coupled with appropriate follow-up and reinforcement directed toward increasing both adherence and persistence with osteoporosis medications should be part of the management strategy for every patient.

Calcium Intake

All patients should achieve a daily intake of dietary calcium of at least 1200 mg, including supplements.[34] Dietary calcium intake can be estimated by multiplying the number of 8-ounce servings of milk and 6-ounce servings of yogurt by 300 mg and the number of 1-ounce servings of cheese by 200 mg and adding this number to 250 mg for the nondairy sources of calcium. Calcium supplements should be taken if this total does not equal or exceed 1200 mg. Calcium supplements most commonly come either as calcium carbonate or calcium citrate. Calcium carbonate should be taken with meals because of better absorption in an acid milieu; calcium citrate can be taken either with or between meals. If the amount of supplements required is greater than 500 mg per day, then the dosage should be divided. Although calcium supplementation has been shown to have a small positive effect on bone mineral density, it has not been shown to have a significant effect on fracture risk reduction.[35]

Fall Prevention

Both the type of fall and the biomechanics of the fall are related to fracture risk in older women.[36] Numerous risk factors for falls have been identified

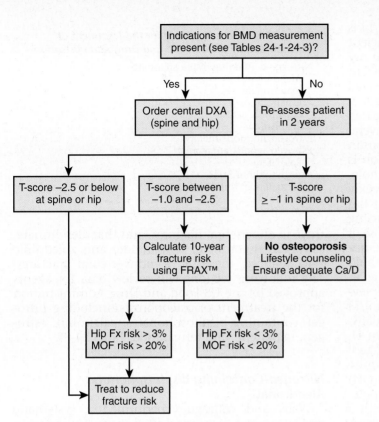

Figure 24-2. Algorithm summarizing use of bone mineral density in determining need for treatment to reduce fracture risk based on National Osteoporosis Foundation recommendations.

Table 24-6. *Laboratory Tests for Identifying Secondary Causes of Osteoporosis*

Routine
Complete blood count
Erythrocyte sedimentation rate
Comprehensive metabolic profile
25-hydroxyvitamin D level
Thyroid stimulating hormone, if patient on thyroid replacement
Serum testosterone level (in men only)
24-hour urine collection for calcium excretion

Optional
Serum parathyroid hormone (PTH)
Serum and urine protein electrophoresis
Biochemical markers of bone turnover

Vitamin D

Sufficiency of vitamin D should be determined in all patients who are being considered for treatment for osteoporosis. Vitamin D status is best assessed by measurement of serum levels of 25-hydroxyvitamin D (25[OH]D) using either the DiaSorin radioimmunoassay (Stillwater, MN) or the gold standard technique of liquid chromatography–mass spectroscopy.

Table 24-7. *Risk Factors for Falls*

Medical Risk Factors
　Older age
　Anxiety and/or depression
　Arrhythmias
　Impaired transfer and mobility
　Kyphosis
　Muscle weakness
　Medications causing oversedation
　Orthostatic hypotension
　Decreased visual acuity
　Poor balance
　Poor contrast sensitivity
　Prior falls and/or fear of falling
　Reduced proprioception
　Diminished cognitive skills and/or mental acuity
　Hypovitaminosis D
Environmental Risk Factors
　Lack of assistive devices in bathrooms
　Loose throw rugs
　Inadequate indoor lighting
　Obstacles in walking path
　Slippery outdoor conditions

(Table 24-7).[37] Because of the multitude of risk factors for falls, a multifactorial approach to fall prevention has been advocated. This approach includes an assessment of the patient by an occupational or physical therapist with instructions in lifestyle modifications and muscle strengthening and balance exercise programs, as well as an assessment of medical conditions and medication use by a nurse or physician with modification of the treatment regimen to eliminate drugs associated with falling. Although this approach has been tested in RCTs and shown to reduce the incidence of falls in elderly individuals,[38] it has not been shown to reduce the incidence of fractures.

A serum 25(OH)D level of 30 ng/mL (75 nmol/L) is considered the minimum of the normal or sufficient range.[39] Patients with 25(OH)D levels below 20 ng/mL (50 nmol/L) are considered vitamin D deficient and should have their vitamin D stores corrected before beginning pharmacologic therapy for osteoporosis, particularly if they are going to be treated with a nitrogen-containing bisphosphonate. Several preparations and protocols are available for vitamin D repletion in these patients; the most common is using either vitamin D_2 (ergocalciferol) or D_3 (cholecalciferol) in doses of 50,000 units orally once weekly for 6 to 8 weeks.[39] An alternative regimen that has been shown to be efficacious and safe in older nursing home residents is the use of ergocalciferol at a dose of 50,000 units three times a week for 4 weeks.[40] Once her vitamin D stores are repleted, the patient should receive 800 to 1000 units of vitamin D_3 (cholecalciferol) orally once daily. Patients whose 25(OH)D levels are between 20 and 30 ng/mL (50 and 75 nmol/L) should receive 2000 units of vitamin D3 orally daily, with the dose reduced to 1000 units of vitamin D_3 once their 25(OH)D level reaches the normal range.[41] Patients with malabsorption syndromes may require higher daily doses to maintain their serum 25(OH)D levels within the normal range. Vitamin D supplementation has been shown to be associated with a reduced incidence of falls and fractures.[42,43] Indeed, there is evidence that the benefits of vitamin D supplementation are greatest when combined with calcium supplementation.[44]

Pharmacologic Modalities

The approach to the choice of a pharmacologic regimen for the individual patient with osteoporosis or increased fracture risk, and to a lesser extent glucocorticoid-induced osteoporosis, is complex because one must consider not only the patient's characteristics but also the benefits and risks of each of the individual drugs. This choice should be based, to the greatest extent possible, on the principles of evidence-based medicine wherein the evidence for efficacy and safety of each drug is derived from systematic reviews of RCTs with meta-analyses providing summary estimates for efficacy as measured by fracture risk reduction for vertebral and nonvertebral, including hip fractures, and tolerability as measured by rates of discontinuation for adverse events.[45] MacLean and colleagues performed a systematic review in 2007 to describe the benefits in terms of fracture risk reduction and the harms from adverse events among and within the various classes of pharmacologic therapies for osteoporosis.[8,9] They included a total of 76 RCTs and 24 meta-analyses in their efficacy analysis and 493 articles in their analyses of adverse events. They reported that, in high-risk groups, there was good evidence that alendronate, calcitonin, estrogen, ibandronate, risedronate, raloxifene, teriparatide and zoledronic acid reduced

Table 24-8. *Drugs Approved for the Treatment of Osteoporosis by the US Food and Drug Administration*

Nitrogen-containing bisphosphonates
  Alendronate
  Ibandronate
  Risedronate
  Zoledronic acid
Calcitonin
Estrogen/hormone therapy
Estrogen agonist/antagonist
  Raloxifene
Parathyroid hormone
  Teriparatide (rhPTH 1–34)

the risk of vertebral fractures, and that alendronate, estrogen, risedronate, teriparatide, and zoledronic acid reduced the risk of nonvertebral fractures. The following sections will review data for agents approved by the US Food and Drug Administration for the treatment of osteoporosis, including nitrogen-containing bisphosphonates, calcitonin, estrogen, raloxifene, and teriparatide (Table 24-8).

Nitrogen-Containing Bisphosphonates
Alendronate

Wells and colleagues performed a systematic review to assess the clinical efficacy of alendronate in the primary and secondary prevention of osteoporotic fractures in postmenopausal women compared with untreated women over a follow-up period of at least 1 year.[46] They identified a total of 11 RCTs that enrolled 12,068 women and fulfilled their prespecified criteria, three were primary prevention trials and eight were secondary prevention or treatment trials (i.e., they enrolled women with either a BMD T-score of −2.0 or below or a prevalent vertebral fracture).

Data on the incidence of vertebral fractures were reported in 8 of the 11 trials; however, only four trials could be pooled for analysis of the effects of the 10 mg daily dose (i.e., the dose that was approved for treatment of women with postmenopausal osteoporosis). There was a significant 45% reduction in risk of vertebral fractures: relative risk (RR) = 0.55 (95% CI, 0.45–0.67); there was no evidence of heterogeneity in the effect across the primary or secondary prevention trials. Data on the incidence of nonvertebral fractures were reported in nine of the 11 trials; however, only five trials could be pooled for analysis of the effects of the 10 mg daily dose. There was a significant 16% reduction in risk of nonvertebral fractures: RR = 0.84 (95% CI, 0.74–0.94). The reduction in risk in the four secondary prevention (treatment) trials was 23% (95% CI, 8%–36%), whereas that in the one primary prevention trial was not significant. Data on hip fractures were reported in six trials that could be pooled for analysis of the effects of the 10-mg daily dose; in these studies, there was a significant 39% reduction in risk: RR = 0.61 (95% CI, 0.40–0.92). The reduction in risk in the five secondary prevention trials was 53% (95% CI, 15%–74%), whereas that in the one primary prevention trial was not significant.

Based on the hypothesis that intermittent administration of the cumulative total dose given at weekly intervals would have the same efficacy as daily dosing, Schnitzer and colleagues showed that increases in bone mineral density and declines in bone turnover markers over 2 years were equivalent between alendronate given at a dose of 70 mg once weekly and 10 mg daily.[47,48] Although the incidence of clinical fractures, reported as adverse events, was similar between the treatment groups in this study, there have been no placebo-controlled studies specifically addressing the antifracture efficacy of the once-weekly dosing regimen. Hence, it is assumed that the antifracture efficacy of the daily dose can also be attributed to the once-weekly dosing regimen.

Risedronate

Wells and colleagues performed a systematic review to assess the clinical efficacy of risedronate in the primary and secondary prevention of osteoporotic fractures in postmenopausal women compared with untreated women over a follow-up period of at least 1 year.[49] They identified a total of seven RCTs that enrolled 14,049 women and fulfilled their prespecified criteria; two were primary prevention trials, and five were secondary prevention or treatment trials.

Data on the incidence of vertebral fractures were reported in four secondary prevention trials; however, only three of these trials could be pooled for analysis of the effects of the 5-mg daily dose. There was a significant 39% reduction in risk of vertebral fractures (RR = 0.61 [95% CI, 0.50–0.76]). Data on the incidence of nonvertebral fractures were reported in all five secondary prevention trials; however, only four secondary prevention trials could be pooled for analysis of the effects of the 5-mg daily dose. There was a significant 20% reduction in risk of nonvertebral fractures (RR = 0.80 [95% CI, 0.72–0.90]). Data on hip fractures were reported in three secondary prevention trials that could be pooled for analysis of the effects of the 5-mg daily dose; there was a significant 26% reduction in risk (RR = 0.74 [95% CI, 0.59–0.94]).

Based on the hypothesis that intermittent administration of the cumulative total dose given at weekly intervals would have the same efficacy as daily dosing, Brown and colleagues showed that increases in bone mineral density and declines in bone turnover markers over 1 year were equivalent between risedronate given at a dose of 35 mg once weekly and 5 mg daily.[50,51] The incidence of radiographic vertebral fractures was similar between the treatment groups at both 1 and 2 years. While the incidence of clinical nonvertebral fractures, reported as adverse events, also was similar between the treatment groups in this study, there have been no placebo-controlled studies specifically addressing the antifracture efficacy of the once-weekly dosing regimen. Hence, it is assumed that the antifracture efficacy of the daily dose can also be attributed to the once-weekly dosing regimen.

Recently, data have been published on the equivalence of a once-monthly regimen of either 150 mg or 75 mg given on 2 consecutive days to the 5-mg daily regimen[52,53]; similar assumptions can be applied for the antifracture efficacy for nonvertebral fractures of the once-monthly regimen as the once-weekly regimen.

Ibandronate

A single placebo-controlled RCT demonstrated that ibandronate at a dose of 2.5 mg orally once daily significantly reduced the risk of new vertebral fractures by 52% (RR = 0.48 [95% CI, 0.32–0.72]); however, there was no evidence that ibandronate reduced the risk of nonvertebral fractures, the cumulative incidence of clinical nonvertebral fractures was 8.2% and 9.1% in the placebo and pooled ibandronate groups, respectively.[54] There was evidence, however, of a significant interaction between baseline femoral neck BMD and effect of ibandronate on risk of nonvertebral fracture; for women with a baseline femoral neck BMD T score of –3.0 or below, there was a signficant risk reduction for nonvertebral fractures with daily oral ibandronate 2.5 mg of 69%.

Harris and colleagues performed an individual patient data meta-analysis using data from four phase III RCTs of ibandronate of at least 2 years' duration in women with postmenopausal osteoporosis.[55] Two of these studies were placebo controlled and 3 years in duration[54,56] whereas the other two compared alternate dosage regimens with the 2.5-mg daily dose and were 2 years in duration.[57-60] Patients were categorized into three stratified groups for analysis based on estimated annual cumulative drug exposure: low, mid, and high.[61] The 2.5-mg daily dose was included within the mid-dose stratum, whereas the 150-mg once-monthly oral dose and both the 2-mg every-2-month IV and the 3-mg every-3-month IV doses were included in the high-dose stratum. A total of 8710 women were included in the overall analysis. The primary outcome was "key" nonvertebral fractures: clavicle, humerus, wrist, hip, pelvis, and leg; all nonvertebral fractures were examined as a secondary outcome. Data were analyzed using Cox proportional hazard models adjusting for baseline age, total hip BMD, and history of prevalent fractures. There was a significant reduction in risk of key nonvertebral and all nonvertebral fractures in the high-dose stratum compared with the placebo group: RR = 0.656 (95% CI, 0.45–0.96) and 0.701 (95% CI, 0.50–0.99), respectively in the all-year models. Cranney and colleagues performed an individual patient data meta-analysis using data from eight RCTs of ibandronate of at least 1 year in duration in women with postmenopausal osteoporosis and compared the cumulative incidence of "key" nonvertebral fractures in women by annual cumulative drug exposure.[62] Based on data from the two noninferiority studies,[57-60] the adjusted RR was 0.634 (95% CI, 0.427–0.943) for women receiving ibandronate in the high- versus low-exposure stratum. Based on data from three RCTs comparing women in the low exposure stratum with women randomized to placebo, there was no evidence of nonvertebral fracture risk reduction. These results do not provide the same strength of evidence as those for alendronate or risedronate because not all of the studies were placebo controlled, individual patient data were pooled across the studies, the high-dose ibandronate–treated patients were followed for a shorter period of time, allowing fewer fractures to accumulate, and only a limited number of variables were controlled for in the analysis. Nonetheless, it appears that ibandronate at a dose of 150 mg orally once monthly is associated with reduction in nonvertebral fracture risk.

Zoledronic Acid

A pivotal double-blind 3-year RCT that enrolled 7765 postmenopausal women with osteoporosis demonstrated that zoledronic acid given as an IV infusion of 5 mg once yearly was associated with a significant 70% reduction in the risk of new vertebral fractures, 25% reduction in risk of nonvertebral fractures, and a 41% reduction in risk of hip fractures: RR = 0.30 (95% CI, 0.24–0.38), 0.75 (95% CI, 0.64–0.87) and 0.59 (95% CI, 0.42–0.83), respectively.[63] A second double-blind, placebo-controlled RCT enrolled 2127 men and women aged 50 years and older who had undergone surgical repair of a hip fracture within the previous 90 days and were unable or unwilling to take an oral bisphosphonate.[64] The median follow-up time was 1.9 years, and the incidence of nonvertebral and hip fractures were two of the secondary endpoints. There was a significant 27% reduction in the cumulative incidence of nonvertebral fractures (RR = 0.73 [95% CI, 0.55–0.98]) and a 30% reduction in the risk of hip fractures (RR = 0.70 [95% CI, 0.41–1.19]). The incidence of radiographic vertebral fractures was not assessed in this latter trial.

MacLean and colleagues examined the safety of these agents.[8,9] The most common adverse event with orally administered bisphosphonates is upper gastrointestinal distress. Careful patient instruction to take the medications on an empty stomach with 6 to 8 ounces of still water and to remain upright without eating for at least 30 minutes (60 minutes for oral ibandronate) reduces the rate of these events to rates similar to placebo in randomized trials. The orally administered bisphosphonates are contraindicated in patients with disorders of esophageal motility, including esophageal strictures and achalasia, and are not recommended in patients with Barrett's esophagus. All bisphosphonates are not recommended in patients with chronic kidney disease and estimated glomerular filtration rates of 35 mL/min or less. Intravenous zoledronic acid was associated with a significantly increased risk for serious atrial fibrillation in one of the two trials noted earlier.[63] Although there was a trend toward an increased risk for atrial fibrillation with alendronate in the Fracture Intervention Trial,[65] a large case-control study failed to demonstrate an association of current use of bisphosphonates with atrial fibrillation or flutter.[66]

Two rare side effects have received increasing amounts of attention in the past few years; these are osteonecrosis of the jaw (ONJ) and the occurrence of atypical low-trauma fractures, including subtrochanteric fractures. A confirmed case of ONJ was defined by the American Society for Bone and Mineral Research as "…an area of exposed bone in the maxillofacial region that did not heal within 8 weeks after identification by a health care provider, in a patient who was receiving or had been exposed to a bisphosphonate and had not had radiation therapy to the craniofacial region."[67] The vast majority of cases have been reported in patients with malignancy who have received high doses of intravenous bisphosphonates; risk factors include recent dental procedures such as extraction, and pre-existing dental or periodontal disease.[68] ONJ is rare in patients with osteoporosis treated with oral bisphosphonates or once yearly infusions of zoledronic acid. The American Society for Bone and Mineral Research published a position paper on the topic in 2007[67]; recommendations for patients initiating oral bisphosphonates are summarized in Table 24-9. The occurrence of atypical fractures, particularly subtrochanteric stress fractures, has been reported in case series of patients receiving long-term alendronate therapy and has been attributed to excessive suppression of bone turnover.[69] Data from the Fracture Intervention Trial Long-term Extension (FLEX) Study, however, failed to demonstrate an increased incidence of such fractures in women who had received alendronate at a dose of 10 mg daily for up to 10 years (Bauer D: personal communication). A causal association between long-term alendronate use and these atypical fractures requires additional study; however, it is prudent to consider whether therapy beyond 5 years is necessary based on results of the FLEX study.[70] A recent case-control study noted an association between the use of oral bisphosphonates and increased odds of nonunion of humerus fractures in older individuals.[71] It is unclear if these results apply to other types of fractures.

Table 24-9. *Recommendations for Prevention of Osteonecrosis of the Jaw (ONJ) in the Patient with Osteoporosis Initiating Oral Bisphosphonate Therapy*

There should be free and complete communication between the health care professional and the patient

All patients starting oral bisphosphonates should be informed of the benefits and risks of bisphosphonate treatment, including the signs and symptoms of and risk factors for developing ONJ

Patients taking bisphosphonates should be encouraged to maintain good oral hygiene and to have regular dental visits

Patients who express concern about ONJ should be encouraged to seek additional information from a dentist or dental specialist

Modified from Khosla S, Burr D, Cauley J, Dempster DW, Ebeling PR, Felsenberg D, et al: Bisphosphonate associated osteonecrosis of the jaw: report of a Task Force of the American Society for Bone and Mineral Research. J Bone Miner Res 2007;22:1479–91.

In summary, the nitrogen-containing bisphosphonates alendronate, risedronate, and zoledronic acid, have been demonstrated convincingly to reduce the risk of vertebral and nonvertebral fractures, including hip fractures, in systematic reviews of RCTs or individual placebo-controlled RCTs. Ibandronate has also been shown to reduce the risk of vertebral fractures; however, data supporting the reduction in nonvertebral fractures for ibandronate are based on a lesser strength of evidence and there are no published data supporting reduction in risk of hip fracture with this agent. Hence, of the agents approved for oral administration, either alendronate at a dose of 70 mg once weekly or risedronate at a dose of either 35 mg once weekly or 150 mg once monthly are preferred over ibandronate for the patient at risk of both vertebral and nonvertebral fractures, including hip fractures; zoledronic acid given intravenously once yearly at a dose of 5 mg can be used in patients who have a contraindication to or are unable to tolerate the orally approved bisphosphonates.

Calcitonin

Cranney and colleagues performed a systematic review to assess the clinical efficacy of salmon calcitonin in the treatment of postmenopausal women with osteoporosis.[72] They identified a total of 30 RCTs that enrolled 3993 women and fulfilled their prespecified criteria; 13 were prevention trials and 16 were treatment trials.

Data on the incidence of vertebral fractures were reported in four treatment trials; there was a significant 54% reduction in risk of vertebral fractures (RR = 0.46 [95% CI, 0.25–0.87]). Data on the incidence of nonvertebral fractures were reported in three treatment trials; there was a nonsignificant 48% reduction in risk of nonvertebral fractures (RR = 0.52 [95% CI, 0.22–1.23]). Because of small sample sizes in three of the treatment trials, high dropout rates in all of the trials, and significant heterogeneity in effect across trials, the authors believed that the data from the PROOF trial were the most reliable. This 5-year RCT enrolled 1255 postmenopausal women with osteoporosis, of whom 78% had one or more prevalent vertebral fractures at baseline. Intranasal calcitonin at a dose of 200 IU daily was associated with a significant 34% reduction in the risk of new vertebral fractures but had no significant effect on the incidence of nonvertebral fractures.[73] Neither the 100 IU nor 400 IU daily dose had a significant effect on the incidence of either vertebral or nonvertebral fractures. Intranasal calcitonin is well tolerated, except for an increased risk for rhinitis. Calcitonin should be reserved for patients who cannot receive any other form of pharmacologic therapy because of either contraindications or lack of tolerability.

Estrogen

Wells and colleagues performed a systematic review to assess the clinical efficacy of hormone therapy in the treatment of postmenopausal women with osteoporosis.[74] They identified a total of 57 RCTs that fulfilled their prespecified criteria; 47 were prevention trials and 10 were treatment trials. Data on the incidence of vertebral fractures were reported in five trials; there was a nonsignificant 34% reduction in risk of vertebral fractures (RR = 0.66 [95% CI, 0.41–1.07]). Data on the incidence of nonvertebral fractures were reported in six trials; there was a nonsignificant 13% reduction in risk of nonvertebral fractures (RR = 0.87 [95% CI, 0.71–1.08]).

Torgerson and Bell-Syer performed two systematic reviews to assess the clinical efficacy of hormone therapy in the prevention of vertebral and nonvertebral fractures.[75,76] In the former meta-analysis, they combined data across 13 trials and found a pooled significant reduction in risk of new vertebral fractures of 33% (RR = 0.67 [95% CI, 0.45–0.98]). In the latter meta-analysis, they combined data across 22 trials and found a pooled significant reduction in risk of nonvertebral fractures of 27% (RR = 0.73 [95% CI, 0.56–0.94]).

More recent data on the antifracture efficacy of hormone therapy come from the Women's Health Initiative (WHI). In the WHI, randomized placebo-controlled trial wherein 8506 women received combined conjugated equine estrogen, 0.625 mg per day, plus medroxyprogesterone acetate, 2.5 mg per day, and 8102 women received placebo, there was a significant 24% reduction in the risk of any fracture (RR = 0.76 [95% CI, 0.69–0.83]) and a significant 33% reduction in the risk of hip fracture (RR = 0.67 [95% CI, 0.47–0.96]).[77] In the WHI randomized placebo-controlled trial of women with prior hysterectomy wherein 5310 received conjugated equine estrogen, 0.625 mg per day, and 5429 women received placebo, there was a significant 29% reduction in the risk of any fracture (RR = 0.71 [95% CI, 0.64–0.80]) and a significant 35% reduction in the risk of hip fracture (RR = 0.65 [95% CI, 0.45–0.94]).[78] Hence, there is consistent and robust evidence that hormone therapy with conjugated equine estrogen is efficacious for fracture risk reduction.

The limitation to the recommendation of using hormone therapy in all postmenopausal women with osteoporosis is the risk of this therapy. MacLean and colleagues, in their pooled analysis that included data from the WHI trials, noted a significant increased risk for stroke and thromboembolic events, including pulmonary embolism, for women using either estrogen alone or in combination with a progestin.[8,9] They noted a paradoxic relationship, however, of hormone therapy with the risk of breast cancer; the risk was significantly increased among women who received combined estrogen-progestin therapy but was significantly reduced among women who received estrogen alone compared with women who received placebo. In an analysis that combined both WHI trials, Rossouw and colleagues[79] failed to demonstrate a harmful effect of hormone therapy on either total mortality or the incidence of coronary heart disease. In a subgroup analysis, women aged

70 to 79 years did have a significantly increased risk for coronary heart disease events if they received combined estrogen-progestin therapy. Therefore, the use of hormone therapy can be recommended only for younger postmenopausal women who are at increased risk for fracture and have concomitant vasomotor symptoms.[80]

Raloxifene

Cranney and colleagues[81] performed a systematic review to assess the clinical efficacy of raloxifene in the treatment of postmenopausal women with osteoporosis. They identified a total of seven RCTs that fulfilled their prespecified criteria; three were prevention trials, and four were treatment trials. Data on the incidence of fractures were reported in only two treatment trials; because of disparate sample sizes and results of these trials, the authors believed it was inappropriate to pool results and that the data from the Multiple Outcomes of Raloxifene Evaluation (MORE) trial were the most reliable.

The MORE study randomized 7705 postmenopausal women with osteoporosis to either placebo or raloxifene 60 mg or 120 mg/day.[82] Women who received raloxifene 60 mg/day, the approved dose, had a 30% reduction in risk of new vertebral fractures (RR = 0.7 [95% CI, 0.5–0.8]). There was no difference in the incidence of nonvertebral fractures, however, between the placebo and combined raloxifene groups: 9.3% and 8.5%, respectively (RR = 0.9 [95% CI, 0.8–1.1]). The results were similar when the data through 48 months of follow-up were analyzed.[83] The lack of effect of the risk of nonvertebral fractures was demonstrated as well in the Raloxifene Use for the Heart (RUTH) trial; herein, the incidence of nonvertebral fractures over a median follow-up of 5.6 years was 16.7 and 17.3 per 1000 woman-years for the raloxifene and placebo groups, respectively (RR = 0.96 [95% CI, 0.84–1.10]).[84]

Raloxifene also has been demonstrated to reduce the risk of invasive estrogen receptor positive breast cancer.[85,86] MacLean and colleagues[8,9] noted a significant increased risk for thromboembolic events, including pulmonary embolism as well as mild cardiac events for women using raloxifene. Raloxifene is also associated with increased risk of hot flashes, peripheral edema, leg cramps and gallbladder disease, and in the RUTH trial, the drug was associated with an increase in mortality from stroke. Raloxifene appears to be most appropriate for postmenopausal women with osteoporosis who are at high risk for breast cancer and have not had a prior thromboembolic event and do not currently have vasomotor menopausal symptoms.

Teriparatide (rhPTH 1-34)

Two systematic reviews have summarized data on the efficacy of teriparatide[87,88]; however, these data are derived from only one RCT.[89] Neer and colleagues[89] randomized 1637 postmenopausal women with prevalent vertebral fractures to either placebo or teriparatide 20 µg or 40 µg administered subcutaneously per day. Women who received teriparatide 20 µg per day, the approved dose, had a 65% reduction in risk of new vertebral fractures (RR = 0.35 [95% CI, 0.22–0.55]) and a 53% reduction in the risk of new nonvertebral fractures (RR = 0.47 [95% CI, 0.25–0.88]). This planned 36-month pivotal phase III trial was terminated early after a median duration of 21 months due to the finding of osteosarcomas in rat carcinogenicity bioassay studies. The development of osteosarcoma in the rats was dose and duration dependent, and occurred after the development of osteosclerosis.[90] To this author's knowledge, there has been only one reported case of osteosarcoma in any patient treated with teriparatide to date.[91]

Teriparatide is generally well tolerated. In the pivotal RCT, patients who received teriparatide had an increased rate of dizziness and leg cramps, and both mild hypercalcemia and hyperuricemia were common but usually did not require discontinuation of treatment.

Teriparatide should not be prescribed in populations at high risk for osteosarcoma, including patients with Paget's disease of bone, patients with prior radiation therapy to the skeleton, and pediatric populations (and young adults) with open epiphyses. Elevations of serum alkaline phosphatase should be evaluated before using teriparatide because of the possibility of Paget's disease and bone tumors. Patients who have bone metastases or a history of skeletal malignancies should not receive teriparatide. Patients with hypercalcemia should be evaluated, and those with hyperparathyroidism should not receive teriparatide. The approved duration of therapy with teriparatide is 24 months; after 24 months, the patient should receive a bisphosphonate to maintain and consolidate the gains in BMD.

Teriparatide is indicated for postmenopausal women and men who are at high risk for fracture who have failed or are intolerant of previous osteoporosis therapy. At present, it is not recommended that teriparatide be administered concomitantly with an antiresorptive agent, because there are conflicting data regarding efficacy as measured by increases in BMD and no data supporting additive effects on fracture risk reduction. There is ongoing debate as to whether teriparatide should be used as the initial pharmacologic agent in patients with osteoporosis at high risk for fracture or whether it should be reserved for those who have either not tolerated or failed to respond to prior bisphosphonate therapy. Data from a secondary analysis of 245 postmenopausal women who received teriparatide 20 µg daily for 2 years in the European Study of Forsteo (EUROFORS) open-label trial, showed that BMD increased to a similar degree irrespective of the previous antiresorptive treatment.[92] Data from the Open-label Study to Determine How Prior Therapy with Alendronate or Risedronate in Postmenopausal Women with Osteoporosis Influences the Clinical Effectiveness of Teriparatide (OPTAMISE) study showed that among postmenopausal women who had been treated with risedronate or alendronate for at least 2 years and then discontinued their bisphosphonate and received open-label teriparatide for 12 months, those who had previously received risedronate had greater increases in BMD than those who had previously received alendronate.[93] Neither of these studies, however, provided data on fracture rates with teriparatide in these clinical situations.

SUMMARY

At this time, nitrogen-containing bisphosphonates remain the first-line pharmacologic therapy for postmenopausal women and men with osteoporosis, including those with glucocorticoid-induced osteoporosis, because of efficacy, overall safety, and cost. Teriparatide is generally recommended as monotherapy for postmenopausal women and men, including those with glucocorticoid-induced osteoporosis, who have had a suboptimal response to bisphosphonate therapy, largely because of the need for daily subcutaneous injections and high cost.

Hormone therapy and raloxifene have a narrow role as pharmacologic agents for treatment of osteoporosis in postmenopausal women. Hormone therapy is particularly useful in younger postmenopausal women with vasomotor symptoms, and raloxifene is particularly useful in postmenopausal women with a high risk of breast cancer. Both have a wide spectrum of adverse events that limit their general use; furthermore, raloxifene has not been shown to be efficacious in the prevention of nonvertebral fractures. Intranasal calcitonin has a receding place in the armamentarium and should be considered only when all other pharmacologic agents are either contraindicated or have failed because of lack of efficacy or tolerability.

References

1. NIH Consensus Development Panel on Osteoporosis. Osteoporosis prevention, diagnosis and therapy. JAMA 2001;285:785-95.
2. Cummings SR, Black DM, Nevitt MC, Bowner W, Cauley J, Ensrud K, et al. Bone density at various sties for prediction of hip fractures. Lancet 1993;341:72-5.
3. World Health Organization Study Group. Assessment of fracture risk and its application to screening for postmenopausal osteoporosis. World Health Organ Tech Rep Ser 1994;843:1-129.
4. Baim S, Binkley N, Bilezikian JP, Kendler DL, Hans DB, Lewiecki EM, et al. Official positions of the International Society for Clinical Densitometry and Executive Summary of the 2007 ISCD Position Development conference. J Clin Densitom 2008;11:75-91.
5. Ensrud KE, Thompson DE, Cauley JA, Nevitt MC, Kado DM, Hochberg MC, et al. Prevalent vertebral deformities predict mortality and hospitalization in older women with low bone mass: Fracture Intervention Trial Research Group. J Am Geriatr Soc 2000;48:241-9.
6. Department of Health and Human Services. Bone health and osteoporosis: a report of the Surgeon General. Rockville, MD: Office of the Surgeon General; 2004.
7. Cranney A, Guyatt G, Griffith L, Wells G, Tugwell P, Rosen C. Meta-analyses of therapies for postmenopausal osteoporosis: IX. Summary of meta-analyses of therapies for postmenopausal osteoporosis. Endocr Rev 2002;23:570-8.
8. MacLean C, Alexander A, Carter J, Chen S, Desai SB, Grossman J, et al. Comparative Effectiveness of Treatments to Prevent Fractures in Men and Women with Low Bone Density or Osteoporosis. Comparative Effectiveness Review No. 12 (Prepared by Southern California/RAND Evidence-Based Practice Center under Contract No. 290-02-0003.). Rockville, MD: Agency for Healthcare Research and Quality. Accessed January 8, 2008 from www.effectivehealthcare.ahrq.gov/reports/final.cfm.
9. MacLean C, Newberry S, Maglione M, McMahon M, Ranganath V, Suttorp M, et al. Systematic review: comparative effectiveness of treatments to prevent fractures in men and women with low bone density or osteoporosis. Ann Intern Med 2008;148:197-213.
10. Reginster J-Y, Felsenberg D, Boonen S, Diez-Perez A, Rizzoli R, Brandi M-L, et al. Effects of long-term strontium ranelate treatment on the risk of nonvertebral and vertebral fractures in postmenopausal osteoporosis: results of a five-year, randomized, placebo-controlled trial. Arthritis Rheum 2008;58:1687-95.
11. Greenspan SL, Bone HG, Ettinger MP, Hanley DA, Lindsay R, Zanchetta JR, et al. Effect of recombinant human parathyroid hormone (1-84) on vertebral fracture and bone mineral density in postmenopausal women with osteporosis: a randomized trial. Ann Intern Med 2007;146:326-39.
12. Cummings SF, Ettinger B, Delmas PD, Kenemans P, Stathopoulos V, Verweij P, et al. The effects of tibolone in older postmenopausal women. N Engl J Med 2008;359:697-708.
13. Ramachandran M, Little DG. Orthopedic surgical principles of fracture management. In: Primer on metabolic bone disease. 7th ed. Washington, DC: American Society for Bone and Mineral Research; 2008. p. 225-7.
14. Clinician's Guide to Prevention and Treatment of Osteoporosis. Washington, DC: National Osteoporosis Foundation; 2008. Available online at www.nofstore.org.
15. LaCroix AZ, Buist DSM, Brenneman SK, Abbott TA. Evaluation of three population-based strategies for fracture prevention: results of the Osteoporosis Population-Based Risk Assessment (OPRA) Trial. Med Care 2005;43:293-302.
16. Kern LM, Powe NR, Levine MA, Fitzpatrick AL, Harris TB, Robbins J, et al. Association between screening for osteoporosis and the incidence of hip fracture. Ann Intern Med 2005;142:173-81.
17. Lydick E, Cook K, Turpin J, Melton M, Stine R, Byrnes C. Development and validation of a simple questionnaire to facilitate identification of women likely to have low bone density. Am J Managed Care 1998;4:37-48.
18. Solomon DH, Morris C, Cheng H, Cabral D, Katz JN, Finkelstein JS, et al. Medication use patterns for osteoporosis: an assessment of guidelines, treatment rates, and quality improvement interventions. Mayo Clin Proc 2005;80:194-202.
19. Delmas PD, Rizzoli R, Cooper C, Reginster J-Y. Treatment of patients with postmenopausal osteoporosis is worthwhile: the position of the International Osteoporosis Foundation. Osteoporos Int 2005;16:1-5.
20. Kanis JA, Johnell O, Oden A, Dawson A, De Laet C, Jonsson B. Ten year probabilities of osteoporotic fractures according to BMD and diagnostic thresholds. Osteoporos Int 2001;12:989-95.
21. Kanis JA, Johnell O, De Laet C, Johansson H, Oden A, Delmas P, et al. A meta-analysis of previous fracture and subsequent fracture risk. Bone 2004;35:375-82.
22. De Laet C, Kanis JA, Oden A, Johanson H, Johnell O, Delmas P, et al. Body mass index as a predictor of fracture risk: a meta-analysis. Osteoporos Int 2005;16:1330-8.
23. Kanis JA, Johansson H, Oden A, Johnell O, de Laet C, Melton LJ, et al. A meta-analysis of prior corticosteroid use and fracture risk. J Bone Miner Res 2004;19:893-9.
24. Kanis JA, Johansson H, Oden A, Johnell O, De Laet C, Eisman JA, et al. A family history of fracture and fracture risk: a meta-analysis. Bone 2004;35:1029-37.
25. Kanis JA, Johnell O, Oden A, Johansson H, De Laet C, Eisman JA, et al. Smoking and fracture risk: a meta-analysis. Osteoporos Int 2005;16:155-62.

26. Kanis JA, Johansson H, Johnell O, Oden A, De Laet C, Eisman JA, et al. Alcohol intake as a risk factor for fracture. Osteoporos Int 2005;16:737-42.

27. Kanis JA, Borgstrom F, De Laet C, Johansson H, Johnell O, Jonsson B, et al. Assessment of fracture risk. Osteoporos Int 2005;16:581-9.

28. Kanis JA. on behalf of the World Health Organization Scientific Group. Assessment of Osteoporosis at the Primary Health Care Level. 2008 Technical Report. University of Sheffield, UK: WHO Collaborating Center; 2008.

29. Tosteson ANA, Melton LJ, Dawson-Hughes B, Baim S, Favus MUJ, Khosla S, et al. Cost-effective osteoporosis treatment thresholds: The U.S. perspective from the National Osteoporosis Foundation Guide Committee. Osteoporos Int 2008;19:437-47.

30. Dawson-Hughes B, Tosteson ANA, Melton LJ, Baim S, Favus MJ, Khosla S, et al. Implications of absolute fracture risk assessment for osteoporosis practice guidelines in the U.S. Osteoporos Int 2008;19:449-58.

31. Kleerekoper M. Overview of osteoporosis treatment. In: Rosen CJ, Compston JE, Lain JB, editors. Primer on metabolic bone diseases and disorders of mineral metabolism. 7th ed. Washington, DC: American Society for Bone and Mineral Research; 2008. p. 220-1.

32. Tannenbaum C, Clark J, Schwartzman K, Wallenstein S, Lapinski R, Meier D, et al. Yield of laboratory testing to identify secondary contributors to osteoporosis in otherwise healthy women. J Clin Endocrinol Metab 2002;87:4431-7.

33. Gold DT. Compliance and persistence with osteoporosis medications. In: Rosen CJ, Compston JE, Lain JB, editors. Primer on metabolic bone diseases and disorders of mineral metabolism. 7th ed. Washington, DC: American Society for Bone and Mineral Research; 2008. p. 254-6.

34. Standing Committee on the Scientific Evaluation of Dietary Reference Intakes FaNBIoM. Dietary Reference Intakes for Calcium, Phosphorus, Magnesium, Vitamin D and Fluoride. Washington, DC: National Academy Press; 1997.

35. Shea B, Wells G, Cranney A, Zytaruk N, Robinson V, Griffith L, et al. Meta-analyses of therapies for postmenopausal osteoporosis: VII. Meta-analysis of calcium supplementation for the prevention of postmenopausal osteoporosis. Endocrin Rev 2002;23:552-9.

36. Nevitt MC, Cummings SR. Type of fall and risk of hip and wrist fractures: The study of osteoporotic fractures. J Am Geriatr Soc 1993;41:1226-34.

37. Berry SD, Miller RR. Falls: Epidemiology, pathophysiology and relationship to fracture. Curr Osteoporos Rep 2008;6:149-54.

38. Province MA, Hadley EC, Hornbook MC, Lipsitz LA, Miller JP, Mulrow CD, et al. The effects of exercise on falls in elderly patients: a preplanned meta-analysis of the FICSIT Trials. JAMA 1995;273:1341-7.

39. Holick MF. Vitamin D deficiency. N Engl J Med 2007;357:266-81.

40. Przybelski R, Agrawal S, Krueger D, Engelke JA, Walbrun F, Binkley N. Rapid correction of low vitamin D status in nursing home residents. Osteoporos Int 2008;19:1621-8.

41. Aloia JF, Patel M, DiMaano R, Li-Ng M, Talwar SA, Mikhail M, et al. Vitamin D intake to attain a desired serum 25-hydroxyvitamin D concentration. Am J Clin Nutr 2008;87:1952-8.

42. Bischoff-Ferrari HA, Dawson-Hughes B, Willett WC, Staehelin HB, Bazemore MG, Zee RY, et al. Effect of vitatmin D on falls: a meta-analysis. JAMA 2004;291:1999-2006.

43. Bischoff-Ferrari HA, Willett WC, Wong JB, Giovannucci E, Dietrich T, Dawson-Hughes B. Fracture prevention by vitamin D supplementation: a meta-analysis of randomized controlled trials. JAMA 2005;293:2257-64.

44. Boonen S, Lips P, Bouillon R, Bischoff-Ferrari HA, Vanderschueren D, Haentjens P. Need for additional calcium to reduce the risk of hip fracture with vitamin D supplementation: evidence from a comparative metaanalysis of randomized controlled trials. J Clin Endocrinol Metab 2007;92:1415-23.

45. Geusens PP, Roux CH, Reid DM, Lems WF, Adami S, Adachi JD, et al. Drug insight: choosing a drug treatment strategy for women with osteoporosis - an evidence-based clinical perspective. Nature Clin Pract Rheum 2008. doi: 10.1038/ncprheum0773 (published online 8 April 2008 at www.nature.com/clinicalpractice).

46. Wells G, Cranney A, Peterson J, Boucher M, Shea B, Robinson V, et al. Alendronate for the primary and secondary prevention of osteoporotic fractures in postmenopausal women. Cochrane Database Syst Rev 2008;(1):CD001155. DOI: 10.1002/14651858.

47. Schnitzer T, Bone HG, Crepaldi G, Adami S, McClung M, Kiel D, et al. Therapeutic equivalence of alendronate 70 mg once-weekly and alendronate 10 mg daily in the treatment of osteoporosis. Alendronate Once-Weekly Study Group. Aging (Milano) 2000;12:1-12.

48. Rizzoli R, Greenspan SL, Bone HG, Schnitzer TJ, Watts NB, Adami S, et al. Two-year results of once-weekly administration of alendronate 70 mg for the treatment of postmenopausal osteoporosis. J Bone Miner Res 2002;17:1988-96.

49. Wells G, Cranney A, Peterson J, Boucher M, Shea B, Robinson V, et al. Risedronate for the primary and secondary prevention of osteoporotic fractures in postmenopausal women. Cochrane Database Syst Rev 2008;(1):CD004523. DOI: 10.1002/14651858.

50. Brown JP, Kendler DL, McClung MR, Emkey RD, Adachi JD, Bolognese MA, et al. The efficacy and tolerability of risedronate once a week for the treatment of postmenopausal osteoporosis. Calcif Tissue Int 2002;71:103-11.

51. Harris ST, Watts NB, Li Z, Chines AA, Hanley DA, Brown JP. Two-year efficacy and tolerability of risedronate once a week for the treatment of women with postmenopausal osteoporosis. Curr Med Res Opin 2004;20:757-64.

52. Delmas PD, McClung MR, Zanchetta JR, Racewicz A, Roux C, Benhamou CL, et al. Efficacy and safety of risedronate 150 mg once a month in the treatment of postmenopausal osteoporosis. Bone 2008;42:36-42.

53. Delmas PD, Benhamou CL, Man Z, Tlustochowicz W, Matzkin E, Eusebio R, et al. Monthly dosing of 75 mg risedronate on 2 consecutive days a month: efficacy and safety results. Osteoporos Int 2008;19:1039-45.

54. Chesnut III CH, Skag A, Christiansen C, Recker R, Stakkestad JA, Hoiseth A, et al. Effects of oral ibandronate administered daily or intermittently on fracture risk in postmenopausal osteoporosis. J Bone Miner Res 2004;19:1241-9.

55. Harris ST, Blumentals WA, Miller PD. Ibandronate and the risk of non-vertebral and clinical fractures in women with postmenopausal osteoporosis: results of a meta-analysis of phase III studies. Curr Med Res Opin 2008;24:237-45.

56. Recker R, Stakkestad JA, Chesnut 3rd CH, Christiansen C, Skag A, Hoiseth A, et al. Insufficiently dosed intravenous ibandronate injections are associated with suboptimal antifracture efficacy in postmenopausal osteoporosis. Bone 2004;34:890-9.

57. Miller PD, McClung MR, Macovei L, Stakkestad JA, Luckey M, Bonvoisin B, et al. Monthly oral ibandronate therapy in postmenopausal osteoporosis: 1-year results from MOBILE study. J Bone Miner Res 2005;20:1315-22.

58. Reginster JY, Adami S, Lakatos P, Greenwald M, Stepan JJ, Silverman SL, et al. Efficacy and tolerability of once-monthly oral ibandronate in postmenopausal osteoporosis: 2-year results from the MOBILE study. Ann Rheum Dis 2006;65:654-61.

59. Delmas PD, Adami S, Strugala C, Stakkestad JA, Reginster JY, Felsenberg D, et al. Intravenous ibandronate injections in postmenopausal women with osteoporosis: one-year results from the dosing intravenous administration study. Arthritis Rheum 2006;54:1838-46.

60. Eisman JA, Civitelli R, Adami S, Czerwinski E, Recknor C, Prince R, et al. Efficacy and tolerability of intravenous ibandronate injections in postmenopausal osteoporosis: 2-year results from the DIVA study. J Rheumatol 2008;35:488-97.

61. Papapoulos SE, Schimmer RC. Changes in bone remodeling and antifracture efficacy of intermittent bisphosphonate therapy: implications from clinical studies with ibandronate. Ann Rheum Dis 2007;66:853-8.

62. Cranney A, Wells GA, Yetisir E, Adami S, Cooper C, Delmas PD, et al. Ibandronate for the prevention of nonvertebral fractures: a pooled analysis of individual patient data. Osteoporos Int 2008. DOI 10.1007/s00198-008-0653-8.

63. Black DM, Delmas PD, Eastell R, Reid IR, Boonen S, Cauley JA, et al. Once-yearly zoledronic acid for treatment of postmenopausal osteoporosis. N Engl J Med 2007;356:1809-22.

64. Lyles KW, Colón-Emeric CS, Magaziner JS, Adachi JD, Pieper CF, Mautalen C, et al. Zoledronic acid and clinical fractures and mortality after hip fracture. N Engl J Med 2007;357:1799-809.

65. Cummings SR, Schwartz AV, Black DM. Alendronate and atrial fibrillation. N Engl J Med 2007;356:1895-6.

66. Sorensen HT, Christensen S, Mehnert F, Pedersen L, Chapurlat RD, Cummings SR, et al. Use of bisphosphonates among women and risk of atrial fibrillation and flutter: opulation based case-control study. BMJ 2008. doi: 10.1136/bmj.39507.551644.BE.

67. Khosla S, Burr D, Cauley J, Dempster DW, Ebeling PR, Felsenberg D, et al. Bisphosphonate associated osteonecrosis of the jaw: report of a Task Force of the American Society for Bone and Mineral Research. J Bone Miner Res 2007;22:1479-91.

68. Woo SB, Hellstein JW, Kalmar JR. Systematic review: bisphosphonates and osteonecrosis of the jaws. Ann Intern Med 2006;144:753-61.

69. Kwek EB, Goh SK, Koh JS, Png MA, Howe TS. An emerging pattern of subtrochanteric stress fractures: a long-term complication of alendronate therapy? Injury 2008;39:224-31.

70. Black DM, Schwartz AV, Ensrud KE, Cauley JA, Levis S, Quandt SA, et al. Effects of continuing or stopping alendronate after 5 years of treatment: The Fracture Intervention Trial Long-term Extension (FLEX): a randomized trial. JAMA 2006;296:2927-38.

71. Solomon DH, Hochberg MC, Mogun H, Schneeweiss S. The relation between bisphosphonate use and non-union of fractures of the humerus in older adults. Osteoporos Int 2009; 25:895-901.

72. Cranney A, Tugwell P, Zytaruk N, Robinson V, Weaver B, Shea B, et al. Meta-analysis of calcitonin for the treatment of postmenopausal osteoporosis. Endocr Rev 2002;23:540-51.

73. Chesnut CH, Silverman S, Andriano K, Genant H, Gimona A, Harris S, et al. A randomized trial of nasal spray calcitonin in postmenopausal women with established osteoporosis. The Prevent Recurrence of Osteoporotic Fractures Study. Am J Med 2000;109:267-76.

74. Wells G, Tugwell P, Shea B, Guyatt G, Peterson J, Zytaruk N, et al. Meta-analysis of the efficacy of hormone replacement therapy in treating and preventing osteoporosis in postmenopausal women. Endocr Rev 2002;23:529-39.

75. Torgerson DJ, Bell-Syer SE. Hormone replacement therapy and prevention of vertebral fractures: a meta-analysis of randomized trials. BMC Musculoskelet Disord 2001;2:7.

76. Torgerson DJ, Bell-Syer SE. Hormone replacement therapy and prevention of nonvertebral fractures: a meta-analysis of randomized trials. JAMA 2001;285:2891-7.

77. Cauley JA, Robbins J, Chen Z, Cummings SR, Jackson RD, LaCroix AZ, et al. Effects of estrogen plus progestin on risk of fracture and bone mineral density: the Women's Health Initiative Randomized Trial. JAMA 2003;290:1729-38.

78. Jackson RD, Wactawski-Wende J, LaCroix AZ, Pettinger M, Yood RA, Watts NB, et al. Effects of conjugated equine estrogen on risk of fractures and BMD in postmenopausal women with hysterectomy: results from the Women's Health Initiative Randomized Trial. J Bone Miner Res 2006;21:817-28.

79. Roussow JE, Prentice RL, Manson JE, Wu LL, Barad D, Barnabei VM, et al. Postmenopausal hormone therapy and risk of cardiovascular disease by age and years since menopause. JAMA 2007;297:1465-77.

80. Estrogen and progestogen use in postmenopausal women: July 2008 position statement of The North American Menopause Society. Menopause 2008;15:584-603.

81. Cranney A, Tugwell P, Zytaruk N, Robinson V, Weaver B, Adachi J, et al. Meta-analysis of raloxifene for the prevention and treatment of postmenopausal osteoporosis. Endocr Rev 2002;23:524-8.

82. Ettinger B, Black DM, Mitlak BH, Knickerbocker RK, Nickelsen T, Genant HK, et al. Reduction of vertebral fracture risk in postmenopausal women with osteoporosis treated with raloxifene: results from a 3-year randomized clinical trial. JAMA 1999;282:637-45.

83. Delmas PD, Ensrud KE, Adachi JD, Harper KD, Sarkar S, Gennari C, et al. Efficacy of raloxifene on vertebral fracture risk reduction in postmenopausal women with osteoporosis: four-year results from a randomized clinical trial. J Clin Endocrinol Metab 2002;87:3609-17.

84. Ensrud KE, Stock JL, Barrett-Connor E, Grady D, Mosca L, Khaw K-T, et al. Effects of raloxifene on fracture risk in postmenopausal women: the Raloxifene Use for the Heart trial. J Bone Miner Res 2008;23:112-20.

85. Martino S, Cauley JA, Barrett-Connor E, Powles TJ, Mershon J, Disch D, et al. Continuing outcomes relevant to Evista: breast cancer incidence in postmenopausal osteoporotic women in a randomized trial of raloxifene. J Natl Cancer Inst 2004;96:1751-61.

86. Moen MD, Keating GM. Raloxifene: a review of its use in the prevention of invasive breast cancer. Drugs 2008;68:2059-83.

87. Stevenson M, Lloyd Jones M, De Nigris E, Brewer N, Davis S, Oakley J. A systematic review and economic evaluation of alendronate, etidronate, risedronate, raloxifene and teriparatide for the prevention and treatment of postmenopausal osteoporosis. Health Tech Assess 2005;9:1-160.

88. Trevisani VFM, Riera R, Imoto AM, Saconato H, Atallah AN. Teriparatide (recombinant human parathyroid hormone 1-34) in postmenopausal osteoporosis: systematic review. Sao Paulo Med J 2008;126:279-84.

89. Neer RM, Arnaud CD, Zanchetta JR, Prince R, Gaich GA, Reginster J-Y, et al. Effect of parathyroid hormone (1-34) on fractures and bone mineral density in postmenopausal women with osteoporosis. N Engl J Med 2001;344:1434-41.

90. Vahle JL, Long GG, Sandusky G, Westmore M, Ma YL, Sato M. Bone neoplasms in F344 rats given teriparatide [rhpth (1-34)] are dependent on duration of treatment and dose. Toxicol Pathol 2004;32:426-38.

91. Harper KD, Krege JH, Marcus R, Mitlak BH. Osteosarcoma and teriparatide? J Bone Miner Res 2007;22:334.

92. Boonen S, Marin F, Obermayer-Pietsch B, Simoes ME, Barker C, Glass EV, et al. Effects of previous antiresorptive therapy on the bone mineral density response to two years of teriparatide treatment in postmenopausal women with osteoporosis. J Clin Endocrinol Metab 2008;93:852-60.

93. Miller PD, Delmas PD, Lindsay R, Watts NB, Luckey M, Adachi J, et al. Early responsiveness of women with osteoporosis to teriparatide after therapy with alendronate or risedronate. J Clin Endocrinol Metab 2008;93:3785-93.

Chapter 25

Regional Disorders of the Neck, Shoulder, Arm, and Hand

Joel A. Block and Sonali Khandelwal

REGIONAL DISORDERS OF THE NECK

CASE STUDY 1

A 45-year-old healthy woman presented with neck pain with gradual onset over 3 to 4 weeks. Pain was described as worse in the lower neck and around the shoulders, and achy in nature. She described a headache intermittently associated with the pain, especially at the end of the day. She had recently begun a job as a receptionist and was spending 7 hours each day working at a computer and using the telephone. Acetaminophen provided minimal relief.

Physical Examination:

Cervical spine was normal to inspection, but with slightly diminished flexion associated with pain; extension was normal. Mild tenderness was present over the inferior cervical spine and at the scapulae, and there was moderate tenderness at the paraspinal musculature including trapezius as well as the sternocleidomastoids. The neurologic examination was normal.

CASE STUDY 2

A 62-year-old woman with a history of rheumatoid arthritis, fibromyalgia, and depression presented with neck pain localized to the posterior neck and occasionally the base of the skull. The pain was worse in the evenings and interfered with the patient's sleep. Ibuprofen provided only minimal relief. There were no paresthesias or symptoms of neuropathy.

Physical Examination:

The cervical spine was normal to inspection. However, there was diminished flexion and extension and these motions reproduced the pain. There was

tenderness over the inferior cervical vertebral bodies. A test for radiculopathy, by neck extension with rotation of the head (Spurling's maneuver), was negative. The neurologic examination was normal, and there were normal deep tendon reflexes in the upper extremities.

Imaging: Lateral radiography of the cervical spine (Fig. 25-1) revealed anterior spondylolisthesis of C3 on C4, and grade 1 spondylosis of the mid and upper cervical spine; odontoid radiographs were normal.

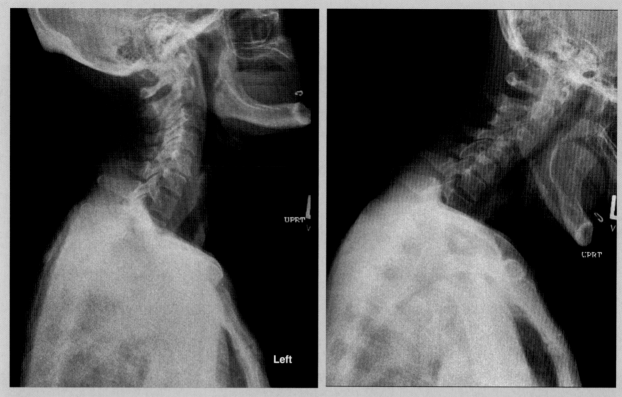

Figure 25-1. Radiography of the cervical spine in extension (*left*) and flexion (*right*), revealing anterior spondylolisthesis of C3 on C4, and grade 1 spondylosis of the mid and upper cervical spine.

CASE STUDY 3

A 37-year-old previously healthy man presented with neck and arm pain of 2 months' duration, which had progressed to a sensation of numbness in the right hand and resulted in him dropping objects occasionally. The pain was constant during the day, worse on the right side, and especially in the right shoulder. There were associated paresthesias of the thumb and second finger, which were exacerbated by active motion of the arm. Analgesics and nonsteroidal anti-inflammatory drugs (NSAIDs), as well as massage and acupuncture, had not provided symptomatic relief. There was no history of trauma or injury, and there were no other neuromuscular complaints.

Physical Examination:

The cervical spine was normal to inspection, but there was slightly decreased flexion and extension, with reproduction of pain at the extremes of both flexion and extension. Paravertebral muscle spasm was noted. Spurling's maneuver reproduced the pain with the head tilted to the right. Shoulder examination was normal without evidence of impingement. Neurologic examination revealed weakness of the right biceps and wrist extensors (4/5), diminished brachioradialis and biceps reflexes on the right, and diminished sensation to pin prick of the right thumb and index finger.

Imaging: T-2 weighted magnetic resonance imaging (MRI) scan of the cervical spine (Fig. 25-2) revealed posterior bulging and herniation of the intervertebral disc at the C5-C6 and C6-C7 levels, causing mild spinal cord impingement.

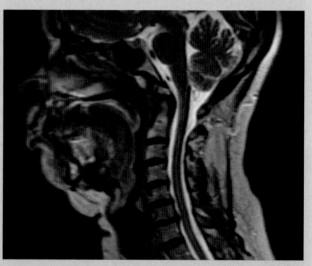

Figure 25-2. T2-weighted magnetic resonance imaging scan of the cervical spine, revealing posterior bulging and herniation of the intervertebral disc at the C5-C6 level and C6-C7 level causing mild spinal cord impingement.

CASE STUDY 4

A 44-year-old woman with a history of depression and hypothyroidism presented with diffuse neck and shoulder pain. The pain had been intermittent for approximately one year, and was described as a chronic ache across the upper back and neck and radiating to both shoulders. The pain had affected the patient's sleep as well as her ability to care for her children and to participate in sports. She reported lack of energy, extreme fatigue, and stiffness of the neck and back in the mornings. There was no history of trauma or injury.

Physical Examination:

The neck and back were normal to inspection and examination except for tender points suboccipitally, as well as at the trapezius, supraspinatus, and paraspinal muscles. Shoulders and upper extremities were normal, and the neurologic examination was unremarkable. There were additional tender points noted at the second costochondral junction, lateral epicondyles, and at the greater trochanters.

Laboratory evaluation, including blood count, comprehensive metabolic profile, and thyroid function, was normal.

Introduction

Neck pain affects individuals of all ages. An understanding of neck anatomy is essential to evaluate the etiology of neck pain. The seven vertebrae of the cervical spine constitute the axial skeleton of the neck and support the neck through its arc of motion. The natural lordosis of the neck, assumed during infancy, enhances the compliance of the vertebral column during weight bearing.[1] The first and second cervical vertebrae, the atlas and axis, respectively, differ anatomically from the other cervical vertebrae and account for approximately half of the ability to rotate the head on the neck; the lower cervical levels contribute the rest.[1] Although the total range of motion of each cervical segment varies from individual to individual,[2] the axis of rotation of each vertebral level may be more constant and has been used as a semiobjective measure of disturbed cervical function.[3] The spinal musculature of the neck consists of the posterior cervical paraspinal muscles, which provide cervical extension; the lateral cervical spine muscles, which rotate and laterally flex the neck; and the anterior cervical spinal muscles, which flex the neck. The trapezius muscles comprise the primary posterior muscles of the neck, whereas the most important lateral cervical muscle is the sternocleidomastoid.

The evaluation of neck pain begins by determining its source; potential sources of neck pain may be categorized as intra-articular, periarticular, age-related degenerative disease, or referred pain from neurovascular processes. Table 25-1 provides a brief differential diagnosis of regional neck pain syndromes. A thorough clinical history, including occupational and recreational activities and a comprehensive physical examination are necessary to distinguish among the various causes of neck pain.

Intra-articular Etiologies

Articular etiologies of neck pain include degenerative spine disease due to osteoarthritis, any of the inflammatory arthritides, including rheuma-

Table 25-1. *Differential Diagnosis of Neck Pain*

Articular disease
  Systemic inflammatory arthropathy (e.g., rheumatoid arthritis, etc.)
  Osteoarthritis or degenerative arthritis
  Spondyloarthropathy
  Fracture
Periarticular disease
  Cervical strain/sprain
  Whiplash
  Myofascial pain
  Spondylosis
  Myalgia or myositis
Neurovascular causes
  Syringomyelia
  Thoracic outlet syndrome
Referred pain
  Thyroid disorders
  Pharyngitis/laryngitis
  Esophageal disorders
  Cardiac disorders
  Carotid artery disorders
Miscellaneous
  Malignancy
  Infections
  Fibromyalgia

toid arthritis and the spondylitides, and infection. These presentations are discussed in detail in separate chapters. In addition, severe neck pain may be a feature of systemic inflammatory conditions, such as polymyositis, dermatomyositis, and polymyalgia rheumatic; however in these cases, neck pain is generally not an isolated finding and often reflects involvement of the muscles rather than the joints.

Periarticular Etiologies

Neck pain emanating from periarticular structures, the focus of this section, can be organized into relatively distinct groups: acute injury, chronic overuse disorders, age-related degenerative changes, and myofascial syndromes. The majority of minor neck pain is nonspecific, and results from muscular strain related to posture, stress, or occupational or sporting activities. As in many periarticular conditions discussed in this Chapter, repetitive activities, overuse, and lifestyle factors greatly contribute. The term *cervical strain* describes injuries to the musculotendonous portions of the neck and *cervical sprain* describes pain related to injury of the ligaments of the neck.[4] Case Study 1 is an example of cervical strain. Neck strain or sprain can result acutely from sports injuries or can develop chronically due to lifestyle factors. A related acute cervical injury is so-called whiplash, which refers to neck strain that results from an acceleration-deceleration injury involving the abrupt extension of the neck during acute trauma, typically during a motor vehicle accident. Although the pathology of this injury is poorly understood, clinical, animal, and cadaveric investigations suggest that mechanical overload injury of the zygoapophyseal joints, with concomitant injury to the articular pillars or the joint capsule, may be a significant source of whiplash pain.[5] The clinical syndrome of whiplash-associated disorders consists of neck pain, neck stiffness, arm pain and paresthesias; in addition, associated temperomandibular joint pain, headache, visual and memory disturbances, and psychological dysfunction are sometimes ascribed to the whiplash injury.[6]

Spondylosis refers to age-related degenerative changes of the spinal column that impinge on the adjacent neurological structures. Cervical spondylosis, as described in Case Study 2, is a common cause of axial neck pain, whereby vertebral osteophytes, or degenerative intervertebral discs, compress nerve roots or the spinal cord.[7] It is important to remember, however, that during normal aging, the intervertebral discs lose much of their viscoelasticity, which causes them to lose height and to bulge posteriorly into the spinal canal[8]; thus, radiographic evidence of cervical spondylosis is common, even in asymptomatic individuals,[9] especially among the elderly, and the distinction between normal aging and disease is usually made on clinical grounds. In addition to neck pain, spondylosis can cause radiculopathy and myelopathy through extrinsic compression of the nerve roots or spinal cord by posteriorly bulging discs or by vertebral osteophytes. In cervical radiculopathy, there is pain, hyperesthesia, or neurologic dysfunction in the distribution of one or more cervical nerve roots, whereas in cervical myelopathy, there are varied neurologic deficits and signs in both the upper and lower extremities due to spinal cord compression. Cervical radiculopathy in young adults typically results from herniation of a cervical disc or by acute trauma damaging a nerve root at the foramen; in contrast, cervical radiculopathy in older patients is more frequently a result of foraminal narrowing from osteophytes, osteoarthritis of the uncovertebral joints anteriorly or of the facet joints posteriorly, or degenerative disc disease with decreased disc height.

Myofascial pain refers to regional pain of soft tissue origin[10] characterized by painful muscles with increased tone and stiffness and with trigger points,[11] and is a common source of muscular pain in the shoulder-neck region[12]; the fibromyalgia syndrome refers to generalized myofascial pain. It has been reported that 72% of patients with fibromyalgia have active trigger points and 20% of patients with myofascial pain syndrome have fibromyalgia.[13] Case Study 4 represents a case of fibromyalgia with myofascial pain of the neck.

Clinical History and Symptoms

The clinical history of patients suffering from neck strain (Case Study 1) includes acute neck pain and stiffness, often with inability to perform daily tasks. There may be an inciting injury or recreational activity that has caused or aggravated the pain; however, strain may result simply from awkward positioning of the neck during the night or while cradling a phone. Patients suffering from neck strain often report only incomplete relief with rest and anti-inflammatory medications.

In contrast to the acute pain of neck strain, cervical spondylosis (Case Study 2) has a more insidious onset, with axial neck pain often referred to the lower part of the head, the shoulder blades or the upper limbs, and which is aggravated by movement.[7] This may be accompanied by paresthesias of the upper limbs and vertigo, which would suggest the presence of radiculopathy or myelopathy. Cervical radiculopathy (Case Study 3) most commonly involves nerve root compression at the C5 to C7 levels, with segmental distribution of shooting pain, hyperesthesia, and numbness.[7] Cervical myelopathy presents with symptoms similar to radiculopathy, but in addition, there are often reports of clumsiness of the hands, gait ataxia, and motor weakness with muscle wasting in the upper and lower extremities; bladder/bowel dysfunction may be present in severe cases.[8]

The presentation of myofascial neck pain tends to be nonspecific with complaints of varied symptoms; however, there is usually a complaint of deep pain of the neck musculature which may fluctuate in severity.[14] The onset is characteristically insidious but can sometimes be traced by the patient to a specific injury. There are often subjective reports of imbalance, dizziness, or tinnitus[15]; however, if these are clearly evident in an objective examination, then an alternative etiology would need to be sought. Finally, it must be remembered that certain symptoms such as nonmechanical neck pain, unintended weight loss, fever, or worsening neurologic deficits may be markers of possible neoplastic or infectious pathology, and urgent evaluation would be warranted.

Physical Examination

The physical examination is primarily directed at excluding structural or mechanical etiologies, because the examination would be expected to be essentially normal with most causes of regional neck pain that are not associated with lateralizing neurologic symptoms.[16] Inspection may reveal obvious bony deformities or soft tissue swelling. Next, palpation starts at the occiput and proceeds inferiorly to include the cervical vertebrae and paraspinal musculature, cervical lymph nodes, as well as the larynx and thyroid. In patients with cervical strain, whiplash, and myofascial neck pain, palpation of the cervical and paraspinal musculature will reproduce pain in varying degrees. Each of the classic cervical trigger points should be assessed, especially if myofascial pain is suspected.

Cervical motion is assessed with active and passive range of motion in extension, flexion, lateral flexion, and rotation. Most patients with regional neck pain have some restriction in range of motion; however, the significance of this is uncertain as studies have shown that there is great variation in range of neck movement even among normal individuals[2]; substantial global loss of motion is suggestive of significant articular disease, as seen in the inflammatory arthritides.

A thorough neurologic evaluation is warranted, especially when there are specific neurologic complaints. In cervical radiculopathy and myelopathy, neurologic examination alone often pinpoints the level of nerve root or spinal cord involvement, and the commonly involved nerve roots result in typical deficits. Radiculopathy of the third cervical root, between the second and third cervical vertebrae, which innervates the suboccipital region, causes pain to the posterior region of the head often extending to the ear.[17] Radiculopathy of the fourth cervical root causes numbness and pain to the neck and superior shoulder; involvement of the fifth cervical root presents with numbness and pain at the superior shoulder to the lateral arm, which often presents as shoulder pain but with normal range of motion. Motor deficits are also common: the deltoid muscle is innervated by the fifth nerve root; the diaphragm is innervated by the third, fourth, and fifth nerve roots; hence, radiculopathy of these roots may result in paradoxical breathing patterns[18]; and the fifth and sixth nerve roots innervate the biceps, thus affecting the biceps reflex when they are involved. Radiculopathy of the sixth cervical nerve root results in pain and numbness from the lateral neck to the lateral arm and to the dorsal web space between the thumb and index finger, and may involve weakness of the wrist extensors and supinators; thus, the brachioradialis and biceps reflexes may both be diminished, as illustrated by Case 3.

The seventh cervical nerve root is the most commonly involved level in cervical radiculopathy.[17]

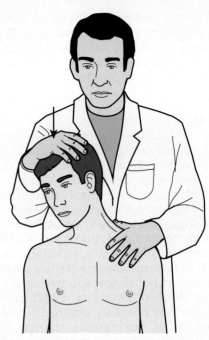

Figure 25-3. The Spurling test is a clinical assessment for nerve root compression. Downward pressure is uniformly applied by the examiner while the head is gently rotated toward the side of the suspected lesion. The test is positive if there is pain or paresthesias radiating to the upper limb.

With involvement at this level, radicular symptoms and pain are felt from the posterior shoulder along the triceps and dorsum of the forearm to the dorsum of the index finger. The triceps, wrist flexors, and finger extensors may be weak, and the triceps reflex may be diminished. The *Spurling test* is a test for nerve root compression (Fig. 25-3). With the patient seated, downward pressure is uniformly applied by the examiner to the patient's cranium while the head is gently rotated toward the side of the suspected lesion. The test is positive if there is immediate pain or paresthesias radiating to the upper limb.

In contrast to radiculopathy, the presentation of cervical myelopathy can be variable. Motor weakness and wasting of the upper and lower extremities is common. Sensory deficits may include diminished pain, temperature, proprioception, and vibration perception. The combination of muscle weakness and sensory loss often results in a broad-based unsteady gait. The confirmatory signs of upper motor neuron lesions include brisk reflexes, clonus, and the presence of pathologic reflexes such as the extensor plantar response and the Hoffman reflex, wherein tapping of the terminal phalanx of the third or fourth finger results in reflex flexion of the terminal phalanx of thumb.

When evaluating pain radiating from the neck to the arm, alternate diagnoses always need to be kept in mind. For example, a suspected case of radiculopathy with reported severe shoulder pain may in fact be due to rotator cuff or glenohumeral joint disease; similarly, peripheral nerve entrapments often mimic radiculopathy. In cases of severe pain radiating down the arm, myocardial infarction, of course, needs to be considered in an at-risk population.

Diagnosis

Individuals presenting with "red flag" symptoms associated with neck pain including trauma, a history of cancer with night neck pain, fever, chills, unexplained weight loss, a history of recent systemic infection or of a recent invasive procedure, progressive neurologic dysfunction, or bowel or bladder dysfunction, require imaging without delay[8]; for other patients with neck pain, especially those with myofascial neck pain, imaging studies are often not a part of the initial diagnostic evaluation. When imaging is deemed necessary, plain radiographs are often the first modality obtained. However, as mentioned earlier, degenerative changes including intervertebral disc space narrowing, osteoarthrosis of facet joints and osteophytes are common in individuals without cervical pain,[9] and therefore, their presence does not necessarily imply a source of pain. The diagnosis of whiplash is made on clinical grounds; imaging studies are not helpful as they are normal in most cases.[6]

Magnetic resonance imaging (MRI) is the test of choice when cervical radiculopathy or myelopathy is a concern; however, there are no objective guidelines defining when such imaging is warranted[19]; reasonable indications for prompt MRI testing include the presence of any "red flag" symptoms, suspicion of cancer or infectious process, or progressive neurologic decline. As is the case with standard radiography, the detection by MRI of abnormalities such as disk herniation and spinal cord impingement and compression are common incidental findings even in asymptomatic patients, and thus do not alone assign a structural etiology to neck pain.[20]

Computed tomography (CT) is useful to evaluate bony conduits through which the neural structures pass and can distinguish the magnitude of bony spurs, foraminal encroachment, or ossification of the posterior longitudinal ligament. CT myelography, the addition of intrathecal contrast material to CT, provides accuracy that is at least comparable to MRI in distinguishing osseous from soft tissue etiologies of impingement and in identifying foraminal stenosis.[21]

Management

Treatment of cervical strain or sprain and of myofascial neck pain is directed at palliating symptoms. Local modalities include electrotherapy, cold or heat application, and local anesthetics.[22]

Conventional pharmacologic therapy for musculoskeletal pain includes nonsteroidal anti-inflammatory drugs (NSAIDs), muscle spasmolytics, antidepressants, and opioid and nonopioid analgesics.[23] NSAIDs have been found to be useful for the treatment of neck pain; however, long-term use for this indication may entail the risk of renal and gastrointestinal adverse effects. There is no evidence that any particular NSAID is superior to others with regard to pain relief, however, patients who are refractory to one NSAID may obtain relief after switching to another NSAID class.[24] Finally, attention to behavioral issues, though often overlooked, may provide important adjunctive relief. For example, lifestyle factors may contribute to a chronic cycle of cervical strain and myofascial pain. Postural and ergonomic modifications, both at home and at work, and stress reduction through biofeedback, meditation or progressive relaxation techniques may be helpful,[14] though there are few controlled studies to support these approaches. There is evidence that stretching exercises, supervised by a physical therapist, may improve pain and function in the myofascial pain syndromes, and have become a primary therapeutic modality for addressing myofascial pain.[25]

Injections of trigger points with lidocaine, or occasionally with glucocorticoids, have been used as second line therapy in conjunction with stretching exercises to augment their effect,[26] though their long-term efficacy is unproven. Most practitioners who employ this modality suggest that their efficacy may be optimized if the injections are preceded and immediately followed by manual muscle trigger point release techniques and stretching exercises.[14] Other less conventional therapies for myofascial pain that have been advocated include botulinum toxin type A injection, which may reduce pain and palpable muscle firmness in individuals with chronic pain,[27] although the literature is conflicting regarding its efficacy,[28] and acupuncture, which has been evaluated in myofascial pain and fibromyalgia,[29] but less extensively in nonspecific neck pain.

Treatment for acute whiplash is focused on palliating symptoms, improving function and preventing chronicity. Conservative measures such as a cervical soft collar, passive physical therapy, and rest have been shown to be inferior to programs that reinforce return to normal activities and active mobilization exercises.[30] There is no consensus regarding whether chronic whiplash exists as a discrete syndrome, nor what the source of chronic pain is in this condition[31]; hence, there is a paucity of controlled studies that evaluate treatment approaches. Nevertheless, there is some evidence that neurotomy of the facet innervation may provide effective pain relief in chronic whiplash,[32] whereas intra-articular injections have been found to be ineffective.[33] There are no data confirming the use of exercise regimens in chronic whiplash, although it is believed to be of significant clinical value.[6]

Initial management of cervical spondylosis is generally conservative, with the goal of reducing pain and inflammation. NSAIDs, opiates, muscle relaxants, and antidepressants have been used empirically, as have soft cervical collars, although clinical studies are lacking.[8] Nonetheless, 45% to 60% of patients with cervical spondylosis and symptoms of neck pain or radiculopathy will have resolution of symptoms with conservative therapy alone.[34] Additional modalities that may be helpful include epidural corticosteroid injections[35] and physical therapy regimens that include isometric exercises and active range of motion maneuvers.[36] In contrast, systematic reviews suggest that cervical traction[37] and acupuncture[38] may be ineffective in cervical spondylosis.

Indications for surgical intervention in spondylosis are often specific to the clinical situation. Patients with progressive or disabling neurologic dysfunction are typically considered for early surgery,[8] whereas uncomplicated disease is usually treated conservatively. In general, operative intervention is appropriate for these patients if they have severe persistent pain that has a significant adverse effect on function or lifestyle and that has failed a reasonable trial of conservative management. The duration of conservative management prior to considering surgery depends on the patient's situation; 12 months may be reasonable in uncomplicated cervical degenerative disease, whereas 3 months may be more appropriate for persistent cervical radiculopathy. It is important to correlate the clinical history and examination with diagnostic imaging when contemplating surgical intervention for neck pain, because the risk-benefit analysis must include the possibility of structural anomalies that are unrelated to symptoms. Finally, damage to the spinal cord, as in myelopathy, is often permanent despite surgical intervention, whereas symptoms may progress after surgery.[7]

Neurovascular and Referred Neck Pain

Syringomyelia and thoracic outlet obstruction are neurovascular conditions in which neck pain may be a prominent feature. Syringomyelia refers to the development of a fluid filled cyst in the spinal cord, and may result from a congenital cerebellar defect, the so-called Chiari I malformation, or from acquired etiologies such as tissue damage from trauma, infection, or tumor. Over time, the syrinx may expand and compromise neurological function. Neck pain and stiffness may be early symptoms of the process, but neurologic deficits become manifest with progression. Diagnostically, MRI is highly sensitive for detecting the presence of a syrinx. Thoracic outlet syndrome occurs when nerves, vessels, or both are compressed due to anatomic abnormalities, trauma, or major changes of body habitus such as weight gain. Neck pain associated with numbness, paresthesias, and occasionally discoloration of the skin of the hands and fingers is frequently associated with thoracic outlet syndrome; this can be differentiated from intra-articular or periarticular etiologies of neck pain because they do not cause vascular changes.

In light of its central location, the neck can be a site of pain referred from the anterior neck, thorax, heart, stomach, and diaphragm. Thyroid disorders, laryngitis, tracheitis, esophageal obstruction or dysmotility, cardiogenic pain from acute coronary syndrome or pericarditis, and carotid artery disorders such as carotidynia or dissection can each be a source of neck pain, and should be considered when the clinical presentation is appropriate.

REGIONAL DISORDERS OF THE SHOULDER

Introduction

Shoulder pain is a malady that affects all ages and occupations. As with all musculoskeletal disorders, the approach to diagnosis and treatment depends on an understanding of the underlying anatomy and on identifying the source of the pain. The shoulder region consists of the glenohumeral and acromioclavicular joints, as well as the scapulothoracic and even the sternoclavicular joints, along with the surrounding musculature and tendons. The shoulder is commonly involved in inflammatory

---

CASE STUDY 5

A 27-year-old woman with no past medical history presented with right lateral shoulder pain. She stated that the pain began three weeks previously and did not resolve with rest and anti-inflammatory medications. The patient assumed that this was a muscle strain and treated herself with a heating pad but without relief. There was no history of injury or sports participation, but the patient had recently painted her apartment. She denied any history of swelling, loss of function or numbness in the arm or shoulder.

Physical Examination:

The right shoulder was normal to inspection. Palpation of the greater tuberosity elicited tenderness. There was no apparent effusion, warmth or erythema of the shoulder. Passive range of motion was full and pain free; active range of motion elicited shoulder pain at abduction above 90 degrees but the patient was able to raise her arm to 160 degrees. Tests of shoulder impingement (Hawkin's and Neer's) were positive, but the drop arm test was negative.

No imaging was performed.

CASE STUDY 6

A healthy 64-year-old man presented with left shoulder pain of 7 months' duration. The patient recalled traveling at the time of onset but denied trauma or any precipitating event. Approximately 4 months previously, radiography of the painful shoulder was reportedly normal. The pain progressed, and at the time of the visit was present at rest, worse at the end of the day, and was waking him at night. He denied symptoms of numbness or swelling. He was substantially limited in his ability to lift heavy objects and to comb his hair with the right hand. Shoulder exercises and ibuprofen provided only mild pain relief.

Physical Examination:

Inspection of the left shoulder revealed mild atrophy posteriorly. Passive flexion yielded audible grating and palpable crepitus. There was no swelling or erythema of the glenohumoral joint. Passive range of motion was mildly limited at the extremes and painful; active range of motion was more limited, with abduction to 90 degrees and external rotation to 60 degrees. Tests of shoulder impingement (Hawkin's and Neer's) and the drop arm test were positive.

Radiography (Fig. 25-4) revealed normal glenohumoral joint space, a subacromial osteophyte, and no apparent soft tissue swelling.

MRI was remarkable for a full-thickness tear of the rotator cuff at the supraspinatus, with impingement of the acromial osteophyte on the supraspinatus.

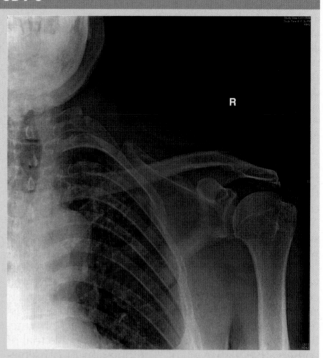

Figure 25-4. Anteroposterior radiograph of the left shoulder revealing normal glenohumoral joint space, a subacromial osteophyte, and no soft tissue swelling.

CASE STUDY 7

A 63-year-old woman with a history of ovarian cancer 10 years previously and of diabetes presented with left shoulder pain that had been present for 6 months and was described as diffuse throughout the shoulder region and radiating to the upper back. She could not lie on the left side because of pain in the shoulder. There was a sensation of increasing "stiffness" during the past 2 months, and she was no longer able to lift the left arm as high as her right arm. She had no history of arthritis or trauma.

Physical Examination:

The left shoulder was normal to inspection. There was mild diffuse tenderness throughout the shoulder, but no palpable effusion. Significant reduction in active and passive range of motion of the left shoulder was appreciated: passive abduction was 40 degrees, passive external rotation was 10 degrees, and passive internal rotation was 15 degrees.

Radiography of the left shoulder was normal.

CASE STUDY 8

A 55-year-old woman with a history of osteoporosis and diabetes presented with anterior left shoulder pain of two months' duration. The pain was described as a chronic, aching pain that was aggravated with minor lifting but was not present at rest. While describing the pain, the patient pointed to one area of the anterior shoulder where the pain was the worst. There was no history of arthritis or trauma, nor had the patient noticed swelling or redness of the shoulder. Ibuprofen provided incomplete relief.

Physical Examination:

Inspection of the left shoulder was normal. There was focal tenderness at the bicipital groove, which was exacerbated by resisted flexion of the elbow. Pain was also present with passive and active shoulder extension, but there was little limitation to motion. Speed's and Yergason's tests were positive.

No imaging was performed.

Table 25-2. *Differential Diagnoses of Shoulder Pain*

Articular disease
  Glenohumeral arthritis
  Acromioclavicular arthritis
  Crystalline arthropathy
  Avascular necrosis
Periarticular disease
  Chronic impingement syndrome
  Rotator cuff tendonitis or tear
  Bicipital tendonitis or biceps tendon tear
  Subacromial bursitis
  Adhesive capsulitis
Neurovascular causes
  Thoracic outlet syndrome
  Acute brachial plexus injury
  Cervical radiculopathy or spondylosis
Referred and miscellaneous causes
  Reflex sympathetic dystrophy
  Polymyalgia rheumatica
  Fibromyalgia
  Angina
  Peritonitis/cholecystitis/hepatitis

polyarthropathies, and intra-articular structural derangement is common; nonetheless, periarticular disorders represent a much more common source of shoulder pain in adults. Periarticular syndromes, the focus of this discussion, may emanate from the structures that comprise the rotator cuff, from the bursae, or may be manifestations of referred pain from peripheral nerve, plexus, nerve roots, or the spinal cord. Table 25-2 is a brief list of differential diagnoses to consider in patients presenting with shoulder pain.

Intra-articular Syndromes

The shoulder may be involved in virtually all of the inflammatory polyarthropathies, and the etiology of the shoulder pain itself is usually obvious from systemic findings; isolated shoulder pain without associated disease is unusual. In all patients who are older, as well as those with a history of inflammatory or degenerative arthritis, articular disease of the glenohumeral and acromioclavicular joints should be considered in the differential diagnosis of shoulder pain. Whereas shoulder involvement in patients with systemic inflammatory disease is not usually subtle, osteoarthritis of the shoulder may be neglected because osteoarthritis is often assumed not to have a predisposition for the shoulder. Nonetheless, *glenohumeral* osteoarthritis is common, especially in the elderly and in individuals with a prior history of significant shoulder trauma. Osteophytes that develop in *acromioclavicular* osteoarthritis may be a source of chronic friction to the overlying rotator cuff, and may be especially common in degenerative rotator cuff disease in the elderly. In cases of osteoarthritis of the shoulder, the presenting history typically includes an insidious

course with gradual worsening of pain over time and with limitation in range of motion and in function. Palpable effusion may be present at the glenohumeral joint, and radiography reveals typical signs of osteoarthritis. Other intra-articular pathologies that must be considered in the differential diagnosis include crystalline arthropathy, avascular necrosis, neuropathic arthropathy, and damage to the articular cartilage such as a torn labrum.

Periarticular Etiologies

Periarticular processes are a major cause of shoulder pain and are the focus of this section. The etiology of periarticular pain may be related to derangement of the soft tissues surrounding the joint, including the bursae, tendons, or muscles, or alternatively it may be of distant origin, with pain referred to the shoulder. The tendons and muscles surrounding the shoulder, in combination with the glenohumeral synovium, form the rotator cuff and the shoulder capsule. The rotator cuff is composed of the interconnecting tendons of four muscles, the supraspinatus, infraspinatus, subscapularis, and teres minor. These muscles surround and stabilize the humeral head against the glenoid fossa, while also functioning to provide rotation and abduction of the arm. Owing to their stabilizing function, these muscles and tendons sustain repetitive action and high loading, and injuries to these structures represent a common source of shoulder pain. Although trauma or overuse cause injury, shoulder pain from apparently spontaneous rotator cuff dysfunction is common.[39] *Rotator cuff tendonitis* occurs when there is disruption or inflammation of the rotator cuff tendons. Clinically, tendonitis is difficult to distinguish from incomplete tears of the rotator cuff, whereas complete rupture has specific clinical findings (see later). In light of the similarity of presentation, the entire spectrum of subacromial space lesions, including partial thickness rotator cuff tears, rotator cuff tendonitis, calcific tendonitis, and subacromial bursitis is sometimes considered as a single syndrome, the *chronic impingement syndrome* or *painful arc syndrome*.[40]

Case Study 5 is a case of rotator cuff tendonitis, and Case Study 6 illustrates a rotator cuff tear. Younger, athletically active individuals may suffer traumatic or acute tears of the rotator cuff, often accompanied by acute pain and local swelling. In contrast, among middle-aged and elderly patients rotator cuff tears most frequently result from age-related tendon degeneration and chronic mechanical impingement.[41] As is the case with all tendons, the rotator cuff tendons are poorly vascularized, which renders them especially susceptible to minor injuries; moreover, during the degenerative processes of aging, the tensile strength of the collagen fibers is diminished, and the tendons may be further impaired by chronic traction over osteophytes at the acromioclavicular joint.[42] Degenerative tears begin as partial thickness and generally originate in the supraspinatus tendon. As they progress anteriorly or posteriorly, they may transform to full-thickness tears, especially among individuals over 60 years of age.[43]

The bursae of the shoulder that are frequently painful and develop bursitis include the subacromial bursa, subdeltoid bursa, and less commonly the scapulothoracic bursa. Bursitis may be diagnosed by exquisite pain elicited by pressure exerted directly over the involved bursa and by pain on active motion across the bursa. Bursitis in the shoulder region is usually idiopathic, and the association between rotator cuff tendonitis and subacromial bursitis is sufficiently strong that the two are often considered to be clinically synonymous; in contrast, secondary bursitis in the shoulder due to trauma, infection, crystalline arthropathy, or rheumatoid arthritis is not as frequently encountered.

Adhesive capsulitis or *frozen shoulder*, as illustrated by Case Study 7, is a process that appears to occur only in the shoulder and involves the progressive restriction of passive and active range of motion in all planes, usually associated with significant pain. The pathogenesis of primary capsulitis remains unclear; however, it is known that synovial cytokine levels are elevated in the capsule of patients with adhesive capsulitis.[44] Adhesive capsulitis associated with an identifiable intrinsic, extrinsic or systemic etiology is referred to as secondary capsulitis; examples of such conditions include trauma, the postsurgical state, prolonged shoulder immobilization,[45] as well as metabolic diseases, such as diabetes[46] and hypothyroidism.[47]

In addition to the shoulder structures themselves, periarticular shoulder pain may stem from tendons that insert at the shoulder but function distally. Case Study 8 demonstrates a case of bicipital (biceps) tendonitis. This syndrome refers to inflammation of the long head of the biceps tendon, generally focused on its course in the bicipital groove of the anterior humerus. Primary isolated bicipital tendonitis typically results from overuse injuries such as repetitive lifting in weightlifting or overhead reaching as in pitching baseballs. These repetitive actions lead to inflammation and microtears. More commonly however, bicipital tendonitis results from chronic subacromial impingement occurring in association with rotator cuff tendonitis and glenohumeral instability.[48] In the setting of a chronically inflamed tendon or in elderly patients, the tendon can rupture spontaneously.

Clinical History and Symptoms

Rotator cuff tendonitis (Case Study 5) in young individuals is frequently a result of a sports-related injury. High-risk activities include those in which the arm is repeatedly held in an overhead position such as basketball, tennis, or swimming. In contrast, among older individuals, a history of repetitive motion above the shoulder level or of recent strenuous unaccustomed arm activity is common, although idiopathic rotator cuff tendonitis may be most common. In both cases, typical symptoms include aching pain in the lateral aspect of the upper arm that cannot be localized to a single site, but is exacerbated by raising the arm over the head or by lying on the affected side.

Individuals with rotator cuff tears (Case Study 6) experience pain and stiffness that are exacerbated with extremes of motion; in addition, pain at night while lying on the affected side is characteristic. Difficulties with daily activities that involve rotation of the shoulder, such as combing one's hair, hooking a bra strap, or reaching into a back pocket, are common. Patients with chronic rotator cuff tears may experience recurrent lateral shoulder pain of several months' duration, usually without a history of trauma; symptoms typically are exacerbated with activity, though the clinical presentation is variable.[49]

Adhesive capsulitis (Case Study 7) typically presents with gradual onset of pain followed by loss of motion. Classic adhesive capsulitis has been classified into three stages, each of approximately 6 months duration: initially, the "freezing" stage is characterized by insidious pain onset and limitation of shoulder range of motion; this is followed by the "frozen" stage, wherein pain subsides but range of motion becomes markedly restricted; finally, during the "thawing" stage, range of motion slowly improves, often requiring 12 to 24 months for full resolution.[45]

Bicipital tendonitis (Case Study 8) presents with anterior shoulder pain that is exacerbated by activities that involve lifting and overhead reaching. The point of maximal tenderness follows the bicipital groove, in contrast to the pain of rotator cuff tendonitis or of tears, which is more laterally focused. However, because there is a strong association of bicipital tendonitis with rotator cuff tendonitis, there may be a great deal of overlap in the clinical history provided by patients with each condition.[48]

Physical Examination of the Shoulder

Inspection of the shoulder begins with an evaluation for abnormal contours, asymmetry, and for the presence of bony prominences. Although no visual abnormalities are expected in cases of acute rotator cuff tendonitis or bicipital tendonitis, chronic rotator cuff tendonitis or tears may present with visible loss of muscle bulk posteriorly, indicating atrophy of the supraspinatus and infraspinatus muscles. Palpation of the clavicle determines whether there is tenderness, swelling, or instability of the acromioclavicular or sternoclavicular joints, as well as yield information about the glenohumeral joint. Palpation of the anterolateral portion of the acromion and of the greater tuberosity of the humerus may reveal tenderness of the subacromial bursa or of the rotator cuff; bursitis may be characterized by point tenderness over the bursa which is exacerbated by exertion of the overlying muscles. The glenohumeral joint should be palpated for evidence of effusion and for tenderness, and the bicipital groove, approximately 2 to 3 cm inferiorly from the anterolateral tip of the acromion, should be examined for tenderness of the bicipital tendon. Finally, the cervical vertebrae and the muscles of the neck should be examined for tenderness and for myofascial pain, as well as for evidence of primary pathology that may refer pain to the shoulder.

Range of motion of each shoulder is evaluated passively and actively for abduction, forward flexion and external and internal rotation (Fig. 25-5A–C). With the elbow placed at the side, the normal maximal external rotation may vary from 45 to 90 degrees and internal rotation from 55 to 80 degrees; with the shoulder abducted to 90 degrees and the elbow flexed at a right angle, both internal and external rotation should be 90 degrees. Typically, passive range of motion is not restricted by periarticular disorders unless there is adhesive capsulitis, whereas active motion is restricted either by pain or by injury to the soft tissues; in contrast, intra-articular pathology is associated with limitations of both passive and active motion. Impingement syndromes may be detected by the presence of a painful arc as the patient raises the arm in abduction; pain onset at abduction angles between 60 and 180 degrees is characteristic of impingement syndrome.

Various maneuvers have been described to assist in the diagnosis of shoulder pain. Two widely used techniques to assess impingement are the Neer impingement sign and the Hawkins impingement test. In the Neer sign, the examiner depresses the patient's scapula with one hand while elevating the arm with the other, thereby compressing the greater tuberosity against the anterior acromion and eliciting pain if rotator cuff tendonitis or a tear is present (Fig. 25-6). The Hawkins test may be more sensitive for detecting impingement syndrome,[50] and is performed by the examiner once again stabilizing the patient's scapula with one hand, while the other hand passively abducts the patient's shoulder to 90 degrees and flexes the elbow to 90 degrees with the arm in neutral position. With the arm thus supported, internal rotation causes impingement of the greater tuberosity against the anterior acromion and results in pain when a rotator cuff tear or tendonitis is present (Fig. 25-7). The drop arm test, when present, is pathognomonic for large tears of the rotator cuff. This is performed by positioning the patient's shoulder to 90 degrees abduction and then having the patient slowly lower the arm from full abduction. The test is positive if the arm involuntarily drops (Fig. 25-8). Yergason's and Speed's tests were developed to evaluate bicipital tendonitis.

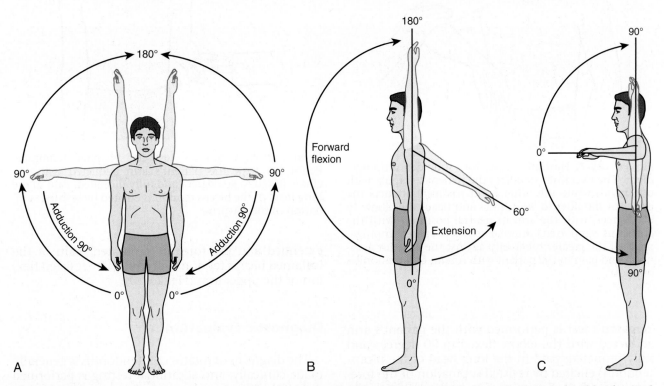

Figure 25-5. Mobility testing of the shoulder. **A,** Active shoulder abduction/adduction. **B,** Active shoulder forward flexion/extension. **C,** Active shoulder internal and external rotation.

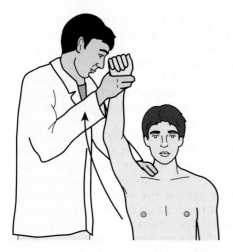

Figure 25-6. Neer's test for shoulder impingement. The examiner depresses the patient's scapula with one hand while elevating the arm with the other, thereby compressing the greater tuberosity against the anterior acromion and eliciting pain if rotator cuff tendonitis or a tear is present.

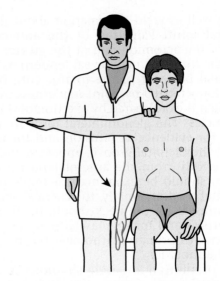

Figure 25-8. Drop arm test for shoulder impingement. This is performed by positioning the patient's shoulder to 90 degrees of abduction and then having the patient slowly lower the arm from full abduction. The test is positive if the arm involuntarily drops.

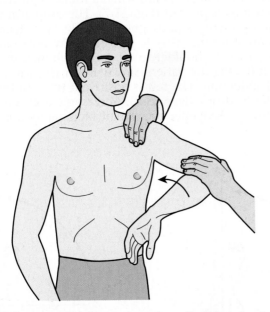

Figure 25-7. Hawkins' test for shoulder impingement. The examiner stabilizes the patient's scapula with one hand, while the other hand passively abducts the patient's shoulder to 90 degrees and flexes the elbow to 90 degrees, with the arm in neutral position. With the arm thus supported, internal rotation causes impingement of the greater tuberosity against the anterior acromion and pain in the patient with rotator cuff tendonitis or a tear.

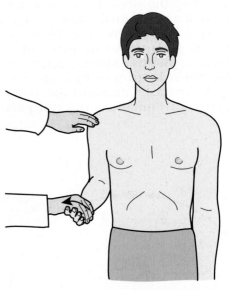

Figure 25-9. Yergason's test for bicipital tendinitis. Performed with the patient's arm adducted with the elbow flexed to 90 degrees and fully pronated. Pain in the long head of the biceps tendon is elicited by resisted supination of the forearm.

extended and the forearm supinated; pain of the inflamed biceps tendon is produced by resisted flexion of the upper arm (Fig. 25-10).

Diagnostic Evaluation

The diagnosis of rotator cuff tendonitis is generally made clinically, and additional testing is performed only if there is a need to exclude other diagnoses. In these instances, imaging may be obtained if there

Yergason's test is performed with the patient's arm adducted with the elbow flexed to 90 degrees and fully pronated; pain in the long head of the biceps tendon is elicited by resisted supination of the forearm (Fig. 25-9). Speed's test is performed with the shoulder flexed to 30 degrees and with the elbow

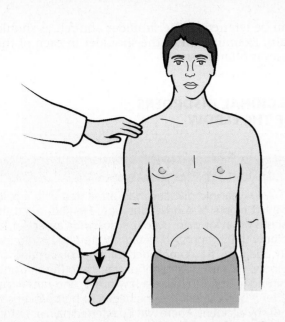

Figure 25-10. Speed's test for bicipital tendinitis. Performed with the patient's shoulder forward flexed to 30 degrees, with the elbow extended and the forearm supinated. Pain of the inflamed biceps tendon is produced by resisted flexion of the upper arm.

are inconsistencies between history and examination or if articular disease is a strong consideration. Both MRI and ultrasonography are useful diagnostic modalities to evaluate the rotator cuff tendons; in experienced hands, both modalities have approximately 90% accuracy for the diagnosis of full-thickness and partial thickness tears.[51] However, conventional radiography remains in widespread use for the initial diagnostic evaluation of rotator cuff tears. Radiographic evidence of chronic rotator cuff rupture includes superior migration of the humeral head towards the acromion and an acromiohumeral distance of less than 7 mm. Radiography obtained at 30 degrees caudal tilt may be more sensitive for rotator cuff pathology than standard shoulder radiography, and may also reveal osteophytes of the inferior surface of the acromion, such as were present in Case Study 2. Similar to the evaluation of rotator cuff tendonitis, the diagnostic evaluation of bicipital tendonitis and of adhesive capsulitis does not generally require radiography, as both would be expected to be unremarkable or to have calcification of the involved structures, and radiography is primarily indicated to exclude other conditions, such as osteoarthritis, destructive calcific periarthritis (so-called *Milwaukee Shoulder*), or other pathology. MRI has acceptable reliability for detecting signal and thickness abnormalities of the synovial capsule in patients with capsulitis,[52] and there is some evidence that thickening of the coracohumeral ligament and of the joint capsule are highly specific for frozen shoulder syndrome.[53] Arthrography has largely been supplanted by MRI in the diagnostic evaluation of shoulder syndromes, although it may retain value therapeutically (see later).

Management

Therapy for periarticular shoulder pain is largely empiric and is generally conservative; there are relatively few well-controlled randomized trials that evaluate the efficacy of most interventions, and true evidence-based therapy is limited. The approach to treatment of these conditions generally rests on adjunctive physical therapy to preserve range of motion and strength, and on analgesics and anti-inflammatory medication for pain relief; in most cases, surgery is reserved either for refractory pain or in cases of acute trauma with rupture of the involved structures. Initial therapy for rotator cuff tendonitis consists of rest, ice, and analgesics or NSAIDs. Physical therapy to maintain and promote shoulder range of motion, and strengthening exercises, have been shown to shorten recovery times and may provide longer term functional benefit,[54] as well as assist in preventing the progression to adhesive capsulitis. Similarly, glucocorticoid injections into the subacromial bursa may provide pain relief and permit improved adherence to physical therapy regimens.

If significant pain persists despite adequate rehabilitation and conservative therapy, then referral to an orthopedic surgeon would be appropriate. Rotator cuff tears that result from acute trauma in young patients are typically repaired surgically, and early attention is preferred, ideally within 6 weeks after injury.[51] In contrast, chronic or degenerative tears of the rotator cuff are generally approached in a manner similar to rotator cuff tendonitis, with rest, ice, analgesia, or NSAIDs, and physical therapy to maintain range of motion and strength. Glucocorticoid injections may be effective for pain relief, but are employed judiciously because of a theoretical concern of propagating the tear. Furthermore, the subacromial corticosteroid injections appear to have only mild and unsustained efficacy.[55] As with rotator cuff therapy, surgery is reserved for patients with significant persistent pain after an adequate trial of rehabilitation and analgesia; moreover, the primary aim of surgery in degenerative rotator cuff tears is pain relief rather than full functional restoration. Factors that favor surgical reattachment of a detached tendon include age younger than 60 years, a traumatic etiology, short duration of symptoms (< 2 months), no history of smoking, absence of previous shoulder surgery, MRI revealing minimal tendon retraction and muscle atrophy, and good general health.[51]

Management of biceps tendonitis is similar to that of shoulder pain in general, because the goals are to relieve pain, reduce inflammation, strengthen the biceps muscle and tendon, and avoid rupture.[54] Initial therapy includes ice and NSAIDs. In addition, patients should be counseled to avoid heavy lifting and over-the-shoulder activities during the acute period due to the risk of rupture. These cautions should be emphasized to patients with a high risk of rupture, such as those with recurrent tendonitis, previous rotator cuff or contralateral biceps tendon rupture, older age (older than 50 years), poor general shoulder conditioning, or systemic inflammatory arthritis. Physical therapy for muscle strengthening is generally initiated after resolution of acute pain, and the regimen typically includes isometric exercises of elbow flexion. For patients in whom pain persists for more than 1 month despite therapy, local glucocorticoid injection may be considered, although care must be taken to avoid direct injection of the tendon, because such injections are associated with tendon rupture, especially in older individuals. The glucocorticoid should be infiltrated along the bicipital groove, or alternatively, into the subacromial bursa, especially in patients at higher risk of rupture. A second injection several weeks later is often helpful in patients who achieve only partial relief; however, chronic pain may be an indication of concomitant shoulder pathology such as impingement syndrome or glenohumeral instability that is undiagnosed.

The natural history of adhesive capsulitis, or frozen shoulder syndrome, may be spontaneous resolution after several months to years[56]; hence, the goal of treatment is primarily to diminish the duration and severity of the pain and functional impairment. An aggressive physical therapy regimen with assisted range of motion exercises is considered to be essential in all stages of the disease, because disuse exacerbates the limitations. In addition to maintenance of range of motion, management should focus on pain reduction; analgesics and NSAIDs are important, and there is evidence that *intra-articular* glucocorticoid injection may be beneficial in adhesive capsulitis.[55] Arthrography with distention of the capsule may also yield short-term functional improvement and pain relief.[57] In refractory cases, manipulation under general anesthesia has long been used; however, this procedure may be complicated by rupture of the inferior capsule.

Neurovascular and Miscellaneous Causes

The presence of neurologic symptoms such as peripheral neuropathies, paresthesias, or neck pain suggests neurovascular compromise. In such cases, thoracic outlet syndrome, brachial plexus involvement, and cervical causes should be considered. Patients with prominent constitutional complaints associated with pain in their shoulder, for example, fatigue, generalized weakness, or myofascial pain, may have a chronic pain syndrome, such as fibromyalgia, but other conditions, including reflex sympathetic dystrophy and polymyalgia rheumatic, should also be considered. Furthermore, pain emanating from the heart, as in angina, or from the superior abdomen, as in hepatitis or cholecystitis, can be referred to the shoulder and felt as shoulder pain. Examination of the shoulder in each of these cases is often normal.

REGIONAL DISORDERS OF THE ELBOW

CASE STUDY 9

A 61-year-old diabetic man presented with a painful left elbow of 4 days' duration. He had noted the acute onset of pain over the posterior aspect of his elbow that progressed to slightly limiting his motion. In addition, he complained of swelling around his elbow. He admitted to minor trauma to the area after hitting it against a table a few times, and noted that after it became swollen, he began to bump it repeatedly by accident. There was no referred pain or history of neuropathy, and he denied having fever or chills. He obtained moderate pain relief with ibuprofen.

Physical Examination:

The left olecranon had visible swelling and a pocket of fluid, with tenderness to palpation. There was minimal erythema and warmth, and full active and passive flexion/extension of the elbow without pain. In addition, there was full wrist flexion and extension.

Aspiration of the olecranon bursa yielded 3 mL of bloody-appearing fluid, which was negative for infection or crystals.

CASE STUDY 10

A 51-year-old man with osteoarthritis and hypertension presented with a 1-month history of right forearm pain and weakness. The pain arose gradually but was worse with activity, especially when lifting. There was no pain at rest. The pain had markedly restricted the patient's ability to lift packages and, therefore, had an impact on his employment as a postal worker. The patient denied having noticed swelling warmth, numbness, or tingling. He received moderate relief with ibuprofen and rest.

Physical Examination:

There were no obvious skin changes or swelling of the right arm, and the shoulder had full range of motion. The elbow was tender to palpation slightly distal to the lateral epicondyle. Active wrist supination, but not pronation, elicited pain at the elbow. Similarly, there was pain with extension of the wrist, which was worse with resistance. Wrist flexion was normal.

Heberden's nodes were noted at the second and third digits, but all other joints of the hands and wrists were normal, as was the neurologic examination.

CASE STUDY 11

An otherwise healthy 45-year-old man presented with right medial forearm pain that had gradual onset but had worsened over a period of 3 weeks. The pain was exacerbated by lifting heavy objects. He denied weakness or paresthesias, and had no recent trauma or injury. Other than coaching his son's baseball team, he did not participate in regular athletics.

Physical Examination:

There were no obvious skin changes or swelling of the right arm, and the shoulder had full range of motion. Pain was noted on palpation slightly distal to the medial epicondyle. In addition, wrist pronation, but not supination, was painful. There was full wrist extension, however pain was noted on flexion and was exacerbated by resistance. Examination of the hand was normal, as was the neurologic examination.

Introduction

Elbow pain may be caused by diverse sources. As with pain localizing in any anatomic site, elbow pain can be due either to local pathology or to pain referred from a distant site. When pain originates at the elbow, it may stem from intra-articular pathology or from the periarticular soft tissues. The elbow is commonly affected in rheumatoid arthritis as well as in other inflammatory arthropathies; however, it is only rarely involved without concomitant disease elsewhere. Osteoarthritis, however, only rarely involves the elbow, except after major trauma. In contrast, *periarticular disorders* of the elbow are common because of the frequent demands on the forearm muscles and the poor soft tissue protection around the elbows. As in any rheumatologic assessment, careful distinction must be made between an articular, periarticular, osseous or neurological source of pain. After considering the history and physical examination, a reasonably directed differential diagnosis can be generated as illustrated in Table 25-3.

Table 25-3. *Differential Diagnoses of Elbow Pain*

Articular disease
   Inflammatory arthropathy (e.g., rheumatoid arthritis)
   Crystalline arthropathy (e.g., gout, pseudogout)
   Infectious arthritis
   Joint neoplasm
   Osteochondritis and loose bodies
Periarticular disease
   Lateral epicondylitis
   Medial epicondylitis
   Olecranon bursitis
Neurovascular and entrapment neuropathy
   Cubital tunnel syndrome
   Pronator teres syndrome
   Radial tunnel syndrome
Referred and miscellaneous
   Cervical radiculopathy
   Shoulder disease
   Reflex sympathetic dystrophy

Monoarthritis and the systemic arthritides affecting the elbow are discussed in separate chapters; hence, this discussion focuses on *periarticular pathology*, which represents the most frequent source of isolated elbow pain. In general, the periarticular soft tissues are frequently affected by overuse due to repetitive occupational or recreational activity. Case Study 9 is a description of olecranon bursitis. The olecranon bursa, located superficially at the extensor angle of the olecranon, is poorly protected by overlying tissue, and thus susceptible to irritation and inflammation. Although the olecranon bursa can be inflamed due to discrete trauma or to infection, bursitis most frequently has insidious onset related to overuse or to an idiopathic etiology. Traumatic olecranon bursitis may result from an acute injury or from repetitive minor trauma, such as frequent leaning on hard surfaces or from striking objects, as occurred to the patient in Case Study 9. In addition, although Case Study 9 appeared to be trauma-related bursitis, it is imperative to exclude septic bursitis before ascribing the inflamed olecranon bursa to trauma; this is especially important in patients who are immunocompromised, have diabetes, or have evidence of systemic symptoms. Case 10 is an example of lateral epicondylitis, so-called "tennis elbow," which typically results from cumulative overuse and mechanical loading of the component of the common extensor tendon derived from the extensor carpi radialis brevi. This muscle is a powerful wrist extensor that is activated to provide hand grip strength. During a power grip, the wrist is in forced extension, which, in turn, produces significant traction at the insertion of the proximal tendon on the lateral epicondyle. Repeated tasks, such as lifting heavy objects, gardening, or classically, playing tennis, may inflame the site of tendon insertion, thereby causing pain. Of note, this process is believed to be degenerative, rather than inflammatory; histological studies have demonstrated a consistent pattern of tissue degeneration with fibroblast and microvascular hyperplasia, but without the presence of inflammatory cells,[58] and in light of the absence of inflammation, some authors have suggested that this condition be referred to as lateral tendinosis, instead of tendonitis,[59] although that appellation is rarely used. Case Study 11 represents medial epicondylitis, so-called "golfer's elbow." This overuse syndrome results from repetitive strain of the portion of the common flexor tendon of the forearm that is derived from the pronator teres and flexor carpi radialis muscles. These muscles are involved in both forearm pronation and wrist flexion. Although medial epicondylitis is less common than lateral epicondylitis,[60] it may be as painful and disabling. Medial epicondylitis typically results from recreational activities, such as swimming, baseball pitching or golfing, or occupationally if repetitive activities with hammers or screwdrivers are required.

Clinical History and Symptoms

The swelling associated with olecranon bursitis can develop either acutely or insidiously, depending on the etiology. Pain is variable but in cases due to acute injury or infection, it can be intense. There is often a report of a "lump" that is tender when touched or bumped against surfaces. In lateral epicondylitis, there is typically a gradual onset of pain in the lateral elbow and forearm during activities that involve wrist extension such as lifting, turning a screwdriver, or hitting a backhand in tennis; as the condition progresses, patients may report pain at rest as well. The pain is usually described as being localized to the lateral epicondyle, although occasionally it may radiate throughout the arm. In contrast, medial epicondylitis typically results in pain over the medial epicondyle, which is exacerbated by wrist flexion and forearm pronation. At times, the patient may have difficulty shaking hands. Ulnar neuropathy may coexist with medial epicondylitis, and a history of paresthesias of the fourth and fifth fingers should be sought.

Physical Examination of the Elbow

Inspection is an especially important component of the physical examination of the elbow because of the relative paucity of overlying soft tissue; hence, alterations of the bony anatomy and soft tissue swelling are often apparent visually. Laterally, a synovial effusion can be detected as fullness in the region of the lateral infracondylar recess. Posteriorly, swelling of the olecranon bursa, as in Case Study 9, or the presence of nodules as in rheumatoid arthritis or tophaceous gout can be detected. Similarly, *palpation* provides abundant information about the superficial structures of the elbow. Attention is focused on the lateral and medial epicondyles and the olecranon tip, and the associated bursae. The olecranon bursa, immediately adjacent to the olecranon, develops tenderness and a boggy mass with olecranon bursitis; in such cases, the dimensions of the bursa can be quantified and monitored to document response to therapy. Tenderness in the region of the lateral epicondyle, as illustrated by Case Study 10, indicates lateral epicondylitis. There is often point tenderness, and at times warmth and swelling, at the origin of the common extensor tendon, approximately 1 cm distally, and the condition is typically accompanied by an aching discomfort in the proximal forearm. In contrast, medial epicondylitis presents with tenderness at the medial epicondyle as well as point tenderness just distal to the epicondyle.

Assessment of mobility of the elbow includes active and passive ranges of motion in flexion, extension, and rotation. The normal range of flexion-extension is 0 to 160 degrees, and it is flexion-extension that is typically affected first in range of motion restrictions due to intra-articular pathology; rotational restrictions generally occur only in advanced disease. In contrast, the most frequent source of reduced range of motion is pain rather

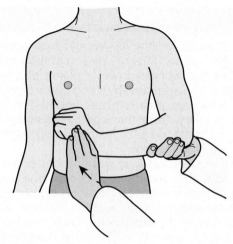

Figure 25-11. Resisted wrist extension test for lateral epicondylitis.

than structural pathology. As with all rheumatologic examinations, passive range of motion tends to be unaffected with periarticular conditions. In olecranon bursitis (Case Study 9), as well as with lateral (Case Study 10) and medial epicondylitis (Case Study 11), complete active and passive range of motion at the elbow tend to be maintained, although there is pain with forced rotation (see later).

Special tests for lateral epicondylitis include
1. Resisted wrist extension: the elbow is placed in full extension, and forced dorsiflexion of the wrist against resistance causes pain when lateral epicondylitis is present (Fig. 25-11).
2. Chair-lift: with the elbow extended and the forearm and hand pronated, the patient lifts a chair; the presence of lateral epicondylitis results in sharp pain at the lateral epicondyle.
3. Resisted supination of the forearm, with the elbow passively at 90 degrees.

Special test for medial epicondylitis: Resisted pronation of the forearm, followed by resisted flexion of the wrist (with the elbow extended) causes pain at the medial epicondyle with medial epicondylitis (Fig. 25-12). It should be remembered that ulnar neuropathy may frequently co-exist with medial epicondylitis, as the ulnar nerve passes through the medial epicondylar notch; therefore attention should be given to potential signs of ulnar neuropathy, such as decreased sensation of the fourth and fifth fingers or weakness of the intrinsic muscles of those digits.

Diagnostic Evaluation

The diagnosis of periarticular etiologies of elbow pain is typically determined solely on the basis of the clinical presentation. Radiography is useful only to evaluate for coexistent articular disease or after trauma to assess bone integrity. In the case of olecranon bursitis, aspiration of the bursa is of both diagnostic and therapeutic value; analysis of the synovial fluid for cells, crystals, Gram's stain, and culture may reveal an underlying infectious or metabolic etiology; similarly,

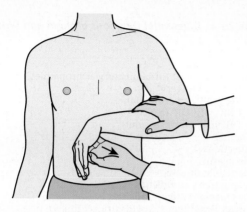

Figure 25-12. Resisted wrist flexion test for medial epicondylitis.

hemorrhagic-appearing aspirates are common in cases of acute or repetitive injury. It is important to maintain a high index of suspicion for septic bursitis in patients who are immunocompromised as well as those with chronic diseases, such as diabetes; in such cases, *Staphylococcus aureus* is the most common organism isolated, followed by *Staphylococcus epidermidis*.[61]

In cases of lateral and medial epicondylitis, other conditions which may mimic condylitis need to be considered. Cervical radiculopathy (see Regional Disorders of the Neck), can produce pain referred to the forearm. Entrapment of the peripheral radial nerve results in radial tunnel syndrome causing lateral arm pain similar to that of lateral epicondylitis, but may be distinguished by the location of the maximal tenderness—4 to 5 cm distal to the lateral epicondyle in radial tunnel syndrome versus 1 cm distally in lateral epicondylitis—and by the maneuvers that elicit pain—resisted thumb and index finger extension in the former versus resisted wrist extension in the latter.[62] Cubital tunnel syndrome is a nerve entrapment syndrome of the ulnar nerve at the groove between the medial epicondyle and the olecranon; the overlying collateral ligament and retinaculum compress the cubital tunnel during elbow flexion, and this may result in neuropathy due to repeated local trauma, constriction, or chronic pressure over the ulnar groove. Although there may be local pain at the medial epicondyle, this syndrome typically presents with paresthesias of the lateral forearm, wrist, and fourth and fifth fingers; hypothenar atrophy may develop if the entrapment becomes chronic.

Management

Therapeutic approaches to periarticular elbow conditions are similar to treatment of soft tissue pathology elsewhere in the body. Treatment for olecranon bursitis depends on the etiology and the severity. In septic bursitis, the bursa is generally aspirated both for diagnosis and for drainage, followed by appropriate antibiotic coverage,[63] although in contrast to septic arthritis, a course of oral antibiotics is generally sufficient. Bursectomy is rarely required, but

may be necessary if the infection fails to resolve or if chronic bursitis persists.[64] For mildly symptomatic bursitis that is not infected, treatment tends to be conservative, with anti-inflammatory medications and activity modification, as appropriate. Large-volume bursitis may respond to a compression bandage, after exclusion of infectious etiologies. If pain is persistent, or if bursal fluid reaccumulates, then glucocorticoid injection of the bursal sac, after aspiration, is often effective. Elbow protection, such as elbow pads, are indicated in cases of bursitis related to occupational or recreational repetitive trauma.

Lateral and medial epicondylitis are managed similarly. Initial conservative therapy consists of reducing repetitive trauma and altering activities that overuse the forearm muscles. Anti-inflammatory medications have been shown to be useful for short-term relief,[65] and adjunctive ice (or heat) and forearm braces or bands are widely considered to be useful, although supportive data are limited.[66] If initial conservative management is insufficient, glucocorticoid injection into the area of maximal tenderness has been demonstrated to be more effective than placebo,[65,67] though it is generally recommended to limit this approach to three injections. Physical therapy is widely recommended, and typically includes assisted gentle stretching and forearm strengthening exercises; manipulation and deep friction massage are also used.[58] Other modalities that may be tried include laser therapy, topical medications, and acupuncture[58]; extracorporeal shock wave therapy, however, has been demonstrated to be ineffective for this indication.[67] Surgery is recommended only after conservative management has failed.

REGIONAL DISORDERS OF THE HAND AND WRIST

CASE STUDY 12

A 74-year-old woman with a 25-year history of rheumatoid arthritis, osteoarthritis, asthma, hypertension, and atrial fibrillation presented with reports that her right third finger locks suddenly, preventing her from fully opening her hand. She noticed some swelling of this finger during the previous 4 days and some pain, especially in the mornings. There was no history of recent injury, and the rheumatoid arthritis had been well controlled.

Physical Examination:

Examination of the right hand revealed mild ulnar deviation and palmar subluxation of the metacarpophalangeal (MCP) joints, as well as Heberden's nodes of the third and fourth distal interphalangeal (DIP) joints, but there was no synovitis. There was point tenderness of the palm at the third MCP joint. A small mobile nodule was palpated, which appeared to move in conjunction with the tendon during passive flexion and extension of the third digit. Full extension of the third finger was inhibited.

CASE STUDY 13

A 46-year-old man with sickle cell anemia, hypertension, and hypothyroidism presented with a 2-month history of pain of his left wrist. He denied antecedent trauma or injury. The pain, not present at rest, occurred with lifting or when making a fist. There was a subjective sensation of mild swelling but no warmth. Radiography performed by his internist was reportedly unremarkable.

Physical Examination:

There was linear tenderness and swelling of the dorsal left wrist that extended from the radial styloid to the base of the thumb. Pain and mild crepitus were noted when the thumb was flexed and extended. Finkelstein's test was positive.

CASE STUDY 14

A 55-year-old hypertensive man presented with tightness and swelling in his hands that he thought may have started over a year previously. He also reported that for the past 2 months he had been unable to fully extend his right ring finger, and this had interfered with his ability to do many tasks. He denied pain or numbness, and there was no history of trauma or injury.

Physical Examination:

Both hands revealed minimal swelling but slightly thickened palmar fascia. Prominent dimpling of the palmar surface near the flexor crease of the right 4th finger was noted, and a painful small nodule was palpable.

CASE STUDY 15

A 36-year-old otherwise healthy primigravid pregnant woman at 30 weeks' gestation presented with aching pain and numbness of both hands. Initially, the numbness occurred only at night and often woke her up; however, it gradually progressed to include daytime symptoms as well, especially while she was driving. The patient reported having symptoms in all fingers, worse in the thumbs and index fingers. She had no paresthesias elsewhere. The pregnancy was otherwise uncomplicated.

Physical Examination:

Both hands exhibited mild generalized swelling. No thenar atrophy was present. Phalen's and Tinel's signs were present.

Introduction

The hand and wrist are critical organs that are uniquely designed for sensory and fine motor activities. For adequate function, a complex interplay between the joints, muscles, and tendons is necessary, and any deviation from normal can lead

Table 25-4. *Differential Diagnosis of Hand and Wrist Pain*

Articular disease
  Arthritis of wrist (inflammatory arthropathies, e.g., RA)
  Arthritis of fingers
    MCP, PIP (e.g., RA, gout)
    CMC, PIP, DIP (e.g., OA)
    DIP (e.g., psoriasis, gout)
  Trauma
  Infectious
  Neoplasm
Periarticular disease
  Dupuytren's contracture
  De Quervain's tenosynovitis
  Finger flexor tenosynovitis (trigger finger)
  Carpal tunnel syndrome
  Synovial cysts (ganglion cysts)
Neurovascular disease
  Carpal tunnel syndrome
  Pronator teres syndrome
  Cubital tunnel syndrome
  Raynaud's phenomenon
  Vasculitis
  Lower brachial plexus (thoracic outlet)
  Cervical radiculopathy
Referred and miscellaneous
  Cervical spine lesions
  Spinal tumors
  Reflex sympathetic dystrophy
  Angina

CMC, carpometacarpal; DIP, distal interphalangeal; MCP, metacarpophalangeal; OA, osteoarthritis; PIP, proximal interphalangeal; RA, rheumatoid arthritis.

to significant pain and functional disability. The differential diagnosis of pain and loss of hand or wrist function includes a wide variety of etiologies, and as with all musculoskeletal issues, can be divided into articular, periarticular, or neurovascular processes, or pain may be referred from more proximal structures such as the elbow, shoulder or cervical spine. Table 25-4 provides a brief list of differential diagnoses to consider in individuals presenting with hand or wrist complaints. The focus of this section is regional disorders of the hand and wrist; disorders related to systemic inflammatory processes or isolated pathology are addressed elsewhere.

Tenosynovitis

Tenosynovitis, or inflammation of the synovial sheath that lines the tendon, is common in areas of repetitive use and may affect any of the tendons of the forearm and hand. However, because of the mechanics of the hand and the demands of modern society, a few tendon sheaths are especially prone to inflammation. Examples include trigger finger (Case 12) and de Quervain's tenosynovitis (Case 13). In addition to overuse and idiopathic etiologies, tenosynovitis may be precipitated by a variety of systemic inflammatory conditions, including rheumatoid arthritis, systemic lupus erythematosus, scleroderma, psoriatic arthritis, reactive arthritis, infection, crystalline arthropathy, amyloidosis, sarcoidosis and pigmented villonodular tenosynovitis.[68]

Flexor digital tenosynovitis or "trigger finger" is often idiopathic, but may also be secondary to the conditions mentioned earlier. Regardless of the cause, chronic inflammation impairs the lubricating function of the synovial sheath of the first annular pulley overlying the MCP joint.[69] This results in a fibrotic reaction of the tendon sheath and, consequently, friction during the sliding motion of the tendon in flexion. As a result, there is pain at the involved finger and impaired mobility of the tendon, resulting in triggering of the finger. Flexor digital tenosynovitis is often restricted to a single digit; the fingers involved, in order of decreasing incidence, are the thumb, ring, middle, little, and index finger. However, when due to chronic inflammatory conditions such as rheumatoid arthritis, simultaneous involvement of multiple fingers is typical.[70] With trigger finger, there is typically a sensation of "catching" upon flexion of the involved finger, along with pain; this sensation is often described by patients as "locking" or "snapping," and may be worse in the morning and associated with swelling and stiffness. In severe cases, the finger may actually be "locked" in the palm. Often, a small lump that moves with flexion and extension of the finger is described in the palm. Physical examination reveals linear tenderness in the palm, and sometimes a palpable nodule at the level of the proximal A1 pulley at the MCP joint. In addition, with passive flexion and extension of the involved finger, locking and tendon crepitus may be appreciated. Typically, resisted movement is painful at the site of tendon inflammation, and the pain may radiate to the proximal interphalangeal joints or to the dorsal aspect of the digit. Full flexion and extension of the involved finger may be impaired.

Occasionally, flexor digital tenosynovitis may progress to stenosing tenosynovitis, with progressive fibrosis of the tendon sheath, interrupting the normal gliding motion of the tendons.[71] This results in "locking" or "catching" of the tendon as it glides through the retinaculum, and may represent an early phase of the spectrum of Dupuytren's contracture, wherein fibrosis and contracture of the palmar fascia result in a flexion deformity of the involved digits, especially the fourth and fifth.

De Quervain's tenosynovitis (Case Study 13) is swelling or stenosis of the tendon sheath of the abductor pollicis longus and extensor pollicis brevis tendons as they pass through the extensor retinaculum of the wrist, which results in pain of the lateral aspect of the wrist and base of the thumb during forced traction across these tendons. This condition is associated with repetitive activity, classically pinching or grasping with the thumb while moving the wrist radially or ulnarly. Although the pathophysiology is poorly understood, repetitive activity may create friction and traumatize the tendon sheath, causing a local inflammatory reaction

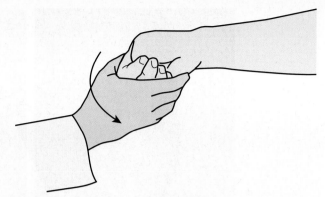

Figure 25-13. Finkelstein test. This test is performed by placing the patient's thumb in full flexion into the palm with the other four fingers flexed over it; if de Quervain's tenosynovitis is present, passive ulnar deviation of the wrist reproduces the pain at the distal radius over the radial styloid.

and subsequent fibrotic reaction during attempted healing. Primary idiopathic de Quervain's tenosynovitis typically occurs in middle aged women,[72] though it is also associated with rheumatoid arthritis, psoriatic arthritis, direct trauma, pregnancy and the postpartum period.[70,73] Characteristically, pain is felt on the radial aspect of the wrist, and at the base of the thumb, and is exacerbated by lifting or grasping; this may be associated with mild swelling. Physical examination reveals swelling and tenderness over the tendons in the first extensor compartment in the region of distal radius, with pain on flexion and extension of the thumb. The *Finklestein* test was described as a diagnostic test for de Quervain's tenosynovitis (Fig. 25-13). This test is performed by placing the patient's thumb in full flexion into the palm, with the other four fingers flexed over it; if de Quervain's tenosynovitis is present, passive ulnar deviation of the wrist reproduces the pain at the distal radius over the radial styloid.

Management of Flexor Digital Tenosynovitis and de Quervain's Tenosynovitis

Both flexor digital tenosynovitis and de Quervain's tenosynovitis are diagnosed on the basis of the clinical presentation, and extensive diagnostic testing or imaging is only useful to exclude other diagnoses. Initial treatment goals, as with other periarticular regional disorders, are to reduce swelling, inflammation, and pain. This includes immobilization via splinting, activity modification, NSAIDs and steroid injections. Extension splinting of the affected digit in tenosynovitis at night prevents painful flexion during sleep. For de Quervain's tenosynovitis, a radial gutter or thumb spica splint (Fig. 25-14) can be used to immobilize

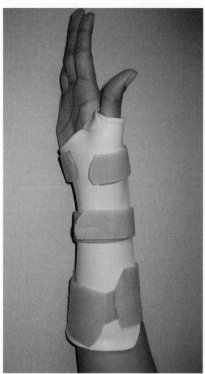
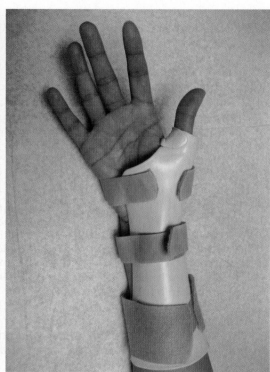

Figure 25-14. Thumb spica splint for de Quervain's tenosynovitis.

the wrist in slight extension and radial deviation to decrease pressure on the tendons of the abductor pollicis longus and extensor pollicis brevis. Nevertheless, corticosteroid injections, with special care not to inject into the tendon itself, have emerged as the mainstay of management for these conditions. The efficacy of corticosteroid injections has been well established in several controlled trials for trigger finger[74-76] and for de Quervain's tenosynovitis.[77,78] Moreover, a retrospective evaluation of steroid injections compared with splinting with anti-inflammatory medications suggested that steroids yielded a significantly better outcome.[79] Some practitioners consider long-acting steroid preparations to be superior to shorter acting steroids, and betamethasone, methylprednisolone, and triamcinolone are each widely used.[80] There is evidence that a history of symptoms of greater than 4 to 6 months and an increased number of injections are associated with a diminished response to corticosteroids,[81] which may be related to fibrocartilaginous metaplasia that develops over time and that is refractory to corticosteroid treatment. The decision to repeat injections or to refer for surgery is case based, and involves a thorough evaluation and discussion of medical comorbidities, disability caused by the condition, and risk of surgical complications. Patients with tenosynovitis related to rheumatoid arthritis, as in Case Study 12, have an increased risk of tendon rupture, and this risk is exacerbated by multiple injections; thus, if relief is not obtained after a single injection, early surgical referral may be indicated.

Dupuytren's Disease

Dupuytren's disease, Case 14, is a fibrotic process characterized by thickening of the palmar fascia, usually accompanied by cord-like structures that extend from the palm into the affected fingers causing contractures of the metacarpophalangeal and proximal interphalangeal joints. The fibrosis is due to fibroblast proliferation and myofibroblast differentiation, with excessive collagen and matrix elaboration resulting in thickening of the palmar fascia, contractures, nodules and cords.[82,83] The etiology of Dupuytren's disease is poorly understood. There is a strong male predominance (approximately nine to one), although later in life, the incidence in women approaches that of men.[84] Age, geography and ethnic origin may also influence disease prevalence, and there is strong evidence for a genetic predisposition[85]; however, inflammation, trauma, and neoplasia may serve as triggering events. Long-standing diabetes is strongly associated with a process similar to Dupuytren's disease, termed diabetic cheiroarthropathy, though the pathophysiology of cheiroarthropathy appears to differ from Dupuytren's and the disease course is typically mild.[86] Epidemiologic studies suggest that the disease is common in Scandinavia, Great Britain, Ireland, Australia, and North America; uncommon in Southern Europe and South America; and rare in Africa and China.[87]

Dupuytren's tenosynovitis typically presents in men older than 40 years and women older than 50 years; disease in younger patients is often more aggressive and may affect sites beyond the palms, including multiple digits and full palm involvement, the plantar fascia (*Ledderhouse's disease*), and the penis (*Peyronie's disease*).[88] The classic presentation of Dupuytren's tenosynovitis, however, is bilateral nodular thickening of the palm with or without contractures of the metacarpophalangeal or proximal interphalangeal joints. The ring finger is the most commonly involved, followed in order by the little finger, the thumb, the middle finger, and the index finger.[88] In patients with diabetes, studies have noted a higher involvement of the ring and middle fingers.[86]

The diagnosis of Dupuytren's is based on the clinical history and physical examination. Examination reveals characteristic palmar fascial thickening, often with skin dimpling due to retraction. Dupuytren's nodules are firm, fixed soft tissue masses either in the palm or in the involved digits; palmar nodules may be palpated adjacent to the distal palmar crease, typically directly proximal to the ring or little finger, whereas digital nodules are usually adjacent to the proximal interphalangeal joints or at the base of the digit. The nodules are often painless but may become painful as they enlarge or if they stimulate an inflammatory reaction in the tendon sheath resulting in stenosing tenosynovitis.[89] Finally, care should be taken to avoid confusing Dupuytren's nodules with other soft tissue processes, such as palmar synovial cysts, callus formations, or pigmented villonodular synovitis.[89]

Management of Dupuytren's Disease

Treatment is primarily aimed at minimizing functional loss. Stretching exercises of the hands and strategies to reduce palmar pressure, such as using padded tools and utensils, may be generally helpful. Cases limited to asymptomatic Dupuytren's nodules or with stable disease and minimal contractures are generally observed without intervention,[88,89] unless the nodules are tender. In such cases, corticosteroids may be injected; however, the efficacy of such injections for this indication is controversial. Novel nonsurgical interventions have generally been disappointing when subjected to controlled trials, and there are currently no treatments that have been demonstrated to interfere with the natural history of the disease; one promising approach is the injection of collagenase, which has appeared to reduce contractures and finger cords in preliminary trials.[90,91] Nevertheless, surgery remains the mainstay of therapy for Dupuytren's contractures that cause significant functional loss. Some clinicians believe that flexion contractures of the metacarpophalangeal joint of more than 30 degrees and of the proximal interphalangeal joint of more than 15 degrees are associated with sufficient dysfunction as to be indications for surgery[89]; however, postoperative recurrences are frequent,[92,93] and surgery is often deferred until absolutely necessary for functional reasons.

Carpal Tunnel Syndrome

Carpal tunnel syndrome (CTS), Case Study 15, is the most common compression neuropathy in the upper extremity, and it occurs when the median nerve is entrapped by the flexor retinaculum at the wrist. This results in pain, weakness and paresthesias in the distribution of the median nerve. Acute CTS is rare, but may occur following trauma, infection, hemorrhage or high pressure injection[94]; in contrast, chronic CTS is common and results from a variety of etiologies, which have been categorized as idiopathic, anatomic, systemic, or exertional.[95] The majority of CTS cases are idiopathic. Women are affected more frequently than men, and incidence increases with aging.[96] CTS can also be caused by space occupying lesions or anatomic anomalies in the carpal canal that cause median nerve entrapment; these include masses, such as synovial cysts, lipomas, or hemangiomas; vascular lesions, such as a thrombosed median artery; or post-traumatic problems like edema, scarring, or hemorrhage.[95] CTS is associated with a large number of systemic conditions, including diabetes, obesity, alcoholism, hypothyroidism, rheumatoid arthritis, primary amyloidosis, and renal failure,[97,98] and is common during all phases of otherwise uncomplicated pregnancy, with resolution after delivery.[99] The etiology in pregnancy is likely related to edema within the carpal tunnel, causing mechanical nerve compression.[100] Finally, exertional causes of CTS have been attributed to repetitive use of the wrists and digits, such as constant computer keyboard use, as well as to repeated impact on the palm, or the operation of vibratory tools.[101,102]

As illustrated by Case Study 15, CTS typically presents with complaints of numbness, burning pain and often nocturnal paresthesias in the thumb and one or more of the radial fingers. Daytime symptoms are often provoked by activities that involve prolonged wrist flexion or holding the wrist in a stationary position, as in driving or reading. Individuals with longstanding CTS can develop persistent hypesthesia, loss of finger dexterity, and thenar wasting causing grip and pinch weakness.[95] Physical examination includes inspection of both hands for evidence of skin changes and atrophy of the thenar and interosseous muscles. As median nerve entrapment may be mimicked by central processes, the physical examination should include complete neurological assessment. Active and passive motion of the cervical spine, shoulders, wrists and hands of both extremities should all be normal, as should strength in the upper extremity muscle groups, unless there is coexistent pathology such as rheumatoid or cervical radiculopathy. In contrast, strength of thumb opposition with the index finger (pinch strength) is often diminished in CTS.

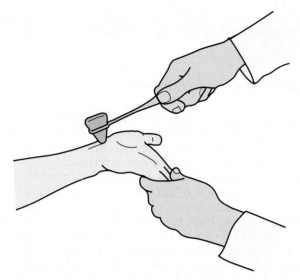

Figure 25-15. Tinel's sign for carpal tunnel syndrome is elicited by gently tapping on the median nerve at the carpal tunnel with a reflex hammer or with the examiner's finger. The sign is present if the patient feels paresthesias in the thumb and one or more radial fingers.

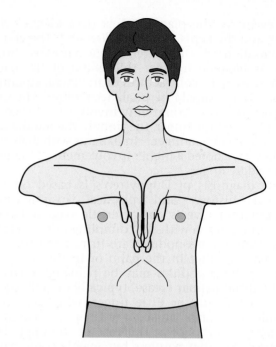

Figure 25-16. Phalen's test for carpal tunnel syndrome is performed by having the patient place the wrists in sustained palmar flexion; paresthesias felt in the distribution of the median nerve within 60 seconds are considered a positive test result.

Specific provocation tests for CTS are not highly sensitive or specific, but when combined with other clinical clues, they may be useful. *Tinel's sign* (Fig. 25-15) is elicited by gently tapping on the median nerve at the carpal tunnel with either a reflex hammer or the examiner's finger; it is present if the patient feels paresthesias in the thumb and one or more radial fingers. *Phalen's test* (Fig. 25-16) is performed by having the patient place the wrists in sustained palmar flexion; a positive test requires the patient to feel paresthesias in the distribution of the median nerve within 60 seconds.

The diagnosis of CTS, like other regional disorders of the hand and wrist, is largely dependent on the clinical history and examination; diagnostic imaging is useful to assess potential secondary causes such as inflammatory arthropathy, but not for uncomplicated idiopathic CTS. Electrodiagnostic testing, electromyography with measurement of nerve conduction velocities, is often not clinically necessary but may be helpful to confirm or to exclude the diagnosis of CTS, and may be useful in guiding the course of treatment.[103]

Management of Carpal Tunnel Syndrome
The primary treatment for CTS includes modification of exacerbating activity, nocturnal splinting with neutral wrist splints (Fig. 25-17), and control of inflammation by the use of NSAIDs; if primary treatment is insufficient, then corticosteroids are generally injected into the carpal tunnel. There are an assortment of options when prescribing wrist splints including neutral versus extension (cock-up) splints, nighttime versus full-time use of the splints, and custom-fabricated versus mass-manufactured splints.[104] Systematic reviews of controlled trials of conservative therapy for CTS suggest that there is strong evidence for the use of local or oral corticosteroids, moderate evidence that splints are effective, and limited or conflicting evidence that NSAIDs, diuretics, yoga, laser or ultrasound are effective.[105,106] In addition, one small randomized controlled trial that compared nocturnal-only to full-time use of neutral splints in patients with CTS reported that there may be a slight advantage at 6 weeks to full-time use, although patients in each group improved.[107] Patients who do not obtain adequate relief with conservative therapy may be candidates for surgical decompression. Surgery has been reported to be more effective for the sustained relief of CTS symptoms than either corticosteroid injections[108] or splinting alone.[109]

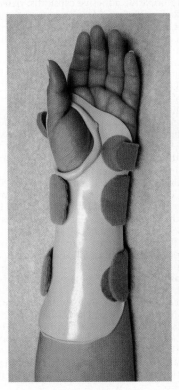
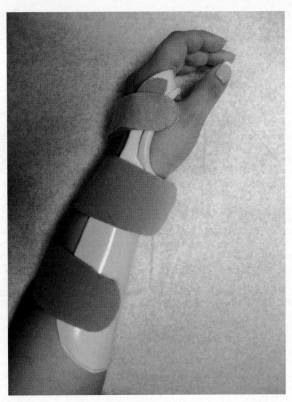

Figure 25-17. A neutral wrist splint positioned to treat carpal tunnel syndrome.

References

1. Bogduk N, Mercer S. Biomechanics of the cervical spine. I: Normal kinematics. Clin Biomech 2000;15:633-48.
2. Van Mameren H, Drukker J, Sanches H, Beursgens J. Cervical spine motion in the sagittal plane (I) range of motion of actually performed movements, an X-ray cinematographic study. Eur J Morphol 1990;28:47-68.
3. Amevo B, Aprill C, Bogduk N. Abnormal instantaneous axes of rotation in patients with neck pain. Spine 1992;17:748-56.
4. Kelley LA. In neck to neck competition are women more fragile? Clin Orthop Rel Res 2000;372:123-30.
5. Barnsley L, Lord S, Bogduk N. Whiplash injury [see comment]. Pain 1994;58:283-307.
6. Rodriguez AA, Barr KP, Burns P. Whiplash: Pathophysiology, diagnosis, treatment, and prognosis. Muscle Nerve 2008;29:768-81.
7. Binder AI. Cervical spondylosis and neck pain. BMJ 2007;334:527-31.
8. Rao RD, Currier BL, Albert TJ, Bono CM, Marawar SV, Poelstra KA, et al. Degenerative cervical spondylosis: clinical syndromes, pathogenesis, and management. J Bone Joint Surg [Am] 2007;89:1360-78.
9. Boden SD, McCowin PR, Davis DO, Dina TS, Mark AS, Wiesel S. Abnormal magnetic-resonance scans of the cervical spine in asymptomatic subjects. A prospective investigation. J Bone Joint Surg [Am] 1990;72:1178-84.
10. Freedman MK, Overton EA, Saulino MF, Holding MY, Kornbluth ID. Interventions in chronic pain management. 2. Diagnosis of cervical and thoracic pain syndromes. Arch Phys Med Rehabil 2008;89(Suppl. 1):S41-6.
11. Simons DG, Travell JG, Simons LS. Travell and Simon's Myofascial Pain and Dysfunction: The Trigger Point Manual, 2nd ed. Baltimore: Williams & Wilkins; 1999.
12. Bliddal H, Danneskiold-Samsoe B. Chronic widespread pain in the spectrum of rheumatological diseases. Best Pract Res Clin Rheumatol 2007;21:391-402.
13. Bendtsen L, Jensen R, Olsen J. Qualitatively altered nociception in chronic myofascial pain. Pain 1996;65:259-64.
14. Borg-Stein J, Simons DG. Focused review: myofascial pain. Arch Phys Med Rehabil 2002;83(Suppl. 1):S40-7, S48-9.
15. Krayback B, Borg-Stein J, Oas J, Dumais D. Reduced dizziness and pain with treatment of cervical myofascial pain. Arch Phys Med Rehabil 1996;77:939-40.
16. Bogduk N. Regional musculoskeletal pain. The neck. Best Pract Res Clin Rheumatol 1999;13:261-85.
17. Rao RD. Neck pain, cervical radiculopathy and cervical myelopathy. Pathophysiology, natural history and clinical evaluation. J Bone Joint Surg 2002;84:1872-81.
18. Cloward RB. Diaphragm paralysis from cervical disc lesions. Br J Neurosurg 1988;2:395-9.
19. Brown BM, Schwartz RH, Frank E, Blank NK. Preoperative evaluation of cervical radiculopathy and myelopathy by surface-coil MR imaging. Am J Roentgenol 1988;151:1205-12.
20. Teresi LM, Lufkin RB, Reicher MA. Asymptomatic degenerative disk disease and spondylosis of the cervical spine; MR imaging. Radiology 1987;164:83-8.
21. Modic MT, Masaryk TJ, Mulopulos GP, Bundschuh C, Han JS, Bohlman H. Cervical radiculopathy: prospective evaluation with surface coil MR imaging, CT with metrizamide, and metrizamide myelography. Radiology 1986;161:753-9.
22. Hou C, Tsai L, Cheng K, Chung K, Hong C. Immediate effects of various physical therapeutic modalities on cervical myofascial pain and trigger point sensitivity. Arch Phys Med Rehabil 2002;83:1406-14.
23. Wheeler AH. Myofascial pain disorders: theory to therapy. Drugs 2004;64:45-62.
24. Argoff CE, Wheeler AH. Spinal and radicular pain disorders. Neurol Clin 1998;4:833-49.
25. Hanten WP, Olson SL, Butts NL, Nowicki AL. Effectiveness of a home program of ischemic pressure followed by sustained stretch for treatment of myofascial trigger points. Phys Ther 2000;80:997-1003.

26. Graff-Radford SB, Reeves JL, Jaeger B. Management of chronic headache and neck pain: effectiveness of altering factors perpetuating myofascial pain. Headache 1987;127:186-90.

27. Cheshire WP, Abashian SW, Mann JD. Botulinum toxin in the treatment of myofascial pain. Pain 1994;59:65-9.

28. Wheeler AH, Goolkasian P, Gretz SS. A randomized, double-blinded, prospective pilot study of botulinum toxin injection for refractory, unilateral, cervicothoracic, paraspinal, myofascial pain syndrome. Spine 2009;23:1662-6.

29. Berman BM, Ezzo J, Hadhazy V, Swyers JP. Is acupuncture effective in the treatment of fibromyalgia? J Fam Pract 1999;48:213-8.

30. Peeters GC, Verhagen AP, De Bie RA, Oostendorp RA. The efficacy of conservative treatment in patients with whiplash injury: a systemic review of clinical trials. Spine 2001;26:64-73.

31. Sterner Y, Gerdle B. Acute and chronic whiplash disorders—a review. J Rehabil Med 2004;36:193-209; quiz 210.

32. Lord SM, Barnsley L, Wallis BJ, McDonald GJ, Bogduk N. Percutaneous radio-frequency neurotomy for chronic cervical zygoapophyseal-joint pain. N Engl J Med 1996;335:1721-6.

33. Barnsley L, Lord SM, Wallis BJ, Bogduk N. Lack of effect of intraarticular corticosteroids for chronic pain in the cervical zygoapophyseal joints. N Engl J Med 1994;330:1047-50.

34. Gore DR, Sepic SB, Gardner GM, Murray MP. Neck pain: A long term followup of 205 patients. Spine 1987;12:1-5.

35. Bush K, Hillier S. Outcome of cervical radiculopathy treated with periradicular/epidural corticosteroid injections: a prospective study with independent clinical review. Eur Spine J 1996;5:319-25.

36. Chiu TT, Lam TH, Hedley AJ. A randomized controlled trial on the efficacy of exercise for patients with chronic neck pain. Spine 2005;30:1-7.

37. Van der Heijden GJ, Beurskens AJ, Koes BW, Assendelft WJ, de Vet HC, Bouter LM. The efficacy of traction for back and neck pain: a systemic blinded review of randomized clinical trial methods. Phys Ther 1995;75:93-104.

38. White AR, Ernst E. A systemic review of randomized controlled trials of acupuncture for neck pain. J Rheumatol 1999;38:143-7.

39. Koester MC, George MS, Kuhn JE. Shoulder impingement syndrome. Am J Med 2005;118:452-5.

40. Silva L, Andreu JL, Munoz P, Pastrana M, Millan I, Sanz J, et al. Accuracy of physical examination in subacromial impingement syndrome. Rheumatology 2008;47:679-83.

41. Tempelhof S, Rupp S, Seil R. Age-related prevalence of rotator cuff tears in asymptomatic shoulders. J Shoulder Elbow Surg 1999;8:296-9.

42. Barr KP. Rotator cuff disease. Phys Med Rehabil Clin North Am 2004;15:475-91.

43. Nho SJ, Yadav H, Shindle MK, Macgillivray JD. Rotator cuff degeneration: etiology and pathogenesis. Am J Sports Med 2008;36:987-93.

44. Rodeo SA, Hannafin JA, Tom J, Warren RF, Wickiewicz TL. Immunolocalization of cytokines and their receptors in adhesive capsulitis of the shoulder. J Orthop Res 1997;15:427-36.

45. Tasto JP, Elias DW. Adhesive capsulitis. Sports Med Arthrosc 2007;15:216-21.

46. Bridgman JF. Periarthritis of the shoulder and diabetes mellitus. Ann Rheum Dis 1972;31:69-71.

47. Wohlgethan JR. Frozen shoulder in hyperthyroidism. Arthritis Rheum 1987;30:936-9.

48. Sethi N, Wright R, Yamaguchi K. Disorders of the long head of the biceps tendon. J Shoulder Elbow Surg 1999;8:644-54.

49. Duckworth DG, Smith KL, Campbell B, Matsen FA III. Self-assessment questionnaires document substantial variability in the clinical expression of rotator cuff tears. J Shoulder Elbow Surg 1999;8:330-3.

50. MacDonald PB, Clark P, Sutherland K. An analysis of the diagnostic accuracy of the Hawkins and Neer subacromial impingement signs. J Shoulder Elbow Surg 2000;9:299-301.

51. Matsen FA III. Rotator cuff failure. N Engl J Med 2008;358:2138-47.

52. Lefevre-Colau MM, Drape JL, Fayad F, Rannou F, Diche T, Minvielle F, et al. Magnetic resonance imaging of shoulders with idiopathic adhesive capsulitis: reliability of measures. Eur Radiol 2005;15:2415-22.

53. Mengiardi B, Pfirrmann CW, Gerber C, Hodler J, Zanetti M. Frozen shoulder: MR arthrographic findings. Radiology 2004;233:486-92.

54. Green S, Buchbinder R, Hetrick SE. Physiotherapy interventions for shoulder pain. Cochrane Database Syst Rev 2008;(4).

55. Buchbinder R, Green S, Youd JM. Corticosteroid injections for shoulder pain. Cochrane Database Syst Rev 2008;(4).

56. Brue S, Valentin A, Forssblad M, Werner S, Mikkelsen C, Cerulli G. Idiopathic adhesive capsulitis of the shoulder: a review. Knee Surg Sports Traumatol Arthrosc 2007;15:1048-54.

57. Buchbinder R, Green S, Youd JM, Johnston RV, Cumpston M. Arthrographic distension for adhesive capsulitis (frozen shoulder). Cochrane Database Syst Rev 2008;(4).

58. Faro F, Wolf JM. Lateral epicondylitis: review and current concepts. J Hand Surg [Am] 2007;32:1271-9.

59. Nirschl RP, Ashman ES. Elbow tendinopathy: tennis elbow. Clin Sports Med 2003;22:813-36.

60. Shiri R, Viikari-Juntura E, Varonen H, Heliovaara M. Prevalence and determinants of lateral and medial epicondylitis: a population study. Am J Epidemiol 2006;164:1065-74.

61. Canoso JJ, Barza M. Soft tissue infections. Clin Rheum Dis 1993;19:293-309.

62. Rinker B, Effron CR, Beasley RW. Proximal radial compression neuropathy. Ann Plast Surg 2004;52:174-80.

63. Stel IM. Septic and non-septic olecranon bursitis in the accident and emergency department—an approach to management. J Accid Emerg Med 1996;13:351-3.

64. Stewart N, Manzanares JB, Morrey BF. Surgical treatment of aseptic olecranon bursitis. J Shoulder Elbow Surg 1997;6:49-54.

65. Green S, Buchbinder R, Barnsley L, Hall S, White M, Smidt N, et al. Non-steroidal anti-inflammatory drugs (nsaids) for treating lateral elbow pain in adults. Cochrane Database Syst Rev 2008;(4).

66. Struijs PAA, Smidt N, Arola H, van Dijk CN, Buchbinder R, Assendelft WJJ. Orthotic devices for the treatment of tennis elbow. Cochrane Database Syst Rev 2008;(4).

67. Buchbinder R, Green SE, Youd JM, Assendelft WJJ, Barnsley L, Smidt N. Shock wave therapy for lateral elbow pain. Cochrane Database Syst Rev 2008;(4).

68. Canoso JJ. Bursitis, tenosynovitis, ganglions, and painful lesions of the wrist, elbow, and hand. Curr Opin Rheumatol 1990;2:276-81.

69. Moore JS. De Quervain's tenosynovitis. Stenosing tenosynovitis of the first dorsal compartment. J Occup Environ Med 1997;39:990-1002.

70. Gray RG, Gottlieb NL. Hand flexor tenosynovitis in rheumatoid arthritis. Prevalence, distribution, and associated rheumatic features. Arthritis Rheum 1920;4:1003-8.

71. Thorson E, Szabo RM. Common tendinitis problems in the hand and forearm. Orthop Clin North Am 1992;23:65-74.

72. Field JH. De Quervain's disease. Am Family Phys 1979;20:103-4.

73. Nygaard IE, Saltzman CL, Whitehouse MB, Hankin FM. Hand problems in pregnancy. Am Fam Physician 1989;39:123-6.

74. Murphy D, Failla JM, Koniuch MP. Steroid versus placebo injection for trigger finger. J Hand Surg [Am] 1995;4:628-31 [erratum appears in J Hand Surg [Am] 1995;20:1075].

75. Lambert MA, Morton RJ, Sloan JP. Controlled study of the use of local steroid injection in the treatment of trigger finger and thumb. J Hand Surg [Br] 1992;17:69-70.

76. Peters-Veluthamaningal C, Winters JC, Groenier KH, Jong BM. Corticosteroid injections effective for trigger finger in adults in general practice: a double-blinded randomised placebo controlled trial. Ann Rheum Dis 2008;67:1262-6.

77. Richie III CA, Briner Jr WW. Corticosteroid injection for treatment of de Quervain's tenosynovitis: a pooled quantitative literature evaluation. J Am Board Fam Practice 2003;16:102-6.

78. Sakai N. Selective corticosteroid injection into the extensor policis brevis tenosynovium for de Quervain's disease. Orthopedics 2002;25:68-70.

79. Lane LB, Boretz RS, Stuchin SA. Treatment of de Quervain's disease: role of conservative management. J Hand Surg [Br] 2001;26:258-60.

80. Ryzewicz M, Wolf JM. Trigger digits: principles, management and complications. J Hand Surg [Am] 2006;31A:135-46.

81. Rhoades CE, Gelberman RH, Manjarris JF. Stenosing tenosynovitis of the fingers and thumb: results of a prospective trial of steroid injection and splinting. Clin Orthop 1984;190:236-238.

82. Rayan GM, Parizi M, Tomasek JJ. Pharmacologic regulation of Dupuytren's fibroblast contraction in vitro. J Hand Surg [Am] 1996;21:1065-70.

83. Tomasek JJ, Haaksma CJ. Fibronectin filaments and actin microfilaments are organized into a fibronexus in Dupuytren's diseased tissue. Anat Rec 1991;230:175-82.

84. Early PF. Population studies in Dupuytren's contracture. J Bone Joint Surg [Br] 1962;44:602-13.

85. Chansky HA, Trumble TE, Conrad EU, Wolff JF, Murray LW, Raskind WH. Evidence for polyclonal etiology of palmar fibromatosis. J Hand Surg [Am] 1999;24:339-44.

86. Noble J, Heathcote JG, Cohen H. Diabetes mellitus in the aetiology of Dupuytren's disease. J Bone Joint Surg 1984;66B:322-5.

87. McFarlane R. On the origin and spread of Dupuytren's disease. J Hand Surg [Am] 2002;27:385-90.

88. Swartz WM, Lalonde DH. MOC-PS(SM) CME article: Dupuytren's disease. Plast Reconstr Surg 2008;121(Suppl.):1-10.

89. Rayan GM. Dupuytren disease: Anatomy, pathology, presentation, and treatment. J Bone Joint Surg [Am] 2007;89:189-98.

90. Badalmonte MA, Hurst LL. Enzyme injection as non-surgical treatment of Dupuytren's disease. J Hand Surg [Am] 2000;25:629.

91. Badalamente MA, Hurst LC. Efficacy and safety of injectable mixed collagenase subtypes in the treatment of Dupuytren's contracture. J Hand Surg [Am] 2007;32:767-74.

92. Trojian TH, Chu SM. Dupuytren's disease: diagnosis and treatment. Am Fam Physician 2007;76:86-9.

93. Townley WA, Baker R, Sheppard N, Grobbelaar AO. Dupuytren's contracture unfolded. BMJ 2006;332:397-400.

94. Szabo RM. Acute carpal tunnel syndrome. Hand Clin 1998; 14:419-29, ix.

95. Cranford CS, Ho JY, Kalainov DM, Hartigan BJ. Carpal tunnel syndrome. J Am Acad Orthop Surg 2007;15:537-48.

96. Mondelli M, Aprile I, Ballerini M, Ginanneschi F, Reale F, Romano C, et al. Sex differences in carpal tunnel syndrome: comparison of surgical and non-surgical populations. Eur J Neurol 2005;12:976-83.

97. Michelsen H, Posner MA. Medical history of carpal tunnel syndrome. Hand Clin 2002;18:257-68.

98. Stevens JC, Beard CM, O'Fallon WM, Kurland LT. Conditions associated with carpal tunnel syndrome. Mayo Clin Proceed 1992;67:541-8.

99. Stolp-Smith KA, Pascoe MK, Ogburn Jr PL. Carpal tunnel syndrome in pregnancy: frequency, severity and prognosis. Arch Phys Med Rehabil 1998;79:1285-7.

100. Padua L, Aprile I, Caliandro P, Carboni T, Meloni A, Massi S, et al. Symptoms and neurophysiological picture of carpal tunnel syndrome in pregnancy. Clin Neurophysiol 2001;112:1946-51.

101. Dias JJ, Burke FD, Wildin CJ, Heras-Palou C, Bradley MJ. Carpal tunnel syndrome and work. J Hand Surg [Br] 2004;29:329-33.

102. Stromberg T, Dahlin LB, Lundborg G. Hand problems in 100 vibration-exposed symptomatic male workers. J Hand Surg [Br] 1996;21:315-9.

103. Jablecki CK, Andary MT, So YT, Wilkins DE, William FH. Literature review of the usefulness of nerve conduction studies and electromyography for the evaluation of patients with carpal tunnel syndrome. Muscle Nerve 1993;16:1392-414.

104. Gravlee JR, Van Durme DJ. Braces and splints for musculoskeletal conditions. Am Fam Phys 2007;75:342-8.

105. Piazzini DB, Aprile I, Ferrara PE, Bertolini C, Tonali P, Maggi L, et al. A systematic review of conservative treatment of carpal tunnel syndrome. Clin Rehabil 2007;21:299-314.

106. Bland JD. Carpal tunnel syndrome. BMJ 2007;335:343-6.

107. Walker WC, Metzler M, Cifu DX, Swartz Z. Neutral wrist splinting in carpal tunnel syndrome: a comparison of night-only versus full-time wear instructions. Arch Phys Med Rehabil 2000;81:429.

108. Ly-Pen D, Andreu JL, de Blas G, Sanchez-Olaso A, Millan I. Surgical decompression versus local steroid injection in carpal tunnel syndrome: a one-year, prospective, randomized, open, controlled clinical trial. Arthritis Rheum 2005;52:612-9.

109. Verdugo RJ, Salinas RS, Castillo J, Cea JG. Surgical versus non-surgical treatment for carpal tunnel syndrome. Cochrane Database Syst Rev 2003;(2):CD001552. [update of Cochrane Database Syst Rev 2002;(3):CD001552; PMID: 12076416].

Chapter 26

Management of Mechanical Lumbar Spine Disease

David G. Borenstein

Mechanical disorders of the lumbar spine are the most common causes of low back pain. These disorders are related to overuse of a normal anatomic structure or secondary to deformity or injury of an anatomic structure. The common mechanical lumbosacral disorders include lumbar strain, herniated intervertebral nucleus pulposus with radiculopathy, osteoarthritis, and spinal stenosis. Recent epidemiologic surveys suggest that the US prevalence of low back pain is 59 million in the last 3 months.[1]

An essential clinical difficulty that exists with mechanical disorders of the lumbar spine is the absence of close correlation between anatomic alterations and the presence of symptoms. The absence of correlation does not negate the legitimate complaints of a proportion of individuals with anatomic abnormalities that do cause pain. In older populations, the presence of anatomic variations from normal is common. Therefore, a large number of individuals report mechanical low back pain, although they represent a minority of all individuals with these common anatomic alterations. These "degenerative" processes start during the adolescence of all individuals.[2] Diminished blood flow to the intervertebral disc in the first half of the second life decade appears to initiate tissue breakdown.[3] Through a variety of factors, both genetic and environmental, the progression is more rapid in some populations than in others. Environmental risk factors, such as smoking, obesity, and heavy physical activity, heighten the potential to develop symptomatic forms of mechanical disorders.

The symptoms of mechanical disorders are characteristically relieved by certain positions and activities and exacerbated by others. The pattern of alleviating and aggravating factors helps localize the disorder to particular portions of the spine. For example, lumbar spine flexion exacerbates intervertebral disc disease and alleviates apophyseal (facet) joint disease. Physical examination is unable to identify the exact location of the source of pain in many circumstances. However, physical examination does identify limitations of function and neurologic deficits. Radiographic evaluation is able to identify anatomic alterations in the spine but does

not necessarily correlate those changes with the patient's symptoms.[4]

The diagnosis of causes of mechanical low back pain is more specific when corresponding abnormalities in the neurologic system are present. For example, the diagnosis of a lumbar radiculopathy can be suspected by characteristic physical findings and may be confirmed with neurophysiologic testing with nerve conduction tests and electromyography. Making a more specific diagnosis of mechanical low back pain is worth the effort. The differential diagnosis is different for the various forms of back pain.[5] In addition, different components of medical therapy are more appropriate for specific forms of mechanical low back pain, such as epidural corticosteroid injections for radicular pain related to intervertebral disc herniation (Table 26-1).

Many mechanical disorders are self-limited in duration, with the majority of patients improving spontaneously. Other disorders wax and wane over longer periods of time. This progression to "natural healing" makes placebo look efficacious in many clinical trials investigating new therapies for low back pain. This situation results in evidence-based reviews of clinically significant therapies revealing very few categories that have a remarkable impact on the improvement of low back pain. Nonetheless, physicians need to make therapeutic choices for their patients despite this relative paucity of evidence. Therapy for mechanical lumbar spine disorders include controlled physical activity, nonsteroidal anti-inflammatory drugs (NSAIDs), skeletal muscle relaxants, local and epidural corticosteroid injections, and long-term pain therapy. Surgical intervention is reserved for patients who have not had improvement with medical therapy and have a surgically correctable abnormality.

LUMBAR SPINE STRAIN

Lumbar spine strain can be defined as nonradiating low back pain with onset associated with a prolonged abnormal position or mechanical stress. This group comprises the greatest number of individuals

Table 26-1. *Mechanical Disorders of the Lumbar Spine*

Characteristics	Muscle Strain	HNP	Osteoarthritis	Spinal Stenosis
Age (y)	20–40	30–50	> 50	> 60
Pain pattern				
Location	Back (unilateral)	Back/leg (unilateral)	Back (unilateral)	Leg (bilateral)
Onset	Acute	Acute	Insidious	Insidious
Standing	I	D	I	I
Sitting	D	I	D	D
Bending	I	I	D	D
Straight leg	–	+	–	+ (stress)
Plain radiographs	–	–	+	+
CT	–	Disc herniation	Joint arthritis	Canal narrowing
MRI	–	Disc herniation	Joint arthritis	Canal narrowing

-, not present; +, present; CT, computed tomography; D, pain decreases; HNP, herniated nucleus pulposus; I, pain increases; MRI, magnetic resonance imaging.

CASE STUDY 1   Acute-Onset Localized Low Back Pain

A 28-year-old man is physically active, playing sports regularly. He was well until last weekend, when while playing racquetball, he rotated his spine to reach a ball and experienced acute right-sided back pain. He had to stop playing immediately and found his back to be very stiff and painful. He comes to your office 3 days later with continued localized low back pain. He had tried acetaminophen with minimal benefit.

Physical examination of the lumbar spine demonstrates decreased flexion to 40 degrees, right lateral flexion to 15 degrees, left lateral flexion to 0 degrees with increased paraspinous muscle contraction, and extension to 5 degrees. Straight-leg raising test is negative for any radicular pain. Neurologic examination reveals normal sensory, motor, and reflex function. Radiographic tests were not ordered.

---

with low back pain. Most people with spinal pain (90%) have it on a mechanical basis.[6] Of patients with mechanical low back pain, back strain may account for 60% to 70% of occurrences.

The cause of lumbar strain is most likely related to muscular, fascial, or ligamentous strain related to a specific traumatic episode or continuous mechanical stress. In proper alignment with good posture, little strain is placed on spinal structures and supporting tissues. These tissues are in a resting state and require little energy to function. Tonic contraction associated with injuries result in relative oxygen deprivation and the development of pain. The lumbar spine and supporting muscles may be damaged when an individual lifts an object beyond the capabilities of those structures to sustain the weight. If the force is too great, the stress is first

transferred to the supporting ligaments. Then intradiscal pressure increases, and forces are transferred to the apophyseal joints (Table 26-2). These damaging forces result in injury to these structures and the subsequent reflexive physiologic responses.

The diagnosis of lumbar strain is determined by a history of localized low back pain associated with a traumatic event and a compatible physical examination demonstrating localized pain with palpation or movement, muscle contraction, and a normal neurologic examination.

Treatment

The course of patients with lumbar spine strain is one of gradual improvement over a 2-week period. At 2 months, 90% of individuals are cured without

---

Table 26-2. *Mechanisms of Muscle Pain*

Muscle strain pain may be related to muscle disruption from indirect trauma, such as excessive tension or stretch. A source of continued risk for recurrent injury is inelastic scar tissue.

Muscle fatigue from overuse is another mechanism. Increased concentrations of lactic acid, a byproduct of anaerobic metabolism, may be associated with increased muscle pain and fatigue. High loads requiring maximal effort of muscles causes ultra structural damage to muscle with a delayed inflammatory response

Persistent muscle contraction is a component of muscle spasm. The absence of blood flow with an accumulation of metabolic byproducts may stimulate pain receptors within blood vessels.

Muscle injury results in paraspinous muscle deconditioning. Radiographic evaluation of cross-sectional views of patients with back pain demonstrated decreased muscle mass in the paraspinous and psoas muscles. Decreased muscle mass results in decreased muscle power. This situation puts individuals at risk for persistent muscle injury.

any residual but an increased risk of a recurrence.[7] The vast majority are at risk for another episode that will be of greater duration and severity. Of occupationally related low back pain, 60% of individuals have recurrent symptoms within a year.

Therapy for lumbar strain includes controlled physical activity, NSAIDs, muscle relaxants, and physical therapy. In regard to controlled physical activity, I ask patients to limit bed rest as much as possible. Studies have demonstrated that regular activity as tolerated has a better outcome than those who have bed rest for as short a period as 2 days.[8] Bed rest is detrimental in causing muscle atrophy and absenteeism from work. As soon as very acute pain is diminished, patients are encouraged to increase physical activity. I describe a "comfort zone" for the patient.[9] I ask them to start by doing one tenth of the activity they did before the event. That would mean one block versus 10 blocks of walking, or 3 minutes of treadmill walking versus 30 minutes. They are encouraged to increase activity incrementally as they improve. Educating the patient about the natural resolution of their pain can have a therapeutic effect.

Non-narcotic analgesics in the form of NSAIDs are helpful in decreasing pain and inflammation in patients with acute lumbar strain. NSAIDs that are analgesic with a more rapid onset of action are preferred. No one NSAID has been specifically tested against others to determine the best agent for this disorder. I tell patients that the NSAID is being used to facilitate function. By decreasing pain, the individual is able to gradually increase physical activity, which is an important component of healing. The exposure to the toxicities of NSAIDs is short term. These agents have little risk in those who are not aspirin sensitive or who do not have severe renal or hepatic dysfunction. NSAIDs are continued until the patient's pain has improved significantly and they have returned to normal function. NSAIDs

have been shown in meta-analyses to be better than placebo in the relief of acute low back pain.[10]

Muscle relaxants may be of use in patients who have palpable spasm or who have difficulty sleeping at night secondary to muscle tightness. These drugs are used to facilitate movement and decrease pain. For example, in a study of 1445 patients with a majority with back pain, a dose of cyclobenzaprine 5 mg tid was more effective than placebo in improving spasm and pain.[11] The 5-mg tablet was as effective as the 10-mg dose with less toxicity. A number of muscle relaxants are available for treatment of acute muscle spasm (Table 26-3).[12] In general, antispasmodics have greater efficacy than anti-spasticity medicines for this form of muscle contraction. I start with the lowest effective dose and increase doses depending on the patient's response. I limit the prescription of muscle relaxants that have abuse potential. The muscle relaxant is continued until muscle tightness has resolved. In most circumstances, I use a combination of an NSAID and a skeletal muscle relaxant to treat lumbar strain. Observational studies have demonstrated this combination to be an effective regimen.[13]

Physical therapy in the setting of acute lumbar spasm is directed at decreasing pain. Modalities in the form of ice massage initially or heat packs subsequently may decrease pain and diminish spasm. Patients are instructed in simple stretching exercises for the lumbar spine. These exercises encourage gradual movement of supporting muscles so that they do not become deconditioned. Exercise therapy is superior to no exercise for the treatment of acute low back pain.[14] Some of the advocated exercise programs include Williams flexion exercises, MacKenzie extension exercises, and aerobic conditioning. It is difficult to determine the exact benefit of exercise because studies examine different types of exercise and added modalities. In most circumstances, it is reasonable to advise patients to return

Table 26-3. *Skeletal Muscle Relaxants (Antispasmodics/Nonbenzodiazepams)*

Agent	Formulations	Recommended Dose	Most Common Toxicities
Carisoprodol	350 mg 250 mg	Four times daily	Dizziness, drowsiness, headache, physical or psychological dependence
Chlozoxazone	250 mg 750 mg	Three to four times daily	Dizziness, drowsiness GI bleeding – rare
Cyclobenzaprine	5.0 mg 7.5 mg 10.0 mg 15.0 mg (ER) 30.0 mg (ER)	From 5 mg three times daily to 30 mg once a day	Drowsiness, dry mouth, urinary retention, increased intraocular pressure. arrhythmias
Metaxalone	800 mg	Three to four times daily	Drowsiness, dizziness, headache, paradoxical muscle cramps
Methocarbamol	750 mg	Four times daily	Mental status impairment
Orphenadrine	100 mg	Two times daily	Drowsiness, dry mouth, urinary retention, increased intraocular pressure

ER, extended release; GI, gastrointestinal.

to normal activities without a referral to a therapist. I recommend a visit to the therapist for individuals who are willing to do exercises to prevent a recurrence of acute back pain.

Myofascial trigger points can cause localized muscle pain with referred pain to the buttocks and lateral thighs. The muscles that may become affected include the quadratus lumborum, gluteus medius, and gluteus maximus. Injection of these areas with anesthetic and semisoluble corticosteroid has modest benefit.[15,16] In general, local injections are more helpful for acute low back pain than for longer duration pain. I will use a local injection of lidocaine and corticosteroid if I can identify a specific tender point that has not responded to oral medical therapy.

Spinal manipulation is also mentioned frequently by patients as a component of therapy for acute low back pain. Manipulation involves abrupt movement of spinal structures beyond their physiologic but not their anatomic range of movement. A number of studies have shown no specific benefit compared with regular medical care. For example, the addition of chiropractic care to an exercise program offers no additional benefit.[17] In fact, the "benefit" of chiropractic care may have nothing to do with movement of the spine. In a study of 467 patients, overall satisfaction was three times greater with chiropractors than with the physicians. Physicians were perceived as being less concerned about the patient's condition and pain. Physicians were also perceived as being less confident about the cause of the patient's pain.[18] I recommend physical therapy as a substitute for chiropractic manipulation for those who want to participate in a movement program.

Case Study 1 Treatment

The patient was placed on naproxen 500 mg twice a day with meals and cyclobenzaprine 5 mg three times a day. The patient was given a list of flexion stretching exercises to complete as his pain improved. He was told to maintain his daily, nonexercise activities as tolerated. The patient took these medicines for two weeks. He gradually decreased cyclobenzaprine first. He then discontinued naproxen therapy. He had resolution of pain by the third week and returned to his sports activities after 4 weeks from the onset of his pain.

Had this patient not improved, he would have been given another NSAID with analgesic properties from a different chemical group. An alternate muscle relaxant would be prescribed if he received no benefit or experienced drug toxicities. A local injection would be considered if he identified a singular location that remained painful and was the source of limited function. Physical therapy would be prescribed at week four if he demonstrated continued muscle contraction and limited motion.

CASE STUDY 2   Acute-Onset Low Back And Leg Pain

A 38-year-old woman has had intermittent low back pain that has resolved spontaneously. She was moving into an apartment carrying a number of boxes. She developed low back pain that quickly expanded into left-sided low back pain that radiated to the big toe. She had great difficulty sitting. She was more comfortable standing or supine in bed. Physical examination demonstrates decreased flexion to 30 degrees, right lateral bending to 15 degrees, left lateral bending to 5 degrees with increased radicular symptoms, and extension to 10 degrees of the lumbar spine. Straight-leg raising test is positive on the left in the seated and supine position. Cross-leg straight leg raising test is negative. Neurologic examination reveals decreased sensory function in L5 distribution, no motor abnormalities, and no reflex abnormalities. Radiographic tests include a magnetic resonance imaging (MRI) scan demonstrating a herniated disc with compression of the left L5 nerve root.

LUMBAR HERNIATED NUCLEUS PULPOSUS WITH RADICULOPATHY

A herniated disc is defined as the extrusion of the nucleus pulposus through the fibers of the annulus fibrosus. Most disc ruptures occur during the third and fourth decades of life when the nucleus pulposus remains gelatinous. The most likely time of day associated with increased force on the disc is in the morning. The morning is the time the disc is distended to its greatest volume from absorbing water throughout the evening. Alterations in the properties of the nucleus pulposus start in the second decade.[3] A number of factors, including excessive force on disc structures, can result in a breach of the annulus fibrosus by material in the nucleus pulposus.

The most common levels for disc herniation are L4-L5 and L5-S1 which account for 98% of lesions. In general, disc herniations at L5-S1 usually compromise the first sacral root, and a lesion at the L4-L5 affect the fifth lumbar root. It is important to remember that disc resorption is part of the natural healing process associated with disc herniation. The enhanced ability to resorb disc contents has the potential for resolving clinical symptoms more rapidly. Tumor necrosis factor is a product that may help to attract phagocytic cells that resorb herniated tissues.

The pathophysiology of disc herniation causing radicular pain is not fully elucidated. Compression of a nerve root by a herniated disc explains only part of the pathophysiology of radicular pain.[19] A variety of inflammatory mediators are released. These mediators are important in the resorption of extruded tissues. At the same time, leakage of these

Table 26-4. *Sensory, Motor, Reflex Distribution of Lumbar Roots*

Root	Cutaneous Area	Muscle Weakness/Movement Affected	Tendon Reflex
L2	Anterior thigh Upper buttock	Hip flexion, adduction	–
L3	Lower anterior thigh Buttock Lateral posterior thigh	Hip adduction Knee extension	Knee jerk
L4	Anterior lower leg Lateral knee Medial ankle	Knee extension Foot inversion, dorsiflexion	Knee jerk
L5	Lateral calf Dorsum of foot Knee flexion Large toe—plantar surface	Hip extension, abduction Foot/toe dorsiflexion	–
S1	Small toe Medial calf Sole of foot	Knee flexion Foot/toe plantar flexion Foot eversion	Ankle jerk

factors may produce excitation of the nerve root and enhancement of pain-producing substances. Tumor necrosis factor recreates the neurophysiologic abnormalities associated with radicular pain in animal models of radiculopathy.[20] Therefore, the generation of the clinical symptoms of disc herniation is related to a varying ratio of mechanical compression and inflammatory mediators.

The diagnosis of a herniated disc is made on the basis of the history and physical examination (Table 26-4).

Plain radiographs of the lumbar spine are obtained if there are other causes of spinal pathology such as an infection or tumor. Other radiographic tests, MRI scan, computed tomography (CT) scan, or myelograms are used to confirm the clinical correlation with clinical complaints and anatomic alterations (Fig. 26-1). Patients with osteoarthritis of the spine may develop facet syndrome that is associated with leg pain. Spinal stenosis patients with radicular pain tend to be older than those in whom herniated discs develop.

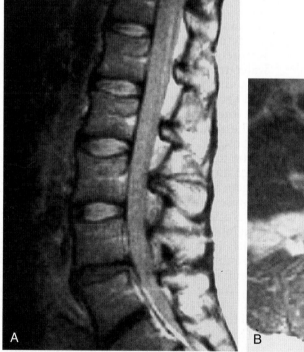
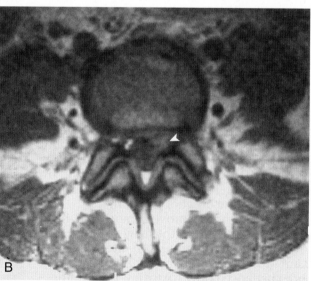

Figure 26-1. Disc hernation. **A,** Herniated intervertebral lumbar disc. Sagittal magnetic resonance imaging (MRI) scan demonstrates a herniated disc with caudal migration of the disc at the L4/5 interspace. **B,** Herniated intervertebral lumbar disc. Axial MRI scan demonstrates a herniated disc (*arrowhead*) blocking the left neural foramen. (From Hochberg M, Silman A, Smolen J, Weinblatt M, Weisman M. Rheumatology. 4th ed. Philadelphia: Elsevier; 2008. p. 609-10. Figures 58.34 and 58.35.)

Treatment

Treatment for most patients with a herniated disc can be nonoperative or surgical depending on the severity of symptoms inasmuch herniated intervertebral discs can resorb spontaneously. Investigators have documented improvement in symptoms at a time before the complete resorption of intervertebral discs.[21] In these patients, the control of inflammatory mediators has a greater effect on the lessening of clinical symptoms. Individuals who have contrast-enhanced extruded discs have a greater opportunity to resorb the herniated portion.[22]

Controlled physical activity is a component of nonoperative therapy for patients with herniated discs. Bed rest is kept to a minimum. When in bed, patients use a semi-Fowler position, with hips and knees comfortably flexed. This position is ideal because it keeps intradiscal pressure down and reduces nerve root tension.

NSAIDs, analgesics, and muscle relaxants are important components of drug therapy for low back and radicular pain. Inasmuch as some of the symptoms of low back and leg pain are inflammatory in nature, as well as mechanical compression, anti-inflammatory medications are indicated. Doses at the upper ranges of therapeutic index are indicated. No specific NSAID is better than another. I choose between chemical classes if the initial drug is ineffective or causes toxicity. I am concerned about gastrointestinal toxicities, although the NSAID is prescribed for a relatively short period of time. I will prescribe a proton pump inhibitor if the patient has gastrointestinal symptoms or is older than the usual younger patient with a herniated disc.

The use of oral corticosteroids as a component of therapy for radiculopathy secondary to a herniated disc is a controversial issue. Although many practitioners admit to prescribing corticosteroids for radiculopathy, clinical trial results demonstrating benefits are nonexistent. In this circumstance, absence of proof is not proof of absence. I do not prescribe large doses of dexamethasone. I prefer prescribing prednisone in doses up to 20 mg per day. I will continue prednisone for a period of about 4 to 6 weeks before deciding if the medicine has been helpful. I will discontinue the medicine if patients have not responded or have developed intolerable toxicities. I will gradually taper the prednisone in 5-mg decrements over a number of weeks monitoring the continued improvement measured in decreased pain and a normalization of neurologic function.

Analgesics are an important component of therapy to improve patient comfort as they heal. Analgesics are adjunctive therapy. Analgesics, in addition to NSAIDs, may include acetaminophen, tramadol, and opioids.[23] The patient should understand that the dose of analgesics should not be increased without discussion with their physician. Increasing doses may offer little benefit but an increased risk of toxicity. Requests for increasing doses of analgesics for control of severe leg pain are indications for consideration of surgical intervention.

Muscle relaxants can help with uncontrolled muscle contraction associated with nerve impingement. The mechanism of action of these agents is unknown. The beneficial effects of this group of drugs were thought to be related to their tranquilizing effects. In a large study of low-dose cyclobenzaprine that demonstrated efficacy, the benefits were unassociated with the presence or absence of somnolence.[11] Muscle relaxants without abuse potential are preferred.

Epidural corticosteroid injections are considered for patients with radiculopathy who are not responding to modified activities, NSAIDs, and muscle relaxants. Carette and coworkers[24] studied the efficacy of epidural corticosteroid injections for sciatica secondary to disc herniation. At 3 weeks, patients receiving 80 mg of methylprednisolone acetate had fewer physical limitations than the control group. At 6 weeks, the improvement persisted. At 3 months, no significant differences were found between groups. At 12 months, the number of disc surgeries was similar in active and placebo groups. Other studies have had less success with periradicular injections.[25] I prescribe three epidural injections to be given over a 6-week period. I evaluate the patient after every injection to determine if additional injections in the series are indicated. Epidural injections can be helpful in relieving leg pain as a temporizing intervention. This therapy is less invasive than discectomy.

Surgical Therapy

Surgical intervention is considered for patients with motor weakness or intractable pain. Patients who have failed conservative therapy are also candidates. Clinical trials have attempted to demonstrate the relative benefit of surgical versus medical therapy for intervertebral disc herniation.[26] In general, patients who undergo discectomy resolve symptoms more rapidly than those treated without surgery. Also earlier surgery tends to have a more timely resolution of symptoms, although delayed surgery of 4 to 6 months continues to have benefits for pain resolution.[27] Discectomy for disc herniation at superior levels of the lumbar spine (L2-L3, L3-L4) may have greater treatment effects. Medical therapy for these upper lumbar herniations may be less effective.[28] Despite these early benefits, when evaluated 2 years after surgery, disc herniation patients have similar improved outcomes whether treated with discectomy or medical therapy. Also of concern are the long-term consequences of spine surgery. Patients who have one surgery may be at greater risk for additional surgery because of re-herniation at the same level, or herniation at neighboring disc levels. A study by Mariconda et al suggests that discectomy patients have a satisfactory self-reported health-related quality of life and continued pain relief up to 25 years after surgery.[29]

Case Study 2 Treatment

The patient was treated with diclofenac 100 mg bid for 2 weeks. The patient had a partial response but continued with mild weakness. The patient received prednisone 20 mg qd. At re-evaluation at 4 weeks, the patient's leg pain was decreased. A physical therapy program with MacKenzie exercises was started. The patient's symptoms improved over the next 4 months. This prednisone was decreased 5 mg every 2 to 4 weeks as her symptoms improved. At month 4 she discontinued diclofenac therapy. She was encouraged to continue strengthening exercises to maintain lumbar spine strength.

Epidural injections would be offered had the patient not responded to oral corticosteroid therapy. Analgesic therapy would be added if the NSAID therapy was inadequate to allow completion of activities of daily living. Surgical consultation would be recommended if weakness or severe pain increased.

CASE STUDY 3   Chronic Localized Low Back Pain

A 57-year-old woman has increasing back pain and stiffness after a meeting where she needed to stand for an extended period of time. She had a history of knee and hip joint replacement for osteoarthritis. She has tried intermittent exercises and occasional NSAID therapy. Her back pain persisted and recurred on a daily basis when she stood. Physical examination of the lumbar spine revealed flexion to 70 degrees, lateral bending to 10 degrees, and extension to 5 degrees with pain in the lumbar spine. Straight-leg raising test is negative. Movement of her leg with her hip replacement caused some minimal discomfort. Neurologic examination reveals no sensory, motor, or reflex abnormalities. Radiographs of the lumbar spine demonstrate intervertebral disc space narrowing at the L5-S1 level, with sclerosis and narrowing of the apophyseal joints at this level.

LUMBAR SPINE OSTEOARTHRITIS

Osteoarthritis is a chronic, noninflammatory joint disease characterized by slowly developing joint pain, stiffness, deformity, and limitation of motion. The lumbar spine is a frequent location of osteoarthritis. Osteoarthritis is one of the leading causes of disability and pain in the elderly.

Development of spinal osteoarthritis is one that occurs gradually over an individual's life.[30] Major changes in the lumbar spine occur between the third and fifth decades of life. The intervertebral discs lose their integrity initially in the nucleus pulposus, then the annulus fibrosus. This disc changes results in disc flattening causing progressive pressures on the apophyseal, or facet, joints.[31] The resulting biomechanical insufficiency results in a transfer of stresses posteriorly to the facet joints and ligaments that are ill suited to assume compressive, tensile, and shear loads. This process may be painless until alterations in facet joint alignment occur. The anatomic alterations associated with these abnormal forces include the generation of traction spurs or osteophytes, redundant ligament flava, and realignment of the planes of motion of the facet joints.

The diagnosis of osteoarthritis of the lumbar spine is suggested by the patient's age and a clinical history of back pain of long duration that increases with mechanical stress, and is documented by radiographic alterations of the lumbar spine (Fig. 26-2). The diagnosis of osteoarthritis is one made by exclusion of other possible diagnoses, such as neoplasms. Individuals with facet joint osteoarthritis that is symptomatic are more likely to have positive single photon emission CT (SPECT) bone scans of the lumbar spine. Dolan and associates[32] studied 58 patients with back pain and clinical findings compatible with facet joint arthritis with SPECT scans. Of the 22 patients with positive scans, 73% had improvement of pain at 3 months after a facet joint block at a positive level compared with none of the 38 with negative scans. Joints with increased activity are more responsive to local anesthetic injections but were not the joints with the greatest degree of osteoarthritis.

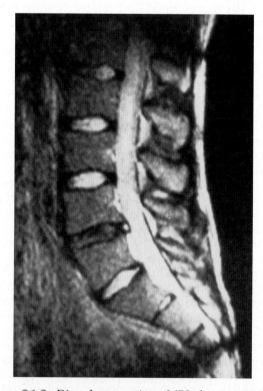

Figure 26-2. Disc degeneration. MRI demonstrating a high-intensity zone lesion in the L4/5 intervertebral disc. (From Hochberg M, Silman A, Smolen J, Weinblatt M, Weisman M. Rheumatology. 4th ed. Philadelphia: Elsevier; 2008. p. 601. Figure 58.14.)

Treatment

Treatment of spinal osteoarthritis includes physical interventions, pharmaceuticals, and local injections. The majority of patients can be treated nonsurgically. NSAIDs are helpful in controlling symptoms. These drugs are helpful for decreasing pain and local inflammation in the low back as they do in the knee, hand, feet, or hip.[33] The toxicities of these agents are more likely to appear in the age group developing symptomatic osteoarthritis. These individuals need to be made aware of the gastrointestinal and cardiovascular toxicities so that ill effects may be mitigated. Patients with gastrointestinal difficulties should take NSAIDs with meals and should ingest gastroprotective therapy such as proton pump inhibitors or misoprostil. Topical therapies in the form of patches and gels are available but indicated for acute musculoskeletal injuries. It is not clear if these therapies are able to direct medicines deep enough into tissues below the skin surface. Theoretically, these therapies would be ideal for older individuals who need to limit systemic exposure but would benefit from local anti-inflammatory effects.

A more specific intervention for the treatment of facet joint arthritis is periarticular or intra-articular joint injections. Intra-articular injections may decrease intra-articular inflammation but have no effect on the medial posterior branches of the lumbar spinal nerves that supply two facet joint levels. Conversely, numbing the medial branches may not have any effect on local intra-articular inflammatory processes. Therefore, injections directed at only one of these components may have only a partial benefit at relieving pain. Gorbach and colleagues[34] described benefits at 3 months in 33% of patients who received facet joint blocks. Other studies have documented the benefit of joint injection in SPECT-positive osteoarthritis patients.[35]

Percutaneous radiofrequency neurotomy is another procedure that prolongs the effects of lumbar medial branch anesthetic injections. Dreyfuss and coworkers[36] completed diagnostic lumbar medial branch blocks in 15 patients with chronic low back pain. The patients underwent neurotomy at the corresponding facet joint and were followed over the next 12 months. Sixty percent of patients obtained at least 90% pain relief at 12 months, with 87% receiving at least 60% pain relief.

Physical therapy is directed at exercises that strengthen flexion muscles of the abdomen. These muscles help stabilize the lumbar spine. Improved strength in the flexor group allows patients to do pelvic tilts that flatten the back and unweight the facet joints. Modalities, primarily heat therapies, are useful to decrease increased muscle tension that limits motion.

No specific surgical procedure has been recognized as effective for the therapy of osteoarthritis of the lumbar spine. Any procedure for this entity would need to be considered experimental. Any individual who decides on surgery for this mechanical disorder should do so only as part of a clinical trial to determine the long-term benefits of the intervention.

Case Study 3 Treatment

She started on long-acting ketoprofen and a flexion exercise strengthening program. Over the next 12 months, she switched NSAIDs from refecoxib, diflunisal, valdecoxib, and back to ketoprofen. Intermittently, she used a lidocaine patch that offered some additional pain relief. She improved for about an 18-month period when she had a recurrence of her low back and right buttock pain. She realized that her back pain was associated with difficulty walking with groin pain. Further evaluation demonstrated instability of her hip replacement. Revision arthroplasty relieved both her buttock and back pain. She required ketoprofen rarely as long as she continued with her flexion exercises.

> ### CASE STUDY 4   Chronic Intermittent Low Back and Leg Pain
>
> An 87-year-old man reported increasing back and leg pain with walking. He has pain down both legs, right greater than left. His pain had been worse in his right knee at the end of the day, even when he was seated. This pain was improved with his right knee replacement. He had hoped that his leg pain with walking would disappear with his joint replacement, but his pain persisted. He has pain radiating from his back to the calves after he walks about three blocks. His pain resolves when takes a seated position. He is otherwise in good physical condition without comorbidities. Physical examination of the lumbar spine demonstrates flexion to 80 degrees, lateral bending of 5 degrees, and extension to 5 degrees with minimal back pain. His pain occurs after he walks six times around the office. Straight-leg raising test after this stress is positive in the seated and supine position. This test returns to normal after he is seated for 5 minutes. He has no sensory deficits. His reflexes are not obtainable. Motor strength is age appropriate. An MRI scan of the lumbar spine demonstrates diffuse canal narrowing with severe involvement at the L4-L5 level.

LUMBAR SPINAL STENOSIS

Lumbar spinal stenosis is caused by insufficient room in the spinal canal for the neural elements. An understanding of the pathogenesis of this disorder is helpful for understanding the potential benefits of different therapies. The pathogenesis of spinal stenosis is reminiscent of the processes that produce osteoarthritis. The loss of integrity of intervertebral discs results in transfer of pressures posteriorly to apophyseal joints and supporting ligaments. The added weight results in the formation of osteophytes on apophyseal joints and redundancy of ligamentum flavum. However, in addition to the development of osteophytes, the area within the spinal canal is encroached by deformed anatomic structures. Different areas of the spinal canal may become narrowed depending on the height of the neural foramina, anteroposterior diameter of the canal, and trefoil canal shape.

Although lumbar spinal stenosis is a common diagnosis, no specific physical finding or radiographic test is thought of as being pathognomonic of the disorder. A recent review of 41 studies concluded that no "gold standard" existed for this diagnosis.[37]

Lumbar spinal stenosis is a clinical diagnosis characterized by specific historical and physical findings with corroboration with MRI or CT that shows compression of nerve root (Fig. 26-3). The loss of volume in the spinal canal for the neural elements is the essential finding that results in the pseudoclaudication closely associated with this clinical problem. A number of spinal disease processes are associated with lumbar stenosis (Table 26-5).[38] These entities can be divided into congenital and acquired disorders. Acquired disorders occur more frequently. For the most past, radiographic evaluation is able to differentiate among these numerous entities.

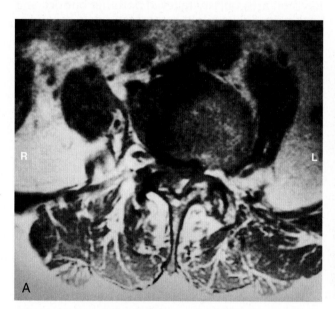

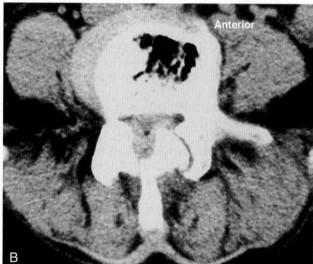

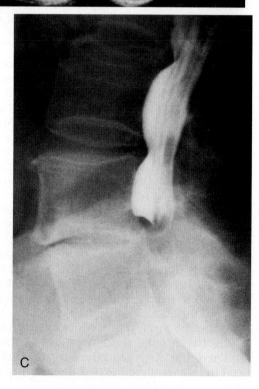

Figure 26-3. Lumbar spinal stenosis. **A,** Magnetic resonance imaging (MRI) scan, axial view, of the L3/4 disc level demonstrating osteophytic overgrowth, disc degeneration, and ligamentous hypertrophy. The cauda equina is compressed in the central area of the canal. **B,** Computed tomography (CT) scan showing thickened ligamentum flavum, facet joint hypertrophy, and posterior disc bulging. Note absence of epidural fat with trefoil deformity of lumbar spinal canal. **C,** Myelogram in extension. Note increased block with marked posterior indentation due to the ligamentum flavum. (From Hochberg M, Silman A, Smolen J, Weinblatt M, Weisman M. Rheumatology. 4th ed. Philadelphia: Elsevier; 2008. p. 610, 612. Figures 58.36, 58.39 and 58.40.)

Table 26-5. *Causes of Lumbar Spinal Stenosis*

Congenital/Developmental
  Metabolic/Genetic
    Achondroplasia
    Morquio's syndrome
    Hypophosphatemic vitamin D-resistant rickets
  Other
    Down syndrome
    Scoliosis
    Short-pedicle syndrome
  Idiopathic
Acquired
  Degenerative
    Spondylosis
    Disc resorption
    Lateral nerve root entrapment
    Spondylolisthesis
    Adult scoliosis
    Calcification of the ligamentum flavum
    Intraspinal synovial cysts
    Spinal dysraphism
  Metabolic/endocrine
    Osteoporosis with fracture
    Acromegaly
    CPPD disease
    Renal osteodystrophy
    Hypoparathyroidism
    Epidural lipomatosis
  Traumatic
    Fracture
  Postoperative
    Postdiscectomy
    Postfusion
    Postlaminectomy
  Miscellaneous
    Conjoined origin of lumbosacral roots
    Amyloid
    Flurosis
    Diffuse idiopathic skeletal hyperostosis
    Paget's disease

CPPD, calcium pyrophosphate dehydrate.

Leg pain is caused by a number of ailments in a geriatric population. Vascular claudication is manifested by leg pain associated with physical activity that radiates proximally from the foot to the thigh. Leg pain that occurs in a seated position while riding a bicycle is frequently caused by vascular claudication. Hip arthritis causes pain with walking that radiates to the knee, but rarely further down the leg. Peripheral neuropathy causes dysesthesias in the feet and lower leg when the individual is supine. The dysesthesias are frequently exacerbated at night.

Osteoarthritis of the apophyseal joints may cause pain in the lumbar spine that radiates in a sclerotomal pattern into the lower extremity (facet syndrome). These symptoms may mimic those of lumbar spinal stenosis. These patients have back pain with extension of the spine. Pain in the buttock and posterior thigh may develop, with prolonged compression associated with standing. These patients may walk in a flexed posture for extended distances without the development of leg pain. Facet syndrome is unassociated with neurologic deficits.

Treatment

The treatment of lumbar spinal stenosis must match the severity of the functional impairment with the benefits and risks of therapy. The clinician needs to decide on whether limitations of cardiac or pulmonary systems are having the greatest impact on function. Aggressive therapy for spinal stenosis is directed to those individuals where their spine is the major health problem.

Medical therapy can be effective for patients with mild to moderate stenosis. The goal of therapy is to maximize the space in the canal by flexing the spine and reversing swelling of soft tissues that have become inflamed. Medical therapy included weight reduction, aerobic exercise in the form of a stationary bicycle or water exercises, and flexion strengthening exercises.[39]

NSAIDs have a role to play primarily because of their anti-inflammatory and analgesic effects.[40] The smallest effective dose is preferred. Gastrointestinal ulcers, hypertension, and peripheral edema are real toxicities in these patients. I offer concomitant medications to reduce side effects in patients who are susceptible.

Opioid analgesics should be used at times when the patient will be doing activities that result in leg pain.[41] Short-acting opioids are prescribed for use prior to walking or standing that causes radicular pain. I limit the use of long-acting opioids to individuals with persistent pain who are poor surgical candidates. Opioids are not well tolerated by older patients. I attempt to use the lowest dose possible to minimize toxic reactions.[42]

Low-dose prednisone (5 to 10 mg qd) may be useful for patients who are not candidates for NSAIDs or opioids. My clinical experience has included a group of elderly patients who take low-dose prednisone who are able to function at a satisfactory level without significant steroid toxicities. Oral steroids are useful in patients who benefit from epidural corticosteroid injections but have difficulty receiving injections on a regular basis (e.g., patients taking warfarin). Intravenous pulse corticosteroid infusions have been studied with modest improvement in radicular symptoms for short periods of time.[43]

Epidural corticosteroid injections are worth a trial prior to surgical intervention.[44,45] I order an injection once every 2 months, as needed. Subsequent injections are delayed until symptoms return in those individuals who are responsive. A total of 3 injections are allowed every 6 months. I have had patients who have received epidural injections for a number of years as the primary therapy to maintain function and control pain.

Surgical decompression is indicated in patients who have failed medical therapy and are physically incapacitated by neurogenic claudication.[46] I recommend surgical evaluation for patients who have neurogenic claudication who have leg pain with standing for 10 to 15 minutes or with walking short distances, a city block or two. A decompression operation relieves leg pain, not back discomfort. A deciding factor for surgery should be the physiologic, not chronologic, age of the patient. Surgical decompression should be considered when your patient is limited by their inability to walk secondary to pain versus dyspnea secondary to congestive heart failure or balance difficulties and dysesthesias related to peripheral neuropathy. A variety of surgical procedures is available for decompression of the lumbar spine (Table 26-6).

The goal of surgery is to obtain adequate decompression without causing instability of the lumbar spine.[47] The difficulty for spine surgeons is identifying the significant stenotic levels, because the degree of narrowing does not specifically identify the most symptomatic level. A local expander of posterior elements may be successful if a single level of narrowing is identified.[48] I rely on the experience of the surgeon to decide on the level and extent of decompression. Accomplishing this is more difficult in those with degenerative spondylolisthesis or scoliosis. The need for spinal fusion with or without instrumentation is a decision finalized by the spine surgeon. The surgical literature remains divided over the benefits of fusion with or without instrumentation as a part of a decompression procedure.

The determination of the eventual outcome of medical versus surgical therapy of lumbar spinal stenosis remains to be determined.[49,50] Investigators have described small groups of nonsurgical spinal stenosis patients with stable symptoms for extended periods of time. Others have described a natural history of slow but steady decrease in function measured in years. Surgical decompression offers better short-term outcomes than medical therapy. Patients with fewer comorbid conditions have a better outcome. Debate is ongoing on the fate of surrounding intervertebral disc spaces and the risk of restenosis.

Table 26-6. Surgical Procedures for Lumbar Spinal Stenosis

Stable Spine
  Wide laminectomy: Decompression of the central canal, lateral recess, and neural foramina
  Hemilaminectomy: Unilateral decompression for single-sided symptoms
  Laminotomy: Removal of the undersurface of the laminae of the posterior elements, partial facetectomy, and neural foramina
  Expansive laminoplasty: Use of bone grafts to enlarge the volume of the spinal canal
  Distraction device: Interspinous process distraction device
Unstable Spine – Degenerative Spondylolisthesis/Scoliosis
  Laminectomy alone: preservation of facet integrity
  Laminectomy with uninstrumented fusion
  Laminectomy with instrumented fusion
  Laminectomy with scoliosis segmental correction with fusion and stabilization of sagittal and coronal scoliosis

---

Chronic pain therapy may also become a mainstay of therapy for individuals with spinal stenosis who forego surgery or who have residual pain postoperatively. Chronic pain therapy has many of the components of care already mentioned in this chapter. Additional oral therapies may include antidepressants and anticonvulsants. Antidepressants that are not epinephrine reuptake inhibitors have greater benefit than selective serotonin reuptake inhibitors.[51] The toxicities of these agents in the elderly tend to limit their utility in this population with chronic low back pain. Antiepileptics, such as gabapentin, have been studied in small clinical trials of patients with chronic low back and radicular pain. The strength of the evidence demonstrating efficacy is modest.[52]

Topical therapies including patches have the benefit of minimal systemic exposure and the associated toxicities. Only a minimal amount of data are available to evaluate the benefit of these therapies for chronic back pain.[53] Acupuncture is another form of therapy that has few adverse toxicities. That is a characteristic in its favor. In clinical trials, acupuncture has demonstrated benefit in pain relief compared with placebo.[54] However, although offering pain relief, acupuncture does not have a greater benefit over other active therapies.[55] I recommend acupuncture as adjunctive to a drug program. Patients need to understand a number of visits, usually ten, are needed to experience the full benefits of acupuncture treatment. Cognitive-behavioral therapy may also be considered for those with time to commit to the therapy and the availability of a program. This psychological therapy program improves pain intensity, and daily functioning.[56]

Case Study 4 Treatment

The patient was treated over a 5-year period. Initially, he was treated with acetaminophen, celecoxib, and a cane to facilitate ambulation. He subsequently took valdecoxib for 18 months with a beneficial effect. He supplemented low-dose tramadol for added pain relief. He had increasing difficulty with severe osteoarthritis of the right knee and had a joint replacement that improved his gait. He had greater difficulty walking longer distances and prednisone 5 mg was prescribed for days he would be walking extensively. After 10 months, he tried an epidural injection. The benefits lasted for 2 months and he had a subsequent injection that lasted for 6 months. He had subsequent injections for the next 12 months. At that time, he had no further benefit from the injections and he experienced leg pain within minutes of standing up. He was evaluated by a spine surgeon, who agreed that he was a good candidate for spinal decompression surgery because he had no significant comorbidities. The patient underwent a two-level decompression and had an excellent result. He has continued to have improvement 2 years after his operation. He is taking no medicine for musculoskeletal pain and uses his cane only for balance purposes.

Experimental Treatment

A number of therapies are available for the treatment of mechanical disease of the lumbar spine. Some therapies have indications for low back pain (intervertebral disc replacement) but are designated for very specific patient populations. Other therapies have been reported in the medical literature but have not received approval through insurance companies, making availability limited.

Tumor Necrosis Factor Inhibitors

Tumor necrosis factor (TNF) is located at the site of nerve injuries associated with disc herniations in animal models. TNF produces wallerian degeneration of nerve fibers and myelin sheath splitting similar to that induced by herniated discs.[20,57] Theoretically, inhibition of TNF would have the benefit of diminishing the symptoms and signs of radiculopathy related to disc herniation.[58] The results of clinical trials have not been promising in support of this hypothesis. A double-blind, placebo-controlled trial of a one-time infusion of infliximab was not better than placebo in resolving lumbar radiculopathy.[59] However, a more recent trial of two adalimumab injections separated by a week's interval did demonstrate improvement in the need for fewer operations compared to placebo.[60] The true benefit of TNF inhibitors for acute sciatica related to disc herniation requires additional study. The parameters for patient selection remain to be determined. For example, TNF may be most important early in the development of sciatica. If this statement was correct, TNF inhibitor therapy would need to be given early to show the greatest effect.

Intradiscal Electrothermal Treatment

Intradiscal electrothermal treatment (IDET) is a technique used in patients with presumed discogenic causes of chronic low back pain. The technique places an electric catheter in a symptomatic disc, and heats and congeals the internal components of the disc. The procedure is proposed as a substitute for interbody fusion with plates or cages for symptomatic disc disease. Discography is the method used to identify symptomatic discs. The catheter is heated to a temperature of 90° F for 13 minutes.[61] Clinical trials concerning this technique have not demonstrated significant benefits compared with placebo In general, patients who undergo IDET procedures may have greater residual back pain than those who follow a natural history of disease without invasive intervention. The procedure is associated with complications including the risk of additional episodes of disc herniation.[62] Major questions remain regarding the utility of IDET for individuals with back pain. Does discogenic pain exist? Is the disc or surrounding tissues the source of pain? Will making the disc stiffer prolong the "spacer" function, or will degeneration occur at a more rapid rate? IDET must be considered an experimental procedure until the answers to these questions are determined.

Other invasive therapies directed toward improvement of disc pain include intradiscal injections, percutaneous discectomy, intradiscal laser discectomy, and nucleoplasty. All of these methods presume that the intervertebral disc without herniation is a source of persistent low back pain. Intradiscal injections with corticosteroids have no predictable benefit.[63] Patient selection is essential in considering the appropriate candidates for these experimental surgical techniques that invade the integrity of the disc.[64]

Sclerosant (Prolotherapy) Injections

Ligamentous structures play an important role in the stability of the spine. Optimal function of the lumbar spine requires mobilization of stiffened structures while strengthening weakened supporting connective tissue. Sclerosant therapy uses a chemical irritant (phenol, dextrose) to induce fibroblastic hyperplasia, causing an increase in collagen formation. The goal of sclerosant therapy is the deposition of increased amounts of normal collagenous material in ligament, fascia, or tendon by provoking a controlled inflammation at the injection site. Exercise therapy is a component of therapy after injection to maximize motion. Clinical trials have not demonstrated the benefits of sclerosant injections compared to saline injections.[65] The injections can be associated with significant toxicities including paralysis and death. Therefore, these injections should be given only by practitioners familiar with the appropriate sites for injections. In any case, sclerosant therapy is an experimental treatment.

Another form of injection therapy for paraspinous soft tissue contraction is botulinum neurotoxin. Open-label trials have demonstrated improvement in about 50% of patients at 2 months. Only a small group less than 10% has a sustained benefit at 6 months.[66] A recent review of botulinum toxin studies suggested only a marginal benefit for these injections.[67]

Artificial Lumbar Disc Replacement

Lumbar spine disc disease can be associated with decreasing motion and increasing pain with unnatural pressures placed on articular elements. The artificial disc replacement has been engineered to maintain motion at a disc level and re-establish normal relationships between anatomic structures of the vertebral segment.[68] The exclusions for this operation is extensive including facet arthritis, spondylolysis, spondylolisthesis, herniated disc with radiculopathy, scoliosis, osteoporosis, or postsurgical pseudoarthrosis among others. In other words, the patients eligible for this operation are few.[69] Surgeons are concerned that the patients who are eligible for the operation may have so few anatomic abnormalities that they would not need the operation. The surgical procedure is more intricate than usual disc surgery.[70] Long-term outcome studies are not available. Failures of the replacement may be related to the implant, osteoporosis of vertebral bone, heterotopic ossification, among others.[71] Although the US Food and Drug Administration has approved disc replacement for placement in patients, the procedure is in its infancy. Much greater research will be needed before the procedure is considered routine.

References

1. Lawrence RC, Felson DT, Helmick CG, Arnold LN, Choi H, Deyo RA, et al. Estimates of the prevalence of arthritis and other rheumatic conditions in the United States. Part II. Arthritis Rheum 2008;58:26-35.
2. Nerlich AG, Schleicher ED, Boos N. 1997 Volvo award winner in basic science studies: Immunologic markers for age-related changes of human lumbar intervertebral discs. Spine 1997;22:2781-95.
3. Boos N, Weissbach S, Rohrbach H, Weiler C, Spratt KF, Nerlich AG. Classification of age-related changes in lumbar intervertebral discs: 2002 Volvo award in basic science. Spine 2002;23:2631-44.
4. Chou R, Qaseem A, Snow V, Casey D, Cross JT Jr, Shekelle P, et al. Diagnosis and treatment of low back pain: A joint clinical practice guideline from the American College of Physicians and the American Pain Society. Ann Intern Med 2007;147:478-91.
5. Borenstein DG, Wiesel SW, Boden SD. Low Back and Neck Pain: Comprehensive Diagnosis and Management. 3rd ed. Philadelphia, PA: Saunders; 2004.
6. Nachemson A. The lumbar spine—an orthopaedic challenge. Spine 1976;1:59-71.
7. Dillane JB, Fry J, Kalton G. Acute back syndrome: a study from general practice. BMJ 1966;3:82.
8. Malmivarra A, Hakkinen U, Aro T, Heinrichs ML, Koskenniemi L, Kuosma E, et al. The treatment of acute low back pain: Bed rest, exercises, or ordinary activity? N Engl J Med 1995;332:351-5.
9. Borenstein D. Back. In: Borenstein D, editor. Control: A Conventional and Complementary Prescription for Eliminating Back Pain. New York: M Evans and Company; 2001. p. 54–62.
10. Chou R, Huffman LH. Medications for acute and chronic low back pain: A review of the evidence for an American Pain Society/American College of Physicians Clinical Practice guideline. Ann Intern Med 2007;147:505-14.
11. Borenstein DG, Korn S. Efficacy of a low-dose regimen of cyclobenzaprine hydrochloride in acute skeletal muscle spasm. Results of two placebo-controlled trials. Clin Ther 2003;25:1056-73.
12. See S, Ginzburg R. Choosing a skeletal muscle relaxant. Am Fam Physician 2008;78:365-70.
13. Cherkin DC, Wheeler KJ, Barlow W, Deyo RA. Medication use for low back pain in primary care. Spine 1998;23:607-14.
14. Chou R, Huffman LH. Nonpharmacologic therapies for acute and chronic low back pain: A review of the evidence for an American Pain Society/American College of Physicians clinical practice guideline. Ann Intern Med 2007;147:492-504.
15. Garvey TA, Marks MR, Wiesel SW. A prospective, randomized, double-blind evaluation of trigger-point injection therapy for low back pain. Spine 1989;14:962-4.
16. Nelemans PJ, deBie RA, deVet HC, Sturmans F. Injection therapy for subacute and chronic benign low back pain. Spine 2001;26:501-15.
17. Hurwitz EL, Morganstern H, Harber P, Kominslei GF, Berhin TR, Yu F, et al. University of California-Los Angeles. A randomized trial of medical care with and without physical therapy and chiropractic care with and without physical modalities for patients with low back pain: 6-month follow-up outcomes from the UCLA low back pain study. Spine 2002;27:2193-204.
18. Cherkin DC, MacCornack FA. Patient evaluations of low back pain care from family physicians and chiropractors. West J Med 1989;150:351-5.
19. Goupille P, Jayson MI, Valat JP, Freemont AJ. The role of inflammation in disk herniation-associated radiculopathy. Semin Arthritis Rheum 1998;28:60-71.
20. Olmarker K, Rydevik B. Selective inhibition of tumor necrosis factor-alpha prevents nucleus pulposus-induced thrombus formation, intraneural edema, and reduction of nerve conduction velocity. Possible implications for future pharmacologic treatment strategies of sciatica. Spine 2001;26:863-9.
21. Komori H, Shinomiya K, Nakai O, Yamaura I, Takeda S, Furuya K. The natural history of herniated nucleus pulposus with radiculopathy. Spine 1996;21:225-9.
22. Komori H, Okawa A, Haro H, Muneta T, Haro H, Shinomiya K. Contrast-enhanced magnetic resonance imaging in conservative management of lumbar disc herniation. Spine 1998;22:67-73.
23. Mahowald ML, Singh JA, Majeski P. Opioid use by patients in an orthopedics spine clinic. Arthritis Rheum 2005;52:312-21.
24. Carette S, LeClaire R, Marcoux S, Morin F, Blaise GA, St-Pierre A, et al. Epidural corticosteroid injections for sciatica due to herniated nucleus pulposus. N Engl J Med 1997;336:1634-40.
25. Ng L, Chaudhary N, Sell P. The efficacy of corticosteroids in periradicular infiltration for chronic radicular pain: A randomized, double-blind, controlled trial. Spine 2005;30:857-62.
26. Weinstein JN, Lurie JD, Tosteson TD, Skinner JS, Hanscom B, Tasteson AN, et al. Surgical vs nonoperative treatment for lumbar disk herniation: the Spine Patient Outcomes Research Trial (SPORT) observational cohort. JAMA 2006;296:2451-9.
27. Peul WC, van Houwelingen HC, van den Hout WB, Brand R, Eekhof JA, Tans JT, et al. Surgery versus prolonged conservative treatment for sciatica. N Engl J Med 2007;356:2245-56.
28. Lurie JD, Faucett SC, Hanscom B, Tosteson TD, Ball PA, Abdu WA, et al. Lumbar discectomy outcomes vary by herniation level in the Spine Patient Outcomes Research Trial. J Bone Joint Surg Am 2008;90:1811-9.
29. Mariconda M, Galasso O, Secondulfo V, Rotonda GD, Milano C. Minimum 25-year outcome and functional assessment of lumbar disectomy. Spine 2006;31:2593-9.
30. Jones TR, Rao R. Pathophysiology of axial low back pain. Semin Spine Surg 2008;20:78-86.
31. Butler D, Trafimow JH, Andersson GB, McNeill TW, Huckman MS. Discs degenerate before facets. Spine 1990;15:111-3.
32. Dolan AL, Ryan PJ, Arden NK, Stratton R, Wedley JR, Hamann W, et al. The value of SPECT scans in identifying back pain likely to benefit from facet joint injection. Br J Rheumatol 1996;35:1269-73.
33. Dieppe P, Brandt KD. What is important in treating osteoarthritis? Whom should we treat and how should we treat them? Rheum Dis Clin North Am 2003;29:687-716.
34. Gorbach C, Schmid MR, Elfering A, Hodler J, Boos N. Therapeutic efficacy of facet joint blocks. AJR Am J Roentgenol 2006;186:1228-33.
35. Ackerman 3rd WE, Ahmad M. Pain relief with intraarticular or medial branch nerve blocks in patients with positive lumbar facet joint SPECT imaging: a 12-week outcome study. South Med J 2008;101:931-4.
36. Dreyfuss P, Halbrook B, Pauza K, Joshi A, Mclarty J, Bogduk N. Efficacy and validity of radiofrequency neurotomy for chronic lumbar zygapophyseal joint pain. Spine 2000;25:1270-7.
37. De Graaf I, Prak A, Bierma-Zeinstra S, Thomas S, Peul W, Koes B. Diagnosis of lumbar spinal stenosis: A systematic review of the accuracy of diagnostic tests. Spine 2006;31:1168-76.
38. Moreland LW, Lopez-Mendez A, Alarcon GS. Spinal stenosis: A comprehensive review of the literature. Semin Arthritis Rheum 1989;19:127-49.
39. Whiteman JM, Flynn TW, Childs JD, Wainner RS, Gill HE, Ryder MG, et al. A comparison between two physical therapy treatment programs for patients with lumbar spinal stenosis. Spine 2006;31:254-9.
40. van Tulder MW, Scholten RJ, Koes BW, Deyo RA. Nonsteroidal anti-inflammatory drugs for low back pain: a systematic review within the framework of the Cochrane Collaboration Back Review Group. Spine 2000;25:2501–13.
41. Martell BA, O'Connor PG, Kerns RD, Becker WC, Morales KH, Kosten TR, et al. Systematic review: Opioid treatment for chronic back pain: Prevalence, efficacy, and association with addiction. Ann Intern Med 2007;146:116-27.

42. Borenstein D. Opioids: To use or not to use? That is the question. Arthritis Rheum 2005;52:6-10.
43. Finckh A, Zufferey P, Schurch M, Balague F, Waldburger M, So AK, et al. Short-term efficacy of intravenous pulse glucocorticoids in acute discogenic sciatica. A randomized controlled trial. Spine 2006;31:377-81.
44. Rydevik BL, Cohen DB, Kostuik JP. Spine epidural steroids for patients with lumbar spinal stenosis. Spine 1997;22:2314-7.
45. Botwin KP, Gruber RD. Lumbar epidural steroid injections in the patient with lumbar spinal stenosis. Phys Med Rehabil Clin N Am 2003;14:121-41.
46. Sengupta DK, Herkowitz HN. Lumbar spinal stenosis. Treatment strategies and indicators for surgery. Orthop Clin North Am 2003;34:281-95.
47. Weinstein JN, Tosteson TD, Lurie JD, Tosteson ANA, Blood E, Hanscom B, et al. Surgical versus nonsurgical therapy for lumbar spinal stenosis. N Engl J Med 2008;358:795-810.
48. Siddiqui M, Smith FW, Wardlaw D. One-year results of X STOP interspinous implant for the treatment of lumbar spinal stenosis. Spine 2007;32:1345-8.
49. Airaksinen O, Herno A, Turunen V, Saari T, Suomlainen O. Surgical outcome of 438 patients treated surgically for lumbar spinal stenosis. Spine 1997;22:227-8.
50. Atlas SJ, Keller RB, Wu YA, Deyo RA, Singer DE. Long-term outcomes of surgical and nonsurgical management of lumbar spinal stenosis. Spine 2005;30:936-43.
51. Staiger TO, Gaster B, Sullivan MD, Deyo RA. Systematic review of antidepressants in the treatment of chronic low back pain. Spine 2003;28:2540-5.
52. Yaksi A, Ozgonenel L, Ozgonenel B. The efficiency of gabapentin therapy in patients with lumbar spine stenosis. Spine 2007;32:939-42.
53. Gimbel J, Linn R, Hale M, Nicholson B. Lidocaine patch treatment in patients with low back pain: results of an open-label, nonrandomized pilot study. Am J Ther 2005;12:311-9.
54. Haake M, Muller H, Schade-Brittinger C. German acupuncture trials (GERAC) for chronic low back pain. Arch Intern Med 2007;167:1892-8.
55. Manheimer E, White E, Berman B, Forys K, Ernst E. Meta-analysis: acupuncture for low back pain. Ann Intern Med 2005;142:651-63.
56. Linton SJ, Nordin E. A 5-year follow-up evaluation of the health and economic consequences of an early cognitive behavioral intervention for back pain. A randomized controlled trial. Spine 2006;31:853-8.
57. Olmarker K, Larrson K. Tumor necrosis factor-alpha and nucleus pulposus-induced nerve root injury. Spine 1998;23:2538-44.
58. Goupille P, Mulleman D, Pintaud G, Watier H, Valat JP. Can sciatica induced by disc herniation be treated with tumor necrosis factor α blockade? Arthritis Rheum 2007;56:3887-95.
59. Korhonen T, Karppinen J, Paimela L, Malmivaara A, Lindgren KA, Bowman C, et al. The treatment of disc herniation-induced sciatica with infliximab; one-year follow-up results of First II, a randomzied controlled trial. Spine 2006;31:2759-66.
60. Genevay S, Viatte S, Zufferey P, Finckh A, Balague F, Cem G. Adalimumab in the treatment of acute severe sciatica, a randomized double blind placebo controlled study. Arthritis Rheum 2008;58:S630.
61. Saal JA, Saal JS. Intradiscal electrothermal treatment for chronic discogenic low back pain. Prospective outcome study with a minimum of 2-year follow-up. Spine 2002;27:966-74.
62. Hulen CA. Nonoperative treatment of low back pain. Semi Spine Surg 2008;20:102-12.
63. Simmons JW, McMillin JN, Emery SF, Kimmich SJ. Intradiscal steroids: a prospective double-blind clinical trial. Spine 1992;17:S172-5.
64. Klein RG, Eek BC, O'Neill CW, Elin C, Mooney V, Derby RR. Biochemical injection treatment for discogenic low back pain: a pilot study. Spine J 2003;3:220-6.
65. Ohnmeiss DD, Guyer RD, Hochschuler SH. Laser disc decompression: the importance of proper patient selection. Spine 1994;19:2054-9.
66. Yelland MJ, Glasziou PP, Bogduk N, Schluter PJ, McKernon M. Prolotherapy injections, saline injections, and exercises for chronic low back pain: a randomized trial. Spine 2004;29:9-16.
67. Ney JP, Difazio M, Sichani A, Monacci W, Foster L, Jabbari B. Treatment of chronic low back pain with successive injections of botulinum toxin a over 6 months: a prospective trial of 60 patients. Clin J Pain 2006;22:363-9.
68. Naumann M, So Y, Argoff CE, Childers MK, Dykstra DD, Gronseth GS, et al. Assessment: Botulinum neurotoxin in the treatment of autonomic disorders and pain (an evidence-based review): report of the Therapeutics and Technology Assessment Subcommittee of the American Academy of Neurology. Neurology 2008;70:1707-14.
69. Randolph GB, Scioscia TN, Wang JC. Lumbar total disc arthroplasty: State of the data. Semin Spine Surg 2006;18:61-71.
70. Zigler JE, Ohnmeiss DD. Patient selection for lumbar arthroplasty. Semin Spine Surg 2006;18:40-6.
71. Tortolani PJ, McAfee PC, Saiedy S. Failures of lumbar disc replacmenet. Semin Spine Surg 2006;18:78-86.

Chapter 27

Mechanisms and Treatment Strategy of Complex Regional Pain Syndromes

Wilfrid Jänig and Ralf Baron

INTRODUCTION

Complex regional pain syndromes (CRPS) are painful disorders typically affecting the limbs that may develop as a consequence of trauma. That the sympathetic nervous system is causally involved in CRPS is based mainly on two observations: (1) the pain is spatially correlated with signs of autonomic dysfunction, that is, with abnormalities in blood flow and sweating, as well as with trophic changes, and (2) temporary blocking the efferent sympathetic supply to the affected part relieves the pain in subgroups of patients with CRPS. CRPS syndromes were originally known under the terms reflex sympathetic dystrophy or causalgia (or several other terms depending on medical speciality and country).[1,2] However, these terms were thought to be inappropriate as a clinical designation: They were sloppily used to describe an extensive range of clinical presentations and the pathophysiologic mechanisms underlying these syndromes were poorly understood. The new terminology is descriptive and based entirely on elements of history, symptoms, and findings on clinical examination, with no implied pathophysiologic mechanism avoiding any mechanistic implications.[3] According to the International Association for the Study of Pain (IASP) Classification of Chronic Pain, reflex sympathetic dystrophy and causalgia are now called Complex Regional Pain Syndromes (CRPS). In reflex sympathetic dystrophy (CRPS type I), minor injuries at the limb or lesions in remote body areas precede the onset of symptoms. CRPS type II (causalgia) may develop after injury of a major peripheral nerve.[4]

Patients with CRPS presenting with exactly the same clinical signs and symptoms can be further divided into two subgroups by the negative or positive effect of sympathetic blockade. The pain component that is relieved by specific sympatholytic procedures is considered sympathetically maintained pain (SMP). Thus, SMP is defined as a *symptom* and *not a clinical entity. The positive effect of a sympathetic blockade is not essential for the diagnosis of CRPS.* On the other hand, the only possibility to differentiate between SMP and sympathetically independent pain (SIP) is the efficacy of a correctly applied sympatholytic intervention.[3]

The mechanisms underlying CRPS remain controversial despite the extensive body of clinical experience and experimentation on patients and animal models. The lack of well-controlled clinical studies has been accompanied by extensive speculations about the underlying pathophysiology. Here we will first present a hypothesis stating that CRPS is a disease of the central nervous system (CNS) involving central and peripheral components and discuss the clinical and experimental data supporting this hypothesis. Based on this concept we will then describe the diagnostic approach and the treatment strategy. The clinical phenomena of CRPS (Table 27-1) are described in detail in references 5 to 8.

COMPLEX REGIONAL PAIN SYNDROME IS A NEURONAL DISEASE INVOLVING THE CENTRAL NERVOUS SYSTEM

CRPS is characterized by sensory, sympathetic, somatomotor, and trophic changes (including swelling) that occur in variable combinations. We have hypothesized that these changes are the result of an altered processing of information in the CNS involving the somatosensory non-nociceptive and nociceptive systems, the endogenous neuronal systems controlling nociceptive impulse transmission, the sympathetic systems, and the somatomotor system. Various levels of integration probably are involved such as spinal cord, brain stem, diencephalon (hypothalamus, thalamus), and telencephalon (cortex and limbic system). Key players in generation and maintenance of CRPS are most likely the nociceptive system and the sympathetic nervous system. But CRPS cannot be reduced to a malfunctioning of one of these systems or components of them alone.[9,10] Here we discuss the arguments supporting that CRPS is a CNS disease. The upper part in Table 27-2 lists clinical and experimental observations made on patients with CRPS that clearly support this contention. The lower part in Table 27-2 lists the peripheral changes observed in patients with CRPS that are also related in some yet unknown way to the central changes.

Table 27-1. *Diagnostic Criteria and Diagnostic Tests in Complex Regional Pain Syndrome (CRPS)*

A. Diagnostic Criteria: Categories of Clinical Signs and Symptoms*

1. Positive sensory abnormalities
   - Spontaneous pain
   - Mechanical hyperalgesia
   - Thermal hyperalgesia
   - Deep somatic hyperalgesia
2. Vascular abnormalities
   - Vasodilation
   - Vasoconstriction
   - Skin temperature asymmetries
   - Skin color changes
3. Edema, sweating abnormalities
   - Swelling
   - Hyperhidrosis
   - Hypohidrosis

4. Motor (M) and trophic changes (T)
   - Motor weakness (M)
   - Tremor (M)
   - Dystonia (M)
   - Coordination deficit (M)
   - Nail or hair changes (T)
   - Skin atrophy (T)
   - Joint stiffness (T)
   - Soft tissue changes (T)

Interpretation
Clinical use
≥1 symptoms of ≥3 categories each AND ≥1 signs at the time of evaluation in ≥2 categories each
Sensitivity 0.85, specificity 0.60
Research use
≥1 symptoms in each of the 4 categories AND ≥1 signs at the time of evaluation in ≥2 categories each
Sensitivity 0.70, specificity 0.96

B. Diagnostic Tests

Test	*Sensitivity*	*Specificity*
1. Plain Radiograph (only chronic CRPS)	0.73	0.57
2. Three phase bone scan (only acute CRPS)	0.97	0.86[†]
3. Quantitative sensory testing	High	Low
4. Temperature differences (during symptom stimulation)	0.76	0.93
5. MRI (e.g., skin, joint)	0.91	0.17
6. Magnet encephalogram, functional MRI (cortical reorganization)	Unknown (prob. not useful)	Probably low

MRI, magnetic resonance imaging.
*These diagnostic criteria have been modified[56-58] compared with the original criteria as defined by Stanton-Hicks and collegues[3] in order to obtain a higher specificity for clinical use (to avoid overdiagnosis of CRPS) and a higher sensitivity for research use.
†Early differentiation from normal post-traumatic states is difficult.
From Baron R. Complex regional pain syndromes. In: Basbaum AL, Kaneko A, Shepherd GM, Westheimer G, Basbaum AI, editors. The Senses: a Comprehensive Reference. Vol 5. Pain. San Diego: Academic Press; 2008. p. 909-18.

The explanatory hypothesis as outlined in Figure 27-1 puts the clinical findings observed in patients with CRPS in relation to the changes in the somatosensory, autonomic and somatomotor systems and postulates that changes in the central representations of these systems must occur in order to explain the clinical findings. The events initiating the clinical symptoms are mostly associated with a trauma at the extremities but sometimes also with trauma in the viscera or in the CNS. The changes developing after these triggering events usually outlast the trauma by orders of magnitude.

An important component of the hypothesis for patients with CRPS with SMP is postulated to be a positive feedback circuit consisting of afferent neurons, central neurons (spinal circuits and their supraspinal controls), sympathetic neurons, and sympathetic-afferent coupling. This circuit would maintain spontaneous pain (sympathetically maintained), hyperalgesia and allodynia and the other associated changes in the peripheral tissues (see 6-8 in Table 27-2 and Figure 27-1).[11,12] This positive feedback circuit does not explain the (peripheral and central) mechanisms in detail and fails to explain

the central changes that must occur in CRPS in view of the clinical changes observed in these patients (see below and Table 27-2). Furthermore, it fails to explain why CRPS I without SMP is clinically entirely indistinguishable from CRPS I with SMP.

Clinical and Experimental Observations Supporting the Hypothesis

Initiating Events

The signs and symptoms in CRPS (see Table 27-1A) are disproportionate to the traumatic events initiating or triggering this syndrome. The local changes generated by the trauma often disappear, yet the syndrome persists. Furthermore, CRPS I in an extremity may be triggered by remote events (e.g., in the viscera) or by events in the CNS (e.g., central lesions) (*1* in Fig. 27-1). It has been proposed that processes in the prefrontal, frontal, and parietal cortices that are related to psychosocial changes enhance the clinical signs and symptoms in CRPS or

Table 27-2. *Arguments for Central and for Peripheral Changes in Complex Regional Pain Syndrome**

Central Changes
Initiating events (1 in Fig. 27-1)
- Out of proportion to finding (minor trauma)
- Events remote from affected extremity (e.g., in the visceral domain)
- Central (e.g., after stroke; related to endogenous control systems?)

Sensory changes (2 in Fig. 27-1)
- Mechanical allodynia (quadrant, hemisensory)
- Hypoesthesias (mechanical, cold, warm; hemisensory, quadrant)
- Bilateral distribution of hypo- and hyperesthesias (mechanical, cold, warm, heat)

Pain relief by sympathetic blocks with local anesthetics (3 in Fig. 27-1)
- Relief of pain *outlasts conduction block* by an order of magnitude (i.e., a temporary block is followed by a *long-lasting* pain relief)
- A few temporary blocks are sometimes sufficient to generate permanent pain relief
- Sympathetic activity maintains a positive feedback circuit (?)

Changes of regulation by sympathetic systems (4 in Fig. 27-1)
- Thermoregulatory reflexes in cutaneous vasoconstrictor neurons reduced
- Respiration elicited reflexes (generated by deep inspiration and expiration) in cutaneous vasoconstrictor neurons reduced
- Changes of activity in sudomotor neurons (sweating)
- Swelling reduced by sympathetic blocks

Somatomotor changes (5 in Fig. 27-1)
- Active motor force and active range of motion reduced
- Physiologic tremor increased
- Poor motor control and coordination of movement; altered gait and posture
- Dystonia
- Sensory-motor body perception disturbance

Peripheral Changes
Sympathetic-afferent coupling (6 in Fig. 27-1)
- After nerve lesion via norepinephrine and adrenoceptors (CRPS II)
- Indirectly via vascular bed and other mechanisms (CRPS I; deep somatic?)
- [Indirectly via inflammatory mediators and neurotrophic factors]
- [Mediated by the adrenal medulla (epinephrine)]

Inflammatory changes and edema (7 in Fig. 27-1)
- Neurogenic inflammation (precapillary vasodilation, venular plasma extravasation), involvement of peptidergic afferents (?)
- Sympathetic fibers mediating effects of inflammatory mediators (e.g., bradykinin) to venules leading to plasma extravasation (?)
- Involvement of inflammatory cells and immune system (?)
- Change of capillary filtration pressure (?)

Trophic changes (8 in Fig. 27-1)
- Long-range consequences of inflammatory changes and edema (?)
- Direct (trophic?) effect of sympathetic and afferent fibers on tissue (?)
- Endothelial damage (?)

*Arguments for central and peripheral changes based on clinical observations and quantitative measurements made in patients with CRPS. In bold are listed the phenomena observed on the patients. The numbers in brackets refer to the explanatory hypothesis outlined graphically in Figure 27-1. Modified from Jänig W, Baron R. Complex regional pain syndrome: mystery explained? Lancet Neurol 2003;2:687-97.

even may initiate them.[15-18] These clinical observations argue (1) that mechanisms operating in CRPS cannot simply be explained to be *caused* by events in the body related to the trauma (e.g., sympathetic-afferent coupling or persistent activation of nociceptive afferents) and (2) that the CNS is important to understand the mechanisms initiating and maintaining the CRPS syndromes.

Somatic Sensations Including Pain

Pain is a salient feature of CRPS, consisting of ongoing pain, hyperalgesia and allodynia* generated by mechanical or cold stimuli. However, it must

---

*Hyperalgesia describes increased pain generated by normally painful mechanical or thermal stimuli. Allodynia (mechanical, cold) describes pain to mechanical or cold stimuli that are normally not painful and excite mechanoreceptors (with Aβ-fibers) or cold receptors but not sensitized receptors.[4]

be kept in mind that about 10% or more of patients with CRPS do not have ongoing pain, that the pain is mostly not restricted to the site of trauma, that the pain is associated with other somato-sensory changes (cold, mechanical, warm hypoesthesias) in 50% of the patients, and that pain (and the other somatosensory changes) persists for long periods of time after the local changes of the trauma have subsided.[19,20] Thus, pain in CRPS must be understood in a wider context in order to understand the therapeutic implications: (1) Ongoing pain and evoked pain (superficial and particular deep mechanical hyperalgesia and allodynia) are mostly entirely out of proportion to the trauma. (2) The anatomic distribution of the changed painful and nonpainful somatosensory perceptions observed in CRPS patients are likely due to changes in the central representation of somatosensory sensations in the thalamus and cortex. This is fully supported by

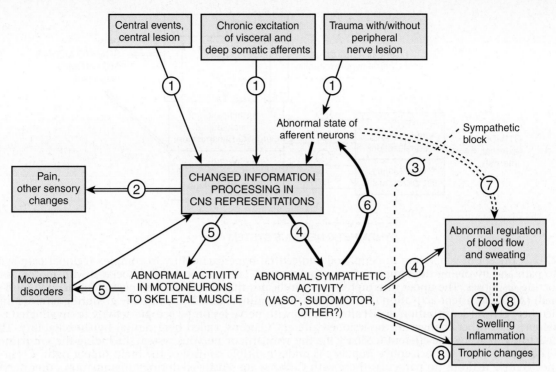

Figure 27-1. General explanatory hypothesis about the neural mechanisms of generation of complex regional pain syndromes (CRPS) I and II following peripheral trauma with and without nerve lesions, chronic stimulation of visceral afferents (e.g., during angina pectoris, myocardial infarction) and of deep somatic afferents and, rarely, central trauma. The clinical observations are put in bold-lined boxes. Note the vicious circle (*arrows in bold black*). An important component of this circle is the excitatory influence of postganglionic sympathetic axons on primary afferent neurons. The numbers indicate the changes occurring potentially in patients with CRPS that have been quantitatively measured or postulated on the basis of clinical observations (see Table 27-2): *1*, changes in sympathetic neurons; *2*, pain, somatosensory changes; *3*, changes in somatomotoneurons; *4*, initiating events; *5*, consequences of sympathetic blocks or sympathectomy (dotted line); *6*, sympathetic-afferent coupling (positive vicious feedback circuit [in bold]); *7*, "antidromically" conducted activity in peptidergic afferent C-fibers (*double dotted arrow*) leading to increase of blood flow (arteriolar vasodilation) and venular plasma extravasation, both hypothetically contributing to increase in blood flow, swelling/inflammation and trophic changes; *8*, sympathetic postganglionic fibers hypothetically contributing to swelling/inflammation and trophic changes. For details see text. (Modified from Jänig W. Causalgia and reflex sympathetic dystrophy: in which way is the sympathetic nervous system involved? Trends Neurosci 1985;8:471-7 and Jänig W. The puzzle of reflex sympathetic dystrophy: mechanisms, hypotheses, open questions. In: Jänig W, Stanton-Hicks M, editors. Reflex Sympathetic Dystrophy: A Reappraisal. Seattle: IASP Press; 1996. p. 1-24 and based on Livingston WK. Pain Mechanisms. A Physiological Interpretation of Causalgia and Related States. New York; Macmillan [reprinted by Plenum Press (1976)]; 1943.)

magnetic encephalographic (MEG) and functional magnetic resonance imaging (MRI) studies showing that changes occur in various cortical areas, including the primary and secondary somatosensory, insular, frontal and parietal cortices[15-18] (for discussion and references see reference 21). In fact, patients with CRPS can exhibit strong body perception disturbances[22,23] and show sensations referred to areas of the body immediately adjacent to the stimulated body sites.[24] (3) Generalized somatosensory deficits are particularly found in patients with chronic CRPS, indicating long-term plastic changes in the telencephalon. To emphasize, these CNS changes occur in patients with CRPS I who have no nerve lesions. (4) CRPS patients mostly locate their spontaneous pain into deep somatic structures of the affected extremity. Furthermore, they have deep somatic mechanical hyperalgesia/allodynia.

Sympathetically Maintained Pain in Complex Regional Pain Syndrome

Pain dependent on activity in the sympathetic neurons called *sympathetically maintained pain* (SMP[3,5]) usually includes both spontaneous and evoked pain (i.e., allodynia evoked by mechanical or cold stimuli) and is present in about 60% of patients with acute CRPS and can persist for years. The concept that the (efferent) sympathetic nervous system is involved in the generation of pain is based on long standing clinical observations.[3,25-27]

In healthy subjects, there is no obvious sign for direct or indirect coupling between the efferent sympathetic systems and the afferent systems in the peripheral tissues leading to pain, discomfort, or other sensations maintained by the sympathetic outflow. This may change after trauma with or without nerve lesion. Now activity in

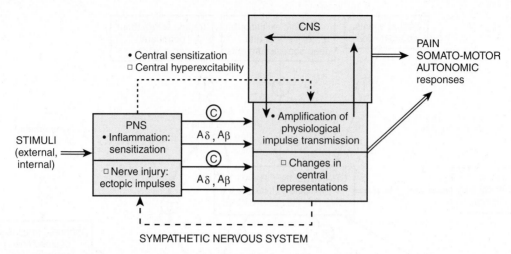

Figure 27-2. Concept of generation of peripheral and central hyperexcitability in complex regional pain syndromes leading to pain and involving the sympathetic nervous system. The pain is always associated with motor, autonomic and endocrine responses. The upper interrupted arrow indicates that the central changes are generated (and possibly maintained) (**A**) by persistent activation of nociceptors with unmyelinated (C-) fibers (e.g., during chronic inflammation) called here central sensitization or (**B**) after trauma with nerve lesion by ectopic activity in myelinated (Aδ-, Aβ-) and C-afferents and other changes in the lesioned afferent neurons, called here central hyperexcitability. The lower interrupted arrow indicates the efferent feedback via the sympathetic nervous system (including the sympathoadrenal system). The transmission of nociceptive impulses is under multiple control of the brain (upper right, CNS). Primary afferent nociceptive neurons (in particular those with C-fibers) are sensitized during inflammation. After nerve lesion, *all* lesioned primary afferent neurons (unmyelinated as well as myelinated ones) undergo biochemical, physiologic, and morphologic changes that become irreversible with time. These peripheral changes entail changes of the central representations (of the somatosensory system), which become irreversible if no regeneration of primary afferent neurons to their target tissue occurs. The central functional changes, induced by persistent activity in afferent nociceptive neurons during chronic inflammation or by ectopic activity in afferent neurons after nerve lesion, are also reflected in the sympathetic efferent feedback system that may establish positive feedback loops to the primary afferent neurons. CNS, central nervous system. PNS, peripheral nervous system. (From Jänig W. Autonomic nervous system dysfunction. In: Mayer EA, Bushnell MC, editors. Functional Pain Syndromes: Presentation and Pathophysiology. Seattle: IASP Press; 2009. p. 265-300.)

sympathetic neurons may lead to SMP. The concept is schematically exemplified in Figure 27-2. During inflammation or following nerve lesion, the efferent (noradrenergic) innervation of the affected tissue may generate feedback to the primary afferent neurons and activate them, enhance their ongoing activity, or enhance their activity to mechanical or thermal stimuli. This, in turn, would amplify the physiologic impulse transmission in the spinal or trigeminal dorsal horn (sensitization of dorsal horn neurons) or would enhance the hyperexcitability of these neurons following nerve lesion.[28]

Cross-talk from sympathetic postganglionic (noradrenergic) neurons to primary afferent neurons may occur in several forms. The mechanisms of coupling as well as transmitter and receptors (mainly norepinephrine and adrenoceptors) involved have been discussed in the literature.[28-30] The physiologic changes in the spinal dorsal horn following peripheral inflammation or nerve injury are also dependent on the supraspinal control (CNS loop in Fig. 27-2) of the nociceptive impulse transmission in the dorsal horn. Thus, SMP in patients cannot be reduced to the sympathetic feedback loop only.

Three groups of experimental studies on patients with CRPS are representative for this extensive work (for detailed literature see Jänig,[28] Baron and Jänig[29]):

1. In patients with CRPS with SMP (CRPS I, II), it has been shown that spontaneous pain, mechanical allodynia, and cold allodynia, that are alleviated by sympathetic ganglion blocks, can be rekindled, under the condition of proximal sympathetic block, or enhanced by injection of noradrenaline into the skin area that is painful or was painful before sympathetic blockade. Intradermal injection of noradrenaline, in physiologic concentrations (0.1–1 μM) in the unaffected contralateral limb or in limbs of healthy subjects does not elicit pain. SMP is significantly reduced by the α-adrenoceptor blocker phentolamine infused intravenously.[31,32]

2. The intensity of spontaneous cutaneous pain and the area of cutaneous mechanical hyperalgesia/allodynia (punctate/dynamic) increase during selective activation of the cutaneous vasoconstrictor outflow to the painful extremity by whole body cooling in patients with CRPS I with SMP but not in patients with CRPS I without SMP, that is, having sympathetically independent pain (SIP).[33] However, about 75% of the SMP in CRPS patients occurs in deep somatic tissues, that is, the coupling between sympathetic postganglionic fibers and afferent neurons occurs in skeletal muscle, joint, fascia, or bone. This corresponds

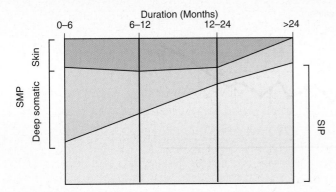

Figure 27-3. Different components of sympathetic maintained pain. The component of pain that depends on the cutaneous sympathetic innervation (skin SMP), on the deep somatic sympathetic innervation (deep SMP) and the pain component that is not maintained by sympathetic activity (SIP; sympathetically independent pain) during the course of the disease of 13 patients with complex regional pain syndromes (CRPS). Note that SMP decreases with time after the initiating event leading to CRPS. (With permission from Schattschneider J, Binder A, Siebrecht D, Wasner G, Baron R. Complex regional pain syndromes: the influence of cutaneous and deep somatic sympathetic innervation on pain. Clin J Pain 2006;22:240-4.)

to the observation that deep somatic tissues are extremely painful in many patients with CRPS. The SMP component is quantitatively significantly higher in early CRPS than in chronic CRPS (Fig. 27-3).[34]

3. Blockade of sympathetic activity to the affected extremity by a local anesthetic applied to the appropriate sympathetic paravertebral ganglia generates pain relief in the affected extremity for significantly longer time periods compared with saline injected close to the same site in the same group of patients with CRPS with SMP (Fig. 27-4A).[35] Thus, the pain relief generated by blockade of sympathetic activity exceeds that produced by a similar placebo block, and the duration of pain relief greatly outlasts the duration of conduction block generated by the local anesthetic. This indicates that the pain-relieving effect of sympathetic blocks observed in CRPS patients with SMP cannot be explained simply by temporary blockade of activity in the sympathetic neurons but that activity in sympathetic neurons, which is of *central origin*, maintains a positive feedback circuit via the primary afferent neurons. Activity in sympathetic neurons maintains a central state of hyperexcitability (e.g., of neurons in the spinal dorsal horn), via excitation of afferent neurons (see Fig. 27-2), which may be initiated by an intense noxious event or by central events. The central state of hyperexcitability is switched off during a temporary block of conduction in the sympathetic chain lasting only for a few hours and cannot be switched on again when the block wears off and the sympathetic

activity, and therefore also the sympathetically induced activity in afferent neurons, returns.

The mechanisms of sympathetic-afferent coupling leading to SMP are discussed in references 28 to 30.

Sympathetic Systems Supplying Skin

Cutaneous Vasoconstrictor Neurons, Skin Temperature, and Skin Blood Flow

One prominent sign in patients with CRPS is the difference in skin temperature between the affected extremity and the contralateral healthy extremity. At thermoregulatory neutral states this temperature difference is maximal and can reach values of up to 10° C. In early acute CRPS, the affected extremity is usually warmer, and in chronic CRPS, cooler than the contralateral extremity. Systematic experimentation on CRPS patients clearly shows that this difference in temperature is related to the failure of regulation of activity in cutaneous vasoconstrictor neurons by the CNS. Patients with CRPS exhibit, in the affected extremity, an impaired regulation of activity in cutaneous vasoconstrictor neurons innervating acral skin areas during whole body cooling or warming[37] or during deep inspiration or expiration.[38] This impaired regulation is reversed after successful treatment of CRPS (see later).

Sudomotor Neurons and Sweating

Clinical observations described in the literature show that sweating is changed in the affected extremity (e.g., hypo- or hyperhidrosis) compared with the unaffected contralateral extremity in patients with CRPS. Activation of sweat glands always occurs only via its cholinergic innervation and not by circulating substances or local mechanisms. Therefore, these changes can only be attributed to central changes, which then lead to changes of activity in sudomotor neurons. Experimentation on animals and humans show that central regulation of activity in cutaneous vasoconstrictor neurons and sudomotor neurons are closely linked to each other. Reflex inhibition in cutaneous vasoconstrictor neurons induced by peripheral or central (warm) stimuli is always accompanied by reflex activation of sudomotor neurons. This reciprocal reflex organization is based on the organization of both systems in the spinal cord, brain stem, and hypothalamus.[39] During mental and emotional stimulation both systems are activated simultaneously in humans, this being related to the control of both systems by the telencephalon.

Somatomotor Changes

About 50% or more of patients with CRPS show a decrease of active range of motion, increased amplitude of physiological tremor, reduced active motor force in the affected extremity, and in the extreme, myoclonus or dystonia.[40-44] These motor changes are unlikely related to a peripheral process (e.g., influence of the sympathetic nervous system on neuromuscular transmission and/or contractility of skeletal muscle) or related to activation of nociceptors with

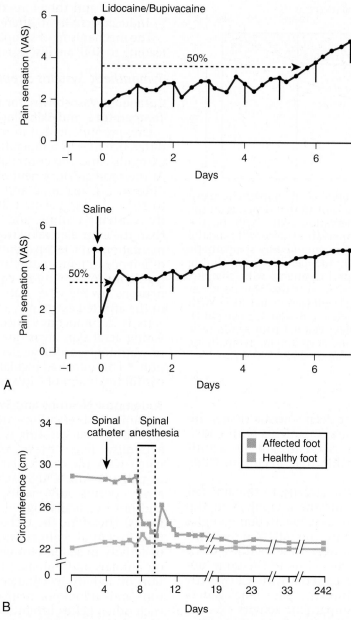

Figure 27-4. Consequences of sympathetic blocks. **A,** Sympathetic blocks with a local anesthetic in patients with complex regional pain syndrome (CRPS) I with SMP leads to a long-lasting significant reduction of pain. The local anesthetic or saline (control) were injected close to the corresponding paravertebral sympathetic ganglia (stellate ganglion in 4 patients, lumbar sympathetic ganglia in 3 patients) in the same group of 7 CRPS I patients. Double-blind crossover study. Pain was measured repeatedly using the Visual Analog Scale (VAS) on the day of the injection and 7 days after the injection. Both interventions produced pain relief (see 50% value of pain relief). However, the duration of the mean relief of pain to injection of the local anesthetic lasted for 6 days and was significantly longer than the mean pain relief following local injection of saline, which lasted for 6 hours (placebo block). The initial maximal peaks of relative analgesia were statistically not different. Means + SEM. (Modified from Price DD, Long S, Wilsey B, Rafii A. Analysis of peak magnitude and duration of analgesia produced by local anesthetics injected into sympathetic ganglia of complex regional pain syndrome patients. Clin J Pain 1998;14:216-26.) **B,** Spinal anesthesia reduces severe edema in a patient with CRPS I. Female patient who is 15 years of age, 3 months after trauma on foot. No spontaneous pain, cutaneous hyperalgesia or allodynia, but deep hyperalgesia. Implantation of spinal catheter at thoracic level T10 on day 4. She underwent spinal anesthesia for 43 hours starting on day 7 with 1.4 mL 0.5% bupivacaine/h. She had an increase of skin temperature of foot to 36° C (indicating complete decrease of activity in cutaneous vasoconstrictor neurons). Significant decrease of edema in 1 day and its complete disappearance with time after termination of the spinal anesthesia, together with other symptoms of CRPS I. The decrease of the edema was considered to be due to decrease of activity in sympathetic neurons. However, it cannot be excluded that antidromically conducted activity in peptidergic primary afferent neurons with unmyelinated axons was blocked. (Modified from Blumberg H, Hoffmann U, Mohadjer M, Scheremet R. Clinical phenomenology and mechanisms of reflex sympathetic dystrophy: emphasis on edema. In: Gebhart GF, Hammond DL, Jensen TS, editors. Proceedings of the 7th World Congress on Pain. Seattle: IASP Press; 1994. p. 455-81.)

pain leading to reflex activation/inhibition of central circuits regulating activity in motoneurons. They have more likely a central origin and are possibly related to plastic changes in the somatosensory, motor, and premotor cortices. A pathologic sensorimotor integration located in the parietal cortex may induce an abnormal central programming and processing of motor tasks.[11,17] It has been postulated by McCabe and coworkers[21,24,45] that an important mechanism underlying somatomotor changes and somatosensory changes (including pain) is a mismatch between motor output (to motoneurons and the spinal motor circuits) and the sensory feedback from the skeletomotor system and the visual system. This incongruence between central motor output and sensory input was hypothesized to be responsible for the body perception disturbance in CRPS.[22] Using the method of graded motor imagery followed by mirror visual feedback from a moving unaffected limb can reduce pain and swelling in patients with chronic CRPS and re-establish the pain-free relationship between sensory feedback and motor execution[21,46-49](see reference 6 and later).

Edema, Inflammation, and Trophic Changes
Edema and Inflammation

Based on observations following sympathetic blocks, it is a long-standing assumption that swelling (edema) in the affected limb of CRPS patients is dependent on activity in sympathetic neurons. Spinal anesthesia or sympathetic blocks may be followed by a decrease of the edema starting within 1 to 2 hours. The edema may disappear within days (see Fig. 27-4B). The edema may also or additionally be related to antidromic activity in peptidergic afferent neurons with unmyelinated (C) and small diameter myelinated (Aδ) fibers (see interrupted arrow in Fig. 27-1). It has been proposed that this antidromic activity is generated by primary afferent depolarization of the central terminals of these peptidergic afferent neurons in the superficial horn of the spinal cord via GABAergic interneurons, generating impulses in these afferent neurons traveling antidromically to the periphery. The antidromically conducted impulses would produce in peripheral tissues arteriolar vasodilation and venular plasma extravasation (for review see reference 50). However, it must be kept in mind that the swelling is present in many CRPS patients in the entire distal extremity, that is, far beyond the territory of the site of the trauma. In any case, *temporary* blockade of the sympathetic activity (and/or possibly of the antidromically conducted activity in afferent neurons) appears to interrupt a vicious circle that maintains the edema (see 6 in Fig. 27-1). The mechanism underlying this vicious circle is unknown.

The idea that patients with CRPS I undergo *inflammatory processes* in the affected extremity, in particular in the deep somatic tissues including bones, goes back to Sudeck[51,52] who believed that this syndrome is an inflammatory bone atrophy ("entzündliche Knochenatrophie"). Accordingly, bone scintigraphy demonstrates periarticular tracer uptake in acute CRPS, and synovia biopsies and scintigraphic investigations with radiolabeled immunoglobulins show protein extravasation, hypervascularity, and neutrophil infiltration. Furthermore, in the fluid of artificially produced skin blisters significantly higher cytokine levels (interleukin-6 [IL-6], tumor necrosis factor-α [TNF-α]) as well as tryptase (a measure of mast cell activity) were observed in the involved extremity of patients with CRPS as compared with the uninvolved extremity.[10,29] This is supported by animal studies, showing that the sympathetic nervous system can influence the intensity of an inflammatory process and clinical studies showing that sympatholytic procedures can ameliorate pain, inflammation, and edema in human patients.[31,53] The mechanisms of initiation and maintenance of inflammatory processes occurring in early CRPS and the role of sympathetic postganglionic neurons in it are unclear and remain to be worked out.

Trophic Changes

The underlying mechanisms of trophic changes, as prominent as they may be, are entirely unclear. However, based on the observation that these changes may ameliorate after sympathetic blocks, argues that they are related to the sympathetic innervation.

Conclusions

Clinical observations, and experimentation on humans and animals indicate that CRPS is primarily a disease of the CNS:

1. Patients with CRPS exhibit functional alterations of the somatosensory system, the sympathetic nervous system, and the somatomotor system reflected in multiple perceptual somatosensory changes, changes of blood flow and sweating, and movement disorders, indicating that the central representations of these systems are changed (see dots in Fig. 27-5 and bold-lined boxes in Fig. 27-1).
2. The peripheral functional changes (sympathetic-afferent coupling, vascular changes, edema/inflammation, trophic changes) cannot be seen independently of the central ones. CNS and peripheral body tissues interact with each other via afferent and efferent signals, yet the nature of this interaction is still a puzzle. We postulate that a mismatch between afferent and efferent signals, occurring at different levels of integration in the afferent and efferent body maps in the CNS causes the changed autonomic, sensory, and somatomotor reactions.[54]
3. This conceptual view will further our understanding why CRPS may be triggered after a trivial trauma, after a trauma being remote from the affected extremity exhibiting CRPS, or following processes in the CNS. It will explain why, in CRPS patients with SMP, a few temporary blocks (and sometimes only one block) of the sympathetic

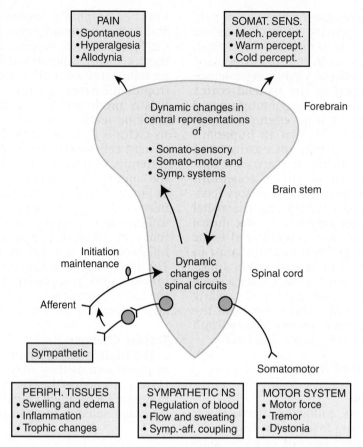

Figure 27-5. Development of CRPS as disease of the central nervous system: a hypothesis. Schematic diagram summarizing the sensory, autonomic and somatomotor changes in patients with complex regional pain syndrome (CRPS) I. The figure symbolizes the central nervous system (forebrain, brain stem, and spinal cord). Changes occur in the central representations of the somatosensory, somatomotor, and sympathetic nervous system (which include spinal circuits) and are reflected in the changes of perception of painful and nonpainful stimuli, of cutaneous blood flow and sweating, and of motor performances. They are triggered and possibly maintained by nociceptive afferent inputs from the somatic and visceral body domains. It is unclear whether these central changes are reversible in chronic patients with CRPS I. The central changes affect the endogenous control system of nociceptive impulse transmission possibly, too. Coupling between sympathetic neurons and afferent neurons in the periphery (see *bold closed arrow*) is one component of pain in patients with CRPS I with SMP. However, it seems to be unimportant in CRPS I patients without SMP. (Modified from Jänig W, Baron R. Complex regional pain syndrome is a disease of the central nervous system. Clin Auton Res 2002;12:150-64; and Jänig W, Baron R. Complex regional pain syndrome: mystery explained? Lancet Neurol 2003;2:687-97.)

supply to an affected extremity sometimes leads to a long-lasting (even permanent) pain relief and to resolution of the other changes present in CRPS.

4. This changed view will bring about a diagnostic reclassification and redefinition of CRPS and will lead to new mechanism-based therapeutic approaches (see later).

DIAGNOSTIC CRITERIA FOR COMPLEX REGIONAL PAIN SYNDROMES AND DIAGNOSTIC TESTS

Clinical Criteria

The diagnosis of CRPS is mainly based on clinical criteria because there are no gold standards to compare with and no absolute diagnostic tests that are specific for CRPS. It is difficult to distinguish CRPS from other extremity pain syndromes. Furthermore, it is difficult, if not impossible, to predict acutely after a trauma to an extremity who is going to develop a CRPS and who is not. Thus, we have no predictor for CRPS. This is not very surprising in view of the hypothesis that CRPS is a disease of the CNS and cannot be causally related in its development to a distinct group of traumatic events, as outlined earlier. In fact, chronic CRPS and other chronic pain syndromes have in common that they cannot be defined mechanistically by peripheral events that are erroneously believed to initiate and maintain them (e.g., by activity in sensitized nociceptors).[55]

A novel diagnostic algorithm that is at least to some extent anchored in mechanisms, was recently proposed (see Table 27-1A).[56–58] In addition to the improved clinical categories it became clear to distinguish between criteria for clinical use and a classification for research purposes. For the clinician and particularly for the patients it is important to have a high sensitivity value combined with a fair specificity (e.g., 0.85 versus 0.60, see Table 27-2). For research purposes, however, it is much more important to have a high specificity in order to perform studies in a precisely diagnosed population (e.g., 0.7 versus 0.96, see Table 27-1A).

Tests That Aid the Diagnosis of Complex Regional Pain Syndromes

Several procedures are often used to support the diagnosis of CRPS (see Table 27-1B).

Bone Scintigraphy

Osseous changes are common in CRPS. Thus, a three-phase bone scintigraphy can provide valuable information. A homogenous unilateral hyperperfusion in the perfusion- (30 sec p.i.) and blood-pool phase (2 min p.i.) is characteristic and will help to exclude differential diagnoses, for example, osteoporosis due to inactivity. Three hours p.i. the mineralization-phase will show an increased unilateral periarticular tracer uptake. A pathologic uptake in the metacarpophalangeal or metacarpal bones is thought to be highly sensitive and specific for CRPS. However, a gold standard to compare with is not known yet but it is useful to rule out pain syndromes of other origin. It should be noted that it only shows significant changes during the subacute period (up to 1 year).

Plain Radiographs and Magnetic Resonance Imaging

Endosteal and intracortical excavation, subperiosteal and trabecular bone resorption, spotty and localized bone demineralization or osteoporosis have been thought to be specific signs of CRPS, but these are only positive in chronic stages. A comparison of radiography and three-phase scintigraphy in early postfracture CRPS showed a lower sensitivity and specificity of the radiography. MRI scans are proposed to be more reliable than radiographic examination and scintigraphy but have to prove their value in further studies.

Skin Temperature Measurements

Because of the abnormal activity in the sympathetic innervation of the skin, the affected extremity is often either warmer or colder than the healthy side. Measurements of differences in skin temperature between both sides have been assessed during a long-term thermoregulatory cycle. Using a special algorithm, a sensitivity and specificity of more than 80% have been calculated.

THERAPY FOR COMPLEX REGIONAL PAIN SYNDROMES

Any therapy of CRPS should be anchored in possible peripheral and central mechanisms underlying this disease. In view of the lack of detailed knowledge about these mechanisms it is not very surprising that many propagated treatment procedures are purely based on practical experience, that is, they are empirical. However, as seen from the mechanisms underlying CRPS as we have discussed them earlier, we can clearly conclude that the therapeutic interventions should occur in the periphery of the body (i.e., at the affected extremity or contralateral to it) and centrally (Fig. 27-6). This applies to interventional, psychological, physical, occupational, and pharmacologic therapies. In fact, some of these therapies are indeed to a certain degree mechanism based. This applies to the mirror image therapy and mirror image program (Fig. 27-7), to sympathetic blocks and to various types of physical therapy. For example, physical therapies acting on peripheral tissues manipulate the different integration centers in the brain (spinal cord, brain stem, hypothalamus,

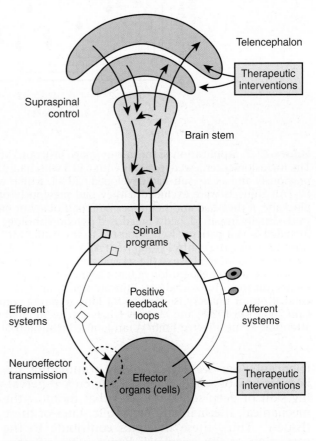

Figure 27-6. Therapeutic interventions: a concept. Therapeutic interventions principally act both at the peripheral body tissues and at the integration centers in the central nervous system (spinal cord, brain stem, hypothalamus, telencephalon). This principally applies to interventional, psychological, physical, occupational, and pharmacologic therapies.

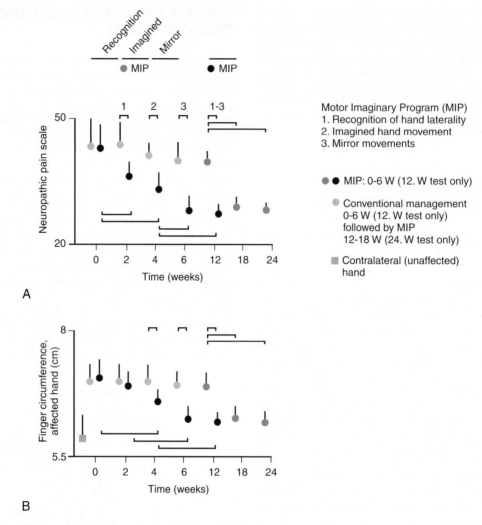

Figure 27-7. Application of the mirror image program (MIP) to patients with complex regional pain syndrome (CRPS) I. The inclusion criteria were patients with CRPS who had sustained a noncomplicated wrist fracture more than 6 months previously and as a result had developed CRPS I, which was diagnosed according to Bruehl and colleagues[56] (see Table 27-1A). Subjects were excluded if they had previously obtained a benefit from an intravenous regional sympathetic blockade, if they had another upper limb pathology or pain, had any neurologic or motor disorder including dyslexia, were visually impaired, had a diagnosed psychopathology or had any invasive analgesic strategy. Thirteen patients were included: seven patients were allocated to the initial MIP and six patients to the control (conventional management). After 12 weeks, the control group was taken in the MIP. **A,** Pain was measured using the Neuropathic Pain Scale.[75] **B,** The circumference of the base of the second and third digits was measured using a hand measuring tape. The MIP consisted of 2 weeks each of recognition of hand laterality (recognition), imagined hand movements (imagined) and mirror movements (mirror). Horizontal bars indicate significance ($P < 0.05$) on post hoc Scheffé tests. (Modified from Moseley GL. Graded motor imagery is effective for long-standing complex regional pain syndrome: a randomised controlled trial. Pain 2004;108:192-8; and Moseley GL. Is successful rehabilitation of complex regional pain syndrome due to sustained attention to the affected limb? A randomised clinical trial. Pain 2005;114:54-61.)

telencephalon; see Fig. 27-6) by stimulating the populations of small diameter afferents innervating skin or deep somatic tissues that monitor the mechanical, thermal, and metabolic states of these tissues.[54] Thus, these therapies contribute to the correction of the mismatch between the afferent inflow from the body tissues (and this includes the nociceptive as well as the non-nociceptive afferent feedback) and the neural programs that regulate the somatomotor and the autonomic motor outflow to the affected tissues. The correction of the mismatch potentially occurs on all central integration levels,

leading to normal somatic sensations (including decrease of pain), normal perception of the affected extremity, normal motor behavior, and normal regulation of autonomic parameters by the sympathetic nervous system (e.g., cutaneous blood flow and sweating, decrease of edema). In fact, a very promising and exciting development is the mirror image therapy and mirror image program as propagated by McCabe and Moseley (see Fig. 27-7).[46-49,59] These studies should be replicated by other groups.

Only few evidence-based clinical trials for CRPS are available. In fact, three literature reviews of outcome studies found discouragingly little consistent information regarding the pharmacologic agents and methods for treatment of CRPS.[60-62] Moreover, the methodology is often of low quality within the studies available. In the absence of more specific information about pathophysiologic mechanisms and treatment of CRPS, one mainly has to rely on outcomes from treatment studies for other neuropathic pain syndromes.

Interventional Therapies

Sympathetic Blockade

At present, two therapeutical techniques to block sympathetic nerves are used: (1) injections of a local anesthetic around sympathetic paravertebral ganglia that project to the affected body part (sympathetic ganglion blocks), and (2) regional intravenous application of guanethidine, bretylium, or reserpine (which all deplete norepinephrine in the postganglionic axons) to an isolated extremity blocked with a tourniquet (intravenous regional sympatholysis [IVRS]).

There are many uncontrolled surveys in the literature reviewing the effect of sympathetic interventions in CRPS. In acute CRPS, about 85% of the patients report a positive effect. The efficacy of these procedures is, however, still discussed controversially and has been questioned in the past. In fact, the specificity, the long-term results, and the techniques used have been rarely adequately evaluated (for discussion and references see reference 5). One controlled study in patients with CRPS I has shown that sympathetic ganglion blocks with a local anesthetic have the same immediate effect on pain as a control injection with saline[35] (see Fig. 27-4A). However, after 24 hours, patients in the local anesthetic group were much better, indicating that "nonspecific" placebo effects are important initially and that evaluating the efficacy of sympatholytic interventions is best done after 24 hours. With these data in mind, the uncontrolled studies mentioned earlier must be interpreted cautiously. Only 10 out of the 24 studies we reviewed assessed long-term effects.

The irreversible sympathectomy may be effective in very selected cases. However, because of the risk of development of adaptive supersensitivity of the vasculature and possibly even nociceptive neurons to catecholamines with consecutive pain increase and prolongation, this procedure is no longer recommended.

There is a desperate need for controlled studies that assess the acute as well as the long-term effect of sympathetic blockade on pain and other CRPS symptoms, in particular motor function. Well-performed sympathetic ganglion blocks should be performed rather than IVRS.

Stimulation Techniques

Epidural spinal cord stimulation (SCS) has shown efficacy in one randomized study in selected chronic CRPS patients[63] that improved pain, and health-related quality of life but not functional outcome assessed 2 years later. Interestingly, these patients had previously undergone unsuccessful surgical sympathectomy. The pain-relieving effect was not associated with peripheral vasodilatation, suggesting that central disinhibition processes are involved. A meta-analysis showed that in selected patients, SCS can relieve pain, allodynia and improve quality of life[64] with an adverse event rate of 34%, but still further studies are warranted. A health economical study revealed that the use of spinal cord stimulation (SCS) in combination with physiotherapy compared with physiotherapy alone is associated with a lifetime cost saving of 58.000 Euro per patient.[65]

Physical Therapy and Occupational Therapy

It should be stressed that clinical experience clearly indicates that physiotherapy is of utmost importance to achieve recovery of function and rehabilitation. Standardized physiotherapy has shown long-term relief in pain and physical dysfunction in children.[66] Physical and, to a lesser extent, occupational therapy are able to reduce pain and improve active mobility in CRPS I.[67] Patients with initially less pain and better motor function are predicted to benefit to a greater degree than others.[68] Recent studies have demonstrated the combination of hand laterality recognition training, imagination of movements, and mirror movements reduces pain and disability in patients with CRPS (see Fig. 27-7).[47-49]

Pharmacologic Therapy

For CRPS, only very few pharmacological treatment options have been evaluated in controlled clinical trials. None are approved for CRPS. One usual approach is to translate the knowledge obtained in other neuropathic pain conditions to the situation in CRPS. In the following summary, these caveats are highlighted.

- Nonsteroidal anti-inflammatory drugs (NSAIDs) have not been investigated in the treatment of CRPS so far. However, from clinical experience they can control mild to moderate pain.

  The use of opioids in CRPS has not been studied. In other neuropathic pain syndromes, compounds like tramadol, morphine, oxycodone and levorphanol are clearly analgesic when compared with placebo. However, there are no long-term studies of oral opioids use for treatment of neuropathic pain, including CRPS.

- Tricyclic antidepressants have been intensely studied in different neuropathic pain conditions but not in CRPS.

- Lidocaine administered intravenously is effective in CRPS I and II regarding spontaneous and evoked pain. Neither carbamazepine nor lamotrigine have been tested in CRPS.

- Intrathecally administered baclofen is effective in the treatment of dystonia in CRPS. No further trials in CRPS are available, and there is no evidence for an analgesic effect of baclofen, valproatic acid, vigabatrine, and benzodiazepines in CRPS.

- One randomized double-blind placebo-controlled trial demonstrated a mild effect of gabapentin on pain and a good effect on sensory symptoms in CRPS I.
- Orally administered prednisone has clearly demonstrated efficacy in the improvement of the entire clinical status up to 75% in acute CRPS patients. In CRPS I following stroke, 40 mg prednisolone for 14 days improved significantly the signs and symptoms compared with piroxicam 20 mg daily.[69]
- Two case reports have reported beneficial results with anti TNF antibodies (infliximab).[70] In a prospective multiple-dose, open label cohort study in patients who suffered from a variety of chronic pain syndromes including CRPS, patients were treated with human pooled immunoglobulins. Pain relief by about 70% was found in all major symptom groups.
- Clinically available compounds that have N-methyl-D-aspartate (NMDA) receptor-blocking properties include ketamine, dextromethorphane, and memantine. A pilot open-label study of the efficacy of subanesthetic ketamine in refractory patients with CRPS shows no effect on pain relief. Another study that used ketamine as an adjuvant in sympathetic blocks for the management of central sensitization indicated a relief in allodynia without significant neuropsychiatric side effects.
- Calcitonin intranasally demonstrated a significant pain reduction in patients with CRPS.[71] Intravenous clodronate and alendronate showed a significant improvement in pain, swelling and movement range in acute CRPS. However, a recent meta-analysis found too little consistent evidence to recommend bisphosphonates in clinical practice.[72] The mode of action of these compounds in CRPS is unknown.
- Free radical scavengers dimethylsulfoxide 50% topically (DMSO) or N-acetylcysteine (NAC) orally were tested in placebo-controlled trials for the treatment of CRPS I.[73] Both drugs were found to be equally effective, whereas DMSO seemed more favorable for "warm" and NAC for "cold" CRPS I. The results were negatively influenced by a longer disease duration.
    - Transdermal application of the α_2-adrenoceptor agonist clonidine, which is thought to prevent the release of catecholamines by a presynaptic action, may be helpful when small areas of hyperalgesia are present.

Therapy Guidelines of Complex Regional Pain Syndromes

Treatment should be immediate and most importantly directed toward restoration of full function of the extremity. This objective is best attained in a

Table 27-3. *Pharmacologic Treatment for Complex Regional Pain Syndromes (Examples): Doses For Adults*

Drug	Dose
Steroids	
Prednisone/prednisolone	100 mg/d (initial dose)
Methylprednisolone	80 mg/d (initial dose)
Antidepressants	
Amitriptyline	25–150 mg/d
Anticonvulsants (Na)	
Carbamazepine	600–1400 mg/d
Anticonvulsants (Ca)	
Gabapentin	1200–3600 mg/d
Pregabalin	150–600 mg/d
Tramadol	Up to 400 mg/d
Opioids	
Morphine	Individual dose titration

comprehensive interdisciplinary setting with particular emphasis on pain management and functional restoration.[74]

In mild cases of CRPS, a pharmacologic treatment regimen in combination with physical and occupational treatment might be sufficient to resolve the symptoms. In these cases, five main classes of oral medications may be used (summarized in Table 27-3): antidepressants with reuptake blocking effect, such as amitryptiline; anticonvulsants with Na-blocking action, such as carbamazepine; anticonvulsants with Ca-modulating actions, such as gabapentin; tramadol; and opioids. In many cases, the initiation of combination therapies with compounds having different mechanisms of action is useful. If signs of inflammation are present, additional oral corticosteroids should be used. Dose ranges for these medications are given in Table 27-3. If there is no substantial improvement of the signs and symptoms after 3 weeks a consultation at a specialized center should be considered.

Severe cases should be referred immediately to a specialized center. The pain specialists should include neurologists, anesthesiologists, orthopedic surgeons, physiotherapists, psychologists, and the general practitioner.

The severity of the disease determines the therapeutic regimen (Fig. 27-8). The reduction of pain is the precondition with which all other interventions have to comply. All therapeutic approaches must not produce pain. At the acute stage of CRPS, when the patient still suffers from severe pain at rest and during movements, it is mostly impossible to carry out intensive active therapy. Painful interventions and particularly aggressive physical therapy at this stage often lead to deterioration. Therefore, immobilization and careful contralateral physical therapy should be the acute treatment of choice, and intense pain treatment should be initiated immediately. First-line analgesics and coanalgesics are opioids, antidepressants, and anticonvulsants. Additionally, corticosteroids should be considered if inflammatory signs and symptoms are predominant. Sympatholytic procedures, preferably sympathetic ganglion blocks, should identify the component

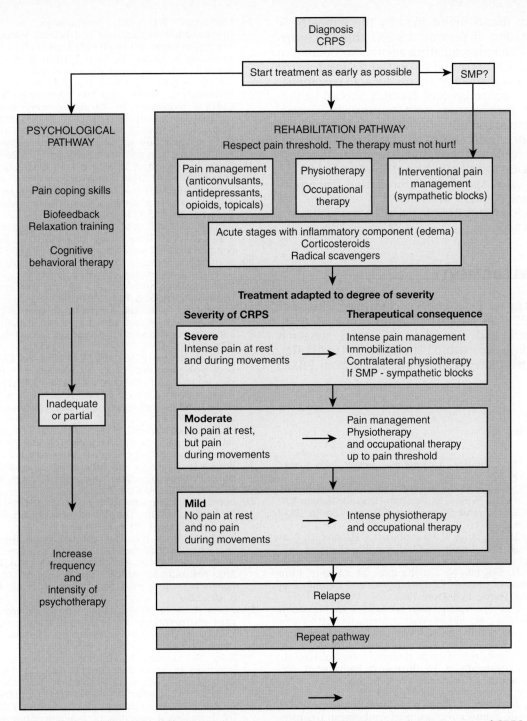

Figure 27-8. Treatment algorithm for complex regional pain syndrome (CRPS). 1. At the acute state of CRPS with severe pain at rest, immobilization and careful contralateral physical therapy should be the treatment of choice. Sympatholytic procedures, preferentially sympathetic ganglion blocks, should identify the component of pain that is maintained by the sympathetic nervous system. 2. If resting pain subsides physical therapy should be performed in combination with sensory desensitization programs and pain therapy. 3. If movement-induced pain subsides, physico- and occupational therapies should be intensified. (Modified from Baron R. Complex regional pain syndromes. In: McMahon SB, Koltzenburg M, editors. Wall & Melzack's Textbook of Pain. 5th ed. Edinburgh: Elsevier Churchill Livingstone; 2006. pp. 1011-27; and Forouzanfar T, Köke AJ, van Kleef M, Weber WE. Treatment of complex regional pain syndrome type I. Eur J Pain 2002;6:105-22.)

of the pain that is maintained by the sympathetic nervous system. If present, a series should be perpetuated. Calcium-regulating agents can be used in cases of refractory pain. If resting pain subsides, first passive physical therapy, then later active isometric followed by active isotonic training should be performed in combination with sensory desensitization programs and mirror training until restitution of complete motor function. Psychological treatment has to flank the regimen to strengthen coping strategies and discover contributing factors. In refractory cases, spinal cord stimulation and epidural clonidine could be considered. If refractory dystonia develops, intrathecal baclofen application is worth considering.

ACKNOWLEDGMENTS

Supported by the Deutsche Forschungsgemeinschaft (DFG Ba 1921/1-3, Jä 240/19-1), the German Ministry of Research and Education, German Research Network on Neuropathic Pain (BMBF, 01EM01/04), and an unrestricted educational grant from Pfizer, Germany.

References

1. Richards RL. Causalgia. A centennial review. Arch Neurol 1967;16:339-50.
2. Wilson PR, Bogduk N. Retrospection, science and epidemiology of CRPS. In: Wilson PR, Stanton-Hicks M, Harden RN, editors. CRPS: Current Diagnosis and Therapy. Seattle: IASP Press; 2005. p. 19-41.
3. Stanton-Hicks M, Jänig W, Hassenbusch S, Haddox JD, Boas R, Wilson P. Reflex sympathetic dystrophy: changing concepts and taxonomy. Pain 1995;63:127-33.
4. Merskey H, Bogduk N. Classification of Chronic Pain: Descriptions of Chronic Pain Syndromes and Definition of Pain Terms. Seattle: IASP Press; 1994.
5. Baron R. Complex regional pain syndromes. In: McMahon SB, Koltzenburg M, editors. Wall & Melzack's Textbook of Pain. 5th ed. Edinburgh: Elsevier Churchill Livingstone; 2006. p. 1011-27.
6. Baron R. Complex regional pain syndromes. In: Basbaum AL, Kaneko A, Shepherd GM, Westheimer G, Basbaum AI, editors. The Senses: a Comprehensive Reference, vol. 5. Pain. San Diego: Academic Press; 2008. p. 909-18.
7. Baron R, Blumberg H, Jänig W. Clinical characteristics of patients with complex regional pain syndrome in Germany with special emphasis on vasomotor function. In: Jänig W, Stanton-Hicks M, editors. Reflex Sympathetic Dystrophy: A Reappraisal. Seattle: IASP Press; 1996. p. 25-48.
8. Wilson PR, Stanton-Hicks M, Harden RN. CRPS: Current Diagnosis and Therapy. Seattle: IASP Press; 2005.
9. Jänig W, Baron R. Complex regional pain syndrome is a disease of the central nervous system. Clin Auton Res 2002;12:150-64.
10. Jänig W, Baron R. Complex regional pain syndrome: mystery explained? Lancet Neurol 2003;2:687-97.
11. Harden RN, Baron R, Jänig W. Complex Regional Pain Syndrome, vol. 22. Seattle: IASP Press; 2001.
12. Jänig W, Stanton-Hicks M. Reflex Sympathetic Dystrophy—a Reappraisal. Seattle: IASP Press; 1996.
13. Jänig W. Causalgia and reflex sympathetic dystrophy: in which way is the sympathetic nervous system involved? Trends Neurosci 1985;8:471-7.
14. Livingston WK. Pain Mechanisms. A Physiological Interpretation of Causalgia and Related States. New York: Macmillan (reprinted by Plenum Press [1976]); 1943.
15. Juottonen K, Gockel M, Silen T, Hurri H, Hari R, Forss N. Altered central sensorimotor processing in patients with complex regional pain syndrome. Pain 2002;98:315-23.
16. Maihöfner C, Handwerker HO, Neundorfer B, Birklein F. Cortical reorganization during recovery from complex regional pain syndrome. Neurology 2004;63:693-701.
17. Maihöfner C, Baron R, DeCol R, Binder A, Birklein F, Deuschl G, et al. The motor system shows adaptive changes in complex regional pain syndrome. Brain 2007;130:2671-87.
18. Pleger B, Tegenthoff M, Schwenkreis P, Janssen F, Ragert P, Dinse HR, et al. Mean sustained pain levels are linked to hemispherical side-to-side differences of primary somatosensory cortex in the complex regional pain syndrome I. Exp Brain Res 2004;155:115-9.
19. Rommel O, Gehling M, Dertwinkel R, Witscher K, Zenz M, Malin JP, et al. Hemisensory impairment in patients with complex regional pain syndrome. Pain 1999;80:95-101.
20. Rommel O, Malin JP, Zenz M, Jänig W. Quantitative sensory testing, neurophysiological and psychological examination in patients with complex regional pain syndrome and hemisensory deficits. Pain 2001;93:279-93.
21. McCabe CS, Blake DR. An embarrassment of pain perceptions? Towards an understanding of and explanation for the clinical presentation of CRPS type 1. Rheumatology (Oxford) 2008;47:1612-6.
22. Lewis JS, Kersten P, McCabe CS, McPherson KM, Blake DR. Body perception disturbance: a contribution to pain in complex regional pain syndrome (CRPS). Pain 2007;133:111-9.
23. Förderreuther S, Sailer U, Straube A. Impaired self-perception of the hand in complex regional pain syndrome (CRPS). Pain 2004;110:756-61.
24. McCabe CS, Haigh RC, Halligan PW, Blake DR. Referred sensations in patients with complex regional pain syndrome type 1. Rheumatology (Oxford) 2003b;42:1067-73.
25. Bonica JJ. Causalgia and other reflex sympathetic dystrophies. In: Bonica JJ, editor. Management of Pain. Philadelphia: Lea and Febiger; 1953. p. 913-78.
26. Bonica JJ. Causalgia and other reflex sympathetic dystrophies. In: Bonica JJ, editor. The Management of Pain. Philadelphia: Lea and Febiger; 1990. p. 220-43.
27. White JC, Sweet WH. Pain and the Neurosurgeon: A Forty Year Experience. Springfield, IL: Charles C. Thomas; 1969.
28. Jänig W. Autonomic nervous system and pain. In: Bushnell MC, Basbaum AI, editors. The Senses: A Comprehensive Reference, vol. 5. Pain. San Diego: Academic Press; 2008. p. 193-226.
29. Baron R, Jänig W. Adrenergic and cholinergic targets in pain pharmacology. In: Beaulieu P, Lussier D, Porreca F, Dickinson AH, editors. Pharmacology of Pain. Seattle: IASP Press; 2009.
30. Jänig W, Levine JD. Autonomic-neuroendocrine-immune responses in acute and chronic pain. In: McMahon SB, Koltzenburg M, editors. Wall & Mezack's Textbook of Pain. 5th ed. Edinburgh: Elsevier Churchill Livinstone; 2006. p. 205-18.
31. Ali Z, Raja SN, Wesselmann U, Fuchs PN, Meyer RA, Campbell JN. Intradermal injection of norepinephrine evokes pain in patients with sympathetically maintained pain. Pain 2000;88:161-8.
32. Torebjörk HE, Wahren LK, Wallin BG, Hallin R, Koltzenburg M. Noradrenaline-evoked pain in neuralgia. Pain 1995;63:11-20.
33. Baron R, Schattschneider J, Binder A, Siebrecht D, Wasner G. Relation between sympathetic vasoconstrictor activity and pain and hyperalgesia in complex regional pain syndromes: a case-control study. Lancet 2002;359:1655-60.
34. Schattschneider J, Binder A, Siebrecht D, Wasner G, Baron R. Complex regional pain syndromes: the influence of cutaneous and deep somatic sympathetic innervation on pain. Clin J Pain 2006;22:240-4.
35. Price DD, Long S, Wilsey B, Rafii A. Analysis of peak magnitude and duration of analgesia produced by local anesthetics injected into sympathetic ganglia of complex regional pain syndrome patients. Clin J Pain 1998;14:216-26.

36. Blumberg H, Hoffmann U, Mohadjer M, Scheremet R. Clinical phenomenology and mechanisms of reflex sympathetic dystrophy: emphasis on edema. In: Gebhart GF, Hammond DL, Jensen TS, editors. Proceedings of the 7th World Congress on Pain. Seattle: IASP Press; 1994. p. 455-81.

37. Wasner G, Schattschneider J, Heckmann K, Maier C, Baron R. Vascular abnormalities in reflex sympathetic dystrophy (CRPS I): mechanisms and diagnostic value. Brain 2001;124: 587-99.

38. Wasner G, Heckmann K, Maier C, Baron R. Vascular abnormalities in acute reflex sympathetic dystrophy (CRPS I): complete inhibition of sympathetic nerve activity with recovery. Arch Neurol 1999;56:613-20.

39. Jänig W. The Integrative Action of the Autonomic Nervous System. Neurobiology of Homeostasis. Cambridge, NY: Cambridge University Press; 2006.

40. Schwartzman RJ, Kerrigan J. The movement disorder of reflex sympathetic dystrophy. Neurology 1990;40:57-61.

41. Deuschl G, Blumberg H, Lücking CH. Tremor in reflex sympathetic dystrophy. Arch Neurol 1991;48:1247-52.

42. Bhatia KP, Bhatt MH, Marsden CD. The causalgia-dystonia syndrome. Brain 1993;116:843-51.

43. van Hilten JJ, Blumberg H, Schwartzman RJ. Movement disorders and dystrophy—pathophysiology. In: Wilson PR, Stanton-Hicks M, Harden RN, editors. CRPS: Current Diagnosis and Therapy. Seattle: IASP Press; 2005. p. 119-37.

44. van Rijn MA, Marinus J, Putter H, van Hilten JJ. Onset and progression of dystonia in complex regional pain syndrome. Pain 2007;130:287-93.

45. McCabe CS, Haigh RC, Halligan PW, Blake DR. Simulating sensory-motor incongruence in healthy volunteers: implications for a cortical model of pain. Rheumatology (Oxford) 2005;44:509-16.

46. McCabe CS, Haigh RC, Ring EF, Halligan PW, Wall PD, Blake DR. A controlled pilot study of the utility of mirror visual feedback in the treatment of complex regional pain syndrome (type 1). Rheumatology (Oxford) 2003a;42:97-101.

47. Moseley GL. Graded motor imagery is effective for long-standing complex regional pain syndrome: a randomised controlled trial. Pain 2004;108:192-8.

48. Moseley GL. Is successful rehabilitation of complex regional pain syndrome due to sustained attention to the affected limb? A randomised clinical trial. Pain 2005;114:54-61.

49. Moseley GL. Graded motor imagery for pathologic pain: a randomized controlled trial. Neurology 2006;67:2129-34.

50. Willis Jr WD. Dorsal root potentials and dorsal root reflexes: a double-edged sword. Exp Brain Res 1999;124:395-421.

51. Sudeck P. Über die akute (trophoneurotische) Knochenatrophie nach Entzündungen und Traumen der Extremitäten [On the acute (trophoneurotic) bone atrophy following inflammation and traumas at the extremities]. Deutsche Med Wschr 1902;28:336-42.

52. Sudeck P. Die trophische Extremitätenstörung durch periphere (infektiöse und traumatische) Reize [The trophic extremity disturbance induced by peripheral (infectious and traumatic) stimuli]. Deutsche Zeitschr Chirurg 1931;234:596-612.

53. Jänig W, Levine JD, Michaelis M. Interactions of sympathetic and primary afferent neurons following nerve injury and tissue trauma. Prog Brain Res 1996;112:161-84.

54. Jänig W. Autonomic nervous system dysfunction. In: Mayer EA, Bushnell MC, editors. Functional Pain Syndromes: Presentation and Pathophysiology. Seattle: IASP Press; 2009. p. 265-300.

55. Mayer EA, Bushnel MC. editors. Functional Pain Syndromes: Presentation and Pathophysiology. Seattle: IASP Press; 2009.

56. Bruehl S, Harden RN, Galer BS, Saltz S, Bertram M, Backonja M, et al. External validation of IASP diagnostic criteria for Complex Regional Pain Syndrome and proposed research diagnostic criteria. International Association for the Study of Pain. Pain 1999;81:147-54.

57. Harden RN, Bruehl S, Galer BS, Saltz S, Bertram M, Backonja M, et al. Complex regional pain syndrome: are the IASP diagnostic criteria valid and sufficiently comprehensive? Pain 1999;83:211-9.

58. Harden RN, Bruehl S, Stanton-Hicks M, Wilson PR. Proposed new diagnostic criteria for complex regional pain syndrome. Pain Med 2007;8:326-31.

59. McCabe CS, Haigh RC, Blake DR. Mirror visual feedback for the treatment of complex regional pain syndrome (type 1). Curr Pain Headache Rep 2008;12:103-7.

60. Forouzanfar T, Köke AJ, van Kleef M, Weber WE. Treatment of complex regional pain syndrome type I. Eur J Pain 2002;6: 105-22.

61. Kingery WS. A critical review of controlled clinical trials for peripheral neuropathic pain and complex regional pain syndromes. Pain 1997;73:123-39.

62. Perez RS, Kwakkel G, Zuurmond WW, de Lange JJ. Treatment of reflex sympathetic dystrophy (CRPS type 1): a research synthesis of 21 randomized clinical trials. J Pain Symptom Manage 2001;21:511-26.

63. Kemler MA, Barendse GA, van Kleef M, De Vet HC, Rijks CP, Furnee CA, et al. Spinal cord stimulation in patients with chronic reflex sympathetic dystrophy. N Engl J Med 2000;343: 618-24.

64. Taylor RS, Van Buyten JP, Buchser E. Spinal cord stimulation for complex regional pain syndrome: a systematic review of the clinical and cost-effectiveness literature and assessment of prognostic factors. Eur J Pain 2006;10:91-101.

65. Kemler MA, Furnee CA. Economic evaluation of spinal cord stimulation for chronic reflex sympathetic dystrophy. Neurology 2002;59:1203-9.

66. Sherry DD, Wallace CA, Kelley C, Kidder M, Sapp L. Short- and long-term outcomes of children with complex regional pain syndrome type I treated with exercise therapy. Clin J Pain 1999;15:218-23.

67. Oerlemans HM, Oostendorp RA, de Boo T, van der Laan L, Severens JL, Goris JA. Adjuvant physical therapy versus occupational therapy in patients with reflex sympathetic dystrophy/complex regional pain syndrome type I. Arch Phys Med Rehabil 2000;81:49-56.

68. Kemler MA, Rijks CP, De Vet HC. Which patients with chronic reflex sympathetic dystrophy are most likely to benefit from physical therapy? J Manipulative Physiol Ther 2001;24: 272-8.

69. Kalita J, Vajpayee A, Misra UK. Comparison of prednisolone with piroxicam in complex regional pain syndrome following stroke: a randomized controlled trial. QJM 2006;99: 89-95.

70. Bernateck M, Rolke R, Birklein F, Treede RD, Fink M, Karst M. Successful intravenous regional block with low-dose tumor necrosis factor-alpha antibody infliximab for treatment of complex regional pain syndrome 1. Anesth Analg 2007;105:1148-51.

71. Gobelet C, Waldburger M, Meier JL. The effect of adding calcitonin to physical treatment on reflex sympathetic dystrophy. Pain 1992;48:171-5.

72. Brunner F, Schmid A, Kissling R, Held U, Bachmann LM. Biphosphonates for the therapy of complex regional pain syndrome I—Systematic review. Eur J Pain 2008;13:17-21.

73. Perez RS, Zuurmond WW, Bezemer PD, Kuik DJ, van Loenen AC, de Lange JJ, et al. The treatment of complex regional pain syndrome type I with free radical scavengers: a randomized controlled study. Pain 2003;102:297-307.

74. Stanton-Hicks MD, Burton AW, Bruehl SP, Carr DB, Harden RN, Hassenbusch SJ, et al. An updated interdisciplinary clinical pathway for CRPS: report of an expert panel. Pain Pract 2002;2:1-16.

75. Galer BS, Jensen MP. Development and preliminary validation of a pain measure specific to neuropathic pain: the Neuropathic Pain Scale. Neurology 1997;48:332-8.

Management of Fibromyalgia and Unexplained Generalized Pain Syndromes

Leslie J. Crofford

CASE STUDY 1   Primary Fibromyalgia

A 34-year-old woman is referred by her primary physician for musculoskeletal pain and stiffness involving joints and muscles which has been present for approximately 1 year, but has worsened to the point that the patient is frequently missing work over the last 2 months. The patient states that she was previously healthy, taking only oral contraceptives and intermittent medications for migraine headaches before the onset of symptoms. She initially developed pain in her neck and shoulders that she associated with her work in an automobile parts assembly plant. She was told that she had a rotator cuff injury and was treated with physical therapy that worsened her symptoms. She states that the pain began to spread to her arms and back, and she now has marked functional impairment related to the pain. She states she has a very difficult time with function in both morning and evening with "a few good hours" in the middle of the day. Exercise worsens her symptoms. Her symptoms do not respond well to over-the-counter analgesic or anti-inflammatory medications. Her primary care physician has given her a prescription for hydrocodone-acetaminophen, which she states provides minimal relief, but its use is associated with nausea.

Review of symptoms reveals debilitating fatigue that she relates to lack of sleep from pain. She complains of pain in the neck, back, shoulders, elbows, and hips but has not identified joint swelling. She states that she is diffusely stiff. Her headaches have increased in frequency and severity. There are no cardiopulmonary complaints, but the patient has frequent bouts of diarrhea. She denies any additional symptoms of connective tissue diseases, including absence of ocular and mucosal symptoms. She complains of anxiety related to her inability to fulfill her responsibilities at work and at home.

Past medical history reveals G2, P2. She has regular menstrual periods while on oral contraceptives, but reports a diagnosis of endometriosis. She was diagnosed with postpartum depression following the birth of her second child 5 years previously. The patient reports no other chronic medical problems.

Regarding her social history, the patient lives with her husband and sons ages 7 and 5. Daycare for her children is provided through her church, and her older son was recently diagnosed with attention-deficit disorder. Her husband works in construction. The patient works full time. She does not smoke, but her husband smokes 1 pack of cigarettes daily. She consumes alcohol on social occasions, but her husband consumes approximately 3 to 4 glasses of beer every evening.

Family history is significant because her mother was frequently "down" with "arthritis in her back" and thyroid disease. Her father passed away due to myocardial infarction at the age of 58. Her four younger siblings are healthy.

Physical examination reveals a pleasant, anxious woman. Vital signs are normal. Body Mass Index (BMI) is 31. Examination of the head and neck are normal. Cardiopulmonary examination is normal. There is mild abdominal tenderness without rebound and there is no organomegaly. Skin shows no rash and examination of the musculoskeletal system reveals limited range of motion in all planes at the cervical spine, tenderness in the cervical and lumbar paraspinal regions and the trapezius musculature, absence of synovitis, and presence of 16 of 18 tender points for fibromyalgia (FM) (Fig. 28-1). The neurologic examination is normal, including muscle strength testing.

Laboratory evaluation demonstrated a normal complete blood count (CBC) and metabolic profile. Thyroid-stimulating hormone (TSH) was normal. Rheumatoid factor (RF) and antinuclear antibody (ANA) drawn by her primary care physician were negative. There was a slightly elevated C-reactive protein (CRP) of 1.3. Erythrocyte sedimentation rate (ESR) was normal.

Discussion of Differential Diagnosis

The features of the above-mentioned case that are frequently observed in patients with FM include the combination of widespread musculoskeletal pain and stiffness worsened by physical activity, fatigue, and sleep disturbance. A triggering pain generator (rotator cuff injury) is identifiable. The patient has a history of a pain syndrome (migraine) that may also serve as a pain generator, and mood disorder (postpartum depression). She has significant emotional

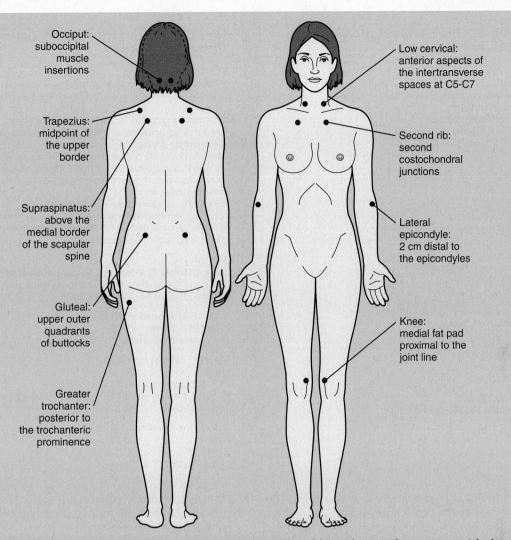

Occiput:
suboccipital
muscle
insertions

Trapezius:
midpoint of
the upper
border

Supraspinatus:
above the
medial border
of the scapular
spine

Gluteal:
upper outer
quadrants
of buttocks

Greater
trochanter:
posterior to
the trochanteric
prominence

Low cervical:
anterior aspects of
the intertransverse
spaces at C5-C7

Second rib:
second
costochondral
junctions

Lateral
epicondyle:
2 cm distal to
the epicondyles

Knee:
medial fat pad
proximal to the
joint line

Figure 28-1. Tender points in fibromyalgia. Tenderness should be addressed using the pressure with the thumbnail at approximately 4 kg/cm^2. In practice, this amount of pressure causes the tip of the thumbnail to turn white.

comorbidity (anxiety) associated with her symptoms and the accompanying inability to fulfill roles and responsibilities. There is significant and ongoing psychosocial stress (son with attention-deficit disorder). There is a family history of chronic pain. Physical examination is negative for features of inflammatory arthritis and connective tissue disease, but evidence of widespread allodynia (as detected using the digital tender point examination to detect diffusely lowered mechanical pain threshold) is present. Laboratory testing does not reveal evidence of significant inflammation, autoimmunity, or endocrine disorder.

Although the patient under discussion appears straightforward, a thorough history and physical examination (H&P) of patients with diffuse, chronic myalgias and arthralgias is essential to avoid missing a diagnosis that requires specific treatment and to avoid overuse of laboratory and radiographic tests. Furthermore, inaccuracy in the referring diagnosis is surprisingly frequent.[1] The differential diagnosis is broad (Table 28-1), but narrowing the possibilities can be done relatively easily with a thorough H&P

and a few laboratory tests. It is imperative to distinguish between a non-FM primary diagnosis and the presence of FM triggered by an alternate diagnosis (Table 28-2). Patients with Lyme disease who need treatment with antibiotics must be distinguished from patients with post-Lyme FM.[2]

One should initially determine if the patient has an autoimmune inflammatory etiology or not. Patients with more than 6 to 12 months of symptoms typically have a relatively easily identifiable autoimmune inflammatory disorder if it is present. If the patient under consideration were older than 50 years of age, then polymyalgia rheumatica should be considered; a normal ESR and CRP significantly reduces the likelihood of that diagnosis. Rheumatoid arthritis is unlikely in this patient given the absence of synovitis, minimal evidence of systemic inflammation, and negative rheumatoid factor. If the patient's symptom profile or laboratory tests were more suggestive of rheumatoid arthritis (RA), an anti-CCP antibody and radiographs should be added to the work-up. More difficult to exclude is a seronegative spondyloarthropathy including inflam-

Table 28-1. *Differential Diagnosis of Diffuse Arthralgias and Myalgias*

Inflammatory
Polymyalgia rheumatica
Inflammatory arthritis: rheumatoid arthritis, spondyloarthritidies
Connective tissue diseases
Systemic vasculitidies

Infectious
Hepatitis C
Human immunodeficiency virus
Lyme disease
Parvovirus B19
Epstein-Barr virus

Noninflammatory
Degenerative joint/spine disease
Fibromyalgia
Myofascial pain syndromes
Metabolic myopathies

Endocrine
Hypothyroidism or hyperthyroidism
Hyperparathyroidism
Addison's disease

Neurologic Diseases
Multiple sclerosis
Neuropathic pain

Psychiatric Disease
Major depressive disorder

Drugs
Statins
Aromatase inhibitors

Table 28-2. *Selected Peripheral Pain Generators/ Triggers in Fibromyalgia*

Musculoskeletal
Osteoarthritis and spondylosis
Other spinal disorders: Disk disease, spinal stenosis, scoliosis
Inflammatory arthritis: Rheumatoid arthritis, spondyloarthritis (psoriatic arthritis, reactive arthritis, ankylosing spondylitis)
Connective tissue diseases: Systemic lupus erythematosus, Sjögren's syndrome, inflammatory myopathies, systemic sclerosis, mixed connective tissue disease
Joint hypermobility
Injuries/Trauma: whiplash, repetitive strain disorders, bursitis, tendonitis, postsurgical
Myofascial pain disorders: Temporomandibular disorders, muscular back pain

Neurologic
Neuropathies: Post-herpetic neuralgia, diabetic neuropathy, sciatica and other peripheral neuropathies
Chronic headache: Migraine, tension

Endocrine Disorders Associated with Chronic Pain
Hypothyroidism
Hyperparathyroidism

Visceral Pain Syndromes
Irritable bowel syndrome
Irritable bladder/interstitial cystitis
Chronic pelvic pain disorders: Endometriosis, vulvar vestibulitis

Infections Associated with Chronic Musculoskeletal Pain
Hepatitis C
Lyme disease

matory bowel disease–associated reactive arthritis. The patient gives a history of back pain and diarrhea with a slight elevation of CRP, a finding common in individuals with a BMI higher than 30. The symptoms, however, are not typical of inflammatory back pain given the lack of clear morning predominance and worsening (rather than improving) with exercise. Of all the inflammatory disorders, spondyloarthropathies are the most frequently overlooked in patients with fibromyalgia-like symptoms.[3] The clinician should evaluate the patient for presence of ocular inflammation, mucosal ulceration, psoriasis, enthesitis, dactylitis, and inflammatory bowel disease. Early sacroiilitis can be difficult to diagnose and if suspicion for a spondyloarthritis is high, plain films or MRI may be needed.

The patient under consideration does not meet criteria for a systemic connective tissue disorder given lack of connective tissue disease (CTD) symptoms and the negative ANA. In this patient, however, careful evaluation for presence of SICCA complaints should be performed and consideration should be given to evaluating antibodies to SSA and SSB if these symptoms are present. No objective proximal muscle weakness was identified. However, if concern for a primary muscle disease is present, measurement of creatine phosphokinase (CPK) and aldolase should be performed. If the patient did have a positive ANA (low-titer), no further testing or evaluation would be required. A high-titer ANA in this patient should be

further evaluated for other autoantibodies that might signal a need for close monitoring for development of a connective tissue disease.

Infectious etiologies that should be considered include Lyme disease, parvovirus B-19, human immunodeficiency virus (HIV), and hepatitis C virus (HCV).[4] Given the relatively high prevalence of HCV, the clinician should inquire into risk factors for HCV and screen when present. Epstein-Barr virus infection can also lead to chronic (> 3 months) symptoms, although other myotropic viruses would be shorter lived.

Noninflammatory conditions include FM, myofascial pain syndromes (a more limited musculoskeletal pain syndrome with significant overlap in symptom domains), and generalized osteoarthritis/spondylosis. Endocrine disorders, particularly hypothyroidism and hyperthyroidism but also including parathyroid and adrenal gland dysfunction, can cause widespread myalgias and arthralgias. Vitamin D deficiency is also associated with these symptoms and questioning the patient about diet and sun exposure followed by screening for at-risk patients is recommended.[5,6] Patients should be screened for major depressive disorder by query for depressed mood (feeling down, depressed, or hopeless) and anhedonia (little interest or pleasure in activities). Drug-induced myalgias are seen in patients taking statins and aromatase inhibitors among many others, and a careful history should be able to determine a temporal association between onset of symptoms and the offending drug.[7-9]

CASE STUDY 2   Secondary Fibromyalgia

A 28-year-old woman with a 4-year history of systemic lupus erythematosus (SLE) presents complaining of a "flare" of her lupus characterized by pain in her shoulders and back with a marked increase in fatigue. She was initially diagnosed following the birth of her first child when she developed a malar rash, alopecia, oral ulcers, Raynaud's phenomenon, arthritis, and serositis. Laboratory evaluation at that time revealed mild normochronic anemia and leukopenia. Her creatinine and urinalysis were normal. ESR was elevated at 46 mm/hr. Serologic testing revealed a positive fluorescent ANA at a titer of 1:640, positive anti-ds-DNA at 1:80, and positive SSA. Complement levels were normal. The patient was treated with prednisone 20 mg daily and hydroxychloroquine 400 mg daily. She responded quickly to this treatment and prednisone was tapered off over the ensuing 3 months.

Over the next several years, the patient had intermittent exacerbations of her symptoms typified by increasing fatigue, malar rash, arthritis in her elbows, wrists, metacarpophalangeal (MCP), and peripheral interphalangeal (PIP) joints, and oral ulcers. She usually responded to reinstitution of prednisone at doses of 10 to 15 mg. No nephritis, central nervous system disease, severe hematologic manifestations, or vasculitis has been identified. Flares were usually accompanied by elevation of ESR, increased anti-ds-DNA, and mild leukopenia.

At the present time, the patient reports a marked increase in her fatigue and musculoskeletal pain in the shoulders and low back. She states that the symptoms are disrupting her attempt to return to school and would like a prescription for prednisone.

On further questioning, the patient denies swelling in her peripheral joints, although she has had a malar flush and a few recent oral ulcers. On physical examination, the vital signs are normal. The patient does not have a visible rash nor mucosal ulcerations. Joints reveal no swelling, but there is diffuse tenderness of the joints and muscles. There was increased tone of the cervical and lumbar paraspinal musculature and the trapezius muscles. FM tender points were positive in 16 of 18 sites. Neurologic examination is normal including muscle strength testing.

The patient reports that she has recently returned to school to complete her bachelor's degree in history and plans to go to law school. She is married and her husband is a physician.

Laboratory testing reveals a white blood cell (WBC) count of 3900, unchanged from her last visit. Urinalysis is normal, ESR is 25 mm/h, anti-ds-DNA is 1:10, and complements are normal.

Discussion of Differential Diagnosis

FM is a frequent comorbid condition with autoimmune inflammatory rheumatic diseases.[10,11] It is thought that the increased incidence relative to the population at large reflects the capacity of these disorders to function as pain generators (see Table 28-2), although the possibility of shared genetic vulnerability between autoimmune diseases and FM (through altered function of the hypothalamic-pituitary-adrenal axis, as is postulated for mood disorders, for example) cannot be excluded. The challenge is to distinguish between exacerbation of the underlying autoimmune inflammatory disease and comorbid FM. In general, it is preferable to assure, as best as possible, that the underlying autoimmune or inflammatory disorder is treated before attributing symptoms to FM. However, in cases in which characteristic FM symptoms are present, concomitant therapy may be beneficial. It is also necessary to evaluate the patient for other new disease, particularly including a new autoimmune disease such as thyroid disease.

In the case under discussion, the patient's clinical manifestations are different from previous flares. She specifically had no signs of arthritis in peripheral joints and rash, and mucosal ulcers were not clinically evident. Laboratory tests were unchanged from her baseline values. It is useful to discuss with the patient the differences between her current symptoms and symptoms of lupus and in this case, it is preferable to treat the patient for FM symptoms without intensifying treatment for SLE.

PRINCIPLES OF TREATMENT

FM has a substantial negative impact on social and occupational function as assessed in a recent qualitative study.[12] Patients reported disrupted relationships with family and friends, social isolation, reduced activities of daily living and leisure activities, avoidance of physical activity, and loss of career or inability to advance in careers or education. This impact should be understood by the clinician and return to function and improved health-related quality of life should be emphasized as the primary treatment goal. Accordingly, it is essential to recognize that multiple symptom domains contribute to the functional deficits experienced by patients with FM. In a recent study designed to determine the relevant symptom domains, patients and clinicians participated in an exercise to achieve group consensus using the Delphi method, a structured process of consensus building via questionnaires together with systematic and controlled opinion feedback.[13] The relevant symptom domains identified included pain, stiffness, fatigue, sleep, cognition, depression, and quality of life. In approaching the treatment of an individual patient with FM, determining the most important symptom domains and functional goals is critical to designing a treatment plan.

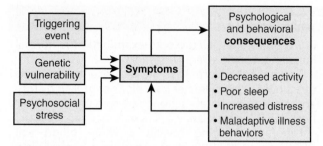

Figure 28-2. Dual approach to treatment. Although medications may be effective for treatment of physiologic alterations, nonpharmacologic approaches are required to address behavioral changes that occur in the context of chronic pain.

In approaching the treatment plan, it is useful to think of the symptoms and their consequences as needing different but complementary approaches (Fig. 28-2). For example, the physiologic alterations that lead to altered pain processing may by amenable to drug treatment, but the decreased activity associated with musculoskeletal pain and postexertional malaise should be approached using nonpharmacologic therapies. In discussing this dual approach to treatment, patients with FM should be engaged as active participants in the treatment program and clearly understand what each treatment is designed to address.

There has been controversy as to whether making a diagnosis of FM or avoiding a diagnostic label is more beneficial to the patient.[14] Studies directly addressing this hypothesis fail to support the assertion that labeling a patient as having FM increases the likelihood of persistent symptoms.[15] Furthermore, absence of a clear diagnosis leads the patient to seek out additional clinicians and treatments, and solidifies maladaptive health behaviors. Recent studies have demonstrated that use of health care resources is decreased significantly following diagnosis of FM, although effective treatment is needed to achieve long-term reductions in the medical costs of FM.[16,17]

Providing a diagnosis is an essential first step in discussion of an intellectual framework by which the patient may understand his or her symptoms and treatment (Table 28-3). This framework can provide increased control and self-efficacy for the patients that may, in turn, improve self-management of

Table 28-3. *Management Strategies in Patients with Fibromyalgia*

Diagnosis
Education
Diagnose and treat associated conditions and pain
  generators
Exercise and other physical strategies
Cognitive behavioral strategies: sleep hygiene, stress
  management, pain coping
Pharmacologic treatment of syndrome symptoms
Treatment of specific symptoms

symptoms.[18,19] Furthermore, there is substantial and growing evidence that physiologic alterations in FM patients can be treated pharmacologically. Explanation of why specific types of treatments are used requires a discussion of the diagnosis and its underpinnings.

It is likely that there are multiple genetic vulnerabilities and triggers that lead to a similar physiology.[4,20,21] This final common pathway leads to patients who can be identified using the current classification criteria for FM.[22] Although not all patients respond to or can tolerate currently available treatments, addressing treatment to the central elements of pain processing pathways (treatments with efficacy in neuropathic pain) has been more effective than approaches directed toward peripheral pain mechanisms (inflammatory pain). This is clearly reflected in evidence-based guidelines published recently that outline proved treatments.[23,24] Additional comprehensive reviews of treatment approaches are available that review large numbers of potential treatments.[25] The following is a distillation of proved therapies for FM and a pragmatic approach to their use.

Nonpharmacologic Approaches

A number of recent systematic reviews of nonpharmacologic therapies for FM have been completed.[26-29] In very general terms, the methodologic quality of the studies are lower than in the more recent studies of pharmacologic treatments, but many of these approaches provide positive treatment effects for at least some of the domains of FM that are equivalent to drug treatment.

Mind-body therapies including education, cognitive behavioral training, relaxation exercises, hypnosis, guided imagery, and biofeedback were evaluated by meta-analysis and provided solid evidence of improved self-efficacy in patients with FM.[26] This did not necessarily translate into improvements in parameters such as pain or physical function, in which exercise interventions fared better. Nevertheless, behavioral therapy can be a useful management tool, although different patients may respond to cognitive-behavioral compared with operant-behavioral interventions and tailored therapy is likely to prove most useful.[30] Cognitive-behavioral approaches can be used in one-on-one or group settings.[31] Behavioral approaches can be aimed at specific symptoms and may be particularly useful for sleep disturbance in FM.[32]

Exercise has been shown to be useful, though significant issues surrounding adherence remain.[33] The most recent meta-analysis of exercise interventions shows significant clinical heterogeneity among studies. There is moderate quality evidence that aerobic-only exercise training at recommended intensity levels has positive effects on global well-being (standardized mean difference [SMD], 0.44; 95%

confidence interval [CI], 0.13 to 0.75) and physical function (SMD, 0.68; 95% CI, 0.41 to 0.95) and possibly on pain (SMD, 0.94; 95% CI, -0.15 to 2.03) and tender points (SMD, 0.26; 95% CI, -0.28 to 0.79). Strength and flexibility training remain underevaluated. The authors conclude that there is solid evidence that supervised aerobic exercise training has beneficial effects on physical capacity and FM symptoms. Strength training may also have benefits on some FM symptoms. Further studies on muscle strengthening and flexibility are needed. Research on the long-term benefit of exercise for FM is still needed.[34] Combination of exercise with education may provide additional benefits.[19]

There are a number of additional treatments that have been tried with mixed results.[25] Acupuncture, for example, has not been found useful compared to sham in rigorously designed clinical studies.[35] However, it is reasonable to work with patients who are interested in trying nonpharmacologic approaches using an "n-of-1" approach, a clinical trial for a single individual patient. Patients should be instructed to assess their symptoms before instituting a particular treatment, then reassess after a period of time. This approach can provide patients an opportunity, as a partner with the clinician, to guide their treatment in a rational manner. It is useful to apply this principal to other complementary and alternative therapies, in addition to pharmacologic approaches.

Pharmacologic Approaches

There are a number of ways to approach pharmacologic treatment for patients with FM that take into account the primary symptoms and functional deficits in each individual patient. Unfortunately, it is not currently possible to predict with certainty which patient will respond best to which treatment approach. The major categories of drugs shown most useful in the management of FM are in the antidepressant and anticonvulsant classes (Table 28-4). From within the antidepressant class, drugs vary with regard to effects on serotonin and norepinephrine (Fig. 28-3). Furthermore, chemical class and pharmacologic profiles also lead to different clinical effects. For example, tricyclic antidepressants (TCAs) and norepinephrine serotonin reuptake inhibitors (NSRIs) exhibit balanced norepinephrine and serotonin reuptake inhibition and provide analgesic effects. However, TCA at the lower doses are typically used in FM to improve sleep, whereas NSRIs are often accompanied by insomnia. These types of effects may provide guidance to assist in initial treatment choice (Table 28-5).

Anticonvulsant drugs that act as ligands for the alpha-2-delta subunit of voltage-gated calcium channels, gabapentin and pregabalin, have efficacy in neuropathic pain syndromes, and have been studied and shown to be effective in short- and long-term studies in patients with FM.[36-40] These agents have the effect of reducing calcium flux and release of transmitters associated with neuronal activation such as excitatory amino acids and substance P. Note that all studies in patients with FM have excluded patients with autoimmune inflammatory diseases, so efficacy in this group of patients has not been defined. In the Gabapentin In Fibromyalgia Treatment (GIFT) study, an investigator-initiated, National Institutes of Health–funded study, gabapentin in patient-optimized doses between 1200 and 2400 mg/day (n = 75) was compared with placebo over 12 weeks.[37] Patients treated with gabapentin (median dose 1800 mg/day) had significantly greater improvement in pain severity than patients treated with placebo ($P < 0.015$). In addition, 51% of gabapentin-treated patients compared with 31% of placebo-treated patients had a greater than 30% reduction in endpoint pain intensity ($P < 0.014$). Gabapentin compared with placebo also significantly improved function, sleep, and vitality, but not tender point pain threshold or depression.[37]

Pregabalin shares mechanism of action with gabapentin, though the pharmacokinetic profile demonstrates a more linear dose-response relationship.[36] Industry-sponsored studies have led to regulatory approval for pregabalin for the treatment of FM in doses of 300 to 450 mg/day in the United States. In an 8-week, multicenter, randomized, dose-finding study, pregabalin was used at doses of 150, 300, and 450 mg/day (n = 529) and compared with placebo. Pregabalin 450 mg/day had a significant beneficial effect on average daily pain ($P < 0.001$). In addition, patients treated with either 300 or 450 mg/day had significantly greater improvement in fatigue, sleep, and health-related quality of life when compared with placebo.[36] Two placebo-controlled, parallel group studies of pregabalin confirmed efficacy in FM.[39,40] A 6-month study evaluated the durability of response in a population enriched with responders to pregabalin in patient-optimized doses of 300, 450, or 600 mg/day. Responders were defined as having a greater than 50% reduction in average daily pain and a rating of much or very much improved. Responders underwent double-blind randomization to continue their optimal dose of pregabalin or to taper pregabalin and change to placebo. Two thirds (61%) of responders maintained on pregabalin had sustained improvement (> 30% reduction from open-label baseline) for 6 months compared with 32% of those patients randomized to placebo ($P < 0.001$).[38] Although pregabalin has anxiolytic effects, the analgesic effect of pregabalin was not dependent on improvements in anxiety or depression.[41] Similar to gabapentin, pregabalin treatment does not result in improvement of tender point pain threshold.

Both gabapentin and pregabalin are associated with a high frequency of dose-dependent dizziness and somnolence.[36-38] Tolerance improves if patients are started on lower doses with an incremental increase to optimal dose. The severity of these adverse effects is generally mild with few discontinuations in clinical trials; however, these and other adverse events, including weight gain and peripheral edema, may limit the utility of these drugs in some clinical settings.

Table 28-4. *Selected Treatments for Fibromyalgia*

Agent	Class	Mechanism	Comments
Gabapentin, Pregabalin	Anticonvulsants	Alpha-2-delta ligands; affects calcium flux and release of excitatory amino acids and neuropeptides	Gabapentin should be used tid and most will require 1200–2400 mg/day; pregabalin is approved by FDA at 300 and 450 mg/day taken in divided doses twice daily; start with lower dose and increase to minimize adverse effects; dizziness and somnolence may limit tolerability
Cyclobenzaprine	Muscle relaxant	Norepinephrine reuptake inhibition, possible central proserotonergic effect	10–30 mg dose; improved sleep may be main mechanism for efficaciousness
Amitryptiline and related tricyclic and heterocyclic compounds	Antidepressants	Norepinephrine and serotonin reuptake inhibitors with additional anticholinergic, antiadrenergic, antihistaminergic, and quinidine-like effects	Doses of 25–50 mg amitryptiline effective; pleotrophic actions increase side effects; should be avoided in the elderly and those with heart problems
Fluoxetine	Antidepressant	Serotonin reuptake inhibitor	Titration between 20 and 60 mg may be needed for effectiveness; has more important effects on mood than on pain, but higher doses may improve analgesic effects; other, more highly serotonin-selective agents have not been effective for relief of pain
Duloxetine	Antidepressant	Balanced norepinephrine and serotonin reuptake inhibition	Approved for treatment of neuropathic pain; no evidence that twice daily dosing provides significant improvement in efficacy; recommend starting with 30 mg dose and increasing to 60, 90 or 120 mg daily; GI effects may limit tolerability; can cause insomnia
Milnacipran	Antidepressant	Balanced norepinephrine and serotonin reuptake inhibition	Likely requires divided dosing and most will require 200 mg/day; GI side effects may limit tolerability
Tramadol with or without acetaminophen	Analgesic	μ-opioid receptor agonist, norepinephrine and serotonin reuptake inhibition	May be associated with withdrawal with discontinuation and may be associated with abuse and dependence; adverse effects include nausea, constipation, dizziness and somnolence

FDA, US Food and Drug Administration; GI, gastrointestinal.

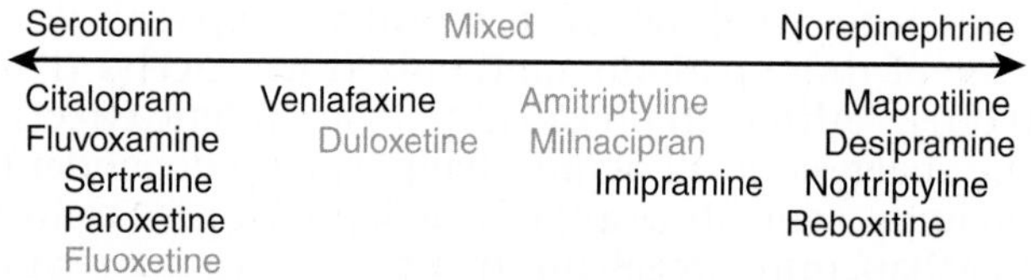

Serotonin		Mixed		Norepinephrine
Citalopram	Venlafaxine	Amitriptyline		Maprotiline
Fluvoxamine	Duloxetine	Milnacipran		Desipramine
Sertraline		Imipramine		Nortriptyline
Paroxetine				Reboxitine
Fluoxetine				

Figure 28-3. Relative serotonin and norepinephrine reuptake inhibition of antidepressants. Studies have demonstrated that inhibition of both of these neurochemicals is most effective for analgesia. Therefore, use of mixed inhibitors or a combination of selective agents is recommended for pain relief.

Table 28-5. *Rational Pharmacologic Approach to Specific Symptom Domains*

Symptom	Treatment
Pain	TCA, α2δ ligand, NSRI, tramadol
Sleep	TCA, α2δ ligand, pramipexole
Depression/Anxiety	NSRI, SSRI
Fatigue	NSRI, SSRI
Cognitive Impairment	NSRI, SSRI
Stiffness	Cyclobenzaprine

TCA, tricyclic antidepressant, e.g., amitriptyline; α2δ ligand, gabapentin, pregabalin; NSRI, norepinephrine serotonin reuptake inhibitor, e.g. duloxetine; SSRI, selective serotonin reuptake inhibitor, e.g., fluoxetine.

NRSIs, chiefly TCAs, have been used clinically for neuropathic and functional pain for many years. Norepinephrine and serotonin are important mediators of descending inhibition of noxious signaling and also are important mediators of the stress-response pathways. Meta-analyses of these agents in patients with FM have demonstrated the efficacy of TCAs.[25,42] A related cyclic heterocyclic, cyclobenzaprine, classified as a muscle relaxant is also effective in FM patients. There is overall improvement, and patients report improvement in some symptoms, particularly sleep.[43]

There has been mixed efficacy of selective serotonin reuptake inhibitors.[27,42] Although these agents improve depression and fatigue, analgesic effects may require higher doses. For example, in a flexible-dose study of fluoxetine, a mean dose of 45 mg was used, resulting in an improvement of multiple domains of FM.[44] Similarly, venlafaxine was ineffective in low doses, but an open-label study of higher doses proved useful.[45] Citalopram, a highly serotonin selective drug was not effective in clinical studies.[42] More recently, newer dual reuptake inhibitors with balanced inhibition of norepinephrine and serotonin lacking the adrenergic, cholinergic or histaminergic receptor activity or effects on sodium channels of TCA have been developed and evaluated in patients with FM.[25,42] These agents, duloxetine and milnacipran, are effective analgesics.

Duloxetine is an antidepressant, but is also effective in neuropathic pain independent of its effects on mood. Two 12-week randomized, double-blind, placebo-controlled trials have evaluated duloxetine in patients with FM.[46,47] In the initial study, men and women stratified for the presence of current major depression were treated.[47] Significantly more women treated with duloxetine (30%) than placebo (16%) had a greater than 50% reduction in pain.[48] Duloxetine-treated male patients failed to improve significantly. A second study limited to women with FM evaluated both a 60 mg twice daily and a 60 mg/day dose in a 12-week, randomized, placebo-controlled study. Again, significantly more patients treated with duloxetine had a reduction in pain severity as measured by the Brief Pain Inventory (BPI) scale, but also more duloxetine-treated (41%) women than placebo-treated (23%) women had a greater than 50% reduction in the BPI average pain scale.[46] A pooled analysis of these two studies demonstrated that the reduction in pain was independent of the effect on mood and the presence of major depressive disorder.[48] A long-term study of duloxetine at doses of 60 or 129 mg/d demonstrated that a beneficial effect of this drug was sustained improvement in pain over a 6-month period.[49] The most frequent treatment-emergent adverse event with duloxetine is nausea, and most side effects were mild to moderate in intensity.[48]

Milnacipran is a second dual norepinephrine and serotonin reuptake inhibitor approved for treatment of depression in Europe, Asia, and elsewhere.[25] A 12-week randomized, placebo-controlled study designed as a dose-finding trial of 25 to 200 mg/day given as a daily or twice-daily regimen milnacipran or placebo during the first 4 weeks, followed by 8 weeks of stable dose has been reported.[50] Most patients titrated to the highest dose of 200 mg/day whether they were dosed once or twice daily. The primary outcome measure of average daily pain score was recorded on an electronic diary, and there was no significant improvement compared with placebo on this measure. However, significantly more patients receiving milnacipran twice daily (37%) than placebo (14%) reported a reduction in the weekly average pain scores. The most frequent adverse effects were headache and gastrointestinal symptoms including nausea. Of interest, pain reduction was greater in nondepressed patients compared with depressed patients.

Development and study of novel drugs with analgesic effects on different types of pain is certainly needed. There are reports of serotonin-receptor antagonists, dopamine receptor agonists, and the sedative-hypnotic agent gamma-hydroxybutyrate that have demonstrated pain reduction in patients with FM.[25]

Practical Approach to the Use of Pharmacologic Agents

In FM, as in other rheumatic diseases, drugs should be approached with a view to understanding their relative benefits and risks. It is particularly important in the treatment of FM because side effects of the drugs can mimic the symptoms of the disorder. For example, NSRIs and SSRIs cause insomnia, and alpha-2-delta ligands can cause somnolence. It is prudent to select an agent based on the symptoms of the given patient (see Table 28-5), start with a low dose, adjust to tolerance, and assess efficacy. For most of the agents, beneficial effects are seen in 1 to 2 weeks. Therefore, a titration in intervals of 2 weeks to efficacious doses is reasonable (see Table 28-4). The patient should be instructed to contact the clinician if side effects develop during the titration and to go back to the previous tolerated dose. If an agent is not useful or poorly tolerated, a drug of a different class should be tried next. It should be possible to identify within 3 to 4 months the class of agent most effective for a given patient, then optimize the dose. The goal should be to use a single agent that treats as many symptoms of FM as possible. However, combining drugs that inhibit serotonin selectively (fluoxetine) with those that inhibit norepinephrine (desipramine) can provide the balanced reuptake inhibition of the newer agents (see Fig. 28-3).

If the initial approach does not resolve some symptoms, combination therapy may be needed. Caution should be taken when combining agents that have proserotonergic effects because the serotonin syndrome can occur, usually with a serotonergic agent and a monoamine oxidase inhibitor, but the condition has been reported with combinations of multiple agents often used in FM. This syndrome includes agitation, tachycardia, hypertension, hyperthermia, diaphoresis, mydriasis, diarrhea, tremor (greater in legs), hyperreflexia, clonus, and muscle rigidity.[51] Combined antidepressant medications and alpha-2-delta ligands have not been studied in clinical trials, but because side effect profiles differ, this approach may be shown useful. For those who require an analgesic effect, tramadol or tramadol with acetaminophen can be recommended. More potent opioids should be avoided except as rescue medication. Nonsteroidal anti-inflammatory drugs do not work for the central pain of FM but may be very useful for treatment of pain generators.

Clinicians should also identify disorders frequently comorbid with FM that may respond well to specific treatments and influence choice of treatment. For example, restless legs syndrome may respond well to dopaminergic agents such as pramipexole and ropinerole, although this syndrome also can be treated with gabapentin.[52] Irritable bowel syndrome can be treated with antidepressants.[53] Clinicians should also identify and treat peripheral pain generators and co-occurring disorders. It is vital to avoid the temptation to attribute every complaint to FM rather than evaluating and treating new complaints objectively. FM patients, for example, can respond very well to injection therapy for rotator cuff or trochanteric bursitis similar to those patients without FM.

Difficult Management Issues

Chronic Opioid Analgesic Use

One of the most difficult management issues surrounds opioid use—often initiated before diagnosis and initiation of more rational treatments for FM. New insights into the actions of opioids reveal the complex issues that surround use of these agents in central pain syndromes. It is now known that in addition to their action as ligand to μ-opioid receptors, opioids bind to toll-like receptor (TLR)-4 on the surface of glia in the dorsal horn of the spinal cord, resulting in an activation phenotype.[54] Glial activation during neuropathic pain is associated with reduced efficacy and increased rebound pain associated with use of opioids. To the extent that central mechanisms associated with FM pain are similar to neuropathic pain, this mechanism may be of importance in the lack of efficacy of these agents. Furthermore, patients with FM have reduced μ-opioid binding capacity in the central nervous system, suggesting that these drugs have limited capacity to provide analgesic effects in usual doses.[55]

From a clinical and therapeutic perspective, these types of studies provide evidence that currently available opioids should not be first-line management for pain not responding to NSAIDs and simple analgesics. Whether this holds true for tramadol with or without acetaminophen, an agent with weak μ-opioid receptor binding combined with dual serotonin and norepinephrine reuptake inhibition is unclear. This agent has been shown to be useful in patients with FM in a randomized, placebo-controlled study.[56]

Although relatively few chronic pain patients develop abuse or addition (~3%), adverse drug related behaviors occur in a larger percentage (~11.5%) more commonly in patients with a prior history of substance abuse.[57] However, with the knowledge that opioids may contribute to persistence of chronic pain and that efficacy may be reduced in patients with FM compared with patients with other causes of chronic musculoskeletal pain, the risk-benefit ratio is not favorable, and this should be clearly explained to patients. From a practical standpoint, opioids can be useful for as-needed pain relief in patients that do not use them chronically. Because patients with FM complain that it is difficult for them to predict when pain will be severe enough to limit function thereby reducing social and workplace function, as-needed opioids can relieve anxiety surrounding the pain.

Poor Medication Tolerance

Many patients with FM develop side effects to multiple medications reducing tolerability. It is essential to avoid the temptation to treat medication side effects (nausea) with other medications (antiemetics) in these patients. The clinician should be very clear that although some medications can be helpful, they are not required to manage FM. This creates anxiety in many patients, but in fact provides an opportunity for clinicians to manage FM with nonpharmacologic treatments. When evaluating the effect size of various treatments, it is clear that nonpharmacologic approaches can be equally effective to pharmacologic treatments.[58] This should be the first message to patients. Second, it should be emphasized that non-pharmacologic treatments should be viewed as seriously as pharmacologic treatments and that the treatment "dose" should be calibrated for maximum benefit.

Using information technology to assist patients with disease self-management can reduce time needed for patient instruction. For example *http://www.med.umich.edu/painresearch/patients/index.htm* assists patients in developing exercise regimens and guides patients through a selection of self-management skills and developing an exercise program.

SUMMARY

Treatment of patients with FM can be challenging and rewarding. Patients must have confidence that their symptoms are heard, understood, evaluated, and treated objectively. The relationship between psychosocial stress and FM symptoms is certainly understood by patients; therefore, this relationship should be known and acknowledged by clinicians. Less clearly understood by patients is the relationship between behaviors (lack of exercise, poor sleep hygiene) and symptoms, which can be explained by clinicians in a manner that provide tools for patients to regain control over their symptoms. There are many social and family issues that the health care system cannot address that may impact patients with FM, acknowledging this limitation is vital. A common understanding of the context of FM forms the basis for a therapeutic relationship that can be the most effective tool for treatment of patients with FM.

References

1. Fitzcharles MA, Boulos P. Inaccuracy in the diagnosis of fibromyalgia syndrome: analysis of referrals. Rheumatology (Oxford) 2003;42:263-7.
2. Dinerman H, Steere AC. Lyme disease associated with fibromyalgia. Ann Intern Med 1992;117:281-5.
3. Fitzcharles MA, Esdaile JM. The overdiagnosis of fibromyalgia syndrome. Am J Med 1997;103:44-50.
4. Buskila D, Atzeni F, Sarzi-Puttini P. Etiology of fibromyalgia: the possible role of infection and vaccination. Autoimmun Rev 2008;8:41-3.
5. Atherton K, Berry DJ, Parsons T, Macfarlane GJ, Power C, Hypponen E. Vitamin D and chronic widespread pain in a white middle-aged British population: evidence from a cross-sectional population survey. Ann Rheum Dis 2009;68: 817-22.
6. Turner MK, Hooten WM, Schmidt JE, Kerkvliet JL, Townsend CO, Bruce BK. Prevalence and clinical correlates of vitamin D inadequacy among patients with chronic pain. Pain Med 2008;9:979-84.
7. Felson DT, Cummings SR. Aromatase inhibitors and the syndrome of arthralgias with estrogen deprivation. Arthritis Rheum 2005;52:2594-8.
8. Presant CA, Bosserman L, Young T, Vakil M, Horns R, Upadhyaya G, et al. Aromatase inhibitor-associated arthralgia and/or bone pain: frequency and characterization in non-clinical trial patients. Clin Breast Cancer 2007;7:775-8.
9. Jacobson TA. Toward "pain-free" statin prescribing: clinical algorithm for diagnosis and management of myalgia. Mayo Clin Proc 2008;83:687-700.
10. Buskila D, Press J, Abu-Shakra M. Fibromyalgia in systemic lupus erythematosus: prevalence and clinical implications. Clin Rev Allergy Immunol 2003;25:25-8.
11. Clauw DJ, Katz P. The overlap between fibromyalgia and inflammatory rheumatic diseases: when and why does it occur? J Clin Rheumatol 1995;1:335-41.
12. Arnold LM, Crofford LJ, Mease PJ, Burgess SM, Palmer SC, Abetz L, et al. Patient perspectives on the impact of fibromyalgia. Patient Educ Couns 2008;73:114-20.
13. Mease PJ, Arnold LM, Crofford LJ, Williams DA, Russell IJ, Humphrey L, et al. Identifying the clinical domains of fibromyalgia: contributions from clinician and patient Delphi exercises. Arthritis Rheum 2008;59:952-60.
14. Ehrlich GE. Pain is real; fibromyalgia isn't. J Rheumatol 2003;30:1666-7.
15. White KP, Nielson WR, Harth M, Ostbye T, Speechley M. Does the label "fibromyalgia" alter health status, function, and health service ulitlization? A prospective, within-group comparison in a community cohort of adults with chronic widespread pain. Arthritis Rheum 2002;47:260-5.
16. Hughes G, Martinez C, Myon E, Taïeb C, Wessely S. The impact of a diagnosis of fibromyalgia on health care resource use by primary care patients in the UK: an observational study based on clinical practice. Arthritis Rheum 2006;54:177-83.
17. Annemans L, Wessely S, Spaepen E, Caekelbergh K, Caubère JP, Lay KL, et al. Health economic consequences related to the diagnosis of fibromyalgia syndrome. Arthritis Rheum 2008;58:895-902.
18. Burckhardt CS, Bjelle A. Education programmes for fibromyalgia patients: Description and evaluation. Bailliere's Clin Rheumatol 1994;8:935-55.
19. Rooks DS, Gautam S, Romeling M, Cross ML, Stratigakis D, Evans B, et al. Group exercise, education, and combination self-management in women with fibromyalgia: a randomized trial. Arch Intern Med 2007;167:2192-200.
20. Markkula R, Järvinen P, Leino-Arjas P, Koskenvuo M, Kalso E, Kaprio J. Clustering of symptoms associated with fibromyalgia in a Finnish Twin Cohort. Eur J Pain 2009;13:744–50.
21. Buskila D, Sarzi-Puttini P. Biology and therapy of fibromyalgia. Genetic aspects of fibromyalgia syndrome. Arthritis Res Ther 2006;8:218.
22. Wolfe F, Smythe HA, Yunus MB, Bennett RM, Bombardier C, Goldenberg DL, et al. The American College of Rheumatology 1990 criteria for the classification of fibromyalgia. Arthritis Rheum 1990;33:160-72.
23. Carville SF, Arendt-Nielsen S, Bliddal H, Blotman F, Branco JC, Buskila D, et al. EULAR evidence-based recommendations for the management of fibromyalgia syndrome. Ann Rheum Dis 2008;67:537-41.
24. Goldenberg DL, Burckhardt C, Crofford L. Management of fibromyalgia syndrome. JAMA 2004;292:2388-95.
25. Arnold LM. New therapies in fibromyalgia. Arthritis Res Ther 2006;8:212-32.
26. Rossy LA, Buckelew SP, Dorr N, Hagglund KJ, Thayer JF, McIntosh MJ, et al. A meta-analysis of fibromyalgia treatment interventions. Ann Behav Med 1999;21:180-91.
27. Arnold LM, Keck Jr PE, Welge JA. Antidepressant treatment of fibromyalgia. A meta-analysis and review. Psychosomatics 2000;41:104-13.
28. Sim J, Adams N. Systematic review of randomized controlled trials of nonpharmacological interventions for fibromyalgia. Clin J Pain 2002;18:324-36.
29. Busch AJ, Barber KA, Overend TJ, Peloso PM, Schachter CL. Exercise for treating fibromyalgia syndrome. Cochrane Database Syst Rev 2007;(4):CD003786.
30. Thieme K, Turk DC, Flor H. Responder criteria for operant and cognitive-behavioral treatment of fibromyalgia syndrome. Arthritis Rheum 2007;57:830-6.
31. Bennett R, Nelson D. Cognitive behavioral therapy for fibromyalgia. Nat Clin Pract Rheumatol 2006;2:416-24.
32. Edinger JD, Wohlgemuth WK, Krystal AD, Rice JR. Behavioral insomnia therapy for fibromyalgia patients: a randomized clinical trial. Arch Intern Med 2005;165:2527-35.
33. Dobkin PL, Da Costa D, Abrahamowicz M, Dritsa M, Du Berger R, Fitzcharles MA, et al. Adherence during an individualized home based 12-week exercise program in women with fibromyalgia. J Rheumatol 2006;33:333-41.
34. Busch AJ, Schachter CL, Overend TJ, Peloso PM, Barber KA. Exercise for fibromyalgia: a systematic review. J Rheumatol 2008;35:1130-44.
35. Mayhew E, Ernst E. Acupuncture for fibromyalgia—a systematic review of randomized clinical trials. Rheumatology (Oxford) 2007;46:801-4.
36. Crofford LJ, Rowbotham MD, Mease PJ, Russell IJ, Dworkin RH, Corbin AE, et al. Pregabalin for the treatment of fibromylagia syndrome: Results of a randomized, double-blind, placebo-controlled trial. Arthritis Rheum 2005;52:1264-73.
37. Arnold LM, Goldenberg DL, Stanford SB, Lalonde JK, Sandhu HS, Keck Jr PE, et al. Gabapentin in the treatment of fibromyalgia: a randomized, double-blind, placebo-controlled, multicenter trial. Arthritis Rheum 2007;56:1336-44.
38. Crofford LJ, Mease PM, Simpson S, Martin SA, Young Jr JP, Haig G, et al. Fibromyalgia relapse evaluation and efficacy for durability of meaningul relief (FREEDOM): A 6-month placebo-controlled, double-blind study with pregabalin. Pain 2008;136:419-31.
39. Arnold LM, Russell IJ, Diri EW, Duan WR, Young Jr JP, Sharma U, et al. A 14-week, randomized, double-blinded, placebo-controlled monotherapy trial of pregabalin in patients with fibromyalgia. J Pain 2008;9:792-805.
40. Mease PJ, Russell IJ, Arnold LM, Florian H, Young Jr JP, Martin SA, et al. A randomized, double-blind, placebo-controlled,

phase III trial of pregabalin in the treatment of patients with fibromyalgia. J Rheumatol 2008;35:502-14.

41. Arnold LM, Crofford LJ, Martin SA, Young JP, Sharma U. The effect of anxiety and depression on improvements in pain in a randomized, controlled trial of pregabalin for treatment of fibromyalgia. Pain Med 2007;8:633-8.

42. Uçeyler N, Häuser W, Sommer C. A systematic review on the effectiveness of treatment with antidepressants in fibromyalgia syndrome. Arthritis Rheum 2008;59:1279-98.

43. Tofferi JK, Jackson JL, O'Malley PG. Treatment of fibromyalgia with cyclobenzaprine: A meta-analysis. Arthritis Rheum 2004;51:9-13.

44. Arnold LM, Hess EV, Hudson JI, Welge JA, Berno SE, Keck PE. A randomized, placebo-controlled, double-blind, flexible-dose study of fluoxetine in the treatment of women with fibromyalgia. Am J Med 2002;112:191-7.

45. Dwight MM, Arnold LM, O'Brian H, Metzger R, Morris-Park E, Keck Jr PE. An open clinical trial of venlafaxine treatment of fibromyalgia. Psychosomatics 1998;39:14-7.

46. Arnold LM, Rosen A, Pritchett YL, D'Souza DN, Goldstein DJ, Iyengar S, et al. A randomized, double-blind, placebo-controlled trial of duloxetine in the treatment of women with fibromyalgia with or without major depressive disorder. Pain 2005;119:5-15.

47. Arnold LM, Lu Y, Crofford LJ, Wohlreich M, Detke MJ, Iyengar S, et al. A double-blind, multicenter trial comparing duloxetine with placebo in the treatment of fibromyalgia patients with or without major depressive disorder. Arthritis Rheum 2004;50:2974-84.

48. Arnold LM, Pritchett YL, D'Souza DN, Kajdasz DK, Iyengar S, Wernicke JF. Duloxetine for the treatment of fibromyalgia in women: pooled results from two randomized, placebo-controlled clinical trials. J Womens Health (Larchmt) 2007;16:1145-56.

49. Russell IJ, Mease PJ, Smith TR, Kajdasz DK, Wohlreich MM, Detke MJ, et al. Efficacy and safety of duloxetine for treatment of fibromyalgia in patients with or without major depressive disorder: Results from a 6-month, randomized, double-blind, placebo-controlled, fixed-dose trial. Pain 2008;136:432-44.

50. Gendreau RM, Thorn MD, Gendreau JF, Kranzler JD, Ribeiro S, Gracely RH, et al. Efficacy of milnacipran in patients with fibromyalgia. J Rheumatol 2005;32:1975-85.

51. Sun-Edelstein C, Tepper SJ, Shapiro RE. Drug-induced serotonin syndrome: a review. Expert Opin Drug Saf 2008;7:587-96.

52. Trenkwalder C, Hening WA, Montagna P, Oertel WH, Allen RP, Walters AS, et al. Treatment of restless legs syndrome: An evidence-based review and implications for clinical practice. Mov Disord 2008;23:2267-302.

53. Ford AC, Talley NJ, Schoenfeld PS, Quigley EM, Moayyedi P. Efficacy of antidepressants and psychological therapies in irritable bowel syndrome: systematic review and meta-analysis. Gut 2009;58:367-78.

54. Watkins LR, Hutchinson MR, Ledeboer A, Wieseler-Frank J, Milligan ED, Maier SF. Norman Cousins Lecture. Glia as the "bad guys": implications for improving clinical pain control and the clinical utility of opioids. Brain Behav Immun 2007;21:131-46.

55. Harris RE, Clauw DJ, Scott DJ, McLean SA, Gracely RH, Zubieta JK. Decreased central mu-opioid receptor availability in fibromyalgia. J Neurosci 2007;27:10000-6.

56. Bennett RM, Kamin M, Karim R, Rosenthal N. Tramadol and acetaminophen combination tablets in the treatment of fibromyalgia pain: a double-blind, randomized, placebo-controlled study. Am J Med 2003;114:537-45.

57. Fishbain DA, Cole B, Lewis J, Rosomoff HL, Rosomoff RS. What percentage of chronic nonmalignant pain patients exposed to chronic opioid analgesic therapy develop abuse/addiction and/or aberrant drug-related behaviors? A structured evidence-based review. Pain Med 2008;9:444-59.

58. Mease P, Arnold LM, Bennett R, Boonen A, Buskila D, Carville S, et al. Fibromyalgia syndrome. J Rheumatol 2007;34:1415-25.

Section VI Selected Topics in the Management of the Patient with Rheumatic Diseases

Chapter 29

The Significance of Behavioral Interventions for Arthritis

Perry M. Nicassio

The last two decades have witnessed an expansion in research on the development and application of behavioral interventions for chronic illness. This research has resulted from an appreciation of the significance and relevance of the biopsychosocial model[1] in understanding the adjustment of patients to medical problems that disrupt quality of life and create functional limitations. Over this same time period, the fields of health psychology and behavioral medicine have fostered the promotion of interdisciplinary methodologies for examining how behavioral, psychological, and social factors can affect health promotion, disease prevention, and adaptational mechanisms in persons with a range of illnesses such as cancer, cardiovascular disease, diabetes, and arthritis. Creative and effective nonpharmacologic treatment approaches have emerged from a broadening of the paradigm for understanding the adjustment process in chronic disease. A wider range of alternatives for managing chronic disease currently exists than has ever existed before, infusing hope and optimism in the delivery of health care services for patients and their families.

It is within this broader context that health care professionals should conceptualize the care of patients with arthritis. A large body of research documents the contribution of psychosocial variables to clinical outcomes in arthritis as well as the efficacy of behavioral treatment strategies that have major relevance for enhancing clinical care.[2] However, it is unclear if such research is affecting the clinical care of arthritis patients. There is also a lack of information regarding the types of obstacles that may be interfering with optimal service delivery. It is possible that, in spite of illustrative research findings, rheumatologists and other arthritis health professionals may not be aware of the value and importance of behavioral interventions in their clinical decision making and patient interactions. Alternatively, clinical settings may lack the capacity to provide optimal biopsychosocial care, even when professionals embrace its value and practical importance. In this chapter, I present support for the empirical and theoretical justification for behavioral interventions, analyze findings on the efficacy of behavioral approaches, and describe future challenges in addressing how behavioral interventions can become more relevant to arthritis patient care.

THE NEED FOR BEHAVIORAL INTERVENTIONS

Although there are a multitude of variables that support the application of behavioral interventions for arthritis, three sets of factors are paramount. First, arthritis often has a significant, deleterious impact on patients' quality of life, emotional functioning, and financial well-being. These problems frequently persist despite efficacious medical treatment, creating frustration for patients and health care providers alike. Second, very high rates of psychiatric comorbidity have been found in persons with arthritis, and myriad psychosocial factors have been shown to affect the long-term adjustment of patients, supporting the need for broader, integrative treatment models and approaches. Third, behavioral interventions recognize the value of patient self-management and empowerment, which are essential to effective functioning in the face of chronic symptoms and illness-related obstacles. Behavioral interventions emphasize the importance of skills of management that are central to coping with difficult symptoms and preventing health risk, changing the way that patients relate to their health care team and reducing their dependency on biomedical treatment as the only means of management. Behavioral interventions promote a collaborative model of care in which patients participate actively with their physicians in managing their arthritis and in clinical decision-making.

THE FUNCTIONAL AND ECONOMIC IMPACT OF ARTHRITIS

Despite ongoing advances in the development of drugs that reduce inflammation and disease activity, arthritis continues to disrupt quality of life and lead to significant disability. The disability associated with arthritis has been the subject of research for many years and has led to the development of several different measures that capture individual variation in functional adaptation.[3-5] Although significant variability between patients exists in such areas as emotional, social, occupation, and physical functioning, the overall impact of arthritis is severe and pervasive. Unfortunately, medical approaches to managing disability are often ineffective because they are not equipped to deal with the range of factors (e.g., socioeconomic, environmental, social, psychological) that affect disability in individual cases. Other approaches are necessary to fill this void.

A recent study by Verbrugge and Juarez[6] has highlighted the extent and nature of arthritis disability. Using data collected as part of the 1994 and 1995 National Health Interview Surveys, the authors compared persons with arthritis (n = 2469) with persons with other forms of disability (n = 14,592) on their responses to questions on personal care (i.e., activities of daily living [ADLs]), household management (i.e., instrumental activities of daily living [IADLs]), physical limitations (PLIM), home, and work. Individuals with arthritis had more disabilities of all types than individuals with other disabilities and experienced more pain and fatigue in carrying out ADLs, IADLs, and PLIM. The study found that differences in physical limitations, the "building blocks" for roles and activities, were the most pronounced. Individuals with arthritis also traveled less and encountered more transportation barriers than their counterparts. The authors note that a distinctive aspect of arthritis disability is its significant social breadth, causing difficulties for patients in leaving their homes for social activities, attending social events, and experiencing pleasure with others.

PSYCHIATRIC COMORBIDITY AND PSYCHOSOCIAL FACTORS

In addition to functional limitations and impairment in quality of life, having arthritis creates an enormous financial burden for many patients and families. Arthritis ranks high among chronic diseases nationally and worldwide in medical costs, lost income, unemployment, and underemployment. Recent findings from Yelin et al.[7] confirm the economic impact of arthritis. Based on data from a national probability sample of the Medical Expenditures Panel Survey in 2003, the authors found that mean patient medical expenditures were $6978, yielding a total of $321.8 billion, and that patients earned $3613 less than persons with no chronic conditions. They also reported that medical expenditures and earnings losses increased from 1997 to 2003, attributing the rise primarily to a higher prevalence of arthritis found in the 2003 sample. Augmenting the financial impact of arthritis are indirect costs resulting from lost productivity, sick days, and early retirement, which are more difficult to quantify and are often underestimated.[8] The emotional impact of such losses and the disruption to family stability due to financial stressors are common, additional burdens.

The psychological impact of arthritis has been known for many years. From data collected as part of a National Institute of Mental Health (NIMH) catchment area study, Wells and colleagues[9] reported a lifetime prevalence rate of psychiatric disorders of 63.6% in persons with arthritis, which is higher than in persons with other medical conditions such as cancer, diabetes, heart disease, and chronic obstructive pulmonary disease. Following this landmark epidemiologic study, investigators have conducted research on the role and prevalence of depression in arthritis. Estimates of the prevalence of depression in arthritis range from 15% to 40%, depending on the diagnostic criteria, sampling procedures, and measurement approaches adopted.[10] These prevalence rates are very high compared with rates of 5% to 8% that are found in samples of individuals without chronic medical problems. However, despite the fact that depression is very common, there is evidence that rheumatologists seldom query patients about their mood during routine office visits. A recent study by Sleath and coworkers,[11] in which more than 200 doctor-patient interactions were audiotaped in several clinics in North Carolina, found that depression was addressed in only 11% of clinical transactions and that in all cases, patients presented their mood problems to their physicians. Physicians did not initiate discussions about depression with patients in any of the interactions. Unfortunately, the reasons for this surprising finding were not examined in this study, and we do not know how typical this problem is across rheumatology practices in other regions. Nevertheless, it is clear that if depression is not explicitly addressed during rheumatology visits, it will not be effectively managed. Unmanaged depression, in turn, may compromise the efficacy of biomedical treatment, cause significance distress, and interfere with patients' quality of life. Health services research that focuses on the variables that either facilitate or inhibit the detection of depression in rheumatology practice is both warranted and critical.[12]

A plethora of research evidence conducted over the past 25 years has substantiated the important contribution of a variety of psychosocial factors to health outcomes in such conditions as rheumatoid arthritis, fibromyalgia, and systemic lupus erythematosus. The breadth of this work is beyond the scope of this chapter and has been carefully reviewed elsewhere.[2,13-15] Illness beliefs such as helplessness (e.g., lacking control over the illness) and catastrophizing (e.g., thinking that the worst will happen), pain coping strategies (passive and active coping), stress, and social support have all been shown to directly affect outcomes such as pain, mood, and disability independently of disease activity and provision of standard medical care. In some instances,

Table 29-1. *Major Psychosocial Processes and Health Outcomes in Arthritis*

Variable	Outcomes Affected
Illness beliefs (e.g., helplessness, catastrophizing)	Mediator of effects of pain depression, anxiety, coping
Coping	
Pain coping	Pain, depression, disability
Resilient coping	Positive mood, less pain
Social support	Enhanced mood, adaptive coping
Stress	Worsens pain, disease activity
Mood disturbance	Worsens pain, disability, significant disease activity

these variables also may serve as mediators of the relationship between biomedical factors and clinical outcomes. Helplessness, for example, has been shown to mediate the effects of arthritis pain on mood.[16] In other instances, these factors may serve as moderators of the effects of disease activity either by dampening or exacerbating its effects. For example, pain coping strategies and social support may buffer the effects of pain or stress on health outcomes such as depression and disability. When pain or stress is high, effective coping or adequate social support may protect the patient. Table 29-1 presents an outline of these factors and their importance and relevance to rheumatology care.

These variables illustrate the importance of adopting the biopsychosocial model in evaluating the adjustment of arthritis patients. These variables affect outcomes in a similar manner across many arthritic diseases and account for a significant amount of variability in such clinical outcomes as pain, disability, mood, and quality of life. Moreover, their effects are robust, clinically significant, and provide added rationale for the use of behavioral strategies. Their relevance to patient care in rheumatology practice deserves careful attention and ongoing assessment. Screening and evaluation procedures can be established in clinical settings to identify problems in psychosocial functioning that can yield major benefits to rheumatologists and patients alike by highlighting the need for complementary behavioral or psychological interventions. Behavioral medicine specialists and other members of the health care team can then intervene to provide ongoing care for psychological issues or disease management.

THE EVOLUTION OF BEHAVIORAL INTERVENTIONS FOR ARTHRITIS

The development of the interdisciplinary field of behavioral medicine in the late 1970s and early 1980s provided the foundation for researchers and clinical scientists to devise behavioral approaches to assist patients in managing the vicissitudes of chronic illness and promote enhanced quality of life. Many leaders in the field of behavioral medicine were clinical psychologists trained primarily in the rigors of behavior therapy and social learning theory, which formed the major groundwork for many contemporary approaches to chronic illness management. At around the same time, but independently of the field of behavioral medicine, psychoeducational programs began to emerge that fostered greater awareness in patients about the importance of self-management and how to work with the health care system in getting the most out of their medical care. The development of the Arthritis Self-Help Program (ASMP) by Kate Lorig and colleagues at Stanford University[17] played a crucial role in promoting this philosophy and contributing to the public health significance of a holistic, integrative approach to arthritis care. Research on the ASMP has substantiated its efficacy on central clinical outcomes such as pain, health care use, and adaptive health behaviors.[2]

The origins of behavioral interventions for arthritis can be traced to the growth of social learning theory and the development of effective behavioral strategies for managing depression, phobias, and other psychiatric disorders. A basic tenet of social learning approaches is that learning processes are fundamental to managing these disorders, including the control of difficult symptoms, the prevention of disability, and the enhancement of quality of life. Because many patients with arthritis have psychiatric comorbidities and problems of this nature, behavioral medicine specialists realized that many of the same models and strategies could apply to managing arthritis. The use of behavioral strategies for managing depression and anxiety, for example, seemed like an appropriate fit for patients with arthritis.

In addition to the broader evolution of social learning theory, specific developments in the treatment and management of patients with chronic pain contributed to the application of behavioral principles and strategies for arthritis. The opportunity for the environment to affect pain increases as patients adjust to the demands of having arthritis over time and develop strategies for managing pain and disability. Operant learning approaches have shown that reports of pain and behavioral limitations in chronic pain patients could be altered by contingencies of reinforcement and extinction. Reports of pain and disability, for example, may continue if attention from others or disability payments follow pain complaints or avoidance of work.[18] Furthermore, pain and disability may come under different contingencies, leading to circumstances in which patients may report little pain but still have considerable behavioral impairment. Despite effective biomedical treatment for arthritis pain, patients may encounter substantial pain-related problems if they receive reinforcement for maladaptive pain coping, poor functional outcomes, or occupying the sick role.

The advent of cognitive behavior therapy, shortly after the operant learning movement, showed that patients' attention and beliefs about their symptoms could affect emotional outcomes and behaviors. The cognitive behavior therapy approach provided a complementary intervention to operant techniques to managing chronic pain by emphasizing the importance of modifying attentional processes and beliefs that exacerbated reports of pain severity, depression, and anxiety. As research evidence on the role of helplessness and pain catastrophizing on adverse outcomes in arthritis patients mounted, the salience of cognitive behavior therapy strategies for managing arthritis pain correspondingly increased. Cognitive behavior therapy techniques such as distraction, imagery, and cognitive restructuring for dysfunctional beliefs were developed and subsequently applied for managing arthritis pain in randomized clinical trials. A substantial body of evidence has accumulated over the last 20 years, documenting the efficacy and role of such techniques in arthritis care.

CONCEPTUALIZING THE ROLE OF BEHAVIORAL INTERVENTIONS IN ARTHRITIS

Figure 29-1 illustrates three different ways of conceptualizing the importance of behavioral interventions in chronic illness and arthritis care. In the first scenario, having a chronic illness creates risk for psychological distress and potential problems with depression, anxiety, and diminished quality of life. The burdens of arthritis, including pain and disability, may lead to psychological distress, adding to the complexity of patient management. The role of behavioral interventions is to reduce disease-related burdens, enhance quality of life, and contribute to greater psychological well-being in patients. The second scenario illustrates the potential role of psychological factors in influencing the disease course in arthritis. For example, depression may interfere with medical compliance and increase inflammation that, in turn, may lead to poor disease control and a worsening in symptoms such as pain and swelling. Behavioral interventions in this framework may be implemented to reduce depression in order to prevent or abate disease progression. The third scenario, a combination of the other two, illustrates a cyclical, recursive process that is typical of chronic illnesses such as arthritis. In this framework, chronic illness leads to psychological dysfunction, which then can aggravate the underlying disease. Behavioral interventions have a dual function in this scenario–to mitigate disease-related burdens on psychological functioning, and to enhance psychological functioning as a means of promoting better disease control and optimal health status.

The first scenario has dominated the major focus of clinical trials that have evaluated behavioral interventions for arthritis in that they have been principally designed to reduce the adverse effects of pain and enhance psychosocial functioning in patients. The role of behavioral interventions has been to complement state-of-the-art medical care aimed at controlling inflammation and disease progression. Importantly, this is a high clinical standard for behavioral interventions, as they must demonstrate an additive effect by contributing to efficacy over and above the role of powerful disease-modifying pharmacologic agents. Whether behavioral interventions can affect disease activity in the second scenario is an especially intriguing concept that reflects their potential in reducing inflammation via the hypothalamic pituitary pathway that communicates with the immune system.[19]

Figure 29-2 illustrates a dominant paradigm for understanding psychosocial adjustment to arthritis and the role of behavioral interventions. The horizontal pathway describes elements of the coping process, starting with disease activity, which leads to symptoms and other illness-related stressors. As a result of experiencing symptoms, patients develop beliefs (appraisals) about their severity and controllability. The beliefs, in turn, affect the choice of coping responses to manage the symptoms. Coping responses, depending on their efficacy, can lead to changes in health status such as increases or decreases in pain, depression, disability, or health-related quality of life. The coping process is dynamic and recursive, subject to change in all of its individual elements, and modifiable by the patient. For example, improvement in pain may lead to more adaptive appraisals that reinforce effective coping responses and maintain positive health outcomes. Importantly, the model takes into account environmental factors

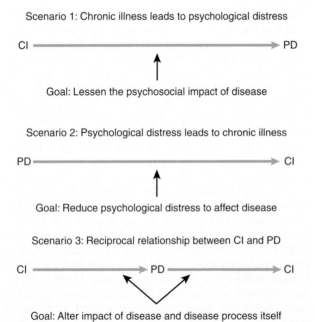

Figure 29-1. A conceptual foundation for the role of behavioral interventions for chronic illness.

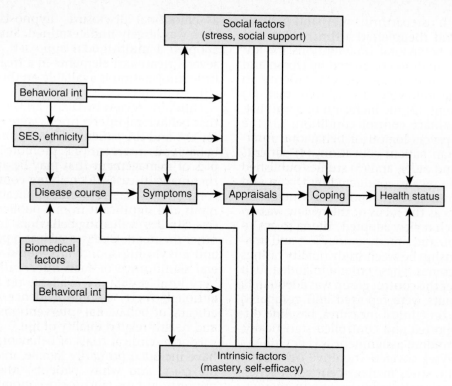

Figure 29-2. General model underlying behavioral approaches for arthritis and chronic illness.

and individual difference variables that can potentially affect the coping process and outcomes in health status directly.

Behavioral interventions in Figure 29-2 can promote improvement in health status in three major ways. First, they can affect the coping process directly by teaching patients, for example, how to restructure faulty thinking about symptoms or to reduce pain. Second, they can alter environmental factors (e.g., stress) that are having a deleterious effect on the coping process or health outcomes directly. Strategies may be used to enhance social support or attenuate the impact of situational (e.g., interpersonal, work) stressors. Third, interventions may be directed at personality characteristics of patients such as dependency or low self-esteem that affect illness appraisals and/or choice of coping responses. It is important to note that behavioral interventions in the model are not aimed directly at reducing disease activity but are focused instead on the cognitive, emotional, and behavioral sequelae of the disease. In contrast, biomedical interventions focus on the amelioration of disease activity but do not address elements of the coping process. Thus, behavioral and biomedical interventions function in a complementary manner and collectively promote an interdisciplinary, behavioral medicine approach to chronic illness management. Psychologists, allied health professionals, and physicians all have their respective roles in this process. As arthritis professionals and colleagues, they all share in the responsibility for helping patients manage the disease process comprehensively and effectively.

THE EFFICACY OF BEHAVIORAL INTERVENTIONS

On both theoretical and empirical grounds, the development of behavioral interventions for arthritis has been justified, and many studies have been conducted to evaluate their efficacy by numerous investigative teams across a wide range of locations. The establishment of efficacy in randomized clinical trials is an essential criterion for determining the potential clinical relevance and value of behavioral interventions to arthritis care. Evidence-based practice (EBP) relies on efficacy studies to guide treatment planning and clinical decision-making for individual cases.[20] However, an important distinction exists between *clinical efficacy* and *clinical effectiveness*. Although efficacy reflects the experimental impact of an intervention on a clinical outcome compared with a control condition to determine its statistical significance, effectiveness is concerned with the degree to which patients derive value from the intervention in helping them manage their arthritis on a daily basis. Patient reports and evaluations by the health care team are used to determine clinical effectiveness. Importantly, effectiveness is dependent on efficacy, but behavioral interventions can be efficacious without being effective. The most valuable interventions are those that possess both clinical efficacy and effectiveness.

Two meta-analytic reviews have been conducted to determine the clinical efficacy of behavioral interventions for arthritis. The first meta-analysis conducted by Astin and colleagues[21] excluded studies with patients with osteoarthritis (OA) and patients with both OA and rheumatoid arthritis (RA) and focused only on behavioral interventions for RA. The second meta-analysis conducted by Dixon and colleagues[22] covered both RA and OA patients. In both reviews, the following criteria were met: (1) random assignment, (2) the inclusion of a wait list, usual care, or contact control condition, (3) the evaluation of a psychological or behavioral intervention other than patient education, (4) patients 18 years of age and older, and (5) studies published in English. In the review conducted by Dixon and colleagues,[22] pain had to be reported as one of the clinical outcomes as the focus of the review was on arthritis pain. Each review adopted criteria to evaluate the quality of study methodology,[23-24] and analyzed the relationship between study quality ratings and clinical outcomes. These criteria included such factors as whether the control group was adequately described, dropouts were reported and compared with completers on clinical measures, baseline differences were reported and controlled statistically, and method of random assignment was described.

The meta-analyses covered cognitive behavioral strategies for pain, stress management approaches, biofeedback, emotional disclosure, group therapy, hypnosis, problem-solving therapy, and psychodynamic therapy. Many of the studies incorporated a multimodal approach, using more than one intervention modality. The most frequently used interventions were cognitive behavioral treatments for pain (n = 23) and stress management approaches (n = 5) whereas the other interventions received much less empirical attention. The efficacy findings, therefore, are heavily weighted to reflect the impact of these interventions. In contrast, the reviews are rather inconclusive regarding the efficacy of such approaches as biofeedback, group therapy, or emotional disclosure.

Both reviews provided consistent evidence for the efficacy of behavioral interventions for arthritis patients, illustrating their potential as complementary treatments. Several important conclusions can be drawn from these reviews that have relevance for future research and clinical practice. First, both Astin and colleagues[21] and Dixon and colleagues[22] found that behavioral interventions were superior to a variety of control conditions on clinical outcomes. Therefore, the behavioral interventions proved to be active treatments, whose effects were not accounted for by attention, group support, expectation for improvement, or simply providing education to patients. The data thus confirmed the efficacy of behavioral interventions as unique, independent treatments.

Second, neither review found a difference in efficacy between specific types of interventions. However, because the preponderance of clinical trials evaluated cognitive behavioral interventions for pain, the comparison between interventions was not meaningful. The clinical value, though, of behavioral treatments for pain was confirmed. The general significance of interventions such

as emotional disclosure, hypnosis, and biofeedback was largely undetermined. Since most studies adopted a multi-modal approach, that combined several treatment elements in a treatment package, little information is available on the efficacy of specific strategies.

Third, the review by Dixon and colleagues[22] found that behavioral interventions were equally effective for OA and RA patients. This finding suggests that behavioral interventions promote general principles of management that may be applicable across rheumatic diseases. Identifying common treatment components that have wide applicability is parsimonious and significant from a public health perspective. Studies evaluating behavioral interventions for other rheumatic diseases such as lupus, scleroderma, and ankylosing spondylitis would clarify the general significance of such intervention approaches. Very limited data are available on these disorders, although there is some evidence confirming the efficacy of behavioral interventions for lupus pain and health-related quality of life.[25]

Fourth, clinical trials of behavioral interventions have included primarily female, middle-aged, middle class, and white patients. Men, members of minority groups, and socioeconomically disadvantaged patients have been grossly underrepresented. The exclusion of these samples could reflect a number of factors, including limited access to care in these populations, recruitment obstacles, lack of outreach strategies into community settings, or lack of initiative on the part of investigators. Thus, little information is available for the efficacy of behavioral interventions for these patients.

Fifth, the studies have varied significantly in methodologic quality, although more recent trials have had higher methodological quality than those conducted earlier. Interestingly, the reviews found that methodological quality was not related to clinical outcomes, suggesting that the findings on efficacy were robust across methodologic limitations and differences, such as sample size, recruitment procedures, randomization, types of outcome measures, and types of controls. Nevertheless, methodological quality is important in determining the internal validity of a trial (e.g., the scientific certainty of being able to attribute differences between groups to experimental interventions) and, therefore, is a highly important criterion in evaluating the merits of individual studies.

Finally, the efficacy of behavioral interventions differed substantially across clinical outcomes. Studies also varied according to the clinical outcomes that were assessed. Pain was a primary outcome in most studies, although secondary outcomes such as functional disability, coping, depression, and anxiety were commonly included. A rather small number of studies incorporated objective measures of disease activity and biological functioning. The outcomes, to a large extent, reflect the clinical objectives of the behavioral interventions and are thus skewed toward functional criteria and away from disease processes. We have scant data on whether behavioral interventions affect disease activity. This remains a question for future researchers to address.

Behavioral interventions have had the most pronounced effect on adaptive coping, with effect sizes in the moderate to large range (.52 to .72). This finding is especially important because coping is a primary target of behavioral interventions and is evidence of treatment validity. Although various measures of coping have been used in clinical trials, behavioral interventions have maximized active coping, which promotes attempts at pain control rather than avoidance and dependent behaviors. Active coping is also postulated as a mechanism through which other clinical outcomes such as pain and disability improve (see Fig. 29-2).

As anticipated, behavioral interventions have led to significant improvements in pain, with modest effect sizes (.18 to .27). The effects on physical disability have been of similar magnitude (.15 to .27). Importantly, these effects have persisted across follow-up, indicating that patients have acquired and implemented effective self-management strategies that may have enduring clinical benefits. Dixon and colleagues[22] pointed out that several studies have not used measures that are specific to arthritis pain and disability and, therefore, may have lacked sensitivity to change and caused treatment effects to be underestimated. Nevertheless, it is important to note that arthritis pain and disability can be refractory to improvement despite the most aggressive biomedical treatments. Even modest improvements can be highly valuable to patients who have been frustrated with other approaches and realize gains within relatively brief treatment periods, lasting on average, 8.5 sessions.[22]

Although the vast majority of behavioral interventions have focused primarily on enhancing pain management, the reviews provided evidence that psychological outcomes also improved. The two most frequently assessed outcomes were depression and anxiety. Astin and associates[21] and Dixon and coworkers[22] reported effect sizes of .15 and .21, respectively, for depression. Dixon and coworkers[22] found an effect size of .28 for anxiety. The reviews found evidence for maintenance of improvement on psychological outcomes through follow-up. As pointed out earlier, depression is commonly ignored in rheumatology practice, and it is encouraging that improvement is obtainable even when behavioral interventions are not explicitly addressing this outcome. Future interventions that directly target mood disturbance in arthritis may yield even more favorable results.

Since relatively few clinical trials have incorporated objective measures of disease activity or biologic markers, little information exists regarding the efficacy of behavioral interventions on these outcomes. Despite some evidence that behavioral interventions may lead to improvement in joint swelling,[26] whether behavioral interventions can alter the production of proinflammatory cytokines and quiet the immune system is unknown at this juncture. This issue remains a subject of speculation and significant theoretical interest on the part of behavioral medicine investigators and rheumatologists alike. Although most researchers would agree that the major purpose of behavioral interventions is to enhance the psychosocial adjustment of patients, for many scientists and arthritis professionals, the potential of behavioral interventions to affect disease is seen as hard evidence of their validity and clinical significance and is of equal or greater value. The counterargument to this view is that it is more important for behavioral interventions to improve symptoms and psychosocial functioning rather than biologic outcomes because the former outcomes are more central to quality of life and drive health care use. Moreover, it can be argued that the advent of increasingly effective disease-modifying medications decreases the relevance of whether behavioral interventions can affect disease as well. Compared with pharmacologic approaches, behavioral interventions may not be efficient or cost effective for this purpose.

Nevertheless, despite some ongoing debate about the importance of behavioral interventions illustrated by the question above, it is clear that behavioral interventions constitute an effective complement to standard, best practices of medical care for patients with arthritis. However, several unaddressed issues remain regarding their efficacy and, importantly, their relevance to patient care. A significant concern is whether behavioral interventions are being incorporated into practice settings and are making a difference in arthritis care. A related concern is how to maximize their use and public health significance. The next section of the chapter highlights some major scientific questions as well as future issues for clinicians who have responsibility for managing arthritis patients, including the use of behavioral interventions in their medical team.

WHY ARE BEHAVIORAL INTERVENTIONS EFFECTIVE? HOW DO THEY WORK?

After determining that behavioral interventions can reliably produce effective results, clinical researchers face the challenge of identifying and understanding the mechanisms of action responsible for their efficacy. Thus far, no clear picture of mediational mechanisms has emerged, leaving a significant void in the clinical trials literature. This is a very important question for the following reasons. First, identifying factors responsible for the effects of treatment promotes a clearer theoretical understanding of the nature of behavioral interventions and, therefore, their proper role in arthritis management. Second, knowledge of mechanisms sheds light on the central factors affecting disease outcomes and, thus, on the etiology of the conditions themselves. Finally, once mechanisms are identified, other treatment approaches could be considered that target mechanisms directly, leading to a more rational and parsimonious treatment focus in the delivery of care.

To identify a treatment mechanism, the following conditions must be met: (1) the treatment must affect the outcome; (2) the mechanism must affect the outcome; (3) the treatment must affect the mechanism, and (4) the mechanism must significantly diminish the effects of treatment on the outcome and, in essence, account for the effects of treatment on the outcome.[27] A limitation of the randomized controlled trials literature for behavioral interventions is that investigators have not specified a model describing the mediational pathways that contribute to treatment efficacy. In the absence of a model, statistical analyses have not been sufficient to identify treatment mechanisms.

Currently, we can only speculate on the factors responsible for the efficacy of behavioral interventions. Table 29-2 lists some potential mechanisms that account for the clinical improvements in pain and disability. Based on the outcome literature, it is more plausible that enhanced coping and improvement in mood may serve as mediators than other factors for the following reasons. The meta-analyses demonstrated effects on these factors, and an abundant literature exists on the importance of these factors in pain and functional outcomes. Because treatment effects on coping have been of the highest magnitude, the potential role of coping as a mediator of treatment should be strongly considered. Theoretically, adaptive coping could influence other outcomes as well such as changes in disease activity, quality of life, and mood. In contrast, because evidence is lacking on the effects of behavioral interventions on improvements in inflammation, health behaviors, sleep, and social support, it is premature to consider these factors as mediators. Future research is needed to determine whether these factors are responsive to change from behavioral interventions before their role as mediators can be evaluated.

Table 29-2. Potential Mechanisms of Action for Behavioral Interventions*

Potential Mediators
Enhanced coping
Improvement in mood
Enhanced sleep quality
Reduced inflammation
Improvement in social support
Improvement in health behaviors (e.g., exercise, diet)
Perceived control of illness
Reduced stress

*Effects of behavioral interventions on health outcomes are *downstream*, or mediated by other psychological, social, and biologic factors.

EXPLORING OTHER TREATMENT APPROACHES

The growth of complementary and alternative medicine has increased public awareness of the value of techniques such as Tai Chi Chih, pilates, and yoga in regulating stress and increasing emotional and physical well-being. Investigators have noted that these methods may contribute to managing arthritis pain, increasing muscle strength, and enhancing endurance.[28,29] However, scientific evidence on complementary alternative medicine (CAM) treatments for arthritis is lacking at present, and it is premature to recommend their use as empirically verified behavioral management strategies. Randomized controlled trials are needed to establish their efficacy for arthritis and whether there are unique advantages to such treatments compared with conventional cognitive behavior therapy and stress management approaches. Owing to their popularity and frequency of use, clinical scientists should take advantage of opportunities to explore the public health significance of CAM treatments to determine their potential role in arthritis care.

A newer form of behavioral treatment, acceptance and commitment therapy (ACT), has stimulated significant interest in the treatment of a variety of disorders, including alcohol addiction, depression, anxiety, and chronic pain.[30] ACT espouses the importance of awareness, acceptance, and committed action as core principles underlying clinical change. It integrates principles of mindfulness and cognitive behavior therapy. Although ACT has not been evaluated in the treatment of arthritis, it could be potentially useful in helping patients accept difficult symptoms and losses associated with their condition and in promoting meaningful, goal-directed activity. Its role in the behavioral medicine treatment arsenal is growing and may prove to be an important intervention for persons with chronic illness.

DISSEMINATION OF BEHAVIORAL INTERVENTIONS

More than two decades of research have shown that behavioral interventions can improve health outcomes for patients with arthritis. An empirical foundation has been established for translating this research into clinical practice settings. Clinical scientists and arthritis health professionals now face the challenge of incorporating behavioral interventions into clinical care and should consider alternate models of service delivery[31] that incorporate effective dissemination practices. Behavioral interventions that have proven efficacy can significantly increase patients' disease management skills and have the potential to contribute to the welfare of thousands of arthritis patients if health care teams have the capacity to implement them at clinic sites. Presently, it is unclear if interventions such as cognitive behavioral treatment for pain, stress management, and strategies to manage mood are making an appreciable difference in arthritis care. Health services researchers have not embraced this issue, contributing to an absence of knowledge regarding how arthritis professionals manage the psychological and behavioral problems of their patients in rheumatology practice settings.

The challenge of integrating empirically supported behavioral interventions into clinical settings is not unique to arthritis care. The gap between research and practice has been an ongoing problem in many areas of health care including medicine, public health, and psychology for decades and has been the focus of study by behavioral scientists that have championed the translational research cause.[32] Several factors associated with the interventions themselves, the clinical setting, the cost of implementing them, and the types of patient populations served can significantly influence the delivery of effective treatments. Owing to the significance and complexity of this problem, it is beyond the scope of this chapter to analyze the factors that either inhibit or facilitate the adoption of behavioral interventions. However, the importance of addressing this problem cannot be stressed enough.

As a starting point, it is important to consider the type of model of care that provides an appropriate conceptual framework for the delivery of behavioral interventions in arthritis clinics and other medical settings. Exclusive reliance on the biomedical model is insufficient for understanding the multiplicity of variables that affect arthritis health outcomes. In contrast, the biopsychosocial approach[1] espouses a holistic, integrative, and interdisciplinary approach to care that is fundamental to applied behavioral medicine practice. The adoption of this framework affects many practical features of rendering care, including diagnostic practices, the management of psychiatric disorders, the choice of treatments, and the kinds of personnel hired to work with patients.

Importantly, health care providers must appreciate the difference between realizing the theoretical or empirical value of a model and making a commitment to putting into practice. A salient question to consider is whether rheumatology embraces this model of care and is willing to support its implementation. It is important for all members of the health care team to promote this model and to understand how to apply it in their clinical decision making and communication with patients. With appropriate education and guidance, the patients themselves will adopt this framework in the development of skills to manage their arthritis and enhance their quality of life. They will understand how psychosocial factors affect their adjustment to arthritis and the importance of behavioral interventions as a complement to best practices medical care. Ideally, there should be congruence between arthritis professionals and patients in their comprehension of the model of care that underlies the delivery of clinical services. A shared understanding will facilitate communication, adherence, and how to address difficult clinical questions. Discordance, on the other hand, can be disruptive to clinical care by creating confusion about the importance of different procedures and the role of patients in managing their medical condition.

WHAT PATIENTS STAND TO BENEFIT FROM BEHAVIORAL INTERVENTIONS?

Although clinical trials have established the general efficacy of behavioral interventions for patients with arthritis, specific guidelines or algorithms for implementing behavioral interventions for individual cases presently do not exist. However, the absence of guidelines should not deter the health care team from using behavioral interventions in rendering service to patients. A range of patient populations may benefit from behavioral interventions. Patients with intractable pain and impaired functioning are primary candidates because behavioral interventions have been chiefly designed to help patients with these problems. In addition, behavioral interventions are appropriate for patients with depression or anxiety, or for those who feel stressed as a result of their medical condition or who have a history of mood disturbance that interferes with adherence to medical treatment or management of pain. Biomedical treatment alone will not be effective for these patients. The type and intensity of care will vary, of course, depending on patients' clinical needs and history. For example, patients with severe pain should receive treatment to help them develop skills to cope with their pain more effectively, whereas other patients who suffer from depression will require specific strategies to enhance mood. Some patients could need assistance in both areas.

The argument can be made, however, that all patients with arthritis should receive some education about the coping process, quality-of-life issues, and knowledge about effective management practices. The disease course in most forms of arthritis is punctuated by episodic increases in symptoms, and even patients who function well most of the time will experience flare-ups that are taxing and interfere with quality of life. Basic skills in the management of pain, stress, and mood could protect patients in such instances and enhance their self-efficacy in managing their medical condition in the future. In this regard, behavioral interventions, if rendered early in the disease process, could help in the prevention of functional declines that afflict the majority of patients over time.[33] This public health approach to management could potentially lead to reductions in morbidity and rising health care costs that have been endemic to arthritis care for several decades.

THE CHALLENGE OF DELIVERING BEHAVIORAL INTERVENTIONS TO UNDERSERVED GROUPS

Black, Asian, Native-American, and Hispanic patients tend to have high rates of conditions such as RA, OA, and lupus, and at the same time, encounter many barriers in gaining access to effective arthritis medical care. This troubling paradox represents a national problem in health care disparities that has grown in severity over the past decade. Socioeconomic deprivation, lack of insurance, geographic barriers, and transportation problems frequently prevent such patients from getting the care that they need. A recent review by McIlvane and colleagues[34] found that clinical trials evaluating behavioral interventions reported sparse data on the recruitment of minority patients, their attrition rates, and their response to treatment. Although there are notable exceptions to this trend,[35,36] investigators have not systemically addressed the challenge of recruiting and retaining minority patients into their clinical trials. This neglect has resulted in a lack of scientific evidence on the efficacy of behavioral interventions for minority patients with arthritis and on how to tailor such treatments in a culturally sensitive manner.

Scientists and arthritis professionals need to be more conscious of the nature and importance of this problem and to work together on an agenda for addressing it. Together, they may consider a number of approaches, including (1) establishing partnerships with professionals and local organizations serving minority individuals, (2) conducting needs assessments with prospective minority research participants to identify adherence issues and clarify the nature of the research process, (3) hiring minority research staff who can identify and help manage the concerns of these patients, and (4) gaining consultation from sociologists and medical anthropologists on methods of conducting research with underserved groups. Collectively, these efforts could lead to different research strategies and creative techniques for delivering behavioral interventions to ethnically and culturally diverse patient groups. Other medical disciplines facing similar challenges may benefit from these efforts as well.

THE IMPORTANCE OF SYSTEMS LEVEL CHANGE

In addition to reducing disease activity, major goals of arthritis care are to control difficult symptoms, enhance quality of life, and prevent psychological distress in vulnerable patients. Behavioral interventions can be very helpful to patients in addressing these goals and have earned a place in arthritis care. However, best practices medical approaches do not as yet incorporate behavioral interventions. As a result, patients may not be receiving the help that

they need to cope with pain and the related illness burdens associated with arthritis.

The health care system should facilitate, rather than inhibit, the use of effective behavioral interventions, increasing their availability to patients in rheumatology practice settings. Barriers (e.g., time, financial) that interfere with, or prevent, psychosocial treatment should be identified and managed with the goal of minimizing their impact. Importantly, clinics should have the capacity to implement behavioral interventions. Professional personnel in the clinic should be available to help patients develop behavioral skills to manage their arthritis. With appropriate training, rheumatology nurses, for example, have the potential to make a significant contribution in rendering behavioral strategies. In addition, rheumatologists may integrate behavioral medicine specialists into clinic operations to develop behavioral management services, render behavioral treatments, and train other personnel. This interdisciplinary model of service delivery for behavioral medicine is efficient and far superior to one in which patients are referred to specialists outside the rheumatology clinic. Integrated care is more difficult in such circumstances, and patients may resist seeing a mental health provider removed from their medical care.

Above all, rheumatologists must see the opportunities that emerge from their partnership and collaboration with behavioral medicine professionals and allied health personnel in the effort to provide comprehensive psychosocial care to patients (Fig. 29-3). The same productive interdisciplinary alliance that facilitated more than two decades of behavioral research in arthritis could also pave the way for significant advances in the clinic setting.

The synergy from this alliance will provide the groundwork for enhanced models of care and creative treatment approaches that will lead to improvement in the quality of life of arthritis patients. The time has arrived for this form of innovation in service delivery. Although there is ample scientific evidence that such change is both justified and necessary, significant leadership from rheumatologists and public health advocacy will be required to ensure that behavioral interventions and related psychosocial treatments are integrated into the clinic and rendered to the arthritis population.

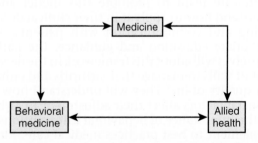

Figure 29-3. Interdisciplinary alliance in arthritis care and research.

References

1. Engel G. The clinical application of the biopsychosocial model. Am J Psychiatry 1980;137:535-44.
2. Nicassio PM, Greenberg MA. The effectiveness of cognitive-behavioral and psychoeducational interventions in the management of arthritis. In: Weisman MH, Weinblatt ME, Louie JS, editors. Treatment of the Rheumatic Diseases. 2nd ed. Philadelphia: W.B. Saunders; 2001. p. 147-61.
3. Fries J, Spitz P, Kraines R, Holman H. Measurement of patient outcome in arthritis. Arthritis Rheum 1980;23:137-45.
4. McElhone K, Abbot J, Shelmerdine J, Bruce I, Ahmad Y, Gordon C, et al. Development and validation of a disease-specific health-related quality of life measure, the lupusqol, for adults with systemic lupus erythematosus. Arthritis Care Res 2007;57:972-9.
5. Meehan R, Gertman P, Mason J. Measuring health status in arthritis: the Arthritis Impact Measurement Scales. Arthritis Rheum 1980;23:146-52.
6. Verbrugge L, Juarez L. Profile of arthritis disability. II. Arthritis Care Res 2006;55:102-13.
7. Yelin E, Murphy L, Cisternas M, Foreman A, Pasta D, Helmick C. Medical care expenditures and earnings losses among persons with arthritis and other rheumatic conditions in 2003, and comparisons with 1997. Arthritis Rheum 2007;56:1397-407.
8. Kvien T. Epidemiology and burden of illness of rheumatoid arthritis. Pharmaceoeconomics 2004;22(Suppl. 1):1-12.
9. Wells K, Golding J, Burnham M. Psychiatric disorders in a sample of the general medical population with and without medical disorders. Am J Psychiatry 1988;145:976-81.
10. Covic T, Tyson G, Spencer D, Howe G. Depression in rheumatoid arthritis patients: Demographic, clinical and psychological predictors. J Psychosom Res 2006;60:469-76.
11. Sleath B, Chewning B, deVellis BM, Weinberger M, deVellis RG, Tdor G, et al. Communication about depression during rheumatoid arthritis patient visits. Arthritis Care Res 2008;59:186-91.
12. Nicassio PM. The problem of detecting and managing depression in the rheumatology clinic. Arthritis Care Res 2008;59:155-8.
13. Goldengerg D, Burckhardt C, Crofford L. Management of fibromyalgia syndrome. JAMA 2004;292:2388-95.
14. Zautra A, Manne S. Coping with rheumatoid arthritis: A review of a decade of research. Ann Behav Med 1992;14:31-9.
15. Seawell A, Danoff-Burg S. Psychosocial research on systemic lupus erythematosus: a literature review. Lupus 2004;13:891-9.
16. Smith T, Peck J, Ward J. Helplessness and depression in rheumatoid arthritis. Health Psychology 1990;9:337-89.
17. Lorig K, Holman H. Arthritis self-management studies: A twelve-year review. Health Educ Q 1993;20:17-28.
18. Fordyce W. Pain and suffering. A reappraisal. Am Psychol 1988;43:276-83.
19. Tracey K. The inflammatory reflex. Nature 2002;420:853-9.
20. Kazdin A. Evidence-based treatment and practice: new opportunities to bridge clinical research and practice, enhance the knowledge base, and improve patient care. Am Psychol 2008;63:146-59.
21. Astin J, Beckner W, Soeken K, Hochberg M, Berman B. Psychological interventions for rheumatoid arthritis: a meta-analysis of randomized controlled trials. Arthritis Care Res 2002;47:291-302.
22. Dixon K, Keefe F, Scipio C, Perri L, Abernethy A. Psychological interventions for arthritis pain management in adults. A meta-analysis. Health Psychol 2007;26:241-50.
23. Abernethy A, Keefe F, McCrory D, Scipio C, Matchar D. Technology assessment on the use of behavioral therapies for treatment of medical disorders: Part 2 - Impact on management of patients with cancer pain (Report to the U.S. Agency for Healthcare Research and Quality). Durham, NC: Duke Center for Clinical Health Policy Research; 2005.
24. Jadad AR, Moore RH, Carroll D, Jenkinson C, Reynolds DJ, Gavaghan DJ, et al. Assessing the quality of reports of randomized clinical trials: Is blinding necessary? Control Clin Trials 1996;17:1-12.
25. Greco CM, Rudy TE, Manzi S. Effects of a stress-reduction program on psychological function, pain, and physical function of systemic lupus erythematosus patients: a randomized controlled trial. Arthritis Care Res 2004;51:625-34.
26. Radojevic V, Nicassio P, Weisman M. Behavior therapy with and without family support for rheumatoid arthritis. Behav Ther 1992;23:13-30.
27. MacKinnon D, Dwyer J. Estimating mediated effects in prevention studies. Evaluation Rev 1993;17:144-58.
28. Vitetta L. Alternative therapies for musculoskeletal conditions. Best Pract Res Clin Rheumatol 2008;22:499-522.
29. Zaman T, Agarwal S, Handa R. Complementary and alternative medicine use in rheumatoid arthritis: An audit of patients visiting a tertiary care centre. Natl Med J India 2007;20:236-9.
30. Powers M, Zum Vörde Sive Vörding M, Emmelkamp P. Acceptance and commitment therapy: A meta-analytic review. Psychother Psychosom 2009;78:73-80.
31. Dzewaltowski D, Glasgow R, Klesges L, Estabrooks P, Brock E. RE-AIM: Evidence-based standards and a Web resource to improve translation of research into practice. Ann Behav Med 2004;28:75-80.
32. Glasgow R, Emmons K. How can we increase translation of research into practice? Types of evidence needed. Annu Rev Public Health 2007;28:413-33.
33. Fries J, Spitz P, Kraines R, Holman H. Measurement of patient outcome in arthritis. Arthritis Rheum 1980;23:137-45.
34. McIlvane J, Baker T, Mingo C, Haley W. Are behavioral interventions for arthritis effective with minorities? Addressing racial and ethnic diversity in disability and rehabilitation. Arthritis Care Res 2008;59:1512-8.
35. Messier S, Loeser R, Miller G, Morgan T, Rejeski W, Sevick M, et al. Exercise and dietary weight loss in overweight and obese older adults with knee osteoarthritis: the Arthritis, Diet, and Activity Promotion Trial. Arthritis Rheum 2004;50:1501-10.
36. Lorig K, Ritter P, Laurent D, Fries J. Long term randomized controlled trials of tailored-print and small-group arthritis self-management interventions. Arthritis Rheum 2004;42:346-54.

Chapter 30

Physical Activity and Exercise in Rheumatic Disease

Christina H. Opava and Kaisa Mannerkorpi

CASE STUDY 1

Presentation

A 54-year-old woman who has had rheumatoid arthritis (RA) for almost 2 years presents at a regular medical check-up with her rheumatologist. She is married and employed as a nurse at a local hospital, but has not been able to work, other than for short periods, since the time of her diagnosis. Her height is 1.65 m, her body weight is 74 kg, and her blood pressure is 160/110 mm Hg. Medication with methotrexate, 20 mg/week, and oral corticosteroids, 5 mg/day controls inflammation well; a few finger joints are still swollen and her Disease Activity Score (DAS28) score is 3.2. Her Visual Analog Scale (VAS) rating of pain and global disease impact are 23 and 25, respectively, her Health Assessment Questionnaire (HAQ) score is 0.50. She reports severe fatigue as the reason for a mainly sedentary lifestyle and her inability to work. This worries her because the family economy has declined as a consequence of her work disability. Other concerns relate to her sedentary lifestyle and overeating, which has made her put on weight, and to her strong heredity for cardiovascular disease because she knows that her RA increases the risk of cardiovascular comorbidity.

Discussion

Further investigation into whether this patient is at risk for developing cardiovascular disease and diabetes type II is warranted because of her strong family history, high blood pressure, medication with corticosteroids and an unhealthy lifestyle.

Assessment by a physical therapist is also indicated in order to test body functions, to survey cognitive-behavioral factors related to lifestyle, and to prescribe an individualized physical activity program that may help reduce not only her fatigue but also the risk of future cardiovascular disease. Body function testing reveals that the patient has reduced grip strength, reduced lower limb function, and poor cardiovascular fitness compared with norm data. Joint motion, particularly that of hands and shoulders, is painful and their range of motion reduced. Metatarsophalangeal joints are tender. Previously the patient used to be physically active with hiking and biking, and she is ready to change her current sedentary lifestyle. Specific goals for changed physical activity behavior are thus discussed and set. The ultimate goal will be daily brisk walks, strength training twice a week, and range-of-motion (ROM) exercises for painful and stiff joints, when indicated. However, this goal will be approached in small steps that are written down and defined as to mode, time, place, frequency, duration, and intensity. Plans for progression as well as for relapse prevention are made. The importance of appropriate footwear, including insoles, is discussed. The patient will keep a physical activity log and regular visits, more frequent during the initial phase, are scheduled with the physical therapist in order to avoid relapse, check progress, and instruct in new exercises. The expected outcome of these interventions, based on evidence from randomized and longitudinal studies, is reduced fatigue and improved body functions, but also reduced risk for cardiovascular disease and diabetes.

CASE STUDY 2

Presentation

A 48-year-old woman with fluctuating pain for 3 years, without any signs of inflammation in joints or muscles, consults a rheumatologist for overall deterioration of functioning. Her pain, along with stiffness, has worsened during the past 5 months, with tangible consequences for employment, household, and leisure time. She describes difficulty in walking

longer than 15 minutes, climbing stairs, standing for a prolonged time, and carrying and lifting objects. She has discontinued all physical exercise and heavier household tasks, because physical activity aggravates her pain. She is a social worker, married, and has two children. During recent months, she has worked only 50% of her regular full-time schedule because of her disabilities. Her height is 1.74 m, her body weight 82 kg, and her blood pressure is 115/70 mm Hg. She rates her pain as 65 on a 100 VAS, whereas pain in the right hip, leg, and lower back from time to time increases to 80 on a VAS. She rates her fatigue as 60 and global disease impact as 65 on a VAS. Her current medication with nonsteroidal anti-inflammatory drugs (NSAIDs) does not alleviate pain. Clinical examination does not show any swollen joints, signs of bursitis, or neurologic origins for her pain, but does reveal a lowered pain threshold at palpation (allodynia) all over the body. Pain localization covers the definition of generalized pain according to the American College of Rheumatology (ACR) criteria for fibromyalgia (FM). A total of 16 positive tender points are found by specific examination of such points. Blood tests do not show any signs of inflammation.

Discussion

A diagnosis of FM is made. Pharmacologic therapy is initiated to alleviate generalized pain and fatigue. She is referred to a physical therapist for further investigation of impairments in the right hip, leg, and lower back and for a comprehensive assessment of body functions, as well as interventions to improve overall body function and to prevent further inactivity. A referral to a patient education program is also considered.

Assessment of the lower extremities and lower back by a physical therapist reveals muscular imbalance involving shortened muscles, reduced muscle strength, increased muscle tension, and pain at various muscles. The pain is aggravated by physical loading, especially in the right leg. The patient expresses being motivated to start exercising, but fears further deterioration of her functioning, because pain affects her working capacity. Short-term and long-term goals for exercise are discussed and set. At this initial phase, starting regular exercise is determined as the first priority, whereas the duration and intensity of exercise are secondary priorities. The patient receives instructions for a home exercise program to increase mobility, blood circulation, and muscle endurance of the lower extremities and the low back, limited to 40% to 50% of the maximal performance capacity, so as not to further increase the pain. The patient is also referred to a supervised exercise program in a temperate pool for a period of time in order to improve muscle function by stretching and strengthening exercises, combined with body awareness and relaxation. In parallel, daily walks, starting with a short duration and at low intensity, are planned and initiated. Information on the risks and benefits of exercise is given. Plans for management of activity-induced pain, modification of the exercises, and a long-term plan to escalate the exercise level in terms of mode, duration, intensity and frequency are discussed and set. The long-term goal is exercise at 60% to 70% of maximum capacity three times a week. Information on generalized pain and FM is given, and written information is forwarded. The patient will keep a physical activity log and regular visits, more frequent during the initial phase, are scheduled with the physical therapist in order to avoid relapse, and to modify and progress the exercise level. The expected outcome of the planned interventions, based on evidence from randomized and longitudinal studies, is improved walking capacity and overall health status including reduced pain. The increased amount of physical exercise is expected to reduce or postpone the risks for disorders associated with inactivity.

The interventions discussed in the present chapter are physical activity and exercise; the latter being a subset of the former (Fig. 30-1).[1] *Physical activity* includes all bodily movement that requires muscle work and results in increased energy expenditure compared to that in a resting position.[2] Thus, physical activity includes all the activities of daily life that are performed without any specific intention to improve functioning or health. *Health-enhancing physical activity* denotes a level of activities that prevents the development of lifestyle related disease.[3] *Exercise* is performed in a planned and structured way, with the aim to improve or maintain body functions.[2] In the rheumatic diseases exercise targets are mainly joint ROM, muscle function, and cardiovascular capacity, whereas adequate levels of physical activity target immediate general physical and psychological well-being and a long-term reduction of

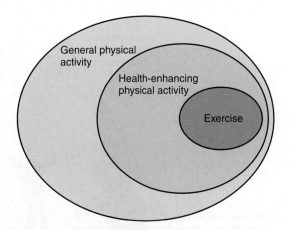

Figure 30-1. Graphical description of definitions of physical activity and related concepts. (Adapted from Hagströmer M. Assessment of health-enhancing physical activity at population level. Thesis for doctoral degree. Stockholm: Karolinska Institutet, 2007. *http://diss.kib. ki.se/2007/978-91-7357-334-4/.*)

risks for lifestyle-related diseases. Although planned and structured exercise interventions aiming at improved body functions have gradually become a self-evident intervention in the rheumatic diseases during the past decades, the importance of health-enhancing physical activity in daily life has received much less attention.

Health-Enhancing Physical Activity

A sedentary lifestyle is one of the most important independent predictors of poor general health and premature death, and it is well known that appropriate physical activity protects against cardiovascular disease as well as against poor health due to other physical and psychological conditions.[4,5] Despite this, it is estimated that approximately half the world's population is mainly sedentary or accumulates too little physical activity to preserve good health. People with rheumatic disease accumulate less physical activity than healthy individuals,[6] but their physical activity behavior does not seem to be determined by disease activity or degree of disability.[7] There are good reasons to believe that physical activity in rheumatic disease would help reduce not only the risk of additional health problems such as stress, anxiety, and depression, but also the risk of future comorbidity and premature death that is related to several of the inflammatory rheumatic diseases.

Public health recommendations include levels of physical activity to prevent poor health not only among the general public,[8] but also in different subpopulations.[9] Recommendations for healthy people aged older than 65 years and for those between 50 and 64 years with a chronic condition such as arthritis are shown in Figure 30-2. Thus, it is recommended that a basis for health-enhancing physical activity consists of either 30 minutes of moderately intense daily physical activity or 20 minutes of high-intensity exercise at least three times a week. This basis should be supplemented with strength training 2 to 3 times a week, and with ROM exercises and balance exercises whenever indicated. An exercise plan is also recommended.[9]

Physical activity intensity is classified as low (< 40% of Vo_2max), moderate (40% to 60% of Vo_2max) or high (> 60% of Vo_2max). In the absence of heart rate monitoring examples of typical activities, age-predicted maximum heart rate (220 – age), or rating of perceived exertion may be used to estimate physical activity intensity. Thus, a brisk walk that increases breathing and induces sweating, but still allows for conversation, corresponds to moderate intensity. A heart rate of 55% to 70% of age-predicted maximum, in a person with normal body weight, and ratings of perceived exertion about 12 to 13 on the Borg RPE scale[10] also indicate moderate intensity. Some caution as to the interpretation of perceived exercise load may be adequate because patients' understanding of this phenomenon may vary greatly.[11]

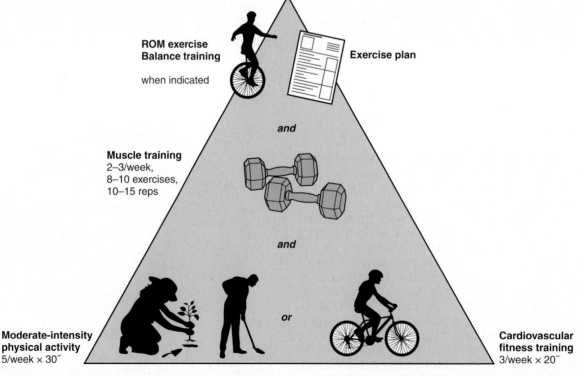

ROM exercise
Balance training

when indicated

Exercise plan

and

Muscle training
2–3/week,
8–10 exercises,
10–15 reps

and

or

Moderate-intensity
physical activity
5/week × 30″

Cardiovascular
fitness training
3/week × 20″

Figure 30-2. Illustration of current recommendations for health-enhancing physical activity for people older than 65 years of age or with chronic conditions such as arthritis. (From Nelson ME, Rejeski WJ, Blair SN, Duncan PW, Judge JO, King AC, et al. Physical activity and health in older adults: recommendations from the American College of Sports Medicine and the American Heart Association. Med Sci Sports Exerc 2007;39:1435-45.)

No scientific evidence has yet been found to support the idea that physical activity prevents comorbidity and premature death specifically among people with rheumatic disease. However, because public health recommendations include people with chronic disease, our present hypothesis should be that they, irrespective of age and disability status, should be recommended health-enhancing physical activity, adapted to their condition, in order to maintain good general health. One important piece of information for individuals who have difficulties to perform 30 minutes of physical activity at one time is that physical activity accumulated in 10-minute bouts during the day and adding up to at least 30 minutes may be equally beneficial for their health.[12]

Joint Range of Motion Exercise

Many rheumatic joint diseases result in reduced ROM in peripheral as well as in spinal joints. In the early course of the disease, stiffness and restricted movement are often related to joint pain, muscle spasm, and swelling. In patients with long-standing disease ROM is more likely to be restricted by soft tissue contractures or by destructions of cartilage and bone. Patients should be recommended to check ROM in affected joints regularly in order to detect signs of reduction and, during periods when ROM is threatened, be advised to perform regular exercise in order to preserve optimal joint function.

ROM exercise may be performed actively, with or without assistance, or passively. Active exercise should be preferred, but if the patient is in too much pain or is too weak or fatigued, it may be necessary to reduce body weight during exercise. Such reduction can be obtained by use of equipment, in water, or manually by a physical therapist. Sometimes passive mobilization of joint structures may be indicated in order to avoid manifest contractures. Such techniques are frequently used in exercises for patients with ankylosing spondylitis (AS) and similar conditions when body weight is used to passively stretch out structures that tend to contract. Specific manual passive mobilization of joints by a physical therapist may also be indicated occasionally.

Muscle Training

Reduced muscle function is common in all kinds of rheumatic diseases.[13,14] In some conditions, endurance is reduced to a greater extent than strength and may be caused by selective type II fiber atrophy. Other causes of reduced muscle function are pain, reflex inhibition, changes in muscle metabolism, reduced numbers of working fibers, poor biomechanical conditions due to damaged bone and cartilage, peripheral nerve injury, and physical inactivity. Patients with rheumatic disease should be recommended to perform muscle training and to continue physical activity in order to preserve or restore muscle function.[12]

Muscle training consists of different components directed toward improved strength, endurance, or balance and coordination. Exercise for strength and endurance may be static or dynamic. Static exercise implies muscle contraction without concomitant joint motion, whereas dynamic exercise is performed by muscle contraction during simultaneous joint motion. Strength training is performed with a relatively higher load and fewer repetitions compared with endurance training. Dynamic training may be performed with a constant load through the whole range of motion or through certain parts of it where increased strength is required. The load may also be isokinetic, which means that it is adjusted to fit the actual strength in different parts of the motion range. Furthermore, the dynamic training may be eccentric or concentric, which means that the muscles involved work during phases of lengthening or shortening respectively. For example, muscles that extend the knees work eccentrically while descending stairs but concentrically while ascending stairs. Balance and coordination exercises are either performed very specifically to increase voluntary muscle control or in situations that simulate daily activities to increase safety and avoid falls.

In sedentary individuals with weak muscles, the output of muscle training is often general, resulting in increased strength as well as improved endurance and coordination, although the training program does not include elements specifically targeting all of them. This might be due to neuromuscular adaption and recruitment of new motor units rather than increased muscle mass. However, the basic rule is that improvement of muscle function is specific, that is, it occurs in the area targeted by the training program, for example, strength or coordination. Thus, it is important that muscle training is preceded by thorough analysis in order to be as effective as possible. In rheumatic disease, additional factors related to risk of injury should be included in the analysis. There are no absolute contraindications toward muscle training in rheumatic diseases. However, a number of relative contraindications exists and should be considered in the prescription of exercise programs. They are related to degree of local inflammation and joint destruction, decreased solidity of bone and soft tissues following previous inflammation, long-term steroid intake and prolonged periods of physical inactivity.

Muscle training may be performed in a number of ways, and individual preferences should be considered when designing the program. It may include training with more or less advanced technical equipment in a clinic or in a public gym; be performed at home with simple devices such as rubber bands, weight cuffs, or resisted by body weight; or take place in a pool using water resistance. The recommended doses of muscle training given in Table 30-1 are based on those used in scientifically evaluated programs resulting in

Table 30-1. *Evidence-Based Recommendations for Muscle Training and Cardiovascular Fitness Training*

Target	Frequency (times/week)	Duration (minutes)	Intensity (% of max)	Load (% of 1 RM)
Increased strength	2–3	-	-	50–80
Increased endurance	2–3	-	-	30–40
Increased cardiovascular fitness	3	30–60	60–85	-

RM, repetition maximum.
From Stenström CH, Minor MA. Evidence for the benefit of aerobic and strengthening exercise in rheumatoid arthritis. Arthritis Rheum 2003;49:428-34.

benefits for patients with rheumatoid arthritis (RA).[15] Thus, the present evidence suggests that principles for dosage of muscle training to patients with RA do not differ much from general dosage principles. However, it is important to bear in mind that 1 repetition maximum (RM), that is, the weight that can be lifted only once, may be lower in an individual with rheumatic disease than in a healthy person and thus the actual training load may be considerably lower for the former. For optimal training results, 1 RM should be tested regularly during a training program and the load adjusted to a recent test value.

Cardiovascular Fitness Training

Cardiovascular fitness, that is, maximal oxygen uptake, may be reduced for several reasons in patients with rheumatic disease. Many try to reduce pain and fatigue by resting it away. This leads to a physically inactive lifestyle that eventually results in reduced fitness. Restricted thoracic movement and subsequently reduced lung volumes in patients with AS may cause poor cardiovascular fitness. The general systemic involvement in several rheumatic diseases may also confer poor function of oxygen-transporting organs. Moreover, exercises targeting cardiovascular fitness may also be helpful in reducing pain and improving function, and are therefore recommended as an intervention for people with rheumatic disease.[12]

The maximum oxygen uptake needs to be determined or estimated before appropriate cardiovascular fitness training can be prescribed. The most valid method for this is a maximum work capacity test. However, submaximal tests on ergometer bicycles or on treadmills are often preferred in clinical practice because they are more convenient.[16] Standardization of the tests is of utmost importance, and sources of error should be eliminated to the greatest extent possible. Thus, patients should be advised not to exercise, eat, or smoke within 1 hour before the test, it should not be performed in a busy environment, and no conversation should be allowed during testing. The exercise load needs to be heavy enough (heart rate >100–120 beats/minute) because psychological effects such as anxiety are then less likely to bias the outcome. On the other hand, loads that are too high demand high motivation and confer a risk of overload on affected joints and muscles. Thorough inquiry and, in case of suspected cardiovascular disease, consultation

with the patient's medical doctor, should precede the testing in order to exclude contraindications for this measurement.

Cardiovascular fitness training can be performed in many ways and may include elements of simultaneous ROM exercise and muscle training.[17] Scientific evidence exists for fitness training in the form of biking, brisk walking, aquaerobics, and different types of circuit training. Thus, exercise modes may vary depending on the patients' preferences, but with the goal in mind to improve cardiovascular fitness, accurate dosage is far more important than mode. The dosage guidelines presented in Table 30-1 are based on scientifically evaluated training programs resulting in positive effects on cardiovascular fitness in patients with RA[15] but do not differ substantially from those targeting the general public.

Rheumatic diseases per se do not represent any absolute contraindications to cardiovascular fitness training. However, it is important to remember that conditions representing relative contraindications, or requiring special attention in relation to fitness training may be more frequent in this population. Furthermore, a number of issues of certain importance to fitness training in rheumatic disease needs to be highlighted:

- The training program should be designed to spare potentially painful joints, bone, and soft tissue that may be less solid, and contracted or unstable joints;
- To avoid increased symptoms and subsequently reduced self-efficacy for exercise, the training should be increased gradually, that is, loads should initially be less, sometimes much less than those recommended to give beneficial fitness effects, and then gradually increased;
- It cannot be expected that training intensity will be consistently increased as in a healthy individual but must always be adjusted to variations in the disease course.

Physical Activity and Exercise in the Patient with Inflammatory Rheumatic Disease

Specific Indications for Exercise

Poor physical fitness has been found to predict mortality[18] and physical inactivity to predict poor general health perception[7] in patients with RA.

Thus, health-enhancing physical activity, as well as planned and structured exercise, is important to maintain or improve body functions, and to reduce the increased risk of comorbidity and the emotional distress caused by an unpredictable short- and long-term disease course. Although the introduction of new drugs has dramatically improved the health of people with rheumatic diseases during the past decade, a large proportion of patients may still have impaired body functions despite well-controlled inflammation.[19] However, the rheumatic diseases may also represent barriers, mental as well as physical, to physical activity and exercise among patients and health professionals.[20,21] Thus, rehabilitation measures may often be limited to those aimed at immediate symptom relief rather than considering them as a help to overcome barriers to a healthy lifestyle. A fear of aggravating symptoms by exercise possibly also still exists. Thus, although there is a strong argument for people with rheumatic disease to be physically active,[12,22] they have repeatedly been reported to have similar or lower activity levels compared with the general population.[6]

Evidence for Physical Activity and Exercise

It was concluded in a meta-analysis that dynamic exercise therapy of moderate intensity is effective at increasing cardiovascular fitness and muscle strength in patients with RA. However, effects on activity limitation and radiologic progression were unclear. No signs of detrimental effects on disease activity and pain were observed in the included studies.[23] It also seems that high-intensity training is safe and beneficial for most patients with RA. Thus, a training program applied twice a week for 75 minutes including cycling at 70% to 90% of maximum heart rate, circuit training, and sports resulted in beneficial effects on cardiovascular fitness, muscle strength, reduced activity limitation, and improved emotional status over the 2-year study period. No detrimental effect on disease activity was found, but a slightly increased radiologic progression among those with considerable baseline damage.[24]

Increasingly higher educational levels and greater access to information among the public, together with improved inflammation control among patients with inflammatory diseases, call for new forms of administering physical activity interventions. Thus, many patients can and should probably be able to accumulate health-enhancing physical activity in their daily life with support from a physical therapist. Two studies on such coaching interventions, including elements of cognitive-behavioral techniques, for patients with RA show promising results.[25,26] In both studies, a few clinical physical therapy sessions were supplemented with individualized coaching over the Internet and telephone, respectively. Beneficial outcomes related to physical activity behavior, general health perception, and body functions were reported. It seems that the attitude of the physical therapist toward exercise-induced pain in RA plays a role in the outcome, and that a focus on exercise goals rather than on exercise-induced pain is more beneficial.[27]

A meta-analysis of exercise studies including patients with AS drew several conclusions. Thus, individual home-based or supervised exercise programs are better than no intervention, that supervised group physiotherapy is better than home exercises, and that combined inpatient spa-exercise therapy, followed by group physiotherapy is better than group physiotherapy alone.[28] It also seems that patients with SLE and Sjögren's syndrome can take advantage of exercise. However, the evidence for this is limited, because few studies have so far been carried out, and more research is needed.[29-31] Increased muscle strength and endurance as well as reduced activity limitation among patients with poly- and dermatomyositis have been reported.[32,33]

Possible Risks

A fear that physical activity and exercise may aggravate the short-term and long-term disease course of the rheumatic diseases still exists. However, so far, in studies with carefully selected patients and exercise programs designed in accordance with the above-mentioned guidelines, no signs of increased local or systemic inflammatory activity have been reported.[23] This also seems to be valid for patients with active inflammation and severe disability.[34,35] Only a few exercise studies have included radiologic assessment. One study on high-intensity exercise in patients with RA reported increased joint destruction after 2 years for a subgroup of patients. The subgroup consisted of those patients, who already initially had severe joint destruction of large joints.[24] However, negative side effects of high-intensity as well as other exercise could probably be avoided if the guidelines given above for the prescription of muscle training and cardiovascular fitness training are followed.

There is a more obvious risk of exercise complications in various organ systems among patients with systemic rheumatic diseases. So far there are only a few studies, many to be considered as pilot studies that report exercise outcomes in patients with, for example, systemic lupus erythematosus (SLE) and polymyositis or dermatomyositis. Strength training in patients with myositis does not seem to confer negative side effects in either the acute nor in chronic phases.[32] Exercise also seems to be safe for patients with SLE. However, it is important to bear in mind that study participants with systemic diseases have been carefully selected in order to avoid negative side effects and, thus, study results can only be generalized to certain subgroups of patients with similar characteristics.

Secondary fibromyalgia in patients with inflammatory rheumatic diseases require specific attention, as described later.

Exercise and Inflammation

In a comprehensive review of randomized controlled trials of exercise in RA, it was noted that six out of the 14 included studies reported signs of reduced inflammation, assessed by swollen joint count, erythrocyte sedimentation rate (ESR), or C-reactive protein (CRP).[15] Similar observations have been reported in exercise studies including patients with polymyositis and dermatomyositis. Although the primary target of physical activity and exercise is not to reduce inflammation, some interesting hypotheses for such effects may be formulated based on results from basic and clinical studies involving healthy subjects as well as patients with chronic disease, including those with rheumatic conditions.[36] Accumulating evidence in these studies suggests that exercise might have beneficial effects on certain molecular processes in skeletal muscle and cartilage, as well as in reducing both local muscle inflammation and systemic inflammation (Fig. 30-3).

Physical Activity and Exercise in the Patient with Fibromyalgia Syndrome and Related Conditions

Specific Indications for Physical Activity and Exercise

Patients with FM commonly report activity limitations in daily life, such as carrying objects and working with the arms in elevated positions,[37] and in walking, prolonged sitting, and standing.[38] Activity-induced pain, together with worries and lack of knowledge about reasons for pain, often leads to physical inactivity and reduced

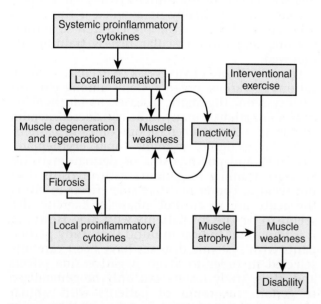

Figure 30-3. From inflammation to disability: a vicious circle. (From Lundberg IE, Nader GA. Molecular effects of exercise in patients with inflammatory rheumatic diseases. Nat Clin Pract Rheumatol 2008;4:597-604.)

overall fitness.[39] In contrast, some patients with FM appear to manage their symptoms by developing constructive strategies that help them to cope with everyday problems.[40] One such strategy is regular exercise, strengthening not only their physical function but also their image of themselves as healthy individuals.[41]

Patients with FM display reduced upper and lower extremity physical performance capacity compared with age- and sex-matched healthy controls.[42,43] Voluntary muscle strength and endurance are usually reduced,[44,45] although some studies have not documented any differences in muscle strength between patients with FM and healthy individuals.[46] Similarly, some studies reported decreased cardiovascular fitness in FM, whereas others have not found any differences between the patients studied and a sedentary reference group.[42,47] Such conflicting results are probably due to varying levels of impairment among patients with FM. Moreover, in patients with FM, objective measurements of body functions by walking capacity, grip strength, and other performance-based tests are only poorly or moderately associated with self-rated activity limitation.[48]

Evidence for Physical Activity and Exercise

Patients with FM demonstrated improvements of body functions and reduction of symptoms when initiating muscle training twice a week, starting at 40% to 60% of their 1 RM voluntary contraction, and gradually increasing the load to 60% to 80%. Thus, a meta-analysis of two studies applying this mode of training calculated the effects by standardized mean difference (SMD) and found improved body function (SMD = 0.52), reduced pain (SMD = 3.00), better well-being (SMD = 1.43), fewer tender points (SMD = 1.52), and less depression (SMD = 1.14).[49] The same meta-analysis also included studies on cardiovascular fitness training in patients with FM and found positive effects regarding improvement of body function (SMD = 0.66), reduced pain (SMD = 0.65), better well-being (SMD = 0.49), and fewer tender points (SMD = 0.23).[49]

Patients who do not manage high-intensity exercise owing to disabling pain, fatigue, distress or fear of exercise-induced pain should initiate exercise at a comfortable level, and cautiously increase their exercise intensity when possible. Walking at self-selected intensity is feasible for most patients. Those who cannot manage walking for 30 minutes may divide their daily walks into two 15-minute sessions.[50] In a systematic review of randomized controlled trials (RCTs) of walking, it was found that walking enhances body function and reduces symptom severity in sedentary patients with FM.[51] Brisk walking was found to improve cardiovascular fitness in sedentary patients, who participated in supervised walking three times a week for 20 weeks. Walking speed was tailored to each patient's condition and gradually increased.[52]

Pool exercise in temperate water is suitable also for patients with severe pain and disability, because it reduces stiffness, alleviates pain, and offloads the body weight. Because movements and exercise load can easily be adjusted to each patient's condition, the risk of exercise-induced pain can be reduced. Studies evaluating the effects of pool exercise have applied different modes of exercise and outcome measurements. In a systematic review of RCTs, it was found that pool exercise improved health status in terms of less pain and distress, and better well-being and walking capacity.[51] If exercise is performed with an intensity of 60% to 80% of the maximum heart rate, cardiovascular fitness can also be improved.[53] Even passive relaxation in temperate water appears to alleviate pain and stiffness among patients with FM.

Pain is often associated with increased muscle tension, shortened muscles, and a deviant movement pattern, which should be considered when planning exercise for patients with FM. By focusing on quality of movement, muscular balance and posture, patients can learn more functional movement patterns. Such aspects can be included in any exercise program but also be taught separately in body awareness training, qigong, or taiji. A study evaluating the effects of body awareness training combined with qigong found improved movement harmony,[54] whereas another study, evaluating the effects of qigong combined with meditation, found reduction of FM symptoms and distress.[55]

Possible Risks

Pain in FM is related to abnormalities in physiologic pain processing mechanisms, including central sensitization and inadequate pain inhibition, which lead to increased sensitivity to painful stimuli, or allodynia. Owing to the lowered pain threshold, exercise-induced pain can be expected among most patients with FM who start a new mode of exercise. Once central sensitization has been established, little additional nociceptive input is required to maintain the sensitized state and chronic pain.[56] Thus, microtrauma during exercise might contribute to postexertional pain in FM.

Reduced muscle strength is not a contraindication to exercise, but adaptation to exercise may take a long time. Local musculoskeletal dysfunctions, for example, tendinitis, trochanteritis, or myofascial pain may become a barrier to exercise. Because peripheral tissues can both initiate and maintain chronic pain,[56] local musculoskeletal dysfunctions have to be taken into account when planning the mode and intensity of exercise and, if possible, be treated using, for example, traditional physical therapy measures such as physical modalities and massage.

Patients with FM of long duration may not achieve the same exercise effects as those with shorter symptom duration.[57] Furthermore, patients with severe symptoms may not be able to exercise at levels required for improvement of muscle strength or cardiovascular fitness, and in these cases, the expectations of beneficial effects should not be raised too highly. However, almost all exercise at an adequate level appears to enhance mood and self-efficacy in patients with FM.[51]

Exercise and Pain

Peripheral tissues are thought to initiate and contribute to maintenance of central sensitization.[56] Metabolic adaptation induced by exercise may, in turn, normalize some of these peripheral tissues, thus contributing to the reduction of pain. Improved muscle function may thus be a reason for exercise, resulting in improved tolerance of physical load during daily activities, reducing the overall pain in FM. Additional factors related to exercise may also contribute to improvement. Thus, learning a more functional movement pattern and relaxation techniques may be of great value for some individuals because it will reduce undesirable overload during daily activities. Furthermore, learning to relax tense muscles may reduce pain among those with high stress levels. Another value of exercise sessions with social interaction is that patients are confronted with their limitations and resources. This may lead to a process involving both body and mind, resulting in a more constructive relationship to pain and the body, as well as to improved self-efficacy for pain control.[41]

Patients with satisfactory baseline body functions can exercise at a moderate-to-high intensity level, like healthy individuals. If the baseline pain is severe, the patient displays severe impairments of body functions, or expresses fear of deterioration, it is wise to start exercise at a low intensity, because adaptation to a new mode of exercise can take up to 3 months. A supervised low-intensive exercise program, during which the patient is taught how to modify the exercise in relationship to his or her own condition so as not to overload the weakened tissues, may be needed in an initial phase (Table 30-2). Exercising in a group may also enhance adherence by providing an opportunity for social interaction and support. If disabling exercise-induced pain is still present for 1 to 2 days, the intensity of exercise should be lowered for a period of time, but it is important to motivate the patient to continue at the same duration and frequency to prevent further reduction of exercise tolerance. Gentle stretching of painful muscles is recommended to enhance blood circulation and reduce muscle tension.

All exercise should be planned with a long-term perspective. Most patients with FM believe that exercise is important for their health, well-being, and peacefulness during and after exercising despite pain.[58]

MOTIVATION AND ADHERENCE

Pain is the most important reason for people with rheumatic disease to seek health care, and most patients probably do not expect prescription

Table 30-2. *Schematic View of Physical Activity Prescription for Patients with Different Severities of Fibromyalgia*

	Severe Pain, Distress and Disability	Mild Pain and Disability
Target	Increased exercise tolerance	Increased muscle strength and/or cardiovascular fitness
Exercise mode	Comfortable intensity Adjusted to condition 30 or 2 × 15 minutes 2–5 times/week	Moderate-to-high intensity 30–45 minutes 3–5 times/week
Strategies	Slow progression Supervision	Moderate progression Supervised and non-supervised programs

of physical activity and exercise as part of the solution to their problems. Modern evidence-based drug treatment targets both immediate symptom reduction and a favorable long-term outcome for the patient. In line with this concept, long-term perspectives should also be held by other health professionals in order to improve their patients' health. Thus, considering the general health benefits that can be expected from physical activity and the existing scientific evidence for positive outcome of exercise programs, there certainly is a case for recommending these interventions as supplements to measures taken mainly to control inflammation and reduce symptoms.

Lifelong diseases, often requiring lifelong treatments, necessitate early and consistent involvement of the patients in decision making and responsibility for their health. This is particularly important when it comes to lifestyle-related behavior. However, pain, fatigue, depressed moods, impaired body functions, and maybe fear of increased symptoms and disease aggravation may represent obstacles to such an approach in patients with rheumatic disease. The medical doctor holds a key role in initiating the idea of incorporating health-enhancing physical activity and exercise in the overall management of their patient's disease.[59] Recommendations from the doctor may sometimes be sufficient in order to make patients adopt and maintain a healthy lifestyle. However, investigation into the patient's thoughts and emotions and interventions tailored to influence cognitions and behavior may often be required to obtain change.

The Transtheoretical Model and Stages of change offers a theoretical framework for cognitive-behavioral intervention.[60] It may thus be useful to identify the patient's readiness for change (Table 30-3) and adjust information and advice to his or her actual stage. Another useful technique may be the decisional balance, that is, a structured discussion and investigation into the perceived pros and cons for maintained and changed behaviors respectively (Table 30-4). Furthermore, identifying and strengthening the patients' self-efficacy for adopting a new behavior may be critical and the application of elements from other cognitive-behavioral theories may also be useful.[61]

A physical therapist is an important resource in this respect as well as in the prescription and implementation of an evidence-based program targeting

Table 30-3. *The Six Stages of Change Described as a Process-Involving Progress in the Transtheoretical Model and Stages of Change*

Stages of Change	Description
Precontemplation	Has no intention to take action within the next 6 months
Contemplation	Intends to take action within the next 6 months
Preparation	Intends to take action within the next 30 days and has taken some behavioral steps in this direction
Action	Has changed overt behavior for less than 6 months
Maintenance	Has changed overt behavior for more than 6 months
Termination	A new healthy behavior is established

From Prochaska JO, DiClemente CC, Norcross JC. In search of how people change. Applications to addicitive behaviors. Am Psychol 1992;47:1102-14.

Table 30-4. *Example of Decisional Balance Reflecting an Individual's Weighing of the Pros and Cons of Changing Behavior from being Sedentary to Adopt Health-Enhancing Physical Activity*

Decision to Adopt Physical Activity	Decision Not to Adopt Physical Activity

Pros
    More energy
    Less risk of comorbidity
Cons
    Certain costs
	Pros
	    More time for watching television
	Cons
	    Medication for high blood pressure and type 2 diabetes necessary
	    Increasing body weight

ROM, muscle function or cardiovascular fitness. The physical therapist also has an important role in assisting their patients in setting specific goals for the behavior change, tailoring interventions to patients' individual preferences and health status, supporting their patients during the process of adopting a new behavior, and assisting in solving problems that may emerge. It is also important that issues related to maintenance of the new behavior are considered and implemented early in the process.[62]

PRESCRIPTION

A written plan or prescription, including the mode, frequency, duration, and intensity of physical activity, is a useful tool in order to make the patients understand what he or she needs to do.[59] Each patient with a rheumatic disease should be recommended health-enhancing physical activity in daily life. If this is impossible for some reason or insufficient, there is a case for planned and structured exercise. The first choice would then often be general fitness training including elements to increase ROM and to improve muscle function and cardiovascular fitness. Local impairments require specific exercise targeting certain muscle groups or joints. Manual techniques and physical treatments including massage, heat, cold, ultrasound, or transcutaneous electrical nerve stimulation, for which scientific, empirical evidence is still weak in patients with rheumatic disease, should preferably be used with the explicit aim to enhance physical activity. This also applies to various kinds of stabilizing orthoses, shoe insoles, and recommendations on appropriate footwear for physical activity.

FOLLOW-UP AND EVALUATION

Measures to follow-up and evaluate physical activity should constantly be on the agenda within health care for patients with rheumatic disease. Specific inquiry at regular medical check-ups into concrete circumstances relating to physical activity and the use of assessments related to negotiated and set exercise goals will help the patient understand the importance of physical activity. Suggestions on assessments of body function tests to assess the outcome of physical activity are given in Table 30-5.[63-72] In addition, questionnaires on activity limitations, exercise self-efficacy or general health perception, and simple rating scales for various symptoms can be used.[73] Body weight and risk factors for comorbidity can be monitored as usual, so that feedback on the results can be discussed in relation to physical inactivity or activity.

Table 30-5. *Suggestions on Outcome Measures to Evaluate Physical Activity and Exercise in Clinical Practice*

Target	Method	Result
Range of motion	Goniometer	Angular ROM, degrees
	EPM-ROM scale[63]	Angular ROM in selected joints, score 0–30
	Shoulder Function Assessment[64]	ROM and pain rating, score 5–30/0–10
	BASMI[65]	ROM, score 0–10
Muscle function	Dynamometer	Strength and endurance, N
	Timed Stands Test[66]	10 timed risings, s
	Index of Muscle Function[67]	13 tasks for strength, endurance and balance/coordination, score 0–40
	Functional Index 2[68]	8 tests of muscle endurance, repetitions, n
	Timed 'Up & Go'[69]	Rise-walk-turn-walk-sit, s
	Balance task in a figure-of-an-eight[70]	Oversteps, n
Cardiovascular fitness	Submaximal work capacity	
	Bicycle ergometer[71]	mlO_2/kg/min
	Treadmill[72]	mlO_2/kg/min

BASMI, Bath Ankylosing Spondylitis Metrology Index; EMP-ROM scale, Escola Paulista de Medicina Range of Motion; ROM, range of motion.

References

1. Hagströmer M. Assessment of health-enhancing physical activity at population level. Thesis for doctoral degree. Stockholm: Karolinska Institutet; 2007. http://diss.kib.ki.se/2007/978-91-7357-334-4/.
2. Caspersen CJ, Powell KE, Christenson GM. Physical activity, exercise, and physical fitness. Public Health Rep 1985;100:125-31.
3. Foster C. Guidelines for health-enhancing physical activity promotion programmes. Tampere, Finland: The UKK Institute for Health Promotion Research; 2000.
4. World Health Organization. The World Health Report 2002. In: Reducing risks, promoting healthy life. Geneva, Switzerland: World Health Organization; 2002.
5. Warburton DE, Nicol CW, Bredin SS. Health benefits of physical activity: the evidence. CMAJ 2006;174:801-9.
6. Sokka T, Häkkinen A, Kautiainen H, Maillefert JF, Toloza S, Mørk Hansen T, et al. Physical inactivity in patients with rheumatoid arthritis: data from twenty-one countries in a cross-sectional, international study. Arthritis Rheum 2008;59:42-50.
7. Eurenius E, Brodin N, Lindblad S, Opava CH. PARA Study Group. Predicting physical activity and general health perception among patients with rheumatoid arthritis. J Rheumatol 2007;34:10-5.
8. Haskell WL, Lee IM, Pate RR, Powell KE, Blair SN, Franklin BA, et al. Physical activity and public health: updated recommendation for adults from the American College of Sports Medicine and the American Heart Association. Med Sci Sports Exerc 2007;39:1423-34.
9. Nelson ME, Rejeski WJ, Blair SN, Duncan PW, Judge JO, King AC, et al. Physical activity and health in older adults: recommendations from the American College of Sports Medicine and the American Heart Association. Med Sci Sports Exerc 2007;39:1435-45.
10. Borg GA. Psychophysical bases of perceived exertion. Med Sci Sports Exerc 1982;14:377-81.
11. Brodin N, Swärdh E, Biguet G, Opava CH. Understanding how to determine the intensity of physical activity—an

interview study among individuals with rheumatoid arthritis. Disabil Rehabil 2009;31:458-65.

12. Minor M, Stenström CH, Klepper S, Hurley M, Ettinger WH. Work Group Recommendations: 2002 Exercise and Physical Activity Conference, St. Louis, Missouri. Session V: Evidence of benefit of exercise and physical activity in arthritis. Arthritis Rheum 2003;49:453-4.

13. Häkkinen A. Effectiveness and safety of strength training in rheumatoid arthritis. Curr Opin Rheumatol 2004;16:132-7.

14. Lohmander LS, Roos EM. Clinical update: treating osteoarthritis. Lancet 2007;370:2082-4.

15. Stenström CH, Minor MA. Evidence for the benefit of aerobic and strengthening exercise in rheumatoid arthritis. Arthritis Rheum 2003;49:428-34.

16. Eurenius E, Brodin N, Opava CH. PARA Study Group. Clinical applicability of two tests of aerobic fitness in patients with rheumatoid arthritis. Adv Physiother 2007;9:97-104.

17. Westby MDA. Health professional's guide to exercise prescription for people with arthritis. A review of aerobic fitness activities. Arthritis Rheum 2001;45:501-11.

18. Sokka T, Häkkinen A. Poor physical fitness and performance as predictors of mortality in normal popuations and patients with rheumatic and other diseases. Clin Exp Rheumatol 2008;26(Suppl. 5):S14-20.

19. Eurenius E, Stenström CH. The PARA Study Group. Physical activity, physical fitness, and general health perception among individuals with rheumatoid arthritis. Arthritis Rheum 2005;53:48-55.

20. Iversen MD, Fossel AH, Daltroy LH. Rheumatologist-patient communication about exercise and physical therapy in the management of rheumatoid arthritis. Arthritis Care Res 1999;12:180-92.

21. Eurenius E, Biguet G, Stenström CH. Attitudes toward physical activity among people with rheumatoid arthritis. Physiother Theory Pract 2003;19:53-62.

22. Ottawa Panel. Ottawa panel evidence-based clinical practise guidelines for therapeutic exercises in the management of rheumatoid arthritis in adults. Phys Ther 2004;84:934-72.

23. Van Den Ende CH, Vliet Vlieland TP, Munneke M, Hazes JM. Dynamic exercise therapy for rheumatoid arthritis. Cochrane Database Syst Rev 2000;(2):CD000322.

24. DeJong Z, Munneke M, Zwinderman AH, Kroon HM, Jansen A, Ronday KH, et al. Is a long-term high-intensity exercise program effective and safe in patients with rheumatoid arthritis? Results of a randomized controlled trial. Arthritis Rheum 2003;48:2415-24.

25. Van den Berg MH, Ronday HK, Peeters AJ, le Cessie S, van der Giessen FJ, Breedveld FC, et al. Using Internet technology to deliver a home-based physical activity intervention for patients with rheumatoid arthritis: a randomized controlled trial. Arthritis Rheum 2006;55:935-45.

26. Brodin N, Eurenius E, Jensen I, Nisell R, Opava CH. PARA Study Group. Coaching patients with early rheumatoid arthritis to healthy physical activity: A multicenter, randomized, controlled study. Arthritis Rheum 2008;59:325-31.

27. Stenström CH. Home exercise in rheumatoid arthritis functional class II: Goal-setting versus pain attention. J Rheumatol 1994;21:627-34.

28. Dagfinrud H, Hagen K. Physiotherapy interventions for ankylosing spondylitis. Cochrane Database Syst Rev 2008;(1):CD002822.

29. Ayán C, Martin V. Systemic lupus erythematosus and exercise. Lupus 2007;16:5-9.

30. Strömbeck B, Jacobsson LT. The role of exercise in the rehabilitation of patients with systemic lupus erythematosus and patients with primary Sjögren's syndrome. Curr Opin Rheumatol 2007;19:197-203 [Erratum in: Curr Opin Rheumatol] 2007;19:403.

31. Strömbeck BE, Theander E, Jacobsson LT. Effects of exercise on aerobic capacity and fatigue in women with primary Sjogren's syndrome. Rheumatology (Oxford) 2007;46:868-71.

32. Alexanderson H, Lundberg IE. The role of exercise in the rehabilitation of idiopathic inflammatory myopathies. Curr Opin Rheumatol 2005;17:164-71.

33. Alexanderson H, Dastmalchi M, Esbjörnsson-Liljedahl M, Opava CH, Lundberg IE. Benefits of intensive resistance training in patients with chronic polymyositis or dermatomyositis. Arthritis Rheum 2007;57:768-77.

34. Van den Ende CHM, Breedveld FC, le Cessie S, Dijkmans BAC, de Mug AW, Hazes JM. Effect of intensive exercise on patients with active rheumatoid arthritis: a randomized clinical trial. Ann Rheum Dis 2000;59:615-21.

35. Marley WP, Santilli TF. A 15-year exercise program for rheumatoid vasculitis. Scand J Rheumatol 1998;27:149-51.

36. Lundberg IE, Nader GA. Molecular effects of exercise in patients with inflammatory rheumatic diseases. Nat Clin Pract Rheumatol 2008;4:597-604.

37. Henriksson C, Gundmark I, Bengtsson A, Ek A. Living with fibromyalgia. Consequences for everyday life. Clin J Pain 1992;8:138-44.

38. Waylonis G, Ronan P, Gordon C. A profile of fibromyalgia in occupational environments. Am J Phys Med Rehabil 1994;73:112-5.

39. Natvig B, Bruusgaard D, Eriksen W. Physical leisure activity level and physical fitness among women with fibromyalgia. Scand J Rheumatol 1998;27:337-41.

40. Mannerkorpi K, Kroksmark T, Ekdahl C. How patients with fibromyalgia experience their symptoms in everyday life. Physiother Res Int 1999;4:110-22.

41. Mannerkorpi K, Gard G. Physiotherapy group treatment for patients with fibromyalgia—an embodied learning process. Disabil Rehabil 2003;25:1372-80.

42. Mengshoel A, Forre O, Komnaes H. Muscle strength and aerobic capacity in primary fibromyalgia. Clin Exp Rheumatol 1990;8:475-9.

43. Burckhardt C, Mannerkorpi K, Hedenberg L, Bjelle A. A randomized, controlled clinical trial of education and physical training for women with fibromyalgia. J Rheumatol 1994;21:714-20.

44. Lindh M, Johansson G, Hedberg M, Grimby G. Studies on maximal voluntary muscle contraction in patients with fibromyalgia. Arch Phys Med Rehabil 1994;75:1217-22.

45. Norregaard J, Bulow P, Lykkegaard J, Mehlsen J, Danneskiold-Samsoe B. Muscle strength, working capacity and effort in patients with fibromyalgia. Scand J Rehab Med 1997;29:97-102.

46. Miller T, Allen G, Gandevia S. Muscle force, perceived effort, and voluntary activation of the elbow muscle flexors assessed with sensitive twitch interpolation in fibromyalgia. J Rheumatol 1996;23:1621-7.

47. Nielens H, Boisset V, Masquelier E. Fitness and perceived exertion in patients with fibromyalgia syndrome. Clin J Pain 2000;16:209-13.

48. Mannerkorpi K, Svantesson U, Broberg C. Relationships between performance-based tests and patients' ratings of activity limitations, self-efficacy and pain in fibromyalgia. Arch Phys Med Rehabil 2006;87:259-64.

49. Busch AJ, Barber KA, Overend TJ, Peloso PM, Schachter CL. Exercise for treating fibromyalgia syndrome. Cochrane Database Syst Rev 2007;(4):CD003786.

50. Schachter C, Busch A, Peloso P, Sheppard M. The effects of short versus long bouts of aerobic exercise in sedentary women with fibromyalgia: a randomized controlled trial. Phys Ther 2003;83:340-58.

51. Mannerkorpi K, Henriksson C. Non-pharmacological treatment of chronic widespread musculoskeletal pain. Best Pract Res Clin Rheumatol 2007;21:513-34.

52. Valim V, Oliveira L, Suda A, Silva L, de Assis M, Neto T, et al. Aerobic fitness effects in fibromyalgia. J Rheumatol 2003;30:2473-81.

53. Jentoft ES, Kvalvik AG, Mengshoel AM. Effects of pool-based and land-based aerobic exercise on women with fibromyalgia/chronic widespread muscle pain. Arthritis Rheum 2001;45:42-7.

54. Mannerkorpi K, Arndorw M. Efficacy and feasibility of body awareness therapy combined with qigong for patients with fibromyalgia. J Rehabil Med 2004;36:279-81.

55. Astin JA, Berman BM, Bausell B, Lee WL, Hochberg M, Forys KL. The efficacy of mindfulness meditation plus

Qigong movement therapy in the treatment of fibromyalgia: a randomized controlled trial. J Rheumatol 2003;30:2257-62.

56. Staud R. Biology and therapy of fibromyalgia: pain in fibromyalgia syndrome. Arthritis Res Ther 2006;8:208.

57. Garcia-Campayo J, Magdalena J, Magallon R, Fernandez-Garcia E, Salas M, Andres E. A meta-analysis of the efficacy of fibromyalgia treatment according to level of care. Arthritis Res Ther 2008;10:R81 [Epub 2008].

58. Mannerkorpi K, Rivano-Fischer M, Ericsson A, Nordeman L, Gard G. Experience of physical activity in patients with fibromyalgia and chronic widespread pain. Disabil Rehabil 2008;30:213-21.

59. Sorensen JB, Skovgaard T, Puggaard L. Exercise on prescription in general practice. A systematic review. Scand J Prim Health Care 2006;24:69-74.

60. Prochaska JO, DiClemente CC, Norcross JC. In search of how people change. Applications to addictive behaviors. Am Psychol 1992;47:1102-14.

61. Gonzalez VM, Goeppinger J, Lorig K. Four psychosocial theories and their application to patient education and clinical practice. Arthritis Care Res 1990;3:132-43.

62. Swärdh E, Biguet G, Opava CH. Views on exercise maintenance. A qualitative study among individuals with rheumatoid arthritis. Phys Ther 2008;88:1049-60 [Erratum in: Phys Ther] 2008;88:1232.

63. Vliet Vlieland TPM, van den Ende CHM, Breedveld FC, Hazes JMW. Evaluation of joint mobility in rheumatoid arthritis: the value of the EPM-range of motion scale. J Rheumatol 1993;20:2010-4.

64. Boström C, Harms-Ringdahl K, Nordemar R. Clinical reliability of shoulder function assessment in patients with rheumatoid arthritis. Scand J Rheumatol 1991;20:36-48.

65. Jenkinson T, Mallorie P, Whitelock H, Kennedy LG, Garrett SL, Calin A. Defining spinal mobility in ankylosing spondylitis. The Bath Ankylosing Spondylitis Metrology Index. J Rheumatol 1994;21:1694-8.

66. Newcomer KL, Krug HE, Mahowald ML. Validity and reliability of the timed-stands test for patients with rheumatoid arthritis and other chronic diseases. J Rheumatol 1993;20:21-7.

67. Ekdahl C, Englund A, Stenström CH. Development and evaluation of the Index of Muscle Function. Adv Physiother 1999;1:45-55.

68. Alexanderson H, Broman L, Tollbäck A, Josefson A, Lundberg IE, Stenström CH. Functional index-2: Validity and reliability of a disease-specific measure of impairment in patients with polymyositis and dermatomyositis. Arthritis Rheum 2006;55:114-22.

69. Podsiadlo D, Richard VS. The Timed 'Up & Go'. A test of basic functional mobility for frail elderly persons. JAGS 1991;39:142-8.

70. Norén AM, Bogren U, Bohlin J, Stenström CH. Balance assessment in patients with rheumatoid arthritis. Applicability and reliability of some clinical assessments. Physiother Res Int 2001;6:193-204.

71. Minor MA, Johnson JC. Reliability and validity of a submaximal treadmill test to estimate aerobic capacity in women with rheumatic disease. J Rheumatol 1996;23:1517-23.

72. Åstrand O, Rodahl K. Textbook of Work Physiology. New York: McGraw-Hill; 1970.

73. Katz P. editor. Patient outcomes in rheumatology. A review of measures. Arthritis Rheum 2003;49(Suppl.):S1-S232.

Management of the Patient with Rheumatic Disease During and After Pregnancy

Lisa R. Sammaritano

INTRODUCTION

Rheumatic diseases disproportionately affect women and, in some patients, may be serious enough to preclude consideration of pregnancy; however, with advances in rheumatology therapies and sophisticated reproductive technologies, increasing numbers of patients with rheumatic disease have the option of pursuing pregnancy. Important considerations for every patient include the effect of pregnancy-related immune changes on underlying disease, the impact of rheumatic disease activity or damage on pregnancy outcome, the effect of maternal autoantibodies on fetal and neonatal health, and potential adverse fetal effects of medications.

NORMAL PREGNANCY

In order to monitor a patient with rheumatic disease through pregnancy, it is critical to have some understanding of normal pregnancy physiology. Immunologic changes in uncomplicated pregnancy are significant, although they are incompletely understood. Cell-mediated immunity is generally depressed with an increase in humoral and innate immune responses, and complement levels are elevated due to an increase in synthesis. Multiple mechanisms for fetal tolerance appear to protect the fetus from a maternal cytotoxic immune response.

Many physiologic adjustments of pregnancy are easily confused with active rheumatic disease, or may worsen existing rheumatic disease symptoms. One critical hemodynamic change is an increase in intravascular volume by 30% to 50%, providing additional stress for patients with renal or cardiac compromise (cardiac output similarly increases by 30%–50%). The glomerular filtration rate also increases by up to 50%, and, as a result, women with pre-existing proteinuria may be expected to have significant increases in urinary protein excretion, particularly during the second and third trimesters.[1]

Hematologic changes are also significant: pregnancy generates a prothrombotic state, with increased plasma levels of fibrinogen, factor II, and other procoagulant proteins and decreased protein S levels and fibrinolytic system activity. This hypercoagulability, in conjunction with venous stasis, compression by the gravid uterus, and bed rest, increases the risk of venous thromboembolism in normal pregnancy by a factor of five. Pregnant women usually become anemic due to hemodilution in the third trimester, and although platelet production usually increases in a compensatory fashion, platelet turnover increases and mild thrombocytopenia ($70–150 \times 10^9$/L) occurs in about 8% of uncomplicated pregnancies. The white blood cell count rises progressively, with a relative increase in neutrophils; the erythrocyte sedimentation rate (ESR) also rises, making both these tests, which are otherwise useful in assessing vasculitis activity, unreliable indicators of inflammation.[1]

Overall, a majority of organ systems experience some degree of change during pregnancy. Thirty to fifty percent of pregnant patients have significant gastroesophageal reflux disease, and patients with pre-existing gastrointestinal motility problems, especially those with scleroderma, are likely to experience an exacerbation of symptoms. Although saliva production is unchanged, gums may swell and bleed, exacerbating dental problems in patients with sicca symptoms. Facial erythema may mimic a lupus or other autoimmune disease rash, and mottled palmar erythema may be confused with cutaneous vasculits. Bland joint effusions and arthralgias due to ligamentous laxity may similarly be confused with mild inflammatory arthritis. Finally, both pregnancy and lactation cause reversible bone loss in healthy women; this loss is increased in women who breastfeed for longer intervals, an issue of potential concern for rheumatic disease patients on long-term corticosteroid therapy.[1]

COMPLICATED PREGNANCY

Distinguishing common disorders of pregnancy from autoimmune disease activity may present a significant challenge. The pre-eclampsia syndrome includes complications that may mimic lupus nephritis, scleroderma renal crisis, or vasculitis: late pregnancy hypertension (blood pressure greater than 140/90 after 20 weeks' gestation), proteinuria (greater than 300 mg/24 hours), edema, and hyperuricemia. When seizures occur, the syndrome is defined as eclampsia. The hemolysis, elevated liver enzymes, and low platelets (HELLP) syndrome is a severe variant of pre-eclampsia, and presents with prominent hepatic enzyme abnormalities, abdominal pain, fever, thrombocytopenia, and encephalopathy.[2] Pre-eclampsia, intrauterine growth restriction (IUGR) (infants weighing less than 10% of weight for age), preterm delivery (< 37 weeks' gestation) and pregnancy loss are complications that are more common in a number of rheumatic diseases.[3-5] Pregnancy loss may occur in any of four major developmental periods: pre-embryonic loss (conception through week 4 of gestation); embryonic loss (weeks 5 through 9); fetal loss (week 10 until delivery); and neonatal loss.

Interactions of pregnancy and specific rheumatic diseases are described later, with particular focus on maternal complications, neonatal outcome, and management recommendations. A detailed summary of medications and their safety in pregnancy follows.

Systemic Lupus Erythematosus

Systemic lupus erythematosus (SLE) is most common during the reproductive years, and patients require thorough evaluation both before and during pregnancy. With appropriate planning, monitoring, and medical therapy, most patients with SLE can undergo successful pregnancies with good fetal outcome.

CASE STUDY 1

A 27-year-old woman with long-standing SLE comes in to discuss plans for pregnancy. She presented with diffuse proliferative glomerulonephritis at age 18 and was treated with cyclophosphamamide for 6 months, followed by 2 years of azathioprine therapy. She is currently on hydroxychloroquine 400 mg/day, enalopril 5 mg/day, and prednisone 7.5 mg/day. Serum creatinine is 1.1 and creatinine clearance is 70 mL/hour, with mild baseline proteinuria of 350 mg/24 hours. Serologies include positive anti-SSA/Ro and anti-SSB/La antibodies, with negative antiphospholipid antibodies (aPLs). Anti-ds DNA antibody is negative, and complement levels (C3, C4) are normal. How does one advise this patient?

Maternal Considerations

Pregnancy in a patient with SLE represents an added risk to an already complex clinical situation. Large-scale epidemiologic studies confirm that despite improvements in overall pregnancy outcome over recent years, maternal morbidity is still high for patients with SLE: hypertensive complications, renal disease, preterm delivery, cesarean section, postpartum hemorrhage and thrombosis, fetal growth restriction, and neonatal death are all more common in SLE pregnancies.[4,5] One national study found maternal mortality to be 20-fold higher among women with SLE; in addition, roughly one third of patients with SLE have cesarean sections, one third deliver prematurely, and one fourth develop pre-eclampsia.[5] Fortunately, identification of particular risk factors can help predict likelihood of complications and aid in risk counseling. Important risk factors include presence of lupus disease activity, renal involvement, aPLs and anti-SSA/Ro and SSB/La antibodies. Pre-pregnancy evaluation involves assessment of level of disease activity, presence of disease damage, review of current medications, and laboratory tests, especially autoantibody status. The algorithm in Figure 31-1 illustrates a general approach

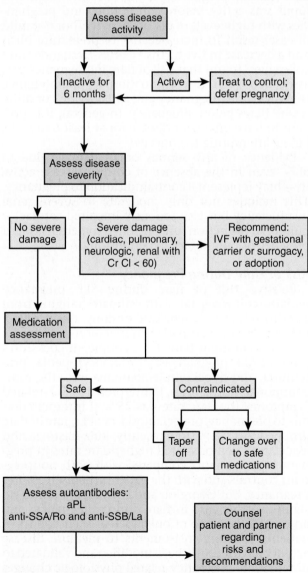

Figure 31-1. Pre-pregnancy evaluation of the rheumatic disease patient.

to evaluation of rheumatic disease patients before pregnancy.

Medication Assessment

Review of medications before conception allows adjustment with careful follow-up to ensure maintenance of disease control. Detailed recommendations appear below. In brief, however, prednisone, methylprednisolone, hydroxychloroquine, azathioprine, cyclosporine, and intravenous immunoglobulin may be continued through pregnancy; in most circumstances, other immunosuppressive medications should be discontinued or replaced. Continuation of hydroxychloroquine is encouraged, because recent data support fetal safety and a lowered risk of maternal disease flare.[6,7]

Disease Activity

The importance of quiescent disease at the time of conception cannot be overemphasized. Risk of flare during pregnancy is significantly higher if lupus was active before conception, and pregnancies with high levels of disease activity (but not mild disease) result in increased risk of premature birth and a decrease in live births.[8] Cortes-Hernandez and colleagues[9] found that risk of flare in pregnancy was associated with discontinuation of maintenance therapy before pregnancy and a history of 3 or more severe flares before pregnancy. In general, it is prudent to have quiescent disease for at least 6 months before attempting to conceive.

Evidence of any serious organ damage due to SLE—even in the absence of current disease activity—may represent a contraindication to pregnancy. This includes not only moderate to severe renal insufficiency but also seriously impaired cardiac or pulmonary function, uncontrolled hypertension, or presence of pulmonary hypertension.

Risk of Flare During Pregnancy

Relative risk of flare during SLE pregnancy remains controversial, with estimates ranging from 13% to 60%.[10-12] Discordant findings likely reflect differences between patient populations and in the definition of lupus flare. For example, in Lockshin's series of SLE pregnancies, thrombocytopenia, proteinuria, and hypocomplementemia were the most common abnormalities. If interpreted as SLE-related symptoms, the flare rate was 25%; if interpreted as due to pregnancy, pre-eclampsia, or aPLs, rate of flare dropped to 13%.[10] More recently, Ruiz-Irastorza and associates[11] demonstrated higher flare rates in pregnant lupus patients compared with both nonpregnant controls and with the patients themselves after pregnancy, but Georgiou and coworkers[12] found no significant increase in flare during pregnancy, and an overall flare rate of only 13% in their cohort of patients. Existing instruments to measure disease activity have recently been modified and validated to differentiate pregnancy-related physiologic changes from lupus activity, and will allow greater comparability between future studies. Pregnancy-specific disease activity indices include the SLE-Pregnancy Disease Activity Index and the Lupus Activity Index Pregnancy Scale.[13]

Despite the varied estimates of precise risk of flare during lupus pregnancy, it is reasonable to counsel patients regarding a small to moderate increased risk of disease exacerbation, even with long-term quiescent disease, which may occur during any trimester or the postpartum period. Prophylactic steroid therapy is not recommended to prevent flare.

Impact of Lupus Nephritis

Renal insufficiency is an important risk factor for poor fetal outcome and for serious renal deterioration during pregnancy.[14] Precise renal histology is less important than the presence of clinical renal dysfunction.[15] Although exacerbation of renal disease may occur in up to 40% of cases, severe or permanent renal deterioration develops in less than 10%.[16] The physiologic stress of pregnancy, even in patients with quiescent nephritis, may accelerate deterioration, especially in those with initial serum creatinine greater than 1.6 mg/dL. Onset of worsening renal function usually occurs in the latter half of pregnancy. In addition to the risk of moderate renal insufficiency, baseline proteinuria presents an independent risk: Moroni and associates[16] demonstrated that proteinuria greater than 500 mg/24 hours is an independent predictor of poor fetal outcome. Fetal loss occurred in 57% of patients with proteinuria versus 10% of those without. Recent active nephritis also increased risk of renal deterioration during pregnancy: risk of renal flare was 5% in those with quiescent nephritis, and 39% in those with recently active nephritis.[16]

Patients with SLE with renal transplants usually have successful pregnancies. McGrory and colleagues[17] compared pregnancy outcomes in renal transplant recipients with (60 pregnancies) and without (374 pregnancies) SLE. Significant hypertension and cesarean sections were less common in patients with SLE, and other maternal conditions and pregnancy outcomes were comparable in both groups.

Differentiation of Systemic Lupus Erythematosus Flare from Pregnancy-Related Complications

In the SLE population, the differential diagnosis for new-onset proteinuria in the second half of pregnancy includes lupus nephritis, pre-eclampsia, or both. Two thirds of patients with SLE entering pregnancy with pre-existing renal disease develop pre-eclampsia, compared with 14% of patients with lupus without kidney disease.[14] It is often not possible to differentiate between SLE nephritis and pre-eclampsia during pregnancy, and frequently, therapy is directed toward both. Clinical signs of active SLE such as inflammatory arthritis or rash, fever, lymphadenopathy, hematuria, leukopenia, erythrocyte casts, and rising anti-DNA antibody favor the diagnosis of lupus glomerulonephritis.

Table 31-1. *Clinical Laboratory Measures/Physical Findings in Preeclampsia Versus Systemic Lupus Erythematosus (SLE) Nephritis*

Clinical Measure	Pre-eclampsia	SLE Nephritis
Complement	Usually normal	Usually low
Urine red cell casts	Rare	Frequent
Liver function tests	May be elevated	Usually normal
Proteinuria onset	Abrupt	Gradual/Abrupt
24-hour protein	Does not differentiate (2–25 g)	Does not differentiate (2–25 g)
Thrombocytopenia	Does not differentiate	Does not differentiate
Hyperuricemia	Does not differentiate	Does not differentiate
Hypertension	Does not differentiate	Does not differentiate
Arthritis	Not present	May occur
Inflammatory rash	Not present	May occur
Fever	Not present	May occur

Thrombocytopenia, hypertension, and hyperuricemia occur in both SLE and pre-eclampsia (Table 31-1). ESR, increased in normal pregnancy, becomes an unreliable measure of lupus activity during pregnancy. Normal serum complement favors a diagnosis of pre-eclampsia. Measures of alternative pathway complement activation (Ba and Bb), are reported to be abnormal in active lupus nephritis and normal in lupus pregnancies with proteinuria not due to active SLE.[18] Seizures may occur due to eclampsia or to neuropsychiatric lupus.

Thrombocytopenia during SLE pregnancy varies in presentation, and may be due to flare, aPLs, HELLP syndrome, or even normal pregnancy itself. Active SLE-related moderate thrombocytopenia (50–120×10^9/L) may be difficult to distinguish from benign (mild) thrombocytopenia of late pregnancy, unrelated to SLE. Although rare, severe lupus-related thrombocytopenia may occur, with counts less than 10×10^9/L.

Pregnancy Outcome
Neonatal Lupus Erythematosus

SLE may influence neonatal outcome by direct or indirect effects on the fetus. Neonatal lupus erythematosus (NLE) reflects a direct effect of transplacental autoantibodies to the SS-A/Ro and SS-B/La antigens, leading to fetal inflammation. Clinical manifestations include photosensitive rash, thrombocytopenia, liver function abnormalities, and rarely, irreversible congenital heart block (CHB). With the exception of CHB, manifestations disappear with clearance of maternal antibody at 6 months. The mortality rate associated with CHB is 20%, and most surviving patients require permanent pacing.[19] The

risk of any manifestation of NLE for the neonate of an anti-SSA/Ro positive woman is 20%, and the risk of CHB less than 3%. Although anti-SSA/Ro antibodies are responsible for NLE, they do not affect other pregnancy outcomes, and the risk of NLE is determined by the presence of the antibody, not the underlying maternal diagnosis. The risk of CHB in offspring of women with a previously affected child is higher, approximately 20%.[20]

Immunoblot patterns of anti-SSA/Ro and SSB/La antibodies are related to the risk of CHB: 75% to 100% of mothers whose children develop CHB show reactivity with recombinant 52-kD SSA/Ro antigen.[20] Because the anti-SSA/Ro 52-kD test is not generally available in clinical laboratories, however, management decisions are usually based on enzyme-linked immunosorbent assay (ELISA) results. Current recommendations suggest fetal echocardiography be done weekly from 16 to 26 weeks for high-risk patients (previous child with any manifestation of NLE) and every 2 weeks from 26 to 34 weeks.[20] Anti-SSA/Ro and/or anti-SSB/La–positive patients without a history of a child affected by NLE are usually followed by fetal echocardiography at more variable intervals of every 2 to 3 weeks: although it is reported that third degree heart block can appear within a period as short as 1 week, no evidence-based guidelines exist. If significantly prolonged PR interval, advanced degree block, or evidence of pericardial or myocardial inflammation is detected, fluorinated corticosteroid treatment is generally instituted, although efficacy is unproven: reversal of complete heart block has not been reported in any pregnancy treated with fluorinated corticosteroid. Steroid therapy is most effective in resolution of pleural effusion, ascites, and hydrops fetalis.[19] Intravenous immunoglobulin (IVIG) and even plasmapheresis have been suggested as potential future therapies.

Prematurity, Intrauterine Growth Restriction, and Other Fetal Complications

IUGR and prematurity are the most common fetal complications of lupus pregnancy. Maternal risk factors for threatened fetal growth and development are active SLE, impaired renal function, and presence of aPL. A retrospective review of 72 SLE pregnancies[3] found that preterm deliveries, observed in 39% of their patients, were associated with aPL and higher prednisone dose. Other authors have similarly identified aPL and corticosteroid use, as well as hypertension, hypocomplementemia, and thrombocytopenia, as predictive of preterm delivery or pre-eclampsia.[9,21,22]

Other complications may be seen. Unexplained elevation of maternal alpha-fetoprotein may occur in patients with SLE in the absence of neural tube defects and is associated with increased risk of fetal death. Elevation correlates with preterm delivery, high prednisone dosage, and presence of aPL.[23] Presumably, abnormalities in the fetoplacental barrier lead to increased transport of alpha-fetoprotein from fetus to mother.

Maternal immunoglobulin G (IgG)–mediated thrombocytopenia may occasionally be transmitted to the fetus, but most infants born of thrombocytopenic mothers with SLE have normal platelet counts. IgG Coombs' hemolytic antibody may cause hemolysis in the fetus and newborn.

Short-term follow-up of offspring of women with SLE suggest children develop normally compared with children of similar prematurity.[24] Long-term follow-up of SLE offspring compared with matched controls found intelligence to be normal but identified a high frequency of learning disabilities, particularly in boys.[25]

Management and Therapy

Treatment of the pregnant patient with SLE does not usually differ from that of the nonpregnant patient. Careful follow-up and monitoring with both the rheumatologist and obstetrician are essential (Table 31-2). Hydroxychloroquine should be continued to prevent disease flare. Clinical flares of skin, joints, blood, kidneys, and nervous system require therapy with (unfluorinated) corticosteroids. Use of immunosuppressive therapies other than corticosteroid is generally limited to azathioprine or cyclosporine (see details later). Corticosteroid should be prescribed for thrombocytopenia if the platelet count drops significantly; life-threatening thrombocytopenia ($< 30 \times 10^9$/L) or imminent delivery requires platelet transfusion, intravenous IgG, or both.

Table 31-2. *Monitoring of the Pregnant Systemic Lupus Erythematosus Patient*

Schedule	Monitoring Test
First visit	Complete blood count with platelets
	Comprehensive metabolic panel
	Urinalysis, creatinine clearance, 24-hour urine protein or spot protein/creatinine ratio
	Anticardiolipin antibody, lupus anticoagulant, anti-β2-Glycoprotein I antibody
	Anti-ds DNA, anti-SSA/Ro and SSB/La antibodies
	Complement levels (C3, C4)
Every 4–6 weeks	Platelet count*; anti-ds DNA antibody; complement levels; urinalysis*
Each trimester	Creatinine clearance with 24-hour protein or protein/creatinine ratio*
Weekly (third trimester)	If aPL positive: Antenatal fetal heart rate testing (nonstress test) or fetal umbilical artery Doppler velocimetry
Weeks 16–34	If anti-SSA/Ro and/or anti-SSB/La positive:
	Weekly fetal echocardiograms weeks 16–26, biweekly weeks 26–34 if high risk (previous child with neonatal lupus erythematosus)
	Every 2–3 weeks fetal echocardiograms if not high risk

*More frequently if abnormal.

The risk of pre-eclampsia is significantly increased in lupus pregnancy. Although low-dose aspirin is used to prevent pre-eclampsia in high-risk women with pre-existing hypertension, renal insufficiency, or history of previous pre-eclampsia, there is as yet no systematic study of the use of aspirin to prevent pre-eclampsia in patients with SLE (with or without aPL), although it is frequently prescribed.

There is general agreement on several key observations regarding risk and outcome of lupus pregnancy: first, inactive disease at the time of conception (and for the 6 months preceding pregnancy) is associated with a lower likelihood of disease exacerbation and better fetal outcome.[12] Second, although precise risk of exacerbation is difficult to quantitate, SLE may flare anytime during pregnancy, including the postpartum period. Third, renal insufficiency and hypertension may worsen during pregnancy, and active renal disease is associated with both unfavorable maternal and fetal outcome.[16] Finally, fetal outcome is related to presence of aPL, renal involvement,[10] and high levels of lupus disease activity.[8]

Antiphospholipid Syndrome

CASE STUDY 2

A 32-year-old woman presents with a recent fetal loss at 18 weeks after several weeks of poor fetal growth during her first pregnancy; past medical history is otherwise unremarkable. Routine laboratories are normal, ANA and anti-ds DNA antibodies are negative, IgG anticardiolipin is greater than 80 GPL units, and lupus anticoagulant is positive. The patient is anxious to conceive again and asks what therapy is advised for a next pregnancy, and what to expect for likelihood of successful pregnancy next time.

Maternal Considerations

Obstetric manifestations of antiphospholipid syndrome (APS) are not restricted to fetal loss. Current APS criteria include pregnancy loss or early delivery due to pre-eclampsia, IUGR, or fetal distress in the presence of persistent moderate to high titer anticardiolipin antibody (aCL), anti-β2-Glycoprotein I antibody (anti-β2GPI), or lupus anticoagulant.[26] Fetal loss (>10 weeks of gestation) is more strongly associated with aPL than are earlier pregnancy losses. Midtrimester loss is considered characteristic; however, up to one half of losses may be in the first trimester.[27] Since pre-embryonic and embryonic losses (< 10 weeks of gestation) are common in the general population, the diagnosis of APS should be made only with three or more consecutive losses in the absence of other identifiable etiologies. The two greatest risk factors for fetal loss are high titer IgG aCL and a history of previous fetal loss: these patients have up to 80% risk of current pregnancy loss if untreated.[28] Although aCL and LA are closely linked to pregnancy loss, the predictive value of anti-β2GPI for pregnancy loss is less well studied.[29] Concordance between types of aPLs are incomplete, so all should be tested if APS is suspected. Antibodies directed against other phospholipids, such as antiphosphatidylserine or antiphosphatidylethanolamine, do not generally identify additional patients and are not usually tested.[30]

Even in the presence of positive aPL antibody, exclusion of confounding conditions is important in patients with pregnancy morbidity, because more than one factor may be present. Gynecologic conditions may include uterine abnormalities, hormonal imbalance (e.g., luteal phase defect), maternal and paternal karyotype abnormalities, or fetal genetic abnormalities.

Other Maternal Complications

In addition to pregnancy loss, associated maternal obstetric complications include pre-eclampsia, eclampsia and HELLP syndrome.[31] Rates of gestational hypertension and pre-eclampsia range from 30% to 50%. Arterial or venous thrombosis and aPL manifestations such as severe thrombocytopenia may occur.[27] A report of cerebral infarction postpartum with discontinuation of aspirin therapy[32] emphasizes the importance of postpartum thromboprophylaxis. Finally, fifteen cases of catastrophic APS developing during pregnancy have been reported, many associated with concomitant HELLP syndrome.[33]

Pregnancy Outcome

Neonatal complications include prematurity and IUGR[34,35]; in one large series, the rate of preterm delivery was 43% and that of IUGR was 31%.[34] Preterm delivery is the strongest risk factor for adverse neonatal outcome[36] and reflects the greatest concern for patients with APS.

IgG aCL can traverse the placenta. Although most large studies of aPL pregnancies do not find fetal or neonatal thrombosis, rare cases of intrauterine thromboembolic stroke, arterial or venous thrombosis, and neonatal seizures have been reported.[37]

Although at least one large study suggests no long-term developmental abnormalities in offspring,[38] the rate of learning disability was increased in a single small series of 17 children of mothers with APS.[39]

Management and Therapy

Low-dose aspirin plus subcutaneous low-dose heparin is the standard prophylactic therapy during pregnancy for patients who have had prior pregnancy events. Untreated patients with high-titer aPL and a history of previous pregnancy loss have a high chance of subsequent fetal loss; with low-dose aspirin and heparin therapy, the likelihood of a full-term delivery rises to 70% to 80%.[27,40] A recent meta-analysis of randomized controlled trials of therapy for aPL-positive patients with pregnancy

loss found that low-dose aspirin and low-dose heparin significantly reduced risk of pregnancy loss compared with aspirin alone (relative risk [RR], 0.46). Aspirin alone did not show a significant reduction in rate of pregnancy loss (RR, 1.05). Prednisone and aspirin treatment increased risk of prematurity (RR, 4.83) but did not significantly decrease the risk of pregnancy loss (RR, 0.85).[40] Although initial studies used unfractionated heparin, most clinicians prefer low-molecular-weight heparin (LMWH) owing to convenience and lower risk of side effects including osteoporosis; recent small studies suggest at least equal efficacy.[41] LMWH dosing is not uniform, but pregnancy-related pharmacokinetic changes suggest LMWH might best be given twice daily, even for pregnancy prophylaxis therapy.[42] LMWH is generally converted to unfractionated heparin several weeks before the expected due date due to the latter's shorter half-life.

There are no clear guidelines in the management of patients in a first pregnancy, or those who have no, one, or two embryonic or pre-embryonic losses; however, low-dose aspirin treatment is often given to these patients because of its low-risk profile. Low-dose aspirin and heparin in therapeutic doses with midinterval partial thromboplastin time (aPTT) or anti-factor-Xa level monitoring must be used in patients with APS with a history of vascular thrombosis. IVIG has been used in addition to aspirin and heparin for those in whom standard therapy has failed, although a small placebo-controlled study showed no benefit.[43] Suggested guidelines for therapy of aPL pregnancies are shown in Table 31-3.

All patients require at least 6 weeks of anticoagulation postpartum, whether with aspirin alone, heparin, or warfarin. The importance of fetal monitoring during pregnancy should also be emphasized. Nonstress tests, biophysical profiles, or fetal umbilical artery Doppler velocimetry starting at 26 to 28 weeks may provide early indications of fetal distress requiring intervention.

During long-term follow-up, long-term low-dose aspirin appears to be protective against development of vascular thrombosis in patients with APS with a history of pregnancy morbidity alone[44] and is generally recommended.

Rheumatoid Arthritis

CASE STUDY 3

A 24-year-old woman with rheumatoid arthritis (RA) presents for evaluation. She just determined that she is 4 weeks pregnant. Her symptoms have been well controlled on etanercept 50 mg weekly and naproxen 500 mg bid. How do you advise her regarding medications and what to expect in terms of disease activity and pregnancy outcome?

Table 31-3. *Suggested Treatment of aPL Antibody in Pregnancy*

Patient/Serology	Obstetric History	Treatment
Low titer aCL/aβ2GPI	First pregnancy and/or no history of loss	None
Low titer aCL/aβ2GPI	1–2 early losses	Ld aspirin
Mod-high titer aCL/aβ2GPI or positive LA	0–2 early losses	Ld aspirin
HTN or abnormal renal function plus any aPL	First pregnancy and/or no history of loss	Ld aspirin (preeclampsia prophylaxis)
Positive aPL	≥ 3 early losses or ≥ 1 fetal loss	Ld aspirin and prophylactic* heparin/LMWH
Positive aPL	Previous IUGR/ Preeclampsia/ Placental infarction/ Other prothrombotic risk/ Special circumstances (e.g., AMA and IVF)	Ld aspirin and prophylactic* heparin/LMWH
Positive aPL and previous thrombosis	Any	Ld aspirin and therapeutic* heparin/LMWH (heparin while trying to conceive)
Positive aPL and Ld aspirin and heparin failure	≥ 3 early losses or ≥ 1 fetal loss	Consider addition of IVIG to low dose aspirin/heparin

aβ2GPI, anti-β2-glycoprotein I antibody; aCL, anticardiolipin antibody; AMA, advanced maternal age; IUGR: intrauterine growth restriction; IVF: in vitro fertilization; IVIG: intravenous immunoglobulin G; LA, lupus anticoagulant; Ld aspirin, low dose aspirin; LMWH, low-molecular-weight heparin.
*See text for dose recommendations:
Early loss: < 10 weeks
Fetal loss: ≥10 weeks

Maternal Considerations

The effect of pregnancy on RA is usually positive: up to 73% of patients experience some degree of clinical remission of symptoms during pregnancy, even in the absence of usual medications. In one series of 308 pregnancies, amelioration in symptoms was detected in about 50% of patients in the first trimester, in an additional 14% in the second trimester, and in a further 6% in the third trimester. Improvement persisted throughout the course of the pregnancy.[45] A prospective study of 140 women with RA during pregnancy demonstrated significant variability in degree of response, however, with about one quarter of patients doing worse, two thirds partially improved and only 16% of patients attaining complete remission.[46]

Regardless of the degree of improvement experienced during gestation, most patients relapse following delivery, many of these within the first 6 weeks, and almost all by 4 months.[45] Although this suggests that pregnancy-related hormones might influence remission, breastfeeding does not appear to change the timing of relapse. Recent work suggests that persistence of active disease during pregnancy may relate to a similarity between maternal and fetal HLA (HLA-DQ system).[47]

The effect of pregnancy on the development of RA is controversial. Pregnancy as well as use of oral contraceptives has been suggested to reduce the risk of disease onset,[48] and an increased risk of disease onset is noted in the postpartum period.[49] A recent study, however, suggests no protective effect of parity but does demonstrate a protective effect of breastfeeding against development of RA.[50]

Pregnancy Outcome

Fertility is not clearly decreased in patients with RA, and no increase in fetal loss has been demonstrated.[4] A slightly increased rate of fetal complications of prematurity and low birth weight has been reported, however, and rates of pre-eclampsia and cesarean section are higher than in the general population.[4,51] A case of marked fetal growth retardation has been described in severe RA with associated vasculitis.[52]

Management and Therapy

Few of the common medications for treatment of RA are considered safe during pregnancy; fortunately, owing to high likelihood of at least partial remission, many patients discontinue medication entirely or can be managed with low doses of corticosteroid.

As with all rheumatic disease patients, the patient with RA should be counseled before attempting pregnancy. The preconception visit should include discussion of the likelihood (but not certainty) of some degree of remission, recommendations for discontinuation of medications as necessary, and the potential adverse effects of any medications that will be continued. Note that testing for presence of anti-SSA/Ro and anti-SSB/La antibodies should be done, and patients with positive results should be counseled and monitored as described earlier in the section on NLE.

Potential fetal effects of medications are discussed in detail at the end of the chapter. In general, NSAIDs are avoided, plaquinil and sulfasalazine may be continued, and methotrexate must be discontinued at least 3 months before conceiving. Leflunomide must be discontinued and "washed out" with a course of cholestyramine. Tumor necrosis factor (TNF) inhibitors have not been proven safe during pregnancy, but reports of immediate pre-pregnancy or early first-trimester use are reassuring,[53] and if required, the fetal risk of continuing these until the diagnosis of pregnancy appears to be quite low. This is especially important for patients with fertility issues: although pregnancy may bring about remission, it may take many months to conceive for some patients. If even young RA patients experience delay in conceiving, aggressive pursuit of fertility therapy may minimize the amount of time their joints are not optimally protected. Low-dose prednisone (with calcium and vitamin D supplementation) is used as necessary throughout pregnancy.

Although uncommon, cervical spine arthritis with atlantoaxial instability requires careful management of the patient under general anesthesia since manipulation of the unstable spine may produce spinal cord compression. Severe cricoarytenoid involvement may also be a relative contraindication to intubation with general anesthesia. Hip range of motion should be assessed for adequacy before anticipated vaginal delivery. Stress dose steroid should be administered if the patient has been on long-term steroid therapy, and prophylactic antibiotics are recommended for patients with prosthetic joints.

A particular concern for the RA patient is the near-certainty of postpartum flare. For patients with severe erosive disease, it may be wise to recommend avoiding breastfeeding and restarting combination therapy immediately postpartum. Patients with mild disease often elect to breastfeed until they flare, then wean and restart medications.

Other Inflammatory Arthritides

Although little in the literature has focused on other types of inflammatory arthritis during pregnancy, juvenile RA patients appear to have similar positive effects on disease activity.[54,55] Psoriatic arthritis also tends to improve during pregnancy, unlike ankylosing spondylitis, in which the majority of patients have unchanged or worsened symptoms.[55]

Systemic Sclerosis

Because systemic sclerosis (SSc) often affects women in later reproductive years, pregnancy during established disease is less common than with SLE or RA.

CASE STUDY 4

A 30-year-old woman was diagnosed with diffuse scleroderma several months ago. Her symptoms of puffy hands, difficulty swallowing, and mild shortness of breath have been present for 1 year. Her blood pressure is 138/94, and renal function is normal. High-resolution chest computed tomography shows changes consistent with interstitial lung involvement. She would like to conceive as soon as possible. How would you advise her?

Maternal Considerations

Early reports of maternal morbidity in scleroderma pregnancy were negative: in a combined analysis of early studies, about one third of patients reported pregnancy-related aggravation of their disease.[56] Ten percent died of pregnancy-related complications, primarily hypertension, renal failure, and cardiovascular complications. Importantly, however, these series included a number of cases described before advances in management.

In contrast, a retrospective case-control study[57] found no difference in the rates of accelerated hypertension or renal failure in parous versus nulliparous scleroderma patients, suggesting that pregnancy may not adversely affect disease course. Incidence of hypertension, pre-eclampsia, or proteinuria was no different in pregnancies after diagnosis as compared with pregnancies before diagnosis of disease. In Steen's prospective studies of 91 pregnancies in 59 patients with systemic sclerosis,[58] maternal outcome was generally good, with worsening of disease during pregnancy in about 20% of patients. Raynaud's phenomenon improved during pregnancy, whereas esophageal reflux became worse. There were three cases of renal crisis during pregnancy, all in women with early diffuse disease.[58,59]

Pregnancy Outcome

Scleroderma patients were initially reported to have both decreased fertility and decreased parity when compared with control populations. Early case-control studies showed twice the rate of spontaneous abortion and three times the rate of infertility compared with controls as well as a significant incidence of IUGR and preterm births that occurred with equal frequency before and after the diagnosis of systemic sclerosis.[60] More recent prospective data, however, show no consistent decrease in fertility[59] or increase in frequency of miscarriage except in the subgroup of patients with long-standing diffuse scleroderma, in which miscarriage rates are as high as 45%.[58] Preterm births occurred in 29% of pregnancies, but neonatal survival was good. Of note, four women in this series had five healthy infants while taking angiotensin-converting enzyme (ACE) inhibitors.[58,59]

Management and Therapy

Preconception evaluation of disease status and organ function is critical in advising patients with systemic sclerosis about pregnancy. Patients with early diffuse disease are advised to delay pregnancy if possible until disease stabilizes, to reduce the risk of renal crisis during pregnancy. ACE inhibitors should be stopped due to risk of fetal toxicity, and other antihypertensives should be substituted. It is prudent to make this change before pregnancy and to observe for a minimum of several months to be confident that blood pressure is adequately controlled. Once pregnant, blood pressure and renal function should be monitored carefully, and include use of home blood pressure monitoring. For true scleroderma renal crisis during pregnancy, a life-threatening complication, ACE inhibitors are the only effective therapy and must be used to protect maternal health.

Skin thickening may be a concern for intravenous access or cesarean section, but wound healing is generally normal. In patients with severe Raynaud's phenomenon, warming the patient throughout labor and delivery with use of blankets, socks, and increased room temperature may minimize symptoms.

Women with severe cardiac, renal, or pulmonary disease for whom pregnancy is contraindicated may consider in vitro fertilization and surrogate pregnancy with a gestational carrier.

Sjögren's Syndrome

Sjögren's syndrome is often secondary to RA and other autoimmune diseases, and relatively little is known about the interaction of pregnancy with the primary syndrome other than the obvious concern of NLE from fetal exposure to anti-SSA/Ro and anti-SSB/La antibodies.

CASE STUDY 5

A 28-year-old woman with primary Sjögren's syndrome wishes to conceive. She has high-titer anti-SS-A/Ro antibody, and mild eye and mouth dryness with occasional arthalgias. She is on no medications other than topical cyclosporine eye-drops. How do you advise her?

Maternal Considerations

Few studies have assessed maternal morbidity in primary Sjögren's syndrome, and many of the reported pregnancies have occurred before the diagnosis of disease because peak onset of disease tends to be in the later reproductive years. Scattered case reports describe rare but severe complications, including onset of Sjögren's syndrome during pregnancy with renal insufficiency requiring hemodialysis and aggressive treatment with steroid and cyclophosphamide,[61] as well as a patient with established Sjögren's syndrome who developed mesangial proliferative glomerulonephritis during pregnancy.[62]

Pregnancy Outcome

Fetal and neonatal outcome have been evaluated in patients with primary Sjögren's syndrome in several studies with inconsistent results.[63,64] One study suggested that pregnancies in patients with the primary syndrome may have an increased risk of fetal loss, unrelated to presence of aPL or anti-SSA/Ro and anti-SSB/La antibodies.[63] Fetal growth retardation appears to be uncommon. A more recent case control study found primary Sjögren's syndrome to have no impact on pregnancy outcome.[64] Of note, most patients in both studies were diagnosed with Sjögren's syndrome after their last birth, which is consistent with the later age of onset in many patients.

The major neonatal risk is that of NLE, described in detail earlier. The risk of development of NLE is related only to the presence of anti-SSA/Ro and anti-SSB/La antibodies and not to the underlying connective tissue disease diagnosis.

Management and Therapy

The most common management issue during pregnancy is appropriate monitoring or treatment for CHB or other inflammatory cardiac manifestations in the fetus, as detailed earlier.

Although many patients choose to discontinue topical cyclosporine eye-drops, this is unnecessary: cyclosporine has little effect on fetal development and may be safely continued during pregnancy. Although uncommon, severe neurologic or renal involvement during pregnancy may be treated with corticosteroids. Immunosuppressives (other than azathioprine) should not be used.

Polymyositis and Dermatomyositis

CASE STUDY 6

A 30-year-old woman with a history of juvenile dermatomyositis (DM) presents at 6 weeks of pregnancy. She has been asymptomatic for the last 4 years and off all medications. She asks what the chances of flare during pregnancy are, and what to expect in terms of pregnancy outcome.

Maternal Considerations

Although polymyositis (PM) and DM are relatively uncommon, a number of reports describe pregnancies in association with these diseases.[65-72] Pregnancies have been reported during both quiescent and active disease, and a fair number of patients have presented with new-onset disease during pregnancy or in the postpartum period.[67,71,72] Disease presenting during pregnancy may be acute and severe, and often improves after delivery. Associated rhabdomyolysis and myoglobinuria have been reported.[65] Overall, the risk of flare during pregnancy for patients in remission is about 25%, and although disease with onset during pregnancy appears to have a more severe course, for most patients, maternal outcome is good and maternal mortality is rare.[70]

Pregnancy Outcome

The presence of active disease appears to have an adverse effect on pregnancy outcome.[65,69,70] Neonatal outcome is worst for patients with new-onset disease during pregnancy, with only 38% survival rate.[73] Neonatal outcome for patients with established diagnoses who are in remission before conception is better, with no increased risk of fetal loss. Of nine patients with established disease in a recent retrospective analysis, the five with quiescent disease had uneventful pregnancies and delivered at term. Of the four patients (seven pregnancies) with active disease at conception, four pregnancies ended in spontaneous abortion, two deliveries were preterm, and only one was uneventful. Mean birth weight was higher in the inactive disease group.[70] Another small series of four patients reported a fetal loss and a spontaneous abortion in the two active patients (one on methotrexate) with successful outcome in the two patients in remission.[69]

In addition to prematurity, other rarer neonatal complications have been described: two infants have been reported with elevated creatine kinase (CK) levels that persisted for several months after birth.[72] In addition, several cases of massive perivillous fibrin deposition in the placenta (a pathology finding generally associated with clinical evidence of placental insufficiency) have been reported in association with polymyositis.[74]

Management and Therapy

As with SLE, timing of pregnancy in relation to disease onset or exacerbation has a significant effect on pregnancy outcome. Prepregnancy evaluation of patients with known PM/DM for assessing disease activity is critical, and patients with active disease should be encouraged to postpone pregnancy until they reach remission. No evidence supports prophylactic corticosteroid treatment of patients in remission; however, prompt diagnosis and corticosteroid therapy of new-onset disease or flare in pregnancy may improve prognosis. Certain steroid-sparing drugs may be used, if necessary, including cyclosporine and azathioprine. Of interest are recent reports of treatment with IVIG,[68] including an unusual case of successful treatment in a high-risk patient with early-onset disease in the first trimester who received steroid and monthly IVIG, resulting in remission and successful term delivery.[71]

Behçet's Disease

CASE STUDY 7

A 26-year-old woman of Turkish descent presents during the first trimester of her second pregnancy. She was diagnosed with Behçet's syndrome 5 years earlier when she presented with recurrent oral and genital ulcerations, arthritis, and mild uveitis. Her first pregnancy 2 years ago was complicated by a flare requiring low-dose corticosteroid treatment in the first trimester. She asks if she should start on steroid now to prevent a flare in her current pregnancy. She is currently at 5 weeks' gestation.

Maternal Considerations

Behçet's disease primarily presents during the reproductive years. Early case reports suggested contradictory findings of pregnancy effect on disease activity,[75–77] with individual case reports documenting both exacerbations and remissions of disease. In one family, a mother and two daughters had severe and prolonged exacerbation of disease during pregnancies.[75] One daughter experienced similar symptoms while on oral contraceptives, and the mother's symptoms remitted with menopause. In another case,[76] a woman with mild manifestations developed severe oral and genital ulcers and iridocyclitis by week 25 of gestation. Postpartum chronic uveitis occurred with visual loss. Other case reports describe dramatic amelioration of all symptoms during pregnancy, with exacerbation in the postpartum period.[77]

Recent studies suggest little or variable effect of pregnancy on the course of Behçet's disease,[78,79] both between patients and within different pregnancies in the same patient. A recent retrospective series of 44 pregnancies in 28 women showed exacerbation in 27% of patients, with remission in 52% and no change in the remaining cases.[78] Finally, a case-control study of 31 women with 135 pregnancies showed an increased rate of remission during pregnancy and postpartum compared with controls, with exacerbations in only one sixth of the patients.[79] Thromboembolic disease, already a potential complication in Behçet's disease, may be increased: one report describes a patient with Behçet's disease with superior vena cava thrombosis and pulmonary embolism during pregnancy.[80]

Pregnancy Outcome

No clear deleterious effect on fetal outcome is demonstrated, although one case-control study identified a significantly increased rate of miscarriage, pregnancy complications, and cesarean section.[79] Overall fetal outcome is generally good, although rare infants with pustulonecrotic skin lesions and other manifestations have been reported.[81] Lesions healed with scarring by 8 weeks. A neonate of a mother with Behçet's disease has been reported who developed generalized seizures and cerebral ischemia at 6 days of life, with no other identifiable etiology; this was suggested to represent neonatal Behçet's disease.[82]

Management and Therapy

Patients with Behçet's disease are generally treated with corticosteroids and, for severe manifestations, immunosuppressive medications. Azathioprine may be continued during pregnancy, if necessary, but other immunosuppressive agents are contraindicated. Prepregnancy counseling should include the unpredictability of pregnancy course, with possible exacerbation or remission related to pregnancy, and the need to discontinue teratogenic medications.

VASCULITIS SYNDROMES

Takayasu's Arteritis

Unlike most vasculitides, Takayasu's arteritis generally affects young women during their reproductive years and presents particular concerns, especially during the peripartum period.

CASE STUDY 8

A 32-year-old woman has a 7-year history of Takayasu's arteritis. Blood pressure is well controlled on atenalol 100 mg daily, and she has a known asymptomatic noncritical stenosis of the left carotid artery. She wishes to conceive but is afraid she will have a stroke. How do you advise her?

Maternal Considerations

Despite a high rate of maternal complications, pregnancy in patients with Takayasu's arteritis generally has a good outcome if blood pressure is aggressively controlled. Potential for maternal complications is most closely related to severity of underlying established vascular disease: there is no evidence of significant relapse in disease activity during pregnancy.[73]

Pre-eclampsia is significantly increased owing to the high prevalence of chronic hypertension.[83,84] In describing the clinical course of 33 pregnancies, Ishikawa and Matsuura[83] found that two thirds of patients developed complications, including hypertension, congestive heart failure, and cerebral ischemia in four patients; worsening renal insufficiency may also occur.[84] A large series included a total of 30 pregnancies in 13 patients both before and after diagnosis: as expected, the 11 pregnancies before disease onset were uneventful. In the 19 pregnancies complicated by Takayasu's, one was electively terminated and three ended in spontaneous abortion. Most of the remaining pregnancies were complicated by pre-eclampsia (11/15), although no

case of eclampsia was seen. More than half of the patients were first diagnosed during their pregnancy. No major obstetric problems were noted other than hypertension, and pharmacologic therapy for hypertension was required in half of the pregnancies.[85] Pregnancy-related hypertension and pre-eclampsia likely increase the risk of neurologic events, including stroke or seizure.[83,84] In addition, severe aortic valvular disease and aortic aneurism are risk factors for maternal morbidity and mortality and represent contraindications to pregnancy.

Pregnancy Outcome

Fetal outcome in Takayasu's arteritis is generally good, although IUGR and premature delivery affect up to 40% of neonates.[73] Changes in placental blood flow may influence outcome: development of IUGR is related to severity of hypertension, extent of abdominal aorta and renal artery involvement, and onset of pre-eclampsia.[85]

Management and Therapy

Usual management during pregnancy includes corticosteroid, if indicated, for active disease; careful monitoring and treatment of hypertension; and aggressive hemodynamic and pharmacologic management in the peripartum period. Cardiac function should be assessed at baseline and periodically throughout the pregnancy, if necessary. Abdominal aortic aneurysms are at risk of rupture or thrombus if compressed by the enlarged uterus.[86]

Aggressive hemodynamic monitoring and management of anesthesia are critical in the peripartum period, because the risk of complications appears greatest around the time of delivery. Both hypertension and hypotension should be avoided due to vessel changes with marked variation in regional blood flow and, potentially, in organ perfusion. Although both general and epidural anesthesia may affect blood pressure, epidural anesthesia is preferred owing to less significant fluctuation and easier assessment of cerebral blood flow in the conscious patient.[86] Cesarean section should be scheduled for patients with extensive vascular involvement or uncontrolled hypertension, because labor itself increases blood pressure significantly and may increase risk of stroke.

Importantly, peripheral blood pressure monitoring may be inaccurate, and central monitoring may be necessary. Tomioka and associates[87] reported a young woman with Takayasu's arteritis and cerebral hemorrhage during a previous normal vaginal delivery. Blood pressure was successfully managed by monitoring central aortic blood pressure at the thoracic aorta during a subsequent uncomplicated delivery. Even more extensive monitoring has been described: a patient with pulseless upper extremities, history of cerebrovascular disease, and severe bilateral carotid artery stenoses was additionally monitored with processed electroencephalography to detect cerebral ischemia during cesarean section.[88] Surgery was uncomplicated. Chronic disease may require vascular surgery intervention even during or immediately following the pregnancy.

OTHER VASCULITIDES

Polyarteritis Nodosa

Maternal Considerations

Pregnancy in association with polyarteritis nodosa (PAN) is relatively uncommon owing to the older mean age at onset and the male predominance of the disease. For the pregnant patient, time of onset of disease affects both maternal and fetal outcomes. Initial presentation of PAN during pregnancy results in significant maternal mortality, with better fetal than maternal outcome.[89,90] Whether pregnancy actually affects the course of PAN is unclear.

In cases of PAN reported in pregnancy, the disease had its onset during pregnancy or in the immediate postpartum period more than half of the time. Few patients who present during pregnancy have been diagnosed and treated at the time of onset. In one series, of the seven cases reported with onset during pregnancy, all seven patients died by postpartum day 42, with diagnosis made at autopsy for six of the seven cases.[89] Outcome is significantly better for patients with established disease who are in clinical remission at the time of pregnancy.[90,91] Pre-eclampsia with malignant hypertension and acute renal failure has been reported in a case of stable PAN, with dramatic improvement after delivery.[92] PAN is a rapidly fatal disease without appropriate therapy, and it is likely that the high maternal mortality seen with new-onset disease in pregnancy reflects at least partly the difficulty in diagnosis, especially when hypertension and renal insufficiency may be interpreted as being due to pre-eclampsia.

Pregnancy Outcome

Fetal outcome has been surprisingly good, probably because most reported cases of PAN with onset during pregnancy have been in the third trimester or immediate postpartum period. In one series, eight of 10 pregnancies produced viable neonates.[89] Several infants have been reported with transient cutaneous vasculitis.[93]

Management and Therapy

The effect of pregnancy on PAN is not clear, because a number of cases reported were not diagnosed until postmortem. Patients in remission before pregnancy report a low rate of exacerbation. Mild manifestations may be treated with corticosteroids, but more severe manifestations require appropriate immunosuppressive therapy. Therapeutic termination of pregnancy may be considered for severe disease presenting in the first trimester. Immunosuppressive therapy with cyclophosphamide is contraindicated owing to risk of teratogenicity in the first trimester, but has been used anecdotally in patients with vasculitis during the second and third trimesters for life-threatening disease.

Churg-Strauss Syndrome

Maternal Considerations

Relapse rate among women with Churg-Strauss syndrome (CSS) who conceive during a period of remission is fairly significant, approaching 50%.[94] The first successful pregnancy described was a 33-year-old woman with a 1-year history of CSS who presented with mononeuritis multiplex, cutaneous vasculitis, and pleuritis at the 24th week of pregnancy. Treated with high-dose corticosteroid, she ultimately delivered a healthy infant with mild IUGR. Numbers are small, but it is likely that maternal mortality rate in CSS pregnancy is less than that seen with PAN.[95] In a review of eight women who conceived while in remission, two developed worsening asthma and two relapsed with mononeuritis and rash.[86] Exacerbation induced by pregnancy is also suggested by one case with relapse of disease in four successive pregnancies, which was fatal in the fourth pregnancy despite aggressive treatment of fulminant vasculitis and cardiac disease.[96] Maternal and fetal prognoses are likely worse when disease onset is during pregnancy.

Pregnancy Outcome

Pregnancy outcome appears fairly successful in the limited number of cases reported, although prematurity and low birth weight are common.[94] A successful twin pregnancy has been reported after treatment with corticosteroid and cyclophosphamide.[97]

Management and Therapy

As with most other rheumatic diseases, pregnancy should be planned, when possible, during a period of quiescence with vigilant monitoring for evidence of relapse. There are reported successful pregnancy outcomes with steroid and azathioprine, and a recent successful pregnancy treated with intravenous immunoglobulin.[98] Bronchospasm may worsen during pregnancy and should be monitored.[86]

Wegener's Granulomatosis

Maternal Considerations

The spectrum of clinical manifestations of Wegener's granulomatosis (WG) appears to be similar in pregnant and nonpregnant patients. As with other vasculitides, it appears that new-onset WG during pregnancy may have a more aggressive course.[99-102] A recent literature review identified 21 pregnancies in 18 patients with WG and pregnancy.[99] Twelve of the 18 patients were initially diagnosed with WG during the course of the affected pregnancy (including postpartum diagnoses). Cases with new diagnosis during pregnancy have had variable presentations, including new onset tracheal stenosis.[102] New diagnosis may occur during any stage of pregnancy including the postpartum period. Diagnosis in the first trimester presents a particularly difficult problem. Palit and Clague[100] reported a woman who presented with arthritis, hemoptysis, dyspnea, and other symptoms at week 7 of pregnancy. Because of concerns regarding teratogenicity of cyclophosphamide, the patient terminated pregnancy. Another patient with arthralgia, cutaneous lesions, hemoptysis, renal insufficiency, and nasal symptoms at 17 weeks of pregnancy was diagnosed on nasal biopsy, and was treated with oral cyclophosphamide, corticosteroid, and hemodialysis during the second and third trimesters, with delivery of a healthy male infant at 33 weeks' gestation.[101] In a review of nine cases of exacerbation of existing disease during pregnancy, there were two relapses during second pregnancies and two maternal deaths.[99]

Overall, patients with active disease at conception or new-onset disease during pregnancy are at high risk for poor maternal outcome; those who conceive during remission have a relapse rate estimated at 25% which may not be different from that expected in nonpregnant patients.[73]

Pregnancy Outcome

Premature delivery is common, especially in patients with active disease, but outcome otherwise appears unremarkable.

Management and Therapy

It may be difficult to distinguish WG renal relapse from pre-eclampsia. Active urine sediment suggests WG, whereas hypertension is more characteristic of pre-eclampsia. Of note, in severely affected patients, subglottic stenosis may complicate delivery and a temporary tracheotomy may be required to protect the airway.[86] Usual medical treatment of WG involves both high-dose corticosteroid and immunosuppressive medication, usually oral cyclophosphamide. Cyclophosphamide is relatively contraindicated during pregnancy especially during the first trimester due to risk of teratogenicity. Ideally, pregnancy should be planned during a period of remission. For patients with active disease presenting during pregnancy, alternative therapy with corticosteroid alone or with azathioprine should be considered. Severe disease requires use of cyclophosphamide: a small number of patients with active disease in the late second or third trimesters have been successfully treated with cyclophosphamide with good neonatal outcome.[101,103,104] In at least one severe case, successful aggressive therapy has included empiric intravenous immunoglobulin and plasma exchange to avoid use of cyclophosphamide.[101]

Microscopic Polyangiitis

Although few cases of pregnancy in patients with microscopic polyangiitis have been reported, successful cases have been described,[105] as well as a maternal death due to methicillin-resistant *Staphylococcal aureus* pneumonia during therapy with corticosteroid and cyclophosphamide.[106] Interestingly, cases of neonatal myeloperoxidase antibody (MPO) antineutrophil cytoplasmic antibody (ANCA)–associated pulmonary-renal syndrome have been described in infants of women with microscopic polyangiitis.[107]

MEDICATIONS DURING PREGNANCY

Rheumatic disease patients frequently require drug treatment during pregnancy to control underlying disease or to promote successful pregnancy outcome. Use of any medication in pregnancy is always a careful consideration of risks versus benefits. Concerns during pregnancy include the risk of inducing fetal malformation or causing fetal organ damage, and the contribution to maternal pregnancy complications such as hypertension, diabetes, or pre-eclampsia.

The US Food and Drug Administraton (FDA) pregnancy categories are largely based on animal data for the more recently released drugs, and so are not necessarily helpful in clinical decision making. What follows is a brief summary of standard use of common rheumatic disease medications in pregnancy (Table 31-4). A recent comprehensive consensus paper on anti-inflammatory and immunosuppressive drugs in reproduction covers this subject in detail.[108]

Aspirin and Nonsteroidal Anti-inflammatory Drugs

Because of greater experience in pregnancy, aspirin is preferred to the relatively newer nonsteroidal anti-inflammatory drugs (NSAIDs), although nonselective NSAIDs, particularly ibuprofen, are occasionally used until the last 8 weeks of pregnancy.[108] After this, they may cause prolonged labor, increased bleeding, impaired renal function, and premature closure of the ductus arteriosus with fetal pulmonary hypertension. Low-dose aspirin (less than 325 mg/day), however, does not increase these risks. There is no consensus as to whether low-dose aspirin must be discontinued before delivery to reduce risk of bleeding with epidural anesthesia. Cyclooxygenase-2 (COX-2) inhibitors are avoided owing to limited experience in pregnancy. Acetaminophen is safe for simple analgesia but can be insufficient to control pain and arthritis; low-dose corticosteroid is preferable to control joint symptoms.

Table 31-4. *Medication Use in Pregnancy*

Medication	FDA	Recommendations
NSAIDs	B or C	Avoid; contraindicated after 32 weeks due to premature closure of the ductus arteriosus

Corticosteroid:
  Prednisolone
  Methylprednisolone
	B or C	Little placental transfer; generally safe

Fluorinated Corticosteroid:
  Dexamethasone
  Betamethasone
	C	Cross placenta well: use for fetal effect only
		(Betamethasone preferred: no indication of adverse developmental effects long term)

Antimalarials: Hydroxychloroquine	C	Maternal benefit in SLE; generally safe
Sulfasalzine	B	Generally safe (maximum dose 2 g/day)
Colchicine	C	Probably safe; consider amniocentesis to rule out chromosomal abnormalities
TNF inhibitors	B	Unknown; data on early limited exposure to infliximab and etanercept reassuring. Recommend stop once conceive.

Immunosuppressives:
  Azathioprine
  Cyclophosphamide
  Methotrexate
  Leflunomide
  Cyclosporine
	D
	D
	X
	X
	C
		Widely used (rare fetal cytopenias)
		Contraindicated; rare use in second or third trimester
		Contraindicated
		Contraindicated (wash-out before conceiving)
		Widely used

Intravenous immunoglobulin	C	Generally safe

Other biologicals:
  Rituximab
  Abatacept
	C
	C
		Unknown: avoid
		Unknown: avoid

Anticoagulants:
  Low dose aspirin
  Heparin and LMWH
  Warfarin
	D
	C
	X
		Generally safe, no risk of ductus closure with low dose
		Safe: no placental transfer
		Teratogenic first trimester; rare use in later trimesters

LMWH, low-molecular-weight heparin; NSAIDs, nonsteroidal anti-inflammatory drugs; SLE, systemic lupus erythematosus; TNF, tumor necrosis factor.

Corticosteroids

In conventional doses, prednisone and methylprednisolone are safe for the fetus due to the extensive placental metabolism, although risk of corticosteroid-induced maternal hypertension, maternal hyperglycemia, and premature rupture of membranes is increased.[109] The fetal effect (plasma level) in a woman taking a maternal dose of prednisone of 20 mg/day or less is considered insignificant, although a small increased risk of oral cleft has been reported with first-trimester corticosteroid exposure.[110] Fluorinated corticosteroids (dexamethasone and betamethasone) easily cross the placenta and should not be used unless the goal is treatment of the fetus; recent recommendations suggest betamethasone as the preferred agent since dexamethasone may negatively affect neuropsychological development of the offspring.[108] High-dose intravenous (pulse) methylprednisolone does reach the fetus, with unknown effects. Patients on chronic corticosteroid therapy should receive stress-dose steroid at the time of delivery, especially if delivery is by cesarean section. Patients with single-joint arthritis or bursitis can be safely treated with intra-articular or intrabursal corticosteroid injections to avoid systemic therapy.

Antimalarial Drugs

Until recently, hydroxychloroquine (HCQ) was often stopped before pregnancy: it is known to cross the placenta, and the theoretical risk of eye and ear abnormalities were a source of concern. Discontinuation of antimalarial drugs immediately before or at the onset of pregnancy, however, can precipitate a lupus flare,[6,7] whereas women who continue HCQ during pregnancy may be maintained on lower average corticosteroid dose.[7] Safety of HCQ in pregnancy was demonstrated in a controlled retrospective study of 133 HCQ-treated pregnancies[6]: rates of live birth and congenital malformations were not significantly different, and short term follow-up (mean 26 months) did not reveal any visual, hearing, or developmental abnormalities.

Sulfasalazine

In general, sulfasalazine may be continued during pregnancy. There have been rare case reports of congenital cardiovascular defects and oral clefts with first trimester exposure. Folate supplementation decreases the risk, and the sulfasalazine dose should not exceed 2 g/day.[108]

Colchicine

Colchicine is commonly used to treat Behçet's disease and autoinflammatory syndromes such as familial Mediterranean fever; safety in pregnancy has been controversial. Anecdotal reports suggested risk of chromosomal abnormalities in offspring (possibly due to inhibition of mitosis), and amniocentesis has been routinely recommended for patients who continue colchicine through pregnancy. Although recent reports are more reassuring, many authorities continue to perform amniocentesis for karyotyping while awaiting more definitive data to establish whether there is a higher risk of chromosomal anomalies in neonates of patients taking this medication during pregnancy.[111]

Tumor Necrosis Factor-α Inhibitors

All three TNF-α inhibitors (etanercept, infliximab, and adalimumab) are rated FDA pregnancy category "B," meaning that animal studies reveal no fetal harm but no adequate human studies are available. Although no studies in pregnant women have been conducted for any of the TNF-α inhibitors, a limited number of case reports in humans have not identified developmental problems.[53] In general, for severe arthritis, it appears to be reasonable to allow patients to continue these drugs until pregnancy is diagnosed; patients with mild arthritis may stop them before attempting to conceive. Continuing TNF-α inhibitors through pregnancy is not generally recommended, although data are limited and several successful cases are reported.[112] A meta-analysis of pregnancy in 108 rheumatology patients exposed to TNF-α inhibitors found no greater incidence of malformations than in the general population; however, only three neonates had mothers who continued treatment with TNF-α blockade throughout pregnancy, and one of these three neonates had a significant malformation.[112] The report, involving a vertebral anomaly, anal atresia, esophageal atresia and/or tracheoesophageal fistula, radial and renal anomalies (VATER) malformation, merits attention: other malformations reported in TNF-α inhibitor–related patients have been suggested to represent a partial VATER syndrome, and a causal relationship has been proposed between etanercept and such malformations through the inhibition of TNF-receptor–associated factor 4. Of note, however, the patient in the case report was treated with an unusually high dose of etanercept (50 mg twice weekly) throughout her entire pregnancy.[113]

Immunosuppressive Medications

More potent immunosuppressive medications are occasionally needed during pregnancy. Azathioprine, widely used in pregnant renal transplant patients for many years, is considered generally safe in pregnancy,

although fetal cytopenias have rarely occurred. Cyclophosphamide is contraindicated in early pregnancy because of its teratogenicity and abortifacient properties. Several women given cyclophosphamide during late pregnancy have had normal infants, but experience is small.[108] Ideally, pregnancy should not be attempted until 3 months after stopping the medication. Protection of gonadal function through the course of cyclophosphamide therapy with concomitant treatment with a gonadotropin-releasing hormone agonist is recommended for women of childbearing age; a common regimen is depot leuprolide acetate 3.75 mg[2] monthly, started at least 10 days before cyclophosphamide exposure.[114]

Methotrexate is contraindicated in pregnancy: it is abortifacient and causes a characteristic fetal syndrome of craniosynostosis and other malformations. Patients receiving methotrexate should not get pregnant until 3 months after stopping the medication, and folate supplementation should continue uninterrupted. Leflunomide is teratogenic in animals, but no human studies exist. Pregnancy should not be attempted until after elimination of the drug by treatment with cholestyramine: the recommended protocol is 8 g of cholestyramine three times per day for 11 days, followed by documentation of a plasma concentration of leflunomide M1 metabolite less than 0.02 mg/L on two separate tests at least 14 days apart.

Cyclosporine may cause significant maternal toxicity, especially nephrotoxicity, but appears to be safe for the fetus. There are limited animal data on mycophenolate mofetil but there are several reports of congenital anomalies in neonates: it is not recommended during pregnancy and should be discontinued 6 to 8 weeks before conception.[115]

Rituximab, anakinra, and abatacept are biologic agents approved for use in RA. No reasonable data are available on safety of use in pregnancy, and it is not recommended that these be used within at least several months of conception or during pregnancy.

Intravenous Immunoglobulin

IVIG may be safely used during pregnancy and may be especially effective for autoimmune thrombocytopenia, refractory aPL-associated pregnancy losses, and inflammatory myositis.

Anticoagulants

Heparin, which does not cross the placenta, is the preferred anticoagulant during pregnancy and is generally used as anticoagulation for the full 8 to 9 months of gestation, most often for patients with aPL. Maternal complications may include excessive bleeding and risk for osteoporosis. Both fractionated and unfractionated heparins are too large to pass through the placenta and so do not reach the fetal circulation. LMWH has been increasingly used owing to the low risk of heparin-induced thrombocytopenia and heparin-induced osteoporosis, and convenience of use. Bone mass at the lumbar spine has been demonstrated to be significantly decreased in patients receiving unfractionated heparin in comparison with those receiving LMWH during pregnancy, even up to 52 weeks' postpartum.[116]

A distinction is generally made in dosing between "prophylactic" or low dose, for pregnancy prophylaxis, and "therapeutic," or higher dose, for treatment of patients with history or presence of established thrombosis. Prophylactic unfractionated heparin is given as 5000 units^2 every 12 hours. Enoxaparin, a commonly used LMWH, is administered prophylactically as 30 mg^2 every 12 hours, or 40 mg^2 once daily (pregnancy-related pharmacokinetics suggest bid dosing may be more effective). Therapeutic unfractionated heparin dosing requires every-8-hour injections, with aPTT measured midway between doses, with a target of aPTT INR ratio of 2.5. Therapeutic LMWH must be given every 12 hours; for enoxaparin, the dose should be initiated at 1 mg/kg every 12 hours and adjusted according to peak and trough levels. Peak anti-Factor Xa levels should be measured 3 to 4 hours after the dose, and should not be greater than 1.2 anti-Xa units; trough levels should be measured within 1 hour of the next dose and should be more than 0.5 anti-Xa units.[42]

Warfarin during pregnancy is associated with a high incidence of fetal loss and congenital malformations, and may also cause fatal hemorrhage in the fetus. The teratogenic effects (fetal warfarin syndrome) include nasal hypoplasia, stippled epiphyses, limb hypoplasia, low birth weight, hearing loss, and ophthalmic anomalies. Warfarin has been used for pregnant patients with mechanical heart valves and in several reported cases of APS pregnancy[117]: it is thought to be fairly safe when instituted after the embryonic period, that is, after week 10 of gestation, although its use is more common in Europe than in the United States.

Other Medications

Other medications frequently used in rheumatic disease patients include antihypertensives and bisphosphonates. Preferred antihypertensives for pregnancy include methyldopa and labetalol. ACE inhibitors are contraindicated throughout pregnancy: in addition to fetal renal damage with second- and third-trimester use, congenital malformations have been reported with use in the first trimester.[118] Angiotensin II receptor blockers are avoided due to their similar mechanism.

Use of bisphosphonates in women of childbearing age is controversial owing to their prolonged half-lives and animal data suggesting decreased fetal bone growth. If use cannot be avoided in young female patients, pregnancy should be postponed for at least 6 months after discontinuation of bisphosphonates with continuation of calcium and vitamin D supplementation.[108] Owing to its shorter half

life, risedronate may be preferable to alendronate for young female patients who have not completed childbearing.

BREASTFEEDING IN RHEUMATIC DISEASE PATIENTS

For patients who are breastfeeding, heparin, warfarin, corticosteroids, hydroxychloroquine, sulfasalazine, aspirin, and certain NSAIDs may be administered; other drugs are discouraged. Most drug transfer to human milk is by passive diffusion. Because of its high molecular weight, heparin is unable to pass through cell membranes. Aspirin and NSAIDs, highly protein-bound weak acids, do not pass easily into breast milk. Passage of prednisone or methylprednisolone is low, and breastfeeding just before ingestion of medication minimizes infant corticosteroid exposure. Antimalarial drugs, as weak bases, are secreted in breast milk; however they are generally thought to be safe.[108] Sulfasalazine use during breastfeeding is generally safe also; however, infants may develop diarrhea. Colchicine levels in breast milk are one tenth the dose administered to the mother, and limited reports do not suggest adverse effects to the neonate.[119] Safety of breastfeeding while on TNF-α inhibitors is unknown and is not recommended, although, in theory, recombinant monoclonal antibodies should be destroyed in the neonatal gastrointestinal tract. Use of immunosuppressives in the breastfeeding mother should follow guidelines similar to those for pregnancy; generally, they are discouraged. If immunosuppressive therapy is required in the postpartum period, it is safest to discontinue breastfeeding before starting medication.

Although it is not known whether breast milk–transmitted autoantibodies are pathogenic, some investigators advise women with anti-SSA/Ro and anti-SSB/La antibodies against breastfeeding due to concern regarding risk of NLE.

Finally, because breastfeeding prolongs the pregnancy-induced decrease in bone mineral density, it may be inadvisable for patients with pre-existing osteoporosis, or those on long-term glucocorticoids or heparin to breastfeed for a significant period of time.

THE ROLE OF EFFECTIVE CONTRACEPTION

Of note, women with rheumatic diseases can and should use effective birth control to allow timing of pregnancy during an appropriate quiescent period. Safety of estrogen-containing oral contraceptive pills (OCPs) has long been a concern for patients with SLE. If patients are aPL-negative, have no history of thrombosis, and have inactive or stable disease, they may take combined OCPs with little or no risk of disease flare.[120] Patients with contraindications to estrogen-containing OCPs, including those with positive aPL, may use progesterone-only contraceptives, which include the progesterone-only pill, depot medroxyprogesterone acetate (DMPA) injections, and the levonorgestel intrauterine system (LNG IUS). The LNG IUS, a progesterone-containing intrauterine device, has few systemic effects but like other intrauterine devices, it should be avoided or used cautiously in patients on significant immunosuppressive therapy. Progesterone-only contraceptives do not increase risk of thrombosis, and usually decrease menstrual blood flow, which is useful for patients on warfarin. Although no data exist, it would seem prudent to avoid estrogen-containing contraceptives in patients with significant or active underlying vascular disease such as Behçet's disease, Takayasu's arteritis, or other less common vasculitides. DMPA, but not the progesterone pill or the LNG-IUS, may lower bone density and should be used with caution in patients with osteoporosis or on concomitant corticosteroids.[121] A summary of the merits and disadvantages of common contraceptives for patients with rheumatic disease appears in Table 31-5.

OVULATION INDUCTION AND IN VITRO FERTILIZATION

Concern about pregnancy and rheumatic disease may begin long before conception in patients undergoing infertility treatments. Fertility is not generally impaired by rheumatic diseases, but in patients treated with cytotoxic agents, fertility may decline early. Improved disease control and the availability of assisted reproductive techniques for couples with infertility make this issue increasingly common in SLE and other rheumatic diseases. Assisted reproductive techniques include ovarian stimulation, with or without in vitro fertilization (IVF) and subsequent embryo transfer.

Most of the limited literature has focused on patients with SLE and APS. The important risks of fertility drugs in these patients include hormone-associated flare or thrombosis. Risk of thrombosis is likely increased for patients with aPL, because high estrogen levels exert an additional prothrombotic effect. Although ovulation induction (OI)/IVF cycles are often successful in patients with SLE, complications are seen. Guballa and associates[122] reviewed histories of 19 women with SLE or APS who underwent 68 cycles of OI/IVF. Four of 19 patients had a flare of SLE, but no thromboses occurred, although it is important to note that most patients were treated prophylacticaly with aspirin or heparin.

Recommendations similar to those regarding pregnancy seem reasonable for rheumatic disease patients undergoing OI/IVF: patients should be evaluated and counseled regarding individual risk versus benefit. OI/IVF should be deferred in patients with active disease. Prophylactic therapy with low-dose aspirin in patients with asymptomatic aPL should be considered. Patients with APS and a history of thrombosis or fetal loss require subcutaneous heparin and low-dose aspirin. For patients with significant organ damage such as severe renal insufficiency or cardiomyopathy who could not safely go through pregnancy, a carefully monitored IVF cycle, followed by embryo transfer to a gestational carrier may allow a couple to have a biologic child while limiting risk to the mother's health.

Table 31-5. *Contraceptive Methods for Rheumatic Disease Patients—Benefits and Disadvantages*

Method of Contraception	Benefits	Disadvantages
Condoms	Lower risk of sexually transmitted disease No prescription needed	Low efficacy
Intrauterine device (IUD): Copper LNG-IUS*	Effective, good compliance Effective for 10 years Decreases menstrual blood flow, cramps, functional cysts (benefit for patients on warfarin)	Question use in nulligravid women Relatively contraindicated in patients on immune-suppressive drugs Often increases menstrual blood flow and cramps
Combined hormonal contraceptives: Oral Vaginal ring Combined patch	Effective; convenient No increased flare in stable SLE patients	Contraindicated in patients with thrombosis or moderate- to high-titer aPL Not evaluated in active SLE Risk of thrombosis with immobilization Possible difficulty with insertion if severe arthritis Greater estrogen exposure (60%)
Progestin contraceptives: Oral DMPA	Little prothrombotic risk and reduces menstrual flow–safe for aPL patients Effective, convenient	Irregular bleeding Must take same time daily Reversible osteoporosis

aPL, antiphospholipid antibodies; DMPA, depot medroxyprogesterone acetate; LNG-IUS, levonorgestrel intrauterine system; SLE, systemic lupus erythematosus.
*Intrauterine device and progestin contraceptive.

References

1. Gordon MC. Maternal physiology. In: Gabbe SG, Niebyl JR, Simpson JL, editors. Obstetrics: Normal and Problem Pregnancies. 5th ed. Philadelphia: Churchill Livingstone Elsevier; 2007. p. 56-84.
2. Sibai BM. Hypertension. In: Gabbe SG, Niebyl JR, Simpson JL, editors. Obstetrics: Normal and Problem Pregnancies. 5th ed. Philadelphia: Churchill Livingstone Elsevier; 2007. p. 864-906.
3. Clarke CA, Spitzer KA, Nadler JN, Laskin CA. Preterm deliveries in women with systemic lupus erythematosus. J Rheumatol 2003;30:2127-32.
4. Chakravarty EF, Nelson L, Krishnan E. Obstetric hospitalizations in the United States for women with systemic lupus erythematosus and rheumatoid arthritis. Arthritis Rheum 2006;54:899-907.
5. Clowse MEB, Jamison M, Myers E, James AH. A national study of the complications of lupus in pregnancy. Am J Obstet Gynecol 2008;199:127.e1-127.e6.
6. Costedoat-Chalumeau N, Amoura Z, Duhaut P, Huong DLT, Sebbough D, Wechsler B, et al. Safety of hydroxychloroquine in pregnant patients with connective tissue diseases: a study of one hundred thirty-three cases compared with a control group. Arthritis Rheum 2003;48:3207-11.
7. Clowse MEB, Magder L, Witter F, Petri M. Hydroxychloroquine in lupus pregnancy. Arthritis Rheum 2006;54: 3640-7.
8. Clowse MEB, Magder LS, Witter F, Petri M. The impact of increased lupus activity on obstetric outcomes. Arthritis Rheum 2005;52:514-21.
9. Cortes-Hernandez J, Ordi-Ros J, Paredes F, Casellas M, Castillo F, Vilardell-Tarres M. Clinical predictors of fetal and maternal outcome in systemic lupus erythematosus: a prospective study of 103 pregnancies. Rheumatology 2002;41:643-50.
10. Lockshin MD. Pregnancy does not cause systemic lupus erythematosus to worsen. Arthritis Rheum 1989;32:665-70.
11. Ruiz-Irastorza G, Lima F, Alves J, Khamashta MA, Simpson J, Hughes GRV, et al. Increased rate of lupus flare during pregnancy and the puerperium: a prospective study of 78 pregnancies. Br J Rheumatol 1996;35:133-8.
12. Georgiou PE, Politi EN, Katsimbri P, Sakka V, Drosos AA. Outcome of lupus pregnancy: a controlled study. Rheumatology 2000;29:1014-9.
13. Ruiz-Irastorza G, Khamashta MA, Gordon C, Lockshin MD, Johns KR, Sammaritano L, et al. Measuring systemic lupus erythematosus activity during pregnancy: validation of the lupus activity in pregnancy scale. Arthritis Rheum 2004;51:78-82.
14. Nossent HC, Swaak TJG. Systemic lupus erythematosus. VI: Analysis of the interrelationship with pregnancy. J Rheumatol 1990;17:771-6.
15. Devoe LD, Loy GL, Spargo BH. Renal histology and pregnancy performance in systemic lupus erythematosus. Clin Exper Hypertens B 1983;B2:325-40.
16. Moroni G, Quaglini S, Banfi G, Caloni M, Finazzi S, Ambroso G, et al. Pregnancy in lupus nephritis. Am J Kidney Dis 2002;40:713-20.
17. McGrory CH, McCloskey LJ, DeHoratius RJ, Dunn SR, Moritz MJ, Armenti VT. Pregnancy outcomes in female renal recipients: a comparison of systemic lupus erythematous with other diagnoses. Am J Transplant 2003;3:35-42.
18. Buyon JP, Cronstein BN, Morris M, Tanner M, Weissman G. Serum complement values (C3 and C4) to differentiate between systemic lupus activity and pre-eclampsia. Am J Med 1986;81:194-200.
19. Friedman DM, Rupel A, Buyon JP. Epidemiology, etiology, detection, and treatment of autoantibody - associated congenital heart block in neonatal lupus. Current Rheum Reports 2007;9(2):101-8.
20. Friedman DM, Kim MY, Copel JA, Davis C, Phoon CKL, Glickstein JS, et al. Utility of cardiac monitoring in fetuses at risk for congenital heart block: the PR Interval and Dexamethasone Evaluation (PRIDE) prospective study. Circulation 2008;117:485-93.
21. Chakravarty EF, Colón I, Langen ES, Nix DA, El-Sayed YY, Genovese MC, et al. Factors that predict prematurity and preeclampsia in pregnancies that are complicated by systemic lupus erythematosus. Am J Obstet Gynecol 2005;192:1897-904.
22. Clowse MEB, Magder LS, Witter F, Petri M. Early risk factors for pregnancy loss in lupus. Obstet Gynecol 2006;107:293-9.
23. Petri M, Ho AC, Patel J, Demers D, Joseph JM, Goldman D. Elevation of maternal alpha-fetoprotein in systemic lupus erythematosus: a controlled study. J Rheumatol 1995;22:1365-8.
24. Pollard JK, Scott JR, Branch DW. Outcome of children born to women treated during pregnancy for the antiphospholipid syndrome. Obstet Gynecol 1992;80:365-8.
25. Ross G, Sammaritano L, Nass R, Lockshin M. Effects of mothers' autoimmune disease during pregnancy on learning disabilities and hand preference in their children. Arch Pediatr Adolesc Med 2003;157:397-402.
26. Miyakis S, Lockshin M, Atsumi T, Branch DW, Brey RL, Cervera R, et al. International consensus statement on an update of the classification criteria for definite antiphospholipid syndrome (APS). J Thromb Haemost 2006;4295-306.
27. Branch DW, Khamashta MA. Antiphospholipid syndrome: obstetric diagnosis, management, and controversies. Obstet Gynecol 2003;101:1333-44.
28. Lockshin MD, Qamar T, Drusin ML, Goei S. Antibody to cardiolipin, lupus anticoagulant, and fetal death. J Rheumatol 1987;14:259-62.
29. Opatrny L, David M, Kahn SR, Shrier I, Rey E. Association between antiphospholipid antibodies and recurrent fetal loss in women without autoimmune disease: a meta-analysis. J Rheumatol 2006;33:2214-21.
30. Branch DW, Silver R, Pierangeli S, van Leeuwen I, Harris EN. Antiphospholipid antibodies other than lupus anticoagulant and anticardiolipin antibodies in women with recurrent pregnancy loss, fertile controls, and antiphospholipid syndrome. Obstet Gynecol 1997;89:549-55.
31. Branch DW, Andres R, Digre KB, Rote NS, Scott JR. The association of antiphospholipid antibodies with severe preeclampsia. Obstet Gynecol 1989;73:541-5.
32. Le Thi Huong D, Wechsler B, Edelman P, Fournié A, Le Tallec Y, Piette JC, et al. Postpartum cerebral infarction associated with aspirin withdrawal in the antiphospholipid syndrome. J Rheumatol 1993;20:1229-32.
33. Gomez-Puerta JA, Cervera R, Espinosa G, Asherson RA, Garcia-Carrasco M, da Costa IP, et al. Catastrophic antiphospholipid syndrome during pregnancy and puerperium: maternal and fetal characterisitics of 15 cases. Ann Rheum Dis 2007;66:740-6.
34. Lima F, Khamashta MA, Buchanan NM, Kerslake S, Hunt BJ, Hughes GR. A study of sixty pregnancies in patients with the antiphospholipid syndrome. Clin Exp Rheumatol 1996;14:131-6.
35. Ruffatti A, Dalla Barba B, Del Ross T, Vettorato F, Rapizzi E, Tonello M, et al. Outcome of fifty-five newborns of antiphospholipid-positive mothers treated with calcium heparin during pregnancy. Clin Exp Rheum 1998;16:605-10.
36. Tincani A, Lojacono A, Taglietti M, Motta M, Biasini C, Decca L, et al. Pregnancy and neonatal outcome in primary antiphospholipid syndrome. Lupus 2002;11:649-51.
37. Boffa MC, Lachassinne E. Infant perinatal thrombosis and antiphospholipid antibodies: a review. Lupus 2007;16:634-41.
38. Brewster JA, Shaw NJ, Farquharson RG. Neonatal and pediatric outcomes of infants born to mothers with antiphospholipid syndrome. J Perinatal Med 1999;27:183-7.
39. Nacinovich R, Galli J, Bomba M, Filippini E, Parrinello G, Nuzzo M, et al. Neuropsychological development of children born to patients with antiphospholipid syndrome. Arthritis Care Res 2008;59:345-51.
40. Empson M, Lassere M, Craig J, Scott J. Prevention of recurrent miscarriage for women with antiphosholipid antibody or lupus anticoagulant. Cochrane Database Syst Rev 2005;18(2):CD002859.

41. Noble LS, Kutteh WH, Lashey N, Franklin RD, Herrada J. Antiphopsholipid antibodies associated with recurrent pregnancy loss: prospective multicenter controlled pilot study comparing treatment with low-molecular weight heparin versus unfractionated heparin. Fertil Steril 2005;83:684-90.

42. Witter FR. Management of the high-risk lupus pregnant patient. Rheum Dis Clin North Am 2007;33:253-65.

43. Branch DW, Peaceman AM, Druzin M, Silver RK, El-Sayed Y, Silver RM, et al. A multi-center, placebo-controlled pilot study of intravenous immune globulin treatment of antiphospholipid syndrome during pregnancy. Am J Obstet Gynecol 2000;182:122-7.

44. Erkan D, Merrill JT, Yazici Y, Sammaritano L, Buyon JP, Lockshin MD. High thrombosis rate after fetal loss in antiphospholipid syndrome—effective prophylaxis with aspirin. Arthritis Rheum 2001;44:1466-7.

45. Cecere FA, Persellin RH. The interaction of pregnancy and the rheumatic diseases. Clin Rheum Dis 1981;7:747-68.

46. Barrett JH, Brennan P, Fiddler M, Silman AJ. Does rheumatoid arthritis remit during pregnancy and relapse postpartum? Results from a nationwide study in the United Kingdom preformed prospectively from late pregnancy. Arthritis Rheum 1999;42:1219-27.

47. Nelson JL, Hughes KA, Smith AG, Nisperos BB, Branchaud AM, Hansen JA. Maternal-fetal disparity for HLA class II allo-antigens and the pregnancy-induced amelioration of rheumatoid arthritis. N Engl J Med 1993;329:500-1.

48. Hazes JMW, Dijkmans BAC, Vandenbroucke JP, de Vries RR, Cats A. Pregnancy and the risk of developing rheumatoid arthritis. Arthritis Rheum 1990;33:1770-5.

49. Silman A, Kay A, Brennan P. Timing of pregnancy in relation to the onset of rheumatoid arthritis. Arthritis Rheum 1992;35:152-5.

50. Karlson EW, Mandl L, Hankinson SE, Grodstein F. Do breast feeding and other reproductive factors affect future risk of rheumatoid arthritis? Results from the Nurses' Health Study. Arthritis Rheum 2004;50:3458-67.

51. Bowden AP, Barrett JH, Fallow W, Silman AJ. Women with inflammatory polyarthritis have babies of lower birth weight. J Rheumatol 2001;28:355-9.

52. Duhring JL. Pregnancy, rheumatoid arthritis, and intrauterine growth retardation. Am J Obstet Gynecol 1970;108:325-7.

53. Skomsvoll JF, Wallenius M, Koksvik HS, Rodevand E, Salvesen KA, Spigset O, et al. Drug insight: anti-tumor necrosis factor therapy for inflammatory arthropathies during reproduction, pregnancy and lactation. Nat Clin Practice Rheumatol 2007;3:156-64.

54. Musiej-Nowakowska E, Ploski R. Pregnancy and early-onset pauciarticular juvenile chronic arthritis. Ann Rheum Dis 1999;58:475-80.

55. Ostenson M. The effect of pregnancy on ankylosing spondylitis, psoriatic arthritis, and juvenile rheumatoid arthritis. Am J Reprod Immunol 1992;28:235-7.

56. Maynon R, Jejgin M. Scleroderma in pregnancy. Obstet Gynecol Surv 1989;44:530-4.

57. Steen VD, Conte C, Day N, Ramsey-Goldman R, Medsger TA. Pregnancy in women with systemic sclerosis. Arthritis Rheum 1989;32:151-7.

58. Steen VD. Pregnancy in women with systemic sclerosis. Obstet Gynecol 1999;94:15-20.

59. Steen VD, Medsger Jr TA. Fertility and pregnancy outcome in women with systemic sclerosis. Arthritis Rheum 1999;42:763-8.

60. Silman AJ, Black C. Increased incidence of spontaneous abortion and infertility in women with scleroderma before disease onset: a controlled study. Ann Rheum Dis 1988;47:441-4.

61. Aslan E, Tarim E, Kilicdag E, Simsek E. Sjogren's syndrome diagnosed in pregnancy: a case report. J Reproduct Med 2005;50:67-70.

62. Adam FU, Torun D, Bolat F, Zumrutdal A, Sezer S, Ozdemir FN. Acute renal failure due to mesangial proliferative glomerulonephritis in a pregnant woman with primary Sjogren's syndrome. Clin Rheum 2006;1:75-9.

63. Julkunen H, Kaaja R, Kurki P, Palosuo T, Friman C. Fetal outcome in women with primary Sjogren's syndrome: a retrospective case-control study. Clin Exp Rheum 1995;13:65-71.

64. Haga HJ, Gjesdal CG, Koksvik HS, Skomsvoll JF, Irgens LM, Ostensen M. Pregnancy outcome in patients with primary Sjogren's syndrome: a case control study. J Rheumatol 2005;32:1734-6.

65. Kofteridis DP, Malliotakis PI, Sotsiou F, Vardakis NK, Vamvakas LN, Emmanouel DS. Acute onset of dermatomyositis presenting in pregnancy with rhabdomyelosis and fetal loss. Scand J Rheumatol 1999;28:192-4.

66. Chopra S, Suri V, Bagga R, Thami MR, Sharma A, Bambery P. Autoimmune inflammatory myopathy in pregnancy. Medscape J Med 2008;10:17.

67. Park IW, Suh YJ, Han JH, Shin YS, Choi JH, Park HS, et al. Dermatomyositis devewloping in the first trimester of pregnancy. Kor J Int Med 2003;18:196-8.

68. Mosca M, Strigini F, Carmignani F, D'Ascanio A, Genazzani AR, Bombardieri S. Pregnant patient with dermatomyositis successfully treated with intravenous immunoglobulin therapy. Arthritis Rheum 2005;53:119-21.

69. Silva CA, Sultan SM, Isenberg DA. Pregnancy outcome in adult-onset idiopathic inflammatory myopathy. Rheumatol 2003;42:1168-72.

70. Váncsa A, Ponyi A, Constantin T, Zeher M, Dankó K. Pregnancy outcome in idiopathic inflammatory myopathy. Rheumatol Int 2007;27:435-9.

71. Williams L, Chang PY, Park E, Gorson KC, Bayer-Zwirello L. Successful treatment of dermatomyositis during pregnancy with intravenous immunoglobulin monotherapy. Obstet Gynecol 2007;109:561-3.

72. Messina S, Fagiolari G, Lamperti C, Cavaletti G, Prelle A, Scardato G, et al. Women with pregnancy-related polymyositis and high serum CK levels in the newborn. Neurology 2002;58:482-4.

73. Doria A, Iaccarino L, Ghirardello A, Briani C, Zampieri S, Tarricone E, et al. Pregnancy in rare autoimmune rheumatic diseases: UCTD, MCTD, myositis, systemic vasculitis and Behcet disease. Lupus 2004;13:690-5.

74. Al-Adnani M, Kiho L, Schimberg I. Recurrent placental massive perivillous fibrin deposition associated with polymyositis: a case report and review of the literature. Pediatr Dev Pathol 2008;11:226-9.

75. Madkour M, Kudwah A. Behcet's disease Letter. Br Med J 1978;11:1786.

76. Hurt WG, Cooke CL, Jordan WP, Bullock JP Jr, Rodriguez GE. Behcet's syndrome associated with pregnancy. Obstet Gynecol 1979;53:315-35.

77. Hamza M, Elleuch M, Zrib A. Behcet's disease and pregnancy. Ann Rheum Dis 1988;47:350.

78. Uzun S, Alpsoy E, Durdu M, Akman A. The clinical course of Behcet's disease in pregnancy: a retrospective analysis and review of the literature. J Dermatol 2003;30:499-502.

79. Jadaon J, Shushan A, Ezra Y, Sela HY, Orzan C, Rojansky N. Behcet's disease and pregnancy. Acta Obstet Gynecol Scand 2005;84:939-44.

80. Kale A, Akyildiz L, Akdeniz N, Kale E. Pregnancy complicated by superior vena cava thrombosis and pulmonary embolism in a patient with Behcet disease and the use of heparin for treatment. Saudi Med J 2006;27:95-7.

81. Stark AC, Bhakta B, Chamberlain MA, Dear P, Taylor PV. Life-threatening transient neonatal Behcet's disease. R J Rheumatol 1997;36:700-2.

82. Jog S, Patole S, Koh G, Whitehall J. Unusual presentation of neonatal Behcet's disease. Am J Perinatol 2001;18:287-92.

83. Ishikawa K, Matsuura S. Occlusive thromboaortopathy (Takayasu's disease) and pregnancy. Clinical course and management of 33 pregnancies and deliveries. Am J Cardiol 1982;50:1293-300.

84. Sharma BK, Jain S, Vasishta K. Outcome of pregnancy in Takayasu arteritis. Int J Cardiol 2000;75(Supp. 1):S159-62.

85. Wong VCW, Wang RYC, Tse TF. Pregnancy and Takayasu's arteritis. Am J Med 1983;75:597-601.

86. Langford CA, Kerr GS. Pregnancy in vasculitis. Curr Opin Rheumatol 2002;14:36-41.

87. Tamioka N, Hirose K, Abe E, Miyamoto N, Araki K, Nomura R, et al. Indications for peripartum aortic pressure monitoring in Takayasu's disease. A patient with a past history of intrapartum cerebral hemorrhage. Japan Heart J 1998;39:255-60.

88. Clark AG, al-Qatari M. Anesthesia for caeserian section in Takayasu's disease. Can J Anesthes 1998;45:377-9.

89. Owen J, Hauth JC. Polyarteritis nodosa in pregnancy: a case report and brief literature review. Am J Obstet Gynecol 1989;160:606-7.

90. Fernandes SR, Cury CP, Samara AM. Pregnancy with a history of treated polyarteritis nodosa. J Rheumatol 1996;23: 1119-20.

91. Reed NR, Smith MT. Periarteritis nodosa in pregnancy: report of a case and review of the literature. Obstet Gynecol 1990;55:381-5.

92. Aya AG, Hoffet M, Mangin R, Balducchi JP, Eledjam JJ. Severe preeclampsia superimposed on polyarteritis nodosa. Am J Obstet Gynecol 1996;174:1659–60.

93. Stone MS, Olsen RR, Weismann DN, Giller RH, Goeken JA. Cutaneous vasculitis in the newborn of a mother with cutaneous polyarteritis nodosa. J Am Acad Dermatol 1993;28:101–5.

94. Hiyama J, Shiota Y, Marukawa M, Horita N, Kanehisa Y, Ono T, et al. Churg-Strauss syndrome associated with pregnancy. Intern Med 2000;39:985–90.

95. Ogasawara M, Kajiura S, Inagaki H, Sasa H, Aoki K, Yagami Y. Successful pregnancy in a Churg-Strauss syndrome patient with a history of intrauterine fetal death. Int Arch Allergy Immunol 1995;108:200-2.

96. Connolly JO, Lanham JG, Partridge MR. Fulminant pregnancy-related Churg-Strauss syndrome. Br J Rheumatol 1994;33:776-7.

97. Barry C, Davis S, Garrard P, Ferguson IT. Churg-Strauss disease: deterioration in a twin pregnancy. Successful outcome following treatment with corticosteroids and cyclophosphamide. Br J Obstet Gynecol 1997;104:746-7.

98. Hot A, Perard L, Coppere B, Simon M, Bouhour F, Ninet J. Marked improvement of Churg-Strauss vasculitis with intravenous gammaglobulins during pregnancy. Clin Rheumatol 2007;26:2149-51.

99. Harber MA, Tso A, Taheri S, Tuck SM, Burns A. Wegener's granulomatosis in pregnancy—the therapeutic dilemna. Nephrol Dialysis Transplant 1999;14:1789-91.

100. Palit J, Clague RB. Wegener's granulomatosis presenting during first trimester of pregnancy. Br J Rheumatol 1990;29:389-90.

101. Fields CL, Ossorio MA, Roy TM, Bunke CM. Wegener's granulomatosis complicated by pregnancy: a case report. J Reprod Med 1991;36:463-6.

102. Pauzner R, Mayan H, Hershko E, Alcalay M, Farfel Z. Exacerbation of Wegener's granulomatosis during pregnancy: report of a case with tracheal stenosis and literature review. J Rheumatol 1994;21:1153-6.

103. Luisiri P, Lance NJ, Curran JJ. Wegener's granulomatosis in pregnancy. Arthritis Rheum 1997;40:1354-60.

104. Dayoan ES, Dimen LL, Boylen CT. Successful treatment of Wegener's granulomatosis during pregnancy: a case report and review of the medical literature. Chest 1998;113:836-8.

105. Milne KL, Stanley KP, Temple RC, Barker TH, Ross CN. Microscopic polyangiitis: first report of a case with onset during pregnancy. Nephrol Dial Transplant 2004;19:234-7.

106. Cetinkaya R, Odabas AR, Gursan N, Selcuk Y, Erdogan F, Keles M, et al. Microscopic polyangiitis in a pregnant woman. S Med J 2002;95:1441-3.

107. Schlieben DJ, Korbet SM, Kimura RE, Schwartz MM, Lewis EJ. Pulmonary-renal syndrome in a newborn with placental transmission of ancas. Am J Kidney Dis 2005;45:758-61.

108. Østensen M, Khamashta M, Lockshin M, Parke A, Brucato A, Carp H, et al. Anti-inflammatory and immunosuppressive drugs and reproduction. Arthritis Res Ther 2006;8: 209-28.

109. Rayburn WF. Glucocorticoid therapy for rheumatic disease. Maternal, fetal, and breast-feeding considerations. Am J Reprod Immunol 1992;28:138-40.

110. Park-Wyllie L, Mazzotta P, Pastuszak A, Moretti ME, Beique L, Hunnisett L, et al. Birth defects after exposure to corticosteroids: prospective cohort study and meta-analysis of epidemiological studies. Teratology 2000;6:385-92.

111. Berkenstadt M, Weisz B, Cuckle H, Di-Castro M, Guetta E, Barkai G. Chromosomal abnormalities and birth defects among couples with colchicine treated familial Mediterranean fever. Am J Obstet Gynecol 2005;193:1513-6.

112. Roux CH, Brocq O, Breuil V, Albert C, Euller-Ziegler L. Pregnancy in rheumatology patients exposed to anti-tumour necrosis factor (TNF)-a therapy. Rheumatology 2007;46:695-8.

113. Carter JD, Valeriano J, Vasey FB. Tumor necrosis factor-alpha inhibition and VATER association: a causal relationship. J Rheumatol 2006;33:1014-7.

114. Somers EC, Marder W, Christman GM, Ognenovski V, McCune WJ. Use of a gonadotropin-releasing hormone analog against premature ovarian failure during cyclophosphamide therapy in women with severe lupus. Arthritis Rheum 2005;52:2761-7.

115. Pisoni CN, D'Cruz DP. The safety of mycophenlate mofetil in pregnancy. Expert Opin Drug Safety 2008;7:219-22.

116. Pettilä V, Leinonen P, Markkola A, Hiilesmaa V, Kaaja R. Postpartum bone mineral density in women treated for thromboprophylaxis with unfractionated heparin or LMW heparin. Thromb Haemost 2002;87:182-6.

117. Pauzner R, Dulitzki M, Langevitz P, Livneh A, Kenett R, Many A. Low molecular weight heparin and warfarin in the treatment of patients with antiphospholipid syndrome during pregnancy. Thromb Haemost 2001;86:1379-84.

118. Cooper WO, Hernandez-Diaz S, Arbogast PG. Major congenital malformations after first-trimester exposure to ACE-inhibitors. N Engl J Med 2006;354:2443-51.

119. Ben-Chetrit E, Levy M. Colchicine: 1998 update. Sem Arthritis Rheum 1998;28:48-59.

120. Petri M, Kim MY, Kalunian KC, Grossman J, Hahn BH, Sammaritano LR, et al. Combined oral contraceptives in women with systemic lupus erythematosus. N Engl J Med 2005;353:2550-8.

121. Sammaritano LR. Therapy insight review: Contraception in women with rheumatic diseases. Nat Clin Pract Rheumatol 2007;3:273-81.

122. Guballa N, Sammaritano L, Schwartzman S, Buyon J, Lockshin MD. Ovulation induction and in vitro fertilization in systemic lupus erythematosus and antiphospholipid syndrome. Arthritis Rheum 2000;43:550-6.

Chapter 32

Economic Considerations in the Treatment of Rheumatic Diseases

Gisela Kobelt

INTRODUCTION

This chapter will address

- the reasons for economic analysis in health care, including health technology assessment (HTA) and reimbursement of treatments
- the methods of economic analysis, including the types of studies and the need for modeling, focusing on the main issues for economic evaluation in rheumatic diseases.

The topics will be illustrated with examples from rheumatoid arthritis (RA) and ankylosing spondylitis (AS) because these conditions have been most widely studied. However, the methodologic issues are similar across all rheumatic diseases, and the difference is generally due to the availability of the relevant data.

The chapter will not provide a comprehensive overview of studies performed, nor will we offer a critique of the different approaches chosen, because the amount of studies is large and reviews are available elsewhere,[1-4] and because such reviews are rapidly outdated in a field as active as rheumatic diseases.

Health Economics, Reimbursement Decisions, Health Technology Assessment

Health Economics

Health economics is the application of the discipline and the methods of economics to the topic "health." Thus, health care is considered to be no different from any other productive sector of the economy: resources are used and investments are made to produce "health." Health economics is then concerned with achieving efficiency in the allocation of resources in health care, a sector in which a large part of the expenses are carried by the public budget (around 70%–75% in Europe, Canada, Australia, around 40%–45% in the United States; www.oecd.org).

Within this frame, economic evaluations of health interventions provide data and estimates of the value for money (cost-effectiveness) of interventions, as part of the information on which decisions can be made. Cost-effectiveness studies thus do not make decisions, nor do they judge the impor-

tance and value of the clinical benefit provided by the treatment studied. Rather, they assess the cost in relation to the benefit, and compare the results to other interventions (Fig. 32-1).

The methods of health economics and economic evaluation apply across the world.[5,6] However, there is great variation in the amount of resources used for health care across countries, owing to general economic factors. Hence, there will be significant variation in access to the newest and most effective treatments. Thus, economic analyses are always country specific, and it impossible to conclude from the results of one study in a given country on the possible situation in another country. The organization of care differs, treatment patterns vary, and the relative and absolute cost of individual resources can be very different.

Today, information about new treatments is widely available. Few patients, for example, with RA ignore the existence of the biologic drugs (e.g., tumor necrosis factor-α [TNF-α] inhibitors). These treatments are highly effective but also come at a high cost. Their price is global (i.e., similar across countries in order to avoid parallel trade), and therefore, economic factors will be a significant source of variations in access to these drugs. Acceptability of their

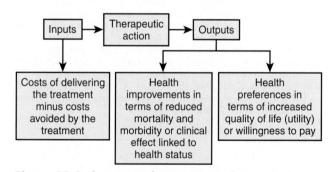

Figure 32-1. Structure of economic evaluation in health care. In economic evaluation, costs of interventions are put into relation with their health effects, and then different interventions are compared. For instance, if a new treatment provides a better outcome but is more expensive than standard therapy and its cost is not off-set by savings in other resources, the question analyzed is how much more we have to pay (incremental cost) for the additional health gain (incremental effect).

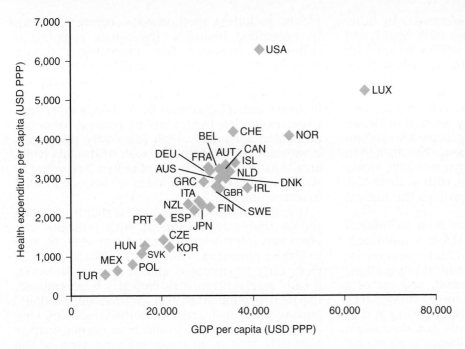

Figure 32-2. Health expenditures per capita in relation to gross domestic product in different countries. Affordability of health care is directly related to the income of a country (gross domestic product [GDP]). Among countries represented in this figure, Turkey has the lowest GDP and consequently also the lowest spending per capita. Within the OECD, the relationship is almost linear, with the only outlier being the USA (essentially due to overall higher prices). (From OECD Health Data 2005.)

cost will be different in the United States with a per capita spending on health care in 2005 of more than $6000 and Turkey with a spending of around $600 (www.oecd.org) (Fig. 32-2).

Payers

Within the relationship between patients (consumers), providers (agents) and payers (Fig. 32-3), the latter group is therefore becoming increasingly important. All payers are interested in opportunities to do something at a lower cost to make room for other payments (cost-containment). They are also concerned about the impact on their budget, that is, the cost of a treatment and the estimated number of treatments (budget impact). However,

particular public payers such as governments in Europe are also interested in cost-effectiveness, asking the question how a given payment will contribute to outcome in terms of survival, quality of life (QoL), and quality of care (value for money). Thus, payers dictate to some extent what treatments can or cannot be used on their budget and how. This is particularly important in RA, in which—without health insurance, be it public or private—few patients will be able to afford the biologic drugs.

Payers, while still demanding innovative treatments, are no longer impressed by fancy new technology, unless it truly improves the outcomes for patients. One could argue that this is clearly the case for the anti-TNF drugs, yet, many restrictions apply to their usage owing to their cost. Cost effectiveness has thus become an important additional criterion for selecting how to use health care resources most efficiently, using economic evaluation as the tool. These studies will provide data in a structured format, but will not make an explicit decision concerning the value of the benefit nor the acceptability of its cost.

Reimbursement and Health Technology Assessment

Most drugs in RA are used in the outpatient setting and are thus subject to formal decisions regarding inclusion in the public reimbursement system. In a number of countries (e.g., Australia, Canada, Belgium, Finland, Netherlands, Norway, Portugal, and Sweden) there has been a formalized process regarding the use of cost-effectiveness studies in the decision-making process for several years. Countries in Eastern Europe and Asia have

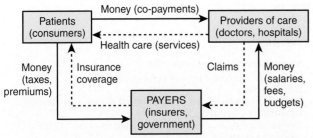

Figure 32-3. Economic relationships in health care. In solidarity-based systems such as in Europe, health care is financed by the population, with mandatory contribution to national health insurances or with taxes to the public budget. In both cases, payments for the services of health care providers thus are via a third party. In this framework, payers decide to some extent what can be used and how on behalf of the population, in order to maximize health within the budget constraints.

recently introduced such requirements. In other countries (e.g., Denmark, France, Italy, Spain, and Switzerland), cost-effectiveness studies are used for pricing and reimbursement decisions, although not as formally. In the United Kingdom and Germany, drugs can be launched immediately after scientific market approval and are theoretically reimbursed. However, drugs are subsequently assessed by health technology assessment (HTA) agencies who recommend when and how to use them. The agency in England and Wales (NICE, www.nice.org) works with a clearly structured process with a direct link to funding and therefore has perhaps the highest visibility, even beyond borders.

Cost-effectiveness studies have been an integral part of HTA for a long time. HTA is a multidisciplinary process of policy analysis that examines the medical, economic, social, and ethical implications of the incremental value, diffusion, and use of a medical technology in health care. Normally, HTA is based on publicly available information and as such often becomes available only at a time when reimbursement decisions have already been made.[7] The impact will thus be on usage, rather than represent a formal decision on access, and study results will often be available some time after introduction of a new treatment.

HTA agencies are linked in an international network (INATHA), the secretariat of which maintains a database of HTA reports, including both ongoing and reported studies (www.inatha.org). Between 1998 and 2006, a total of 85 reports related to RA were published, most of them from 2002 onward. This clearly reflects the need for assessment of the novel but high-priced biologic therapies.

In the field of rheumatology, most reimbursement decisions or HTA recommendations have introduced limitations to the use of the biologic drugs. In general, patients have to show an inadequate response to at least two standard treatments, including methotrexate, before they can be prescribed biologics. Inadequate response is defined as disease activity exceeding a certain level. Treatment can be continued only if a certain response is obtained. These restrictions are triggered by economic considerations due to the cost of the biologics, averaging around Euro 12-15,000 per year. Using expensive treatments in patients who can be treated adequately with less costly treatments is wasteful, as is continuing such treatments when an adequate response is not obtained. According to economic thinking, such funds are better allocated to something else.

One issue with this argument is that it has been shown that early treatment with biologics can often halt joint destruction and may even be able to induce remission. Thus, from a clinical point of view, early treatment is almost a must. However, if early intervention with biologics is generalized, the treated population will increase substantially, putting additional strain on limited resources. One way to deal with this would be a normal market approach, that is, to lower prices in view of the increased volume. Another approach, and the one currently pursued, is better targeting of treatment by improving the time to diagnosis and identifying patients with active disease and a bad prognosis early on.

Formal Guidelines for Economic Evaluation

Guidelines for economic evaluation in countries where these are a formal part of reimbursement decisions are similar from a methodological point of view. This indicates that methods for economic evaluation are well developed, with only a number of methodologic issues still considered a research topic. Differences in these guidelines often relate to these topics. Table 32-1 lists the criteria that are addressed in these guidelines, as well as the topics that can differ.

Table 32-1. *Criteria Addressed in Guidelines for Economic Evaluations*

Topic	Similar Across Guidelines	Different Across Guidelines	Definition
Viewpoint for the analysis		X	Societal versus payer perspective
Outcome evidence		X	Systematic literature review versus trial data
Choice of comparator	X		Gold standard
Patient group	X		Patients likely to receive the treatment, subgroups allowed
Form of economic evaluation	X		Cost-utility preferred
Measurement and valuation of costs and benefits	X		Opportunity costs and quality-adjusted life years (QALYs) whenever possible
Incremental analysis	X		Additional costs for the additional benefit
Time horizon		X	Relevant episode versus lifetime
Discounting	X		Costs and benefits discounted, discount rate differs (3%–5%)
Uncertainty		X	Extensive sensitivity analysis versus probabilistic analysis
Modeling	X		All types of models (decision trees, Markov models, discrete event simulation, regression models) accepted
Presentation of results	X		All details of the analysis

ECONOMIC STUDIES

Type of Studies, Structure of Economic Evaluation, Methods

We distinguish two basic types of economic analyses in health care: descriptive and evaluative (Table 32-2).[5,6]

Descriptive Studies

Cost of illness or burden of illness studies provide information on how much is spent on a given disease. They can be prevalence or incidence based. Prevalence studies will inform about the total amounts spent, and their distribution on different resource types, during a defined time frame (most often a year) and in a defined geographic area (most often a country). Costs can be expressed as average costs for a patient, or total costs for all patients with the disease. A recent study estimated these costs for patients in different countries, using an economic model to impute costs from countries with existing data to countries without data.[8] Table 32-3 shows mean costs per patient and total costs for the estimated prevalence in some selected countries. From these estimates, it also becomes obvious that spending on disease differs between countries with different incomes, illustrating the issue of affordability mentioned above.

Table 32-4 lists the typical resources that are relevant for studies in rheumatic diseases, whereas Table 32-5 indicates some sources for differences in published studies. Figure 32-4 illustrates the cost structure in a sample of around 1500 RA patients in France.[9]

Costs can also be estimated for patients at different stages of the disease. This is particularly important for chronic progressive disease in which the goal of treatment is to prevent patients from

Table 32-3. *Mean Annual Cost Per Patients and Total Annual Cost in Selected Countries*

Country or Area	Mean Annual Cost/Patient (£, 2006)
Belgium	17,400
Denmark	17,300
France	21,900
Germany	22,500
Italy	16,400
Netherlands	12,600
Sweden	12,900
United Kingdom	16,500
Western Europe	*17,100*
Eastern Europe	*4,900*
Australia	15,900
Canada	10,500
Turkey	5,500
USA	21,100

Adapted from Lundkvist J, Kastang F, Kobelt G. The burden of rheumatoid arthritis and access to treatment: health burden and costs. Eur J Health Econ 2008;(Suppl 2):S49-60.

developing severe disease, or slow the progression to severe disease. In diseases such as RA or AS, but likely also other rheumatic diseases, costs increase steadily and substantially as the disease gets more severe. Figure 32-5A illustrates the increase in costs with decreasing functional capacity measured with the Health Assessment Questionnaire (HAQ)[10] in France.[9]

Figure 32-5A also shows that it is essentially costs outside the health care system, such as family help (informal care), investments to enable activities of daily living (ADLs), and productivity losses that make up for most of the cost increase. When only those costs that occur to public payers are included (health care, community care, sick leave compensation, and invalidity pensions), the increase is far less steep, providing less opportunities for cost savings (Fig. 32-5B). Hence, the

Table 32-2. *Types of Economic Analysis in Health Care*

Type of Analysis	Effectiveness Measure	Use
Descriptive Studies		
Cost of illness study	None	Description of all costs related to a disease. Policy information and basis for economic evaluation
Economic Evaluations		
Cost-Effectiveness Analyses		
Cost-minimization	Not measured, as it assumes that the effect of the alternatives is identical	Comparison of treatments within the same clinical indication
Cost-effectiveness	Unidimensional disease-specific measure (e.g., patients cured, life-years saved, disease-free time)	Comparison of treatments within the same clinical indication
Cost utility	Multidimensional outcome measure combining quality of life and life expectancy	Comparison across clinical indications
Cost-Benefit Analysis		
Cost benefit	Health benefit expressed in monetary terms (e.g., willingness to pay by individuals and society for specified benefits)	Comparison across different sectors of the economy

Table 32-4. *Typical Resources Collected in Studies in Rheumatology*

Type of Resources	Details of Items Included (Nonexhaustive)
Direct medical costs	Inpatient admissions (including surgery and prostheses)
	Outpatient admissions (including surgeries and prostheses)
	Rehabilitation (in- and outpatient)
	Medical consultations (rheumatologist, general practitioner, gastroenterologist, surgeon, psychiatrist)
	Nurse visits (at clinic, medical center, or home visits)
	Paramedical consultations (physiotherapist, psychologist, ergo-therapist, podiatrist, acupuncturist)
	Examinations (blood analyses, x-rays, scans)
	Drugs (antirheumatic, other symptomatic drugs)
	Home care
Direct nonmedical costs	Devices (wheelchairs, walking aids, technical devices)
	Investments (changes to the house or the car)
	Community help (home help, meals on wheels)
	Transportation (ambulance, taxi, private means)
	Informal care (help from family and friends due to the disease)
Production losses	Short and long-term sick leave (potentially loss of productivity while working)
	Early retirement (invalidity)
	Premature mortality

Table 32-5. *Sources of Differences in the Results of Published Cost of Illness Studies*

Topic		Differences
Perspective of costs	Societal perspective (all costs regardless of who pays, i.e., direct and indirect costs)	Payer perspective (only costs that are covered by the specific payer, generally only direct costs)
Definition of sample	Population sample (representative of the entire patient population in a geographic area)	Specific sample (e.g., by disease severity, by age, by point of care)
Definition of relevant costs	Consumption of patients with RA (all consumption of a patient with the disease)	Consumption for RA (only RA-related care and consumption)
Mode of data collection	Top-down (from national statistical data bases)	Bottom-up (from medical charts and patients)
	Prospective (following a sample of patients over time)	Retrospective (consumption in the past 1, 3, and 12 months)
Valuation	Tariffs (costs fixed by an insurance)	Opportunity costs (costs in their next best alternative)

RA, rheumatoid arthritis.

major economic opportunity with disease-modifying treatments lies outside the health care system which, however, has to finance the treatment. Costs of treatment occur in one part of our economy, whereas the benefits occur in another. This argues for adopting a societal perspective and put away the restricted budget mentality inherent in our health care organization. Despite this, many countries will consider only health care costs (direct medical costs) when deciding on reimbursement of new treatments, an approach that can considerably underestimate the benefit of treatment, in particular in terms of contribution to the economy (productivity).

Early in most rheumatic diseases, productivity losses will come from short- and medium-term sick leave due to episodes of severe inflammation and pain. As the disease progresses, up to half of the patients with RA have to leave the workforce permanently. Figure 32-6 shows the gap in workforce participation among patients below retirement

age, with decreasing functional capacity, compared with the general population.[9]

All estimates of how costs progress with the disease so far were based on functional capacity, which is indeed by far the strongest predictor of resource consumption. However, inflammation cannot be ignored as a cost driver, as illustrated in Figure 32-7 for AS.[11-13] Inflammation and function cannot be dissociated. However, the effect of disease activity on costs is much more limited than the one of function, most likely because inflammation can be periodical and reversible or controlled.

Much more clearly than on costs, function and disease activity have an independent effect on patients' QoL. A number of cross-sectional studies have shown that, at the same level of HAQ, QoL is different for patients with high or low disease activity. In all of these studies, QoL has been measured as utility, a generic preference weight for given states of health best thought of as a type of index for QoL. Utility

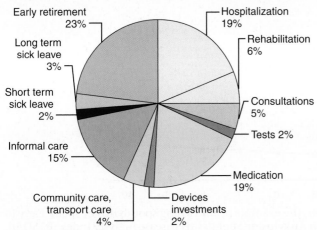

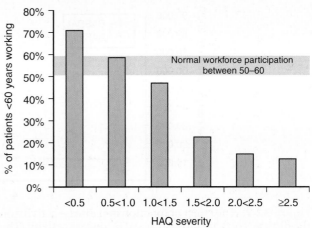

Figure 32-4. Structure of costs in rheumatoid arthritis, using an example from France. The figure illustrates the proportions of cost falling on the different resources in the societal perspective where all costs, regardless of who pays, are included and indirect costs are represented as productivity losses, not as sick leave compensation or invalidity pensions. In this study, almost one quarter of patients were treated with biologic drugs, which explains the high proportion represented by medication. (Adapted from Kobelt G, Woronoff AS, Richard B, Peeters P, Sany J. Disease status, costs and quality of life of patients with rheumatoid arthritis in France: the ECO-PR Study. Joint Bone Spine 2008;75:408-15.)

Figure 32-6. Decreasing workforce participation with increasing disease severity in France. At low levels of functional impairment, early in the disease process and at a younger age, workforce participation is at the normal population level. When Health Assessment Questionnaire (HAQ) reaches 1.0, the possibility to work starts to decline, particularly for work involving physical activity, and the effect is extremely strong at HAQ levels exceeding 1.5. Above HAQ 2.0, only around 12% to 13% of patients below 60 (the official retirement age in France) are still working. (Adapted from Kobelt G, Woronoff AS, Richard B, Peeters P, Sany J. Disease status, costs and quality of life of patients with rheumatoid arthritis in France: the ECO-PR Study. Joint Bone Spine 2008;75:408-15.)

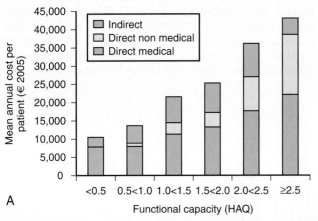

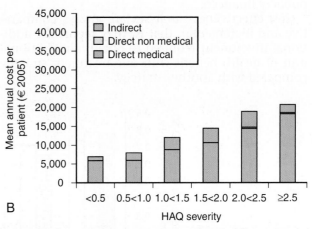

Figure 32-5. Cost of rheumatoid arthritis with progressing disease in the societal perspective and to public payers in France.[9] Total average cost per patient increases steeply in the societal perspective as function declines and patients lose the ability to work and to perform activities of daily living without help (**A**). These costs are around double those paid for by public payers (**B**), where the increase is much less pronounced.

scores are expressed as a value on a scale anchored between 0 (death) and 1 (perfect health). They can be measured directly using techniques from decision analysis (standard gamble, time trade off)[14] or derived from health status systems (tariffs) such as those developed for the EQ-5D, the Health Utility Index (HUI), or the Short Form-36 (SF36).[15-18] Figure 32-8 highlights how in RA utilities are affected by both

HAQ and disease activity, in a sample of patients in Sweden.[19] Economic evaluations of treatments must thus incorporate both measures, particularly because treatment is targeted primarily at inflammation.

Evaluative Studies

Economic evaluations follow a different structure from cost of illness studies (see Table 32-2 for types

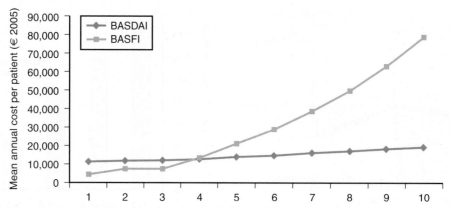

Figure 32-7. The effect of function and disease activity on costs, the example of ankylosing spondylitis in Spain. Early in the disease, costs are mostly caused by disease activity (The Bath Ankylosing Spondylitis Disease Activity Index [BASDAI], 1–10), but when functional capacity (The Bath Ankylosing Spondylitis Functional Index [BASFI], 1–10) starts to decline, costs increase up to eightfold. (Adapted from Kobelt G, Sobocki P, Mulero J, Gratacos J, Pocovi A, Collantes-Estevez E. The burden of ankylosing spondylitis in Spain. Value Health 2008;11:408-15.)

of studies). They relate to social choice and attempt to answer the question "what if." They evaluate what might happen if we change something in the way we are providing care, at a time when we have no definite data. This can concern introduction of a new treatment, changing the sequence of treatments, and introducing criteria for when to start and when to stop treatment. The underlying objective is to maximize social utility (the outcome for the population as a whole), and therefore, such studies are most appropriate in settings in which health care is publicly financed.

Cost-effectiveness analyses are always comparative and incremental, that is, they report the additional investment required to obtain an additional unit of health benefit with one treatment strategy compared with another strategy.

Costs and Health Effects

Within this framework (see also Fig. 32-1), costs are defined as resources used (health care, investments, time) and resources lost (productivity) multiplied with their price and compared between the alternatives evaluated.

Health effects can be expressed with different measures, disease specific or generic, depending on the study question. For instance, if we compare two treatments for severe infection, we might use "% cure" (within a given timeframe), which is very specific to the infection evaluated or we might use "life-years saved," which, although being more general, is still only relevant for this particular case. The QoL of the years of life saved with an intervention may indeed differ between diseases. Hence, to make these estimates useful for

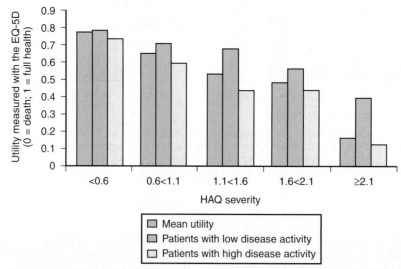

Figure 32-8. Quality of life (utility) of patients with RA by functional level and high/low disease activity. At the same levels of functional impairment, quality of life is differently affected by high or low disease activity (cut-off global Visual Analog Scale [VAS] 4.0, corresponding to Disease Activity Scale [DAS28] of 3.2). Utility was measured in a population-based cross-sectional study including 616 patients in Sweden. (Adapted from Kobelt G, Lindgren P, Lindroth Y, Jacobson L, Eberhardt K. Modelling the effect of function and disease activity on costs and quality of life in rheumatoid arthritis. Rheumatology (Oxford) 2005;44:1169-75.)

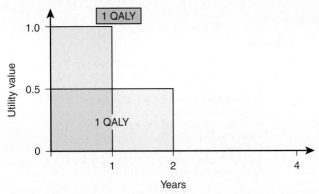

Figure 32-9. Quality-adjusted life years (QALYs) are estimated by weighing life years with a quality index (utility). In this example, living 2 years with a utility of 0.5 results in a QALY. This is the same as living 1 year in full health (utility 1.0). With this outcome measure, it is possible to compare treatments that increase life-expectancy with treatments that improve quality of life.

decisions on resource allocation within a health care budget, the health benefit must be expressed with a generic measure that is comparable across diseases. This is not obvious in RA, where a number of disease-specific measures are used to express the effect of the disease and the effectiveness of treatment: Swollen and tender joints, disease activity, joint damage, functional capacity, and % changes according to the American College of Rheumatology (ACR 20/50/70). None of these are directly usable in economic evaluation performed for policy purposes. This is not different from what happens in a number of other diseases. The concept of the quality-adjusted live year (QALY) has specifically been developed to overcome this problem, as an outcome measure in economic evaluation regardless of the disease analyzed. The QALY combines life expectance and QoL by weighing life-years with a quality index called utility (Fig. 32-9).[14] For instance, living 2 years with a utility of 0.5 will correspond to 1 QALY, which is equivalent to living 1 year with a utility of 1.

As we have discussed earlier, in RA and AS, both costs and QoL (utility) correlate significantly with function (HAQ, The Bath Ankylosing Spondylitis Functional Index [BASFI]) and disease activity (DAS28/The Bath Ankylosing Spondylitis Disease Activity Index [BASDAI]). Thus, when estimating potential changes that might occur with a new treatment that controls disease activity and improves function in the short term, it is rather straightforward to use these two disease measures in economic evaluation. The issue, however, is that treatment is preventive, with the goal to prevent function from deteriorating in the long term, and clinical trials will be too short to allow measuring this. The need to adopt a long-term view makes modeling unavoidable.

Modeling

In chronic progressive diseases costs increase and quality of life decreases as the disease worsens over time, as shown in Figure 32-10. The economic hypothesis is that a treatment that succeeds in changing the speed of progression will change the slopes of these curves, and the area between the two curves will represent cost savings and health gains. Cost-effectiveness will depend on how much these curves can be changed, and how large the investment to obtain the change. It will take a long time before these effects can be observed. Indeed, they may never be observable, because patient management is changed continuously as new data or new treatments become available.

In chronic diseases, models are used to combine different types of data from different sources to overcome the lack of directly observable data. Clinical trial data are incorporated directly, and then combined with epidemiologic data on long-term disease progression and mortality, as well as data on costs and utility. Again, this may not be straightforward. Long-term epidemiologic cohorts are often inception cohorts, with few of the patients having progressed to very advanced disease. They may be too small to produce reliable estimates of progression. Also, with more potent treatments available,

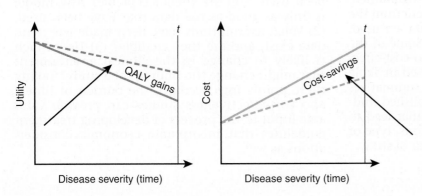

Figure 32-10. Hypothesis behind economic evaluation in rheumatic diseases. As the disease progresses, the patient's quality of life decreases and costs increase. If progression can be slowed, these curves are changed, providing quality-adjusted life years (QALY) gains and cost-savings (areas between the curves) that may or may not offset the cost of the intervention. (With kind permission of Annals of Rheumatic Diseases.)

Table 32-6. *Sources of Differences in Results of Economic Evaluations*

Topic		Differences
Outcome measure	Disease specific (e.g., proportion reaching ACR20)	Generic (e.g., quality-adjusted life years [QALY])
Underlying data	Primary data	Summary data from the literature
Perspective	Society	Health insurance (payers)
Definition of sample	Specific clinical trial population	General sample from clinical practice
Costs	Tariffs versus opportunity costs	Opportunity costs
	Human capital approach for indirect costs	Friction cost method for indirect costs
Time horizon	Short (within trial)	Medium (5–10 years)
		Lifetime
Assumptions	Extrapolation beyond the clinical trial	Extrapolation beyond the clinical trial
	Treatment of missing information	Treatment of missing information

the disease course may have changed since the start of these follow-ups. More recent databases, such as registries, although often much larger, have a short follow-up. Part of the disease progression may thus have to be based on average annual progression rather than on actual patient level data. Costs and utilities by disease severity are much easier to incorporate, provided obviously that adequate recent data from relatively large and representative samples of patients are available.

Models are a structured representation of what we know about an often complicated environment and allow investigating the effects of different hypotheses at a time when limited data are available. Modeling has become the standard methodology for economic evaluation in rheumatology over recent years. Unfortunately, however, as the methodology has developed and computing power increased, models have become more sophisticated and communicating them to a nonspecialist audience has become more difficult.[20] Hence, we will not discuss these techniques in detail in this chapter, but refer the reader to specialized publications.[5,6,21] The specific modeling technique used is secondary and is generally only chosen for convenience (i.e., best adapted to the question to be analyzed or the data at hand). All models should give the same result if they use the same data for the same country, the same assumptions, and are correctly programmed. Differences in published models thus stem from the underlying data and the way these data are used, rather than from the techniques.[1–3,4,20] Some of the points listed in Table 32-5 also apply to cost-effectiveness analyses; further points are listed in Table 32-6. For further illustration, Table 32-7 summarizes results from a non-exhaustive list of published studies in RA and highlights main points that lead to different results: perspective, interventions, type of patients, time-horizon, country, and year of study.

SUMMARY

Where does this leave the rheumatologist?

The burden of illness studies are easy to understand and easy to use, and they provide an important "snapshot" on what we are currently spending on a disease. Within scientific societies, this information can also be used to identify where we may do too much or too little. Over time, it is possible to evaluate changes that occur.

Cost-effectiveness studies are different. First of all, the objective of cost-effectiveness analyses should always be remembered: to maximize the health outcome for the population. They are hence not destined to be used directly for decisions regarding individual or small groups of particular patients. Nevertheless, they can provide helpful information in general economic terms to the practicing physician as well, with a number of caveats: it is clear that a study done in one country has limited relevance for another country, and within countries, assessments will change over time. Some of the issues driving differences in published studies mentioned earlier can also easily be spotted and taken into account. However, the key to understanding is to carefully verify three key points: (1) What types of data have been used, and are they acceptable? Any model is only as good as the data that have been used. (2) What assumptions have been made where no data exist, and are they credible? (3) How much is likely to change in the clinical environment that might change the findings of a study? Taking these points into account, the burden of illness and cost-effectiveness studies can provide valuable input to the process of developing treatment guidelines that incorporate economic considerations as well.

Table 32-7. Results from Published Cost-Utility Analyses in Rheumatoid Arthritis

Country	Perspective	Interventions Compared	Patients Included (baseline HAQ)	Time Horizon	Result	Currency and Year
United States	Health insurance	ETA/LEF/MTX/SSZ/no second-line agent	Early MTX naïve	6 months	$41,900 per patient reaching ACR20 with ETA	US$ 2001
United Kingdom	NHS/PSS	LEF/SSZ; LEF/MTX	Advanced active RA (HAQ 1.3–1.6)	10 years	No difference	GB£ 2002
United Kingdom	NHS/PSS Societal	INF + MTX/MTX	Advanced active RA (HAQ 1.8)	10 years	34,800 £/QALY 29,900 £/QALY	GB£ 2002
Sweden	Societal	INF + MTX/MTX	Advanced active RA (HAQ 1.8)	10 years	16,100 /QALY	2002
United Kingdom (NICE)	NHS/PSS	INF/DMARD sequence; ETA[44]/DMARD sequence	Advanced RA	Lifetime	89,970 £/QALY 64,880 £/QALY	GB£ 2004
Sweden	Societal	INF and ETA/compared with baseline	Advanced RA (HAQ 1.5)	1 year	43,400 /QALY	2003
United States	Societal	INF + MTX/MTX	Advanced active RA (HAQ 1.8)	Lifetime	30,500 $/QALY	US$ 2002
United Kingdom	NHS/PSS	ETA/DMARD sequence	Advanced active RA	Lifetime	16,330 £/QALY	GB£ 200
Sweden	Societal	ADA + MTX/DMARD sequence	Advanced active RA	Lifetime	40-44,000 /QALY	2004
Sweden	Societal	ETA + MTX/MTX	Advanced active RA (HAQ 1.8)	10 years	37-46,000 /QALY	2004
United Kingdom	*NHS/PSS*	*ETA, INF, ADA/DMARD sequence (Registry)*	*Advanced active RA (HAQ 2.1)*	*Lifetime*	*23,900 £/QALY*	*GB£ 2006*

ADA, adalimumab; DMARD, disease-modifying arthritic drugs; ETA, etanercept; HAQ, Health Assessment Questionnaire; INF, infliximab; LEF, leflunomide; MTX, methotrexate; RA, rheumatoid arthritis; SSZ, sulfasalazine,
Reprinted from Kobelt G, Jonsson B. The burden of rheumatoid arthritis and access to treatment: outcome and cost-utility of treatments. Eur J Health Econ 2008;(Suppl. 2):95-106.

References

1. Drummond MF, Barbieri M, Wong JB. Analytic choices in economic models of treatments for rheumatoid arthritis. What makes a difference? Med Decis Making 2005;25:520-33.
2. Kobelt G. Health economic issues in rheumatoid arthritis. Scand J Rheumatol 2006;35:415-25.
3. Bansback NJ, Regier DA, Ara R, Brennan A, Shojania K, Esdaile JM, et al. An overview of economic evaluations for drugs used in rheumatoid arthritis: focus on tumour necrosis factor-alpha antagonists. Drugs 2005;65:473-96.
4. Kobelt G, Jonsson B. The burden of rheumatoid arthritis and access to treatment: outcome and cost-utility of treatments. Eur J Health Econ 2008;(Suppl. 2):95-106.
5. Drummond M, O'Brien B, Stoddart G, Torrance G. Methods for the Economic Evaluation of Health Care. Boston: Kluwer Academic Publishers; 1997.
6. Kobelt G. Health Economics: Introduction to Economic Evaluation. 2nd ed. London: Office of Health Economics; 2002.
7. Drummond MF, Schwartz JS, Jonsson B, Luce BR, Neumann PJ, Siebert U, et al. Key principles for the improved conduct of health technology assessments for resource allocation decisions. Int J Technol Assess Health Care 2008;24:244-58; discussion 362-8.
8. Lundkvist J, Kastang F, Kobelt G. The burden of rheumatoid arthritis and access to treatment: health burden and costs. Eur J Health Econ 2008;(Suppl. 2):S49-60.
9. Kobelt G, Woronoff AS, Richard B, Peeters P, Sany J. Disease status, costs and quality of life of patients with rheumatoid arthritis in France: the ECO-PR Study. Joint Bone Spine 2008;75:408-15.
10. Fries J, Spitz P, Kraines R, Holman H. Measurement of patient outcome in arthritis. Arthritis Rheum 1980;23:137-45.
11. Kobelt G, Andlin-Sobocki P, Brophy S, Jonsson L, Calin A, Braun J. The burden of ankylosing spondylitis and the cost-effectiveness of treatment with infliximab. Rheumatology 2004;43:1158-66.
12. Kobelt G, Andlin-Sobocki P, Rousseau C, Maksymowych W. Cost and quality of life of patients with ankylosing spondylitis in Canada. J Rheumatol 2006;33:289-95.
13. Kobelt G, Sobocki P, Mulero J, Gratacos J, Pocovi A, Collantes-Estevez E. The burden of ankylosing spondylitis in Spain. Value Health 2008;11:408-15.
14. Torrance G. Measurement of health state utilities for economic appraisal. A review. J Health Econ 1986;5:1-30.
15. EuroQol Group. Euroqol—a new facility for the measurement of health-related quality of life. Health Policy 1990;16:199-208.
16. Dolan P, Gudex C, Kind P, Williams A. A social tariff for EuroQol: Results from a UK general population survey. Report No.: Discussion Paper 138. York: Centre for Health Economics, University of York; 1995.
17. Torrance G. Multi-attribute value and utility functions for a comprehensive health status classification system. Toronto: McMasters University; 1992.
18. Brazier J, Roberts J, Deverill M. The estimation of a preference-based measure of health from the SF-36. J Health Econ 2002;21:271-92.
19. Kobelt G, Lindgren P, Lindroth Y, Jacobson L, Eberhardt K. Modelling the effect of function and disease activity on costs and quality of life in rheumatoid arthritis. Rheumatology (Oxford) 2005;44:1169-75.
20. Kobelt G. Thoughts on health economics in rheumatoid arthritis. Ann Rheum Dis 2007;66(Suppl. 3):iii35-9.
21. Briggs A, Sculpher M. An introduction to Markov Modelling for Economic Evaluation. Pharmacoeconomics 1998;13:397-409.

Chapter 33

Introduction of a Biologic Agent into the Clinic

Vibeke Strand and Jeff Smith

Over the last decade, biologic agents have revolutionized the treatment of rheumatoid arthritis (RA) and seronegative spondyloarthropathies. Although many promising interventions failed, these new therapies have taught us much, not only about the underlying immunopathophysiology of inflammatory arthritis but also about their pragmatic use in clinical practice. Future interventions hold promise for addressing the remaining unmet need in inflammatory arthritis, and also systemic lupus erythematosus (SLE), systemic sclerosis (SSc), Sjögren's syndrome (SS), vasculitis, and inflammatory myopathies.

The introduction of a biologic agent into the clinic poses challenges that are different from those posed by a traditional "small molecule" therapeutic. As proteins or peptides, they require more complex manufacturing and characterization processes. Biologics are "designer" drugs whose mode of action in an underlying disease pathophysiology is frequently well understood. Their target specificity means that data derived from animal models can support a more rational clinical development program, facilitating better predictions of dosing, efficacy, and safety profiles compared with small molecule therapeutics.[1,2] Nonetheless, preclinical data and relevant toxicology studies may not be possible in two species, as required by International Conference on Harmonisation (ICH) guidelines, owing to lack of sufficient homology of the target between species. Also, toxicology studies may be limited in duration[3] owing to immunogenicity observed in the species used (usually primate), resulting in increased clearance of the biologic agent and reduced exposure in the animals. Throughout the development program of a biologic agent, guidances are available from the US Food and Drug Administration (FDA), which offer useful information regarding most aspects (Tables 33-1 and 33-2).

CHARACTERIZATION OF THE PRODUCT

Because of their targeted mechanisms of action, means of manufacture, and species specificity, biologic agents must be well characterized by potency, identity/quality, purity, and stability. Typically, ex vivo assays are used to assess potency, and it can be challenging to adapt one or multiple assays to be practical or feasible for routine use in a commercial manufacturing process. Requirements for identity and purity must be well defined, and these as well as stability may change as the manufacturing process is refined. Because of the potential variability introduced by changes in the working cell bank, it is ideal to define the process and initiate scale-up of manufacturing as soon as proof of concept of clinical activity has been obtained. Finally, formulation and route of administration should be decided early in the development process. FDA may allow manufacturers of biologic products to make manufacturing changes without conducting additional clinical efficacy studies but only if "comparability" data demonstrate that the product after the manufacturing change is still identical by assays for purity, potency, and biologic activity.[4] Changes in either formulation or manufacturing process may force "bridging" studies to demonstrate that the newer product is not only identical by potency, purity, and identity as well as pharmacokinetic (PK) profile, but that it also performs similarly in the clinic. Such bridging studies may introduce significant delays in clinical development programs.

Manufacturing Process

Although manufacturing and testing practices typically evolve during product development, scale up is risky if it changes the product characteristics. Often a source of regulatory concern, it should be performed sooner rather than later, for example, before phase 3, and must be dealt with proactively (Fig. 33-1).

Glycosylation occurs in the endoplasmic reticulum and Golgi apparatus as a post-translational modification of protein production. It is absent in *Escherichia coli* but present in yeast and highly conserved among mammalian cells (mouse myeloma, baby hamster, Chinese hamster ovary [CHO] and human), according to the cell line selected for manufacture and working cell bank. Of the tumor

Table 33-1. *Differences Between Biologic Agents and Synthetic Therapeutics*

Traditional Products	Biologic Agents
Low molecular weight (<1 kDa)	High molecular weight
Typically well-defined physicochemical properties	Complex physicochemical properties; tertiary structure; glycosylation
Chemically synthesized	Produced recombinantly in engineered cells
Stable; not heat sensitive	Heat and shear-sensitive, may aggregate
Well characterized; typically homogeneous; High chemical purity with standards well established	Characterization may be challenging; typically heterogeneous composition; Need to define potency, purity, identity, stability
Mechanism of action often not known	Hypothesized mechanism of action usually well characterized
Generic and related products are common	Typically unique based on binding epitope, cell line and FcγR structure
Rapidly enter systemic circulation through blood capillaries	Larger molecules, primarily reach circulation through lymphatic system; May undergo proteolysis during interstitial and lymphatic transit
Distribution to organs/tissues	Distribution usually limited to plasma and/or extracellular fluids
Oral administration typical	Parenteral administration: intravenously, subcutaneously, or intraarticularly
Linear dose response	Nonlinear dose response which may be relatively flat or inverted
Species-independent	Species-specific
Metabolized to nonactive and active metabolites	Catabolized to endogenous amino acids
Cyp 450 involvement	Typically Cyp450 independent
Toxicities may be "off target", e.g., not associated with primary pharmacologic effect	Receptor-mediated or mechanistically related toxicity; toxicities may be species specific "pharmacologic" and "industrial strength" dosing
Nonimmunogenic	Immunogenic
Typically a single analytical method required for pharmacokinetic studies	Multiple assays to assess pharmacokinetics (bioassay, enzyme-linked immunosorbent assay, and ligand-binding assay)

Table 33-2. *Examples of US Food and Drug Administration and International Conference on Harmonisation Guidances for Industry: Selected Guidelines Relevant to Biologic Agents from 1995–2008*

Draft Guidance for Industry: Potency Tests for Cellular and Gene Therapy Products - 10/9/2008

International Conference on Harmonisation (ICH); Guidance for Industry: S1C(R2) Dose Selection for Carcinogenicity Studies (PDF - 185 KB) - 9/17/2008

Concept Paper: Animal Models — Essential Elements to Address Efficacy Under the Animal Rule (PDF) - 9/9/2008

Draft Guidance for Industry: Integrated Summary of Effectiveness - 8/27/2008

Guidance for FDA Reviewers and Sponsors: Content and Review of Chemistry, Manufacturing, and Control (CMC) Information for Human Somatic Cell Therapy Investigational New Drug Applications (INDs) - 4/9/2008

Guidance for FDA Reviewers and Sponsors: Content and Review of Chemistry, Manufacturing, and Control (CMC) Information for Human Gene Therapy Investigational New Drug Applications (INDs) - 4/9/2008

International Conference on Harmonisation (ICH); Guidance for Industry: E15 Definitions for Genomic Biomarkers, Pharmacogenomics, Pharmacogenetics, Genomic Data and Sample Coding Categories - 4/7/2008

International Conference on Harmonisation (ICH); Draft Guidance: S2(R1) Genotoxicity Testing and Data Interpretation for Pharmaceuticals Intended for Human Use - 3/25/2008

Draft Guidance for Industry: Validation of Growth-Based Rapid Microbiological Methods for Sterility Testing of Cellular and Gene Therapy Products - 2/11/2008

International Conference on Harmonisation (ICH); Draft Guidance: Q8(R1) Pharmaceutical Development Revision 1 - 1/10/2008

International Conference on Harmonisation (ICH); Guidance for Industry - Q8 Pharmaceutical Development - 5/19/2006

Guidance for Industry: Providing Regulatory Submissions to the Center for Biologics Evaluation and Research (CBER) in Electronic Format - Lot Release Protocols - 11/27/2007

Draft Guidance for Industry: Drug-Induced Liver Injury: Premarketing Clinical Evaluation - 10/24/2007

Guidance for Industry: Manufacturing Biological Intermediates and Biological Drug Substances Using Spore-Forming Microorganisms - 9/6/2007

Table 33-2. *Examples of US Food and Drug Administration and International Conference on Harmonisation Guidances for Industry: Selected Guidelines Relevant to Biologic Agents from 1995–2008–cont'd*

Draft Guidance for Industry: Pharmacogenomic Data Submissions - Companion Guidance - 8/28/2007
Guidance for Industry: Pharmacogenomic Data Submissions - 3/22/2005
Attachment to Guidance on Pharmacogenomic Data Submissions - 3/22/2005
Guidance for Industry: Regulation of Human Cells, Tissues, and Cellular and Tissue-Based Products (HCT/Ps) - Small Entity Compliance Guide - 8/24/2007
Guidance for Industry: Eligibility Determination for Donors of Human Cells, Tissues, and Cellular and Tissue-Based Products (HCT/Ps) - 8/8/2007
Guidance for Industry: Exports Under the FDA Export Reform and Enhancement Act of 1996 - 7/24/2007
Draft Guidance for Industry: Cooperative Manufacturing Arrangements for Licensed Biologics - 7/20/2007
International Conference on Harmonisation (ICH); Draft Guidance: Q10 Pharmaceutical Quality System - 7/12/2007
Draft Guidance for Industry: Preparation of IDEs and INDs for Products Intended to Repair or Replace Knee Cartilage - 7/6/2007
Draft Guidance for Industry: Integrated Summaries of Effectiveness and Safety: Location Within the Common Technical Document - 7/2/2007
Draft Guidance for Industry: Providing Regulatory Submissions in Electronic Format - Receipt Date - 6/5/2007
Guidance for Industry: Computerized Systems Used in Clinical Investigations - 5/10/2007
Draft Guidance for Industry: Protecting the Rights, Safety, and Welfare of Study Subjects - Supervisory Responsibilities of Investigators - 5/10/2007
Draft Guidance for Clinical Investigators, Sponsors, and IRBs: Adverse Event Reporting - Improving Human Subject Protection - 4/17/2007
Draft Guidance for Industry: Dosage and Administration Section of Labeling for Human Prescription Drug and Biological Products - Content and Format - 4/9/2007
Guidance for Industry: Gene Therapy Clinical Trials - Observing Subjects for Delayed Adverse Events - 11/28/2006
Guidance for Industry: Biological Product Deviation Reporting for Licensed Manufacturers of Biological Products Other than Blood and Blood Components - 10/18/2006
Draft Guidance for Industry: Drug Interaction Studies - Study Design, Data Analysis, and Implications for Dosing and Labeling - 9/11/2006
International Conference on Harmonisation (ICH); Guidance for Industry: S8 Immunotoxicity Studies for Human Pharmaceuticals - 4/12/2006
Guidance for Clinical Trial Sponsors: Establishment and Operation of Clinical Trial Data Monitoring Committees - 3/27/2006
Guidance for Industry: Using a Centralized IRB Review Process in Multicenter Clinical Trials - 3/15/2006
Draft Guidance for Industry: Patient-Reported Outcome Measures: Use in Medical Product Development to Support Labeling Claims - 2/2/2006
Guidance for Industry: Adverse Reactions Section of Labeling for Human Prescription Drug and Biological Products - Content and Format - 1/18/2006
Guidance for Industry: Clinical Studies Section of Labeling for Human Prescription Drug and Biological Products - Content and Format - 1/18/2006
Draft Guidance for Industry: Warnings and Precautions, Contraindications, and Boxed Warning Sections of Labeling for Human Prescription Drug and Biological Products - Content and Format - 1/18/2006
Draft Guidance for Industry: Labeling for Human Prescription Drug and Biological Products - Implementing the New Content and Format Requirements - 1/18/2006
Guidance for Industry: Fast Track Drug Development Programs - Designation, Development, and Application Review - 1/11/2006
Guidance for Industry: Collection of Race and Ethnicity Data in Clinical Trials - 9/19/2005
International Conference on Harmonisation (ICH); Guidance for Industry: Q5E Comparability of Biotechnological/Biological Products Subject to Changes in Their Manufacturing Process - 6/29/2005
Reviewer Guidance: Evaluating the Risks of Drug Exposure in Human Pregnancies - 4/27/2005
International Conference on Harmonisation (ICH); Guidance for Industry: E2E Pharmacovigilance Planning - 3/31/2005
Guidance for Industry: Good Pharmacovigilance Practices and Pharmacoepidemiologic Assessment - 3/25/2005
Guidance for Industry: Continuous Marketing Applications: Pilot 2 - Scientific Feedback and Interactions During Development of Fast Track Products Under PDUFA - 10/6/2003
Guidance for Industry: Sterile Drug Products Produced by Aseptic Processing -- Current Good Manufacturing Practice - 9/29/2004
Draft Guidance for Industry and FDA: Current Good Manufacturing Practice for Combination Products - 9/29/2004 - (PDF - 134 KB)
Guidance for Industry: Available Therapy - 7/21/2004
Draft Guidance for Industry: Information Program on Clinical Trials for Serious or Life-Threatening Diseases and Conditions (Revision 1) - 1/26/2004
Guidance for Industry: Information Program on Clinical Trials for Serious or Life-Threatening Diseases and Conditions - 3/18/2002
Draft Guidance for Industry: Comparability Protocols - Protein Drug Products and Biological Products - Chemistry, Manufacturing, and Controls Information - 9/3/2003
Guidance for Industry: Exposure-Response Relationships - Study Design, Data Analysis, and Regulatory Applications - 5/5/2003
Guidance for Industry: Source Animal, Product, Preclinical, and Clinical Issues Concerning the Use of Xenotransplantation Products in Humans - 4/3/2003
Draft Guidance for Industry; Comparability Protocols - Chemistry, Manufacturing, and Controls Information - 2/20/2003
Draft Guidance for Industry and Reviewers on Estimating the Safe Starting Dose in Clinical Trials for Therapeutics in Adult Healthy Volunteers - 1/15/2003
Draft Guidance for Industry: Drugs, Biologics, and Medical Devices Derived from Bioengineered Plants for Use in Humans and Animals - 9/6/2002
Guidance for Industry: Container Closure Systems for Packaging Human Drugs and Biologics; Questions and Answers - 5/13/2002
Guidance for Industry: Container Closure Systems for Packaging Human Drugs and Biologics; Chemistry, Manufacturing, and Controls Documentation - 7/7/1999
Guidance for Industry: IND Meetings for Human Drugs and Biologics; Chemistry, Manufacturing and Controls Information - 5/25/2001
ICH Guidance for Industry: E 10 Choice of Control Group and Related Issues in Clinical Trials - 5/11/2001

(Continued)

Table 33-2. *Examples of US Food and Drug Administration and International Conference on Harmonisation Guidances for Industry: Selected Guidelines Relevant to Biologic Agents from 1995–2008–cont'd*

Guidance for Industry: Q & A Content and Format of INDs for Phase 1 Studies of Drugs, Including Well-Characterized, Therapeutic, Biotechnology-Derived Products - 10/3/2000

Guidance for Industry: Content and Format of Investigational New Drug Applications (INDs) for Phase 1 Studies of Drugs, Including Well-Characterized, Therapeutic, Biotechnology-derived Products - 11/1995

ICH Guidance on Specifications: Test Procedures and Acceptance Criteria for Biotechnological/Biological Products - 8/18/1999 - (PDF - 58 KB)

ICH Guidance on the Duration of Chronic Toxicity Testing in Animals (Rodent and Nonrodent Toxicity Testing); Availability - 6/25/1999 - (PDF - 22 KB)

Guidance for Industry: For the Submission of Chemistry, Manufacturing and Controls and Establishment Description Information for Human Plasma-Derived Biological Products, Animal Plasma or Serum-Derived Products - 2/17/1999

Guidance for Industry: Population Pharmacokinetics - 2/10/1999

Draft Guidance for Industry: General Considerations for Pediatric Pharmacokinetic Studies for Drugs and Biological Products - 11/30/1998

ICH Guidance on Viral Safety Evaluation of Biotechnology Products Derived From Cell Lines of Human or Animal Origin - 9/24/1998 - (PDF - 89 KB)

ICH Guidance on Quality of Biotechnological/Biological Products: Derivation and Characterization of Cell Substrates Used for Production of Biotechnological/Biological Products - 9/21/1998 - (PDF - 47 KB)

Guidance for Industry: Providing Clinical Evidence of Effectiveness for Human Drugs and Biological Products - 5/15/1998

Guidance for Industry - Changes to an Approved Application: Biological Products - 7/24/1997

Guidance for Industry - Changes to an Approved Application for Specified Biotechnology and Specified Synthetic Biological Products - 7/24/1997

International Conference on Harmonisation (ICH); Guidance for Industry: S6 Preclinical Safety Evaluation of Biotechnology-Derived Pharmaceuticals (PDF) - 7/1997

Guidance for Industry for the Submission of Chemistry, Manufacturing, and Controls Information for a Therapeutic Recombinant DNA-Derived Product or a Monoclonal Antibody Product for In Vivo Use - 8/1996 - (PDF - 44 KB)

International Conference on Harmonisation: Final Guidance on Stability Testing of Biotechnological/Biological Products - 7/10/1996 - (PDF - 26 KB)

FDA Guidance Concerning Demonstration of Comparability of Human Biological Products, Including Therapeutic Biotechnology-Derived Products - 4/1996 - (PDF - 25 KB)

Points to Consider in the Manufacture and Testing of Therapeutic Products for Human Use Derived from Transgenic Animals - 1995

International Conference on Harmonisation (ICH); Guideline for Industry: E1A The Extent of Population Exposure to Assess Clinical Safety: For Drugs Intended for Long-term Treatment of Non-Life-Threatening Conditions (PDF) - 3/1995

International Conference on Harmonisation (ICH); Guideline for Industry: S3A Toxicokinetics: The Assessment of Systemic Exposure in Toxicity Studies (PDF) - 3/1995

International Conference on Harmonisation (ICH); Guideline for Industry: S3B Pharmacokinetics: Guidance for Repeated Dose Tissue Distribution Studies (PDF) - 3/1995

necrosis factor-α (TNF-α) inhibitors, adalimumab and etanercept are manufactured in CHO cells, whereas the aglycosylated F(ab)'-PEG product, certolizumab pegol, is manufactured in *E. coli*.

LESSON 1: DIFFERENCES IN GLYCOSYLATION PATTERNS DUE TO PRODUCTION IN MICROBIAL VERSUS MAMMALIAN CELL LINES: GRANULOCYTE MACROPHAGE/ GRANULOCYTE COLONY STIMULATING FACTOR

Five different granulocyte macrophage (GM)/ granulocyte colony stimulating factor (G-CSF) molecules have been produced in various expression systems. Bacterial expression (*E. coli*) yields aglycosylated molecules (molgramostim and filgrastim), yeast expression (*Saccharomyces cerevisiae*) yields O-glycosylated molecules (sargramostim) and mammalian expression (CHO cell line) yields fully glycosylated molecules (regramostim and lenograstim).

- In prospective randomized placebo controlled trials, only glycosylated CSFs have been associated with improved patient survival (sargramostim and lenograstim).[5-7]
- In vitro and in vivo data generated from comparative studies have documented differences in biologic activity among CSFs.[8-11]
- A literature review of clinical trials evaluating sargramostim (glycosylated) and molgramostim (aglycosylated) concluded that molgramostim was associated with a higher incidence of adverse effects than sargramostim,[12] as shown in the following table.

Adverse Effect	Pooled Median Frequency (%)	
	Sargramostim	Molgramostim
Fluid retention	8.3	18.4
Dyspnea	13.4	55.2
Fever	21.7	40.7
Myalgia/bone pain	16.0	28.5
Rash	14.3	12.5

Other manufacturing platforms include transgenic plants and animals as well as live animal platforms such as mammary glands of living goats.[13] Glycosylation largely determines tertiary,

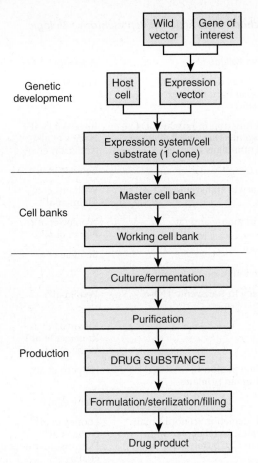

Genetic development

Expression system/cell substrate (1 clone)

Cell banks

Master cell bank

Working cell bank

Culture/fermentation

Purification

Production

DRUG SUBSTANCE

Formulation/sterilization/filling

Drug product

Figure 33-1. Flow diagram for manufacturing processes of biologic agents.

even quaternary structure; binding to the selected epitope as well as immunogenicity. Several examples exist in which changes in the working cell bank due to scale up issues resulted in products with differing glycosylation profiles, resulting in loss of efficacy despite identity by high performance liquid chromatography (HPLC) and other in vitro assays.

LESSON 2: RISKS OF CHANGING MANUFACTURING PROCESSES DURING CLINICAL DEVELOPMENT: PRIMATIZED ANTI CD4 MONOCLONAL ANTIBODY AND LENERCEPT

Monoclonal antibody (mAb) effector function and clearance are affected by glycosylation patterns, which depend on the production cell line [working cell bank] and culture media.

- This was illustrated with a nondepleting primatized anti-CD4 mAb following a change in the working cell bank due to scale up requirements, as well as removal of products of bovine and human origin in the manufacturing process. Although the inserted coding construct remained identical, a new CHO cell line adapted to growth in cell-free media was used,

resulting in sustained rather than transient T-cell depletion, infusion reactions, and less efficacy.[14,15]

- Similarly, attempts to improve manufacturing yield of the p55 soluble TNF-α receptor I (sTNF RI-Fc) construct lenercept resulted in inter-batch differences in glycosylation patterns with loss of efficacy, despite identity in assays of purity, potency, and specificity.[16,17]
- Differences in glycosylation patterns accounted for rapid initial phases of clearance, altering the half life and analytical ultracentrifugation (AUC) of the molecule.[18,19]
- Production processes can also affect immunogenicity, when aggregates form after lyophilization (see Lesson 3).

Changes in manufacturing processes, and even the final formulation, may also introduce variability, which is exemplified by the alterations in final manufacture of erythropoietin, which resulted in cases of pure red cell aplasia ascribed to increased immunogenicity of the altered product.

LESSON 3: SUBTLE CHANGES IN MANUFACTURING PROCESSES CAN SIGNIFICANTLY AND DETRIMENTALLY ALTER IMMUNOGENICITY, DEMONSTRATED BY AGGREGATE FORMATION WITH RECOMBINANT ERYTHROPOIETIN

Since 1998, approximately 200 suspected cases of pure red cell aplasia (PRCA) due to neutralizing antibodies have been reported in patients with chronic renal failure receiving erythropoietin treatment.[20] The majority of cases were associated with the use of epoetin alfa distributed outside of the United States, manufactured at a different site than that distributed within the United States. Immunogenicity of this preparation appeared to occur when polysorbate 80 and glycine were substituted for human serum albumin in the formulation to comply with new regulations from the European regulatory authorities.

It is believed that the new formulation was less stable, so that aggregates might form under adverse storage circumstances, such as prolonged exposure to increased temperatures. The presence of aggregates increase the likelihood of antibody formation following subcutaneous administration, and antierythropoietin antibodies observed in patients with PRCA appear to be directed against the protein moiety of the molecule. It is not known whether subtle differences between the carbohydrate moieties of epoetin alfa and beta have had any impact on this observed immunogenicity.

Preclinical Data

With a well-characterized mechanism of action, animal models are considered to have high relevance to clinical use of biologic agents. Nonetheless they must be viewed with caution in terms of their

Table 33-3. *Examples of In Vivo Validation in Animal Models of Mechanisms of Action of Representative Biologic Agents in Rheumatology*

Compound	Mode of Action	Clinical Phase	In vivo Validation	Reference
HuMax-CD4	Anti CD4 mAb	Discontinued	CD4 T cell depletion and function in nonhuman primates	Fishwild et al[22]
Kelixumab	Anti CD4 mAb	Discontinued	CD4 function in human CD4 transgenic mice; renal allografts in cynomolgus monkeys	Bugelskil et al[23] Hersyk et al[24] Anderson et al[25]
Anakinra	IL-1ra	Approved	CIA	Bendele et al[26]
Infliximab	Anti–TNF-α mAb	Approved	Efficacy in transgenic TNF-α mice	Williams et al[27] Maini et al[28]
Etanercept	sTNF-α RII-IgG1	Approved	CIA in mouse and rat	Wooley et al[29] Piguet et al[30]
sTNFα RII-IgG1	sTNFα RI-IgG1	Discontinued	CIA	Bendele et al[31]
Adalimumab	Anti-TNF-α mAb	Approved	None found on this agent	
Certolizumab pegol	TNF-αF(ab')PEG	Approved in CD	Efficacy in transgenic TNF-α mice	Weir et al[32]
Abatacept	CTLA 4-Ig Fc	Approved	CIA	Kliwinski et al[33] Knoerzer et al[34] Webb et al[35]
Belimumab	Anti-Blys mAb	Phase 3 in SLE	B-cell depletion in nonhuman primates	Halpern et al[36]
Atacicept	TACI Ig	Phase 2 in SLE	CIA	Wang et al[37]
Rituximab	Anti-CD20 mAb	Approved	B-cell depletion in nonhuman primates; B-cell depletion in human CD20 transgenic mice; CIA	Looney et al[38] Gong et al[39] Dumussi-Joannopoulos et al[40]
TRU-015	Anti-CD20 SMIP	Phase 2	B-cell depletion in nonhuman primates	Trubion[41]
HuMax-CD20 (Ofatumumab)	Anti-CD20 mAb	Phase 2	B-cell depletion in laboratory tests and animal studies	Genmab[42]
Tocilizumab	Anti IL-6R	Phase 3 completed in RA	CIA	Alonzi et al[43] Fujimoto et al[44]
AVE9897 (MLN 3897)	CCR1 antagonist	Discontinued	CIA	Amat et al[45]

CD, cluster of differentiation; CIA, collagen-induced arthritis; RA, rheumatoid arthritis; SLE, systemic lupus erythematosus; TNF-α, tumor necrosis factor-α.
Modified from Hegen M, Keith JC, Collins M, Nickerson-Nutter CL: Utility of animal models for identification of potential therapeutic for rheumatoid arthritis. Ann Rheum Dis 2008;67;1505–15.

interpretability and predictive value to human disease. Owing to the lack of species homology for many products, murine-specific analogs may be used in disease models in rodents. With sufficient homology regarding target binding or mechanism of action, pharmacodynamic (PD) effects in primates may be informative. Clearly, differences in the underlying immune systems may result in unexpected or difficult to interpret findings. Most products designed for treatment of RA have been studied in adjuvant-induced (AIA) or collagen-induced (CIA) arthritis in murine systems: rat or mouse. CIA in rhesus monkey offers the potential opportunity to use the human product, but the arthritis in this model is often unpredictable and very severe—and forces use of a valuable animal resource. Gene therapy products have been extensively studied in antigen-induced arthritis in rabbits; B-cell targeted therapies by demonstrating B-cell depletion in nonhuman primates (Table 33-3).[21-45]

Epitope binding of monoclonal antibodies may have significant influence upon their biologic effects and Fc gamma receptor (FcγR) function. Studies in human CD20 transgenic mice have elegantly demonstrated that peripheral B cell depletion may be attributed to both complement-dependent (CDC) and antibody-dependent cytotoxicity (ADCC), the former requiring Kupffer cell function in the liver and the latter abrogated by depletion of macrophages.[29] In comparison to monoclonal antibodies (mAbs) derived from murine systems, such as rituximab, human anti CD20 mAbs developed in immunoglobulin transgenic mice recognize a unique extracellular region that appears to result in more effective complement 1q (C1q) activation and CDC, which cannot be ascribed solely to an expected slower off rate due to superior binding.[46]

Furthermore, most animal models may not reflect the same mechanisms of action predominant in man, nor those which result in perpetuation of disease.[47] An example is the CIA model in which impressive results reported with inhibitors of IL-1 such as anakinra were not duplicated in trials in patients (see Table 33-3). In animal models, it is apparent that IL-1β mediates synovitis and TNF-α erosive disease, whereas in humans, elevated TNF-α levels are responsible for both inflammation and bone erosions.[48] More recently, transgenic overexpression of TNF-α or IL-1β, which causes arthritis and joint destruction, have been used to test cytokine inhibitors and transgenic CD20 mice for B cell inhibitors.[49] Assessment of safety pharmacology may also be limited by species homology.[50]

The relevance of the PK and PD profile of biologic therapeutics in nonhuman primates may be limited. Nonetheless they must be well characterized in hopes of identifying dose and exposure response relationships, whether useful biomarkers exist, and selection of initial doses for phase 1—designed to define the minimum anticipated biologic effective level (MABEL), as well as the maximally tolerated dose (MTD).[51] In July 2005, the FDA issued guidance for estimating the maximum recommended starting dose (MRSD) of a new molecular entity in adult healthy subjects, detailing a standard algorithm comprising four major steps.[52] The no observed adverse effect level (NOAEL) is determined from animal data and is converted to a human equivalent dose (HED) using an appropriate scaling factor. Third, the most appropriate animal species is identified, and fourth, the MRSD is determined by applying a safety factor specifically to the HED of the NOAEL from the most appropriate animal species. A fifth step may be added, depending on the toxicity profile of the agent, for example, if it has an exaggerated pharmacologic effect upon administration, such as vasodilation.[53] Although cross-species PK information is relevant for small synthetic molecules, in comparison monoclonal antibodies that engender both high affinity for the biologic target and PD effect have limited cross-reactivity, primarily to nonhuman primates. An example of the challenges faced in trying to predict human PD effects was exemplified by work with the human mAB to CD4, in which differing cell binding and depletion patterns were observed in cynomolgus versus rhesus monkeys.

LESSON 4: DIFFERENCES IN PHARMACODYNAMIC EFFECTS BETWEEN RHESUS AND CYNOMOLGUS MONKEYS: HUMAX CD4

Chimpanzees are phylogenetically close to humans and share similar circulating lymphocyte population number and subsets, with the exception of enhanced expression of the CD4 antigen on peripheral monocytes.

HuMax CD4 or HM6G was a fully human IgGκ anti CD4 monoclonal antibody, isolated from a human immunoglobulin transgenic mouse. Before introduction into the clinic, PD and PK effects of this mAb were studied in nonhuman primates: chimpanzees and cynomolgus monkeys.[22]

- In chimpanzees, the mAb did not deplete peripheral CD4+ T cells, inhibited ex vivo immune function assays, and was cleared rapidly;
- In cynomolgus monkeys, following rapid infusion at doses 0.6 mg/kg or more, depletion of CD4+T cells occurred in a dose-dependent fashion, for up to 6 months at doses 2.0 mg/kg or more;
- In contrast, slower administration of mAb over 30 minutes or more in cynomolgus monkeys did not result in CD4+ T-cell depletion, despite little alteration in PK parameters
- Neither bolus or prolonged infusions of mAb were associated with alterations in ex vivo immune function assays in cynomolgus monkeys, compared with chimpanzees;
- Duration of mAb binding to CD4+ T cells, for example "coating," was dose dependent.

Subsequent trials in humans in RA were not associated with peripheral CD4+ T-cell depletion, nor with efficacy.[54]

Toxicology Studies

Toxicology studies of biologic agents typically require a "single definitive study in one relevant species." Before determining which species to use, the relative potency of the human therapeutic should be tested against rodent and primate versions of the target antigen. Without manufacture of a murine version of a product, most consider that homology differences will make standard species toxicology studies irrelevant to clinical use. Furthermore, murine-specific but human-irrelevant binding, metabolic activation or degradation question the relevance of such toxicology studies to work in humans. For these reasons, the majority of toxicology studies of biologic agents are performed in cynomolgus or rhesus monkeys. Owing to homology differences, scientific rigor may require use of chimpanzees, an unfortunate requirement to utilizing a limited but valuable animal resource. Allometric scaling based on NOAEL and PK simulations of area under the curve concentrations are used to define 'target' human dose ranges.[55] Generally the starting dose is considered to represent one tenth of maximally tolerated doses (MTD) in milligrams per square meter in the most sensitive species in toxicology studies.[56] However, due to the possibility of a bell shaped response curve, it may be necessary to perform preclinical assessment across a spectrum of doses to obtain an optimal biological dose (OBD).

Length of studies and frequency of administration are based on intended human use, and will be 6 to 12 months in duration, with dosing as frequent as weekly or biweekly to support chronic administration in humans on a monthly or biweekly basis. In addition to in vivo toxicology studies, an in vitro tissue cross-reactivity study is essential to determine that the organ distribution of target binding is the same in the toxicology species as it is in humans. Demonstrated tissue cross-reactivity may also require specific monitoring for anticipated (or unanticipated) "off-target" effects.

Immunogenicity may determine the length of preclinical studies because once antibodies are identified, dosing in the toxicology study should be discontinued; antibodies typically alter PK by increasing clearance and potential biologic effects (if neutralizing) of the product.[57] Preclinical studies, even conducted in macaques, frequently over-predict immune responses in humans, likely owing to inherent differences in how foreign recombinant proteins are viewed immunologically by different species.[58]

Reproductive and carcinogenicity studies are now required earlier in development, especially in targeted disease populations such as RA and SLE, in which the majority of patients are women of childbearing age.[59] Currently, the approval of tocilizumab has been delayed in the United States until a reproductive study has been performed. Since introduction of genetically engineered p53+/- mouse and the rasH2 mouse, use of models for accelerated carcinogenicity testing has steadily grown.[60] These models, rather than wild-type mice, improve testing performance by reducing the number of mouse-specific and human-irrelevant false-positive results by approximately 50% without compromising test sensitivity for outcomes relevant to humans. However, species specificity of the biologic agent may require a murine homolog of the human therapeutic to be used in carcinogenicity studies. Reproductive studies have been performed in cynomolgus monkeys with adalimumab,[61] rats and rabbits with etanercept,[62] and in rats with murine homologs of infliximab[63] and certilizomab pegol.[64]

Route of Administration and Dosing Regimen

Route of administration and dosing regimen may significantly affect the interrelationship between PK and PD effects of biologic agents. This is well illustrated by two pegylated derivatives of interferon-α: a 40-kilo Dalton (kDa) branched polyethylene glycol interferon-α-2a (PEG-IFNα2a) and PEG-IFNα2b, a 12-kDa linear polyethylene glycol (PEG). Both have slower absorption, smaller volumes of distribution, and lower elimination rates following subcutaneous injection than nonpegylated IFN-α. Consequently,

concentrations appropriate to inhibit hepatitis C viral replication are maintained for longer periods of time, allowing once-weekly dosing. Avoidance of multiple weekly injections and achievement of more consistent therapeutic blood levels also reduced adverse effects associated with more frequent dosing, related to excessive Cmax levels.[65] Unanticipated effects may also be related to single versus multiple dose regimens. An early phase 2 study of recombinant human interleukin-12 (rhIL-12) revealed profound toxicity secondary to interferon-γ (IFN-γ) production, which was not predicted by phase 1 data. Of importance, the phase 1 study used single ascending doses of IL-12, followed 2 weeks later by consecutive daily dosing. This 'priming' dose attenuated IFNγ release and protected mice and cynomolgus monkeys from the acute toxicity and mortality subsequently observed with daily dosing.[66,67]

Immunogenicity of biologic agents is determined by epitope, tertiary, and quaternary structure, in which glycosylation patterns or lack thereof may play a significant role. Fcg receptor functions may also enhance immunogenicity as well as contributing to infusion reactions. Route of administration and dosing regimen may also contribute to immunogenicity. Monoclonal antibodies that result in cell lysis after administration, such as alemtuzumab (CAMPATH 1 H) and rituximab, are associated with significant immunogenicity.[57] Use of low-dose background immunosuppressive agents, such as methotrexate, azathioprine, leflunomide, and mycophenolate mofetil, as well as regular dosing with maintenance of measurable blood levels, decrease the likelihood of development of a host immune response to a foreign protein.

First in Man Studies

The use of healthy volunteers in initial phase 1 studies of biologic agents is often more limited than with synthetic products. As with any therapeutic, it is unacceptable to use healthy subjects in phase 1 studies if the biologic agent is suspected to cause major toxicity but also immunogenicity. Theoretically, biologics that are almost identical to naturally derived peptides or proteins could elicit an immune response in healthy subjects to their own natural peptide or protein, a potentially catastrophic effect that could persist for their lifetime. If little or no immunogenicity has been observed in preclinical studies, single-dose or limited multiple-dose phase 1 studies may be performed in healthy volunteers. However, their relevance to subsequent dosing in patients with the targeted disease may be limited. PK and PD profiles may also differ considerably in patients with chronic autoimmune diseases with elevated cytokine levels, naturally occurring anticytokine autoantibodies, and abnormal immune circuitry, which perpetuate the inflammatory process.

Biologic agents, especially humanized or fully human monoclonal antibodies, have very long elimination half lives such that any healthy volunteer or patient participating in a phase 1 study should be followed for safety for many months until they have fully cleared the biologic agent. A good rule of thumb is that surveillance should be continued for at least five half-lives of the product. Presence of measurable levels of biologic agent for a prolonged period of time after a single administration thus poses a challenge when designing phase 1 single- and multiple-dose studies—and also limits the use of normal volunteers in early trials.

Initial introduction into the clinic of a new therapeutic requires a full clinical development plan, a detailed protocol and an investigators brochure. Although expected to change as a product progresses through phases 1 and 2, it is still prudent to plan its progression through clinical trials to approval—outlining trial designs and duration, efforts to determine MABEL and MTD in phase 1, selection of the appropriate dose and dose schedule in phase 2, and demonstrating efficacy and acceptable safety in phase 3. Plans to prospectively analyze data regarding dose individualization and pharmacogenomics are increasingly important.

Regulatory issues and strategy have become increasingly important in the last several years, prompted by the safety concerns exemplified by the cyclooxygenase-2 (COX-2) selective agents and the recent first in man trial of an activating anti CD28 molecule in normal volunteers.

LESSON 5: LACK OF SPECIES HOMOLOGY MAY FAIL TO PREDICT IN VIVO EFFECTS IN MAN: SUMMARY OF THE TEGENERO EXPERIENCE

CD28-Super-mAb (TGN 1412) was an activating (super-agonist) anti-CD28 monoclonal antibody, for treatment of autoimmune diseases.[68] The ligand for TGN1412, CD-28, is present on all T-cell subsets and is a costimulatory molecule for T-cell activation. TGN1412 promotes T-cell proliferation, cytokine production, resistance to apoptosis, and expansion of the T-cell population.

- In preclinical rodent models with murine homologs, FcγR cross-linking of the epitope on the CD28 molecule led to expansion of Treg cells; with beneficial effects.[69]
- Administration of the human therapeutic mAb, a fully human IgG4 isotype, to primates was not reported to have adverse effects.[70]
- The mAb was administered by IV infusion (duration of 3 to 6 minutes) to six healthy subjects at a starting dose of 0.1 mg/kg. This dose was reported to be 1/500th of the safe animal dose. When the first dose was administered to six in an initial cohort of eight healthy volunteers, men aged 19 to 34, approximately 10 minutes apart, all became acutely ill with "cytokine storm" - a consequence of extensive T-cell

activation resulting in multiorgan failure associated with disseminated intravascular coagulation and prolonged lymphopenia, and monocytopenia.[71]

- These effects were reminiscent of extreme first-dose reactions following administration of muromonab CD3 in allograft rejection, also due to T-cell activation induced by FcγR-mediated cross-linking of CD3.[72-74]
- The question is whether these reactions could have been predicted or attenuated, and certainly indicates that extra precaution should be used with mAbs that are designed as agonists.[75]
- Homology between primate and human epitopes were close but not sufficient to predict
  - Differences in binding of the variable region of the mAb to CD28, and
  - FcγR interactions, thereby resulting in extensive cross-linking, cell activation, and cytokine release
- Failure to recognize these potential differences may be a lesson in 'retrospective analyses'; nonetheless:
- "First in man" trials should recognize these potential limitations, and
  - Define initial doses to be at least one tenth of MTD in the most sensitive toxicology species
  - Dose each healthy volunteer or patient within a dose cohort individually, with sufficient time between subjects to carefully observe any untoward or obvious clinical effects; and their resolution before subsequent dosing of another individual
  - Require careful monitoring until all potential clinically related effects, including PK or PD consequences, are fully resolved within each subject before another subject is dosed.

Writing a package insert early, especially including proposed "claims" and "clinical indications" can be very helpful in interpreting clinical data as a product progresses through development. It is important to view phase 1 studies as "first in man" trials and predominantly safety trials, with determination of initial PK and PD profiles. It is important to think broadly about safety issues of a new therapeutic, especially those characterized for other products in its class or in recent FDA guidance documents. It is important to keep clinical trial designs simple, and avoid too many assumptions such as the width of the dose range or multiple endpoints, so that primary and secondary objectives are well defined. Empiric observations should drive development, and data from previous trials should be used to inform decisions and trial designs in subsequent ones.

Attempting to truncate the time of clinical development has often resulted in increased time to approval rather than more efficiency. Proof of concept trials in RA generally require 3 months duration, based on experience with multiple therapeutics, including p38 MAP kinase inhibitors and TNF-α convertase inhibitors, which showed promising benefit at 1 month with loss of effect over 2 to 3 months of treatment.[76-79] If full-dose ranging as well as dose schedule selection have not been completed in phase 2, sponsors may be forced to go back and do such in phase 3 before approval, as exemplified in the development program for abetimus sodium in SLE.[80] And truncating phase 2 exposure may fail to identify important safety signals that ultimately will result in discontinuation of development of a product.[81]

In view of the economic pressures and inequality in access to medical care, costs of biologic agents remain an important issue. Initial cost of goods at the time of marketing approval are based not only on the more expensive manufacturing processes employed to make biologic agents, but costs accrued during their extensive development program. Nonetheless after approval, even if competitive agents become available, traditionally costs of biologic agents have increased over time, despite broader use. Thus, there is an increasing interest in "biosimilars," or "generic biologic agents." Certainly these are possible for hormones [recombinant insulin] and growth factors.

LESSON 6: BIOSIMILARS OR FOLLOW ON BIOLOGICS

There are tremendous economic and political pressures to increase the number of follow-on biologics (FOBs) available on the market. FOBs have already been approved in the European Union and the United States. Examples are erythropoietin analogs, human growth hormone, and G-CSF. However, there are still many issues to resolve regarding FOBs:

- FOBs may have a different immunogenicity profile to the reference product, leading to reduced efficacy and/or safety issues.

It is unlikely that the current regulatory framework for the approval of FOBs will cover monoclonal antibodies or other large glycosylated proteins. Different production methods for monoclonal antibodies can alter the glycosylation profile. This can effect the amount of ADCC and CDC that an antibody can produce. These changes in antibody function can affect both the efficacy and safety profile of an FOB compared with the reference mAB.[82-85]

It is doubtful whether this will soon be possible for mABs or soluble receptors until the effects of glycosylation can be better understood and characterized. Because of the complexity of biologic agents, formal efficacy studies with biosimiliar products should be performed before approval. The need for less expensive therapies is essential, but we should not compromise clinical efficacy and possible safety by adopting biosimilars without appropriate blinded efficacy or safety studies.

Given the extensive costs and time required to characterize promising new therapeutics prior to their introduction into clinical trials, the FDA introduced the Critical Path Initiative in 2004 and issued a guidance on exploratory investigational new drug (IND) studies in 2006.[86] These exploratory studies are designed to screen and identify promising new candidates for treatment of cancer and autoimmune diseases, without requiring the extensive dose characterization and dose escalation involved in traditional phase 1 studies. Such "exploratory INDs" are designed to examine "microdose" studies, for example, single, less than 1/100th of pharmacologically active doses in a small number of patients, based on animal data, to identify PD, distribution, or imaging effects. Once these early studies yield promising information confirming an hypothesized mechanism of action, then resources may be sought to support larger more traditional clinical development. It is hoped such approaches will be increasingly tried to stimulate development of novel therapeutics.

The era of biologic agents has certainly changed clinical rheumatology and the expected outcome for our patients. Development of these agents has brought both new promise and new challenges to drug development. In addition to challenges faced by those in preclinical and clinical development, there are additional challenges to those who will ultimately implement these agents in clinical practice. Pre-clinical studies and clinical trials address safety and efficacy in limited and controlled environments. The challenge of calculating risk benefit ratios and communicating these to patients exposed to these agents will require increasing cooperation between those performing research and those treating patients in daily practice. Now more than ever, an understanding of these two arenas, each with its own science and uncertainty, will be required for the promising potential of current and future biologic therapies to be fully realized.

Acknowledgments

The authors would like to acknowledge the helpful comments and edits from Joy Cavagnaro, PhD, and Jeremy Sokolove, MD.

References

1. Lacana E, Amur S, Mummanneni P, Zhao H, Frueh FW. The emerging role of pharmacogenomics in biologics. Clin Pharm Ther 2007;82:466-71.
2. Baumann A. Early development of therapeutic biologics—pharmacokinetics. Curr Drug Metab 2006;7:15-21.
3. Cavagnaro J. Preclinical safety evaluation of biotechnology-derived pharmaceuticals. Nat Rev Drug Discov 2002;1:469-75.
4. FDA Guidance Concerning Demonstration of Comparability of Human Biological Products, Including Therapeutic Biotechnology-derived Products. April 1996. Accessed July 13, 2009 from www.fda.gov/Drugs/GuidanceComplianceRegulatoryInformation/Guidances/ucm122879.htm.
5. Rowe JM, Andersen JW, Mazza JJ, Bennett JM, Paietta E, Hayes FA, et al. Phase III randomized placebo-controlled study of granulocyte-macrophage colony stimulating factor in adult patients (>55-70 years) with acute myelogenous leukemia (AML): a study of the Eastern Cooperative Oncology Group (ECOG). Blood 1993;82(Suppl. 1):329a.
6. Rowe JM, Andersen JW, Mazza JJ, Bennett JM, Paietta E, Hayes FA, et al. A randomized placebo-controlled phase III study of granulocyte-macrophage colony stimulating factor in adult patients (>55 to 70 years of age) with acute myelogenous leukemia: a study of the Eastern Cooperative Oncology Group (E1490). Blood 1995;86:457-62.
7. Thatcher N, Girling DJ, Hopwood P, Sambrook RJ, Qian W, Stephens RJ. Improving survival without reducing quality

of life in small-cell lung cancer patients by increasing the dose-intensity of chemotherapy with granulocyte colony-stimulating factor support: results of a British Medical Research Council multicenter randomized trial. J Clin Oncol 2000;18:395-404.

8. Hussein AM, Ross M, Vredenburgh J, Meisenberg B, Hars V, Gilbert C, et al. Effects of granulocyte-macrophage colony-stimulating factor produced in Chinese hamster ovary cells (regramostim), Escherichia coli (molgramostim) and yeast (sargramostim) on priming peripheral blood progenitor cells for use with autologous bone marrow after highdose chemotherapy. Eur J Haematol 1995;54:281-7.

9. Martin-Christin F. Granulocyte colony stimulating factors: how different are they? How to make a decision. Anticancer Drugs 2001;12:185-91.

10. Bonig H, Silbermann S, Weller S, Kirschke R, Körholz D, Janssen G, et al. Glycosylated vs non-glycosylated granulocyte colony-stimulating factor (G-CSF)—results of a prospective randomised monocentre study. Bone Marrow Transplant 2001;28:259-64.

11. Beveridge RA, Miller JA, Kales AN, Binder RA, Robert NJ, Heisrath-Evans J, et al. Randomized trial comparing the tolerability of sargramostim (yeast-derived rhugm-CSF) and filgrastim (bacteria-derived rhug-CSF) in cancer patients receiving myelosuppressive chemotherapy. Support Care Cancer 1997;15:289-98.

12. Dorr RT. Clinical properties of yeast-derived versus Escherichia coli-derived granulocyte-macrophage colony-stimulating factor. Clin Ther 1993;15:19-29.

13. Dingermann T. Recombinant therapeutic proteins: Production platforms and challenges. Biotechnol J 2008;3:90-7.

14. Yocum DE, Solinger AM, Tesser J, Gluck O, Cornett M, O'Sullivan F, et al. Clinical and immunologic effects of a primatized anti CD4 monoclonal antibody in active rheumatoid arthritis. J Rheumatol 1998;25:1257-62.

15. Mason U, Aldrich J, Breedveld F, Davis CB, Elliott M, Jackson M, et al. CD4 coating, but not CD4 depletion, is a predictor of efficacy with primatized monoclonal anti-CD4 treatment of active rheumatoid arthritis. J Rheumatol 2002;29:220-9.

16. Rau R, Sander O, van Riel P, van de Putte L, Hasler F, Zang M, et al. Intravenous human recombinant tumor necrosis factor receptor p55-Fc IgG1 fusion protein Ro 45-2081 (lenercept): a double blind, placebo controlled dose-finding study in rheumatoid arthritis. J Rheumatol 2003;30:680-90.

17. Furst DE, Weisman M, Paulus HE, Bulpitt K, Weinblatt M, Polisson R, et al. Intravenous human recombinant tumor necrosis factor receptor p55-Fc IgG1 fusion protein, Ro 45-2081 (lenercept): results of a dose-finding study in rheumatoid arthritis. J Rheumatol 2003;30:2123-6.

18. Jones AJS, Papac DI, Chin EH, Keck R, Baughman SA, Lin YS, et al. Selective clearance of glycoforms of a complex glycoprotein pharmaceutical caused by terminal N-acetylglucosamine is similar in humans and cynomolgus monkeys. Glycobiology 2007;17:529-40.

19. Keck R, Nayak N, Lerner L, Raju S, Ma S, Schreitmueller T, et al. Characterization of a complex glycoprotein whose variable metabolic clearance in humans is dependent on terminal N-acetylglucosamine content. Biologicals 2008;36:49-60.

20. Eckardt K, Casadevall N. Pure red-cell aplasia due to antierythropoietin antibodies. Nephrol Dial Transplant 2003;18:865-9.

21. Hegen M, Keith JC, Collins M, Nickerson-Nutter CL. Utility of animal models for identification of potential therapeutic for rheumatoid arthritis. Ann Rheum Dis 2008;67:1505-15.

22. Fishwild D, Hudson D, Deshpande U, Kung A. Differential effects of administration of a human anti-CD4 monoclonal antibody, HM6G, in nonhuman primates. Clin Immunol 1999;92:138-52.

23. Bugelski PJ, Herzykl DJ, Rehm S, Harmsen AG, Gore EV, Williams DM, et al. Preclinical development of keliximab, a primatized anti-CD4 monoclonal antibody, in human CD4 transgenic mice: characterization of the model and safety studies. Hum Exp Toxicol 2000;19:230-43.

24. Herzyk DJ, Bugelski PJ, Hart TK, Wier PJ. Practical aspects of including functional endpoints in developmental toxicity studies. Case study: immune function in hucd4 transgenic mice exposed to anti-CD4 mab in utero. Hum Exp Toxicol 2002;21:507-12.

25. Anderson D, Chambers K, Hanna N, Leonard J, Reff M, Newman R, et al. A primatized MAb to human CD4 causes receptor modulation, without marked reduction in CD4+ T cells in chimpanzees: in vitro and in vivo characterization of a MAb (IDEC-CE9.1) to human CD4. Clin Immunol Immunopathol 1997;84:73-84.

26. Bendele A, McAbee T, Sennello G, Frazier J, Chlipala E, McCabe D. Efficacy of sustained blood levels of interleukin-1 receptor antagonist in animal models of arthritis: comparison of efficacy in animal models with human clinical data. Arthritis Rheum 1999;42:498-506.

27. Williams RO, Feldmann M, Maini RN. Anti-tumor necrosis factor ameliorates joint disease in murine collagen-induced arthritis. Proc Natl Acad Sci U S A 1992;89:9784-8.

28. Maini R, Feldmann M. How does infliximab work in rheumatoid arthritis? Arth Res 2002;4(suppl 2):S22-8.

29. Wooley PH, Dutcher J, Widmer MB, Gillis S. Influence of a recombinant human soluble tumor necrosis factor receptor FC fusion protein on type II collagen-induced arthritis in mice. J Immunol 1993;151:6602-7.

30. Piguet PF, Grau GE, Vesin C, Loetscher H, Gentz R, Lesslauer W. Evolution of collagen arthritis in mice is arrested by treatment with anti-tumour necrosis factor (TNF) antibody or a recombinant soluble TNF receptor. Immunology 1992;77:510-4.

31. Bendele AM, McComb J, Gould T. Comparative efficacy of sTNFRI, a novel monomeric recombinant soluble TNF type I receptor, to dimeric sTNF-RI and sTNF-RII IgG1 Fc fusion proteins in animal models of rheumatoid arthritis. In: Proc. Int. TNF Congr. Hyannis, Massachusetts; 7 May, 1998.

32. Weir N, Athwal D, Brown D, Foulkes R, Kollias G, Nesbitt A, et al. A new generation of high-affinity humanized pegylated Fab' fragment anti-tumor necrosis factor a monoclonal antibodies. Therapy 2006;3:535-45.

33. Kliwinski C, Kukral D, Postelnek J, Krishnan B, Killar L, Lewin A, et al. Prophylactic administration of abatacept prevents disease and bone destruction in a rat model of collagen-induced arthritis. J Autoimmun 2005;25:165-71.

34. Knoerzer DB, Karr RW, Schwartz BD, Mengle-Gaw LJ. Collagen-induced arthritis in the BB rat. Prevention of disease by treatment with CTLA-4-Ig. J Clin Invest 1995;96:987-93.

35. Webb LM, Walmsley MJ, Feldmann M. Prevention and amelioration of collagen-induced arthritis by blockade of the CD28 co-stimulatory pathway: requirement for both B7-1 and B7-2. Eur J Immunol 1996;26:2320-8.

36. Halpern WG, Lappin P, Zanardi T, Cai W, Corcoran M, Zhong J, et al. Chronic administration of belimumab, a blys antagonist, decreases tissue and peripheral blood B-lymphocyte populations in cynomolgus monkeys: pharmacokinetic, pharmacodynamic, and toxicologic effects. Toxicol Sci 2006;91:586-99.

37. Wang H, Marsters SA, Baker T, Chan B, Lee WP, Fu L, et al. TACI-ligand interactions are required for Tcell activation and collagen-induced arthritis in mice. Nat Immunol 2001;2:632-7.

38. Looney RJ. Treating human autoimmune disease by depleting B cells. Ann Rheum Dis 2002;61:863-6.

39. Gong Q, Ou Q, Ye S, Lee WP, Cornelius J, Diehl L, et al. Importance of cellular microenvironment and circulatory dynamics in B cell immunotherapy. J Immunol 2005;174:817-26.

40. Dunussi-Joannopoulos K, Hancock GE, Kunz A, Hegen M, Zhou XX, Sheppard BJ, et al. B-cell depletion inhibits arthritis in a collagen-induced arthritis (CIA) model, but does not adversely affect humoral responses in a respiratory syncytial virus (RSV) vaccination model. Blood 2005;106:2235-43.

41. Trubion Pharmaceuticals. TRU-015 Factsheet: TRU-015. A novel compound in Phase 2 development for rheumatoid arthritis. Accessed September 2, 2008 from http://www.trubion.com/pdf/Trubion_TRU-015_Fact_Sheet.pdf.

42. Genmab. Accessed September 2, 2008 from http://www.genmab.com/ScienceAndResearch/ProductsinDevelopment/HuMax-CD20.aspx.

43. Alonzi T, Fattori E, Lazzaro D, Costa P, Probert L, Kollias G, et al. Interleukin 6 is required for the development of collagen-induced arthritis. J Exp Med 1998;187:461-8.

44. Fujimoto M, Serada S, Mihara M, Uchiyama Y, Yoshida H, Koike N, et al. Interleukin-6 blockade suppresses autoimmune arthritis in mice by the inhibition of inflammatory Th17 responses. Arthritis Rheum 2008;58:3710-18.

45. Amat M, Benjamin CF, Williams LM, Prats N, Terricabras E, Beleta J, et al. Pharmacological blockade of CCR1 ameliorates murine arthritis and alters cytokine networks in vivo. Br J Pharmacol 2006;149:666-75.

46. Teeling HL, Mackus WJM, Wiegman LJJM, van den Brakel JH, Beers SA, French RR, et al. The biological activity of human CD20 monoclonal antibodies is linked to unique epitopes on CD20. J Immunol 2006;177:362-71.

47. Bendele A, Mccomb J, Gould TY, McAbee T, Sennello G, Chlipala E, et al. Animal models of arthritis: Relevance to human disease. Toxicol Pathol 1999;27:134-42.

48. Williams RO, Marinova-Mutafchieva L, Feldmann M, Maini RN. Evaluation of TNF-alpha and IL-1 blockade in collagen-induced arthritis and comparison with combined anti-TNF-alpha/anti-CD4 therapy. J Immunol 2000;165:7240-5.

49. Arnett HA, Viney JL. Considerations for the sensible use of rodent models of inflammatory disease in predicting efficacy of new biological therapeutics in the clinic. Adv Drug Deliv Rev 2007;59:1084-92.

50. Dempster AM. Nonclinical safety evaluation of biotechnologically derived pharmaceuticals. Biotech Ann Rev 2000;5:221-58.

51. Agoram BM, Martin SW, vander Graaf PH. The role of mechanism-based pharmacokinetic-pharmacodynamic (PK-PD) modelling in translational research of biologics. Drug Disc Today 2007;12:1018-24.

52. Food and Drug Administration. Guidance for industry: estimating the maximum safe starting dose in initial clinical trials for therapeutics in adult healthy volunteers. Rockville, MD: Center for Drug Evaluation and Research (CDER), Food and Drug Administration (FDA); 2005.

53. Mascelli MA, Zhou H, Sweet R, Getsy J, Davis HM, Graham M, et al. Molecular, biologic, and pharmacokinetic properties of monoclonal antibodies: Impact of these parameters on early clinical development. J Clin Pharm 2007;47:553-65.

54. Baslund B, Skjoedt H, Klausen T. A phase I double blind, randomized, placebo controlled study of a non-depleting fully human anti-CD4 monoclonal antibody (humax CD4/HM6G) in patients with active rheumatoid arthritis. Arthritis Rheum 2000;43:S89.

55. Black LE, Bendele AM, Bendele RA, Zack PM, Hamilton M. Regulatory decision strategy for entry of a novel biologic therapeutic with a clinically unmonitorable toxicity into clinical trials: Pre IND meetings and a case example. Toxicol Pathol 1999;27:22-6.

56. Kinders R, Parchment RE, Ji J, Kummar S, Murgo AJ, Gutierrez M, et al. Phase 0 clinical trials in cancer drug development: from FDA guidance to clinical practice. Mol Interv 2007;7:325-34.

57. Strand V, Kimberly R, Isaacs JD. Biologic therapies in rheumatology: lessons learned, future directions. Nat Rev Drug Discov 2007;6:75-92.

58. Bugelski PJ, Treacy G. Predictive power of preclinical studies in animals for the immunogenicity of recombinant therapeutic proteins in humans. Curr Opin Mol Ther 2004;6:10-6.

59. Henck JW, Hilbish KG, Serabian MA, Cavagnaro JA, Hendrickx AG, Agnish ND, et al. Reproductive toxicity of therapeutic biotechnology agents. Teratology 1996;53:185-95.

60. Sistare FD, DeGeroge JJ. Preclinical predictors of clinical safety: Opportunities for improvement. Clin Pharmacol Ther 2007;82:210-4.

61. Abbott. Remicade label. 2009.

62. http://www.fda.gov/cder/biologics/review/etanimm110298r5.pdf [accessed January 8, 2009].

63. Treacy G. Using an analogous monoclonal antibody to evaluate the reproductive and chronic toxicity potential for a humanized anti-tnfα monoclonal antibody. Hum Exp Toxicol 2000;19:226-8.

64. http://www.fda.gov/cder/biologics/review/etanimm110298r5.pdf [accessed January 8, 2009].

65. Medina J, Garcia Buey L, Moreno Monteagudo JA, Trapero Marugan M, Moreno Otero R. Therapeutic advantages of pegylation of interferon alpha in chronic hepatitis C. Rev Esp Enferm Dig 2003;95:568-74, 561-7.

66. Sacco S, Heremans H, Echtenacher B, Buurman WA, Amraoui Z, Goldman M, et al. Protective effect of a single interleukin-12 (IL-12) predose against the toxicity of subsequent chronic IL-12 in mice: role of cytokines and glucocorticoids. Blood 1997;90:4473-9.

67. Coughlin CM, Wysocka M, Trinchieri G, Lee WM. The effect of interleukin 12 desensitization on the antitumor efficacy of recombinant interleukin 12. Cancer Res 1997;57:2460-7.

68. Hunig T, Dennehy K. CD28 superagonists: mode of action and therapeutic potential. Immunol Lett 2005;100:21-8.

69. Beyersdorf N, Gaupp S, Balbach K, Schmidt J, Toyka KV, Lin CH, et al. Selective targeting of regulatory T cells with CD28 superagonists allows effective therapy of experimental autoimmune encephalomyelitis. J Exp Med 2005;202:445-55.

70. Marshall E. Drug trials. Violent reaction to monoclonal antibody therapy remains a mystery. Science 2006;311:1688-9.

71. Suntharalingam G, Perry MR, Ward S, Brett SJ, Castello-Cortes A, Brunner MD, et al. Cytokine storm in a Phase 1 Trial of the Anti-CD28 Monoclonal Antibody TGN1412. N Engl J Med 2006;355:1018-28.

72. Wilde MI, Goa KL. Muromonab CD3: a reappraisal of its pharmacology and use as prophylaxis of solid organ transplant rejection. Drugs 1996;51:865-94.

73. Chatenoud L, Ferran C, Bach JF. The anti-CD3-induced syndrome: a consequence of massive in vivo cell activation. Curr Top Microbiol Immunol 1991;174:121-34.

74. Tax WJ, Tamboer WP, Jacobs CW, Frenken LA, Koene RA. Role of polymorphic Fc receptor Fc□RIIa in cytokine release and adverse effects of murine IgG1 anti-CD3/T cell receptor antibody (WT31). Transplantation 1997;63:106-12.

75. Investigations into adverse incidents during clinical trials of TGN1412. London: Medicines and Healthcare products Regulatory Agency (MHRA). Accessed August 11, 2006 from http://www.mhra.gov.uk/home/idcplg?IdcService=GET_FILE&d DocName=CON2023821&RevisionSelectionMethod=LatestReleased.

76. Damjanov N, Kauffman R, Spencer-Green GT. Safety and efficacy of VX-702, a p38 MAP kinase inhibitor, in rheumatoid arthritis. Ann Rheum Dis 2008;67(Suppl. II):125.

77. Genovese MC, Cohen SB, Wofsy D, Weinblatt ME, Firestein GS, Brahn E, et al: A randomized, double-blind, placebo-controlled Phase 2 study of an oral p38a MAPK inhibitor, SCIO-469, in patients with active rheumatoid arthritis. Arthritis Rheum 2008;58(suppl):S431-2.

78. Kaul S, Hess H, Ping J, Latek R, Kollia G, Xu X, et al. Anti-inflammatory effect of BMS-582949, a P38 mitogen activated protein kinase (MAPK) inhibitor, during experimental endotoxemia in healthy male subjects. Arthritis Rheum 2008;58(suppl):S297.

79. Fleischmann R, Genovese M, Keystone EM, Pavelka L, Durez P, Pavlik-Gaylord S, et al. Lack of efficacy with 3 oral dose levels of TMI-005 (Apratastat), in subjects with active rheumatoid arthritis on a background of methotrexate - a phase 2 double-blind, placebo-controlled, parallel, randomized study. Ann Rheum Dis 2006;65(Suppl. II):339.

80. Hahn B, Anderson M, La Cava A. The anti-DNA Iq consensus peptide pcons facilitates regulatory T cell activity in SLE patients. Arthritis Rheum 2007;56(suppl):S546.

81. Keystone EC. Abandoned therapies and unpublished trials in rheumatoid arthritis. Curr Opin Rheum 2003;15:253-8.

82. Declerck PJ. Biotherapeutics in the era of biosimilars what really matters is patient safety. Drug Safety 2007;30:1087-92.

83. Genazzani AA, Biggio G, Caputi AP, Del Tacca M, Drago F, Fantozzi R, et al. Biosimilar drugs: concerns and opportunitie. Biodrugs 2007;21:351-6.

84. Wurm FM. Manufacturing of biopharmaceuticals and implications for biosimilars. Kidney Blood Press Res 2007;30:S6-8.

85. Roger SD, Goldsmith D. Biosimilars: it's not as simple as cost alone. J Clin Pharm Ther 2008;33:459-64.

86. Jacobsen-Kram D, Mills G. Leveraging exploratory investigational new drug studies to accelerate drug development. Clin Cancer Res 2008;14:3670-4.

Index